Widmann's
Clinical
Interpretation
of Laboratory
Tests

edition **11**

RONALD A. SACHER,

MB, BCh, DTM&H, FRCPC, FASCP, FCAP

Professor of Medicine, Oncology, and Pathology
Chairman, Department of Laboratory Medicine
Georgetown University Medical Center
Washington, DC

and

RICHARD A. McPHERSON, MD

Professor of Pathology
Chairman, Division of Clinical Pathology
Medical College of Virginia Hospitals
Virginia Commonwealth University
Richmond, Virginia

with

JOSEPH M. CAMPOS, PhD

Director, Microbiology Laboratory and Laboratory Informatics
Children's National Medical Center
Professor, Departments of Pediatrics, Pathology, and Microbiology/
   Immunology
George Washington University Medical Center
Washington, DC

Widmann's
Clinical Interpretation of Laboratory Tests

edition **11**

F. A. DAVIS COMPANY   Philadelphia

F. A. Davis Company
1915 Arch Street
Philadelphia, PA 19103

Printed in the United States of America

Last digit indicates print number: 10 9 8 7 6 5 4 3 2

Acquisitions Editor: Robert W. Reinhardt
Senior Developmental Editor: Bernice M. Wissler
Production Editor: Elena Coler
Cover Designer: Louis J. Forgione

As new scientific information becomes available through basic and clinical research, recommended treatments and drug therapies undergo changes. The author(s) and publisher have done everything possible to make this book accurate, up to date, and in accord with accepted standards at the time of publication. The authors, editors, and publisher are not responsible for errors or omissions or for consequences from application of the book, and make no warranty, expressed or implied, in regard to the contents of the book. Any practice described in this book should be applied by the reader in accordance with professional standards of care used in regard to the unique circumstances that may apply in each situation. The reader is advised always to check product information (package inserts) for changes and new information regarding dose and contraindications before administering any drug. Caution is especially urged when using new or infrequently ordered drugs.

Library of Congress Cataloging in Publication Data

Sacher, Ronald A.
    Widmann's clinical interpretation of laboratory tests.— Ed. 11/Ronald A. Sacher and Richard A. McPherson, with Joseph M. Campos.
        p. ; cm.
    Includes bibliographical references and index.
    ISBN 0-8036-0270-7
    1. Diagnosis, Laboratory. I. McPherson, Richard A. II. Campos, Joseph M. III. Widmann, Frances K., 1935- IV. Title.
    [DNLM: 1. Laboratory Techniques and Procedures. QY 4 S1212w 2000]
RB37 .S225 2000
616.07′5—dc21
99-059044

To Heather, Greg, and Sassy.
Thanks for the love and many hours of
support as well as cups of tea that
have sustained me through the
writing of this book.
This book is dedicated to you.
R.A.S.

To Stephanie, Jennifer, and Marianne.
R.A.M.

Preface

This 11th edition is built on the framework of previous editions, aiming to incorporate the changes in laboratory medicine and in the practice of medicine as a whole. We continue to update, expand, and modify the elements of the book based on our personal experiences in the practice of laboratory medicine at Georgetown University Medical Center and at the Virginia Commonwealth University/Medical College of Virginia.

Some of the significant changes in many aspects of laboratory medicine are highlighted throughout this edition. Chapter 1 includes a discussion of point-of-care testing (also called near-patient testing) and of the changes in organ-specific panels and sequential multichannel analyzers. Chapter 1 also presents a theoretical background for the interpretation of laboratory test results and has been expanded to include receiver operating characteristic (ROC) curves, which are universally important for assessing the diagnostic utility of new versus old procedures. Substantial revision of Section Two, Hematology, reflects the advances in diagnostics and therapeutics, especially the new dimensions of molecular testing and flow cytometry.

Chapter 7 introduces more material on immunologic methods and interpretations of results to measure both cellular and humoral immunity and aberrations that lead to autoimmune and other diseases. The changes in Chapter 8 reflect new tests and methods being applied in blood banking and immunohematology, as well as some of the advances that have been made in histocompatibility.

The chapters in Section Four, Clinical Chemistry, have been widely updated to cover such topics as modern approaches to evaluating chest pain and diagnosis of myocardial infarction, newly understood etiologies of liver disease (including hepatitis), strategies for cardiac risk assessment, and many other emerging themes in medicine that rely on laboratory support for diagnosis and patient management. The section on endocrinology places additional emphasis on hormonal mechanisms of action and laboratory analyses. New illustrations have been added to help understanding in the endocrinology chapters and in Chapter 18, Therapeutic Drug Monitoring and Toxicology.

Section Five, Clinical Microbiology, focuses on new testing methods, in particular the molecular techniques. These chapters have been updated to include substantial advances in diagnostics and the identification of newly discovered organisms.

The Appendices have also been updated, particularly regarding advances in nutritional screening and cancer diagnosis using laboratory testing. The table of reference ranges in this edition is taken from those used at Georgetown University Medical Center. The values listed include only the analytes more commonly ordered. They are provided as examples and guidelines for educational purposes and clearly should not be used to interpret results from other laboratories. Typically (and by the regulations of CLIA 88), each laboratory must establish its own reference ranges, taking into account its specific methods, populations, and other influences.

In this book we have tried to present a practical approach to the understanding of pathophysiology and the application of laboratory testing in clinical diagnosis. We have used the approaches and explanations that we have employed while teaching introductory courses in the fundamentals of laboratory medicine as well as advanced training for residents. The book is intended to be an easy-to-read and informative text, more sophisticated than short handbooks that simply list disorders and tests but much more approachable than the comprehensive texts that nevertheless serve as essential reference sources. We believe that it will be a useful addition to the personal libraries of busy clinicians, medical students, laboratory workers, and paramedical personnel who wish to understand the tests and methods used in clinical laboratory medicine.

RONALD A. SACHER, MB, BCh, DTM&H, FRCPC, FASCP, FCAP
RICHARD A. MCPHERSON, MD

Contents

Section One   General Principles

Chapter 1   Principles of Interpretation of
              Laboratory Tests   3

Section Two   Hematology

Chapter 2   Hematologic Methods   31
Chapter 3   Diseases of Red Blood Cells   102
Chapter 4   Diseases of White Blood Cells   167
Chapter 5   Hemostasis and Tests of
              Hemostatic Function   236
Chapter 6   Disorders of Hemostasis   284

ix

Section Three   Immunology

| Chapter 7 | Principles of Immunology and Immunology Testing | 325 |
| Chapter 8 | Transfusion Medicine | 365 |

Section Four   Clinical Chemistry

Chapter 9	General Chemistry	445
Chapter 10	Acid-Base and Electrolyte Regulation	499
Chapter 11	Enzymes and Other Markers of Tissue Dysfunction	533
Chapter 12	Tests of Liver Function	562

Section Five   Clinical Microbiology

Chapter 13	Principles of Clinical Microbiology	603
Chapter 14	Systematic Clinical Microbiology	661
Chapter 15	Serologic Diagnosis of Infectious Diseases	700

Section Six   The Endocrine System

| Chapter 16 | Laboratory Interpretation of Endocrine Tests | 739 |
| Chapter 17 | Reproductive Endocrinology | 825 |

Section Seven   Miscellaneous

Chapter 18   Therapeutic Drug Monitoring and
                   Toxicology   873
Chapter 19   Laboratory Assessment of Body
                   Fluids   924

Appendixes

Appendix A   Disorders of Nutrition   1015
Appendix B   Tumor Markers   1031
Appendix C   Perinatal Laboratory Testing   1048
Appendix D   Neonatal Laboratory Testing   1053
Appendix E   Normal Reference Laboratory
                   Values   1059

Index   1067

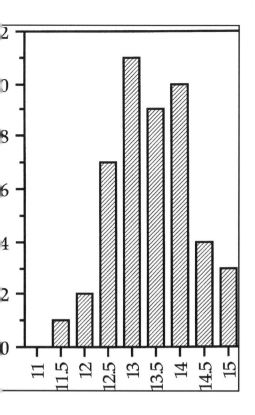

Section One

General Principles

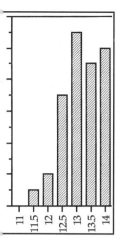

Principles of Interpretation of Laboratory Tests

Laboratory measurements and examinations provide the hard scientific data used to deal with problems identified by the clinical evaluation and are an essential part of the information that contributes to the patient data base. Indications for ordering laboratory tests constitute the most important considerations of laboratory medicine. Approximately 10 to 15% of the national health budget in the United States goes to laboratory testing, and for hospitalized patients, this constitutes 15 to 20% of each bill. Laboratory information can be used diagnostically or to confirm a preliminary diagnosis made during the history and physical examination. Laboratory analysis is also an integral part of health screening and preventive medicine. This chapter reviews how laboratory procedures are involved in the diagnostic process to define the patient's medical problem and its management.

The disciplines of laboratory medicine include several major areas:

1. *Hematology* with examination of the cellular elements of blood and also its clotting factors
2. *Chemical pathology,* including the measurement of over 200 substances in serum and body fluids
3. *Blood banking and transfusion medicine,* involving blood donor screening and testing, blood component preparation, and compatibility testing

3

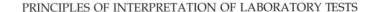

4. *Medical microbiology,* entailing diagnostic bacteriology, mycology, virology, parasitology, and serology
5. *Medical microscopy* for the examination of urine and other body fluids
6. *Immunoassays* for endocrine testing, therapeutic drug monitoring, several toxicology assays, and other special procedures
7. *Immunology,* involving both quantitative and qualitative determinations of humoral and cellular immunity, and immunochemistry

ACCURACY AND PRECISION

When using the data obtained through a laboratory measurement, one must be familiar with the limitations and applications of the data, in particular with the terms **accuracy** and **precision.** Accuracy refers to how closely the measurement approaches the true value of the substance being analyzed. Accuracy is synonymous with correctness. Precision describes how closely together repeat measurements of the same substance in the same sample fall. Precision is synonymous with reproducibility and measures the inherent variability of a test. Some laboratory measurements may have less than ideal accuracy but still have very good precision. For purposes of monitoring patient care, it is probably better to have greater precision than accuracy, since this enables a good (consistent) evaluation of treatment response or changes in the course of a patient's illness. In this regard, a change in the patient is more likely to account for a variation in the measured value than is an analytic variation when using modern automated chemistry systems.

To illustrate the significance of accuracy versus precision, consider the example of repeat measurements of glucose on a single sample in which the glucose is known to be 100 mg/dL. Method A yields the following values on five separate measurements:

109, 110, 112, 108, and 111 (average 110) mg/dL.

On the same material, method B yields the values:

90, 110, 120, 80, and 100 (average 100) mg/dL.

Method A is much more reproducible (precise) than method B because the values do not vary much, but method B may have greater accuracy since the average value is closer to true glucose than that of method A. However, the wide deviations of method B would make it unsuitable for clinical use. Although method A has a positive bias in its results, a physician user could easily compensate for that type of error and be comfortable in relying on method A.

SPECIFICITY AND SENSITIVITY

We shall assume that individuals with a disease have values of an analyte that are generally higher than values in healthy persons (Fig. 1–1A). A

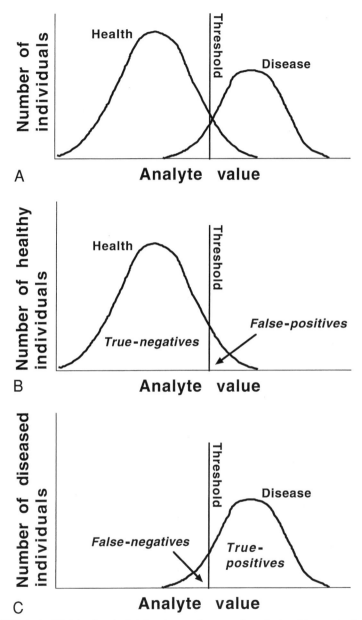

FIGURE 1–1. *(A)* Idealized distributions of an analyte in healthy and diseased individuals. The threshold is chosen to achieve optimal separation of the two populations. *(B)* Categories of true-negatives and false-positives in healthy individuals based on threshold value. *(C)* Categories of true-positives and false-negatives in diseased individuals based on threshold value.

good example of such an analyte is serum alkaline phosphatase, which is present in everyone's blood but is elevated in patients with cancer metastatic to liver or bone. By picking some threshold value, we can distinguish most of the healthy (lower than threshold, false-positives) (Fig. 1–1B) from the diseased (higher than threshold, true-positives) (Fig. 1–1C). However, the distributions of healthy and diseased persons almost always overlap with the result that some healthy persons have values above the threshold (false-positive) (Fig. 1–1B), and some diseased persons have values below the threshold (false-negative) (Fig. 1-1C).

Appreciation and correct utilization of laboratory data require an understanding of the terms **specificity** and **sensitivity.** Specificity means how good a test is at detecting only those individuals that have a disease as opposed to falsely labeling some healthy persons as having disease. In more technical terms, the specificity of a test reflects its ability to detect true-negatives with very few false-positive results. It is expressed mathematically as:

$$\frac{\text{true-negatives}}{\text{true-negatives} + \text{false-positives}} = \text{specificity}$$

where these negative and positive results refer to values obtained on individuals with a particular disease under investigation. Ideally high specificity means that only patients with that disease will demonstrate positive values by that test.

Sensitivity means how well a test detects disease without missing some diseased individuals by falsely classifying them as healthy. Thus it measures the proportion of individuals with a disease. In technical terms, the sensitivity of a test indicates its ability to generate more true-positive results and few false-negative ones. Its mathematical expression is:

$$\frac{\text{true-positives}}{\text{true-positives} + \text{false-negatives}} = \text{sensitivity}$$

Any increase in false-positive results (normal people falsely testing positive for a disease) will decrease a test's specificity, whereas an increase in false-negative results (sick people falsely testing negative for the disease) will diminish the test's sensitivity.

The ideal measurement would have both specificity and sensitivity equal to 100%. Unfortunately, no actual laboratory test meets these criteria completely. In order to detect disease, one requires maximum sensitivity, but often at the expense of specificity. With a very sensitive test that has a low threshold for abnormality, a patient may be falsely labeled as having a disease when in fact the disease is not present. An example of a circumstance in which high sensitivity is mandatory is in the screening of blood donors for hepatitis. It is much better to exclude all true carriers of the disease from donating their blood for transfusion even though some healthy individuals will be incorrectly excluded as well because of the high sensitivity of the testing for hepatitis. Conversely, when dealing with a known illness (or in situations in which there has already been made a strong presumptive diagnosis based on clinical state or screening tests), it is preferable to have very high specificity. For example, when a patient is admitted to the hospital with chest pain and there is suspicion of myocardial infarction, it is desirable to utilize a test with very high specificity for myocardial damage (creatine kinase isoenzyme MB).

In general, tests that are highly sensitive have relatively low specificities, and tests that are highly specific have relatively low sensitivities. This statement is equivalent to moving the threshold for abnormal results to the left to include more cases of disease (high sensitivity, maximize true-positives) or to the right to exclude more cases of healthy individuals (high specificity, maximize true-negatives).

PREDICTIVE VALUES

The **predictive value** of a laboratory measurement is useful to a physician when attempting to determine whether or not a patient has a particular disease based on a specific laboratory result (or combination of results). The predictive value takes into account the prevalence of a disease in the population or community. Thus the predictive value of the same test can be markedly different when applied to different geographic locations or to people of differing age, sex, or other demographics. The predictive value of a positive test result indicates the likelihood that the individual has the disease, whereas the predictive value of a negative test result reflects the likelihood that the individual is free of that disease. In general, the higher the prevalence of a disease (i.e., the percentage of people who have the disease) within the population, the greater is the predictive value of a positive test result. The mathematical expressions for predictive values are:

$$\text{predictive value (positive result)} = \frac{TP}{TP + FP}$$

where TP = true-positives
   FP = false-positives

$$\text{predictive value (negative result)} = \frac{TN}{TN + FN}$$

where TN = true-negatives
   FN = false-negatives

Figure 1–2 presents a useful way to diagram all the possible events of positive and negative test results in a population with a particular disease prevalence. The following probabilities are readily calculated by tracking each path down the arms of this scheme:

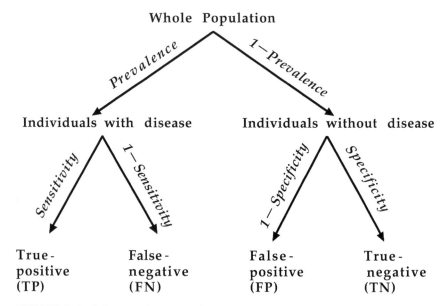

FIGURE 1–2. Scheme of test results in a population with a particular disease prevalence.

Event	Probability		
TP	prevalence	×	sensitivity
FN	prevalence	×	(1 − sensitivity)
FP	(1 − prevalence)	×	(1 − specificity)
TN	(1 − prevalence)	×	specificity

To make this example quantitative, we will choose test characteristics such that, of all persons with the disease, 95% will give a true-positive result and 5% will give a false-negative result (sensitivity = 95%); of all persons who do not have the disease, 5% will give a false-positive result and 95% will give true-negative results (specificity = 95%). At first glance, these numbers seem to be reasonably in favor of making a diagnosis perhaps simply on the basis of this one test. However, the prevalence of disease in the population will really establish just how useful the test will be. Let us consider three particular prevalence rates. For a prevalence of 1% (i.e., 0.01),

$$TP = 0.01 \times 0.95 = 0.0095 \text{ (or 0.95\% of the total results)}$$
$$FN = 0.01 \times 0.05 = 0.0005$$
$$FP = 0.99 \times 0.05 = 0.0495$$
$$TN = 0.99 \times 0.95 = 0.9405$$

At this low prevalence, most test results in the entire population will be true-negative (94.05%). However, the predictive value of a positive result is $TP/(TP + FP) = 0.0095/(0.0095 + 0.0495) = 0.161$. This indicates that only 16.1% of positive results occur in individuals with the disease, whereas 83.9% of positive results occur in the absence of disease. Therefore, a positive result is greater than five times more likely to be in error than it is to predict disease.

As the prevalence of disease changes, the predictive value can change quite dramatically. For a prevalence of 5%, the figures become:

$$TP = 0.05 \times 0.95 = 0.0475$$
$$FN = 0.05 \times 0.05 = 0.0025$$
$$FP = 0.95 \times 0.05 = 0.0475$$
$$TN = 0.95 \times 0.95 = 0.9025$$

In this instance, most results are still true-negative, but the predictive value of a positive result becomes much better: $0.0475/(0.0475 + 0.0475) = 0.50$ or 50%. If the prevalence is higher still (set to 20%), the results are:

$$TP = 0.2 \times 0.95 = 0.19$$
$$FN = 0.2 \times 0.05 = 0.01$$
$$FP = 0.8 \times 0.05 = 0.04$$
$$TN = 0.8 \times 0.95 = 0.76$$

The predictive value of a positive result is $0.19/(0.19 + 0.04) = 0.826$ or 82.6%. Of course, all these calculations would be modified if the test sensitivity and specificity were altered as well, and one approach to dealing with this problem of high false-positives is to change the cut-off point of the reference range (see below). This maneuver of course leads to loss of sensitivity and consequent failure to detect some true-positives. A more acceptable strategy is to consider results of two or more different tests that corroborate and substantiate one another. For example, combined quantitation of serum myoglobin and creatine kinase MB is superior to that of either measurement alone in the diagnosis of myocardial infarction.

There is an analogous formulation of the predictive value of a negative test result as it indicates absence of disease. However, its use is more typically confined to ruling out disease rather than to the particular diagnosis of abnormality. The power of the predictive value of a negative test result then is its ability to exclude disease, allowing the physician to explore other more promising diagnoses.

Another significant test characteristic is its **efficiency,** or ability to detect correctly both true-positives and true-negatives, expressed as:

$$\text{efficiency} = \frac{TP + TN}{TP + FP + TN + FN}$$

or

$$\text{efficiency} = \frac{\text{true results}}{\text{all results}}$$

As false-positive and false-negative results are minimized, the efficiency of a test approaches 100%. A high efficiency indicates that a test is very good at correctly categorizing results as true-positive or true-negative.

RECEIVER OPERATING CHARACTERISTIC (ROC) CURVES

Moving the threshold of abnormality along the entire range of analyte values theoretically generates an infinite number of combinations of sensitivities and specificities (Fig. 1–3A). The areas under the curves and to the right of each threshold (a, b, c, d, and e) yield paired values for true-positive (equivalent to sensitivity) and false-positives (equivalent to [1 – specificity]). Plotting these paired values against one another yields a **receiver operating characteristic (ROC) curve** (Fig. 1-3B).

ROC curves are used to compare how well different assays can distinguish disease from health. Consider assays I and II that have different characteristics of separating healthy and diseased persons (Fig. 1–4A) and give rise to distinct ROC curves (Fig. 1–4B). The behavior of assay II is superior to that of assay I in diagnosing this particular disease. The ROC curves lead to this conclusion by demonstrating better sensitivities and specificities for all thresholds using assay II. ROC curves that lie higher and to the left are judged better than those that fall lower and to the right. If the ROC takes the form of a straight line with slope 1 from lower left to upper right, then that assay has essentially no power to distinguish disease from health. Examination of the ROC curve also facilitates choosing a threshold to optimize assay sensitivity and specificity jointly. Claims by manufacturers for improved assay sensitivity or specificity should not be based on a single point but rather on ROC curves that examine a complete range of possible values.

REFERENCE RANGES (NORMAL VALUES)

Whenever laboratory test results are reported, there is also a notation as to the range of expected values for the substances analyzed. These ranges are values to be found in normal or healthy individuals. To establish such ranges characteristic of health, the laboratory measurements are performed on a large number of normal persons, and the values obtained are plotted in a distribution graph. Figure 1–5 shows an example of such a graph for the distribution of total protein concentration in the serum of a group of healthy medical students. In this instance, the values are centered about 7.2 g/dL with a nearly symmetrical scatter of values both

text continues on page 13

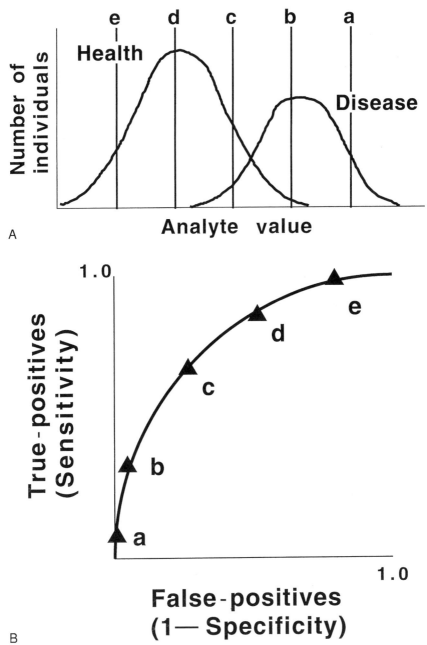

FIGURE 1–3. *(A)* Different thresholds (a, b, c, d, and e) are used to determine paired values of true-positive (area under disease curve to the right of each threshold) and false-positive (area under health curve to the right of each threshold). *(B)* ROC curve obtained from A.

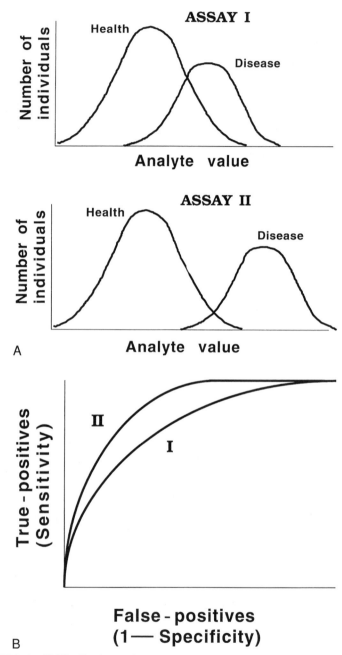

FIGURE 1–4. *(A)* Distributions of results in healthy and diseased individuals using assay I (substantial overlap) and assay II (good separation). *(B)* The ROC curves reflect better sensitivities and specificities with assay II for a wide range of possible threshold choices.

Total Protein Distribution

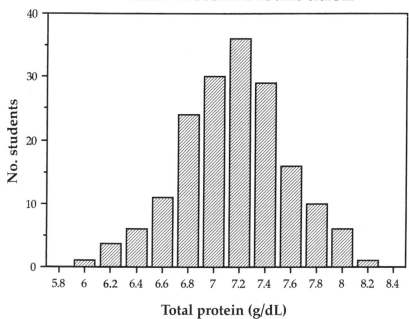

FIGURE 1–5. The distribution of total serum protein values in 173 healthy medical students. This plot is symmetric and appears to follow a Gaussian (normal) mathematical distribution.

above and below that central value. From inspection of this graph, we are inclined to accept the healthy range of total serum protein as 6.0 to 8.2 g/dL. However, the end results have low frequencies and could reflect overlap with values obtained on sick populations. To assist in applying specific guidelines in setting the limits of normal, we can resort to statistical analysis of these data. Since the distribution of total protein has the general configuration of a bell-shaped curve, it is convenient to apply the mathematical formulation for a Gaussian or normal distribution.

It should be recognized that the word "normal" has two different meanings. In the mathematical sense, it refers to a specific mathematic formula that fits data in such a bell-shaped distribution. In the medical sense, normal refers to a state of health. It is not always true that laboratory test results from a "normal" healthy population follow a "normal" Gaussian mathematical distribution. However, for convenience and for uniformity of application, the statistical values of **mean** and **standard deviation (SD)** of laboratory data are calculated using the formula for a normal distribution. By this convention, it is true that slightly more than 95% (actually 95.4%) of healthy results (or normal) will fall within the range ±2 SD of the mean value (i.e., two standard deviations on either side of the mean) and approximately 5% of healthy results will fall outside this range.

The range of normality depends upon the reference group chosen. It would be scientifically incorrect to assume that this range of total protein obtained on young healthy adult medical students can be applied to all other *age groups* (newborn, children, elderly). In fact, it is most desirable to establish this range for each age group separately. We refer to these age-specific ranges as **reference ranges** or **reference intervals** to denote that they reflect more appropriately the demographic group against which a given patient should be compared. Many analytes show a great degree of variability with age. For example, the enzyme alkaline phosphatase is much higher in the blood of children who have growing bones than in adults. In fact, a normal healthy value for alkaline phosphatase in a child would be distinctly abnormal in an adult. Many other substances also show age-related differences, many of which have greatest variation during the change from childhood to adulthood.

There are also reference ranges based on other groupings, such as sex. We know that women tend to have lower levels of red blood cells and of hemoglobin than do men. Figure 1–6 is a comparison of the hemoglobin values in female versus male medical students. There is an obvious difference in hemoglobin of almost 3 g/dL lower in the women students than in the men. This difference is due in part to a woman's loss of blood by menstruation and also to a correlation with lean body mass, which is different between men and women. Whatever the reason, it is most appropriate to judge hemoglobin and other red blood cell measurements in terms of the age- and sex-specific reference interval.

A serum analyte that demonstrates a strong sex-related reference range is uric acid (Fig. 1–7). Men tend to have higher values than do women by almost 2 mg/dL. The distribution of uric acid in male medical students (Fig. 1–7) also illustrates the interesting point of some very low values (1.0 and 1.5 mg/dL) that did not occur in the women studied. These very low values appear to be separate from the bulk of the distribution and are termed "outliers." They are probably due to some inherent differences in the way those two individuals' kidneys excreted uric acid when compared with excretion plus reabsorption of uric acid in most normal people. Although there is no real clinical significance to these very low values, they could be excluded from consideration in establishing the statistics for a reference range because they are obvious outliers.

Other factors can lead to alteration of the expected values in healthy individuals. These include degree of exercise, pregnancy, diet (vegetarian versus meat-eating), tobacco use, and many other subcategories that could even be based on occupation, altitude, distance from an ocean, medications, and so on. For practical purposes, all of these additional factors cannot be accounted for by the laboratory. It is common laboratory practice to report reference ranges that are specific for age and sex and to

text continued on page 17

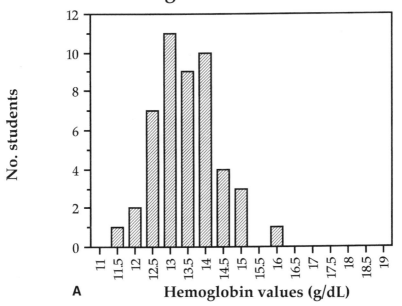

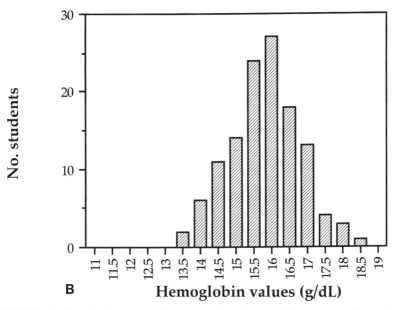

FIGURE 1–6. Distribution plots of hemoglobin in female *(A)* and male *(B)* medical students illustrating sex-related reference ranges.

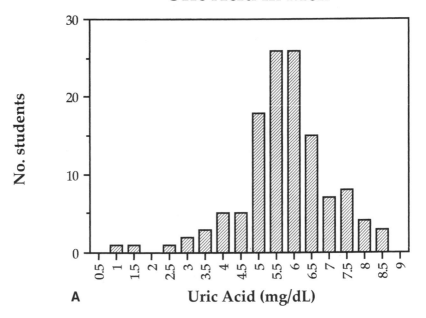

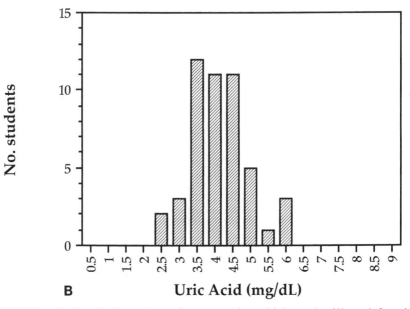

FIGURE 1–7. Distribution plots of serum uric acid in male *(A)* and female *(B)* medical students, illustrating sex-related reference ranges.

let the physician interpret the results further in light of other specific factors (such as diet, activity and medications).

SOURCES OF ERROR

In addition to physiologic and population-based variations in the levels of analytes, there must also be considered the potential for analytic variation due to methodology. This type of variability is relatively easy to quantify by performing multiple repeat measurements of the same substance on the same sample. For example, repeat measurements of serum creatinine may give the values 1.3, 1.4, 1.5, 1.4, 1.3, and 1.4. This level of variability is acceptable since it does not alter clinical assessment. If the variability were 1.0, 1.5, 2.0, 1.7, and 2.1, it would be unacceptable for the practice of monitoring changes in renal function, since significant pathologic changes could be smaller than the analytic ones. To compare methods and establish their validity, we calculate the **coefficient of variation (CV)** of a method as the standard deviation obtained from multiple measurements on the same sample divided by the mean value. Modern instrumentation has become so reproducible in performance due to standardized equipment and reagents that most automated methods can be expected to have CVs in the range of only a few percent, whereas methods with manual pipetting steps usually have CVs of 10 to 15% or more.

Other factors that can affect the quality and variation of laboratory tests are outlined in Table 1–1. For substances that fluctuate in the circulation with a *diurnal variation,* timing of collection can be very important so as not to be measuring a valley when you think you are measuring a peak (e.g., cortisol, iron). Recent ingestion of food is also very important for evaluating glucose and triglycerides and for lipid fractionation. In addition, other substances can have minor alterations after food ingestion (phosphorus, uric acid, alkaline phosphatase). The technique of venipuncture is also critical in obtaining good quality specimens. Too long an application of the tourniquet will result in acidosis in the specimen and also hemoconcentration. The proper sequence of tubes must be maintained with serum clot tubes drawn before those with additives so that no anticoagulant (e.g., with high potassium) may accidentally contaminate the serum. Care must also be exercised to prevent hemolysis of the sample and to obtain whole blood samples free of minor clots for performance of the complete blood count and of plasma clotting studies. In addition, blood samples should be transported promptly and handled appropriately to prevent deterioration of some constituents.

Human error can also account for laboratory variation. This includes errors in the performance of testing (usually minimized by the use of automated equipment), selecting a specimen to analyze from the wrong

TABLE 1-1. FACTORS AFFECTING THE QUALITY OF LABORATORY DATA

Patient Preparation
Time of day
Fasting/nonfasting

Specimen Collection
Venipuncture technique
Proper tube for blood, plasma, or serum
Correct labeling of sample
Overfilling or underfilling sample tubes (e.g., coagulation testing)

Specimen Handling
Transport
Processing
Storage

Analysis
Method precision (coefficient of variation)
Method accuracy (calibration)
Manual versus automated method

Reporting
Calculation
Transcription
Hard copy versus verbal report

patient, transcriptional mistakes, and virtually any action along the whole chain of collecting, processing, analyzing, and reporting. Laboratories that take time to track down errors of this nature can generally eliminate or minimize systematic problems. However, it is a common experience in many institutions that the incidence of mislabeling patient specimens frequently exceeds the rate of errors actually occurring in the laboratory in the analytic phase. Therefore, it is essential that the medical personnel obtaining blood and other samples correctly label those specimens, preferably at the side of the patient, so that no confusion will later arise as to the correct identity of the sample. Many laboratories perform quality control checks on serial samples to ensure that they are from the correct patient. Automation and computerization have made this procedure (called a *"delta check"*) both practical and efficient. For example, hematology samples from a single patient should have roughly the same red cell mean cell volume (MCV) from day to day. If the MCV suddenly shifts from one day to the next, it is likely that the patient's label was placed on a tube of blood from another patient. This suspicion can be confirmed by typing the red cells in both the old and new samples.

Similar checks are prompted by abrupt changes in chemical parameters as well (e.g., glucose, creatinine, enzymes).

INDICATIONS FOR ORDERING LABORATORY MEASUREMENTS AND EXAMINATIONS

Laboratory measurements and examinations are ordered for five major reasons:

1. To confirm a clinical impression or to make a diagnosis (e.g., blood glucose for diabetes mellitus, hemoglobin for anemia)
2. To rule out a disease or diagnosis (e.g., pregnancy test to rule out an ectopic pregnancy in a case of acute abdominal pain)
3. To provide prognostic information (e.g., serum levels of aspartate amino transferase and alanine amino transferase to determine the severity of hepatitis)
4. To provide therapeutic guidance (e.g., prolongation of the prothrombin time in anticoagulant therapy)
5. To screen for disease

Laboratory screening is perhaps the least valid reason to perform measurements widely and with no previous clinical suspicion or indications. However, there are some important applications of screening, including the premarital test for syphilis (Venereal Disease Research Laboratory [VDRL] or rapid plasma reagin [RPR]) and the assessment of newborns for phenylketonuria and for hypothyroidism as mandated by law. In addition, it is standard practice to screen donated blood units prior to transfusion for the presence of potential transfusion-transmitted infections such as hepatitis and the human immunodeficiency virus of acquired immune deficiency syndrome (AIDS).

PROFILE OR PANEL TESTING

A collection of different measurements related to a particular organ, organ system, or disease is referred to as a profile or panel grouping. A "health profile" refers to general measurements of multiple substances that reflect the function of several organ systems (i.e., SMAC-type profiling, Chem 20, etc.). These profiles are facilitated by performance on a single instrument that is capable of doing all the measurements. An organ panel need not be limited to a particular instrument for analysis because it may reflect many different functions of the organ. The design of an organ panel should take into account the needs of the medical staff of a hospital for maximizing both sensitivity and specificity by use of appropriate combinations of determinations. One potential bad aspect of these panels is that after a correct diagnosis is made, the panel may be ordered routinely as a standing order without consideration as to whether monitoring of the disease state requires all the repetition of confirmatory data on a daily basis. Although a single instrument may be capable of performing all or the bulk of those determinations, there is nevertheless a sizeable cost in aggregate to continue to perform all of those repeat tests, some of which may not be useful at all in the making of further clinical decisions. Examples of organ panels are liver function tests that include several enzymes and bilirubin and also the complete blood count, both of which have been widely used for years.

The chemistry profile of roughly 20 tests can be thought of as an amalgam of several different but overlapping organ panels. Thus the screening of many organs can be done by reviewing all of these results collectively, as indicated in Table 1–2. In addition to the organ associations noted in that table, there are many others with highly specific connections such as high calcium and hyperparathyroidism, electrolyte abnormalities and endocrine disease, and enzyme elevations and malignancy. With experience, a physician becomes accustomed to recognizing patterns of abnormalities that are very useful in directing the diagnostic work-up toward more conclusive procedures based on these screening tests. This practice can be very useful in the initial evaluation of a new patient when there is not a large data base on which to make clinical judgment.

There are also arguments against extensive use of profile and panel testing; in particular, the mere use of the profile might (falsely) identify

TABLE 1–2. CHEM 20 HEALTH PROFILE WITH SOME ORGAN ASSOCIATIONS OF EACH ANALYTE

Glucose *F,R**	Bilirubin, direct *L*
BUN *K,L,F*	Bilirubin, total *L*
Creatinine *K,F*	LDH *L,M*
Uric acid *K*	SGOT (AST) *L,M*
Sodium *K,F*	SGPT (ALT) *L*
Potassium *K,F*	Alkaline phosphatase *L,B*
Chloride *K,F*	Albumin *N,L,K*
Bicarbonate *K,F*	Total protein *N,L*
Calcium *B,F*	Cholesterol *N,R*
Phosphorus *K,B*	Triglycerides *N,R*

K = kidneys, *L* = liver, *B* = bone, *N* = nutrition, *M* = muscle, *R* = cardiac risk assessment, *F* = fluid and electrolyte balance.

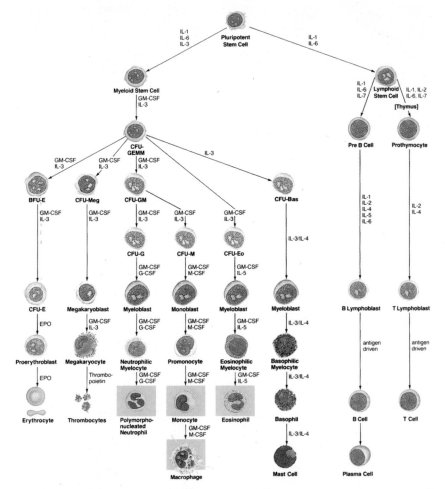

COLOR PLATE 1. Regulation of hematopoiesis by cytokines. **GM-CSF**=granulocyte monocyte/macrophage colony-stimulating factor; **BFU-E**=burst-forming unit—erythroid; **CFU-E**=colony-forming unit—erythroid; **EPO**=erythropoietin; **G-CSF**=granulocyte colony-stimulating factor; **M-CSF**=monocyte colony-stimulating factor; **CFU-Meg**=colony-forming unit—megakaryocyte; **CFU-Bas**=colony-forming unit—basophil; **CFU-GEMM**=colony-forming unit—granulocyte, erythroid, monocyte/macrophage, megakaryocyte; **CFU-Eo**=colony-forming unit—eosinophil; **CFU-M**=colony-forming unit—monocyte; **CFU-G**=colony-forming unit—granulocyte; **Meg-CSF**=megakaryocyte colony-stimulating factor. (Reprinted from Sandoz Pharmaceuticals Corporation and Schering-Plough, with permission.)

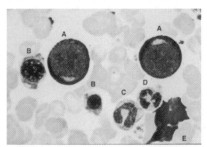

COLOR PLATE 2. Developing red blood cells showing **(A)** basophilic erythroblasts; **(B)** polychromatophilic erythroblasts; **(C)** orthochromatic erythroblasts; **(D)**, **(E)** polymorphonuclear leukocytes. (From Pittiglio, DH, and Sacher, RA: Clinical Hematology and Fundamentals of Hemostasis. FA Davis, Philadelphia, 1987, Fig. 25, with permission.)

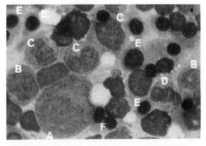

COLOR PLATE 3. Normal bone marrow showing developing white blood cells and red blood cells; leukocyte series—**(A)** promyelocyte; **(B)** myelocytes; **(C)** metamyelocytes; **(D)** bands. Developing erythroid series—**(E)** polychromatophilic erythroblasts; **(F)** orthochromatic erythroblasts.

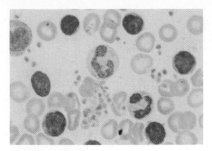

COLOR PLATE 4. Peripheral blood showing normal lymphocytes, neutrophils, and platelets.

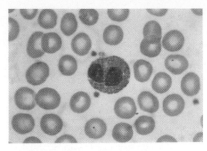

COLOR PLATE 5(A). Segmented eosinophil. (From Pittiglio and Sacher, Fig. 36, with permission.)

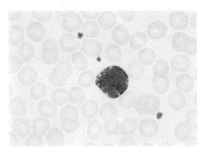

COLOR PLATE 5(B). Basophil (center). (From Pittiglio and Sacher, Fig. 38, with permission.)

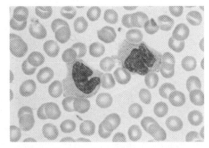

COLOR PLATE 5(C). Monocytes. (From Pittiglio and Sacher, Fig. 40, with permission.)

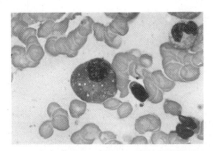

COLOR PLATE 6(A). Marrow showing large and small plasma cells. (From Pittiglio and Sacher, Fig. 53, with permission.)

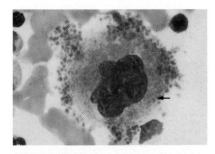

COLOR PLATE 6(B). Megakaryocyte with platelets. (From Pittiglio and Sacher, Fig. 60, with permission.)

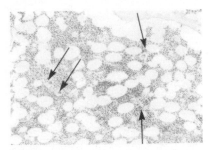

COLOR PLATE 7. Normal bone marrow biopsy showing approximately 50% marrow cellularity. Note the megakaryocytes (low power) (arrows). (From Pittiglio and Sacher, Fig. 79, with permission.)

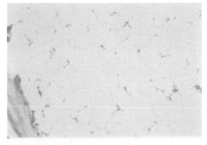

COLOR PLATE 8(A). Hypocellular marrow biopsy from a patient with aplastic anemia. (From Pittiglio and Sacher, Fig. 80, with permission.)

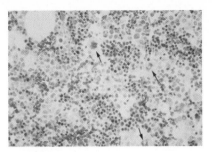

COLOR PLATE 8(B). Hypercellular marrow biopsy taken from a patient with megaloblastic anemia (arrows indicate megakaryocytes).

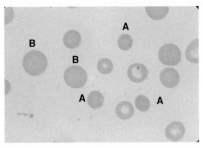

COLOR PLATE 9. Peripheral blood showing **(A)** spherocytes; **(B)** reticulocytes—from a patient with hereditary spherocytosis.

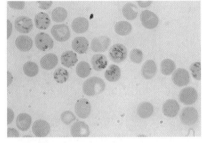

COLOR PLATE 10(A). Peripheral blood showing reticulocytes. (From Gower Medical Publishing, London, with permission.)

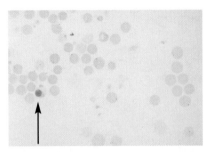

COLOR PLATE 10(B). Heinz body preparation from a patient with glucose-6 phosphate dehydrogenase deficiency. (From Gower Medical Publishing, London, with permission.)

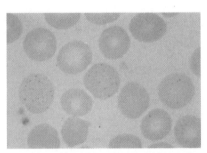

COLOR PLATE 10(C). Basophilic stippling—lead poisoning. (From Gower Medical Publishing, London, with permission.)

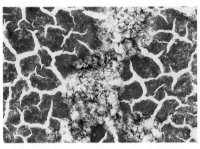

COLOR PLATE 11(A). Bone marrow showing normal iron stores stained with Prussian blue stain, which stains iron blue.

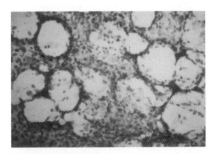

COLOR PLATE 11(B). Absent iron stores from a patient with iron deficiency anemia.

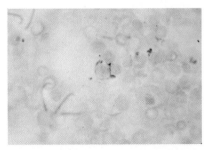

COLOR PLATE 12(A). Sideroblastic anemia bone marrow showing ring sideroblasts.

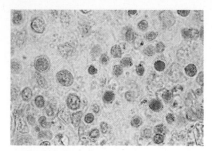

COLOR PLATE 12(B). Bone marrow showing nonring sideroblasts in developing red blood cells from a patient with hemochromatosis.

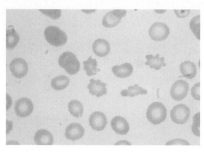

COLOR PLATE 13. Peripheral blood from renal disease patient showing burr cells. (From Pittiglio and Sacher, Fig. 123, with permission.)

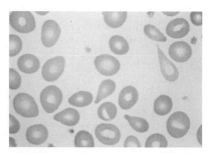

COLOR PLATE 14. Peripheral blood showing teardrop poikilocytes from a patient with myelofibrosis.

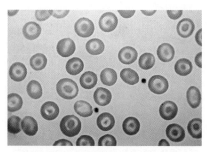

COLOR PLATE 15. Hemoglobin C disease. Peripheral blood showing numerous target cells.

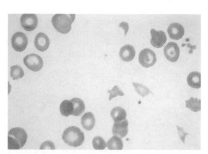

COLOR PLATE 16. Peripheral blood from a patient with cardiac valve hemolysis showing schistocytes.

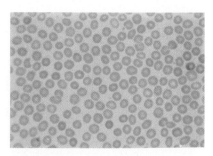

COLOR PLATE 17. Normochromic, normocytic erythrocytes from normal peripheral blood.

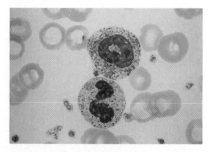

COLOR PLATE 18. Toxic granulation (peripheral blood). Note the prominent dark-staining granules. (From Pittiglio and Sacher, Fig. 136, with permission.)

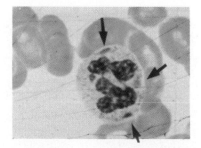

COLOR PLATE 19. Döhle bodies (arrows). Note the large bluish bodies in the periphery of the cytoplasm. (From Pittiglio and Sacher, Fig. 137, with permission.)

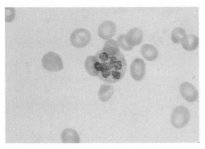

COLOR PLATE 20. Peripheral blood showing neutrophil hypersegmentation (folic acid deficiency).

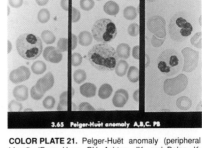

COLOR PLATE 21. Pelger-Huët anomaly (peripheral blood). (From Hyun, BH, Ashton, JK, and Dolan, K: Practical Hematology: A Laboratory Guide with Accompanying Filmstrip. WB Saunders, Philadelphia, 1975, with permission.)

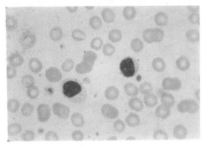

COLOR PLATE 22. Normal large lymphocyte with azurophilic granules (left) and normal small lymphocyte (right). (From Pittiglio and Sacher, Fig. 143, with permission.)

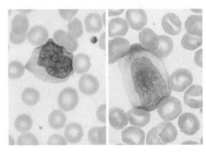

COLOR PLATE 23. Peripheral blood showing atypical lymphocytes from a patient with infectious mononucleosis.

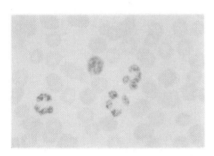

COLOR PLATE 24(A). Leukocyte alkaline phosphatase low in chronic myelogenous leukemia. (From Pittiglio and Sacher, Fig. 177, with permission.)

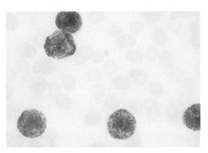

COLOR PLATE 24(B). Leukocyte alkaline phosphatase strongly positive in leukemoid reaction. (From Pittiglio and Sacher, Fig. 182, with permission.)

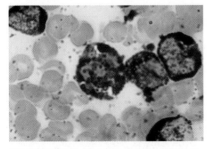

COLOR PLATE 25. Bone marrow myeloblasts showing Sudan black staining in acute myelogenous leukemia.

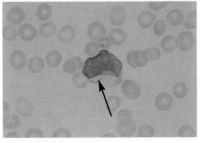

COLOR PLATE 26. Peripheral blood showing Auer rod in myeloblast from a patient with acute myelogenous leukemia. (From Pittiglio and Sacher, Fig. 149, with permission.)

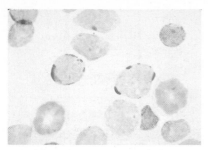

COLOR PLATE 27. Periodic acid-Schiff positivity in acute lymphoblastic leukemia. Note the "block" staining pattern. (From Pittiglio and Sacher, Fig. 154, with permission.)

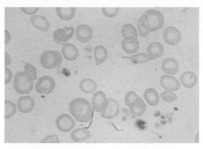

COLOR PLATE 28(A). Peripheral blood: iron deficiency anemia. Note the hypochromic, microcytic cells with target cells and teardrop forms.

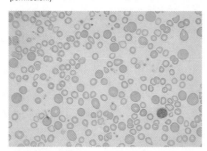

COLOR PLATE 28(B). Peripheral blood: iron deficiency after iron therapy. Note numerous polychromatophilic cells (reticulocytes).

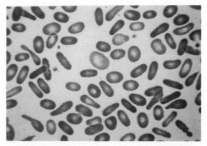

COLOR PLATE 29. Hereditary elliptocytosis (peripheral blood). Note the high percentage of elliptocytes or ovalocytes. (From Pittiglio and Sacher, Fig. 88, with permission.)

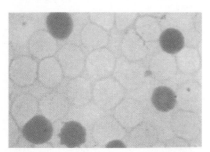

COLOR PLATE 30. Fetal hemoglobin: Kleihauer-Betke stain of newborn blood. Red cells containing hemoglobin F maintained red staining color; clear-staining cells contain hemoglobin A. (From Listen, Look and Learn. National Committee for Careers in the Medical Laboratory.)

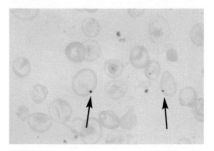

COLOR PLATE 31. Blood film in thalassemia. Note hypochromic, microcytic RBCs and Howell-Jolly bodies (arrows).

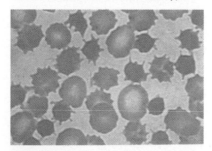

COLOR PLATE 32. Acanthocytosis (patient with abetalipoproteinemia). (From Hyun, BH, Ashton, JK, and Dolan, K: Practical Hematology: A Laboratory Guide with Accompanying Filmstrip. WB Saunders, Philadelphia, 1975, with permission.)

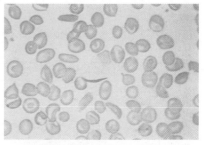

COLOR PLATE 33. Sickle thalassemia syndrome (peripheral blood). Note the sickle cells and target cells. (From Pittiglio and Sacher, Fig. 105, with permission.)

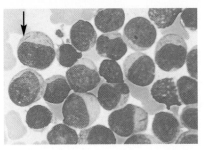

COLOR PLATE 34. Bone marrow: acute myeloblastic leukemia without maturation (FAB—M1). Note Auer rod (arrow).

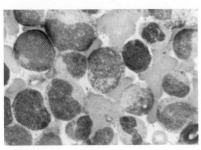

COLOR PLATE 35. Bone marrow: acute myeloblastic leukemia with limited maturation (FAB—M2).

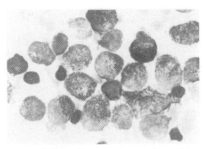

COLOR PLATE 36. Bone marrow: acute promyelocytic leukemia (FAB—M3). (From Pittiglio and Sacher, Fig. 162, with permission.)

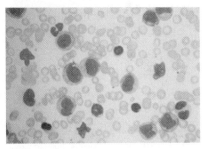

COLOR PLATE 37. Peripheral blood: acute myelo-monocytic leukemia (FAB—M4).

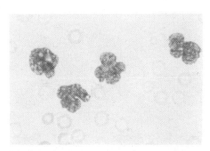

COLOR PLATE 38. Peripheral blood: acute monocytic leukemia, well-differentiated (FAB—M5b). (From Pittiglio and Sacher, Fig. 168, with permission.)

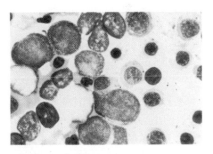

COLOR PLATE 39(A). Bone marrow: acute erythroleukemia (FAB—M6). Note megaloblastoid dyserythropoiesis. (From Pittiglio and Sacher, Fig. 169, with permission.)

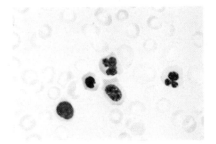

COLOR PLATE 39(B). Peripheral blood: acute erythroleukemia. Note dysplastic nuclei in nucleated red blood cells. (From Pittiglio and Sacher, Fig. 170, with permission.)

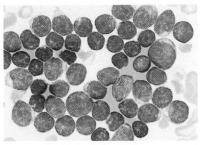

COLOR PLATE 40. Acute lymphoblastic leukemia (FAB—L1). (From Pittiglio and Sacher, Fig. 157, with permission.)

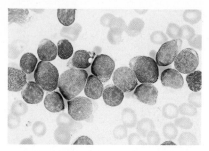

COLOR PLATE 41. Acute lymphoblastic leukemia, L2, bone marrow. (From Pittiglio and Sacher, Fig. 158, with permission.)

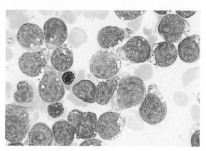

COLOR PLATE 42. Acute lymphoblastic leukemia, L3, bone marrow. (From Pittiglio and Sacher, Fig. 159, with permission.)

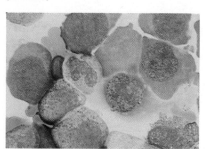

COLOR PLATE 43. Bone marrow from pernicious anemia showing numerous megaloblastic erythroid precursors and abnormal large myeloid precursors.

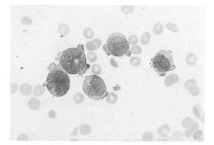

COLOR PLATE 44. Acute megakaryoblastic leukemia (AmegL), M7. (From Perkins, ML, Odell, JM, and Braziel, RM: Introduction to leukemia and the acute leukemias. In Harmening, DM (ed): Clinical Hematology and Fundamentals of Hemostasis, ed 3. FA Davis, Philadelphia, 1997, p. 312, with permission.)

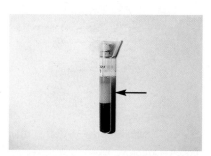

COLOR PLATE 45(A). Blood sample from a patient with chronic myelogenous leukemia (after standing) showing exaggerated "buffy coat" (white central zone—see arrow); white cell count 300,000/μL.

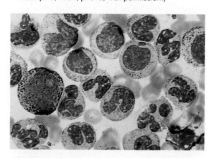

COLOR PLATE 45(B). Bone marrow showing myeloid hyperplasia with all myeloid precursors present in abundance in a patient with chronic myelogenous leukemia.

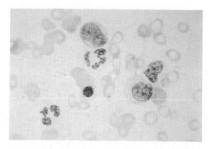

COLOR PLATE 46(A). Peripheral blood showing typical leukoerythroblastic reaction. Note immature white cells and red precursors in the peripheral blood. (From Pittiglio and Sacher, Fig. 131, with permission.)

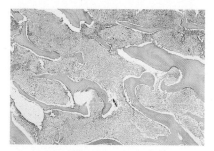

COLOR PLATE 46(B). Bone marrow biopsy showing fibrosis replacing normal marrow elements in a patient with idiopathic myelofibrosis.

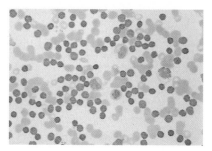

COLOR PLATE 47. Peripheral blood: chronic lymphocytic leukemia—small, regular, mature-appearing lymphocytes.

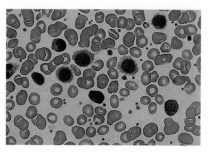

COLOR PLATE 48. Peripheral blood showing hairy cell leukemia. Note hairy projections from lymphoid cells.

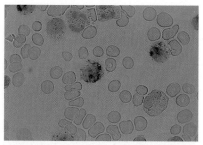

COLOR PLATE 49. Peripheral blood: positive tartrate-resistant acid phosphatase (TRAP) in hairy cell leukemia.

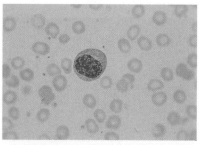

COLOR PLATE 50. Plasmacytoid lymphocyte from a patient with Waldenström's macroglobulinemia. (From Pittiglio and Sacher, Fig. 143, with permission.)

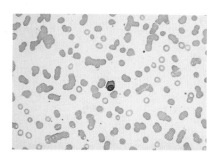

COLOR PLATE 51(A). Peripheral blood from a patient with multiple myeloma showing extensive rouleaux and a circulating plasma cell. (From Pittiglio and Sacher, Fig. 193, with permission.)

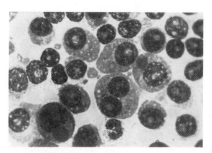

COLOR PLATE 51(B). Bone marrow from a patient with multiple myeloma, showing masses of large plasma cells with prominent nucleoli, including a binucleated plasma cell. (From Pittiglio and Sacher, Fig. 188, with permission.)

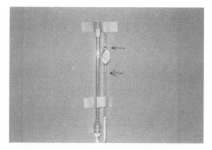

COLOR PLATE 51(C). Viscosimeter to measure serum viscosity. Arrows indicate distance of fluid flow. The time taken to measure rate of flow of serum compared with water gives the relative viscosity.

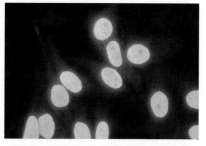

COLOR PLATE 52(A). Antinuclear antibody (ANA) patterns by indirect immunofluorescence on Hep2 cells: homogeneous.

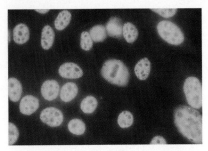

COLOR PLATE 52(B). Antinuclear antibody (ANA) patterns by indirect immunofluorescence on Hep2 cells: speckled.

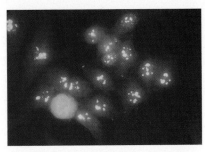

COLOR PLATE 52(C). Antinuclear antibody (ANA) patterns by indirect immunofluorescence on Hep2 cells: nucleolar.

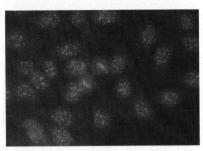

COLOR PLATE 52(D). Antinuclear antibody (ANA) patterns by indirect immunofluorescence on Hep2 cells: centromere.

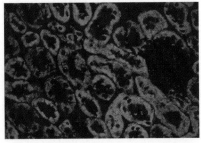

COLOR PLATE 53. Antimitochondrial antibody by indirect immunofluorescence on mouse kidney tubules.

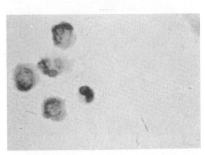

COLOR PLATE 54. Gram-stain smear of cerebrospinal fluid (CSF) from a patient with *Haemophilus influenzae* meningitis (gram-negative pleomorphic bacilli). Note the varied length of the bacilli.

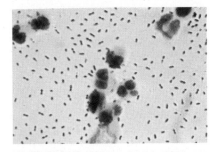

COLOR PLATE 55. Gram-stain smear of CSF from a patient with *Streptococcus pneumoniae* meningitis (gram-positive diplococci).

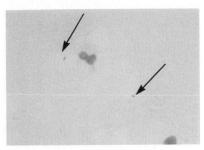

COLOR PLATE 56. Gram-stain smear of CSF from a patient with *Neisseria meningitidis* meningitis (gram-negative diplococci; see arrows). (From Roche Laboratories, Nutley, NJ, with permission.)

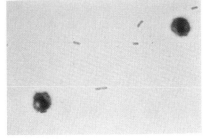

COLOR PLATE 57. Gram-stain smear of urine from a patient with *Escherichia coli* urinary tract infection (gram-negative bacilli).

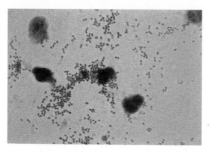

COLOR PLATE 58. Gram-stain smear of pus from a patient with *Staphylococcus aureus* wound infection (gram-positive cocci in clusters).

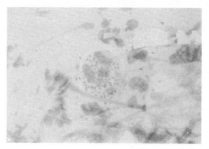

COLOR PLATE 59. Gram-stain smear of discharge from a patient with *Neisseria gonorrhoeae* (gram-negative diplococci; note intracellular distribution).

COLOR PLATE 60. Gram-stain smear of *Campylobacter jejuni*. Note curved gram-negative bacilli.

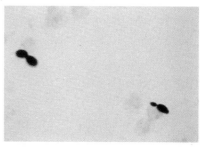

COLOR PLATE 61. Gram-stain smear of discharge from a patient with *Candida albicans* vaginitis (gram-positive oval budding yeast).

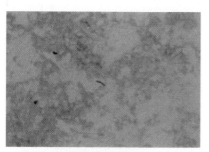

COLOR PLATE 62. Kinyoun-stained smear of sputum from a patient with *Mycobacterium tuberculosis* pneumonia (acid-fast bacillus).

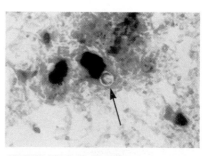

COLOR PLATE 63. Modified Kinyoun-stained smear of stool from a patient with *Cryptosporidium* enteritis (see arrow).

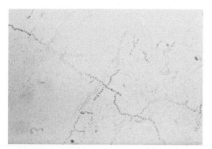

COLOR PLATE 64. KOH preparation of scrapings from a patient with skin ringworm. Note string-like fungal hyphae. (From Gower Medical Publishing, London, with permission.)

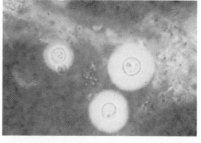

COLOR PLATE 65. India ink preparation of CSF from a patient with cryptococcal meningitis. Note the halo-like capsule. (From Gower Medical Publishing, London, with permission.)

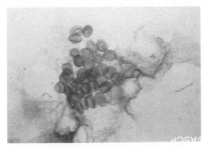

COLOR PLATE 66. Toluidine blue stain of *Pneumocystis carinii* in bronchial alveolar lavage fluid. (From the American Society for Clinical Pathologists, Chicago, with permission.)

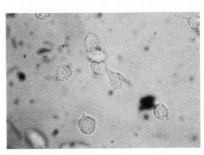

COLOR PLATE 67. Trichrome stain of stool from a patient with *Giardia lamblia* infection.

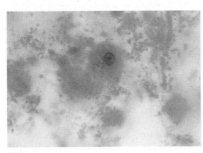

COLOR PLATE 68. Trichrome stain of stool from a patient with *Entamoeba histolytica* infection. Note the trophozoite with single prominent nucleus.

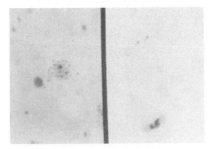

COLOR PLATE 69. Giemsa-stained smears of peripheral blood from patients with malaria. Giemsa stain showing *Plasmodium vivax* malarial trophozoites. On left, *Plasmodium vivax* (thick smear). On right, *Plasmodium falciparum* (thin smear). (From MEDCOM, Inc., with permission.)

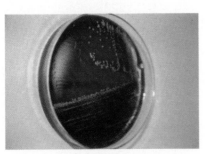

COLOR PLATE 70. Four-quadrant streaking method for obtaining isolated colonies.

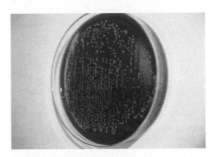

COLOR PLATE 71. Colony-count streaking method for quantitating microorganisms.

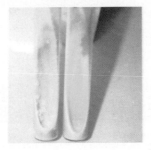

COLOR PLATE 72. Cultures of mycobacteria growing on Lowenstein-Jensen medium.

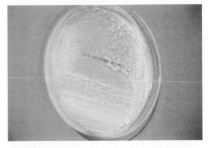

COLOR PLATE 73(A). Growth of *Candida albicans* on Sabouraud-dextrose agar.

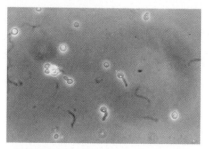

COLOR PLATE 73(B). *Candida albicans* showing germ tube formation. (From Gower Medical Publishing, London, with permission.)

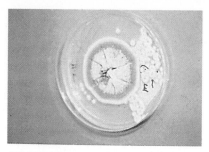

COLOR PLATE 74. Growth of *Aspergillus fumigatus* on Sabouraud-dextrose agar.

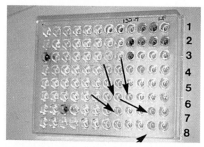

COLOR PLATE 75. Broth microdilution antimicrobial susceptibility test (Combo tray). Rows 1-3 contain biochemical identification test wells. Rows 4-8 contain antimicrobial dilutions. The greenish growth in several wells (arrows) indicates antimicrobial resistance.

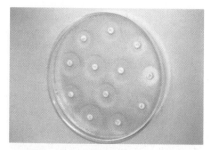

COLOR PLATE 76. Agar disk diffusion antimicrobial susceptibility test. Note circular zones of growth inhibition around antibiotic-impregnated filter paper disks.

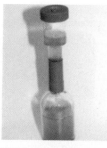

COLOR PLATE 77. Blood culture method. Microbial growth is evidenced by turbidity of the broth, and with this system, by manometric displacement of broth into the reservoir attached to the top of the bottle.

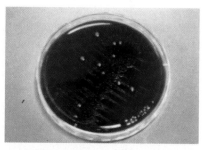

COLOR PLATE 78. Lysis centrifugation/direct plating. Growth of bacteria following plating of lysed blood to agar. (From E.I. DuPont de Nemours and Co., Wilmington, DE, with permission.)

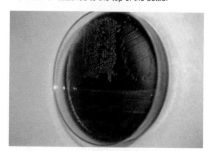

COLOR PLATE 79. Growth of *Haemophilus influenzae* on chocolate agar, showing mucoid colonies.

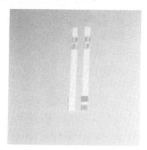

COLOR PLATE 80. Urine dipstick results. A positive leukocyte esterase result is indicated by purple color in the filter paper pad at the bottom of the dipstick. A positive nitrite result is indicated by red color in the filter paper pad immediately above the leukocyte esterase test pad.

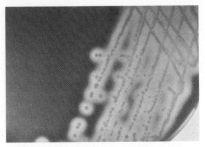

COLOR PLATE 81. Beta hemolysis on 5% sheep blood agar exhibited by group A streptococci following growth in an anaerobic environment. (From Marion Laboratories, Kansas City, MO, with permission.)

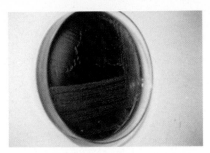

COLOR PLATE 82. Growth of *Neisseria gonorrheae* on modified Thayer-Martin agar.

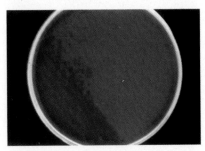

COLOR PLATE 83. Alpha hemolysis on 5% sheep blood agar exhibited by *Streptococcus viridans.*

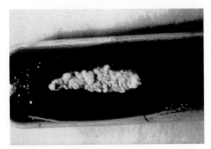

COLOR PLATE 84(A). Growth of dimorphic fungus *Histoplasma capsulatum*—yeast phase. (From Gower Medical Publishing, London, with permission.)

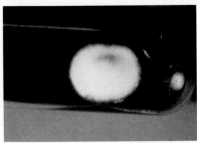

COLOR PLATE 84(B). Growth of dimorphic fungus *Histoplasma capsulatum*—mold phase. (From Gower Medical Publishing, London, with permission.)

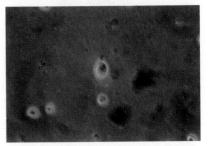

COLOR PLATE 85. Wet mount of vaginal discharge showing a *Trichomonas vaginalis* trophozoite. (From Gower Medical Publishing, London, with permission.)

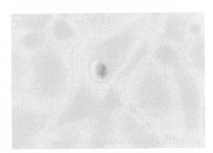

COLOR PLATE 86. Cervical scraping showing iodine-stained intracytoplasmic inclusion bodies of *Chlamydia trachomatis.* (From Gower Medical Publishing, London, with permission.)

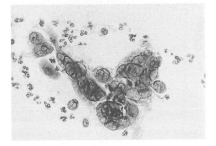

COLOR PLATE 87. Tzanck preparation showing multi-nucleate cells from a herpes simplex genital infection.

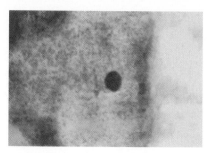

COLOR PLATE 88. Gram-stain smear of vaginal discharge showing "clue cells," epithelial cells coated with large number of gram-variable rods.

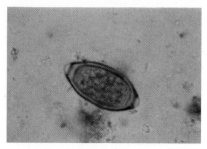

COLOR PLATE 89(A). Wet mount of a *Trichuris trichiura* egg in formalin-preserved stool.

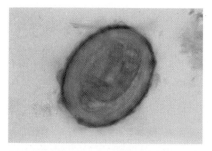

COLOR PLATE 89(B). *Ascaris lumbricoides* egg in stool.

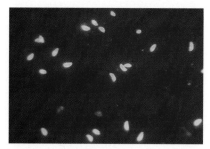

COLOR PLATE 90. Indirect immunofluorescence assay for *Toxoplasma gondii*. (Courtesy of Dr. S. Peters.)

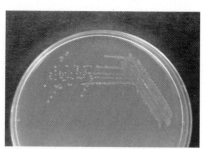

COLOR PLATE 91. Growth of *Shigella sonnei* on desoxycholate citrate agar demonstrating lack of lactose fermentation. (From Gower Medical Publishing, London, with permission.)

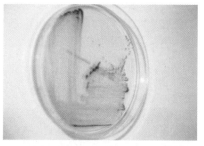

COLOR PLATE 92. Growth of *Salmonella enteritidis* on salmonella-Shigella (SS) agar. Note black colonies indicating hydrogen sulfide production.

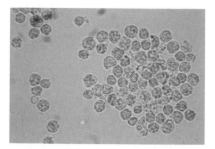

COLOR PLATE 93. Urine: white blood cells. (From Strasinger, SK: Urinalysis and Body Fluids. FA Davis, Philadelphia, 1985, Color Plate 1, with permission.)

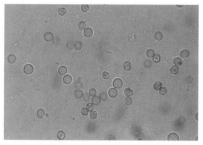

COLOR PLATE 94. Normal red blood cells in urine (×400). (From Strasinger, SK: Urinalysis and Body Fluids, ed 3. FA Davis, Philadelphia, 1994, Color Plate 1, with permission.)

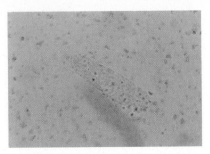

COLOR PLATE 95. Hyaline cast (×400). (From Strasinger, ed 3, Fig. 16, with permission.)

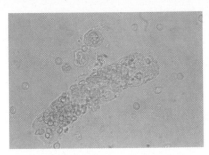

COLOR PLATE 96. Red blood cell cast (×400). Notice the presence of hypochromic and dysmorphic free red blood cells with blebs. (From Strasinger, ed 3, Fig. 17, with permission.)

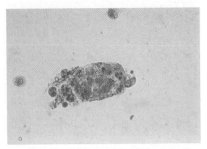

COLOR PLATE 97. Stained white blood cell cast (×400). (From Strasinger, ed 3, Fig. 19, with permission.)

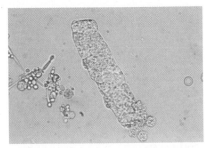

COLOR PLATE 98. Broad granular cast becoming waxy (×400). (From Strasinger, ed 3, Fig. 27, with permission.)

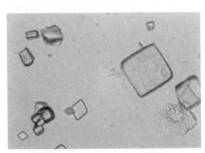

COLOR PLATE 99(A). Uric acid crystals (×400). (From Strasinger, ed 3, Fig. 29, with permission.)

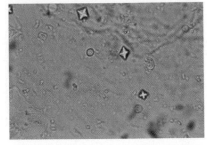

COLOR PLATE 99(B). Calcium oxalate crystals (×400). (From Strasinger, ed 3, Fig. 31, with permission.)

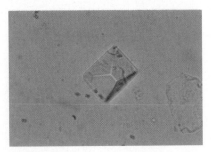

COLOR PLATE 99(C). Triple phosphate crystal (×400). (From Strasinger, ed 3, Fig. 33, with permission.)

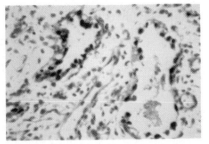

COLOR PLATE 100. In situ DNA hybridization for detection of adenovirus (blue-black inclusions) infecting the airway lining cells of human lung (red counter stain with safranin).

TABLE 1–3. PROBABILITIES OF NORMAL AND ABNORMAL RESULTS ON MULTITEST PANELS

Number of Tests	Probability of Being within Reference Range	Probability of at Least 1 Result Being out of Range
1	$0.95^1 = 0.95$	$1 - 0.95 = 0.05$
2	$0.95^2 = 0.9025$	$1 - 0.9025 = 0.0975$
3	$0.95^3 = 0.8574$	$1 - 0.8574 = 0.1426$
4	$0.95^4 = 0.8145$	$1 - 0.8145 = 0.1855$
•	•	•
•	•	•
•	•	•
10	$0.95^{10} = 0.5987$	$1 - 0.5987 = 0.4013$
•	•	•
•	•	•
•	•	•
20	$0.95^{20} = 0.3585$	$1 - 0.3585 = 0.6415$

laboratory values that are outside of the reference range in a normal individual. The more laboratory parameters performed, the more likely that one or more results will be outside the reference range. As an example, let us assume that the reference range for each analyte of a Chem 20 is set to include 95% of a healthy population. Then the probability of a healthy person having a normal result on any one test is 95% or 0.95 and the probability of having an abnormal result is $1 - 0.95 = 0.05$. The probability of that person having normal results on two tests is $0.95 \times 0.95 = 0.9025$ and the probability of having one or two abnormal results is $1 - 0.9025 = 0.0975$. This mathematical progression continues as illustrated in Table 1–3. The probability that a person will have normal results on all 20 tests is $0.95^{20} = 0.3585$. Thus the probability that the healthy person will have one or more out-of-range results is $1 - 0.3585 = 0.6415$. This is a fairly high probability of falsely calling someone abnormal and is the major theoretical limitation of widespread profile testing, because of the extremely high likelihood of incidental out-of-range results.

MEDICAL NECESSITY FOR LABORATORY TESTING

The United States government recently established extensive guidelines for the ordering of laboratory tests on outpatients covered by Medicare and Medicaid health insurance. These regulations are to be updated every year in an effort to eliminate fraud and abuse by ensuring that tests that are ordered meet criteria of medical necessity for each patient. Every test has a CPT (Current Procedural Terminology) code number, which must match with an approved diagnosis code (International Classification of Diseases, 9th Revision: ICD-9) for the test to be reimbursed by Medicare or Medicaid.

One of the changes imposed by these new federal regulations is the elimination of customized panels and large panels (20 or more tests ordered as one panel), based on the opinion that all such tests would almost never be medically necessary. Instead the Health Care Finance Administration (HCFA) and the American Medical Association (AMA) have formulated five panels intended for use in the outpatient arena. They are the electrolyte panel, basic metabolic panel, comprehensive metabolic panel, hepatic function panel, and renal function panel (Table 1–4). These panels will probably be modified or added to in coming years. For example, the carbon dioxide test was recently added to the comprehensive metabolic panel following requests by physicians.

TABLE 1–4. COMPOSITION OF AMA/HCFA–APPROVED CHEMISTRY PANELS FOR 2000

Test	Electrolyte Panel	Basic Metabolic Panel	Comprehensive Metabolic Panel	Hepatic Function Panel	Renal Function Panel
Sodium	Na	Na	Na	—	Na
Potassium	K	K	K	—	K
Chloride	Cl	Cl	Cl	—	Cl
Carbon dioxide	CO_2	CO_2	CO_2	—	CO_2
Glucose	—	Gluc	Gluc	—	Gluc
Urea nitrogen	—	Urea	Urea	—	Urea
Creatinine	—	Creat	Creat	—	Creat
Calcium	—	Ca	Ca	—	Ca
Albumin	—	—	Alb	Alb	Alb
Total protein	—	—	T prot	T prot	—
AST (SGOT)	—	—	AST	AST	—
ALT (SGPT)	—	—	ALT	ALT	—
Alkaline phosphatase	—	—	ALP	ALP	—
Bilirubin, total	—	—	Bili T	Bili T	—
Bilirubin, direct	—	—	—	Bili D	—
Phosphorus, inorganic	—	—	—	—	Phos

PRIORITY REPORTING: STAT AND PANIC VALUES

In the setting of acute care medicine in hospitals, there is frequently need for immediate turnaround of laboratory results to the physician within one hour or less of drawing the specimen in order to modify therapy. This type of priority is designated **stat** for the Latin word *statim* meaning "immediately." Tests that fall into this category include glucose in diabetic ketoacidosis, some drug levels such as theophylline, amylase in suspected pancreatitis, creatine kinase in suspected myocardial infarction, hematocrit, blood gases, and potassium. In fact, there may be a need for many other determinations under a variety of clinical situations in which a clinical decision of medical management will be made.

Sometimes the results of a test are so far out of expected range that it may be life-threatening. In that situation, it should be the responsibility of the laboratory to contact the physician or other medical personnel to communicate that result immediately. This should be done whether the test was ordered stat or not. To comply with this policy, each laboratory should establish a procedure to include the threshold levels that mandate this action. These levels are termed **critical values** or **panic values** and are confined to a list of analytes that truly do have the potential to be lethal if left unchecked for a short period. Examples of critical values are listed in Table 1–5. As a matter of good medical practice, the laboratory should keep a log of each critical value call, to include the doctor or other person contacted, the patient's name, the value of the analyte, the time and date called, and the name of the caller.

ANCILLARY (POINT OF CARE) TESTING

Ancillary or **point of care testing** refers to those analyses that are performed outside the physical facilities of a centralized clinical laboratory. Examples frequently performed on general medical wards are fingerstick blood analysis for glucose, urine glucose and other urine dipstick tests, fecal occult blood, gastric aspirate for pH and occult blood, and pregnancy testing. Critical care units often perform coagulation studies to adjust heparin doses and arterial blood gas analyses for patients on respirators or undergoing surgery.

The obvious advantages of such programs include immediate access to analytic data that enable medical and therapeutic decisions to be made. Limitations on these tests relate largely to training of personnel, quality control, and documentation. It is essential that such tests be subjected to external proficiency testing at each ancillary (ward) site. Common

TABLE 1–5. CRITICAL VALUES THAT REQUIRE IMMEDIATE COMMUNICATIONS

Test	Critical Value
Hematology	
Hct	<14%
	>60%
WBC	<2000/µL on a new patient or a 1000 difference from previous, if less than 4000/µL
	>50,000/µL on a new patient
Smear	Shows leukemic cells (progranulocytic or blast)
	Shows abnormal leukemoid reaction
	Positive for malaria or other parasites
Platelets	<20,000/µL and not previously reported
	>1 million/µL
Reticulocyte	>20%
Prothrombin time	>40 seconds
Chemistry	
Serum bilirubin	>18 mg/dL (newborn)
Serum calcium	<6 mg/dL
	>13 mg/dL
Serum glucose	<40 mg/dL
	>500 mg/dL
Serum phosphate	<1 mg/dL
Serum potassium	<2.5 mEq/L
	>6.5 mEq/L
Serum sodium	<120 mEq/L
	>160 mEq/L
Serum bicarbonate	<10 mEq/L
	>40 mEq/L
Arterial or capillary PO_2	<40 mmHg
Arterial or capillary pH	<7.2
	>7.6
Arterial or capillary P_{CO_2}	<20 mmHg
	>70 mmHg
Microbiology	
Blood culture	Positive
Gram stain on CSF and any body fluids (pleural, synovial, peritoneal, etc.)	Positive

problems encountered with such tests include the use of expired reagents, inconsistent quality control using test materials with different lot numbers, and lack of maintenance and proficiency testing. Personnel performing such tests should also be trained and assessed annually for their ability to both perform and interpret these tests. These expectations are now included in standards of the Joint Commission on Accreditation of Health Care Organizations and are formalized in federal regulations by the Clinical Laboratories Improvement Act of 1988.

An extension of point of care testing has generated small satellite laboratories that are capable of measuring blood gases, electrolytes, and basic hemoglobin and coagulation profiles. Instrumentation has advanced to become very user friendly and allow analysis on whole blood specimens. Such instruments are not uncommonly found in intensive care units, operating rooms, and emergency departments. These instruments are also used in physician offices where they offer laboratory data with a rapid turnaround time.

LABORATORY ECONOMICS AND DIAGNOSTIC ALGORITHMS

Laboratory testing has costs directly attributable to the following phases:

1. Collecting, transporting, and processing a specimen (preanalytic phase)
2. Testing the specimen and related quality control and proficiency testing (analytic phase)
3. Reporting the results (postanalytic phase)

Although many people think that the analytic phase constitutes greatest laboratory costs, for automated analyses the other components may be more costly because they are so labor-intensive and involve multiple transactions between different medical personnel. Once the costs of acquiring and delivering a specimen to the laboratory are accounted for, the actual expense per test can be very low if performed on a multichannel chemistry or hematology analyzer. Thus the least costly tests (on an individual basis) are those that are bundled into profiles and panels performed on the same instrument. If the specimen must be split to perform assays on a different instrument or with manual manipulations, then the costs go up accordingly (e.g., HDL-cholesterol, iron-binding capacity, cortisol, or phenytoin measurement added onto a Chem 20 panel). Of course some assays do have high reagent costs owing to a combination of proprietary methods for some instruments (e.g., cyclosporine immunoassay) or relatively low usage (e.g., aldolase), both of which preclude being on multichannel analyzers. In general, immunoassays should be expected to cost more than routine chemistry assays, and coagulation factor assays cost more than prothrombin times or other coagulation screening assays. Highly manual procedures are always among the most costly: microbiologic cultures, histocompatibility testing, and type and cross of red blood cells for transfusion.

Assays that are performed in a central laboratory generally have potential advantages of cost reduction by testing in batches or other high-volume strategies that increase efficiencies of reagents, instruments, and labor. However, the time of specimen transportation from patient to central laboratory may be too long for clinical needs, thus leading to near patient testing for selected critical analytes (arterial blood gases, potassium, hemoglobin, activated partial thromboplastin time). Such testing is always more expensive (often several times) than the cost of the same testing in a busy central laboratory because of the purchase price of the reagents, as well as that of the instrument, which remains unused most of the time; the inherent inefficiency of one person (nurse or doctor) performing only one test at a time; the proportionately higher cost of quality control and proficiency testing when the actual number of patient samples is low; and manual methods of result reporting that are not interfaced with the patient's electronic medical record. Despite these shortcomings, the clinical need may demand very quick response, which can ultimately save other costs (e.g., near patient coagulation testing on which to base the use of fresh frozen plasma in transfusion of a surgical patient).

Many medical institutions are now establishing guidelines for the use of cost-effective laboratory, radiology, and other diagnostic procedures in standardized sequences that are termed **critical pathways** or **diagnostic algorithms.** Diagnostic algorithms are series of steps used in diagnosing and treating a disease. Laboratory strategies can be formulated as diagnostic algorithms in which preliminary test results serve as the basis on which to order further laboratory tests in an orchestrated hierarchical manner. The intention is to recommend those procedures that are known to carry the most meaningful diagnostic information in both acute and convalescent care and to avoid excessive ordering of tests that convey merely redundant or marginal additional information. The impetus for this process is decreasing reimbursements for medical care in which payments to hospitals are based on capitation (a fixed amount per patient per year for all medical treatments) or diagnosis and not on how many medical procedures are done. Thus medical centers now are striving to standardize the testing pathways by which new patients are assessed—in emergency rooms, in chest pain protocols, in acute care units. They are also using recommendations for lesser-acuity care such as preoperative screening for elective surgery (e.g., below a certain age, no chest x-ray, no measurements of electrolytes, hemoglobin, or coagulation unless the patient has a history of abnormality) and in postoperative care (no daily chemistry or hematology panels; only continue monitoring those analytes that have been abnormal previously). Laboratorians have a crucial role to play in helping their institutions choose the most effective diagnostic tests and then provide those tests in a timely and low-cost manner.

In summary, to use laboratory measurements properly, it is necessary to appreciate the technical validity (accuracy and precision) of a test, its diagnostic value (sensitivity, specificity, predictive value), optimal specimen collection, potential sources of error, costs of collecting and analyzing specimens, and its ultimate clinical usefulness for screening, diagnosing, or monitoring disease.

SUGGESTED READING

Balenstein, PN: Evaluating diagnostic tests with imperfect standards. Am J Clin Pathol 93:252–258, 1990.

College of American Pathologists Conference XXVIII: Alternate site testing. Arch Pathol Lab Med 119:861–983, 1995. This entire issue is devoted to point-of-care testing.

Creer, MH, and Ladenson, J: Analytic errors due to lipemia. Lab Med 14:351–355, 1983.

Fraser, CG, et al: Biologic variation of common hematologic laboratory quantities in the elderly. Am J Clin Pathol 92:465–470, 1989.

Lundberg, GD: Using the Clinical Laboratory in Medical Decision-Making. American Society of Clinical Pathologists Press, Chicago, 1983.

Watts, NB: Medical relevance of laboratory tests. Arch Pathol Lab Med 112:379–382, 1988.

Weig, NH: Evaluation of the clinical accuracy of laboratory tests. Arch Pathol Lab Med 112:383–386, 1988.

Zweig, MH, and Campbell, G: Receiver-operating characteristic (ROC) plots: a fundamental evaluation tool in clinical medicine. Clin Chem 39:561–577, 1993.

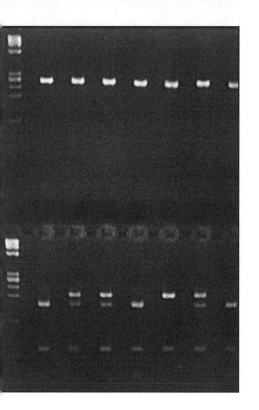

Section Two

Hematology

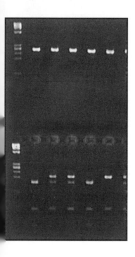

2

Hematologic Methods

Hematology is the study of the blood and the blood-forming tissues that comprise one of the largest organ systems of the body. Blood constitutes 6 to 8% of the total body weight and consists of blood cells suspended in a fluid called **plasma.** The three main types of blood cells are the red blood cells **(erythrocytes),** white blood cells **(leukocytes),** and platelets **(thrombocytes).** The fluid plasma forms 45 to 60% of the total blood volume; the red blood cells (RBCs) occupy most of the remaining volume. White blood cells and platelets, although functionally essential, occupy a relatively small proportion of the total blood mass. The proportion of cells and plasma is regulated and is kept relatively constant.

The principal function of circulating blood is transportation; red blood cells remain within the circulatory system and contain the oxygen-transporting pigment **hemoglobin.** White blood cells are responsible for the body's defenses and are transported by the blood to the various tissues where they perform their physiologic roles. Platelets are responsible for preventing blood loss from hemorrhage and exert their main effects at the blood vessel wall. The plasma proteins are important transporters of nutrients and metabolic byproducts to the respective organs for storage and excretion. Many of the large proteins suspended in plasma are also of interest to the hematologist, especially those proteins concerned with the prevention of hemorrhage by coagulation. The hematology laboratory is concerned with defining normal and abnormal blood cells or blood pigments and determining the nature of the abnormalities. The coagulation laboratory is concerned with evaluating people with abnormal hemostasis, either excessive bleeding or abnormal coagulation or thrombosis. Hematology laboratory studies are often extremely important in appreciating the overall well-being of the patient and are frequently used in health screening tests. Chapter 3 will discuss blood disorders that correspond to most tests discussed in this chapter.

HEMATOPOIESIS

Hematopoiesis refers to the formation and development of all types of blood cells from their parental precursors. Blood cells in normal adults are manufactured in the marrow of the bones, forming the axial skeleton. From infancy to adulthood there is a progressive change in productive marrow to occupy the central skeleton, especially the sternum, ribs, vertebral bodies, pelvic bones, and the proximal portions of the long bones. During fetal development, hematopoiesis is first established in the yolk sac and later transfers to the liver and spleen and finally to the bony skeleton (Fig. 2–1). Hematopoiesis gradually decreases in the shafts of the long bones, and after the age of 4 years, fat cells begin to appear. Generally, hematopoiesis is regulated by both cell-to-cell regulation **(contact phase)** and humoral regulation **(glycoprotein growth factors),** and also according to the demands of the body. In the contact phase, stromal and microenvironmental influences control cell behavior; the glycoprotein humoral factors control progenitor cell proliferation (Color Plate 1 and Table 2–1). Therefore, blood cell production is kept relatively constant but has the capacity to increase with increasing demand. Organs that were capable of sustaining hematopoiesis in fetal life always retain this ability should the demand arise.

The marrow is a special environment for hematopoietic growth and development. In the bone marrow, hematopoiesis occurs in the extravascular part of the red marrow, which consists of a fine supporting reticulin framework interspersed with vascular channels and developing marrow cells. A single layer of endothelial cells separates the extravascular marrow compartment from the intravascular compartment. When the hematopoietic marrow cells are mature and ready to circulate in the peripheral blood, the cells leave the marrow parenchyma by passing through fine "windows" in the endothelial cells and emerge into the venous sinuses. This process can also be stimulated by a number of releasing factors, such as fragments of the third component of complement, glucocorticoid hormones, androgenic steroids, and endotoxins. The process is also facilitated by a number of adhesion molecules that are expressed on the surface of the cells prior to their egress. These molecules initially maintain attachment to the endothelial cells and subsequently migrate through these windows. The molecular basis of this adhesion molecule expression and then down-regulation is providing insight into the highly regulated release of cells from the normal marrow.

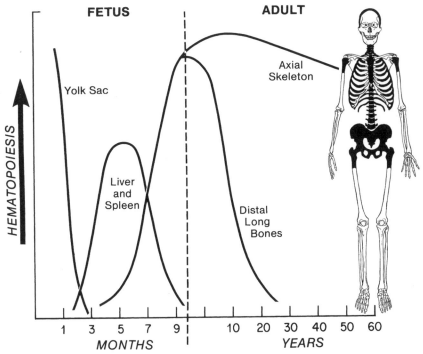

FIGURE 2–1. Location of active marrow growth in the fetus and adult. During fetal development, hematopoiesis is established in the yolk-sac mesenchyme, moves to the liver and spleen, and finally is limited to the bony skeleton. From infancy to adulthood, there is a progressive restriction of productive marrow to the axial skeleton and proximal ends of the long bones *(shaded areas)*. (From Hillman, RS, and Finch, CA: Red Cell Manual, ed 7. FA Davis, Philadelphia, 1996, p 2, with permission.)

Most of the cells in the circulating blood are incapable of further division, are relatively short-lived, and are replaced constantly from the bone marrow. The main blood cell groups—including the red blood cells, white blood cells, and platelets—are derived from a pluripotent hematopoietic stem cell. This stem cell is the first in a sequence of regular and orderly steps of cell growth and maturation (see Color Plate 1). The pluripotent stem cell may mature along morphologically and functionally diverse lines, depending on conditioning stimuli and mediators, and may either produce other stem cells and self-regenerate or mature in two main directions. Stem cells may become committed to the lymphoid cell line for lymphopoiesis, or toward the development of a multipotent stem cell capable of sustaining myelopoiesis, erythropoiesis, and platelet production **(CFU-GEMM)** (see Color Plate 1). Morphologically, these multipotent and pluripotent stem cells appear as small cells that resemble a

TABLE 2–1. HEMATOPOIETIC GROWTH FACTORS AND CYTOKINES

Factor	Hematopoietic Target Cells
Lineage Restricted	
Erythropoietin	Erythrocytes
G-CSF	Granulocytes (predominantly neutrophils)
M-CSF	Monocytes
Thrombopoietin (c-mpl ligand)	Megakaryocytes (Platelets)
Multilineage	
GM-CSF	Granulocytes, Monocytes, Megakaryocytes ($\pm$) Erythrocytes ($\pm$)
IL-3 (multi-CSF)	Granulocytes, Monocytes, Megakaryocytes, Stem cells ($\pm$), Erythrocytes ($\pm$)
c-kit ligand (stem cell factor)	Stem cells (+), Pre-B Cells
IL-1 α and β	Fibroblasts/Stem Cells
IL-2	T Cells, Activated B Cells
IL-4	T Cells, B Cells (+)
IL-5	Eosinophils (+), B Cells
IL-6	Stem Cells, B Cells, Granulocytes, Monocytes
IL-7	T Cells, Pre-B Cells
IL-9	T Cells (helper)
IL-11	Megakaryocytes, B Cells, Mast Cells

CSF = colony-stimulating factor
G = granulocyte
GM = granulocyte and macrophage
IL = interleukin
$\pm$ = limited activity
+ = major activity

mature lymphocyte. Normally approximately $1/10^6$ cell is a stem cell. Factors that regulate proliferation are shown in Table 2–1. Proliferation of pluripotent cells is directed by growth factors such as stem cell factor (c-kit ligand), interleukin-3 (IL-3), IL-6, or IL-11. Multipotent progenitors are directed by other factors such as granulocyte macrophage colony-stimulating factor (GM-CSF) and IL-3. Committed progenitors are influenced by more lineage-specific growth factors such as granulocyte CSF (G-CSF), erythropoietin IL-5, IL-6, and macrophage-CSF (M-CSF). Suppressor factors also influence growth and proliferation. For example, tumor necrosis factor alpha (TNF-alpha) and interferon-γ (derived from activated T cells) may directly suppress hematopoiesis. Yet these cytokines and IL-1 can also amplify hematopoietic proliferation by their activation of accessory marrow cells (fibroblasts and monocytes) (see Table 2–1).

Most stem cells remain in a resting (G_o) state from which they can be recruited to meet an emergency situation such as hemorrhage, infection, or bone marrow injury. The hematopoietic stem cells evolve as **growth units** under the influence of **growth factors.** Red cell development, or **erythropoiesis,** is sustained by the multipotent stem cell maturing into a **burst-forming unit–erythroid** (BFU-E) controlled by a **burst-promoting activity (BPA).** A single BFU-E is capable of producing a colony of more than 1000 developing red cells. This now constitutes a **colony-forming unit–erythroid** (CFU-E). Growth and maturation of the BFU-E is under the influence of hormonal factors, especially the hormone erythropoietin. The hematopoietic stem cell may also give rise to other colony-forming units (CFUs), which grow and mature to granulocytes, monocytes, eosinophils, basophils, and megakaryocytes under the influence of specific **colony-stimulating factors (CSFs)** (see Color Plate 1 and Table 2–1). Bone marrow growth may be studied in the laboratory using *in vitro* culture methods. Colonies may be formed on culture media containing the specific growth factors derived from extracts of supporting marrow cells or purified by recombinant DNA technology, and their effects in sustaining marrow cell growth may be analyzed in culture.

ERYTHROPOIESIS

Erythrocytes are derived from the committed erythroid precursor cells, as described above, through a process of mitotic growth and maturation. The level of tissue oxygenation regulates the production of red cells that transport oxygen to the tissues (effective erythropoiesis). **Erythropoietin** is a hormone produced largely by the kidney peritubular interstitial cells. It stimulates the CFU-E progenitor cells to speed up growth and enhance maturation. The specific pathways regulating tissue oxygen fluctuations with changes in erythropoietin levels are not understood. Although erythropoietin is not stored in the kidneys, renal function and oxygen levels are the main factors controlling erythropoietin release. Normally, only minute (picomolar) quantities are present in the circulating blood. The normal erythropoietin range is 9 to 26 units/mL.

Anything that lowers tissue oxygen delivery increases erythropoietin levels, provided the individual has adequately functioning kidneys. Low blood hemoglobin levels, impaired oxygen release from hemoglobin, impaired respiratory oxygen exchange, and poor blood flow are common causes of tissue hypoxia (see the section on Polycythemia in Chapter 3). Erythropoietin concentration is therefore high in most anemias, hemoglobin disorders, pulmonary diseases, and severe circulatory defects.

The capacity of erythropoietin to produce erythropoiesis depends on an adequate supply of nutrients and minerals (particularly iron, folic acid, and vitamin B_{12}) to the marrow. If the marrow has the capacity to respond, red cell production increases. In many anemias and hemoglobin disorders, the nature of the disease limits an appropriate erythropoietic response. Patients without kidneys do produce red cells, but at a lower than normal rate. In severe renal failure, or in people who have had both kidneys surgically removed, a stable but severely anemic state exists that is limited in its response to hypoxic stimuli. The liver produces whatever erythropoietic factor is functioning in this case.

Erythropoietin accelerates nearly every stage of red cell production. The rate at which the committed stem cells (BFU-E and CFU-E) divide and differentiate toward cell production is especially increased. Under appropriate conditions, erythropoiesis may increase up to 20- to 30-fold. Erythropoietin also increases the rate of cell division, speeds the incorporation of iron into the developing red cells, shortens the time of cell maturation, and hastens (and increases) entry of immature red cells (reticulocytes) into the circulation (Color Plates 2, 3, and 10A). This capacity may be measured in the laboratory by a reticulocyte count. The erythron is the term used to describe the total population of mature erythrocytes and their precursors in the blood and bone marrow. Normally, 10 to 15% of developing red cells die within the marrow. This phenomenon, called ineffective erythropoiesis, may be increased in certain disease states.

GRANULOPOIESIS

The whole blood concentration of circulating white blood cells (leukocytes) is kept relatively constant, despite a large number that die every day. These leukocytes are replaced by cell division. The production of new white cells in the marrow is termed granulopoiesis. Amplification of leukocytes occurs by mitosis, a process of sequential cell growth and division. The stem cells are capable of self-reproduction and development into mature white cells in an orderly sequence of maturation, and are then released from the bone marrow into the circulation. A process of differentiation occurs, whereby the immature white cells gradually develop and exhibit characteristics of mature functional leukocytes.

Developing white cells may be divided into various physiologic compartments: (1) the proliferating pool, (2) the maturation pool and storage pools, (3) the circulating pool, and (4) the marginating pool (Fig. 2–2). These will be described below in the section on Myeloid Growth and Distribution. Under certain physiologic and pathologic stimuli, granulocytes may be released from the storage and marginating pools within minutes, followed somewhat later by enhanced granulocyte production. Unlike erythropoiesis, no single substance comparable to erythropoietin has been found, although total granulocyte mass seems to influence leukocyte production. Nevertheless, cell-cell interaction and the release of the humoral growth factors (CSFs) described later do control both the

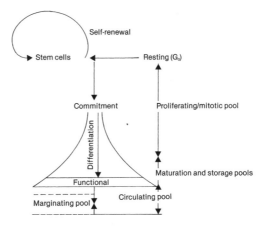

FIGURE   2–2. Granulocytic compartments.

production and maturation of white cells. White cell production is also substantially influenced by chemical mediators **(cytokines and chemokines)** released as part of inflammatory and immune responses.

Growth Factors

The factor that can influence maturation of a stem cell to granulocyte, monocyte and, to a lesser extent, megakaryocyte production is called **colony-stimulating factor for granulocytes and monocytes** (GM-CSF). This is a differentiation-promoting growth factor that allows and stimulates production of granulocytes and monocytes. The process of differentiation represents a process of repression or expression of genetic material. Therefore, granulocytes share with the monocytes a common progenitor cell termed the CFU-GM, or **colony-forming unit–granulocyte, monocyte.** Exposure of this unit to GM-CSF will facilitate the growth of granulocyte and monocyte colonies. Another factor, G-CSF, promotes differentiation more preferentially to granulocytes. A number of cytokines liberated from marrow stromal cells, activated lymphocytes, and monocytes also influence maturation and differentiation. These **interleukins** (e.g., IL-1, IL-3, IL-6, IL-11) can influence myelopoiesis and indeed hematopoiesis at many levels (see Table 2–1). The intermediate cells during the process of differentiation are also shown in Color Plate 1. (Once the granulocytes are mature, they are released into the peripheral blood and subsequently circulate and leave the blood to enter the tissues.) Under normal conditions, the rate of production of granulocytes and their rate of egress from the marrow is constant. However, under conditions of increased demand (e.g., infection or inflammation) their rate of production may increase 20-fold.

Myeloid Growth and Distribution

Granulopoiesis is a continuous evolution from the earliest myeloid precursor to the myeloblast and finally to the most mature cell, the neutrophil (see Color Plates 3 and 4). This process requires 7 to 11 days. Myeloblasts, promyelocytes, and myelocytes all are capable of division and comprise the **proliferating** or **mitotic pool.** Beyond this stage no mitosis occurs, and the cells mature through several phases. This phase is now termed the **maturation pool.** It comprises metamyelocytes, bands, and segmented neutrophils. An excess of these cells may remain in the marrow for release when needed. This population constitutes the **storage pool.** The storage pool cells may remain in the marrow for approximately 10 days, serving as a reservoir when needed. The peripheral blood granulocytes are distributed in two main phases, the **circulating pool** (approximately 50%) and cells that are closely aligned to the blood vessel wall, called the **marginating pool.** Cells may distribute between the circulating and the marginating pools in response to various inflammatory, infectious, or drug stimuli. The granulocytic compartments are diagrammatically represented in Figure 2–2.

The major functions of neutrophils are (1) host defense involving migration to areas of infection and inflammation, (2) recognition and processing of foreign antigens, (3) phagocytosis and killing, and (4) digestion of tissue debris and microorganisms. Phagocytosis is enhanced by processing, opsonization, or preparation of the antigen or microorganism (see the section on Peripheral Blood: White Cells later in this chapter). There are three main types of mature granulocytes: **neutrophils, eosinophils,** and **basophils** (see Color Plates 4 and 5). The process of production is similar, except toward the later maturation phases, where typical intracellular granules become evident. The staining characteristics of these granules in peripheral blood define the cell types. Eosinophils contain red-pink granules, basophils contain blue-black granules, and neutrophils have a less pronounced neutral staining. Each cell has specific functions that will be discussed later. The major thrust of myelopoiesis is, however, directed toward the neutrophil series.

Neutrophils remain in the circulation approximately 7 to 10 hours, and as these cells migrate to the tissues, they are replenished in the blood by cells released from the bone marrow. Release from the bone marrow into the venous sinuses occurs through fine endothelial pores, similar to those described in erythropoiesis. Neutrophils exit the circulation by moving between the blood vessel endothelial cells into the tissues. This egress probably requires the expression of **cellular adhesion molecules** both on the surface of the neutrophil and on the endothelial cells. The neutrophils' ability to focus in at a site of infection or inflammation is also governed by attracting stimuli called **chemotactic factors,** which are released from damaged tissue or bacteria. The neutrophil cell membrane has receptors for these factors, which evoke metabolic changes within the neutrophil.

Neutrophil degradation products, microbial products, and cellular breakdown products all seem to influence granulocyte kinetics. As a result of these various stimuli, the numbers of circulating granulocytes rise, and immature granulocytes may be released into the peripheral blood. Normally, no more than 5% of the circulating granulocytes are immature, and by far the majority of these are at the band stage (see Color Plates 1 and 3 [D]). Under intense granulocytic stimulation, large numbers of **band cells** (immature neutrophils), some **metamyelocytes,** and occasionally even **myelocytes** find their way into the circulation.

The other major direction of differentiation of the CFU-GM is toward monocyte production. **Monocytes** are actively phagocytic leukocytes that also play a major role in defense from pathogenic organisms and antigens. The earliest cell produced, the **monoblast,** matures through the **promonocyte** to the mature monocyte (see Color Plate 5C). The monocytic precursors are usually inconspicuous in normal marrow. Monocytes leave the marrow when mature and enter the venous sinusoids to circulate in the peripheral blood. They circulate for approximately 12 to 14 hours before migrating to the tissue sites.

LYMPHOPOIESIS

Lymphopoiesis is the growth and maturation of lymphocytes (see Color Plates 1 and 4). The **lymphocyte** is the second most abundant white cell circulating in the peripheral blood. Lymphocytes are primarily concerned with the immune defense system. Normal marrow may be composed of up to 20% developing lymphocytes. Lymphocytes are also derived from the marrow stem cell, but the control of lymphocyte production within the marrow is not well understood. Following maturation, the lympho-cytes enter the peripheral blood, circulate for a variable length of time depending on the nature of the cell, and subsequently repopulate the lymph nodes or lymphatic organs. The earliest lymphoid cell is a **lymphoblast,** which is generally indistinct and inconspicuous in normal marrow. Lymphocytes are conditioned by two main organ systems, the thymus (T-lymphocytes) or the bone marrow (B-lymphocytes). Morpho-logic criteria are not useful in determining the subtype or functional characteristics of lymphocytes. B-lymphocytes may differentiate further to produce plasma cells, which comprise less than 4.5% of the normal marrow differential count. Plasma cells have a characteristic morphology with an eccentric cell nucleus, a juxtanuclear halo, and a chromatin pattern described as a cartwheel (see Color Plate 6A). Plasma cells manufacture antibody (immunoglobulin). (See also Chapter 7.)

MEGAKARYOPOIESIS

The characteristic giant cells, the **megakaryocytes,** are precursors of the blood platelets. Platelets prevent bleeding by forming small platelet plugs into defects in capillary walls and also facilitate blood coagulation. The process of platelet development from megakaryocytes is termed **mega-karyopoiesis.** The **megakaryocyte** is the largest cell in the bone marrow and also arises from the multipotent stem cell (see Color Plates 1, 6B, and 7). It is believed that a hormone similar to erythropoietin, termed **thrombopoietin (TPO),** may control proliferation and maturation of megakaryocytes. TPO has only recently been discovered. It induces both megakaryocyte differentiation and platelet production. The TPO gene has been cloned from both humans and animals and appears to be the same molecule that has variously been called "TPO," "c-mp1 ligand," and "megakaryocyte growth and development factor (MGDF)." A number of other cytokines (such as stem cell factor, IL-3, IL-6, and IL-11) also exert controlling influences in megakaryopoiesis. The earliest precursor of the megakaryocyte is termed a **megakaryoblast.** During the stage of megakaryocyte maturation, the nucleus undergoes multiple divisions without corresponding divisions in the cell. Therefore, a multinucleate cell is formed (see Color Plate 6B). As the cell matures, abundant cytoplasm accumulates. Platelets are formed by the development of demarcation membranes within the cytoplasm, and individual platelets are extruded through the endothelial cells of the marrow sinusoids into the venous sinuses. Mature circulating platelets, like mature red cells, have no nucleus. A single megakaryocyte can release several thousand platelets. Following platelet release, the bare nucleus of the megakaryo-cyte is sometimes seen in marrow preparations. Platelets vary in size from 1 to about 4 μm in diameter but may occasionally be larger. They stain light blue and have multiple cytoplasmic granules (see Color Plates 4 and 6B). These granules contain functional constituents that are important in the control of bleeding (see Chapter 5). The circulating platelet count is kept within a narrow range and appears to be controlled by factors that include absolute platelet mass within the body and the release of thrombopoietin. Platelet production can increase at least 3-fold in response to stress.

LABORATORY EVALUATION OF HEMATOPOIESIS

DIRECT MARROW SAMPLING

The elements of hematopoietic activity can be evaluated both quantita-tively and qualitatively. The amount of functional bone marrow can be most simply determined by direct microscopic evaluation. Bone marrow function can also be determined by cell labeling with specific radioisoto-pic tracer elements, which are incorporated within the developing erythroid precursors. In this manner, the use of radioactive iron can be used to evaluate hemoglobin production and sites of erythropoiesis. Other tracer elements can be used to determine the quantity and distribution of bone marrow activity (indium or technetium) or the survival of red blood cells (chromium or indium).

Bone Marrow Aspiration and Biopsy

Microscopic examination of aspirated bone marrow tissue is usually the simplest method of assessing both the amount of bone marrow and the nature of cell growth and maturation.

A bone marrow aspirate is performed by the introduction of a needle through the outer bony layers into the marrow cavity and the withdrawal of a sample of marrow "juice" for examination. Sites for bone marrow aspiration are the posterior iliac crest of the pelvis, the sternum, and the anterior iliac crest. In young children, the proximal portion of the tibia may be used.

The detail and relationship of the developing marrow cells to one another, as well as the pattern of maturation, is best assessed by microscopic examination of the aspirated marrow tissue. Hematopoietic bone marrow contains fat and other connective tissue as well as the blood-forming cells. It is fluid enough to be aspirated through the needle, but only the first few drops should be used for examination because in the later aliquots, peripheral blood dilutes the marrow material. Tiny fragments of connective tissue as well as free-floating cells will be withdrawn. The morphology of these free cells provides the information on the maturation sequence of the cells (see Color Plates 2 and 3).

Bone Marrow Biopsy

In this test, a trephine needle is inserted through the outer portion of the bone (cortex) and the internal trochar is removed, producing a hollow bore. A small portion of the bone is beveled by cutting and rotating into the bone tissue. The specimen then is broken off and removed. It is placed in histologic fixative and submitted to the histology laboratory. Bone marrow biopsies are usually performed from the iliac crests since these provide a large area of bone from which a core biopsy can be removed.

In general, the bone marrow aspirate provides valuable information about the cytologic and morphologic detail, whereas the bone marrow biopsy provides important information regarding the bony structures and the relationship of the cells to one another and to other connective tissue elements. In particular, cellularity of the marrow, abnormal cellular elements, metastatic cancer, and fibrous tissue scarring can best be assessed by the bone marrow biopsy (see Color Plate 8).

For both aspiration and biopsy, a meticulous aseptic technique is necessary because infectious material can be introduced into the bone marrow and can then rapidly reach the entire circulation. The skin and subcutaneous tissues are anesthetized by local injection, which is also infiltrated into the periosteal bone. Despite adequate local anesthetic infiltration, pain is usually elicited following aspiration because the interstices of the bone marrow cannot be anesthetized. These areas are exquisitely sensitive to pressure, and suction similarly elicits pain. Suction or aspiration pain is a normal phenomenon, and its absence on occasion is indicative of infiltrative bone marrow disease.

Following removal of the tissue, an antibiotic-impregnated dressing is applied with pressure over the area for approximately 5 minutes. With attention to aseptic detail, as well as care and local pressure dressing application, bone marrow aspirates and biopsies can be performed even in patients with bleeding disorders. The technique provides very useful information for understanding the nature of many hematologic diseases, as well as metastatic malignancy.

Bone Marrow Cellularity and Myeloid:Erythroid Ratio

Bone marrow cellularity, the relationship of developing hematopoietic cells to the fat spaces within the marrow, is present as a relatively fixed proportion. Normally, the ratio of marrow cells to marrow fat is between 1:1 and 2:1 (see Color Plates 7 and 8). A cell-to-fat ratio greater than 2:1 constitutes *hypercellularity.* This may occur when any or all of the marrow elements are present in abundance. The nature of the cell line that is more abundant can give important clues as to mechanisms of anemia or leukocyte abnormalities. Table 2–2 lists the normal values of bone marrow precursor cells.

Although circulating blood contains 500 to 1000 times as many red cells as white cells (5 million red cells/microliter as compared with 5000 to 10,000 white cells/microliter), nucleated white cells in the bone marrow outnumber the nucleated erythrocytic cells by 3:1. This is called the **myeloid:erythroid ratio** or M:E. Many factors contribute to this disproportion:

- Red cells require 5 to 6 days for bone marrow development, but the nucleus disappears after 2 to 3 days. Maturing red cells enter the circulating blood very promptly, even before the last maturational events have occurred. Red cells remain in the circulation for about 120 days before senescence and destruction.
- Nucleated granulocytic cells are numerous in the marrow because granulocytes have conspicuous nuclei throughout the 5 to 7 days of marrow development, and large numbers of mature cells remain within the marrow as a storage pool.
- On the average, granulocytes spend 7 to 24 hours in the circulating blood and have a total lifespan of only 9 to 15 days.

The combination of massive granulocyte turnover, persistence of the nucleus, and marrow retention of mature cells makes the myeloid series

TABLE 2–2. DIFFERENTIAL COUNTS OF NUCLEATED BONE MARROW CELLS*

	Range of Mean Values[+]
Myeloblast	0.3–2.0
Promyelocyte	1.4–5.0
Myelocyte	4.2–8.9
Metamyelocyte	6.5–22.0
Band	13.0–24.0
Mature granulocyte	
Neutrophil	15.0–20.0
Eosinophil	0.5–2.0
Basophil	0.0–0.2
Lymphocyte	14.0–16.0
Monocyte	0.3–2.4
Plasma cell	0.3–1.3
Pronormoblast	0.2–0.6
Basophilic normoblast	1.4–2.0
Polychromatophilic normoblast	6.0–21.0
Orthochromic normoblast	1.0–3.0
M:E ratio	2.3–3.5 to 1.0

*Figures for adults are taken from several series as reported in Williams, WJ, et al (eds): Hematology. McGraw-Hill, New York, 1990; and in Wintrobe, M, et al: Clinical Hematology, ed 8. Lea and Febiger, Philadelphia, 1981.

[+]Values are expressed as percent of nucleated cells present.

the predominant nucleated form when marrow is examined. The normal M:E is 2:1 to 3.5:1.

CYTOLOGIC EVALUATION OF BONE MARROW

The aspirated marrow is smeared onto a cover slip or glass slide and evenly spread. Hematopoietic cells form trails or spreads amongst the marrow **spicules** (the particles of marrow seen under microscope). Cellularity is evaluated within the spicules, whereas the cytologic detail is determined in the spread marrow trails (see Color Plates 2, 3, 7, and 8). This evaluation encompasses the following:

- The orderly sequence of erythropoiesis is determined, as is the orderly sequence of myelopoiesis. In this manner, a bone marrow differential count can be obtained and the maturation is appreciated.

- The quantity of cells (activity), as well as the presence of all maturation elements, is evaluated.
- The relationship of the myeloid to the erythroid cells is determined as indicated above.
- Any abnormal nonhematopoietic cells are noted.
- Some of the less abundant marrow elements, such as lymphocytes and plasma cells, are assessed.
- Special stains may be performed on the marrow to determine iron status (see Chapter 3).

Table 2–2 indicates the range of normal values for cells in aspirated marrow. Paraffin-embedded tissue biopsy sections are unsuitable for detailed morphologic differential counts. The number of megakaryocytes or platelet precursors can be evaluated within both marrow aspirates and marrow biopsies quite easily (see Color Plate 7). On occasion, aspirated material cannot be obtained despite adequate technique. This condition is termed a "dry tap" and occurs when:

- the hemopoietic activity is so sparse that virtually no marrow cells exist to be withdrawn (with severe hypocellularity or marrow aplasia)
- the marrow contains tightly packed, sticky, highly immature cells that cannot be aspirated (in some cases of acute leukemia)
- marrow fibrosis (scar tissue) or metastatic cancer are present

Under these circumstances, the marrow biopsy is much more helpful than aspiration because it determines the absence of marrow cells or the nature of the infiltrating cellular elements.

LABORATORY EVALUATION OF ERYTHROPOIESIS

MARROW CYTOLOGY

In the developmental morphology of erythrocyte precursor cells (Color Plates 2 and 3 [E and F]), the earliest precursor is the **proerythroblast,** a large, immature cell with multiple nucleoli and a deeply basophilic cytoplasm. This cell matures into the **basophilic erythroblast** (Color Plate 2[A]). With increasing synthesis of hemoglobin, the cytoplasm of the cell takes on a pinkish hue (on Giemsa stains), and the nucleus becomes more pyknotic and clumped, producing a **polychromatophilic erythroblast** (2[B]). Further maturation is associated with more nuclear clumping and continued cytoplasmic hemoglobinization in the **orthochromatic erythroblast.** Finally, the nucleus is extruded, leaving the cell with residual cytoplasmic RNA-producing polychromasia and the morphologic appearance of a **reticulocyte** (an RNA-rich cell slightly larger than the mature cell).

RETICULOCYTE COUNT

Approximately 2 million new red cells are produced each second in adults. As red cells mature, several days are needed for the hemoglobin-containing cells to rid themselves of residual cytoplasmic RNA after the nucleus has been expelled. Part of this process occurs in the bone marrow and part in the circulation. During this last phase of maturation, the RNA-containing reticulocyte is slightly larger than the mature cell; it contains miscellaneous fragments of mitochondria and other organelles as well as ribosomal RNA. These reticulocytes, can often be distinguished on Wright-stained peripheral blood smears by their larger size and slightly gray or purple appearance. The reticulofilamentous material that gives these cells their name is seen only after supravital staining, but it is also responsible for several staining abnormalities seen on routine smears. **Polychromasia** is diffuse grayish or blue discoloration, and **basophilic stippling** is the punctate form of blue discoloration mentioned earlier (see Color Plates 9[B], 10A, and 10C).

Normal cells spend 1 to 2 days circulating as reticulocytes and 120 days circulating in the mature form; approximately 0.5 to 2.5% of circulating red cells are reticulocytes. The reticulocyte count is usually reported as a percentage of circulating erythrocytes. However, interpretation of this count varies, in correspondence with other factors. For example, a reticulocyte count of 0.5 to 2.5% indicates normal marrow activity *if the hemoglobin level is normal.* An elevated reticulocyte count in the presence of normal hemoglobin levels indicates that the red cells are being lost or destroyed, but the marrow has increased erythrocyte production to compensate. With low hemoglobin levels, a reticulocyte count of 0.5 to 2.5% indicates that the response to anemia is inadequate. This can result from defective or decreased bone marrow production or a reduced amount of erythropoietin. If an individual has anemia, the number of circulating erythrocytes falls and therefore a "normal" reticulocyte percentage (0.5 to 2.5%) will increase. The reticulocyte count is therefore corrected for the anemia, normalizing the percentage to a standard hematocrit of 0.45 (45%). Thus the reticulocyte count may then be corrected for anemia as follows:

$$CR = \frac{OR \times \text{Patient's Hematocrit}}{\text{Mean Normal Hematocrit (45)}}$$

where:

CR = Corrected Reticulocyte Count
OR = Observed Reticulocyte Count

When the marrow is healthy and has adequate stores of iron and other precursors, the degree of reticulocytosis parallels the degree of blood loss or red cell destruction. Patients with defects of cellular maturation or hemoglobin production sometimes have ineffective erythropoiesis. In these conditions, erythroid production is greatly increased (hyperplastic), but the reticulocyte count is disproportionately low because many cells never mature sufficiently to enter the peripheral blood. Pernicious anemia and thalassemia are prime examples of ineffective erythropoiesis (see Color Plate 8B).

After blood loss or effective therapy for certain anemias such as iron deficiency anemia, a rising reticulocyte count indicates that the marrow is responding by making more erythrocytes. A single hemorrhagic episode causes reticulocytosis, beginning within 24 to 48 hours and reaching a peak at 4 to 7 days. Normal levels resume when the hemoglobin concentration stabilizes. Persistent reticulocytosis or a second rise in the reticulocyte count indicates continuing or recurrent blood loss.

In iron deficiency, and especially in anemia resulting from prolonged blood loss, therapeutic iron administration produces a reticulocyte response within 4 to 7 days. The reticulocyte count remains elevated until normal hemoglobin values are achieved. Vitamin B_{12} replacement therapy for pernicious anemia also causes a prompt, continuing reticulocytosis. This is often used as a challenge test when physiologic doses of vitamin B_{12} are given to people suspected of having vitamin B_{12} deficiency. If reticulocytosis fails to occur, the diagnosis should be suspect.

The reticulocyte count is commonly used as a measure of marrow erythroid production. This is only valid if the reticulocyte maturation time is known, and some laboratories report a *reticulocyte production index* per day. This value, however, has very little practical utility. Often the absolute reticulocyte count is expressed in reticulocytes per microliter.

Reticulocyte counting is still mostly a visual assessment of cells stained with supravital stains exhibiting the reticulum strands. This is at best a semiquantitative assessment of reticulocyte number. Automated counters using flow cytometry or laser light scattered by residual RNA are being used, but these methods require more standardization. Their advantage is that many more cells are counted, thus giving a more accurate quantitative measurement of reticulocytes.

ERYTHROPOIETIN ASSAY

As already mentioned, erythropoietin is the hormone that preferentially increases erythrocyte-committed progenitors and decreases the maturation time of erythrocytes within the marrow (see Color Plate 1). Erythropoietin also increases the absolute reticulocyte count, which, to some extent, is a reflection of erythropoietin production. Erythropoietin can, however, be measured, and current assay systems use either radioimmunoassays or enzyme-linked immunosorbent assay (ELISA) techniques (reference ranges 9 to 26 units/mL). Formerly, erythropoietin was measured only by a bioassay that is now outmoded. Erythropoietin values can be extremely helpful in differentiating primary polycythemia, with uncontrolled marrow production (unregulated by erythropoietin) and low erythropoietin levels, from secondary erythrocytosis, with a controlled excess of erythroid production stimulated by tissue hypoxia and mediated through erythropoietin. In these latter conditions, erythropoietin values are high (see Chapter 3).

HEMOGLOBIN PRODUCTION AND CONTROL

As outlined above, the erythron, which comprises developing red cell precursors as well as circulating mature erythrocytes, is regulated by erythropoietin and oxygen tension. The major function of the erythrocytes is to transport oxygen to the tissues, and to do so the red cell must be deformable enough to negotiate the small capillaries in the microcirculation. In addition, the red cell must contain adequate amounts of the oxygen-binding pigment *heme,* which is neatly packaged within a protein envelope called *globin.* The delicate structure of the erythrocyte, therefore, is geared to the transport of oxygen and the maintenance of hemoglobin in a functional state. The synthesis of both heme and globin is also finely controlled. The heme portion of hemoglobin consists of a porphyrin ring structure into which iron is precisely suspended (Fig. 2–3). The globin portion is a protein comprising two pairs of amino acid chains termed alpha and non-alpha (beta, gamma, delta, etc.). Adult hemoglobin A consists of two alpha chains and two beta chains. Raw materials necessary for the production of hemoglobin, and indeed red cells, must be in constant supply because a large number of erythrocytes are synthesized daily. Vitamins and minerals as well as amino acids need to be provided. Deficiencies of these components can lead to a reduced number of erythrocytes or decreased amounts of hemoglobin pigment. This state is termed *anemia* (see Chapter 3).

HEME SYNTHESIS

The two parts of the hemoglobin molecule (heme and globin) have very different synthetic pathways. Each hemoglobin molecule has four identical heme moieties attached to the four globin protein chains. Thus a pair of alpha chains are arranged on top of a pair of non-alpha chains (beta chains in adult hemoglobin) (Fig. 2–4). The heme moieties consist of four symmetrically ringed 4-carbon structures called pyrrole rings, which constitute a molecule of *porphyrin.* This porphyrin ring is also seen in

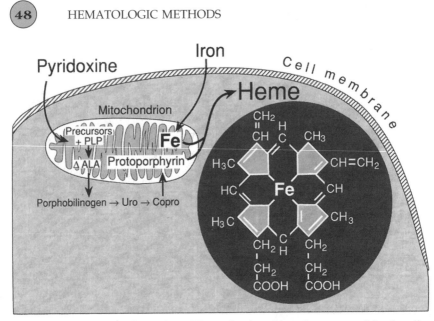

FIGURE 2–3. Heme formation. The mitochondrion is responsible for the synthesis of protoporphyrin, a stepwise process beginning with the formation of delta-aminolevulinic acid from glycine and succinyl-CoA, with pyridoxal-5-phosphate (PLP) as an essential cofactor. The sequence of porphobilinogen, uroporphyrin, and coproporphyrin formation then occurs in the cytoplasm, followed by an intramitochondrial assembly of protoporphyrin and iron to form heme. The structure of the final product, the heme molecule, is shown. It consists of four porphyrin moieties assembled in a ring structure around a central iron molecule. (From Hillman, RS and Finch, CA: Red Cell Manual, ed 7. FA Davis, Philadelphia, 1996, p 10, with permission.)

other proteins in addition to hemoglobin, including myoglobin and other enzymes (catalase, cytochromes, and peroxidase). The rings are suspended as heme pockets within the protein structure. Biosynthesis of heme involves stepwise production of a porphyrin framework, followed by the insertion of iron into each of the four heme groups (see Fig. 2–3).

Synthesis of the porphyrin requires construction of a straight line chain of carbon-containing groups that is closed into a single pyrrole ring. Four pyrroles linked together, after several changes and exchanges of substituent groups, form the final iron-free compound *protoporphyrin.*

The constituent carbon groups constituting this chain are derived from the amino acid glycine and a coenzyme, succinyl coenzyme A. Heme synthesis starts with these compounds and proceeds in a fairly predictable pattern, as follows:

• Initially, these two compounds—glycine and succinyl coenzyme A—are condensed to form the compound *aminolevulinic acid (ALA).* This straight line compound is the first precursor distinctively associated with heme synthesis. The enzyme catalyzing this reaction, *ALA-synthetase,* appears to be a rate-limiting enzyme in this metabolic pathway. *Pyridoxal phosphate* (vitamin B_6) is a coenzyme for this reaction. The reaction is stimulated by the presence of the hormone erythropoietin and inhibited by the manufacturing of heme (negative feedback control). This pathway is initiated in the mitochondria and cytoplasm of the developing cell.

- Two molecules of ALA combine to form *porphobilinogen,* a single-ring molecule.
- Subsequently, four molecules of this compound condense to form a four-ringed (tetrapyrrole) compound, *uroporphyrinogen.*
- This compound is converted to *coproporphyrinogen.*
- Coproporphyrinogen is converted to protoporphyrin.
- Finally, protoporphyrin is coupled with iron in the presence of another rate-limiting enzyme, *ferrochelatase* (heme synthetase), to form the oxygen-carrying pigment heme. Unused coproporphyrin and uroporphyrin are excreted in the urine and feces. If heme synthesis is impaired, abnormal quantities of these compounds and other precursors may be excreted. Identification and measurement will be discussed in the section on Porphyrias in Chapter 3.

Therefore, the clinical states associated with abnormal heme production may include anemia and the genetic or acquired enzyme disorders that produce abnormal accumulation of the porphyrins (porphyria).

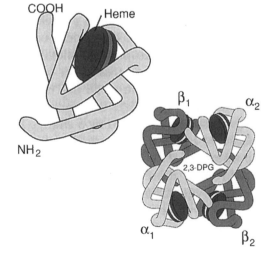

FIGURE 2–4. Hemoglobin structure. Hemoglobin molecules are composed of four subunits: two α chains *(light shading)* and two β chains *(dark shading).* Each of the globin chains provides a pocket for a heme molecule and therefore has the capacity of binding up to four molecules of oxygen. 2,3-DPG binds to the two β chains to stabilize the molecule when it is in the deoxygenated state. (From Hillman, RS, and Finch, CA: Red Cell Manual, ed 7. FA Davis, Philadelphia, 1996, p 18, with permission.)

The insertion of four heme molecules into the four globin molecules constitutes the final synthesis of hemoglobin. Heme is synthesized in the mitochondria, and globin incorporation occurs in the cytoplasm of the developing erythrocyte. (see also Fig. 2–4).

GLOBIN SYNTHESIS

Globin synthesis is also discussed in Chapter 3, in the discussion of thalassemias and hemoglobinopathies. Normal adult hemoglobin (HbA) (95% of adult hemoglobin) consists of four polypeptide chains comprising two alpha chains and two beta chains (α_2, β_2), each with its own attached heme group. Normally, alpha and beta chains are produced in equal proportions. Other minor chains are also synthesized in the adult and include a delta (δ) chain and a fetal gamma (γ) chain, which constitute the two minor adult hemoglobins:

- alpha-2 gamma-2 constitutes hemoglobin F or fetal hemoglobin (<2.5%)
- alpha-2 delta-2 constitutes hemoglobin A_2 (<2.5%)

Presumably the synthesis of globin is also under the control of erythropoietin, although its molecular site of action is uncertain. Globin synthesis is also induced by free heme. Globin synthesis mainly occurs in the early, or basophilic, erythroblast and continues to a limited extent even in the anucleate reticulocyte. It has been estimated that as much as 15 to 20% of hemoglobin is synthesized during this later stage. The genes for globin synthesis are located on chromosomes 11 (gamma, delta, and beta chains) and 16 (alpha) (see Fig. 3–4). Some embryonic hemoglobins are also encoded on these chromosomes. The regulation of DNA expression with subsequent formation of RNA and protein synthesis is now well elucidated. Anemias may occur because of abnormalities at the DNA level, defects in interpreting the template RNA, or because nonsense messenger codes are not translated or expressed during protein synthesis. These problems will be discussed in Chapter 3. Because each individual chromosome is inherited from each parent, genetic expression is clearly dependent on which gene is transferred to the offspring. Inherited disorders of hemoglobin production may cause serious anemias. Globin messenger RNA, harvested from reticulocytes, forms a suitable *in vitro* cell system in which to study globin synthesis in the research laboratory. These genetic codes have been elucidated, and direct the assembly of 141 amino acids into the alpha chain and 146 amino acids into the non-alpha chains.

During fetal life, embryonic chains subsequently switch over to the major fetal hemoglobin (α_2 γ_2, hemoglobin F). This represents the dominant hemoglobin in late fetal and early neonatal life. Conversion of fetal hemoglobin to adult hemoglobin (α_2 β_2) is completed by 3 to 6 months of age. The actual mechanisms controlling the switch are as yet undetermined (see also Fig. 3–4).

ADDITIONAL FACTORS ESSENTIAL FOR HEMOGLOBIN SYNTHESIS

VITAMIN B_{12} AND FOLIC ACID

Vitamin B_{12} consists of a porphyrin ring attached to a nucleotide base (Fig. 2–5). The porphyrin ring is very similar to heme, except that cobalt is substituted for iron. The metabolism of vitamin B_{12} (cyanocobalamin) and folic acid (pteroylglutamic acid) (Fig. 2–5B) is vitally involved in the synthesis and intermolecular exchanges of 1- and 2-carbon fragments. These reactions affect the synthesis of purines and pyrimidines, and thus influence DNA synthesis (Fig. 2–6). Deficiency states cause defective DNA production, abnormal nuclear and cytoplasmic development, and the production of large, dysmature, megaloblastic cells (see the section on Vitamin B_{12} and Folic Acid Deficiency in Chapter 3).

Metabolism of Vitamin B_{12} and Folic Acid

Vitamin B_{12} is synthesized in nature by microorganisms. Humans cannot synthesize vitamin B_{12} and acquire their supplies by eating animal tissues. The normal human diet consists of 5 to 30 µg of vitamin B_{12} daily, of which 1 to 5 µg are absorbed. Normal body stores consist of 3000 to 5000 µg, of which 1000 µg are stored in the liver. Absorption of vitamin B_{12} occurs in the terminal ileum under the influence of a substance produced in the parietal cells of the stomach called **intrinsic factor.** Intrinsic factor is essential for the absorption of vitamin B_{12} in the terminal ileum. Intrinsic factor is a bivalent glycoprotein that preferentially binds to B_{12} and to receptors on the terminal ileum cells. Since vitamin B_{12} is abundant in nature, deficiencies are mostly the result of malabsorption or a deficiency of intrinsic factor. Following absorption, vitamin B_{12} is transported by plasma proteins termed *transcobalamins* (Fig. 2–7). There are three types of transcobalamins, termed transcobalamin I, II, and III. Transcobalamins I and III are storage proteins for vitamin B_{12}, and transcobalamin II is the transport protein. The storage transcobalamins are synthesized in granulocytes and tend to increase in instances where the granulocyte mass is exaggerated, such as myeloproliferative diseases or leukocytosis.

There are two major natural forms of vitamin B_{12}—*cyanocobalamin* and *hydroxycobalamin.* In the body, these are converted into the functional cobalamins methylcobalamin and 5′-deoxyadenosylcobalamin. Normal body stores are sufficient to withstand a year or more of zero intake; however, states of rapid growth or cell turnover increase vitamin B_{12} requirements. Although an obligate substance for normal human metabolism, vitamin B_{12} is unequivocally required for relatively

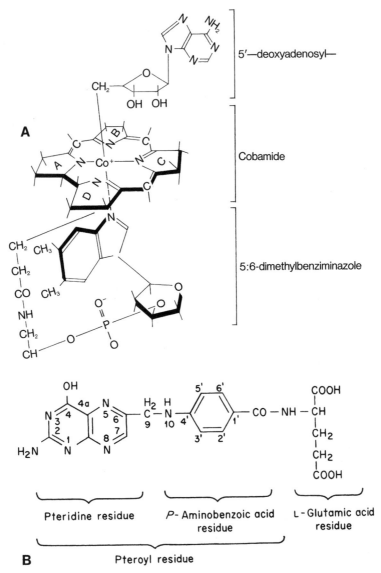

FIGURE 2–5. *(A)* Structure of vitamin B_{12} (5′ deoxyadenosyl cobalamin). (Redrawn from Chanarin, I: The Megaloblastic Anemias. Blackwell Scientific Publications, Boston, with permission.) *(B)* Structure of folic acid (pteroylglutamic acid). (From Williams, WJ, et al: Hematology, ed 3. McGraw-Hill, New York, 1983, p 320, with permission.)

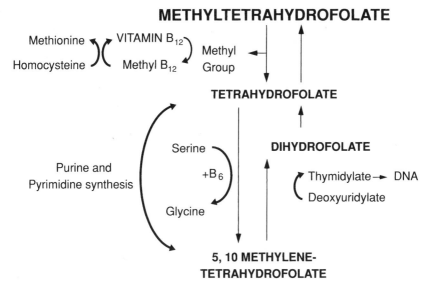

FIGURE 2–6. Metabolic relationships of methyltetrahydrofolate and vitamin B_{12}. Methyltetrahydrofolate is the methyl group donor for the formation of methyl B_{12}, an essential cofactor in the conversion of homocysteine to methionine. This generates tetrahydrofolate, which is the essential substrate for purine and pyrimidine synthesis and the conversion of deoxyuridylate to thymidylate for normal DNA synthesis. Tetrahydrofolate is also the natural substrate for the formation of folate polyglutamate in the liver. (From Hillman, RS, and Finch, CA: Red Cell Manual, ed 7. FA Davis, Philadelphia, 1996, p 8, with permission.)

few reactions. One important reaction is the *methylation of the amino acid homocysteine to the amino acid methionine,* a conversion that not only generates methionine but also the functional folate cofactor *tetrahydrofolate.*

A deficiency of vitamin B_{12} produces failure to regenerate tetrahydrofolate from N^5-methyltetrahydrofolic acid and may lead to megaloblastic anemia.

The key reaction may be represented by the equation:

$$\text{homocysteine} + N^5\text{-methyl-FH4} \overset{\text{methyltransferase}}{\underset{\text{methylcobalamin}}{\longleftrightarrow}} \text{tetrahydrofolate} + \text{methionine}$$

Folic acid is a collective term for a group of compounds derived from green, leafy foliage. These compounds consist of three moieties (see Fig. 2–5B):

- a *pteridine ring*
- *para-amino-benzoic acid*
- one of a number of glutamic acid units

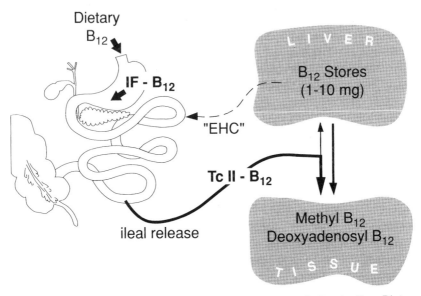

FIGURE 2–7. The absorption, transport, and storage of vitamin B_{12}. Dietary vitamin B_{12} is liberated by peptic acid digestion and then bound to intrinsic factor (IF-B_{12}) produced by the gastric parietal cells. This protects the vitamin B_{12} until it reaches the terminal ileum, where it is released from the intrinsic factor and bound to transcobalamin II (Tc II) for transport to liver and tissues. In normal individuals, 1–10 mg of vitamin B_{12} is stored in the liver. These B_{12} stores may be released and transported directly to tissues or to a lesser extent secreted into bile for reabsorption, an enterohepatic cycle (EHC). (From Hillman, RS, and Finch, CA: Red Cell Manual, ed 7. FA Davis, Philadelphia, 1996, p 99, with permission.)

The first two moieties are collectively termed *pteroyls,* and are further named according to the number of glutamic acid residues that are present, for example, pteroyl monoglutamate or pteroyl polyglutamates. A normal diet consists of 500 to 700 g of folate, of which 50 g/day are absorbed, and the body has one month's supply of storage folate. Folates are absorbed throughout the small intestine, and a deficiency of folic acid usually occurs in situations of excess demand and poor dietary supply.

Metabolically active folate is derived by the reduction of the pteroyl group to dihydrofolate, and subsequently to tetrahydrofolate, in the presence of the enzyme dihydrofolate reductase. Tetrahydrofolic acid is the reduced form of folic acid and is the catalytic, self-regenerating compound that mediates 1-carbon transfers. One-carbon fragments can be bound to the pteroyl groups and transferred in intermediary metabolism involving DNA synthesis. Like vitamin B_{12}, folic acid cannot be synthesized by mammals. The major effect of folic acid deficiency is impairment of thymidine synthesis. Thymidine is part of DNA but not

RNA; thus, altered *thymidine metabolism* specifically affects DNA and leaves RNA production unaffected (see Fig. 2–7). In the presence of folic acid, 1-carbon fragments are transferred from deoxyuridine to deoxythymidine on the pteroyl group. Folic acid is also involved in other pathways involving 1-carbon transfers, and its deficiency also impairs *histidine catabolism.* This abnormality produces no clinical disability but does cause large quantities of the metabolite *formiminoglutamic acid (FIGLU)* to accumulate after a histidine load is given to a folate-deficient subject. This previously formed the basis for documenting folic acid deficiency. Normal values for vitamin B_{12} and folate metabolism are shown in Table 2–3.

Laboratory Determinations of Vitamin B_{12} and Folic Acid

Serum vitamin B_{12} and serum folate may be assayed by several techniques that are discussed in Chapter 3. The usual assay system is enzyme immunoassay.

Cobalamin deficiency is almost always due to vitamin B_{12} malabsorption. Pernicious anemia is the most common cause and is due to a lack of intrinsic factor. Intrinsic factor is normally produced by the parietal cells of the gastric mucosa and is deficient in any condition depleting this production, such as atrophic gastritis or gastrectomy. Intestinal malabsorption syndromes, veganism, or intestinal bacterial overgrowth with organisms requiring vitamin B_{12} may also produce deficiency.

Laboratory Determination of B_{12} Absorption (Schilling Test)

Vitamin B_{12} and folic acid deficiency may be differentiated by measuring serum levels. Vitamin B_{12} deficiency is confirmed by testing B_{12} absorption using the urinary excretion of radiolabeled B_{12} after an oral dose given with or without intrinsic factor **(Schilling test).** The Schilling

TABLE 2–3. NORMAL VALUES FOR VITAMIN B_{12} AND FOLATE METABOLISM

Folic acid	
Serum	3–20 ng/mL
Red cells	165–600 ng/mL
FIGLU	Urinary excretion up to 17 ng/day
Methylmalonate	Urinary excretion up to 10 ng/day
	<5 µg/mg creatinine
Schilling test	15–40% of 0.5-µg dose
	5–40% of 1.0-µg dose
Vitamin B_{12} (serum)	200–900 pg/mL

test is used to establish whether the vitamin B_{12} absorption is defective, and if so, whether the etiology is intrinsic factor deficiency.

With normal absorption, the body receives far more vitamin B_{12} than it needs, and the excess is excreted in the urine. Urinary excretion increases if vitamin B_{12} requirements have already been met. In impaired absorption, the orally administered vitamin does not reach the circulation and therefore does not appear in the urine. Vitamin B_{12} labeled with ^{57}Co is used to follow the absorption and excretion in the urine of the orally administered (0.5–1.0 µg) vitamin B_{12}. Initially, a parenteral loading dose of unlabeled vitamin B_{12} (1000 µg) is administered to saturate the body stores so that when labeled B_{12} is absorbed, a significant amount is subsequently excreted in the urine. Normal subjects will excrete 7% or more of the radioactivity taken orally in their urine, whereas patients with pernicious anemia or other causes of vitamin B_{12} malabsorption will excrete less than 5%. Complete collection of the urine is extremely important, for the test depends on measuring the absolute amount of radioactivity excreted. Because this test depends on urinary excretion, its interpretation may be impaired in cases of renal insufficiency because of reduced urinary output. In this case, the test may be prolonged to a 48- to 72-hour collection.

The second part of the Schilling test is performed with the addition of intrinsic factor. The test is repeated with 60 µg of intrinsic factor administered orally along with vitamin B_{12}. If the megaloblastic anemia is due to lack of vitamin B_{12} from intrinsic factor deficiency (*pernicious anemia*), malabsorption will be corrected by the oral administration of vitamin B_{12} coupled to intrinsic factor. The labeled vitamin B_{12}–bound intrinsic factor will be received by the terminal ileal cells and will be absorbed, and the labeled B_{12} will be excreted in the urine. The second phase of the test assesses the functional integrity of the terminal ileum (i.e., whether there are blocking factors within the lumen of the intestine, preventing vitamin B_{12} absorption). Therefore, if urinary ^{57}Co excretion rises to normal when intrinsic factor is added, the diagnosis of intrinsic factor deficiency is established. A second low excretion indicates some other malabsorptive state.

Before performing the Schilling test, it is imperative that other causes of megaloblastosis, such as folic acid deficiency (by serum folate determination), have been investigated because the parenteral loading dose of vitamin B_{12} may confuse this investigation.

Methylmalonic Acid (MMA)

Ancillary tests of vitamin B_{12} deficiency include serum or **urinary methylmalonic acid (MMA)**, plasma homocysteine, and the deoxyuridine suppression test. Of these, the MMA has found most utility, especially in cases of borderline deficiency or in elderly subjects. This test is based on the accumulation of excessive amounts of MMA in the urine of deficient subjects, since vitamin B_{12} is needed for conversion of MMA to succinic acid.

IRON METABOLISM

Iron is the most abundant trace element in the body. About 65% of the body's normal 4000 mg of iron (60 mg/kg in men and 50 mg/kg in women) is bound to heme. One milliliter of iron is required for each milliliter of red cells produced. Each day, 20 to 25 mg of iron are needed for erythropoiesis, of which 95% is recycled iron salvaged from normal red blood cell turnover and hemoglobin catabolism. Only 1 mg/day (representing 5% of the iron turnover) is newly absorbed to balance minimal iron loss incurred by fecal and urinary excretion. Figure 2–8 illustrates the continuous process of **daily iron turnover.** The remaining body iron, representing one third of total iron content, is stored within the liver, spleen, and bone marrow, or is carried in myoglobin and coenzymes of the cytochrome electron transport proteins. Storage iron exists in the form of hemosiderin or ferritin. Normal values for iron metabolism are shown in Table 2–4.

Iron Absorption

Absorption of iron is regulated by the intestines, which admit just enough iron to cover losses without permitting excessive absorption. Normal dietary iron intake is 10 to 20 mg/day. The amount of iron absorbed from the diet varies greatly, depending on several factors including the amount and type of iron ingested, gastric acidity, the activity of the bone marrow, and the state of the body iron stores. Although the entire small intestine has the capacity to absorb iron, maximal absorption occurs in the duodenum and upper jejunum, owing to the presence of optimum conditions of pH. In the state of severe iron deficiency, the body can increase absorption to up to 30% of the dietary intake to compensate for the depletion.

Elemental iron is biologically active in the ferrous (Fe^{2+}) and ferric (Fe^{3+}) states. In general, an acidic or lower pH favors the ferrous state and iron absorption, whereas a neutral or alkaline pH favors the ferric state and decreased iron absorption.

Iron Transport and Storage

Iron is transported from the mucosal cells of the intestine to the blood, where it is then bound to a specific iron transport protein, **transferrin,** a plasma beta-globulin. Transferrin's capacity to bind iron in normal plasma is 240–360 µg/dL. Transferrin attaches to the receptors of the developing erythrocyte membrane and releases free iron into the erythrocyte for incorporation into heme within the mitochondria. Approximately 10–20% of the total body iron is stored as *ferritin,* a

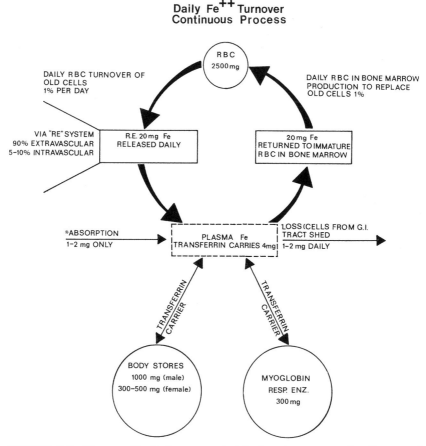

FIGURE 2–8. Diagram illustrating normal daily iron turnover and pathways of internal iron exchanges. (From Pittiglio, DH, and Sacher, RA: Clinical Hematology and Fundamentals of Hemostasis. FA Davis, Philadelphia, 1987, p 42, with permission.)

TABLE 2–4. NORMAL VALUES FOR IRON METABOLISM

Serum iron (Fe): 50–150 µg/dL
Total iron-binding capacity (TIBC): 240–360 µg/dL
Percent saturation: 20–45%
Serum ferritin: 12-300 µg/L
Free erythrocyte protoporphyrin: 15–18 µg/L

spherical molecule consisting of an *apoferritin* shell and an interior ferric oxyhydroxide core (constituting 0.3–1.0 g). When iron is absorbed in excess of the ferritin storage, iron is deposited in lysosomal membranes as a pseudocrystalline complex. This amorphous iron is termed *hemosiderin* and is readily visible on light microscopy by Prussian Blue staining.

Laboratory Evaluation of Iron Status

Peripheral Blood Smear

Examination of a stained peripheral smear is the most simple, cost-effective method of characterizing iron status and getting qualitative information on the degree of hemoglobinization. Iron-deficient cells are characterized by less hemoglobin, termed *hypochromia,* and a smaller cell size, termed *microcytosis* (see Red Blood Cell Morphology in Chapter 3) (see also Color Plate 28).

Serum Iron

Iron is usually measured colorimetrically following the development of a complex with a color-producing compound (chromogen). Blood levels for iron estimation should routinely be drawn in the morning after a 12-hour fast with the exclusion of all iron supplements for 12 to 24 hours. The normal range for serum iron is 50 to 150 µg/dL, averaging 125 µg/dL in men and 100 µg/dL in women. In the elderly, the serum iron levels decrease to 40 to 80 µg/dL. Serum iron levels vary in response to various physiologic disorders: they decrease in iron deficiency, chronic infections, and malignancy; and increase in iron poisoning, intravascular hemolysis, hepatic necrosis, pernicious anemia, and hemochromatosis.

Total Iron-Binding Capacity (TIBC)

The capacity of serum transferrin to bind to iron is obtained by this test. The test is performed in the same way as serum iron, except that excess iron is added to the sample to saturate all *transferrin-binding sites,* and the unbound iron is removed prior to assay. Therefore, the total ability of transferrin to bind iron is assessed by the determination of the total iron bound. This assay does not measure the serum transferrin (protein) level directly, but measures the amount of Fe bound to this protein. The normal range for TIBC in adults is 240 to 360 µg/dL, and tends to decrease with age to approximately 250 µg/dL in people older than 70 years. Total iron-binding capacity is increased in the presence of iron deficiency and pregnancy, but may be normal or low in chronic disease states and malnutrition.

Transferrin Saturation

Transferrin saturation is not directly measured, but is obtained as a ratio:

$$\text{Percentage Saturation} = \frac{\text{Serum Iron}}{\text{TIBC}} \times 100$$

With normal iron stores and protein metabolism, transferrin is usually 30 to 35% saturated. The normal range is between 20 and 45% saturation. Saturation levels follow a diurnal pattern, being highest in the morning and lowest in the late afternoon and early evening. Percentage saturation is low in iron deficiency and chronic disease states, and high in sideroblastic anemia, iron poisoning, and intravascular hemolysis and hemochromatosis (see Table 3–4).

Serum Ferritin

Ferritin is present in the plasma and serum and is in equilibrium with virtually all ferritin-producing tissues. Serum ferritin is a protein devoid of iron and is in a low concentration relative to tissue ferritin. Because it is in equilibrium with tissue ferritin, it can be a very good indicator of iron stores. Serum ferritin is measured by an immunoradiometric assay (IRMA) or enzyme-linked immunosorbent assay (ELISA), and normal ranges are 20 to 250 µg/mL in men and 10 to 200 µg/mL in children and premenopausal women. Each 1 µg/liter of ferritin represents 8 to 10 mg of storage iron. The measurement of serum ferritin can be particularly useful in distinguishing iron deficiency from other causes of hypochromic microcytic anemia (see Table 3–4). Serum ferritins are generally below 10 ng/mL in iron deficiency. Serum ferritin levels are elevated in inflammation, liver disease, malignancy, and other chronic diseases. In iron overload, serum ferritin may increase to as much as several thousand ng/mL.

Free Erythrocyte Protoporphyrin (FEP)

As was discussed under Heme Synthesis (see Fig. 2–3), the enzyme ferrochelatase inserts ferrous iron into protoporphyrin in the final step of heme synthesis. Protoporphyrin without iron is not incorporated into hemoglobin. Erythrocytes normally produce a slight excess of protoporphyrin over what is needed for heme synthesis, but when iron is deficient, protoporphyrin increases several-fold. Ferrochelatase is a rate-limiting enzyme step in heme synthesis, and the insertion of iron into protoporphyrin facilitates a negative feedback (see Fig. 2–3). Measurement of FEP provides a sensitive early indicator of iron deficiency. It is also elevated in chronic disease states and lead poisoning, both of which produce disturbances in iron metabolism. Free erythrocyte protoporphyrin is usually measured by direct fluorescence. Normal values depend on the method and laboratory, but range from 15 to 18 µg/dL of RBCs. This test is useful in diagnosing iron deficiency, even after iron therapy has been instituted.

A variant of this test, *zinc protoporphyrin (ZPP)*, is also used as a screening test for iron deficiency. Both FEP and ZPP provide an assessment of iron incorporation.

Tissue Iron Determination

Iron stores must occasionally be directly estimated for diagnosis. This may be achieved by biopsy of the liver, or more commonly of the bone marrow. Bone marrow iron can be appreciated directly in unstained preparations of aspirates as the golden refractile granules of hemosiderin. Generally, however, bone marrow iron stores are assessed by a reaction with Prussian Blue, which renders the hemosiderin deep blue (see Color Plate 11A). Histologic grading correlates reasonably well with the iron content of the sample. This estimation of iron stores represents the most accurate determination of the body content of iron; however, information can usually be obtained using the other tests listed above.

Morphologically, hemosiderin in small granules reflects intracytoplasmic aggregates of ferritin. Erythroblasts (normoblasts) containing such granules are termed **sideroblasts** (Color Plate 12). In normal marrow, approximately 30% of the erythroblasts contain such granules, and the percentage of sideroblasts in the marrow corresponds closely to the percentage saturation of transferrin. Normally, only two small granules are found per erythroblast. These granules may become more numerous in iron overload states. Occasionally the granules may be arranged in a ring around the nucleus, and these sideroblasts are termed *ring sideroblasts* (see Color Plate 12A). Defects in heme biosynthesis in the mitochondria appear to be responsible for this distribution.

Marrow evaluation of iron stores can yield falsely normal iron estimates in patients who have recently received parenteral iron therapy or blood transfusions because the iron is immediately taken up by macrophages (reticulo-endothelial cells), which are major sites of tissue storage iron. Quantitative iron determination can be made on liver biopsy material by flameless atomic absorption spectrophotometry.

RED BLOOD CELL AND HEMOGLOBIN CONCENTRATION

The factors responsible for red blood cell production (erythropoiesis) and hemoglobin synthesis were discussed earlier in the chapter. For development of the functional mature erythrocyte, which circulates in the peripheral blood and delivers oxygen to the tissues, an intricate balance of porphyrin synthesis, iron supply, and globin synthesis neatly packaged in a deformable red cell membrane must be achieved so that the erythrocyte can traverse tiny capillaries within the tissues. Defects in any of these stages may be responsible for deficient oxygen supply to the tissues. Tests are available for quantitation of erythrocytes and for evaluating their oxygen-carrying capacity. The morphologic appearance of the red cell may also give clues about erythrocyte membrane defects. Laboratory evaluation of these parameters is useful in assessing erythrocyte structure and function and gives an appreciation of red blood cell diseases, which will be covered in the next chapter.

The three primary variables are the amount of *hemoglobin* present in whole blood (in grams per deciliter); the proportion of red cells in whole blood—*packed cell volume* or *hematocrit*—and the *absolute number* of red cells in whole blood, usually expressed as millions of cells per microliter. **Corpuscular indices,** also called **red cell indices,** are calculations that allow the characterization of *average size* and hemoglobin content in individual erythrocytes (Table 2–5).

DIRECT MEASUREMENT OF RED CELL AND HEMOGLOBIN CONCENTRATION

Hemoglobin is the main oxygen-carrying pigment and is distributed in erythrocytes. Hemoglobin is a red pigment and maximally absorbs light at a wavelength of 540 nm. If a fixed concentration of red cells is lysed, hemoglobin is liberated and can be determined spectrophotometrically at this wavelength, with the concentration being proportional to the optical density. All forms of hemoglobin, including oxyhemoglobin, deoxyhemoglobin, methemoglobin, and carboxyhemoglobin, are converted into a single stable form. Conversion to **cyanmethemoglobin** is the method most widely used because reagents and instruments can be controlled most easily against stable and reliable standards. Limitations of this technique lie in accurate sample dilution and reagent preparation, as well as careful calibration of instruments. For adult men, normal levels are 13.5 to 18.0 g/dL. The normal range for women is 12 to 16 g/dL. Hemoglobin may be measured using spectrophotometers available in physicians' offices or in most general laboratories; however, the most

TABLE 2–5. NORMAL VALUES FOR COMPLETE BLOOD COUNT IN ADULTS

	Men	Women
Hematocrit	40–54%	38–47%
Hemoglobin	13.5–18 g/dL	12–16 g/dL
Red cells/μL	4.6–6.2×10^6	4.2–5.4×10^6
White cells/μL	4.5–11×10^3	4.5–11×10^3
Platelets/μL	150–450×10^3	150–450×10^3
Mean corpuscular volume (MCV)	80–98 fL	81–99 fL
Mean corpuscular hemoglobin (MCH)	26–32 pg	26–32 pg
Mean corpuscular hemoglobin concentration (MCHC)	32–36%	32–36%
Red cell distribution width (RDW)	11.6–14.6%	11.6–14.6%
Reticulocyte count	0.5–2.5%	0.5–2.5%

widely practiced method employs automated cell counters that directly measure hemoglobin in the red cell channel.

A qualitative estimation of hemoglobin concentration may be obtained by assessing the specific gravity of whole blood. This method is used as a screening technique to determine whether a person can safely donate blood. In this way a minimum safe level can be ascertained. These levels are 1.053 for women (corresponding to a hemoglobin level of approximately 12.5 g/dL) and 1.055 for men (corresponding to 13.5 g/dL). The test consists of allowing a drop of whole blood to fall through a copper sulfate solution made up to a specific gravity of 1.053 or 1.055. If the drop sinks, its specific gravity equals or exceeds that of the copper sulfate solution; if the drop rises to the top, its specific gravity is less. Inaccuracies arise if the copper sulfate solution changes its specific gravity, either through contamination or evaporation, or if there is anything besides hemoglobin in the blood that significantly affects specific gravity. Myeloma proteins, other abnormal globulins, and radiograph contrast materials are the most likely offenders.

HEMATOCRIT (PACKED RED CELL VOLUME)

Packed red cell volumes can be measured on venous or capillary blood with a macro- or micro-capillary technique. In the macro-capillary technique, venous blood is sampled into a 100-mm–long graduated tube and centrifuged at 2260*g* for 30 minutes. The volume of packed red cells and plasma is read directly from the millimeter marks along the sides of the tube. This method is no longer commonly employed.

The **microhematocrit** method uses either venous or capillary blood to fill a capillary tube approximately 7 centimeters long and 1 millimeter in diameter. The filled tube is centrifuged from 4 to 5 minutes at 10,000*g*, and the proportions of plasma and red cells are determined by means of a calibrated reading device. This method is rapid and simple; however, the centrifuge must be controlled for optimal centrifugal force, and the tube must be carefully positioned and read out against the read-out scale. These techniques allow visual estimation of the volume of white cells and platelets that constitute the buffy coat between the red cells and the plasma (see also Color Plate 40A). The supernatant plasma should also be observed for jaundice or hemolysis. The hematocrit can also be determined using the automated electronic instruments, where it is calculated from the mean cell volume and red cell count.

RED CELL COUNT

Counting the red cells in a small volume of enormously diluted blood is inaccurate and rarely performed. Instead, red cell counts are directly and accurately measured by electronic counters to give reliable and reproducible results. These instruments are programmed to give rapid computation of the corpuscular indices, which have now become a routine part of the complete blood count.

CORPUSCULAR INDICES

The **mean cell volume (MCV), mean cell hemoglobin (MCH),** and **mean cell hemoglobin concentration (MCHC)** are sometimes referred to as the "absolute red cell values" and are calculated from the hematocrit (PCV), hemoglobin estimation, and red cell count. These values have been widely used in the classification of anemia. Using the automated methods, the absolute values are calculated simultaneously with measured values, with the exception of the hematocrit, which is also a calculated value in the automated instruments. Hemoglobin or hematocrit values are commonly used to express the degree of anemia. These two determinations usually have a constant relationship—one hemoglobin unit in grams per deciliter is equivalent to three hematocrit units in percentage points. If, however, the erythrocyte is abnormal in size or shape or if hemoglobin manufacture is defective, there may be a disproportionate ratio.

The Mean Corpuscular Volume (MCV)

This represents the average volume of the red cells. With electronic counters, the MCV is measured directly, but it may be calculated by dividing the hematocrit by the red cell count expressed in millions per microliter and multiplied by 1000. The answer is expressed in femtoliters (fL) per red cell (fL = 10^{-15} liters). The normal range is 80 to 98 fL.

Mean Corpuscular Hemoglobin (MCH)

This is automatically calculated in electronic counters but may also be determined if the hemoglobin and red cell count are known. It is expressed in picograms and may be calculated by dividing the amount of hemoglobin per liter of blood by the number of red cells per liter. The normal range is 26 to 32 picograms (pg = 10^{-12} grams, or micromicrograms).

Mean Corpuscular Hemoglobin Concentration (MCHC)

This is also calculated by the electronic counters following measurement of the hemoglobin and calculation of the hematocrit. It may be manually determined by dividing hemoglobin per deciliter of blood by the hematocrit. Reference values range from 32 to 36%.

The size (MCV) and hemoglobin content (MCH) of individual cells are important in evaluating anemias and other hematologic abnormalities. Cell size may be described as *normocytic* with a normal MCV, *microcytic* with a less than normal MCV, or *macrocytic* with a greater than normal MCV. The degree of hemoglobinization of the cells can be appreciated by measuring the MCH and may be described as having normal mean hemoglobin *(normochromic)* or less than normal mean amounts of hemoglobin *(hypochromic)*.

Certain disorders are associated with an abnormally wide variation in red cell size, but an unremarkable *average* size. The resulting normal MCV may be misleading. Examination of the blood smear will detect this, but it can be electronically quantitated as the red cell distribution width (RDW) (defined in the following section, Red Cell Distribution Width). The normal range is 11.6 to 14.6, with higher values indicating greater size variability (anisocytosis).

There is considerable variation in the hemoglobin content of the red cells at different periods of life. At birth, the hemoglobin value is higher than at any other time and falls in the immediate postnatal period. A value of 10 to 11 g/dL is normal for an infant of 3 months of age (see also Appendix C, Tables C–2, C–3).

Red Cell Distribution Width

The **red cell distribution width (RDW)** is the ratio of the width of the distribution curve (histogram) to the mean red cell volume (Fig. 2–9). The RDW is also calculated from the Coulter counter and is an index of the cell size variation. Normally, the RDW value is between 11.6 and 14.6. Inspection of the size distribution curve provided by the automated counter may reveal the presence of a distinct population of red cells of different cell volume. The example demonstrated in Figure 2–10 shows a population of cells of normal distribution width as well as a small population of cells giving a much wider RDW. The higher the RDW, the greater the variation in cell size. This variation may be caused either by abnormally large or abnormally small cells, a mixture of the two, or cell fragments.

RED BLOOD CELL MORPHOLOGY ON THE PERIPHERAL BLOOD SMEAR

Much diagnostic information can be gained by examining red cells on a well-prepared Wright-Giemsa–stained peripheral blood film. The best area is that at which the cells just touch without overlapping. The normal red cell is a biconcave disc, 6 to 8 μm in diameter. Hemoglobin imparts a reddish-orange appearance to the stained cell. The staining is deeper at the periphery of the cell, gradually lightening as the center is approached (see Color Plate 6). These outer portions of the cell stain more deeply than

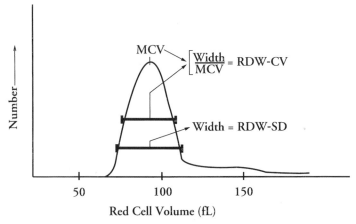

FIGURE 2–9. Red cell distribution width (RDW) measurements. As part of the CBC, electronic cell counters provide two measurements of the relative distribution of red cell size, the RDW-CV and the RDW-SD. The RDW-CV is calculated as the ratio of the red blood cell histogram width at one standard deviation divided by the MCV. The RDW-SD is simply the histogram width at the 20% frequency level. (From Hillman, RS, and Finch, CA: Red Cell Manual, ed 7. FA Davis, Philadelphia, 1996, p 47, with permission).

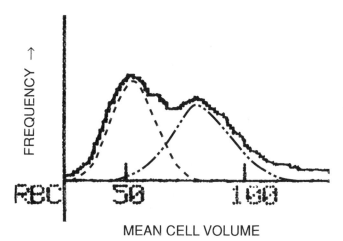

FIGURE 2–10. Size distribution curve for distinct populations of red cells. Inspection of the size distribution curve provided by the automated cell counter may reveal the presence of distinct populations of red cells of different cell volume. This example shows a curve for a patient with a population of extremely small cells *(dashed line)* mixed with a population of near-normal–sized cells *(broken line)*. (From Hillman, RS, and Finch, CA: Red Cell Manual, ed 7. FA Davis, Philadelphia, 1996, p 48, with permission.)

66

the center because there is a greater depth of hemoglobin solution around the periphery than in the flattened center. In addition to being pale, the central area of a normal cell occupies approximately one-third of the diameter.

As discussed earlier, cells that have a normal concentration of hemoglobin are described as normochromic. In the normal smear there is very little variation in size, shape, and staining characteristics (normocytosis). Anisocytosis, a variation in the size of the cells, may mean an increase in the number of small or large cells or a mixture of both. A variation in the shape of the cells, poikilocytosis, may be important in the differential diagnosis of disease states, as discussed in the section on red cell diseases. Alterations in the shape include those that are listed in Table 2–6 and shown in Figure 2–11 (see also Color Plates 11 to 15).

Hypochromia, again, is a decrease in the intensity of the hemoglobin staining that occurs when the area of central pallor occupies more than one-third of the diameter of the cell (see Color Plate 32). Hypochromia, when seen in the blood film, is nearly always associated with a decrease in the MCHC.

Red cells with a diffuse light blue or grayish tint in the cytoplasm are described as having diffuse basophilia (polychromasia) (see Color Plate 11[B]). These cells are young erythrocytes (reticulocytes) that have not yet completely lost their ribonucleic acid. They may be stained by supravital stains in reticulocyte preparations (see Color Plate 17A) and normally constitute less than 2% of the red cell population. Reticulocyte counts should be performed in any patient who has a prominent diffuse polychromasia. These cells are larger than normal and may raise the mean cell volume, producing an apparent macrocytosis (see also the section on Reticulocyte Count).

RED BLOOD CELL INCLUSIONS AND STAINED FRAGMENTS

Basophilic Stippling

Basophilic RNA may also occur as fine stippling. This stippling can occur in association with extensive diffuse polychromasia or in toxic states such as lead poisoning and disorders of hemoglobin production (megaloblastic anemia and thalassemia) (see Color Plate 10C).

Howell-Jolly Bodies

These are fragments of nuclear DNA that appear as circumscribed, densely staining purple particles near the periphery of the cell (see Color Plate 31). The spleen normally removes inclusions of this sort. Cells containing Howell-Jolly bodies are almost always present after splenec-

TABLE 2–6. RED BLOOD CELL ABNORMALITIES SEEN ON STAINED SMEAR

Descriptive Term	Observation	Significance
Macrocytosis	Cell diameter > 8 μm MCV > 100 fL	Megaloblastic anemias Severe liver disease Hypothyroidism
Microcytosis	Cell diameter < 6 μm MCV < 80 fL MCHC < 27%	Iron deficiency anemia Thalassemias Anemia of chronic disease
Hypochromia	Increased zone of central pallor	Diminished hemoglobin content
Polychromatophilia	Presence of red cells not fully hemoglobinized	Reticulocytosis
Poikilocytosis	Variability of cell shape	Sickle cell disease Microangiopathic hemolysis Leukemias Extramedullary hematopoiesis Marrow stress of any cause
Anisocytosis	Variability of cell size	Reticulocytosis Transfusing normal blood into microcytic or macrocytic cell population
Leptocytosis	Hypochromic cells with small central zone of hemoglobin ("target cells")	Thalassemias Obstructive jaundice
Spherocytosis	Cells with no central pallor, loss of biconcave shape MCHC high	Loss of membrane relative to cell volume Hereditary spherocytosis Accelerated red blood cell destruction by reticuloendothelial system
Schistocytosis	Presence of cell fragments in circulation	Increased intravascular mechanical trauma Microangiopathic hemolysis
Acanthocytosis	Irregularly spiculated surface	Irreversibly abnormal membrane lipid content Liver disease Abetalipoproteinemia
Echinocytosis	Regularly spiculated cell surface	Reversible abnormalities of membrane lipids High plasma-free fatty acids Bile acid abnormalities Effects of barbiturates, salicylates, etc.
Stomatocytosis	Elongated, slit-like zone of central pallor	Hereditary defect in membrane transport of sodium Severe liver disease
Elliptocytosis	Oval cells	Hereditary anomaly, usually harmless

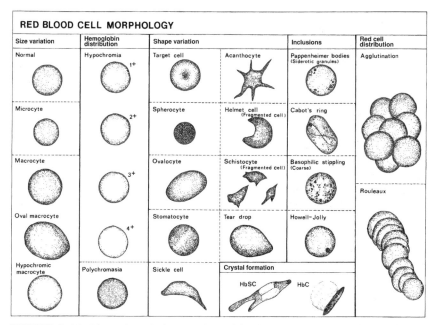

FIGURE 2–11. Normal and abnormal red blood cell morphology. (From Ciesla, BE: Morphological changes associated with disease. In Harmening, DM: Clinical Hematology and Fundamentals of Hemostasis, ed 3. FA Davis, Philadelphia, 1997, p 82, with permission.)

tomy but may also occur with intense or abnormal erythrocyte production resulting from hemolysis or ineffective erythropoiesis.

Siderotic Granules

These are iron-containing granules not normally seen in *mature* erythrocytes; however, they can be present in situations associated with iron overload syndromes or after splenectomy. Special staining of these cells with Prussian Blue stain for iron may demonstrate these siderotic granules. When they are visible on Wright-Giemsa–stained smears, they are called **Pappenheimer bodies.**

Heinz Bodies

Despite the fact that these masses of denatured hemoglobin are invisible on Wright-Giemsa–stained smears, they can be seen easily with phase microscopy or supravital staining (see Color Plate 10B). They represent denatured hemoglobin precipitates occurring with severe oxidative stress (especially in patients with glucose 6-phosphate dehydrogenase deficiency), or with the excess globin chain production that may occur in thalassemias. Heinz bodies may also be seen following splenectomy because the normal spleen removes all intraerythrocyte inclusions.

Nucleated Red Blood Cells

Normally, maturing red cells lose their nuclei well before they leave the bone marrow. However, if erythropoietic stress is intense, less mature cells may also enter the circulation. In addition to numerous young reticulocytes, nucleated precursors may be seen occasionally. Their presence in the peripheral blood indicates either intense erythropoietic activity in the bone marrow, a damaged bone marrow due to infiltrative disease, or the existence of erythropoiesis in the spleen and other nonmarrow sites where there is less control over erythrocyte release into the blood stream—**extramedullary hematopoiesis** (see Color Plates 39B and 46A).

RED CELL METABOLISM

To perform its main function of oxygen transport, the erythrocyte must meet several criteria: first, it must maintain its biconcave structure for maximal gas exchange; second, it must be deformable to negotiate the small microcirculatory capillaries; and finally, it must have a constant internal environment to keep hemoglobin in a reduced form so that it can transport the oxygen. In addition, red cell survival must be normal, and its physical and chemical characteristics must be maintained within a narrow spectrum. To do this, erythrocyte metabolism must provide energy and chemical compounds capable of limiting excess oxidation. Abnormalities of these aspects of metabolism produce a shortened red cell survival (hemolysis), and investigation involves categorizing the nature of these metabolic defects.

THE RED CELL MEMBRANE

The erythrocyte membrane consists of an integral layer of lipids, including phospholipids and cholesterol, which contain an intimate association of proteins. These proteins may be internal or peripheral proteins (Fig. 2–12). This protein-lipid composition is important in maintaining the integrity of the red cell membrane, which resists an uncontrolled influx of sodium ions (present in higher concentration in the

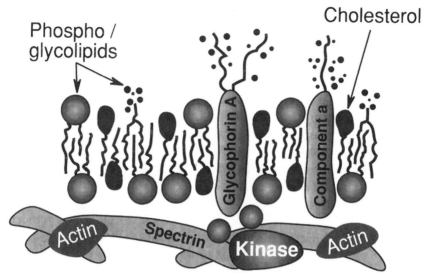

FIGURE 2–12. Structure of the red cell membrane. The adult red cell membrane consists of a lipid sheath two molecules thick, which is affixed to a reticular protein network made up of two major components, spectrin and actin. The external surface is relatively rich in phosphatidylcholine, sphingomyelin, and glycolipid, whereas the inner lipid layer contains mostly phosphatidylserine, phosphatidylethanolamine, and phosphatidylinositol. These phosphoglycolipids are present in an equimolar ratio with cholesterol. In addition, glycophorin A and component a *(band 3)*, two integral proteins, penetrate the bimolecular lipid sheath and are in contact with the aqueous phase on either side. The membrane proteins provide a negative charge to the surface of the cell and help in the diffusion of glucose and anions across the membrane. (From Hillman, RS, and Finch, CA: Red Cell Manual, ed 7. FA Davis, Philadelphia, 1996, p 13, with permission.)

plasma) and an efflux of potassium ions (present in higher concentration within the red cell). Instead, the membrane supports an active transport of sodium ions out of, and potassium ions into, the red cell. This process is critically dependent on an adequate energy source in the form of glucose. The principal *peripheral* membrane protein, **glycophorin,** is a glycosylated protein that contains the majority of the red blood cell antigens. It is probably also responsible for supporting the red blood cell membrane cytoskeleton. The major *internal* protein is called **spectrin** and is assisted by a second protein, **actin,** in forming a lattice structure that is attached to the cytoplasmic ends of the integral proteins, thereby fixing their positions and creating a cell skeleton (see Fig. 2–12). Spectrin is also an important constituent of normal RBC membrane integrity and is responsible for strengthening the membrane and resisting sheer stress from the circulatory system. The integrity of spectrin is maintained by providing energy in the form of adenosine triphosphate (ATP). A defective phosphorylation of spectrin is associated with loss of membrane integrity and decreased deformability. It is believed that this is the defect that occurs in hereditary spherocytosis. Loss of the red cell membrane is associated with the production of a *spherocyte* (see Color Plate 9[A]). An increase in membrane calcium also causes an increase in membrane rigidity. Spherocytes cannot traverse the small pores in the sinusoids of the spleen and are sequestered prematurely or have parts of their membranes removed, which causes their characteristic appearance.

Laboratory Assessment of Red Cell Fragility (Membrane Function)

Structural abnormalities, as well as some metabolic defects, may make red cells abnormally susceptible to in vitro hemolysis as well as *in vivo destruction.* In particular, in the disorder **hereditary spherocytosis,** the spherocytes are particularly fragile when exposed to osmotic stress. The test for **osmotic fragility** exposes red cells to increasingly dilute saline solutions to determine the point at which the internal flow of water into the erythrocyte causes the red cells to swell and rupture (see Fig. 3–2). Normal disc-shaped cells can imbibe water and swell significantly before membrane capacity is exceeded. Red cells with relatively less surface-area-to-volume ratio (spherocytes) will lyse after much smaller amounts of fluid enter. Spherocytes and other cells that have undergone membrane damage burst when exposed to saline solutions only slightly less concentrated than normal saline. This increased osmotic fragility is enhanced still further by incubating the cells at 37°C for 24 hours before exposing them to hypo-osmolar saline. Osmotic fragility is increased in autoimmune hemolytic anemia, presumably because the cells are more rigid than normal and undergo gradual membrane loss. By contrast, in *thalassemia, iron deficiency anemia,* and *sickle cell disease,* red cells have excess membrane and are more than normally resistant to osmotic damage.

Autohemolysis

Normal red cells readily survive 48 hours of incubation at 37°C without any exogenous energy source. Red cells with defective ion transport or energy generation tend to hemolyze after 48 hours in their own defibrinated plasma with no added nutrients. The *autohemolysis test* can be used as a screening test for hereditary spherocytosis because the markedly increased autohemolysis is virtually abolished by incubating the cells with an energy source (glucose or ATP). In the enzyme defect *glucose-6-phosphate dehydrogenase (G-6-PD) deficiency,* autohemolysis is modestly increased, and neither ATP nor glucose has any effect. Cells with the enzyme deficiency *pyruvate kinase (PK) deficiency* show marked autohemolysis that is partially alleviated by ATP, but not by glucose. For both G-6-PD deficiency and PK deficiency, however, better screening tests are readily available, as will be discussed later.

ERYTHROCYTE METABOLIC PATHWAYS

Embden–Meyerhof Pathway

The majority of the energy needed by RBCs is provided by the *Embden-Meyerhof glycolytic pathway.* Through this pathway, each molecule of glucose is metabolized to produce two molecules of ATP (Fig. 2–13). This pathway functions anaerobically, and therefore glucose is not fully metabolized to yield the maximum number of ATP molecules. The red cell requires energy for several metabolic functions, which include the following:

- maintenance of hemoglobin as a respiratory pigment
- maintenance of the electrolyte gradients between plasma and the erythrocyte cytoplasm
- maintenance of the oxidation-reduction metabolic pathways
- the synthesis of lipids and nucleotides

The defective production of energy can affect any or all of these pathways, which may then lead to shortened red cell survival.

Pentose Phosphate Pathway

As already mentioned, the Embden-Meyerhof pathway provides a net of two molecules of ATP and is probably the major energy source of the erythrocyte. Another major erythrocytic metabolic pathway is the *pentose phosphate pathway,* in which glucose is converted into *6-phosphogluconate* in the presence of the enzyme *glucose-6-phosphate dehydrogenase (G-6-PD).* A pyridine nucleotide cofactor, **nicotinamide adenine dinucleotide phosphate (NADP),** is converted in this process to a reduced $NADPH + H^+$ form. This reduced cofactor provides reducing potential in the form of hydrogen ions for a compound called *glutathione,* which is the major reservoir of reducing potential in the erythrocyte. A series of intermediary steps are involved in this process, which is a self-rejuvenating process in the presence of several enzymes (see Fig. 2–13). The deficient production of reduced glutathione and NADP, which may occur in G-6-PD deficiency, is associated with increased oxidative stress on the erythrocyte membrane and many internal proteins. In particular, the globin chains of hemoglobin may become oxidized and lose the ability to keep ferrous iron (Fe^{2+}) in the

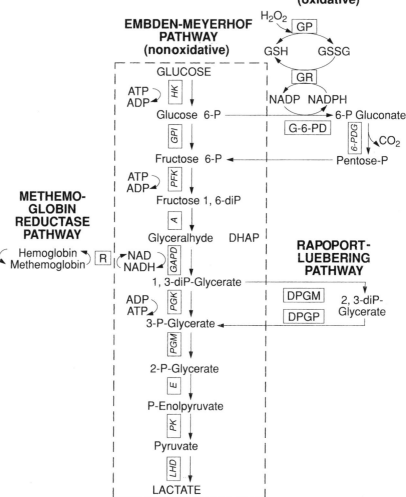

FIGURE 2–13. Red cell metabolic pathways. The enucleated red cell depends almost exclusively on the breakdown of glucose for energy requirements. The Embden-Meyerhof pathway (nonoxidative or anaerobic pathway) is responsible for most of the glucose utilization and generation of adenosine 5′-triphosphate. In addition, this pathway plays an essential role in maintaining nucleotides in a reduced state to support methemoglobin reduction (the methemoglobin-reductase pathway) and 2,3-diphosphoglycerate (2,3-DPG) synthesis (the Rapoport-Luebering pathway). The phosphogluconate pathway couples oxidative metabolism with pyridine nucleotide and glutathione reduction. It serves to protect red cells from environmental oxidants. (From Hillman, RS, and Finch, CA: Red Cell Manual, ed 7. FA Davis, Philadelphia, 1996, p 15, with permission.)

reduced state. This allows the development of oxidized ferric (Fe^{3+}) iron and an unstable hemoglobin, which then cannot function as a respiratory pigment. The net result is shortened red cell survival and hemolysis. Approximately 5 to 10% of glucose is metabolized by the pentose phosphate pathway. An inability to neutralize oxidant stress produced by drugs or genetic deficiencies of the various enzymes can cause the accumulation of hydrogen peroxide and other oxidants. This can be visualized on supravital stains as the appearance of denatured globin aggregates *(Heinz bodies)* (see Color Plate 10B).

The most common disorder associated with defective oxidative neutralization is deficiency of the enzyme glucose-6-phosphate dehydrogenase. This enzyme is pivotal to the generation of NADPH, is remarkably polymorphic, and is inherited through the X chromosome. More than 50 structural variants are known in addition to the normal variants, type A and type B. Type A migrates faster than type B on electrophoresis, and it is found predominantly in blacks. Type B is found more commonly in whites. Many other structural variants have been found that may have normal or near normal activity; however, other variants may be dysfunctional or deficient. Because inheritance is X linked, abnormalities are more commonly seen in men.

Tests to Evaluate the Pentose Phosphate Pathway

Clinically apparent dysfunction occurs only when the G-6-PD enzyme activity is less than 25% of normal. Defective function is uncovered by exposing red cells to an oxidizing stress. Keep in mind, however, that nucleated erythrocytes and reticulocytes may still have the capacity to generate enough G-6-PD to resist oxidant stress in some forms of G-6-PD deficiency. For example, in type A G-6-PD deficiency, only the mature erythrocyte is deficient in the enzyme.

The Ascorbate–Cyanide Test

This test challenges hemoglobin with hydrogen peroxide generated from sodium cyanide and sodium ascorbate. After incubation for 1 or 2 hours, brown methemoglobin is seen with the following—G-6-PD deficiency, PK deficiency, paroxysmal nocturnal hemoglobinuria, and unstable hemoglobins—whereas normal blood remains bright red. The ascorbate-cyanide test is sensitive enough to detect the minimally reduced activity that occurs in G-6-PD heterozygotes and in homozygotes with temporarily increased activity levels; it is not, however, *specific* for G-6-PD deficiency.

The NADPH Fluorescent Test

By contrast, this test is specific for G-6-PD deficiency and its effect on NADP. If G-6-PD is present, its reduction activity stimulation converts NADP to fluorescent NADPH, which appears as a readily visible spot under ultraviolet light. Blood samples up to several weeks old are suitable for use, and the results are moderately sensitive.

The Methylene Blue–Methemoglobin Test

Muddy brown methemoglobin evolves from the transparent red hemoglobin solution if G-6-PD is severely deficient in the presence of methylene blue. This test can detect deficiencies in homozygous women or hemizygous men, but is not sensitive enough to detect female heterozygotes.

Specific enzyme assays and electrophoretic characterization permit the definitive diagnosis of G-6-PD deficiency. Except in rare cases or for characterizing unusual genetic variants, the above screening tests provide all the information needed for clinical diagnosis. The oldest procedure, now rarely used, induces Heinz bodies by incubating the blood with the oxidant drug acetylphenylhydrazine. The screening tests mentioned above are, however, better screening procedures and use chemical endpoints to demonstrate whether or not there is sufficient G-6-PD to generate protective reducing activity.

Young cells have higher G-6-PD levels than older ones, regardless of the genetic variant that is present. If the enzyme is defective, older cells are preferentially destroyed during a mild to moderate hemolytic event. The resultant reticulocytes generated to replace these lost cells have higher activity levels. False-negative test results often occur if blood is examined just after a hemolytic episode, because the reticulocytes and nonhemolyzed remaining cells are, by definition, those with adequate levels. Newly generated reticulocytes have still higher levels, and this can affect the results for 3 to 10 days after a hemolytic episode. The ascorbate–cyanide test is usually sensitive enough to detect reduced activity under these circumstances, but the test should be repeated after red cell production is stabilized.

Methemoglobin Reductase Pathway

Other pathways that are important in red cell metabolism are the NAD^+ and $NADP^+$ *methemoglobin reductase pathways.* NAD^+ and particularly $NADP^+$ are responsible for the maintenance of hemoglobin in a reduced or ferrous state. The ferrous hemoglobin is an oxygen transporter by virtue of the maintenance of heme iron in the reduced, or ferrous, state (Fe^{2+}). These two pathways are also responsible for the reduction of NAD^+ and $NADP^+$ and require specific methemoglobin reductase enzymes. In the absence of these enzymes, there is accumulation of methemoglobin, which is the oxidized form of heme (ferric heme, Fe^{3+}). This form of hemoglobin, *methemoglobin,* has lost its ability to combine with respiratory oxygen.

The Formation of 2,3-Diphosphoglycerate (2,3-DPG)

Another integral pathway crucial to normal hemoglobin function is the Luebering-Rapaport shunt, which is responsible for the production of 2,3-DPG (see Fig. 2–13). This organic phosphate compound is important because it enhances oxygen displacement from hemoglobin and thus facilitates the delivery of oxygen to tissues where there is a low oxygen tension. This compound is present in the red cell in higher concentrations than in any other cell. It has an especially high affinity for hemoglobin A and does not combine with some other hemoglobins, particularly fetal hemoglobin (hemoglobin F). This compound is thus responsible for shifting the hemoglobin dissociation curve to the right (see Fig. 10–1), and is important when considering the age of stored blood for transfusion.

ERYTHROCYTE SENESCENCE AND HEMOGLOBIN CATABOLISM

During its life span of 120 days, the erythrocyte travels approximately 200 to 300 miles. In the process of aging, there is a slow metabolic downgrading of the red cells. Many enzymes show reduced function, and the cells become more sensitive to osmotic lysis. Approximately 1% of the red cells are removed from circulation daily by the reticuloendothelial system. These cells are replaced by reticulocytes from the bone marrow. In addition to the metabolic changes, the loss of the red cell membrane leads to less deformability. As these senescent red cells are removed in the extravascular reticuloendothelial system, the hemoglobin molecule is broken down into its component parts. Approximately 5 to 7 g of hemoglobin are catabolized daily. The iron is salvaged, as previously discussed. The globin portion of the hemoglobin molecule is broken down into amino acids that are recirculated to the amino acid pool. The porphyrin component of the heme molecule is broken down by a series of catabolic steps into a compound called **bilirubin,** which is a brownish-yellow pigment. Bilirubin is bound to albumin and transported to the liver. In the liver it is conjugated by the addition of glucuronides to form a *diglucuronide compound,* which is water soluble and excreted in the bile (see Chapter 12). A small proportion of this compound is reabsorbed and re-excreted (Fig. 2–14). By bacterial action in the bowel, the bilirubin conjugate is further broken down into *urobilinogen* and *stercobilinogen* and excreted in the stool. A small amount of these compounds is reabsorbed through the enterohepatic circulation and excreted in the urine.

Measurement of Red Cell Survival

The red cell life span can be measured by several techniques. The most commonly used technique is the **random method,** where a radioactive

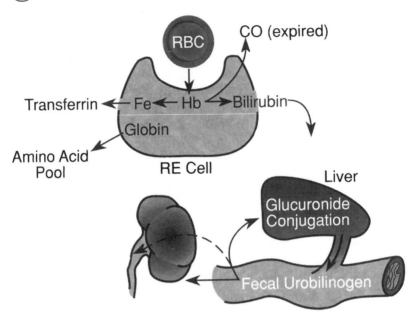

FIGURE 2–14. Red cell destruction by the reticuloendothelial system. Normally, senescent red cells are phagocytized by reticuloendothelial cells, and the hemoglobin is broken down into its essential components. The iron recovered is returned to transferrin for new red cell production, and the amino acids from the globin portion of the molecule are returned to the general amino acid pool. The protoporphyrin ring of heme is broken at the alpha methene bridge and its alpha carbon exhaled as carbon monoxide. The remaining tetrapyrole leaves the reticuloendothelial cell as indirect bilirubin and travels to the liver, where it is conjugated for excretion in the bile. In the gut, the bilirubin glucuronide is converted to urobilinogen for excretion in stool and urine. (From Hillman, RS, and Finch, CA: Red Cell Manual, ed 7. FA Davis, Philadelphia, 1996, p 22, with permission.)

label (either ^{51}Cr or ^{111}In) is attached randomly to red cells of all ages after removal of an aliquot of blood from the patient. The rate at which the label disappears corresponds to the progressive destruction of an unselected cell population. The usual endpoint is the half-disappearance time, which under normal conditions is 28 to 35 days (with ^{51}Cr). With accelerated destruction, the endpoint may be less than a week or even a matter of hours. Radioactive chromate is an effective red cell label because it binds specifically to hemoglobin. Its biologic half-life is not excessively long; it emits an easily counted high-energy gamma ray, and it does not affect the survival of the cell that incorporates it. Chromium labeling can be used to measure the survival time of the patient's own cells or that of transfused, homologous cells in the patient. After introduction of the labeled cells, the baseline radioactivity level indicates the proportion of the total circulating cells that bear the label. This figure is necessary for later comparisons and, with suitable calculation of dilution, it demonstrates the patient's red cell volume (see the section on Erythrocytosis, p. 160).

Survival is measured by observing blood samples at intervals in order to determine the amount of radioactivity remaining in the circulation. Normally, half of the initial dose will have disappeared in 28 to 35 days. This figure is often used inaccurately as the half-life of red cells. The half-life of normal red cells is 60 days. ^{51}Cr half disappearance time is less because 1% or more of the radioactive label escapes from the red cells every day and is lost to counting. A ^{51}Cr half-time ($T_{1/2}$) of less than 25 days indicates accelerated destruction. This can be as low as 3 to 5 days in severe intrinsic hemolytic conditions, or can be measured in minutes or hours if there is antibody-mediated destruction.

With markedly accelerated destruction, the ^{51}Cr label from hemolyzed cells accumulates at the site of cell damage. It has been shown that the spleen is responsible for most hemolysis in some intrinsic hemolytic conditions and is responsible for the removal of damaged cells in other conditions. The accumulation of radioactivity in the liver or spleen can give an insight into the different pathogenetic mechanisms. Intravascular hemolysis occurs with strong complement-binding antibodies such as anti-A and anti-B, or with toxic, chemical, or physical damage to the cells.

Hemoglobin Release and Degradation

Free Hemoglobin

Only 5 to 10% of normal red cell destruction occurs in the vascular system through the process of intravascular hemolysis. When red cells are destroyed within the bloodstream, hemoglobin enters the plasma. Here it dissociates into alpha and beta dimers and complexes with **haptoglobin,** an alpha$_2$ globulin normally present in concentrations of 30 to 200 mg/dL. This quantity is sufficient to dispose of up to 100 mg of free hemoglobin per 100 mL of plasma. This complex is transported to the liver cell for further catabolism, promoting conservation of the iron in heme and preventing renal losses. Haptoglobin levels, therefore, fall, and the reduction of measurable haptoglobin is one important laboratory sign of *intravascular hemolysis.* Haptoglobin may also drop when the reticuloendothelial system is the site of hemolysis (extravascular hemolysis), since hemoglobin may leak from the spleen or other sinusoids into the bloodstream or following large extravascular hemorrhage (e.g., retroperitoneal bleeding). As little as 1 to 2 mL of RBC hemolysis in the intravascular compartment can totally deplete plasma haptoglobin. Another plasma protein, **hemopexin,** also augments the capacity of the plasma to conserve hemoglobin, binding preferentially to heme. Low or absent haptoglobins are often found in any chronic hemolytic process and typically return to normal a week after the cessation of hemolysis.

Haptoglobin

Haptoglobin levels are measured either chemically or (more easily) by immunologic techniques (see Chapter 7). Once the binding capacity of haptoglobin has been exceeded, free hemoglobin appears in the plasma. Since free hemoglobin is a small molecule, it can be excreted in the urine. **Hemoglobinemia** and **hemoglobinuria** occur when the haptoglobin capacity for binding hemoglobin dimers is saturated.

Other Tests of Intravascular Hemolysis

Urinary Hemosiderin

With chronic intravascular hemolysis and hemoglobinuria, pigment is reabsorbed by the renal tubules and may ultimately appear as iron granules within renal cells. Some renal tubular cells are desquamated as a normal process. A sample of urine can be collected, centrifuged, and stained for iron. The presence of intracellular iron granules within the desquamated renal tubular cells is indicative of chronic intravascular hemolysis with iron loss in the urine.

Methemalbumin

With intravascular hemolysis and the release of pigment into the plasma, the plasma color may change depending on the type of hemoglobin present. Oxyhemoglobin is bright red, and methemoglobin is dark brown. Similarly, the color of the serum or urine depends on the nature of the pigment released into the plasma. Methemoglobin is the oxidized version of hemoglobin with iron converted into the ferric state (Fe^{3+}). Free metheme may be bound to the other transport conservation protein, hemopexin (mentioned above), and transported to the liver for further catabolism. Hemopexin has the capacity to bind 50 to 100 mg/dL of heme. Once this capacity is exceeded, metheme binds to albumin. The various hemoglobin compounds may be detected by spectroscopic analysis of the plasma and show specific absorption spectra. Methemalbumin has a typical absorption peak at 630 nm and forms a characteristic hemochromogen color at 558 nm after the addition of ammonium sulfide as performed in the **Schumm's test.** This test becomes positive 1 to 6 hours after intravascular hemolysis of 100 mL of blood. Both the presence of methemalbumin and a positive Schumm's test are indicative of intravascular hemolysis. Methemalbumin remains stable in the plasma until more hemopexin is synthesized to activate transport molecules. Therefore, methemalbumin is more indicative of a chronic intravascular hemolysis (Fig. 2–15).

The catabolism of iron following disassembly in senescent red cells has been discussed under the section on Iron Metabolism earlier in this

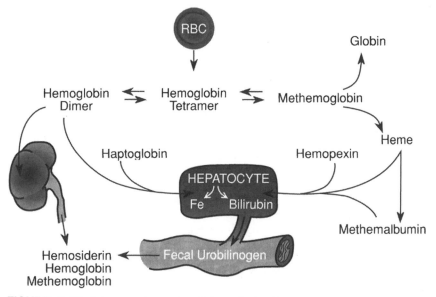

FIGURE 2–15. Intravascular red cell hemolysis. Red cells can also undergo intravascular hemolysis with the release of hemoglobin into circulation. The free hemoglobin tetramer is unstable and rapidly dissociates into alpha-beta dimers, which bind to haptoglobin and are removed by the liver. Hemoglobin may also be oxidized to methemoglobin and dissociate into its globin and heme moieties. To a limited extent, free heme can be bound by hemopexin and/or albumin for subsequent clearance by hepatocytes. Both pathways help recover heme iron for the support of hematopoiesis. Once haptoglobin is depleted, unbound hemoglobin dimers are excreted by the kidney as free hemoglobin, methemoglobin, or hemosiderin. (From Hillman, RS, and Finch, CA: Red Cell Manual, ed 7. FA Davis, Philadelphia, 1996, p 23, with permission.)

chapter. A more complete discussion of the clinical disorders responsible for shortened red cell survival and hemolysis is presented in Chapter 3.

Lactic Dehydrogenase (LDH)

With rupture (hemolysis) of the erythrocyte, its internal enzymes are released and may be measured in the bloodstream. Lactic dehydrogenase is one such enzyme, particularly isoenzymes I and II, and it is usually elevated in clinically significant hemolysis (see Chapters 3 and 12).

Indirect Bilirubin

In significant hemolysis, bilirubin (especially the unconjugated or indirect fraction), the breakdown product of heme catabolism, also usually accumulates prior to its delivery to the liver for conjugation and excretion (see Chapters 3 and 12).

PERIPHERAL BLOOD: WHITE CELLS

Circulating blood contains approximately 4000 to 11,000 white cells per microliter. The normal peripheral blood white cells comprise, morphologically and functionally, distinct populations of three main types: granulocytes, lymphocytes, and monocytes. These cells constitute the normal leukocyte population, but a small number of circulating white cells may be in the penultimate stage of maturation. The morphologic characteristics of the nucleus and cytoplasm of these cells define the specific categories and level of maturation, and the relative percentage of these cells may provide information on different disease states. The absolute numbers of the different types of cells may also provide clues as to whether a primary marrow disorder is present, or whether abnormalities are reactive to a secondary disease process.

WHITE BLOOD CELL COUNT

White cells are distinguished from circulating red cells by the presence of a nucleus (see Color Plates 4, 5, and 17). Automated counting procedures enumerate all nucleated cells as white cells. If large numbers of nucleated red cells are present, they too are counted, and the white cell count may have to be suitably corrected. In spite of this, the total white count is usually determined without difficulty. The **differential white count** gives the proportions of the different cell types that constitute the total number of white cells. Differential counts are sometimes omitted if the total count is normal and there is no clinical or laboratory evidence of hematologic abnormality. However, many neoplastic, inflammatory, and immunologic conditions alter cellular proportions despite a normal level for total white cells.

Like red cell counts, white cell counts use a small sample of diluted blood and are subject to sampling and dilutional errors. Because blood contains far fewer white than red cells, the dilution is less, and a larger volume of blood is examined than in red cell counting. Most laboratories use automated methods for white cell counting, either by electronic particle counting or by light-scattering principles. Manual dilution and visual examination of hemocytometer counts remain reliable when carefully performed. Manual methods are usually performed to corroborate exceedingly high or low electronic white cell counts.

Visual examination of stained blood films remains the mainstay of differential white cell counting, but automated procedures are gaining acceptance. Two different automated approaches are in use. In one of these, a sophisticated computer program for pattern recognition is linked with a lens that scans the stained blood film. This is fundamentally the same approach as that of the human eye and brain. The count is usually done on 100, 200, or 500 cells. A completely different technology separates the various kinds of white cells by manipulating the chemical properties of the medium in a continuous flow system and then enumerates the individual populations by light-scattering and absorbence techniques. Much larger numbers of white cells are sampled in the automated approach (10,000 cells).

GRANULOCYTES

In adults, half or more of circulating white cells are granulocytes, the cytoplasm of which contains readily visible granules of various chemical and enzymatic compositions. As previously discussed, there are three main types of granulocytes: neutrophils, eosinophils, and basophils (see Color Plates 4 and 5). The staining characteristics of the granules define the cell type: specifically, neutral staining characterizes neutrophils; reddish (eosinophilic) (Color Plate 5A) staining characterizes eosinophils; and bluish staining define basophils (Color Plate 5B). The myeloblast is the earliest cell recognizably committed to granulocytic identity (see Color Plates 1, 3, and 34) and typically contains no granules. Specific granules are first seen in the promyelocytes (Color Plate 3[A]), the next developmental phase after differentiation from a myeloblast. In health, maturation occurs only within the bone marrow. Granulocytes normally develop and mature at no other site and, once released from the marrow, cannot reproduce. With intense stimulation to increase circulating granulocytes, immature cells of this series may appear in the blood. Immature or abnormal granulocytes sometimes enter the circulation if bone marrow control mechanisms are deranged by malignant processes or when hematopoietic activity occurs outside of the marrow, as may happen in neoplastic myeloproliferative diseases.

Neutrophils

The cytoplasmic granules of neutrophils react with both basic and acidic stains, producing "neutral" or light purple granules on the most commonly used Wright-Giemsa stain preparations. In the mature cell, nucleochromatin is condensed into discrete lumps or lobes connected by thin strands of material. These cells are called **polymorphonuclear leukocytes** because there are so many **(poly-)** possible forms **(morph-)** that these flexibly linked nuclear lumps can assume. Acceptable shortened terms for this polysyllabic description are "PMNs" and "polys." Less mature neutrophils have larger nuclei that are not separated into lobes. The state that precedes maturity is called a **band cell** because its nucleus is shaped like a curved band (see Color Plate 3[D]).

Neutrophils are actively motile, and large numbers can congregate at sites of tissue injury within a short time. They are attracted to sites of injury and inflammation by a process called *chemotaxis.* Microbial products, the products of cellular injury, and many plasma proteins can exert a chemotactic effect on neutrophils. Neutrophils constitute the body's first line of defense when tissue is damaged or foreign material gains entry into the body. Their function is closely aligned to other defense systems of the body, including antibody production (immunoglobulins) and activation of the *complement system* (see Chapter 7). The interaction of these systems with neutrophils enhances their ability to **phagocytize** and degrade particles of many sorts. They are capable of releasing enzymes into their own cytoplasm, destroying ingested or phagocytized material, and they also can release enzymes into the surrounding medium. One way to identify abnormal or ambiguous immature cells as members of the neutrophil series is to elicit these enzyme reactions with cytochemical techniques (see section on Cytochemical Staining). The neutrophil granules may be divided into **primary granules,** which appear at the *promyelocyte stage,* and **secondary granules,** which appear at the *myelocyte stage* and predominate in the mature granulocytes. The primary granules contain **myeloperoxidase** and **acid phosphatase,** as well as other acid hydrolytic enzymes, whereas the secondary granules contain *alkaline phosphatase* and the enzyme *lysozyme.* The terminally differentiated cells (metamyelocyte, band and neutrophil), contain primary and secondary granules in the ratio of 1:2.

The principal function of neutrophils is the phagocytosis and removal of debris, particulate material, and bacteria, as well as the killing of microbial organisms. Neutrophils can also kill antibody-bound cells by a process called **antibody-dependent cellular cytotoxicity (ADCC).** Their only proven useful role is preventing invasion by pathogenic microorganisms, and localizing and killing them following successful invasion. The circulating neutrophils released from the bone marrow may align themselves closely to the blood vessel *(marginating neutrophils)* or may remain within the circulating bloodstream (see Fig. 2–2). It is probably the marginal neutrophils that are released to tissue sites when needed. Normally the rate at which new cells enter the blood from the bone marrow is equal to the rate at which cells egress to the tissues. Egress from the circulation by neutrophils is random, and a mature neutrophil remains in the bloodstream for approximately 7 to 10 hours before it exits to the tissues and body cavities. There is no evidence that neutrophils ever return to the bone marrow from the blood, and therefore this functional pathway may be considered to proceed in one direction only. The abnormalities in production and distribution within the bloodstream will be considered in Chapter 4.

Eosinophils

Eosinophils are granulocytes with a two-lobed nucleus and moderately large, refractile granules that stain deep red with the acidic dye eosin (see Color Plate 5A). Although capable of phagocytosis, eosinophils are not bactericidal. The eosinophil contains several enzymes that inactivate mediators of acute inflammation and, like the neutrophil, it also contains **histaminase.** The biologic role of eosinophils seems to be the modulation of cellular and chemical activities in immunologically mediated inflammation. These cells proliferate in the bone marrow under the influence of granulocyte macrophage colony–stimulating factor, interleukin-3, and interleukin-5. IL-5 is also known as **eosinophil differentiation factor** and was originally discovered to be a humoral response to parasitic antigens. IL-5 can influence both eosinophilic function and migration. Although during development these cells resemble developing neutrophils, they have distinct terminal stem cells as well as differing chemistries, kinetics, and functions. The normal range for eosinophils is 0 to 700 cells per microliter. Unlike the neutrophil, the eosinophil probably returns from tissues to blood and from blood to marrow under normal circumstances. It may also respond to the same chemotactic stimuli as neutrophils. The eosinophil is more sluggish and inefficient in phagocytosis and the killing of bacteria. In inflammation much of their function is unknown. Eosinophils also have a unique ability to damage larvae of certain helminth parasites.

Basophils

Basophils constitute less than 1% of normal circulating leukocytes. Their large, coarse cytoplasmic granules stain deeply with blue basic dye and are brilliantly stained by metachromatic dyes (see Color Plate 5B). The granules contain acid-mucopolysaccharides, hyaluronic acid, and large amounts of histamine. Basophils in the circulation serve no known function. Cells very similar to blood basophils are plentiful in skin, in the mucosa of the respiratory tract, and in connective tissue. These cells, called **mast cells,** contain histamine, acid mucopolysaccharides (including heparin), and other materials in their granules responsible for causing allergic tissue reactions. Tissue basophils, but not blood basophils, have immunoglobulin E (IgE) receptors adherent to the cell membrane; these receptors react with allergens and IgE to induce the release of vasoactive mediators, which have many different effects. These mediators are also released by interaction with anaphylotoxins derived from the third and fifth component of complement (i.e., C3a and C5a). The massive release of granule contents may evoke sudden death (anaphylactic shock). Many of the mediators cause smooth muscle contraction and increase vascular permeability. Basophils also release chemotactic factors and other chemical mediators of inflammation.

ABNORMAL GRANULOCYTE MORPHOLOGY

It is abnormal for more than 8 to 10% of the circulating neutrophils to be band forms or for any earlier precursors at all to exist in the peripheral blood. Certain morphologic abnormalities may be seen in mature granulocytes that may be indicative of an acquired or hereditary abnormality.

Acquired Abnormalities

Toxic Granulation

In the cytoplasm of neutrophils from severely ill or infected patients or from those in whom tissue destruction or inflammation has occurred, more prominent, coarsely staining cytoplasmic granules can be seen (Color Plate 18). These are thought to be abnormally activated, enzyme-containing granules rather than inclusion bodies or phagocytized material. Frequently, the cytoplasm of these stimulated cells is vacuolated or takes a more basic stain than normal. Cytoplasmic vacuolization is another abnormal finding that, together with toxic granulation, is often seen accompanying bacterial sepsis.

Döhle Bodies

Neutrophils may sometimes contain large, round, pale blue masses in the periphery of the cytoplasm called **Döhle bodies** (Color Plate 19). These may occur with severe infections, burns, malignancies, or extensive cell lysis, but may also be found in normal pregnancy. The masses seem to be aggregated, rough endoplasmic reticulum. Their presence reflects the same metabolic alterations that stimulate rapid neutrophil degranulation and toxic granulation.

Azurophilic Granules

As granulocytes and other leukocytes develop, they may have numerous small, smoothly rounded, red cytoplasmic granules that contain a variety of lysosomal enzymes. As specific granules develop, these azurophilic granules decline sharply, but a few may persist in the cytoplasm of mature lymphocytes, monocytes, or granulocytes. They may have no pathologic significance.

Hypersegmentation and Macropolycytes

Disorders of folic acid or vitamin B_{12} metabolism produce many morphologic abnormalities, of which megaloblastic red cell development is the most conspicuous. Other rapidly proliferating cells also manifest abnormal developmental changes. Granulocytic cells tend to be abnormally large, especially metamyelocytes in the marrow (giant metamyelocytes) and neutrophils in the peripheral blood. These neutrophils have nuclei with seven or eight lobes, instead of the normal three to five lobes, and an abundant but morphologically normal cytoplasm. Cells with similar morphologic abnormalities may also be seen in myeloproliferative disorders (see Chapter 4) (Color Plate 20).

Hereditary Abnormalities

Alder-Reilly Anomaly

In this disorder, the neutrophils contain giant, dark-staining granules filled with polysaccharides. Patients with this disorder have systemic abnormalities of mucopolysaccharide metabolism leading to gargoylism in Hunter's syndrome, Hurler's syndrome, and other mucopolysacchari-doses.

May-Hegglin Anomaly

These neutrophils contain large blue or pinkish bodies, resembling Dohle bodies, that distort the cytoplasm of myeloid and monocytic cells. Moderate thrombocytopenia and abnormal platelet morphology often accompany leukopenia in this condition, but the patients generally remain in good health.

Pelger-Huet Phenomenon

Two forms of this morphologic anomaly may occur, the acquired and the inherited variety. The inherited disorder represents a purely morphologic aberration in which the neutrophils have a bilobed or monolobed nucleus and coarse chromatin but are functionally normal (Color Plate 21). In the acquired disorder, a similar morphology may be seen in persons with myeloproliferative diseases. These mature neutrophils are often mistaken for immature or band forms.

Chediak-Higashi Anomaly

Chediak-Higashi syndrome is a rare autosomal recessive disorder of lysosomal function and structure, leading to the accumulation of giant lysosomes containing various hydrolases and other enzymes. This change is most conspicuous in neutrophils, but it also affects many epithelial cells, nerve cells, and the pigment-containing melanocytes in the skin, hair, and eyes. Anemia, thrombocytopenia, decreased leukocyte counts, and increased susceptibility to infection characterize a frequently downhill clinical course. Aleutian mink, prized for the color of their fur, suffer from a similar form of partial cutaneous albinism and severe susceptibility to infection, caused by abnormal leukocytes.

LYMPHOCYTES

Lymphocytes constitute the second most numerous leukocyte in the peripheral blood. These cells are essential components of the immune defense system; their primary function is to interact with antigens and mount an immune response. This immune response may be (1) *humoral,* in the form of antibody production; (2) cell mediated, with elaboration of *lymphokines* by lymphocytes; or (3) cytotoxic, with the production of *cytotoxic killer lymphocytes.* Not only are the absolute quantities of these cells important, but so are the relative proportions of their different subclasses. This is well demonstrated in the devastating acquired immunodeficiency syndrome (AIDS), in which the infecting virus selectively attacks one lymphocyte subtype (CD4 lymphocytes). The role of the lymphocyte in immune function is discussed in the section devoted to Immunology in Chapter 7.

Circulating blood lymphocytes constitute a tiny fraction (<5%) of the total lymphocyte pool. Dense concentrations are found in the lymph nodes, the spleen, and the mucosa of the alimentary and respiratory tracts, whereas diffuse numbers exist in the bone marrow, liver, skin, and chronically inflamed tissue. There is a continuous circulation of lymphocytes from one compartment to another, which is normally maintained in equilibrium. There are two primary subtypes, T-lymphocytes and B-lymphocytes, each performing unique immunologic functions (see Color Plate 1). In healthy adults, about 75 to 80% of the circulating lymphocytes are T cells and 10 to 15% are B cells; the remainder exhibit neither characteristic and are "null" cells. *T-lymphocytes* are responsible for *cell-mediated immunity* and modulating *immune responsiveness.* *B-lymphocytes* are largely responsible for *humoral immunity* and *antibody production.* T-lymphocytes appear to recirculate much more widely than do their B-lymphocyte counterparts and have a longer life span (months or years compared with weeks or months). Most lymphocytes in the blood and lymphatic tissues are small cells less than 10 μm in diameter. They have deep-staining nuclei that are round or slightly indented, and coarse, ill-defined aggregates of chromatin (see Color Plates 4, 22, 23). Nucleoli are usually not present. The cytoplasm often stains intensely blue, and in most cases is seen as a scanty rim around the nucleus. Larger lymphoid cells occur less frequently, constituting approximately 10% of the circulating lymphocytes. These cells are between 12 to 16 μm in diameter with an abundant cytoplasm, often containing azurophilic granules. These large granular lymphocytes may represent natural killer–cytotoxic lymphocytes (see Color Plate 22), and probably represent active, antigenically stimulated cells.

Lymphocyte Subpopulations

The process of T- and B-lymphocyte development may be studied in the laboratory by quantitating secretory products (lymphokines or antibodies), or by using specific reagents to identify the cell surface characteristics (phenotypic or immunologic). The use of monoclonal antibodies specifically directed against single cell membrane receptors has enabled the characterization of several lymphocyte subpopulations whose functional diversity is only now becoming appreciated. The role of these cells in immune function and their laboratory detection are discussed in the section on Immunology in Chapter 7.

Atypical Lymphocytes

Most immune activities occur outside of the bloodstream, but altered immune responsiveness sometimes produces characteristic changes in circulating lymphocytes. The **atypical lymphocyte, or Downey cell,** is a T-lymphocyte in a state of immune activation and is classically associated with **infectious mononucleosis.** In this disorder the inciting agent is the Epstein-Barr virus (EBV), but other viral stimuli such as the cytomegalovirus (CMV) may also stimulate immune responsive (atypical) lymphocytes (see Color Plate 23).

MONOCYTES

Monocytes constitute 5 to 8% of circulating blood leukocytes. Only small numbers of monocytes circulate at any one time. These cells share a stem cell with neutrophils, but their maturation pathways subsequently diverge (see Color Plate 1). Their precursor cells **(monoblasts)** are well demonstrated by staining with *esterase stains.* The mature monocyte circulates only briefly in the peripheral blood and then enters the tissues to become a macrophage. Known by many names, it appears that "fixed" and "wandering" macrophages, histiocytes, the Kupffer cells of the liver, sinusoidal macrophages in the spleen and lymph nodes, peritoneal macrophages, and the macrophages that line the pulmonary air spaces all originate from the same primordial cell population. Their placement within the tissues seems to influence subsequent maturation and function. For example, the enzymatic compositions of pulmonary and peritoneal macrophages are quite different. Within the tissues, these macrophages may fuse into one another and become multinucleated giant cells that are especially prominent in *granulomatous inflammation.* Inflammation may stimulate monocytes to migrate from the blood into the tissues, but at a slower rate than neutrophils. They are particularly evident in subacute and chronic inflammation. These cells play a vital role in many host defense mechanisms. They are particularly active in the phagocytosis and killing of microorganisms, as well as many complex interactions with immunogens and with the cellular and protein constituents of the immune system. They may initiate and regulate the magnitude of the immune response. They are also responsible for antigen recognition and processing. By processing and presenting antigens to responsive T- and B-lymphocytes, monocytes initiate both cell-mediated and humoral immune responses. They also secrete various soluble, biologically active substances called *monokines,* among them interleukin-1 (see Color Plate 1). This factor promotes the proliferative response and expression of T cell membrane receptors. Their interaction with lymphocytes, in particular T-lymphocytes, is highly integrated and complex (see Chapter 7).

Blood monocytes characteristically are large (16 to 20 μm), with delicate

TABLE 2–7. CONDITIONS CAUSING NEUTROPHILIA (>8000 PMNs/μL)

Physiologic Response to Stress
Physical exercise
Exposure to extreme heat or cold
Following acute hemorrhage or hemolysis
Acute emotional stress
Childbirth

Infectious Diseases
Systemic or severe local bacterial infections
Some viruses (smallpox, chicken pox, herpes zoster, polio)
Some rickettsial diseases (especially Rocky Mountain spotted fever)
Some fungi, especially if there is acute tissue necrosis

Inflammatory Diseases
Rheumatoid arthritis
Acute rheumatic fever
Acute gout
Vasculitis and myositis of many types
Hypersensitivity reactions to drugs

Tissue Necrosis
Ischemic damage to heart, abdominal viscera, extremities
Burns
Many carcinomas and sarcomas

Metabolic Disorders
Uremia
Diabetic ketoacidosis
Eclampsia
Thyroid storm

Drugs
Epinephrine
Lithium
Histamine
Heparin
Digitalis
Many toxins, venoms, and heavy metals

nuclear chromatin. They have elongated, indented, or folded (kidney-shaped) nuclei and abundant, grayish-blue, translucent-looking cytoplasm (see Color Plate 5C). More immature forms, which circulate under conditions of monocytic stress or abnormal marrow proliferation, have a larger nucleus, sometimes a nucleolus, and more basophilic cytoplasm with more azurophilic granules than the mature forms. It is not clear how conditions such as tuberculosis or other inflammatory or immunologic events influence monocyte production, but bone marrow response can clearly be demonstrated.

ABNORMAL DIFFERENTIAL WHITE CELL COUNTS

Since the differential white count is reported in percentages, the total white count must be known in order to understand the pathophysiologic significance of the differential. Proportions change, either because there is a true increase in the numbers of preponderant cells *(absolute increase)* or because of a decline in the numbers of one cell type, which makes the remaining cells appear increased *(relative increase)*.

Circulating white cell counts are remarkably volatile. Absolute and relative values can change within minutes or hours of stimulation. The most dramatic variations in the differential count occur following the release of corticosteroid hormones. These corticosteroids cause lymphocytes and eosinophils to disappear from the circulation within 4 to 8 hours. Circulating granulocytes increase somewhat later, probably because of reduced egress from the bloodstream. Epinephrine, the hormone of the adrenal medulla, causes granulocytosis within minutes, probably by mobilizing mature neutrophils from "storage," or noncirculating, locations. Most of the physiologic stimuli that induce neutrophil leukocytosis (e.g., exercise, emotional stress, exposure to extreme temperatures) appear to act by stimulating epinephrine output. Still unexplained is how a localized, acute, inflammatory stimulus induces the bone marrow toward sustained increases of neutrophil production and release. Tables 2–7, 2–8, and 4–4 list conditions that affect neutrophil numbers.

Lymphocyte proportions often reflect relative changes caused by absolute alterations in granulocyte levels. Conditions that increase absolute lymphocyte numbers are shown in Table 2–9. Relative lymphocytosis

---

TABLE 2–8. CONDITIONS CAUSING NEUTROPENIA (<1500 PMNs/μL)

Chemical and Physical Agents

Dose-related, universal marrow depressants (radiation, cytotoxic drugs, benzene)
Idiosyncratic drug reactions (numerous)

Infectious Diseases

Some bacteria (typhoid, tularemia, brucellosis)
Some viruses (hepatitis, influenza, measles, mumps, rubella, infectious mononucleosis)
Protozoa (especially malaria)
Overwhelming infection of any kind

Hypersplenism

Liver disease
Storage diseases

Other Disorders

Some collagen-vascular diseases, especially lupus erythematosus
Severe folic acid or vitamin B_{12} deficiency

TABLE 2–9. CONDITIONS AFFECTING LYMPHOCYTE COUNTS

Lymphocytosis (>4000 Lymphocytes/μL in Adults; >7200/μL in Children)

Infectious diseases
  Bacterial (whooping cough, brucellosis, sometimes tuberculosis, secondary syphilis)
  Viral (hepatitis, infectious mononucleosis, mumps, many exanthems, cytomegalovirus)
Other disorders (infectious lymphocytosis, toxoplasmosis)
Metabolic conditions
  Hypoadrenalism
  Hyperthyroidism (sometimes)
Chronic inflammatory conditions
  Ulcerative colitis
  Immune diseases (serum sickness, idiopathic thrombocytopenic purpura)

Lymphocytopenia (<1000 Lymphocytes/μL in Adults; <2500/μL in Children)

Immunodeficiency syndromes
  Human immunodeficiency virus
  Congenital defects of cell-mediated immunity
  Immunosuppressive medication
Adrenal corticosteroid exposure
  Adrenal gland hyperactivity
  ACTH-producing pituitary gland tumors
  Therapeutic administration of steroids
Severe, debilitating illness of any kind
  Congestive heart failure
  Renal failure
  Far-advanced tuberculosis
Defects of lymphatic circulation
  Intestinal lymphangiectasia
  Disorders of intestinal mucosa
  Thoracic duct drainage

is common in acute viral syndromes and other infectious conditions that cause neutropenia. In some acute leukemias, a relative preponderance of lymphocytes may be noted in the peripheral blood when the neutrophil count is decreased because of disease or chemotherapy. Conditions affecting other circulating white cells are shown in Table 2–10.

The Shift to the Left

When immature granulocytes become prominent in the differential white count, the condition is sometimes called a "shift to the left." The term derives from early studies that used tabular headings to report the number of each cell type. The cell types were listed across the top of the page, starting with blasts on the left and progressing to mature

---

TABLE 2–10. CONDITIONS AFFECTING OTHER CIRCULATING WHITE CELLS

Monocytosis (>800 Monocytes/μL in Adults)

Infections (tuberculosis, subacute bacterial endocarditis, hepatitis, rickettsial diseases, syphilis)
Granulomatous diseases (sarcoid, ulcerative colitis, regional enteritis)
Collagen-vascular diseases (lupus, rheumatoid arthritis, polyarteritis)
Many cancers, lymphomas, and myeloproliferative disorders

Eosinophilia (>450 Eosinophils/μL)

Allergic diseases (asthma, hay fever, drug reactions, allergic vasculitis, serum sickness)
Parasitic infections (trichinosis, echinococcus, hookworm, schistosomiasis, amebiasis)
Skin disorders (some psoriasis, some eczema, pemphigus, dermatitis herpetiformis)
"Hypereosinophilic" syndromes (systemic eosinophilia associated with pulmonary infiltration and sometimes cardiovascular disturbances)
Neoplastic diseases (Hodgkin's disease, extensive metastases or necrosis of solid tumors)
Miscellaneous (collagen-vascular diseases, adrenal cortical hypofunction, ulcerative colitis)
L-tryptophan eosinophilic myalgia (TEM) syndrome

Basophilia (>50 Basophils/μL)

Chronic hypersensitivity states in the absence of the specific allergen (exposure to the allergen triggers cell lysis and rapid drop in basophil count)
Systemic mast cell disease
Myeloproliferative disorders

---

neutrophils on the right. Large numbers of immature cells provoked entries in the left-hand columns, normally empty except for a few bands. Numbers thus shifted to the left-hand columns when immature cells were numerous. The causes and significance of altered white cell levels are shown in Tables 2–7 through 2–10.

ERYTHROCYTE SEDIMENTATION RATE

This test determines the rate at which erythrocytes fall to the bottom of a vertical tube of anticoagulated blood within a specified period. Measurement of the distance from the top of the column of sedimented erythrocytes to the top of the fluid level in a given period determines the **erythrocyte sedimentation rate (ESR).** Anticoagulated blood placed in a vertical, small-bore tube exhibits settling (sedimenting) of the red cells at a rate determined largely by the relative density of the red cells with respect to the plasma. The actual rate of fall is greatly influenced by the ability of the erythrocytes to form into **rouleaux** (see Color Plate 51A). Rouleaux are clumps of red cells joined not by antibodies or covalent bonds, but merely by surface attraction. This quality represents the ability of red cells to aggregate. If the proportion of globulin to albumin increases, or if **fibrinogen** levels are especially high, rouleaux formation is enhanced and the sedimentation rate increases. A high concentration of asymmetric macromolecules in the plasma also reduces the mutually repellent forces that separate suspended red cells and enhance the formation of rouleaux. Other factors that affect the sedimentation rate include the ratio of red cells to plasma and the plasma viscosity. Table 2–11 is a list of the plasma factors and red cell factors that influence the ESR.

In normal blood, relatively little settling occurs because the gravitational pull of individual red cells is almost balanced by the upward current generated by the displacement of plasma. If the plasma is extremely viscous or cholesterol levels are very high, the upward trend may virtually neutralize the downward pull of individual or clumped red cells.

MEASUREMENT OF ESR

In the **Wintrobe method** for ESR, undiluted anticoagulated blood is allowed to stand for one hour in a tube 100 mm tall and 2.8 mm in diameter. Normal values are up to 8 mm/hour for men and 15 mm/hour

---

TABLE 2–11. FACTORS INFLUENCING ERYTHROCYTE SEDIMENTATION RATE

Plasma Factors (Factors that Reduce the Zeta Potential)

Fibrinogen concentration
Globulin concentration, particularly gamma globulins
Serum cholesterol

Red Cell Factors

Increased ESR
- Anemia (particularly hematocrit range 0.3–0.4)
- Red cell surface area: microcytes sediment more slowly than macrocytes
- Rouleaux: decreased surface area
- Sickle cells fail to form into rouleaux and therefore have a low ESR

Conditions causing increased ESR
- Pregnancy
- Hyperglobulinemia
- Hyperfibrinogenemia

for women. The **Westergren technique** uses a 200-mm column in which the anticoagulated blood, diluted 20% with saline or sodium citrate solution, is allowed to settle for one hour. Normal values are up to 15 mm/hour for men and 20 mm/hour for women, rising somewhat in both sexes after the age of 50. As a rough guideline, the ESR in men should be half the patient's age and in women, half the patient's age plus ten. The Westergren method is generally recommended as the standard method because of its simplicity and reproducibility.

INTERPRETATION OF ESR

Nonspecific increases in globulins and increased fibrinogen levels occur when the body responds to injury, inflammation, or pregnancy. A rise in ESR accompanies most inflammatory diseases, whether localized or systemic, and occurs when smoldering chronic inflammatory processes flare up.

The observed rate of settling varies as the concentration of red cells in plasma changes. Controversy exists over reporting ESR results in a "corrected" form that takes hematocrit level into account. Hematocrit has a much greater potential effect on the Wintrobe method. The Westergren technique is less affected by hematocrit because, in this method, the blood is substantially diluted.

Erythrocyte sedimentation rate really has three main uses: (1) as an aid in detecting an inflammatory process, (2) as a monitor of disease course or activity, and (3) as a screen for occult inflammatory or neoplastic conditions. The test, however, is relatively nonsensitive and nonspecific because it is influenced by many technical factors. Nevertheless, it remains a useful test and is widely employed. It must be emphasized that a normal ESR cannot be used to exclude organic disease; however, most acute and chronic inflammatory and neoplastic conditions are associated with an increase in sedimentation rate. The elevated ESR with pregnancy returns to normal by the third or the fourth week postpartum. Sedimentation rates of greater than 100 mm/hour are seen in plasma cell dyscrasias such as multiple myeloma, where high immunoglobulin concentrations cause increased RBC rouleaux. This can also be seen in collagen-vascular diseases, malignant diseases, and tuberculosis.

SPECIAL LEUKOCYTE STUDIES

LEUKOCYTE CYTOCHEMISTRY

White cells on a freshly made blood film retain enzyme activity and can alter added substrates. This is most useful when cells are morphologically so abnormal that it becomes difficult to detect their cell line of origin. Enzyme studies are also useful in assessing cellular maturation and in evaluating departures from normal differentiation. The development of monoclonal antibody technology has also facilitated the identification of cell origin, particularly that of immature hematopoietic cell precursors, and to a large extent has superseded traditional cytochemistry (see Leukemias in Chapter 4). These are also useful when categorizing immature or undifferentiated cells in acute leukemia.

Leukocyte Alkaline Phosphatase

Among the enzymes in neutrophilic granules is a phosphatase capable of hydrolyzing phosphate-containing substrates into a product that binds to highly colored dyes. Leukocyte alkaline phosphatase (LAP) can be roughly quantitated by scoring the size and intensity of the stained granules. Normal levels fall between 10 and 130 out of a maximum of 400. Generally, 100 cells are counted, and the intensity of the staining is graduated from 0 (no staining) to 4 (heavy and intense staining). LAP increases in polycythemia vera and myelofibrosis and decreases in chronic myelogenous leukemia (CML) and paroxysmal nocturnal hemoglobinuria (PNH). It is normal or elevated in leukemoid reactions to infections. Because all of these conditions have increased the numbers of immature circulating neutrophils, LAP scores can be helpful in distinguishing among them. LAP is unrelated to serum alkaline phosphatase (see also Color Plate 24).

Leukocyte Peroxidase

Myeloid and monocytic cells have cytoplasmic granules that contain enzymes with peroxidase activity capable of transferring hydrogen from a donor compound to hydrogen peroxide. Lymphoid and erythroid cells lack these enzymes. There is little clinical use in testing mature cells for myeloperoxidase content, but stains to demonstrate cytoplasmic peroxidase are extremely useful in distinguishing immature myeloid cells from immature lymphoid cells. In acute myelocytic leukemia, especially M1 (see Chapter 4), more than 75% of the blasts will be peroxidase positive; whereas in acute lymphocytic leukemia, a similar disease morphologically (L2-ALL) (see Chapter 4), very few (if any) of the blasts have peroxidase activity.

Sudan Black B

Sudan Black stains neutral fats and other lipids that, in circulating leukocytes, tend to be most conspicuous in the same cytoplasmic structures that have peroxidase activity. In the acute leukemias, intense Sudan Black staining, either generalized or clumped, is characteristic of acute myelocytic leukemia (Color Plate 25). The monocytic and monoblastic cells of M4 and M5 leukemias usually have fine, scattered granules, and in the lymphoblastic leukemias very few, if any, cells take the Sudan Black stain.

Leukocyte Esterases

Myeloid and monocytic cells contain numerous enzymes that hydrolyze ester bonds. By selecting appropriate substrates and reaction conditions, hematologists can distinguish monocytic cells from myeloid cells. This is most useful in classifying the acute leukemias, in which abnormal maturation and morphology reduce the usefulness of the usual differentiating criteria. Chloroacetate esterase is normally present only in promyelocytes but is sometimes present in leukemic myeloblasts and is characteristically present in Auer rods (Color Plate 26). Monocytic and lymphoid cells lack this esterase; for these cells the substrate used is naphthol AS-D chloroacetate. Chloroacetate esterase activity is not affected by prior fluoride treatment.

Nonspecific Esterase

Nonspecific esterase is most abundant in monocytic cells, but may be weakly present in granulocytes, lymphocytes, or even normoblasts. The discriminating feature, besides the intensity and distribution of the reaction, is that sodium fluoride inhibits the strong esterase activity of monocytes but does not reduce the stain reactivity of granulocytes or other cells. The usual substrate used in testing is alpha-naphthyl acetate.

Periodic Acid-Schiff

In the periodic acid-Schiff (PAS) stain, compounds that can be oxidized to aldehydes are localized by brilliant fuchsin staining. Many elements in multiple tissues are PAS positive, but in blood cells, the PAS-positive material of diagnostic importance is cytoplasmic glycogen. Early granulocyte precursors and normal erythroid precursors are PAS negative. Mature red cells remain PAS negative, but granulocytes acquire increasing PAS positivity only with maturation. Monocytes and lymphocytes may have scattered granules and give a positive test.

In acute granulocytic leukemia, myeloblasts and monoblasts are either negative or weakly positive in a finely granular pattern. Leukemic lymphoblasts, especially in childhood acute lymphoblastic leukemia, often have coarse clumps or masses of PAS-positive material in a block granular fashion within their scant cytoplasm. The staining pattern is usually heterogeneous, with some cells containing PAS-positive chunks and others virtually unstained (see Color Plate 27).

Erythroid precursors contain PAS-positive material in erythroleukemia (see Chapter 4) and in scattered cases of thalassemia and anemias. Conspicuous PAS staining in the erythroid line, however, creates a strong likelihood of erythroleukemia.

Terminal Deoxynucleotidyl Transferase

Terminal deoxynucleotidyl transferase (TdT) is an enzyme marker for immature lymphoid cells. This enzyme is a DNA polymerase that is found in immature lymphoid precursors and also in the majority of patients with acute lymphoblastic leukemia. The test is performed on fixed cell preparation smears by using a labeled antibody to TdT, labeled either with an enzyme or a fluorescent marker. The enzyme is normally present in the nucleus of the immature cells, which would show either positive fluorescence or cytochemical staining if present.

CHROMOSOME STUDIES

The normal human chromosomal karyotype consists of 22 pairs of autosomes and one pair of sex chromosomes. Chromosome studies can be performed on cells that are capable of division by inducing mitosis. If the cell division is arrested at a phase in mitosis and the nuclei of the cells are lysed by osmotic swelling, preparations of these paired chromosomes can be made and photographed. The cut-out photographs of the individual chromosomes can then be arranged in order of decreasing size and compared with one another and with standard morphologic nomenclature (Fig. 2–16). In addition, these chromosomes can also be stained by various methods, producing several bands. Depending on the location of the band and the intensity of the staining, the bands are subclassified. Breakpoints, exchanges of genetic material between chromosomes, and other abnormalities can then be analyzed. Excess chromosomal material can also be seen. Specific abnormalities of chromosomal material can be used diagnostically (e.g., the Philadelphia chromosome in chronic myelogenous leukemia) or prognostically (4;11 translocations in acute lymphoblastic leukemia have a worse prognostic feature; inv 16 in acute myelogenous leukemia has a better prognosis), or to follow therapy and diagnose relapse in leukemia. Chromosomal markers have become an integral part of the investigation of many malignant hematologic disorders. Chromosomal studies can also be used to assess bone marrow engraftment following bone marrow transplantation. The usefulness of chromosomal methods in hematologic diseases is discussed more fully in the section on white cell disorders. The expansion of chromosomal

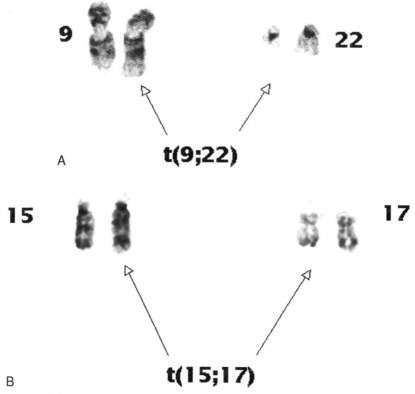

FIGURE 2–16. *(A)* Human chromosomal preparation showing Philadelphia chromosome. Arrows denote t(9;22). *(B)* Human chromosomal translocation involving the retinoic acid receptor (RAR) and promyelocytic leukemia locus (PML). Arrows denote translocation t(15;17). (Photograph kindly supplied by Dr. Jeanne Meck, Ph.D.)

analyses by using molecular and genetic probes has characterized breakpoints on specific chromosomes that may be important in understanding the development of disease, specifically cancer (oncogenes). Recent studies have shown that oncogenes can be relocated and activated as a result of chromosomal translocations. In addition, several chromosomes contain fragile sites that may be important breakpoints in permitting unregulated cell growth. In the future, analysis of the chromosomal constitution of affected cells in many disorders may provide clues to diagnostic, prognostic, and etiologic aspects of malignant disorders. The banding techniques have clearly outlined subchromosomal structure and permitted more refined chromosomal mapping. Molecular probe analysis has remarkably expanded the application of chromosomal studies in disease, primarily in the area of leukemia diagnosis and prognosis.

Chromosomal abnormalities or clonality can also be analyzed by molecular probes labeled with marker reagents (e.g., fluorescent substrates in the process of fluorescent in situ hybridization [FISH] analysis). Sophisticated computer-assisted analysis can now allow rapid karyotyping of chromosomal preparations that facilitate electronic storage and enhanced graphics. Newer leukemia classifications will presumably be based not only on morphology, but also on cytogenetic and immunologic characterizations. In this way, subcategories of leukemia with more refined, precise prognostic and therapeutic implications will be outlined.

SUGGESTED READING

Beutler, E: Red Cell Metabolism, A Manual of Biochemical Methods, ed 3. Grune and Stratton, Orlando, 1984.

Bunn, HF: Hemoglobin structure, function and assembly. In Embury, SH, et al (eds): Sickle Cell Disease, Basic Principles and Clinical Practice. Raven Press, New York, 1994.

Ciesla, BE: Morphological changes associated with disease. In Harmening, DM: Clinical Hematology and Fundamentals of Hemostasis, ed 3. FA Davis, Philadelphia, 1997, pp 80–94.

D'Angelo, A, and Selhub, J: Homocysteine and thrombotic disease. Blood 90:1, 1997.

Dacie, JV, and Lewis, SM: Practical Haematology, ed 6. Churchill Livingstone, Edinburgh, 1985.

Dacie, JV: The Haemolytic Anaemias, Vol I, II, ed 3. Churchill Livingstone, Edinburgh, 1985.

Erslev, AJ: Erythropoietin, N Engl J Med 19:1339–1344, 1991.

Fairbanks, VF, and Klee, GG: Biochemical aspects of hematology. In Burtis, CA, and Ashwood, ER (eds): Tietz Textbook of Clinical Chemistry, ed 2. WB Saunders, Philadelphia, 1994, pp 1974–2042.

Green, R, and Jacobsen, DW: Clinical implications of homocysteinemia. In Bailey, L (ed): Folate in Health and Disease. Marcel Dekker, New York, 1995, pp 75–122.

Handin, RI, Lux, SE, and Stossel, TP (eds): Basic Principles and Practice of Hematology. JB Lippincott, Philadelphia, 1995.

Hillman, RS, and Finch, CA: Red Cell Manual, ed 7. FA Davis, Philadelphia, 1996.

Jacques, PF, et al: Relation between folate status, a common mutation in methylenetetrahydrofolate reductase, and plasma homocysteine concentrations. Circulation 93:8, 1996.

Lindenbaum, J, et al: Diagnosis of cobalamin deficiency II. Relative sensitivities of serum cobalamin, methylmalonic acid and total homocysteine concentrations. Amer J Hematol 34:99, 1990.

Metcalf, D: The colony-stimulating factors: Discovery, development, clinical applications. Cancer 65:10, 2185–2195, 1990.

Mohandas, N, and Chasis, JA: Red cell deformability, membrane material properties and shape. Regulation by transmembrane, skeletal and cytostatic proteins and lipids. Semin Hematol 30:171, 1993.

Nathan, DG, and Oski, FA (eds): Hematology of Infancy and Childhood. WB Saunders, Philadelphia, 1993.

Spivak, JL: Fundamentals of Clinical Hematology, ed 3. Johns Hopkins Univ Press, Baltimore, 1993.

Williams, WJ, et al: Hematology, ed 5. McGraw-Hill, New York, 1995.

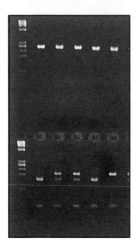

3

Diseases of Red Blood Cells

ANEMIA: DEFINITION AND CLASSIFICATION

The main function of the erythropoietic marrow is production of erythrocytes capable of transporting the respiratory pigment hemoglobin to the tissues for oxygen delivery. Adequate numbers of erythrocytes must be produced, and their hemoglobin must be quantitatively normal and maintained in a functional state for oxygen delivery. The red cell concentration must be kept within normal limits; therefore, red cell destruction must be balanced by red cell production. Furthermore, the red cell membrane must be deformable by passage through the microcirculation. Internal red cell metabolism has been developed to maintain hemoglobin in a state capable of transporting oxygen. Other metabolic activities of the cells are directed at maintaining the cell's deformability and survival in the peripheral blood. Abnormalities of these functions may be associated with disorders of erythrocyte development or distribution and may produce accelerated erythrocyte destruction. **Anemia,** a decrease in the concentration of hemoglobin, is often the result of these abnormalities.

Anemia may also be thought of as a reduction in the red cell mass, producing decreased oxygen-carrying capacity to meet tissue demands. This reduction in red cell mass may occur if the production of red cells is defective or if their destruction or loss exceeds the capabilities of the bone marrow to replace them. Anemias may be classified on the basis of the degree of *hemoglobinization* of the red cells (*hypochromic* or **normochromic**), the *size of the red cells* (**microcytic, normocytic,** or **macrocytic**), or *the category of disorder that is responsible* for the anemia. There are three main categories:

* Disorders of red cell formation
  * Deficiency diseases
  * Hypoproliferative anemias—reduced or absent functional marrow
  * Ineffective erythropoiesis—refractory anemia
* Excessive loss of red cells
  * Hemorrhage
  * Hemolysis
* Abnormal distribution of red cells

Characterization of the type and severity of anemia is achieved by the performance of the **hemoglobin concentration,** or **hematocrit,** and the **red cell indices** mentioned in Chapter 2. Effective red cell production is determined by the **reticulocyte count,** which assesses the number of functional erythrocytes made by the marrow. One of the most important laboratory tests in evaluating any patient with anemia is the examination of the **peripheral blood smear.** This gives many clues as to the etiology of the anemias. However, in many instances a **bone marrow specimen** also must be examined to enable categorization of the type of anemia. Specialized tests help define the exact etiology. The laboratory tests that will be ordered are dependent on the classification of the anemia and its possible cause, as will become apparent in this chapter.

DISORDERS OF RED CELL FORMATION

ANEMIAS DUE TO DEFICIENCY STATES

Iron Deficiency and the Hypochromic Anemias

Deficiencies of the essential minerals and nutrients required for erythropoiesis commonly produce anemias. The most prevalent worldwide cause of anemia is iron deficiency. Iron metabolism is discussed in Chapter 2. Iron deficiency anemia commonly produces **hypochromic, microcytic** erythrocytes. The mean cell hemoglobin is usually below 27 pg/liter, and the mean cell volume is below 80 fL. These cells are microcytic because of the continued synthesis of erythrocytes. There is little incorporation of iron into protoporphyrin, and the rate-limiting enzyme heme synthetase (ferrochelatase) requires iron to switch off heme synthesis (see Fig. 2–3). If iron is deficient, cell division will continue for several additional cycles, producing smaller cells. Because inadequate amounts of iron are present, less hemoglobin is also present per individual red cell, producing the hypochromia. There are four main conditions associated with hypochromic, microcytic anemia. These are:

- iron deficiency anemia
- thalassemia syndromes
- anemia of chronic disease
- sideroblastic anemia

Iron Deficiency Anemia

Iron deficiency is by far the most common cause of anemia. The usual causes of iron deficiency are (1) blood loss (all ages, especially menstruating women), (2) nutritional deficiency (infants), and (3) increased iron demand (pregnancy, lactation, adolescence) (Table 3–1). Iron metabolism is delicately balanced in the body to prevent excessive iron absorption because iron is an abundant element in nature (see Chapter 2). Consequently, iron deficiency generally ensues because the body can only moderately adapt to iron deficiency due to blood loss (particularly continuing blood loss). As was mentioned in Chapter 2, the normal diet contains 10 to 15 mg of iron per day. Normally the body can absorb 10% of this iron, and this balances the amount of iron lost through desquamation of cells, particularly from the gastrointestinal tract and skin. To maintain this steady state, 1 mg of iron needs to be absorbed per day. In

TABLE 3–1. MAJOR CAUSES OF IRON DEFICIENCY

Dietary inadequacy
Malabsorption
  Gastrectomy
  Achlorhydria
  Steatorrhea
  Celiac disease
Increased iron loss
  Menstruation
  Gastrointestinal bleeding
  Hemoptysis
  Hematuria
  Hemodialysis
Increased iron requirements
  Infancy
  Adolescence
  Pregnancy
  Lactation

situations of excess bleeding or, for that matter, normal bleeding in menstruation, iron loss from hemorrhage needs to be replaced. Because the average menstrual cycle is associated with 60 mL of blood loss per month, this translates to 30 mg of iron, and consequently, women require an extra milligram of iron per day to be absorbed to maintain the steady state. In times of depletion, the maximal iron absorption can climb as high as 25% of the dietary iron; women can absorb up to this amount to maintain the steady state. However, young menstruating women, particularly those with heavy blood losses, are commonly iron depleted. A normal pregnancy also depletes the body of 600 to 700 mg of iron. Because the body stores contain 500 to 1500 mg of iron, one pregnancy can deplete the body's stores, especially if iron supplements are not given.

Iron deficiency anemia is especially common during times when iron demands are greatest, as in infancy, during the adolescent growth spurt, and in pregnancy. Chronic blood loss can occur at any age but is particularly prevalent in older adults, especially from gastrointestinal and genitourinary sources. In particular, malignancies of the gastrointestinal tract are associated with iron deficiency anemia.

When negative iron balance occurs, iron deficiency anemia develops only after depletion of the body stores. Following this depletion, serum iron falls and plasma iron-binding capacity increases. Consequently, hemoglobin synthesis is reduced, and defective hemoglobinization of the developing red cells occurs, resulting in red cells that are *pale (hypochromic)* and *small (microcytic)* (Color Plate 28). The red cell indices of hemoglobin concentration (namely the mean cell hemoglobin and mean cell hemoglobin concentration) are reduced. When iron deficiency anemia is severe, tissue iron depletion also occurs and is associated with changes in various tissues, particularly the nails **(koilonychia)** and tongue **(glossitis)** and produces marked fatigue due to depletion of the muscle enzymes and myoglobin, the muscle respiratory pigment (Fig. 3–1).

Dietary depletion of iron is an uncommon cause of deficiency in adults; however, in infants it is more common. The newborn infant begins life with 350 to 500 mg of iron; all further increments come from the diet. Iron requirements are greatest in the first year of life when expanding red cell production requires daily intake of 1 mg/kg to keep pace with growth. Adolescence, pregnancy, and lactation also impose severe stress on iron balance. The most common victims of inadequate dietary intake are small children whose diet consists largely of milk. In the United States, fortified food products and generally varied diet make poor intake alone a rare cause of iron deficiency in older children and adults. A borderline iron balance may occur, however, under conditions of increased requirement such as rapid growth spurts, onset of menstruation, or repeated pregnancies. Adult men and postmenopausal women almost never become iron deficient from diet alone, no matter how poor their diets, unless other problems coexist. In less-developed countries, the combination of poor diet, frequent parasitic infestations, and repeated pregnancies make iron deficiency anemia a widespread and severe health problem.

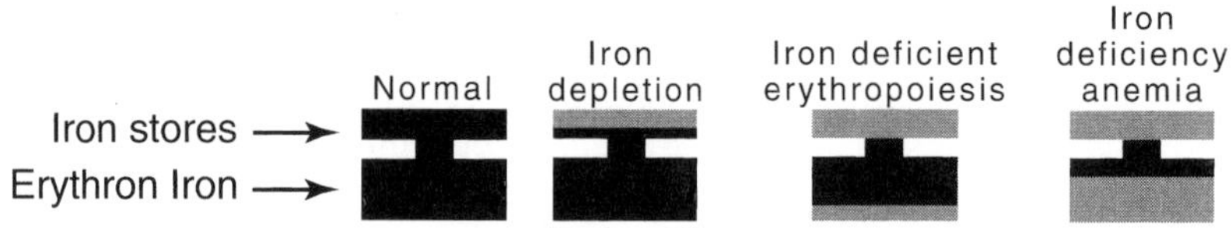

	Normal	Iron depletion	Iron deficient erythropoiesis	Iron deficiency anemia
Iron stores ⟶				
Erythron Iron ⟶				
RE marrow Fe	2 - 3 +	0 - 1 +	0	0
Transferrin IBC (μg/dL)	330 ±30	360	390	410
Serum ferritin (μg/mL)	100 ±60	20	10	<10
Iron absorption (%)	5 - 10	10 - 15	10 - 20	10 - 20
Serum iron (μg/dL)	115 ±50	115	<60	<40
Transferrin saturation (%)	35 ±15	30	<15	<10
Sideroblasts (%)	40 - 60	40 - 60	<10	<10
RBC protoporphyrin (μg/dL RBC)	30	30	100	200
Erythrocytes	Normal	Normal	Normal	Micro/Hypo

FIGURE 3–1. Sequential changes in the development of iron deficiency. Indicators of iron store depletion include the visual inspection of marrow reticuloendothelial iron stores, the total iron-binding capacity (TIBC), the serum ferritin level, and the percent of iron absorbed from an oral iron test dose. With the onset of iron-deficient erythropoiesis, the serum iron, percent saturation of transferrin, percent sideroblasts observed on the marrow iron stain, and erythrocyte protoporphyrin become abnormal. At this point, anemia appears. When anemia has been present for some time, red cells become microcytic and hypochromic. (From Hillman, RS, and Finch, CA: Red Cell Manual, ed 7. FA Davis, Philadelphia, 1996, p 72, with permission.)

Chronic bleeding, often unnoticed, may occur from the gastrointestinal tract. Peptic ulcer, gastritis, hiatal hernia, diverticulitis, and neoplasms are the usual causes. In many cases the patient is asymptomatic or, at the very least, unaware of blood loss. Heavy use of alcohol or aspirin may cause painful gastritis, but the patient may not notice the small, continuous blood loss.

Excessive menstrual loss is a common cause of iron deficiency in women. In adolescent girls, with their frequently erratic diets and often irregular, heavy menstrual periods, the pubertal growth spurt may tip iron balance into a deficiency state. Consecutive pregnancies also exert a cumulative effect by depleting iron stores.

The *urinary tract* is another avenue of loss. Tumors, stones, or inflammatory disease affecting kidneys, ureters, or bladder may cause blood loss in the urine. A rare cause of urinary-related iron deficiency is excretion of large amounts of hemosiderin in patients with chronic intravascular hemolytic states, such as occurs with prosthetic heart valves.

A person may have reduced body iron without being anemic (Fig. 3–1 shows the sequential changes in development of iron deficiency). Many individuals with normal hemoglobin levels are chronically iron depleted but do not develop iron deficiency anemia until some stress—for example, increased demand, repeated blood donation, or acute and chronic hemorrhage—accentuates the negative iron balance. In a largely white population of middle to lower income status, 20% of menstruating women were found to be iron deficient, but less than half of these women had iron deficiency anemia. Of the anemias found in the entire study population, half were due to iron deficiency alone. Table 3–2 lists the laboratory findings in iron deficiency. Iron deficiency may easily be differentiated from the other three conditions by the markedly *reduced serum iron* and markedly *elevated total iron-binding capacity* (Table 3–3). The *saturation of transferrin* is usually below 5% in iron deficiency anemia, and the **serum ferritin,** a test reflecting iron stores, is less than 10 ng/mL, indicating markedly reduced or absent iron stores. The **free erythrocyte protoporphyrin,** which represents the substrate for iron incorporation into heme, is markedly increased because heme synthesis is reduced and therefore the precursor product accumulates. Tests of tissue iron such as *bone marrow iron* show absent iron stores in iron deficiency anemia. Table 3–3 lists laboratory findings characteristic of iron deficiency anemia compared with the other causes of hypochromic, microcytic anemias—namely thalassemia, anemia of chronic disease, and sideroblastic anemia.

TABLE 3–2. LABORATORY FINDINGS IN IRON DEFICIENCY

Blood Count

Microcytic, hypochromic red cells if Hgb < 12 g/dL (men), < 10 g/dL (women)
Leukopenia possible
Platelets high with active bleeding
Reticulocytes lower than expected for degree of anemia

Bone Marrow

Erythroid hyperplasia
Stainable iron very low or absent

Other

Serum iron very low, iron-binding capacity high, percent of saturation very low
Serum ferritin < 10 ng/mL
Free erythrocyte protoporphyrin high
RBC survival time slightly low
RDW high

Hgb = hemoglobin; RBC = red blood cells; RDW = red cell distribution width.

TABLE 3–3. DIFFERENTIAL DIAGNOSIS OF HYPOCHROMIC MICROCYTIC ANEMIA

	Serum Iron	TIBC	Serum Ferritin	FEP	HbA$_2$	HbF	RDW
Iron Deficiency	Low	High	Low	High	Nl	Nl-low	High
Alpha-Thalassemia	High	Nl	High	Nl	Nl	Low	
Beta-Thalassemia	High	Nl	High	Nl	High	High (varies)	High
Anemia of Chronic Disease	Low	Low	High	High	Nl	Nl	Nl
Sideroblastic Anemia	High	Nl	High	Low	Nl	Nl	High

TIBC = total iron-binding capacity; FEP = free erythrocyte protoporphyrin; Nl = normal; HbA$_2$ = hemoglobin A$_2$; HbF = hemoglobin F; RDW = red cell distribution width.

Iron deficiency anemia is a symptom, not a primary disease entity. The cause of the iron deficiency anemia always needs to be established and specific treatment directed to this cause. However, correction of iron deficiency requires replacement of therapeutic doses of iron continuous enough to replenish the body's stores. This may require iron replacement therapy for 3 to 6 months. The iron-deficient patient who receives therapeutic iron develops reticulocytosis within 2 to 3 days, which often spuriously increases the mean cell volume. The reticulocytosis is visible as a polychromatophilia on examination of a peripheral blood smear (see Color Plate 28[B]).

Anemia of Chronic Disease

Because chronic disorders may present with a hypochromic, microcytic anemia, it is important that these conditions be distinguished from iron deficiency anemia. Chronic infections, inflammatory processes, and malignant neoplasms can present with hypochromic, microcytic anemias. The basic defect is in the iron utilization for erythropoiesis. There appears to be a blockage in delivery of iron from the reticuloendothelial iron stores to the developing red cell. Consequently, the red cells are deficient in iron, whereas the body stores have abundant iron. Usually the peripheral blood smear shows a normochromic, normocytic picture, but with advanced states the cells may be hypochromic and microcytic. Microcytosis is usually not as severe as with iron deficiency anemia, and mean cell volume values of less than 70 to 75 fL are rare. Anemias are usually of moderate severity, with hemoglobins in the 7 to 11 g/dL range.

Table 3–3 shows the profile of iron studies in the anemia of chronic disease. Typically, the serum iron values are low, as is the total iron-binding capacity. This latter point differentiates this form of hypochromic anemia from that of iron deficiency anemia. The percentage saturation of transferrin is usually higher than that seen with iron deficiency anemia and is in the 7 to 15% range. A major discriminating feature, of course, is the fact that the serum ferritin value is increased with values of 50 to 2000 ng/mL. This point can be used to discriminate between chronic disease and iron deficiency anemia because serum ferritin values are less than 10 ng/mL in iron deficiency states.

Sideroblastic Anemias

The sideroblastic anemias are a group of disorders characterized by abnormalities of heme metabolism. The diagnostic feature of these disorders is the presence of nucleated red cells with iron granules (*ringed sideroblasts*) in the marrow and the appearance of a *dimorphic peripheral blood picture,* found particularly in the primary types (Table 3–4 and Color Plate 12A). In the sideroblastic anemias, the body has adequate, even abundant, iron but is unable to incorporate it into hemoglobin. The iron enters the developing red cell but accumulates in the perinuclear mitochondria of normoblasts in primary sideroblastic anemia. The dimorphic pattern in the peripheral blood shows two apparent popula-

---

TABLE 3–4. CLASSIFICATION OF SIDEROBLASTIC ANEMIAS

Inherited
  Rare sex-linked
Acquired
  Primary (idiopathic) (myelodysplasias)

  Secondary
    Associated with other myeloproliferative syndromes (leukemias, polycythemia vera)

    Pyridoxine-deficient or responsive anemias
      Vitamin B_6 deficiency
      Drugs: isoniazid, cycloserine
      Alcoholism

    Disorders of hemoglobin synthesis
      Folate deficiency, B_{12} deficiency
      Lead poisoning
      Erythropoietic porphyria

From Pittiglio, DH, and Sacher, RA: Clinical Hematology and Fundamentals of Hemostasis. FA Davis, Philadelphia, 1987, p 51, with permission.

tions of erythrocytes, with one population of fairly normal cells and another population of hypochromic, irregularly shaped, generally small erythrocytes. Consequently, the red cell distribution width (RDW) is increased. The bone marrow shows an increased erythropoietic activity and is therefore hypercellular, but circulating reticulocyte counts are generally not elevated. As previously mentioned, this reflects ineffective erythropoiesis.

Several conditions can produce this apparent abnormality, in which iron is trapped in the mitochondria and cannot be fully utilized in hemoglobin synthesis. These are listed in Table 3–4. In general, the sideroblastic anemias are associated with more than 15% ringed sideroblasts and may be classified as having congenital and acquired causes. Once the secondary disorders listed in the table are excluded, the condition is termed idiopathic or primary. This disorder represents a clonal disturbance of erythropoiesis and is discussed in the disorders classified as the myelodysplastic syndromes (see Chapter 4). Specifically, however, primary or idiopathic sideroblastic anemia is characterized by abnormal erythropoietic maturation (dyserythropoiesis) and abnormal iron utilization with the typical ringed sideroblasts. Ringed sideroblasts may be less prominent in the secondary disorders.

The laboratory data reflect impaired iron utilization with normal or increased iron stores. The red cell indices may vary, depending on which population of cells predominates. Consequently, the MCV may be low, normal, or even increased. The MCH and MCHC are often low but may be normal. White cell abnormalities may also be seen. With defects in the synthesis of porphyrin or the ring insertion of iron, regulation of iron absorption is disturbed and systemic accumulation of iron may develop. The serum iron is usually greater than normal, with a high percentage saturation of transferrin. Serum ferritin values are also markedly elevated. Serum B_{12} and folic acid levels are normal. Other laboratory tests are also reflective of ineffective erythropoiesis, with an elevated lactate dehydrogenase.

Treatment is usually aimed at correcting a secondary cause; however, in the primary disorders, patients are usually unresponsive to the various vitamin supplements, particularly pyridoxine.

Thalassemia Syndromes

These will be discussed in the section on Hemolytic Anemias.

Lead Poisoning

Anemia and disordered heme synthesis accompany lead poisoning and provide the major diagnostic clues for this common, preventable disorder. In adults, lead exposure is usually occupational. In children, the most common cause is **pica,** a tendency to consume inedible materials. Lead-containing paint, formerly a cause of this problem, has largely been eliminated. Children are also sensitive to the lead levels in polluted atmospheres.

Lead depresses enzyme activity at the beginning, middle, and end of heme synthesis. Defective delta-amino-levulinic dehydratase activity causes **delta-aminolevulinic acid (ALA)** to accumulate. Urine ALA levels have long been used as a rough screening test for lead toxicity. Coproporphyrin metabolism is depressed, and the insertion of ferrous iron into protoporphyrin is inhibited because lead also inhibits heme synthetase (see Fig. 2–4). Depression of heme synthetase causes red cells to accumulate excessive protoporphyrin; *elevated red cell protoporphyrin levels* constitute the best laboratory test for quantifying lead toxicity. Table 3–5 lists the laboratory findings in lead poisoning.

Vitamin B$_{12}$ and Folic Acid Deficiency

Although vitamin B$_{12}$ and folic acid deficiencies are the most common causes of **megaloblastic anemia,** diagnosis and therapy of this condition require an understanding of the differential diagnosis and laboratory evaluation of other causes of anemia with macrocytic red cells.

As was mentioned in Chapter 2, **macrocytosis** occurs when the mean cell volume (MCV) is greater than 100 fL. Erythrocytic macrocytosis can easily be determined with the aid of an automated electronic particle

---

TABLE 3–5. LABORATORY FINDINGS IN LEAD POISONING

Anemia

Hemoglobin 9–11 g/dL
MCHC moderately low
Reticulocytosis 2–7%

RBC Changes

Ratio of protoporphyrin to hemoglobin > 5.5 µg/g (>17 in severe cases)
Basophilic stippling
Moderate anisocytosis and poikilocytosis
Diminished osmotic fragility

Blood Lead Usually > 40 µg/mL

Bone Marrow

Erythroid hyperplasia
Ringed sideroblasts

Urine

ALA excretion > 20 mg/L
Coproporphyrin III > 0.5 mg/L
Porphobilinogen normal

MCHC = mean corpuscular hemoglobin concentration; ALA = delta-aminolevulinic acid.

counter, which gives an accurate and reproducible value for the MCV. The finding of macrocytic indices does not imply megaloblastic anemia, since other conditions can produce macrocytosis (Table 3–6). An elevated MCV, however, is an abnormal finding and may precede, by months or years, the onset of a megaloblastic anemia. Megaloblastic anemia may be masked in the presence of complicating infections, inflammatory disease, or iron deficiency.

Spurious macrocytosis can occur with automated measurements, and the finding of an elevated MCV must always be corroborated by examination of the peripheral blood smear. The earliest sign of megaloblastic anemia reflected in the peripheral blood is hypersegmentation of the polymorphonuclear leukocytes. Red cell morphology can also help distinguish the other causes of macrocytosis from megaloblastic anemia. In liver disease, the macrocytosis is usually associated with the presence of *round macrocytes*. B_{12} or folate deficiency (megaloblastic anemia) is associated with *oval macrocytes;* reticulocytosis, with *basophilic round macrocytes;* and altered red cell morphology can also help distinguish the macrocytosis of other myeloproliferative disorders (see Color Plate 12). In general, a bone marrow examination is essential to establish whether megaloblastic anemia is present, although examination of the bone marrow cannot distinguish vitamin B_{12} deficiency from folic acid deficiency. Clinical features are, however, often helpful in differentiating pernicious anemia from folic acid deficiency (Table 3–7). Table 3–8 outlines the laboratory findings in megaloblastic anemias.

TABLE 3–6. DIFFERENTIAL DIAGNOSIS OF MACROCYTOSIS (MCV > 100 fL)

Actual

Megaloblastic anemias
Liver disease
Reticulocytosis
Myeloproliferative diseases (leukemia, myelofibrosis)
Metastatic disease of bone marrow
Multiple myeloma
Hypothyroidism
Aplastic anemia
Drugs (post-chemotherapy, alcohol)

Spurious

Autoagglutination/cold agglutination disease

From Sacher, RA: Pernicious anemia and other megaloblastic anemias. In Rakel, RE (ed): Conn's Current Therapy. WB Saunders, Philadelphia, 1994, p 343, with permission.

TABLE 3–7. SEVEN CLINICAL "P"S OF PERNICIOUS ANEMIA

1. Pancytopenia
2. Peripheral neuropathy
3. Posterior spinal column neuropathy
4. Pyramidal tract signs
5. Papillary (tongue) atrophy
6. pH elevation (gastric fluid)
7. Psychosis (megaloblastic madness)

Adapted from Sacher, RA: Pernicious anemia and other megaloblastic anemias. In Rakel, RE (ed): Conn's Current Therapy. WB Saunders, Philadelphia, 1994, p 343, with permission.

TABLE 3–8. LABORATORY FINDINGS IN MEGALOBLASTIC ANEMIA

Blood Count

Severe anemia
Macrocytosis (MCV 100–140 μm^3) with anisocytosis
Ovalocytes and macro-ovalocytes numerous
WBCs, platelets often low
Hypersegmented neutrophils >5%
Reticulocytes disproportionately low for anemia

Bone Marrow

Marked erythroid hyperplasia
Megaloblastic nuclear appearance in all 3 cell lines
Storage iron normal or high

Blood Chemistry

Bilirubin high (indirect)
Serum iron high
LDH very high
Serum gastrin high (pernicious anemia)

Other Studies

Schilling test abnormal (<2% excretion) (pernicious anemia)
Antibodies to gastric cells, intrinsic factor (pernicious anemia)
Serum (<100 pg/mL), RBC levels of vitamin B_{12} low (vitamin B_{12} deficiency)
Urine methylmalonate high (>10 mg/24 hours) (vitamin B_{12} deficiency)
Serum (<3 pg/mL), RBC (<100 pg/mL) levels of folate low (folic acid deficiency)
Histamine-fast achlorhydria (pernicious anemia)

MCV = mean corpuscular volume; LDH = lactate dehydrogenase; WBC = white blood cells; RBC = red blood cells.

Causes of Megaloblastosis

The two most common problems leading to megaloblastic anemia are vitamin B_{12} (cobalamin) deficiency and a deficiency of folic acid. As was discussed in Chapter 2, cobalamin deficiency is almost always due to vitamin B_{12} malabsorption. Pernicious anemia is the most common cause and is due to lack of **intrinsic factor,** the essential cofactor needed for vitamin B_{12} absorption in the terminal ileum. Intrinsic factor is normally produced by the parietal cells of the gastric mucosa and is deficient in any condition that decreases its production, such as atrophic gastritis and gastrectomy. Occasionally, B_{12} deficiency may result from dietary deficiency (veganism), altered metabolic states, or bacterial overgrowth with organisms requiring intestinal B_{12} for their metabolism, which compete for available B_{12} with the host. These conditions may be differentiated, as was discussed in Chapter 2, by testing vitamin B_{12} absorption using the Schilling test.

Megaloblastic anemia due to folic acid deficiency may have many different causes (Table 3–9). In general, a deficiency of folic acid is nearly always due to a dietary cause. Stores of folic acid are only sufficient for 3 months. These can rapidly be depleted in conditions of excess folic acid

TABLE 3–9. CAUSES OF FOLATE DEFICIENCY

Dietary

Infancy
Pregnancy and lactation
Malnutrition
Alcoholism

Intestinal Malabsorption

Malabsorption syndromes
Drug interaction: phenytoin, oral contraceptives

Increased Demand

Infancy and adolescence
Pregnancy and lactation
Increased cellular turnover
   Chronic hemolytic anemias
   Psoriasis/exfoliative dermatitis

Excess Loss

Hemodialysis
Peritoneal dialysis

Defective Synthesis

Liver disease
Antifolate drugs
Alcoholism

demand such as pregnancy, rapid growth in adolescence and infancy, rapid cell turnover that may occur with hemolytic anemias, poor folate intake, and alcoholism. Folic acid deficiency may also occur with malabsorption syndromes, and its absorption may be competitively inhibited by means of concomitant drugs such as birth control pills and some anticonvulsants. Sprue and other enteropathies often depress absorption of both vitamin B_{12} and folic acid. Many drugs cause megaloblastosis by interfering with DNA synthesis, some as antagonists of folic acid or as inhibitors of purine or pyrimidine synthesis, and others, especially alcohol, through less clearly defined pathways. Several rare, genetically determined enzyme defects (e.g., Lesch-Nyhan syndrome, orotic aciduria) cause megaloblastosis in addition to other signs and symptoms.

Pernicious Anemia

Classic or "Addisonian" **pernicious anemia** is a chronic disease with an apparent familial predisposition. The disease complex includes atrophy of the gastric mucosa, megaloblastic blood cell changes caused by vitamin B_{12} deficiency (see Color Plate 43), a high incidence of autoimmune phenomena, and neurologic manifestations. Clinical features are often most helpful in differentiating pernicious anemia from folic acid deficiency. Table 3–7 lists the seven clinical "P"s of pernicious anemia, which are helpful with this distinction. Dysplastic changes of the oral mucous membranes and tongue are also common. The atrophic gastric mucosa secretes neither intrinsic factor nor hydrochloric acid; therefore the gastric secretions of individuals with pernicious anemia are associated with a lack of acidity and a higher pH. Neither the red cell morphology of the peripheral blood nor the bone marrow examination will distinguish between the megaloblastic anemia of B_{12} deficiency and folic acid deficiency. This distinction is initially made by performing a serum B_{12} or folic acid level; however, the Schilling test is the foundation for the laboratory diagnosis of pernicious anemia once megaloblastic anemia has been diagnosed. More recently, ancillary tests such as urinary methylmalonic acid can help with early diagnosis of marginal B_{12} deficiency (see Chapter 2).

Pernicious anemia becomes apparent in middle adulthood or later. The incidence is highest in persons of northern European origin. No clear pattern of genetic transmission exists, but blood relatives of an affected patient are at a higher risk for part or all of the disease complex. Patients with pernicious anemia as well as their hematologically normal relatives frequently have autoantibodies against stomach parietal cells and intrinsic factor (IF), as well as related thyroid autoantibodies.

Therapy for pernicious anemia is simple and effective. Vitamin B_{12} is given by injection, bypassing the absorption defect and permitting the resumption of normal hematopoiesis. Injected vitamin B_{12} corrects the neurologic symptoms but affects neither the patient's stomach acidity nor the increased liability (about three times normal) to develop gastric carcinoma. Thyroid and adrenal hypofunction are more prevalent in these patients than in the general population.

Other Causes of Impaired Absorption of Vitamin B₁₂

Gastrectomy, either total or partial, causes intrinsic factor deficiency and may lead, in months or years, to vitamin B_{12} deficiency. Prolonged IF deficiency can cause such severe atrophy of the ileal absorption site that therapeutic administration of IF takes some time to promote adequate vitamin B_{12} absorption. **Resection of the ileum,** or ileal diseases such as *celiac disease* and *regional enteritis,* are associated with inflammatory damage to the site of absorption. Organisms within the intestine occasionally use luminal vitamin B_{12} stores for their own use. This can occur with bacterial overgrowth owing to altered intestinal flow patterns ("blind loop" syndrome) or with manifestations of the fish tapeworm, *Diphyllobothrium latum.* This tapeworm problem is largely confined to northern Scandinavia, where incompletely cooked fish is consumed by a population with a high genetic disposition to pernicious anemia.

Folic Acid Deficiency

The specifics of folic acid metabolism were discussed in Chapter 2. In general, folic acid deficiency usually is a result of dietary deficiency or drug-induced antagonism. Dietary deficiency is particularly noticeable at times of increased demand. Table 3–9 outlines causes of folic acid deficiency.

The Effects of Drugs *Alcohol* is undoubtedly the most common pharmacologic cause of folic acid deficiency, but the mechanisms are complex and poorly understood. Alcohol seems to impair absorption and also to interfere with folate-dependent enzymatic reactions. In addition, chronic alcoholics often have defective diets, multiple vitamin deficiencies, reduced hepatic function, and poor or absent tissue stores of folic acid. Because alcohol also influences iron absorption and pyridoxine pathways, it is not surprising that alcoholics so often have complex and severe hematologic problems.

Folic acid antagonists are pharmacologic agents given precisely because they interfere with folate-dependent steps in cell multiplication. Methotrexate is a cytotoxic agent widely used for treating leukemias and other malignancies (lymphomas). Its depressive effects on the marrow and other tissues can sometimes be prevented by simultaneously administering *leucovorin (folinic acid).* Folinic acid is a reduced form of folic acid that bypasses the antifolate activity of methotrexate. It is usually administered parenterally to "rescue" systemic antifolate effects of the drug, enabling a higher antimitotic dose to be given.

Oral contraceptives, phenytoin and related *anticonvulsants,* as well as the *antituberculosis drug cycloserine,* seem to reduce folic acid absorption. Patients taking these drugs should be observed for the development of megaloblastic anemia. Principles of treatment of folic acid deficiency involve reversal of the initial effects of the deficiency by supplementation, replenishment of folate stores, and subsequent maintenance of sufficient dietary intake to ensure adequate folate nutrition.

HYPOPROLIFERATIVE ANEMIAS AND SYNDROMES OF BONE MARROW FAILURE

Anemia resulting from the quantitative reduction of functional bone marrow may occur because of a decrease in the absolute number of stem cells or because of qualitatively abnormal stem cells. The result is a deficiency in the number of committed cell precursors oriented toward erythroid development. Obviously abnormalities of stem cells may affect other cell lines as well, producing leukopenia and thrombocytopenia. Decreased proliferation (hypoproliferation) may support production of some marrow cells, and the severity of the specific cytopenia is reflective of the amount of functional bone marrow. When platelets, white cells, and red cells are all decreased in the peripheral blood, the condition is called **pancytopenia.** Aplastic anemia represents the most severe disease of the spectrum of the hypoproliferative anemias and is characterized by a peripheral blood pancytopenia in association with a reduction or depletion of the hemopoietic stem cells in the marrow. Cellular marrow is replaced by fat, producing marked marrow hypocellularity (see Color Plate 8A). Occasionally, the disorder may start with an isolated anemia, leukopenia, or thrombocytopenia, and mild to moderate forms of the disease do occur. The severe form, however, is characterized by a hematocrit of less than 20% with marked reticulocytopenia, a granulocyte count of less than 500/μL, and a platelet count of less than 20,000/μL. Table 3–10 lists a differential diagnosis of pancytopenia.

Aplastic Anemia

Aplastic anemia is a serious, but fortunately rare, disorder with an incidence of approximately 1 case per 100,000 population. In some cases an association has been seen with drug exposure (chloramphenicol and phenylbutazone), and a long list of other drugs. In other cases, the condition may have been preceded by some infection, in particular viral infections including hepatitis B, cytomegalovirus, Epstein-Barr virus, and parvovirus B-19. Exposure to other toxins such as chemical solvents, benzene, irradiation, or cytotoxic drugs is also associated with aplastic anemia. Irradiation tends to produce rapid aplasia, and exposure to the cytotoxic drugs in cancer treatment may produce variable aplasia with variable recovery, depending on the drug used. These agents are expected to produce marrow hypoplasia, which is usually dose dependent and self-limiting. Aplastic anemia associated with drugs not ordinarily

TABLE 3–10. CAUSES OF PANCYTOPENIA

Marrow Failure Syndrome

Quantitative reduction of hematopoietic tissue (bone marrow deficiency)

1. Hypoproliferative and aplastic anemias
   Fanconi's anemia
   Idiopathic anemia
     Viral infections
       Hepatitis B virus
       Epstein-Barr virus
       Cytomegalovirus
       Parvovirus
     Bacterial (tuberculosis)
     Neoplasms
       Clonal hematopoietic diseases
       Secondary (metastatic) malignancies
         Carcinomas
         Lymphomas
       Myelodysplastic syndromes
     Toxic
       Drugs
         Chloramphenicol
         Phenylbutazone
         Chemotherapy
         Others (idiosyncratic)
       Irradiation
     Autoimmune disease
       SLE
       Rheumatoid arthritis
       Autoimmune pancytopenia

2. Bone marrow replacement
   Myelofibrosis
     Idiopathic
     Secondary (metastatic malignancy, TB)
     Lymphomas
     Granulomatous disease

Ineffective Hematopoiesis

   Megaloblastic anemias
   Myelodysplastic syndromes

Hemodilution

Hypersplenism/Splenomegaly

Immune Destruction (Autoimmune Diseases)

expected to produce hypoproliferative anemia is thought to be an idiosyncratic reaction.

Other conditions known to be associated with hypoproliferative anemias include autoimmune diseases such as lupus erythematosus. Antibodies against stem cells or T-cell inhibition of stem cells are suspected as immune mediators of injury. Some patients have a truly inherited disposition to aplasia, as occurs with Fanconi's anemia. Children with this disorder appear to have a deficiency in cellular DNA repair. This condition is associated with other constitutional abnormalities including abnormal kidneys, digits, and facial characteristics. Aplasia or hypoplasia of the thumb is a common association. Other skeletal malformations occur in approximately two-thirds of patients. Aplastic-hypoplastic anemia also occurs in association with other clonal hematologic neoplasms. It may herald the onset of an acute leukemia by months or even years and may also be associated with paroxysmal nocturnal hemoglobinuria (PNH).

Laboratory Findings

Patients with aplastic anemia usually have pancytopenia with reticulocytopenia; however, a deficiency of a specific cell line can predominate (e.g., anemia, leukopenia, or thrombocytopenia). A bone marrow study must always be performed and shows hypocellularity of all elements, with a relative predominance of supporting marrow cells (plasma cells, lymphocytes, and reticulum cells) (see Color Plate 8A). If immature cells are seen, a myelodysplastic process should be suspected (preleukemia). If many lymphocytes predominate, a collagen-vascular disorder may be suspected as a co-association. Chromosomal studies are important to exclude Fanconi's anemia, especially in children. The acidified serum test and leukocyte alkaline phosphatase (LAP) test should be performed to exclude PNH. In PNH, the LAP score is low (see Chapters 2 and 4).

Prognosis

Severe aplastic anemia has been fatal in most patients, but improved results have been seen following bone marrow transplantation and immunosuppressive treatment. Patients classified as having severe aplasia have three of the four following criteria:

1. neutrophil count of less than 500/µL
2. platelet count of less than 20,000/µL
3. reticulocyte count of less than 10,000/µL
4. a markedly hypocellular marrow with less than 20% hematopoietic cells remaining for longer than 3 weeks

The disease used to be associated with a 50% 6-month mortality, but many patients now survive longer because of improved clinical support measures. If the patient is less than 40 years of age and has an HLA-matched sibling bone marrow donor, the prognosis is very much better, with a high likelihood of cure following bone marrow transplantation. The prognosis is especially better for children and young adults. Patients who have been multiply transfused appear to have a worse prognosis, although the overall results of bone marrow transplantation in aplastic anemia show a 70 to 80% recovery.

Bone Marrow Replacement

Pancytopenia may also occur when the bone marrow is replaced by nonhematopoietic cells, as occurs in secondary or metastatic malignancy, or when there is an abnormal growth of hematopoietic cells replacing the normal bone marrow (e.g., leukemia, multiple myeloma) (see Chapter 4). When neoplastic cells infiltrate the hematopoietic marrow, pancytopenia develops if the process is extensive, but red cell production is depressed before other cell lines are affected. Leukemias, multiple myeloma, lymphoma, and carcinomas of the prostate, lung, and breast are the most common tumors involved. Diagnosis rests on demonstrating the presence of malignant cells, but the presence of bizarre or randomly immature blood cells in the circulation tends to raise suspicion, especially if there are suggestive roentgenogram changes.

Myelofibrosis is replacement of hematopoietic marrow by fibrous connective tissue elements. Myelofibrosis is discussed in more detail under the section on The Myeloproliferative Syndromes in Chapter 4. In this condition, because of either a primary clonal hematologic disease or a secondary malignancy, the bone marrow is replaced by fibrous tissue. Hematopoietic development is usually taken over by other reticuloendothelial organs, particularly the spleen and the liver. Since those organs are less discriminating in preventing abnormal cells from being released into the bloodstream, numerous misshapen and bizarre erythroid elements are seen in the peripheral blood in these conditions.

Hypoproliferative Anemia Associated with Other Diseases

Chronic infections, noninfectious inflammatory diseases such as rheumatoid arthritis and lupus erythematosus, slowly progressive neoplasms, and long-standing renal failure all depress bone marrow function by mechanisms not clearly understood. The laboratory findings are of a normochromic, normocytic anemia, usually of moderate degree (7 to 11 g/dL hemoglobin) with normal or near normal red cell survival, reduced serum iron and transferrin levels, and normal or increased storage iron in the marrow (see the earlier section on Anemia of Chronic Disease). The bone marrow may be somewhat less cellular than normal, but those cells that are present have a normal appearance and are in normal proportions. Treatment is aimed at correction of the underlying disease, which, if achieved, is associated with improvement in the hematologic parameters.

Bone marrow aplasia sometimes follows hepatitis B infections; other viral infections have also been implicated in sporadic cases (parvovirus B-19). Tuberculosis may depress bone marrow function, but its other possible hematologic effects include pancytopenia caused by splenomegaly, or leukocytosis so severe as to resemble leukemia. Hypothyroidism may also be associated with a macrocytic anemia. Because metabolic activity is low, the low hemoglobin level does not cause tissue hypoxia; thus, erythropoietin is not stimulated, and the bone marrow adjusts to lowered equilibrium.

Pure Red Cell Aplasia

In this disorder, there is hypoplasia of the erythrocyte precursors only, producing a severe anemia with reticulocytopenia. A bone marrow aspirate shows absence of erythroid precursors with normal myeloid and platelet elements. Peripheral blood indices usually show normochromic, normocytic red cells; however, occasionally macrocytosis may be seen. This disorder may occur transiently in association with other hemolytic anemias (e.g., sickle cell disease or spherocytosis) and may be caused by an infection from a parvovirus. This type of crisis has been termed **aplastic crisis,** and may be associated with an acute drop in hemoglobin or hematocrit. Patients may require blood transfusions if recovery does not occur within a short period. *Red cell aplasia* has also been seen in association with certain drugs, and may also occur with vitamin deficiency (particularly pyridoxine and riboflavin). In addition, a more common association of pure red cell aplasia with a tumor of the thymus gland (thymoma) is recognized. The condition is often corrected with removal of the thymus, or may respond to corticosteroid treatment. A congenital form of red cell aplasia presents with severe anemia in infancy, but is not associated with suppression of the white cell or platelet counts or skeletal abnormalities, as is seen in Fanconi's anemia. A condition termed *transient erythroblastopenia of childhood (TEC)* occurs as an acquired self-limited condition in early infancy. The origin is also thought to be a parvovirus infection, but may be immune-mediated. It is usually self-limiting in several weeks, but may require transfusion therapy or corticosteroid treatment.

REFRACTORY ANEMIA AND INEFFECTIVE ERYTHROPOIESIS

Refractory Anemia

The refractory anemias constitute a group of disorders that are characterized by abnormal red cell production, generally unresponsive to any treatment. These disorders are often considered "preleukemic syndromes," a term that is inaccurate because the majority of these disorders do not evolve into acute leukemia. However, the more unstable the bone marrow growth and the more abundant immature cells, particularly blasts, are in the bone marrow, the greater the likelihood for leukemic transformation. These conditions are more appropriately classified as **myelodysplastic syndromes** and include the following conditions in which refractory anemia is often a major feature (see section on Myelodysplasias and Preleukemic Syndromes in Chapter 4):

- idiopathic refractory anemia
- refractory anemia with ring sideroblasts
- refractory anemia with excess blasts
- refractory anemia with excess blasts in transformation

The hallmark of these conditions is ineffective erythropoiesis in which the marrow is usually markedly hypercellular and shows an abundance of abnormal erythroid precursors. In many instances, the red cell precursors show megaloblastic features. These conditions are clonal abnormalities of marrow precursor cells, and consequently leukopenia and thrombocytopenia may coexist. In addition, cytogenetic abnormalities occur in almost half the patients with myelodysplastic syndromes involving, most commonly, chromosomes 5, 7, or 8 (see Chapter 4).

Paroxysmal Nocturnal Hemoglobinuria

Paroxysmal nocturnal hemoglobinuria (PNH) is a rare, acquired disorder characterized by the proliferation of an abnormal clone of hematopoietic cells in the bone marrow, producing erythrocytes with increased sensitivity to complement fixation and intravascular hemolysis. Despite the name, the majority of patients manifest with chronic intravascular hemolysis characterized by the presence of hemosiderin in the urine and not frank hemoglobinuria. Half of the cases of PNH develop between the ages of 20 and 40. In some cases, a similar PNH-like defect may occur in association with other hematologic malignancies such as leukemia, myelofibrosis, and aplastic anemia. Despite the descriptive name, episodic urinary excretion of hemoglobin after a night's sleep occurs in only 25% of cases.

Cellular Defects

The pathognomonic feature of PNH is a strikingly increased susceptibility to complement-mediated red cell lysis. Not every circulating cell is equally affected. Blood from PNH patients contains cells with three different degrees of complement sensitivity: 25 to 30 X normal, 3 to 5 X normal, and normal. The relative proportions of these populations determines how severely the patient is affected. Severity differs markedly from patient to patient but tends to follow an episodic, gradually worsening course in the majority of affected individuals.

The membrane of PNH cells has both morphologic and chemical

abnormalities. Scanning electron microscopy reveals strange pits and protuberances on the red cell surface. Chemical analysis reveals deficient acetylcholinesterase activity and the presence of abnormally constituted glycoproteins. It is probable that both acetylcholinesterase deficiency and complement sensitivity are manifestations of some underlying, still undefined causal phenomenon rather than having a cause-and-effect relationship with each other.

Laboratory Findings

Paroxysmal nocturnal hemoglobinuria is diagnosed by demonstrating that red cells experience excessive hemolysis when exposed to low-ionic–strength solutions (sugar or sucrose lysis test). This test is often used as a screening test; however, the definitive test of PNH is the demonstration of excessive hemolysis when exposed to complement-containing serum at low pH (Ham's acid hemolysis test). The acid hemolysis test is less sensitive but more specific than the sugar water test; therefore, the latter is usually performed as a screening test. Patients with PNH usually have chronic, compensated hemolysis; however, unlike most patients with ongoing hemolysis, they have low iron stores and may be frankly iron deficient. Iron depletion occurs because hemoglobin and hemosiderin are excreted in the urine after complement-mediated intravascular hemolysis releases hemoglobin into the plasma (see Chapter 2).

Bone marrow aplasia is a common presenting symptom in PNH, causing leukopenia and thrombocytopenia, along with depressed red cell production. PNH-like red cells may be seen in 15% of patients with aplastic anemia. Thrombotic and infectious manifestations are other common presenting events and like aplastic crises, they may occur episodically throughout the disease. Reticulocytosis remains disproportionately low for the degree of hemolysis, even between frankly aplastic episodes. Hemolysis may be exacerbated during sleep, or by drug or dietary exposure; however, no clear pattern of inciting substances can be described. Transfusion of blood products containing even small amounts of plasma precipitates hemolysis reliably. If red cell transfusions are necessary, washed or deglycerolized frozen cells should be used to eliminate all the complement-containing plasma.

ANEMIAS CAUSED BY EXCESSIVE RED CELL LOSS

HEMORRHAGIC ANEMIA

A sudden drop in hemoglobin or hematocrit is associated with either acute blood loss or acute destruction of erythrocytes. This distinction is quite easy when bleeding is clinically apparent. The identification of hemolysis is also evident when laboratory criteria for hemolysis are present (see section on Hematologic Methods, Chapter 2). Internal bleeding may be more difficult to detect and may be associated with laboratory features compatible with extravascular hemolysis because extravasated blood is also removed by the reticuloendothelial system (see Chapter 2). Laboratory data usually found in hemolytic anemia, including elevated bilirubin, elevated LDH, and decreased haptoglobin, are more usually associated with hemolysis than bleeding. Reticulocytosis, however, is commonly seen in hemorrhage and hemolysis.

Excessive Loss of Red Cells

Hemorrhage

Acute, massive blood loss does not cause immediate anemia. Rapid hemorrhage acutely decreases the intravascular blood volume and stresses the compensatory circulatory adjustments. Enough hemoglobin may remain to sustain life, but if circulatory mechanisms fail, hemoglobin cannot get to the tissues, and oxygenation is impaired. After acute blood loss, the body adjusts by maintaining circulation through the most vital vascular beds by speeding up heart rates and expanding circulatory volume at the expense of the extravascular fluid. It is this volume adjustment that causes anemia. As extravascular fluid enters the bloodstream, it dilutes the remaining cells and the hematocrit drops over the next 48 to 72 hours.

Hematologic Response to Acute Blood Loss

Acute blood loss stimulates the bone marrow immediately. The platelet count and the number of circulating granulocytes increase before the hematocrit falls. Thrombocytosis between 600,000 and 800,000 per microliter and leukocytosis between 10,000 and 30,000 per microliter may occur within a few hours, accompanied in extreme cases by an outpouring of immature platelets and neutrophils. Since there is no storage reservoir of erythrocytes in the bone marrow, it may take up to several days or weeks to replenish the erythrocytes lost during hemorrhage. Erythropoietin levels rise within 6 hours, and reticulocytosis becomes apparent within 24 hours, reaching a peak in 7 to 10 days. If the hemorrhage is severe enough, "shift reticulocytes" and the presence of later stage normoblasts may be seen in the bloodstream.

If iron stores are normal, the rate of red cell production increases twofold to threefold. Iron-deficient patients cannot increase hematopoiesis appropriately when the hematocrit falls. Patients who receive therapeutic iron to supplement an erratic, inadequate, or borderline supply may show fourfold to sevenfold rises in erythropoietic activity. Reticulocytosis ceases when lost red cells are restored, usually within 30 days if no further bleeding occurs. Persistently elevated reticulocyte counts suggest continuing blood loss or red cell destruction.

If blood is shed into the body cavities, the lumen of the alimentary tract, or the soft tissues, nonviable red cells and hemoglobin accumulate and must be degraded. These changes may cause elevation of blood urea and bilirubin levels. Blood loss to the exterior does not, of course, have this effect. Chronic blood loss due to continuous low-level bleeding does not disrupt the blood volume since fluid adjustments occur automatically. However, as red cells are lost, also lost is the iron in their hemoglobin, and chronic blood loss commonly induces a state of iron deficiency anemia.

HEMOLYTIC ANEMIAS

Hemolytic anemia is a disorder that is associated with a shortened red cell survival. Usually there is either an *intracorpuscular* or *extracorpuscular* abnormality that limits the erythrocyte life span. The extent and severity of the anemia are dependent on the rate of destruction and removal of red cells and balanced by the compensatory increase in bone marrow erythrocyte production. The normal bone marrow is capable of increasing its work activity by sixfold to eightfold, so that an anemia may not be apparent until the red cell life span is shortened to approximately 20 days. Hemolytic anemias may be classified into disorders associated with an *intrinsic defect* (intracorpuscular) or those associated with an *extrinsic abnormality* (extracorpuscular). Table 3–11 lists conditions characterized by hemolysis.

INTRINSIC HEMOLYTIC ANEMIAS

Hereditary Defects

Abnormalities of the Red Cell Membrane

An appreciation of the pathophysiology of hemolysis due to abnormalities of the erythrocyte membranes requires a basic understanding of the structure of the red cell membrane (see Chapter 2). The membrane has a skeletal component that consists of a protein chain adjacent to the cell membrane. The structural integrity of the erythrocyte is dependent on its ability to withstand shear forces during its passage through the microcirculation. It is the membrane's skeletal proteins that enable the erythrocyte to withstand such forces, and disorders of these proteins are associated with shortened red cell survival, that is, hemolysis. The erythrocyte should be deformable and have an appropriate cell surface-area-to-volume ratio to withstand shear forces and osmotic stress. The chemical composition of the membrane is one of a lipid bilayer consisting of cholesterol and phospholipids—forming approximately 50% of the

TABLE 3–11. CLASSIFICATION OF HEMOLYTIC ANEMIAS

Intrinsic Defects

Hereditary defects
　Abnormalities of the red cell membrane
　　Hereditary spherocytosis
　　Hereditary elliptocytosis
　　Hereditary pyropoikilocytosis
　　Hereditary stomatocytosis
　　Hereditary xerocytosis
　Inherited erythrocyte enzyme disorders
　　Glucose-6-phosphate dehydrogenase deficiency
　　Other enzyme deficiencies
　　　Pyruvate kinase deficiency
　　　Pyrimidine-5'-nucleotidase deficiency
　Disorders of hemoglobin production
　　Hemoglobinopathies
　　　Sickle cell syndromes
　　　　Sickle cell disease
　　　　Sickle cell trait
　　　　HbS beta-thalassemia syndrome
　　　　Hemoglobin C disease
　　　　Hemoglobin SC disease
　　　　Methemoglobins/hemoglobin M
　　　　Unstable hemoglobin
　　　Thalassemia syndromes
　　　　Alpha-thalassemia
　　　　Homozygous beta-thalassemia
　　　　Heterozygous beta-thalassemia
　　　　Thalassemia heterozygotes with other hemoglobinopathies
Acquired defects
　Paroxysmal nocturnal hemoglobinuria

Extrinsic Defects

Nonimmune destruction
　Microangiopathic and macroangiopathic hemolytic anemia
　Chemical and toxic agents
　Infections causing hemolysis
　Hypersplenism
　Systemic disorders
Immune hemolytic anemias
　Primary
　Secondary (associated with chronic lymphocytic leukemia, lymphomas, and
　　carcinomas)
　Drug-induced
　Infectious

chemical structure—arranged in close apposition with the membrane proteins. Some membrane proteins traverse the lipid layer, whereas others are internally distributed and some are distributed only on the periphery of the membrane lipids. The **integral proteins** traverse the lipid membrane, whereas the **peripheral proteins** are situated on the internal aspect of the cell membrane. The skeletal proteins of the membrane comprise several proteins called *spectrin, actin,* and some other proteins (see Chapter 2). The cytoskeleton is anchored to the plasma membrane via a protein called *ankyrin.* These proteins may be separated by electrophoretic methods and are classified according to their molecular weight and migration on electrophoretic gels. Although classification will probably be more refined and will be categorized on the basis of the molecular defect, current classifications outlining the hereditary defects of the red cell membrane are morphologic and include five main disorders listed in Table 3–11.

Hereditary Spherocytosis

Hereditary spherocytosis (HS) is a fairly common hemolytic condition that is usually transmitted as an autosomal dominant trait in white people. In 25% of cases, no inheritance pattern is identified, and these persons are thought to have developed this disorder because of a spontaneous mutation. Recently, molecular abnormalities of the skeletal proteins have been identified in some cases of HS (e.g., deficient synthesis of spectrin). In many cases, however, the molecular defect has not been identified. In the United States, HS affects approximately 2.2 per 10,000 whites, but the anemia is relatively mild and sometimes goes undiagnosed until late adulthood. Patients with HS, like those with other chronic hemolytic anemias, have marked susceptibility to formation of bilirubin stones in the gallbladder. Often it is the gallbladder, not the blood problem, that causes patients to seek medical attention.

Cellular Changes   The basic defect in the erythrocyte is loss of membrane, resulting in decreased surface area. This produces a cell with the lowest surface-area-to-volume ratio, namely the *spherocyte* (see Color Plate 9[A]). As previously described, the reduced surface-area-to-volume ratio makes these cells more susceptible to osmotic lysis and consequently increases osmotic fragility (see Chapter 2). These cells are also less deformable and cannot easily negotiate the microcirculation. The reason for the loss of membrane is still unexplained; however, it is thought to occur in passage through the splenic sinusoids. The primary defect, however, is probably an abnormality in the skeletal protein, producing a defect of deformability. As the cells negotiate the splenic sinusoids, more and more membrane is removed with each circulatory passage (microspherocytes formed) until the cell is ultimately sequestered. A formerly held belief now in doubt claimed that cells in HS were metabolically depleted because of extra ATP consumption and problems with sodium and calcium influx. Although this now seems unlikely, it is possible that calcium may interact adversely with spectrin to produce defective deformability.

As mentioned in Chapter 2, a spherocyte is the structure that has the lowest surface area compared with volume and is consequently extremely sensitive to any increase in intracellular fluid (osmotic fragility). Further understanding of the molecular structure of the red cell membrane will enable a more precise classification to be developed, and it is apparent that deficiencies of membrane proteins may lead to spherocytic, elliptocytic, or other morphologic abnormalities in red cell shape, characterized in most cases by shortened red cell survival, that is, hemolysis. Hereditary spherocytosis is the most common of these disorders.

Clinical Features The condition may present a clinical spectrum characterized particularly by varying degrees of anemia, jaundice, and splenomegaly, and the presence of spherocytosis and stomatocytosis in the peripheral blood. Since spherocytes are sequestered and destroyed in their passage through the spleen, the majority of cases benefit substantially by removal of the spleen (splenectomy). Patients may have a mild hemolytic state and be relatively compensated; however, with physical and infectious stress they may manifest an exaggerated anemia *(hemolytic crisis).* Some patients may have a severe hemolytic anemia requiring red cell transfusions. In addition, in response to fever, infections, and stress, patients may experience a sudden decrease in marrow production and manifest with an exaggerated anemia *(aplastic crisis).* Other clinical manifestations of hereditary spherocytosis include skeletal abnormalities due to a continuous marrow hyperproliferation, and chronic leg ulcers and gallstones, which may occur in other hemolytic conditions as well (notably sickle cell disease). A small percentage of patients also have a history of neonatal jaundice.

Laboratory Findings—Red Cell Morphology The laboratory findings in hereditary spherocytosis are listed in Table 3–12. The characteristic cells seen in the peripheral smear are spherocytes (see Color Plate 9[A]), which are uniformly round cells with more intensely staining hemoglobin and with an absence of the central pale area usually seen in a normal red cell. In addition, there is an increased, diffuse **polychromatophilia,** which represents the marrow erythropoietic (reticulocyte) response and is often proportional to the degree of anemia. Since the spherocyte has a normal hemoglobin content but smaller surface area, the mean cell hemoglobin concentration (MCHC) is increased. Other features of a hemolytic process are also present, including an elevated indirect serum bilirubin, an elevated lactate dehydrogenase (LDH), and a decreased serum haptoglobin.

Definitive diagnosis of hereditary spherocytosis is confirmed by demonstrating an abnormal *osmotic fragility test* (Fig. 3–2) which, as was mentioned in Chapter 2, assesses red cell membrane function.

TABLE 3-12. LABORATORY FINDINGS IN HEREDITARY SPHEROCYTOSIS

Blood Count

Mild anemia (Hgb 9–12 g/dL)
MCV normal or slightly low, MCHC high
Spherocytes in peripheral blood
Platelets slightly low if spleen present
Reticulocytes 5–7%

Red Cell Studies

Osmotic fragility very high
Autohemolysis after 48 hr at 37°C 10–50% (normal < 4%)
Glucose or ATP abolishes high autohemolysis

Chemistry

Bilirubin slightly high (indirect)
Urine urobilinogen high
Haptoglobin low

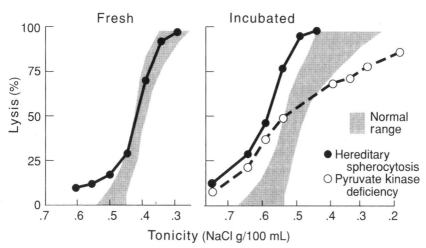

FIGURE 3–2. Osmotic fragility test. This test may be used to identify patients with defects in red cell membrane (i.e., hereditary spherocytosis) or intracellular metabolism (i.e., pyruvate kinase deficiency). The osmotic fragility test involves subjecting the red cells to the stress of increasingly hypotonic salt solutions. When the test is performed on a fresh blood sample, the hereditary spherocytic curve is displaced to the left, representing increased susceptibility to hemolysis. Often this is limited to a small tail of cells that are unusually susceptible to lysis. After incubation, the defect is magnified. In contrast, pyruvate kinase-deficient blood shows a mix of sensitive cells and cells resistant to osmotic lysis. (From Hillman, RS, and Finch, CA: Red Cell Manual, ed 7. FA Davis, Philadelphia, 1996, p 123, with permission.)

Autohemolysis is often markedly increased, especially after incubation at 37°C for 24 to 48 hours. This may be corrected by the addition of glucose (see Chapter 2, p. 72).

Treatment In symptomatic patients, splenectomy is the treatment of choice because it removes the major source of red cell sequestration and destruction. Patients should be maintained on folic acid as a prophylaxis against aplastic crises. Splenectomy does not cure the defect but removes the site of sequestration.

Hereditary Elliptocytosis

This condition is also an inherited disorder associated with a defective membrane protein skeleton structure. The condition is associated with a morphologic abnormality in the peripheral blood smear and the presence of elongated, *elliptical cells* (Color Plate 29). It is inherited as an autosomal dominant trait in most cases. A variant of this condition is another disorder called **hereditary pyropoikilocytosis.** The erythrocytes show marked variation in shape (poikilocytosis) with many teardrop forms, spherocytes, and microspherocytes, as well as fragmented cells. There is also a heat instability. When heparinized patient blood is subjected to a temperature of 45°C, the morphologic changes are exaggerated. Several variants are categorized by the degree of hemolysis and the type of morphologic abnormality. These conditions are often clinically insignificant and represent a "cosmetic" abnormality on the peripheral blood smear. Patients with mild hereditary elliptocytosis usually have normal osmotic fragility and autohemolysis. These tests may be abnormal in the more severe cases.

Hereditary Stomatocytosis and Hereditary Xerocytosis

Two other rare disorders of red cell membrane permeability are **hereditary stomatocytosis** and **hereditary xerocytosis,** characterized by red cell morphologic abnormalities. In hereditary stomatocytosis, the number of stomatocytes is increased, and mean cell volume is elevated. The number of target cells is increased in hereditary xerocytosis.

Inherited Erythrocyte Enzyme Disorders

Deficiency of erythrocyte enzymes (enzymopathies) may be associated with abnormal metabolic functions that may decrease erythrocyte survival. The spectrum of hemolysis produced is dependent on the nature of the enzyme deficiency and its importance in erythrocyte function. Erythrocyte metabolic pathways are discussed in Chapter 2. Although many enzymes are important for normal erythrocyte function, except for glucose-6-phosphate dehydrogenase deficiency, other enzyme deficiencies are extremely uncommon.

Glucose-6-Phosphate Dehydrogenase Deficiency

Glucose-6-phosphate dehydrogenase (G-6-PD) is the initial enzyme involved in the pentose phosphate pathway of erythrocyte metabolism. It catalyzes the removal of hydrogen from glucose-6-phosphate to produce 6-phosphogluconate (6-PG) and requires cofactors nicotine-adenine-dinucleotide phosphate (NADP), which is reduced to NADPH (see Fig. 2–13). This is an important reaction because NADPH is a source of reducing potential for the erythrocyte to resist oxidant stress. Deficiency of this enzyme is associated with an inability to neutralize oxidation stress, which produces instability of the hemoglobin molecule and consequent hemolysis. This is especially provoked by oxidant drugs. NADPH is an electron donor that is active in many biologic systems. Its reducing capacity is important for the red cell's glutathione system, the main reservoir of protection of hemoglobin against oxidative stress and irreversible denaturation.

A gene on the X chromosome determines the structure of G-6-PD, which exhibits remarkable polymorphism in human populations. A mutant expression of the X chromosome is fully expressed in the male *(hemizygote),* who inherits this mutant gene. Female heterozygotes are usually normal, but homozygous females with two mutant X chromosomes can exhibit G-6-PD deficiency and clinical disease. A heterozygote female may exhibit partial expression of the disorder, depending on which X chromosome is inactivated. Since only a single X chromosome is operative in any single cell, random inactivation of the second X chromosome occurs in females *(Lyon hypothesis).* Depending on the degree of inactivation of a normal X chromosome, a mutant X chromosome may be expressed in heterozygous females.

Normal G-6-PD is termed the *B variant,* and is present in 99% of the whites in the United States. A variant G-6-PD that differs from the B variant by a single amino acid is found in approximately 16% of American black males and is called *A variant.* A common defective variant of A, called A⁻, occurs in 9 to 13% of American blacks. This variant is called A⁻ because the functional expression of G-6-PD is generally decreased. The amino acid difference between A and B variants creates differing electrophoretic mobilities, which can be demonstrated in the laboratory. Approximately 20% of black females are heterozygous for the G-6-PD A variant. Nearly all heterozygotes have functionally adequate red cells. There is a relationship between the possession of G-6-PD, type A, and resistance to malaria, for reasons similar to those discussed under the section on Sickle Cell Disease. Most persons with the A⁻ variant do have comfortably adequate activity levels, except when subjected to oxidant drug stress. The function of G-6-PD is assessed clinically by subjecting red cells to oxidative stress (see Chapter 2). Specific variants can be characterized by their *electrophoretic mobility, thermal stability,* and other enzyme *kinetic studies.* **Isoenzymes** are enzymes with the same biologic function but differing physical or chemical properties, including electrophoretic mobility. Of the many isoenzymes of G-6-PD that have been described, the A and B variants are the most common.

Clinical Patterns Glucose-6-phosphate dehydrogenase deficiency may have a varied clinical presentation. The most common clinical patterns are (1) neonatal jaundice, (2) congenital hemolytic anemia, (3) drug-induced hemolysis, and (4) favism.

Patients with the A$^-$ enzyme experience no difficulty under normal conditions. Most remain unaware that hematologic abnormality exists, except that the A$^-$ enzyme has about 15% of normal activity—enough for most purposes. Red cell number, function, and survival are normal unless and until some acute oxidative stress occurs. Activity of G-6-PD declines as the red cell ages, no matter what variant is present. When the enzyme is defective, the effects of this decline become more noticeable. Aging red cells are especially susceptible to oxidative challenge by drugs, systemic infection, metabolic acidosis, and other stresses. Oxidative stress induces rapid intravascular destruction of susceptible cells, leading to hemoglobinemia, hemoglobinuria, and a sudden drop in hematocrit. The hemolytic crisis is self-limited because eventually the only cells left are those younger cells with sufficient enzyme levels to withstand the stress. Prompt erythropoietic response results in reticulocytosis and the introduction of still more young cells that are well supplied with active enzyme. Thus, drug-induced hemolysis is the most common clinical manifestation of G-6-PD deficiency and is usually self-limiting.

Drugs that hemolyze G-6-PD deficient cells are those that either act as direct oxidants themselves or produce peroxide activity. **Primaquine,** an antimalarial drug, is notable in this respect; an older term for the red cell defect G-6-PD deficiency is "primaquine sensitivity." Primaquine is a drug that was used for malarial prophylaxis in the Korean War. Since many black patients were treated with the drug, the association was quickly made between acute hemolysis and the antimalarial oxidant drug primaquine. Hence the term "primaquine sensitivity" and the association with black patients. The severity of the hemolysis depends on the nature of the G-6-PD variant and the degree of deficiency. The signs of intravascular hemolysis occur approximately 3 days after taking the drug, when the patient presents with anemia, jaundice, and hemoglobinuria. Many sulfa drugs, quinine derivatives, nitrofurans, and antipyretic-analgesic drugs can induce hemolysis in G-6-PD–deficient patients. Susceptibility seems to vary among different individuals. The presence of coexistent fever, metabolic disease, or hepatic or renal failure increases the likelihood that symptoms will occur.

Another G-6-PD variant is the **Mediterranean enzyme variant.** This occurs in whites, especially those of Greek, Italian, and some Jewish populations. The Mediterranean variant has severely reduced activity, so that even very young cells have little capacity to generate NADPH. Hemolytic episodes are more severe, are triggered by a greater variety of stimuli, and are less likely to be self-limited than in patients with the A^- variant. Infants with the deficiency may present with severe neonatal jaundice. **Favism,** a susceptibility to massive hemolysis after exposure to the fava bean, occurs especially in persons with the Mediterranean type G-6-PD deficiency. Serum factors and immune mechanisms are involved in this type of hemolysis, although the exact pathogenesis is not clearly understood. Patients with this variant and other more unusual severe variants may have a **chronic hemolytic anemia** associated with chronic intravascular hemolysis. Laboratory findings in this case include a chronic intravascular hemolytic anemia with decreased haptoglobin, increased LDH and bilirubin, an elevated reticulocyte count, and the presence of hemosiderin in the urine, which is indicative of a chronic intravascular hemolysis. See Chapter 2 for assessment of the phosphate pentose pathway and G-6-PD.

Typically, following drug exposure, hemoglobin and hematocrit drop acutely. This is associated with a brisk elevation of the reticulocyte count. Reticulocyte counts may go as high as 50% or more. Screening tests during the acute intravascular hemolytic phase may be normal with the A^- deficiency because of the presence of the high reticulocyte count. During the asymptomatic phase, however, they will be abnormal and will indicate deficiency. The nature of the G-6-PD can be confirmed by gel electrophoresis. Enzyme studies can then identify the specific abnormality and will facilitate quantitation of the deficiency.

During the acute intravascular hemolytic event, the peripheral blood may show fragmented red cells and, more typically, the "blister cell." Because of oxidative denaturation of hemoglobin, the hemoglobin appears to separate from the superficial erythrocyte membrane, which appears as a clear "blister." Since hemoglobin has become denatured and oxidized, Heinz bodies will also be detected (see Color Plate 10). Other laboratory findings indicative of acute intravascular hemolysis, as outlined in Chapter 2, can also be seen during acute crisis, particularly in the Mediterranean type.

Other Enzyme Deficiencies

Pyruvate Kinase Deficiency The next most common defect, representing approximately 95% of the remaining enzyme abnormalities other than G-6-PD, is **pyruvate kinase deficiency.** The rest of the defects are metabolic curiosities involving the entire range of available enzymes. Pyruvate kinase is the enzyme that catalyzes the conversion of 2-phospho-enol-pyruvate into pyruvate, and represents an energy-producing final step of the glycolytic pathway (see Fig. 2–13). The effect of pyruvate kinase deficiency would also be considered to be more profound in older red cells that lack the oxidative phosphorylation metabolic capability. This step, therefore, represents the major source of energy production for nonreticulocyte red blood cells. It is associated with the generation of two molecules of adenosine triphosphate (ATP). Pyruvate kinase-deficient cells are also more preferentially removed in the spleen, and patients have a chronic hemolytic anemia. The clinical features, however, may vary considerably. Failure to generate sufficient ATP results in defective control of ions, so that excessive sodium and calcium enter the cell, and membrane phospholipids may sustain damage.

Defective PK and other glycolytic enzymes may induce hemolytic anemia, which is characterized by increased autohemolysis after incubation at 37°C, and increased indirect bilirubin. The major clinical features are anemia, jaundice, and splenomegaly. The anemia is a nonspherocytic hemolytic anemia, since spherocytes are not seen. Pyruvate kinase deficiency is inherited as an autosomal recessive trait, so both sexes are affected equally.

Pyrimidine-5′-Nucleotidase Deficiency This condition, which is associated with deficiency of the enzyme responsible for metabolism of pyrimidine residues in the developing red cell, is associated with a chronic, congenital hemolytic anemia, whose striking feature is the presence of marked basophilic stippling (see Color Plate 10C). These patients may also present with anemia, jaundice, and splenomegaly, which may be quite prominent. Patients may benefit from the removal of the spleen. This is a rare disorder, and diagnosis is made by special enzyme assays, usually performed by a reference laboratory.

Disorders of Globin Synthesis (Hemoglobinopathies)

Normal Maturational Changes

In the earliest embryonic stages, unique hemoglobins are produced by the yolk-sac derivatives. By 6 weeks, fetal cells begin producing hemoglobin F, which dominates the oxygen-carrying mechanism until birth. Beta chain production can be detected by the sixth month of intrauterine life. At birth, up to 30% of the hemoglobin in each red cell is hemoglobin A, and the change from fetal to adult hemoglobin progresses rapidly. At 6 months of age, 80 to 90% of the hemoglobin present is hemoglobin A, and from 1 year onwards, hemoglobin F constitutes less than 2% of the total. Delta chain production is insignificant before birth. Adult red cells contain 1 to 2% hemoglobin A_2, a level achieved at about 1 year. Each red cell in a given individual contains the same proportions of the same hemoglobins. Figure 3–4, later in the chapter, shows the sequence of hemoglobin chain development.

Hemoglobin Variants

The most common abnormal hemoglobin is hemoglobin S or *sickle hemoglobin,* in which the normal glutamic acid at the sixth position in the beta chain is replaced by the neutral amino acid valine. Hemoglobin S is by far the most common hemoglobinopathy. Amino acid no. 6 occurs at the outer surface of the richly intertwining globin chain configuration, at the area where alpha and beta chains shift position during oxygenation and deoxygenation. Other substitutions can and do occur within the folded globin chain at contact points between the other globin chains, or near the heme insertion. Each substitution produces a different hemoglobin, of which several hundred have been discovered.

Substitutions within the globin chains may cause altered solubility, altered ability to withstand oxidation, instability, increased propensity for methemoglobin production, or increased or decreased oxygen affinity. Some substitutions produce very little in the way of clinical abnormalities.

Genes determining globin chain structures are codominant; this means that the gene product is detectable no matter which allele is on the opposite chromosome. Heterozygotes with two different genes for globin structure will have two kinds of hemoglobin. Heterozygous subjects with hemoglobinopathies, then, will usually have hemoglobin A and the other abnormal substituted variant. People who have two different abnormal alleles have red cells that contain two different abnormal hemoglobins (double heterozygotes) and no normal hemoglobin A at all (e.g., sickle cell [SC] disease). If the same abnormal allele is present on both chromosomes, the individual is homozygous for the hemoglobinopathy, and all the hemoglobin is the same type, expressing the same abnormality.

The existence of a hemoglobinopathy is demonstrated by **hemoglobin electrophoresis.** For the common hemoglobin abnormalities, no further diagnostic proof is needed. More detailed study becomes necessary with rare abnormal hemoglobins and may include hemoglobin synthesis, protein characterization, and physical properties.

Sickle Cell Syndromes

Sickle cell syndromes include all the conditions in which sickle hemoglobin (HbS) is present: heterozygous AS, homozygous SS, the presence of S with other beta chain abnormalities such as SC disease, and the presence of hemoglobin S in association with defective expression of globin chains (e.g., S thalassemia).

Sickle Cell Disease   Sickle cell disease is a disorder in which the patient lacks a normal hemoglobin A and hemoglobin S is present. Therefore, an individual with sickle cell disease has a homozygous expression of S hemoglobin. The sickle cell gene frequency is high among American blacks and is reminiscent of their equatorial African heritage. The gene frequency in equatorial Africa ranges between 5 and 20%. The frequency of the carrier state in the United States is approximately 8% among all American blacks, with the incidence of the homozygous state at birth being 0.16%. Possession of the sickle gene is believed to confer some advantage against (falciparum) malaria infection.

Pathophysiology   When hemoglobin A releases its oxygen, one alpha and one beta chain change their relative positions. They resume their previous positions when reoxygenation occurs. Hemoglobin S has the hydrophobic amino acid valine in place of the hydrophilic amino acid glutamic acid at the sixth position on the beta chain. In the deoxygenated configuration, this substitution assumes critical importance. The valine residue represents a key-like surface structure that just fits into a complementary site on an adjacent, deoxygenated molecule. As one molecule locks into the next, the deoxygenated hemoglobin forms filaments that intertwine into elongated, cable-like, polymeric masses that are insoluble at high concentrations. The initial shape change is reversible. If oxygen is restored, the adjacent sites unlock, the beta chain returns to the oxygenated configuration, and solubility resumes.

Deoxygenated hemoglobin S can link with adjacent molecules of hemoglobin A or other abnormal hemoglobins, but the association is not long-lasting. Whether or not insoluble aggregates will form depends on the proportion of hemoglobin S to other hemoglobins, on the absolute concentration of hemoglobin S, and on the degree of deoxygenation. The presence of hemoglobin A guards, to a modest extent, against polymerization; hemoglobin F exerts a very strong protective effect. Persons heterozygous for hemoglobin S and hemoglobin A have only 30 to 40% hemoglobin S in each cell. The high concentration of hemoglobin A is a deterrent to sickling. Except in nonphysiologic conditions of extreme deoxygenation (in laboratory testing), the cells do not sickle, even though individual molecules may undergo the shape change. High intracellular levels of hemoglobin F can protect even homozygous hemoglobin S from sickling.

It is likely that erythrocytes of patients with sickle cell disease undergo intravascular sickling and unsickling many times as they circulate. Initially sickling may be a reversible effect, but with repeated episodes of sickling, the cells become so-called "irreversibly sickled cells." These cells are less flexible and less deformable to the physical demands of the circulation. Some cells gradually lose their mechanical and osmotic resistance and undergo intravascular dissolution, whereas others withstand individual stresses but are destroyed at an above-normal rate by the reticuloendothelial system. Red cells in hemoglobin S disease experience a chronically shortened lifespan.

The likelihood of sickling increases with low oxygen tensions (hypoxia), lowered pH (acidosis), and increased body temperature (fever). In addition, sickling becomes a danger in those parts of the circulation where blood flow is slow, tissue oxygen levels are low, or metabolic waste products accumulate. Sickle cells pass poorly through tiny vessels. This causes blood viscosity to rise and blood flow to become more stagnant, which in turn aggravates the problems of poor tissue perfusion, increased acidity, and decreased oxygenation.

Clinical Considerations Persons homozygous for hemoglobin S (SS) suffer from **sickle cell anemia,** a lifelong, variably severe, hemolytic anemia punctuated by superimposed episodes of exaggerated hemolysis (hemolytic crisis), bone marrow aplasia (aplastic crisis), and painful vaso-occlusive episodes. Continuous hemolysis causes erythropoietic hyperplasia of such magnitude that the bones may be deformed by the mass of proliferating erythroid marrow. Sickle cell anemia rarely becomes clinically apparent before 6 months of age because protective amounts of hemoglobin F remain in each cell. Intrauterine development is usually normal because hemoglobin F is not affected by abnormalities of beta chain production.

The most common clinical manifestation of sickle cell anemia is the vaso-occlusive crisis, which probably occurs as a result of impairment of blood flow from the irreversibly sickled cells and is perpetuated by deoxygenation and devitalization of the tissues affected. Consequently, depending on which vessels are affected, clinical features may vary tremendously, but the most common manifestations are bone pain and tenderness from micro-infarcts in the bones. Ischemia and infarction can occur in many other sites involving parenchymal organs such as the lungs, liver, spleen, and kidney, and the central nervous system and eyes. In childhood the spleen may be enlarged; however, because of recurrent vaso-occlusive crisis involving this organ, the spleen gradually becomes fibrosed and atrophied. Consequently, persons with sickle cell anemia have functional asplenia and are prone to infections from capsulated organisms, particularly pneumococcus and *H. influenzae*. In children, infarctive crises affecting the developing bones are common, as well as skeletal abnormalities from hyperproliferation of the bone marrow in response to the chronic hemolytic state. With successive episodes of infarction involving parenchymal tissues, there is loss of tissue reserve, and symptomatic disease of that organ may occur. In adults, pulmonary involvement is very common and patients often present with infections and pneumonia.

Inexplicable episodes of marrow aplasia occur, some secondary to parvovirus infection, during which hemolysis continues and erythropoiesis ceases. There is a remarkable drop in the hematocrit and reticulocyte count, which leads to a dangerous level of anemia. The aplastic crises can occur from folic acid deficiency, and patients must be maintained on continuous folic acid for life.

The exaggerated hemolytic crises are difficult to differentiate from the chronic hemolytic state, especially since an increase in jaundice may be secondary to gallstones. Gallstones are very common in patients with any chronic hemolytic anemia, and the clinical features may be very similar to acute intravascular hemolytic crises. In acute intravascular sickling, the hematocrit drops, but the reticulocyte count rises, as do the other laboratory parameters of intravascular hemolysis (Table 3–13 shows the characteristic laboratory findings in sickle cell anemia).

Sickle Cell Trait   Heterozygotes, with one hemoglobin S gene and one hemoglobin A gene, have sickle cell trait but usually have no clinical disease. The heterozygous hemoglobin SA state appears to offer

---

TABLE 3–13. LABORATORY FINDINGS IN SICKLE CELL ANEMIA (HEMOGLOBIN S DISEASE)

Blood Count

Hgb low (usually 6–10 g/dL)
Marked poikilocytosis, inclusion bodies
Irreversibly sickled cells 6–18% of RBCs on smear
WBCs 10–20 × 10^3/μL
Platelets high
Reticulocytes 10–20% (except in aplastic crises)

Bone Marrow

Marked erythroid hyperplasia
Storage iron high

Blood Chemistry

Bilirubin high (especially indirect)
Serum iron high, iron-binding capacity normal, % saturation high

Other Tests

Sickle prep (solubility test) positive (Note: if anemia is severe, it may be necessary to remove some plasma)
Hgb electrophoresis shows Hgb S
Red cell survival low
Erythrocyte sedimentation rate abnormally low

Hgb = hemoglobin; RBCs = red blood cells; WBCs = white blood cells.

significant protection against malarial infection with *Plasmodium falciparum*. This apparently beneficial effect may explain why this otherwise deleterious gene has persisted with such high incidence in areas where malaria is endemic. Patients also have generally no hematologic symptoms and a normal life expectancy with normal patterns of morbidity and mortality. The presence of the gene, however, has potential implications with regard to anesthesia and air travel in unpressurized aircraft. Reduction of oxygen tension can cause the development of sickling. For such patients, oxygen tension needs to be sustained at greater than 100 mm Hg during anesthesia.

Persons with sickle cell trait usually have normal hematologic values with a normal peripheral blood smear. A sickle solubility test is positive, and hemoglobin electrophoresis reveals 55 to 60% hemoglobin A and 35 to 45% hemoglobin S.

Hemoglobin S/Beta-Thalassemia Syndrome This condition occurs as a result of the inheritance of one sickle gene and one beta-thalassemia gene. The severity of the clinical disease will depend on the amount of normal beta chain synthesized. These individuals manufacture normal amounts of alpha chains but, depending on the degree of impairment of the beta chains, may express varying proportions of hemoglobin A or hemoglobin S. Consequently, patients may have a mild disorder or may express a clinical severity similar to sickle cell anemia (see also the section on Thalassemia Syndromes).

Hemoglobin C Disease   Hemoglobin C resembles hemoglobin S with an amino acid substitution at the sixth position on the beta chain. In this case, glutamic acid is replaced by lysine. Hemoglobin C is less soluble than hemoglobin A because the positive charge on the lysine interacts with adjacent negatively charged groups. It is not clear whether in vivo crystallization occurs, but red cells with hemoglobin C as a dominant molecule are more rigid and more liable to fragmentation than normal red cells. About 2 to 3% of American blacks carry the hemoglobin C gene. This heterozygous state (HbC trait) does not cause anemia or shortened red cell lifespan. Although target cells may be seen in the blood smears, there is no anemia and no shortening of red cell survival.

Among American blacks, 1 in 6000 is homozygous for hemoglobin C (CC). This causes a mild, hemolytic anemia with striking red cell morphologic abnormalities (see Color Plate 15). There are numerous target cells, microspherocytes, and intracellular crystals (tactoids), but hemoglobin levels remain in the range of 8 to 12 g/dL. The biochemical findings of hemolysis exist to a modest extent. Because the disease has few intrinsic complications and does not interact adversely with other diseases, patients often remain unaware of their condition until it is detected during hemoglobin screening programs or during medical care for some other condition.

Hemoglobin SC Disease   This condition is a chronic hemolytic anemia associated with the inheritance of one abnormal gene carrying the C trait and another gene carrying the S trait. Consequently, individuals with SC disease are double heterozygotes. This condition occurs with a gene frequency of up to 0.25% of the population in Western Africa and occurs in the United States in approximately 1 in 833 blacks. Clinical features can be very similar to those of patients with SS disease, but they tend to be milder. Curiously, patients with SC disease tend to develop more aseptic necrosis of the femoral head, a common arthritic complaint of this disorder.

The hematologic features of SC disease generally show a mild anemia with reticulocytosis and numerous target cells in the peripheral smear. Occasional sickle cells may also be seen.

Hereditary Persistence of Fetal Hemoglobin

This condition is generally a benign disorder, which manifests a persistence of fetal hemoglobin synthesis into adult life. The regulation of beta-gamma switching is unknown; however, different degrees of persistence of the gamma globin gene activity occur. The homozygous condition is associated with 100% of fetal hemoglobin and usually manifests with erythrocytosis (discussed later in this chapter). Occasionally the presence of this gene may coexist with other hemoglobin abnormalities such as hemoglobin S and hemoglobin C. In the case of the persistence of fetal hemoglobin in the presence of hemoglobin S, the clinical expression of S-hemoglobin is attenuated and may exhibit a mild clinical disease.

The presence of fetal hemoglobin is easily detected in the laboratory by the fact that it is resistant to acid and alkali denaturation, whereas adult hemoglobin (hemoglobin A) is not. Consequently, a smear that is made and placed in an acid or alkaline medium will lyse the hemoglobin A-containing cells, whereas the hemoglobin F-containing cells will remain intact. Staining will identify hemoglobin F inside the intact red cells (Color Plate 30). In hereditary persistence of fetal hemoglobin, there is homogeneous distribution of HbF (present uniformly in all cells). In other conditions in which fetal hemoglobin is increased, such as in thalassemia, there is a heterogeneous distribution. Table 3–14 lists the conditions associated with elevated fetal hemoglobin.

Other Hemoglobinopathies

Genetic disorders causing substitution of internal nonpolar amino acids of the globin chains can produce significant alterations of structure or function of the hemoglobin molecule. These variants may alter the affinity of the hemoglobin molecule for oxygen or may allow oxidation of the iron from the ferrous to the ferric state; on the other hand, they may

---

TABLE 3–14. CONDITIONS ASSOCIATED WITH ELEVATED FETAL HEMOGLOBIN (HbF)

Congenital
Normally elevated at birth
Inherited
Hereditary persistence of fetal hemoglobin (HPFH)
Acquired
Erythropoietin stress
    Acute hemolysis
    Immediately postphlebotomy
    Recovery from transient erythroblastopenia of childhood
    Following bone marrow transplantation
Induced by drug therapy
    Hydroxyurea
    5-Azacytidine
    Recombinant erythropoietin

produce hemoglobin molecules that are unstable and precipitate to form Heinz bodies. In general, these diseases are found in the heterozygous state, since homozygosity is usually incompatible with life.

Methemoglobins/Hemoglobin M As was mentioned in Chapter 2, methemoglobinemia occurs when hemoglobin is oxidized to the ferric form of iron (Fe^{3+}). Since this molecule is unable to effectively transport oxygen, the patient presents with cyanosis and hypoxemia. In general, these patients do not have a hemolytic anemia. They do, however, have an abnormal hemoglobin that can be detectable on hemoglobin electrophoresis.

Unstable Hemoglobin Inheritance of a gene that produces a defect in the structural component of the globin chains can result in instability of hemoglobin. This produces Heinz bodies, which are removed in the spleen, producing an inherited Heinz body hemolytic anemia (see Color Plate 10B). The severity of the disorder is dependent on the nature of the amino acid substitution. The clinical features are those of a hemolytic anemia that is confirmed by laboratory data. Hematologic indices may vary; however, spherocytes are generally not seen in the peripheral blood smear. Laboratory tests for unstable hemoglobins include a heat stability test or exposure to certain drugs such as isopropanol. In unsplenectomized patients, Heinz bodies are sometimes difficult to detect; but following splenectomy they may be quite prominent. Oxidant drugs may precipitate episodes of hemolysis in these patients.

Thalassemia Syndromes

The term **thalassemia** derives from a combination of the Greek words *thalassa* (sea) and *haima* (blood). An early name for the severest form of the disease was *Mediterranean anemia* because Mediterranean populations were the first ones known to be afflicted. The thalassemia syndromes are characterized by a decreased rate of production of the globin chains. They are classified according to which globin chain is affected: *alpha-thalassemia*, where there is a decreased production of alpha chains, and *beta-thalassemia*, where beta chain production is decreased. These are the most common thalassemic syndromes and also occur in a geographic distribution very similar to that of malaria. Rarer types of thalassemia do occur, affecting some other minor globin chains (e.g., the delta chain), and occasional hybrid forms may occur (the so-called beta-delta-thalassemia or hemoglobin Lepore syndromes). The difference between the thalassemia syndromes and the disease-producing hemoglobin variants is that, in most cases, all the chains that are synthesized have a normal structure, although the amount is decreased.

Molecular Biology of Globin Synthesis As was mentioned in Chapter 2, the genetic codes for globin synthesis are located on chromosome 11 (epsilon, gamma, delta, and beta chains) and chromosome 16 (alpha and embryonic chains). Figure 3–3 shows a diagram of progression from the genetic code to the protein polypeptide. For alpha chain synthesis, each chromosome 16 has two subloci, making a total of four functioning subloci in diploid cells of normal people. The genes that control beta, gamma, and delta chain synthesis form a cluster that has been shown in a well-defined sequence on chromosome 11. The control of globin production is achieved by ubiquitous and lineage specific transcriptional factors with *cis*-active regulatory sequences. A powerful regulatory element is located 15–20 Kb upstream of the epsilon gene on chromosome 11 that activates the beta globin domain and insulates this gene from surrounding chromatin influences. This element is termed the **locus control region (LCR).** The fundamentals of globin synthesis have been discussed in Chapter 2. Thalassemia syndromes may occur as a result of abnormalities in the coding sequence, transcription, or processing, or defects in gene translation. The consequence is defective or absent globin chain production. Deletion of all four alpha chain loci causes complete absence of messenger RNA (mRNA) for alpha chain synthesis. Deletion or severe abnormality of two genes slightly reduces levels of mRNA, with mild or no reduction in chain synthesis.

Genes for the beta chain are more variable. One form, called **beta⁺ thalassemia,** results in markedly deficient but still measurable levels of mRNA, whereas the **beta° thalassemia** gene produces no mRNA at all. In both these conditions, the DNA present on the chromosome determines the defective activity. A third possibility can occur when chain production

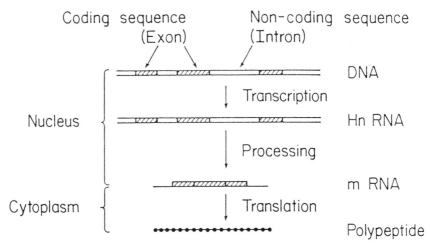

FIGURE 3–3. Diagram of the progression from gene to peptide. (From Pittiglio, DH, and Sacher, RA: Clinical Hematology and Fundamentals of Hemostasis. FA Davis, Philadelphia, 1987, p 122, with permission.)

involves deletion of the gene itself, with absence of any DNA code for beta chain synthesis. A similar situation can exist for delta chains.

Hemoglobin Products   Defective alpha chain production affects all the hemoglobins except those yolk sac-derived embryonic hemoglobins with unique, separately regulated chains. In red cell precursors with grossly deficient alpha chain supplies, four gamma chains may unite as a gamma tetramer, producing hemoglobin Barts. Similarly, four beta chains may unite as a tetramer, producing an abnormal hemoglobin (hemoglobin H). In persons with defective alpha chain production, hemoglobin Barts (gamma^4) is conspicuous during fetal existence when gamma is the dominant non-alpha chain. Hemoglobin H (beta^4) becomes predominant in postuterine life, when beta chain production takes over.

The fetus suffers very little if beta chain genes are defective because hemoglobin F (alpha$_2$ gamma$_2$) is perfectly normal. In extrauterine life, inadequate supplies of beta chains cause excess alpha chains to accumulate (Fig. 3–4). Synthesis of gamma or delta chains may rise to compensate for the deficiency of beta chains and produces increased amounts of hemoglobin A$_2$ (alpha$_2$ delta$_2$) and hemoglobin F (alpha$_2$ gamma$_2$). These hemoglobins support oxygen transport to some extent, although they are less efficient at oxygen delivery than hemoglobin A. The level of compensatory hemoglobin F depends on how completely the switch from gamma synthesis to beta chain production occurs. Massive compensatory delta chain production never occurs, so hemoglobin A$_2$ values are only marginally elevated. Nevertheless, elevation of hemoglobin A$_2$ is an important laboratory finding in beta-thalassemia, although the values never exceed 7% of the total hemoglobin.

Alpha-Thalassemias   Each chromosome 16 has two alpha globin genes (see Fig. 3–4). Thus, each normal person has four alpha genes. Alpha-thalassemia is classified by the relative output of these genes. The designations of alpha° and alpha$^+$ haplotypes describe absent or decreased alpha globin production on each chromosome. Therefore, in alpha° thalassemia, one chromosome has two inactive genes. The heterozygous state is then – –/alpha alpha (alpha° thalassemia trait) and the homozygous state is – –/– –, which produces the hemoglobin Barts *hydrops fetalis syndrome,* a condition causing intrauterine fetal death in mid-pregnancy because the fetus can survive on embryonic hemoglobins only until the second trimester. Once the gamma chain occurs, hemoglobin Barts (gamma × 4) evolves from all the unpaired gamma chains. This has such high oxygen affinity that although blood reaches the tissues, almost no oxygen is released, and the fetus dies from anemia and congestive heart failure (hydrops fetalis).

Alpha$^+$ thalassemia has one active gene and one inactive gene and is designated alpha–. Heterozygosity for this condition is designated alpha–/alpha alpha, and homozygosity alpha–/alpha–. Alpha° and alpha$^+$ complex heterozygotes can also exist (alpha–/– –). This condition

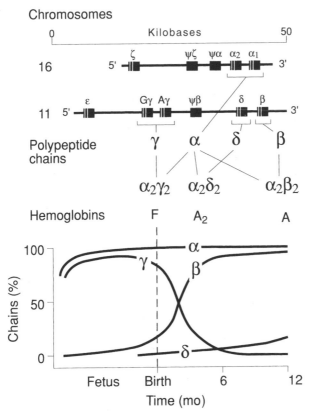

FIGURE 3–4. Changes in hemoglobin with development. Sequential suppression and activation of individual globin genes in the immediate postnatal period result in a switch from fetal hemoglobin (hemoglobin F: two alpha and two gamma chains) to adult hemoglobin (hemoglobin A: two alpha and two beta chains). A small amount of hemoglobin A_2 (two alpha and two delta chains) is also present in the adult. (From Hillman, RS, and Finch, CA: Red Cell Manual, ed 7. FA Davis, Philadelphia, 1996, p 11, with permission.)

produces the syndrome of hemoglobin H disease, which produces a serious, although less severe, hemolytic anemia **(thalassemia interme- dia).** Adult cells have 4 to 30% hemoglobin H; erythropoiesis is inefficient, and anemia is moderately severe. Cord blood has up to 25% hemoglobin Barts.

Heterozygotes for alpha-thalassemia have two or three functioning alpha chain genes and suffer no clinical disability (Table 3–15). In certain American black populations, as many as 2% may be heterozygous for alpha-thalassemia. The diagnosis is best made on cord blood, which has up to 5% hemoglobin Barts. Adult blood in alpha-thalassemia heterozygotes does not contain hemoglobin H, and the hematologic findings are mild and nonspecific. The red cells, however, are hypochromic and microcytic, reflecting the defective hemoglobin synthesis, and the morphology is very similar to that seen in iron deficiency anemia (see Table 3–3). Obviously, since these patients are not iron deficient, they do not respond to iron supplementation, and diagnosis can be established on family studies or more sophisticated alpha-beta synthesis tests. Occasionally, hemoglobin H bodies may be seen on supravital stain smears.

Homozygous Beta-Thalassemia   Each chromosome 11 has a single beta globin locus (see Fig. 3–4). Heterozygotes will have one affected and one normal gene. Homozygotes will have two abnormal genes, but it is possible that some limited beta gene output can occur; this is designated $beta^+$. When no beta gene product is synthesized, then the gene defect is designated $beta^\circ$.

Beta-thalassemia will not manifest itself clinically at birth since the predominant hemoglobin is hemoglobin F (alpha$_2$ gamma$_2$). When the switch to beta chain production occurs at 3 to 6 months after birth (see Fig. 3–4), the defective rate of beta synthesis manifests itself as ineffective red cell production with intramedullary hemolysis. The decreased synthesis of beta chains is partially compensated by an increase in gamma chain synthesis, producing an *elevation of hemoglobin F* (alpha$_2$ delta$_2$) and

---

TABLE 3–15. CLINICAL MANIFESTATIONS OF ALPHA-THALASSEMIA

Demographics

α° thalassemia is limited to the Mediterranean region and parts of Southeast Asia, particularly southern China, Thailand, and Vietnam.

α^+ thalassemia occurs in tropical Africa, the Middle East, parts of India, and throughout Southeast Asia.

Clinical Classification of Thalassemias

Minor: Symptomless, carrier state or trait.

Intermedia: Anemia, more severe than the anemia that may be associated with alpha-thalassemia minor.

Major: Severe anemia (e.g., α thalassemia hydrops fetalis).

Clinical Phenotypes of α Thalassemias

Hb Barts hydrops fetalis syndrome (α thalassemia hydrops fetalis)
Hb H disease
Hb Constant Spring, homozygous state
α thalassemia minor and silent carrier states

From Stomatoyannopoulos, G, et al: The Molecular Basis of Blood Diseases, ed 2. WB Saunders, Philadelphia, 1994, with permission.

an increase in delta chain synthesis, producing an *increase in hemoglobin A_2* (alpha$_2$ delta$_2$).

When both beta chain genes are defective, patients suffer from a severe, lifelong anemia called **thalassemia major (Cooley's anemia** or **Mediterranean anemia)** (Table 3–16). Hemoglobin ranges from 2 to 6 g/dL. Red cells are small, pale, and misshapen, and there is enormous hemolysis and ineffective red cell production. Reticulocytosis runs 15% or more. Nucleated red cells are numerous, and severe splenomegaly and moderate jaundice are present. As alpha chains are produced normally, there is a huge excess of alpha chains that pair with one another and form alpha tetramers. These accumulate and precipitate in the form of intracellular inclusions (Heinz bodies) that interfere with intramedullary maturation and induce intrasplenic destruction of those cells that enter the circulation. Splenectomy can permit somewhat enhanced red cell survival, but leads to an increased risk of sudden, overwhelming bacterial infections (see Color Plate 31).

The severe anemia retards growth and causes marrow expansion with skeletal abnormalities due to the widening of productive bone marrow. This is an attempt at compensatory erythroid production. The over-

TABLE 3–16. LABORATORY FINDINGS IN BETA-THALASSEMIA

	Homozygous	Heterozygous
Hemoglobin	2–6 g/dL	9–11 g/dL
RBC Morphology	Pronounced poikilocytosis Basophilic stippling Target cells Nucleated RBCs Heinz bodies	Small hypochromic cells MCH 20–22 pg MCV 50–70 fL
Reticulocytosis	≥15%	Mildly elevated
Platelets, WBCs	Low if splenomegaly present	Normal
Bone Marrow	Erythroid hyperplasia so marked that bones are deformed	Mild to moderate erythroid hyperplasia
Hemoglobin A_2	Variable	3.5–7%
Hemoglobin F	10–90% of Hgb present	Slight increase in 50% of patients
Storage Iron	Greatly increased, hemosiderosis often fatal	Normal or slightly increased

RBCs = red blood cells; WBCs = white blood cells; MCH = mean corpuscular hemoglobin; MCV = mean corpuscular volume.

whelming marrow hyperplasia is induced by exaggerated erythropoietin levels. Anemia is not the only stimulus to erythropoietin secretion. Hemoglobins F and A_2, produced to compensate for absent hemoglobin A, yield oxygen to the tissues less readily than does hemoglobin A. This leads to tissue hypoxia greater than would occur with normal hemoglobin at the same concentration. Because there is such a brisk erythropoiesis, large quantities of iron are absorbed from the gastrointestinal tract. Iron utilization, however, is poor, and large quantities of storage iron accumulate, first in the reticuloendothelial system and later in parenchymal cells, especially the cells of the heart and liver.

Current treatment strategies for severe thalassemia syndrome (major or some intermedia types) include *hypertransfusion* to suppress ineffective erythropoiesis, and *iron chelation therapy,* which is only partially effective and tedious. Transfusion therapy ameliorates the anemia and suppresses marrow hyperplasia (decreasing skeletal abnormalities) by diminishing erythropoietic production. However, each unit of red cells adds 250 mg of additional iron to the body's already excessive supply. Careful transfusion therapy can restore patients with thalassemia major to a relatively normal existence, but death usually occurs before age 20 because iron overload induces myocardial failure. Therapy with chelating agents and other drugs to mobilize iron excretion has extended the limited lifespan of these patients well into the third, and occasionally the fourth, decade. Other problems of chronic transfusion therapy also occur (see Chapter 8).

Bone marrow transplantation is being evaluated, and gene therapy is not yet practical, but both offer promise for the future.

The syndromes caused by beta$^+$ and beta$^\circ$ thalassemia genes are clinically similar, although on electrophoretic analysis they differ in the proportions of hemoglobin A_2 and F. Thalassemia caused by complete deletion of the gene segment controlling both beta and delta chain production is somewhat less disastrous. Absence of the delta-beta segment seems to allow compensatory gamma chain production, and these patients have markedly elevated hemoglobin F values. These patients also have a less severe clinical syndrome of thalassemia intermedia.

Heterozygous Beta-Thalassemia Patients with one normal and one abnormal beta chain gene have relatively few clinical problems. The laboratory findings vary, depending on which abnormal gene is present. Both beta$^+$ and beta$^\circ$ heterozygotes have hemoglobin A_2, levels raised to about 7% of total hemoglobin, and hemoglobin F is variably increased. Heterozygotes for delta-beta thalassemia have normal hemoglobin A_2, but hemoglobin F values that may constitute 5 to 20% of the total. The hemoglobin F in these syndromes is distributed heterogeneously in erythrocytes. All three types of heterozygotes manifest the syndrome of **thalassemia minor,** characterized by abnormally small, hypochromic red cells with numerous target cells, basophilic stippling, and increased resistance to osmotic lysis. Anemia, however, is mild (hemoglobin levels are usually 9 to 11 g/dL), and erythropoiesis is only mildly inefficient. If the spleen is removed, Heinz bodies become apparent in circulating red cells. Serum iron and transferrin saturations are normal, but may be elevated (see Table 3–16).

The biggest problem with thalassemia minor comes in distinguishing it from iron deficiency anemia (see Table 3–3). Both conditions cause hypochromic, microcytic anemias, often of comparable degree. Measuring serum iron level or examining the bone marrow for storage of iron allows the distinction to be made. Patients with thalassemia minor can, however, also be iron deficient. When iron levels are low, the characteristic increase in hemoglobin A_2 tends to disappear. This removes the distinctive clue for thalassemia, and the patient seems only to be iron deficient. After iron repletion, total hemoglobin fails to achieve normal values, but the abnormal hemoglobin A_2 levels return, and more complete diagnosis can be made.

Thalassemia Heterozygotes with Other Hemoglobinopathies Genes for globin chain structure and for rate of globin synthesis seem to occupy virtually the same genetic locus. It is not clear how functional distinction occurs. The result, however, is that thalassemia genes and hemoglobinopathy genes behave as alleles. The individual with a beta^s allele on one chromosome and a beta$°$-thalassemia allele on the other will have no hemoglobin A but often has more hemoglobin A_2 and F than that seen in homozygotes for hemoglobin S. Still another allele that causes gamma chain production to continue throughout adult life can be paired with normal, thalassemia, or hemoglobin variant genes. In the latter case, a heterozygous state of sickle hemoglobin and the hereditary persistence of fetal hemoglobin (HPFH) will protect the cells against many hemoglobin S-related problems, so the absence of hemoglobin A causes little difficulty. Furthermore, the finding of coexistent thalassemia genes and sickle genes is not infrequent and not surprising considering the geographic distribution of these two populations.

Acquired Thalassemia Syndromes Defects in globin chain production, involving particularly the alpha chain locus, can occur in some *myelodysplastic* and *preleukemic* syndromes (see Chapter 4). These defects may be in gene deletion or in transcription and result in defective amounts of alpha chain being synthesized by the abnormal clone. The clinical features are very similar to hemoglobin H disease, and the patient presents with a hypochromic, microcytic anemia. Bone marrow shows exuberant erythroid response with ineffective erythropoiesis. Hemoglobin electrophoresis confirms the presence of an abnormal hemoglobin, which is fast migrating in the distribution of hemoglobin H (Fig. 3–5). Hemoglobin H bodies are seen on supravital stains of the erythroid cells. This condition is usually rapidly progressive to acute leukemia. Since it is an acquired form, it can easily be distinguished by previously normal blood counts and presentation at an elderly age.

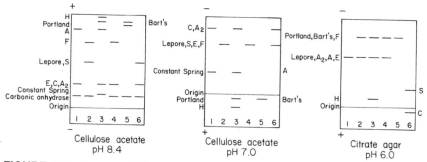

FIGURE 3–5. Diagram of the migration of different hemoglobins at different pH values. (From Harrison, CR: Thalassemia. In Harmening, DM (ed): Clinical Hematology and Fundamentals of Hemostasis, ed 3, FA Davis, Philadelphia, 1997, p 207, with permission.)

Laboratory Investigation of the Hemoglobinopathies

Although clinical features are obviously extremely important in ascertaining the nature of a chronic hemolytic anemia, laboratory tests ultimately reveal whether an abnormal hemoglobin is present and consequently define the disorder.

As with the investigation of any anemia, examination of the peripheral blood smear provides important clues in characterizing a hemoglobinopathy. Red cells are usually normochromic and normocytic, except in the thalassemia syndromes, where they are hypochromic and microcytic. Diffuse polychromatophilia, representing a reticulocytosis, is variably present. Specific morphologic changes are often present in the specific disorders. Irreversibly sickled cells may be seen in sickle cell anemia, and hemoglobin C crystals and clam-shaped cells indicate the presence of hemoglobin C (see Color Plates 10, 15, 31–33). Hemoglobin C disease is also associated with abundant target cell formation (see Color Plate 15). Target cells are also often seen in thalassemias and, in addition, basophilic stippling in this disorder gives a clue about the disordered hemoglobin production (see also Color Plate 10C). Spherocytes are usually not a feature of the hemoglobinopathies, unless splenectomy has been performed (e.g., thalassemia).

Initial laboratory tests must include documenting the presence and the degree of the hemolytic anemia, as was outlined in Chapter 2. Although hemoglobin screening tests are performed prior to genetic counseling, laboratory evaluation of hemoglobinopathies should be supported by a strong suspicion of a hemolytic anemia. In general, a bone marrow examination is not necessary. **Hemoglobin electrophoresis** on cellulose acetate, or starch gel electrophoresis at an alkaline pH of 8.6, is the most convenient laboratory test demonstrating the presence of an abnormal hemoglobin (see Fig. 3–5). Hemoglobin separated by this method may be quantified by elution and spectrophotographic analysis or densitometry scanning. Most of the more important hemoglobins are separated by this method. Unfortunately, the method does not discriminate between hemoglobins A and F, and therefore hemoglobin F must be quantitated by another method. Since hemoglobin F is acid and alkali-resistant, whereas hemoglobin A is denatured, particularly at low pHs, this forms the principle of the **acid-resistant hemoglobin assay for hemoglobin F.** Hemoglobin F can therefore be quantitated by treatment with acid, representing the resistant hemoglobin present. This test forms the basis of the **Kleihauer-Betke test** for the presence of fetal cells in the maternal circulation during pregnancy (see the section on Hemolytic Disease of the Newborn, Chapter 8).

In alpha-thalassemia, the decreased synthesis of alpha chains causes an excess of beta chains. These beta chains may form tetramers, which can easily be demonstrated on supravital staining by the presence of **hemoglobin H crystals.** They produce a "golf ball" morphologic appearance of the red cells, and this is a test for hemoglobin H inclusions. In addition, hemoglobin H migrates differently on hemoglobin electrophoresis and is one of the fast-migrating hemoglobins (see Fig. 3–5).

Clearly the position of a hemoglobin band on hemoglobin electrophoresis can direct the laboratory investigation. The presence of a hemoglobin band in a sickle position can be followed up by performing a *sickle cell screening test,* which is more commonly used prior to hemoglobin electrophoresis. The principle of this test is that a sample of blood placed on a blood smear, covered by a cover slip, and sealed with paraffin or subjected to a reducing agent such as *sodium metabisulfite* is rendered oxygen deficient. Since sickle blood is sensitive to oxygen depletion, sickle cells are formed after approximately half an hour of incubation. This is a screening test for a sickle hemoglobin, and hemoglobin S is subsequently confirmed by hemoglobin electrophoresis.

Unstable hemoglobins can be demonstrated by the presence of Heinz bodies (see Color Plate 10B) or by performing an **unstable hemoglobin test.** In most cases, unstable hemoglobins are sensitive to heat and precipitate after exposure to higher temperatures. This forms the basis of the **heat stability test.** The **isopropanol denaturation test** is another method to enable detection of unstable hemoglobins, which precipitate after exposure to this reagent. Test selection clearly must follow a pattern of suspicion, documentation of a hemolytic anemia, and, most often, the demonstration of an abnormal hemoglobin on hemoglobin electrophoresis. In most cases, more refined testing is unnecessary; however, in difficult cases, amino acid analysis and determination of the hemoglobin synthesis ratios of the alpha and non-alpha chains may be needed. Hemoglobin synthesis ratios are valuable in a research setting to confirm milder cases of thalassemia by comparing the relative synthesis of the two chains. Molecular biologic techniques are currently performed in the research setting to define DNA abnormalities or alterations of messenger RNA expression. These tools are becoming available for use in antenatal testing and may increase in applicability in the routine laboratory.

Acquired Defects

Paroxysmal Nocturnal Hemoglobinuria

This condition was already discussed in the section on Refractory Anemia and Ineffective Erythropoiesis. The condition is a clonal hematologic disorder characterized by abnormal marrow growth and membrane sensitivity to complement-mediated lysis.

EXTRINSIC HEMOLYTIC ANEMIAS

Cases of hemolysis from extracellular causes may be broadly categorized into those that are **immune-mediated** (mediated through an immune antibody) and the *nonimmune hemolytic anemias.* The immune hemolytic anemias are also discussed in Chapter 8.

Nonimmune Destruction

Erythrocytes may have a shortened intravascular survival if subjected to the harmful effects of abnormal or unusual physical or chemical stress, or forces within the circulation that may cause erythrocyte damage. The cell membrane may be damaged by heat, radiation, chemicals, enzymes, and toxins. Internal forces form within the red cells, or parasitic infestations in the erythrocyte may cause the cell to rupture. These processes are acquired hemolytic anemias that do not require the presence of or cooperation with the humoral antibody system or complement activation. The mechanisms of red cell damage are listed in Table 3–17.

Physical Trauma (Angiopathic Hemolytic Anemia)

Red cells that encounter physical obstacles within the vascular bed lose small parts of their membranes and undergo continuous reduction in their surface areas, causing a change in the surface-to-volume ratio. Cracks or other defects in prosthetic heart valves induce a chronic hemolytic process because of damage to passing red cells *(macroangiopathic hemolytic anemia).* Patients whose capillaries are partially occluded by tiny fibrin strands and clots may experience *microangiopathic hemolytic anemia (MAHA),* an acute hemolytic process in which red cells show morphologic evidence of fragmentation. These *schistocytes* are fragments of red cells produced by the mechanical injury as cells pass through and are "chopped" and destroyed (see Color Plate 16). Microangiopathic hemolytic anemia occurs particularly in conditions associated with the syndrome of *disseminated intravascular coagulation (DIC),* where there is a diffuse intravascular clotting process with deposition of fibrin strands (see Chapter 6). Microangiopathic hemolytic anemia also occurs in the rare disorder *thrombotic thrombocytopenic*

TABLE 3–17. EXTRACORPUSCULAR (NONIMMUNE) MECHANISMS CAUSING HEMOLYTIC ANEMIA

Mechanism	Pathogenesis
Mechanical pressure	
In heart and great vessels	Artificial valves
In microcirculation	Hemolytic uremic syndrome (HUS)
	Thrombotic thrombocytopenic purpura (TTP)
	Disseminated intravascular coagulation (DIC)
Membrane disorders	
Loss of membrane	Hypersplenism
Lipid peroxidation	Oxidant drugs
Lipid dissolution	*Clostridium perfringens (Welchii)*
Thermal damage	Burns
Intracellular pressure	
Parasites	Malaria
Water (osmotic)	Drowning
Altered energy production	Lead poisoning

purpura (TTP) (also in Chapter 6). Hemolysis is an integral part of this syndrome and occurs as a result of mechanical fragmentation within the microcirculation.

Typically, in the syndromes of MAHA, the platelet count is often decreased, whereas in fragmentation associated with prosthetic valves, the platelet count is normal. Thrombocytopenia and MAHA also occur in *hemolytic uremic syndrome,* another condition, characterized by renal insufficiency. Microangiopathic hemolytic anemia may also occur in association with some epithelial malignancies, particularly gastric carcinoma, and following drug therapy with the agent mitomycin-C.

A mild mechanical hemolytic state may occur in long distance runners or those who have been marching strenuously. The hemolysis results from repetitive traumatic stress exerted upon the vascular channels of the foot. Called *march hemoglobinuria,* it also can occur with karate exercises and bongo drumming. In most of these conditions, plasma haptoglobin declines and plasma-free hemoglobin accumulates. The urine may contain free hemoglobin and, in chronic intravascular hemolytic states, contains the iron-containing compound hemosiderin.

Chemical and Toxic Agents

Thermal Damage Severe burns cause thermal damage to red cells circulating at the time of injury. As many as 20 to 30% of the red cells may be lysed within the first 24 to 48 hours, leading to massive hemoglobinemia and hemoglobinuria. Clinically, this may be disastrous because it contributes to the renal damage initiated by the blood pressure changes, fluid loss, and circulation of other cellular breakdown products, in particular myoglobin.

Drugs and Chemicals　Most drug-related hemolysis has an immune basis (see Chapter 8), or produces hemolysis in G-6-PH-deficient patients (discussed earlier). Some agents, however, damage red cells directly. Accidental introduction of distilled water into the circulation causes rapid osmotic lysis. Arsene gas, sometimes generated during industrial processes, causes severe hemolysis, as do copper salts.

Oxidizing drugs, notably nitrites, nitrates, and aromatic amino and nitroso compounds, cause methemoglobinemia and, in severe cases, red cell destruction as well.

Hemolysis Associated with Infection

Malaria is the most dramatic and most common infectious cause of intravascular hemolysis. The protozoan ruptures red cells as part of its life cycle. The periodic chills and fever that characterize the disease occur as parasitized erythrocytes burst to release a new generation of organisms. The attachment of the parasite to erythrocytes, and its subsequent ability to enter the red cell, depends on normal cell membrane structures, in particular glycophorin, and the Duffy antigen system (see Chapter 8). Erythrocytes lacking the Duffy antigen fail to be parasitized by *Plasmodium vivax.* Hemolytic anemia in malaria occurs because of mechanical rupture by the parasite but can also occur in association with immunologic mechanisms *(Blackwater fever).* Malarial infection is also discussed in Chapter 13.

Hemolysis can also occur due to parasitization by the protozoan *Babesia,* which has been reported from Nantucket Island off the New England coast of the United States (babesiosis). Other infectious diseases causing hemolytic anemia include clostridial infections, in which lecithinase enzymes damage the lipids of the red cell membrane and may lead to massive hemolysis, sometimes complicating fatal septic episodes. Hemolysis is also produced by organisms such as the *Streptococcus* species and *Hemophilus influenzae.* A toxin produced by the bite of the brown recluse spider produces acute hemolysis of a milder sort, possibly mediated through a hypersensitivity reaction.

Hypersplenism

The normal spleen destroys red cells as they age at the rate of 1/120 of the circulating cells each day. Abnormal red cells undergo accelerated destruction in passing through a normal spleen. By contrast, an abnormally large spleen tends to destroy excessive numbers of red cells, even perfectly normal cells. Any condition that increases spleen size can shorten red cell survival; white cells and platelets may also be affected. These conditions include liver disease with portal hypertension, chronic congestive heart failure, infiltrative diseases such as leukemias and lymphomas, and protozoal infections such as schistosomiasis. All of these may increase spleen size, leading to increased red cell sequestration and decreased red cell survival. Thus, **hypersplenism** is the sequestration of cells by the spleen in conditions associated with an increasing spleen size.

Systemic Disorders Associated with Nonimmune Hemolytic Anemia

Lipid Disorders   Alterations in blood lipid concentrations can produce abnormalities of the erythrocyte membrane lipid composition. This produces shortened red cell survival in a condition called **spur cell anemia.** In hyperlipidemia and liver disease, the peripheral blood shows abundant, sharp, spiculated red cells, or *Zieve's syndrome.* In another condition associated with lipid disorders, **abetalipoproteinemia,** or **hereditary acanthocytosis,** the red cells show multiple, blunted projections in association with a very low blood cholesterol. This is due to the deficiency of the blood transport protein betalipoprotein (a betalipoproteinemia). These individuals may have a concomitant hemolytic anemia.

Renal Disease   Abnormal capillaries in renal glomerular disease can cause mechanical distortion of red cells as they flow through these channels. Typically, in renal disease, the erythrocytes show burr cell formation. Fibrin deposition in the glomerular channels is associated with MAHA.

Immune-Mediated Hemolytic Anemia

Immune-mediated red cell destruction occurs as a result of specific antibody attack against the antigens on the erythrocyte membrane and results in membrane damage and lysis of the cell. This hemolysis may occur *intravascularly* or *extravascularly,* depending on the nature of the immune antibody and whether or not complement is activated. The characteristics of anti-erythrocyte antibodies are discussed in Chapter 8. These compounds are gammaglobulin proteins that are produced by a stimulating antigen. Antibodies can be directed against antigens on red cells, white cells, or platelets, or against protein constituents. These antibodies are capable of producing hemolytic disease—for example, when an individual with preformed natural antibodies or immune antibodies is exposed to foreign red cells, as occurs with an incompatible blood transfusion. When preformed antibodies are directed against erythrocytes from another member of the same species, the process is called *alloimmunity.* The antibodies produced are termed *alloantibodies.* In a hemolytic transfusion reaction, antibodies in the recipient's circulation rapidly destroy transfused cells as they enter the bloodstream. Antibodies against A and B antigens usually cause prompt intravascular hemolysis with rapid liberation of free hemoglobin. Rh antibodies against

Rh antigens, and many other antibodies, attach themselves to the surface of circulating red cells, causing the antibody-coated cells to be removed in the spleen *(extravascular hemolysis).*

Clinical complications from both types of hemolysis include shock, coagulation abnormalities, and renal failure, but the severity of clinical response varies astonishingly among different patients exposed to the same immunologic situations. Diagnosis depends on documenting that the transfused cells possess an antigen to which the patient has a specific antibody directed, thus causing RBC destruction (see Chapter 8). The types of immune hemolytic anemia are listed in Table 3–18.

Autoimmune Hemolytic Anemia (AIHA)

Autoimmune hemolytic anemia occurs when the patient develops antibodies directed against antigens present on the *patient's own erythrocytes,* producing shortened red cell survival. The reasons for this autodestructive phenomenon are not understood. The cell surface characteristics may be modified sufficiently by a virus or a drug that appears "foreign" to the host's immune system. Autoimmune phenomena often accompany other diseases, notably collagen vascular diseases, chronic lymphocytic leukemias and lymphomas, and some non-hematologic solid tumor malignancies. In addition, autoantibodies may accompany several infectious processes such as infectious mononucleosis, mycoplasma, pneumonia, syphilis, and other viral syndromes such as rubella and varicella. The clinical conditions associated with autoimmune hemolysis may be classified as primary (idiopathic), where there is no apparent cause, or secondary, where associated diseases are present.

In many instances, drugs may be incriminated in the development of autoantibodies directed to the red cell (see Table 3–18). The drug may complex with a preformed antibody in the patient's plasma-binding complement, which destroys the red cells by an *innocent bystander* or paraphenomenon. Complement is secondarily adsorbed onto the red cell membrane, which is subsequently destroyed. Drugs eliciting hemolysis through this mechanism include *quinidine* and *quinine derivatives.* Three types of drug-induced hemolysis may occur; two are illustrated in Figure 3–6.

The drug may combine with the red cell membrane and is itself altered or alters the erythrocyte membrane, rendering it foreign to the host *(hapten mechanism).* An antibody response then is elicited against the erythrocyte, producing erythrocyte damage or sequestration. Drugs of the *penicillin* class are more commonly associated with this type of hemolytic mechanism.

Occasionally a true immune response against the drug occurs that in some way cross-reacts with the erythrocyte membrane antigens. The immune response does not require the presence of the drug once the antibody is formed, and a cycle of erythrocyte destruction can then ensue. This true immune type of drug-induced hemolysis occurs with the antihypertensive alpha-methyldopa (Aldomet) and L-dopa.

TABLE 3–18. CLASSIFICATION OF THE CAUSES OF IMMUNE HEMOLYTIC ANEMIAS

	Antibody	Thermal Range of Antibody	Antibody Specificity
Autoimmune			
Primary/Idiopathic	IgG	W	Panspecific
Infections			
Mycoplasma pneumoniae	IgM	C	Anti-I
Epstein-Barr viral syndrome (infectious mononucleosis)	IgM	C	Anti-i
Varicella, rubella	IgG	C/W	Anti-P
Syphilis	IgG	C/W	Anti-P
Neoplasms			
Carcinomas, lymphomas, and chronic lymphocytic leukemia	IgG, IgM (occasionally)	W, C	Panspecific (usually), I/i/other
Collagen vascular disease (lupus erythematosus, etc.)	IgG	W	Panspecific
Drugs			
Quinidine/quinine group	Immune complexes	W	Nonspecific
Penicillin group	Haptenic IgG	W	Panspecific
Aldomet, L-Dopa	IgG	W	Panspecific
Alloimmune			
Hemolytic transfusion reactions	IgM & IgG	C or W	Specific*
Hemolytic disease of the newborn	IgG	W	Specific*

W = warm; C = cold.
*Differing specificities.

Thus, autoimmune hemolytic anemias may be classified according to their cause—primary, secondary, or drug-induced. Another classification of immune-mediated red cell destruction is based on the specific characteristics of the antibody. It is customary to classify AIHA by the thermal optimum of the antibody as determined by serologic testing (see

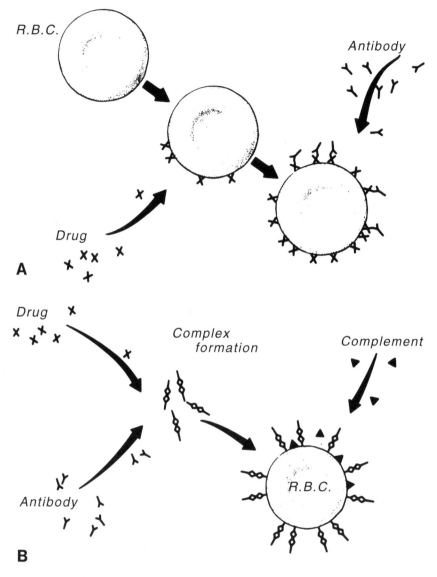

FIGURE 3–6. Two mechanisms of drug-induced hemolysis. *(A)* Drug adsorption mechanism. Antidrug antibody binds with drug bound to the red cell surface. Antidrug antibody does not bind to "drug-free" red cells. *(B)* Immune complex mechanism. Complexes of the drug and antidrug antibody attach to the red cell surface, where they initiate complement activation. (From AABB Technical Manual, ed 9. American Association of Blood Banks, Bethesda, MD, 1985, pp 258–259, with permission.)

Chapter 8). *Warm antibodies* are usually clinically significant at temperatures greater than 30°C. *Cold antibodies* have a thermal optimum between room temperature (22°C) and 4°C.

Warm Autoimmune Hemolytic Anemia Warm AIHA is more common and causes more severe problems than the cold variety. Intravascular lysis does not occur; instead, cells that are coated with antibody circulate and are prematurely removed by the spleen. The rate of splenic destruction varies with the specificity and concentration of the antibody, the presence or absence of complement attachment, and the functional capacity of the spleen. Autoimmune hemolysis can range from a mild, compensated condition with normal hemoglobin levels to a severe anemia compromising life. The laboratory findings in this condition would include a severe anemia, often an elevated mean cell volume reflecting a high percentage of young erythrocytes (reticulocytes), hyperbilirubinemia of the indirect or unconjugated variety, an elevated lactate dehydrogenase, and decreased haptoglobin. Hemoglobinemia and hemoglobinuria are extremely uncommon in warm autoimmune hemolytic anemia. The *antiglobulin test (direct Coombs test)* will establish the presence of an antibody coating the red cells and facilitate the diagnosis of an immune hemolysis. The nature of the antibody and the thermal characteristics are then evaluated, usually in the blood bank (see Antiglobulin Testing in Chapter 8). Diagnosis depends on demonstrating the presence of antibody or complement on the circulating red cells using the antiglobulin test. Antibody sometimes exists free in the serum, but this is not necessary to diagnose AIHA. The clinical syndromes associated with warm AIHA include the secondary causes discussed above, such as collagen vascular disease or lymphomas, drugs, and occasionally infections. Many cases of warm AIHA are idiopathic. Occasionally a patient may develop a characteristic clinical syndrome of warm autoimmune hemolytic anemia, but the direct antiglobulin test and serum screen are negative. In these patients, a highly avid antibody may produce rapid clearance of red cells, and yet may be undetectable because of decreased sensitivity of the antiglobulin reagent. These cases are called *Coombs-negative immune-mediated hemolytic anemia.*

Corticosteroid treatment is usually instituted for warm AIHA. Responses to be assessed include an increasing hematocrit, decreasing reticulocyte count, bilirubin, and LDH. The direct antiglobulin test may remain positive well after the disease is under control.

The finding of a positive direct antiglobulin test in a patient who is otherwise clinically stable and is not anemic does not warrant treatment unless other laboratory parameters indicate hemolysis or symptomatic anemia increases. Very few patients with Aldomet-associated positive AHG tests have significant hemolysis despite the undoubted presence of immunoglobulin on the red cell surface, and fewer still become anemic. In most of the other drug-related hemolytic conditions, antibody is directed against drugs rather than against cells, and in these cases treatment is specifically aimed at elimination of the drug. Furthermore, hemolysis (if it occurs) is associated with the presence of the drug.

Cold Autoantibody Hemolytic Syndromes　Antibodies reactive only at low temperatures cause no clinical problems at the usual body temperatures. Cold autoantibodies that cause clinical illness may work best at 25°C, 18°C, or 4°C, but retain some activity at 37°C. These cold antibodies may also be of clinical importance in patients undergoing heart procedures with the use of cold solutions for cardioplegia. Most cold antibodies activate the complement sequence when they combine with antigen, and it is complement that actually damages the circulating cells. Very rarely, powerful cold-reacting antibodies cause agglutination in the cooler superficial parts of the vascular bed such as the fingers and toes, or with open-heart procedures. This phenomenon may produce the clinical syndrome of **acral cyanosis** and may be associated with ischemia to the hands and vasospasm (Raynaud's phenomenon). Cold antibody-induced hemolysis may be chronic or episodic, but hemoglobin levels rarely fall below 8 or 9 g/dL and often remain within the normal range. Symptomatic cold AIHA is relatively rare, usually occurring after viral infections, in particular in association with *Mycoplasma pneumoniae* (anti-i antibody) or *infectious mononucleosis* (anti-i antibody) (see Table 3–18). Spontaneous or idiopathic cold agglutinin disease sometimes occurs in elderly people. It may be necessary for them to wear gloves, avoid cold exposure, or move to warmer climates, but the disease is usually not life threatening.

Cold Agglutinin Disease　This disorder is due to monoclonal auto-antibody directed against erythrocyte antigens and reactive at low temperatures. The antibody is usually an IgM antibody and more commonly exhibits the kappa light chain type. This syndrome may be idiopathic or secondary, particularly in association with lymphoprolifera-tive disorders. Hemolysis is usually mild and self-limiting. The direct antiglobulin test usually shows the presence of complement only on the erythrocyte membrane, and hemolysis, when it occurs, is usually intravascular. Occasionally chronic intravascular hemolysis may occur, producing hemosiderin in the urine and even iron deficiency anemia.

Paroxysmal Cold Hemoglobinuria　This condition is caused by an IgG antibody that is more reactive in the cold temperature. In actual fact, this antibody has a dual thermal optimal reactivity, reacting with erythrocytes and binding complement in the cold temperature and then completing the complement binding at body temperature, resulting in intravascular hemolysis. This type of antibody syndrome is seen, particularly in viral infections, and was formerly more commonly seen in association with syphilis. Hemolysis may be severe, producing hemoglobinemia and hemoglobinuria following cold exposure on return to warm tempera-tures. The direct antiglobulin test usually shows the presence of complement only on the red cell membrane, and the biphasic nature of the antibody and antibody characteristics can be demonstrated by the Donath-Landsteiner test. Usually these IgG antibodies have specificity for the P blood group system (see also Chapter 8 for serologic techniques and a description of the antiglobulin test).

ERYTHROCYTOSIS

The foregoing discussion concentrated on erythrocyte disorders, in which the ultimate effect was a decrease in erythrocytes in the circulating blood. Certain conditions are also associated with an excess production of red cells, termed *erythrocytosis.* In *primary* erythrocytosis, an uncontrolled growth of red cells produces an excess for no apparent purpose. The main condition associated with this problem is *polycythemia vera,* which will be discussed in Chapter 4. In other instances, an excess erythroid mass is appropriate; it is stimulated by erythropoietin because of decreased oxygen tension. Conditions such as chronic hypoxia, respiratory or cardiovascular disease, living at high altitudes, or high-affinity hemoglobins that fail to deliver oxygen to the tissues may all stimulate excess red cell production. This is considered an appropriate response because there is an increased demand for red cells due to deficient oxygen delivery. These conditions will also be mentioned in Chapter 4. Table 3–19 lists the differential diagnosis of erythrocytosis.

DISORDERS OF HEME SYNTHESIS: PORPHYRIAS

Porphyrin metabolism has been discussed in the section on heme synthesis (Chapter 2). Porphyrins are an integral part of the hemoglobin molecule, with four porphyrin rings between which iron is suspended to produce *heme. Porphyrias* are diseases in which there is usually a genetically acquired inborn error of metabolism associated with impairment or deficiencies of enzymes involved in the porphyrin-heme biosynthetic pathway. Deficiencies of these crucial enzymes are associated with an excessive build-up of the precursor compounds, which produce the biochemical abnormalities and clinical features characteristic of this group of diseases. The major precursors that accumulate and are excreted in excess include the compounds *delta-aminolevulinic acid (ALA)* and *porphobilinogen (PBG),* or the later porphyrin compounds (*uroporphyrin, coproporphyrin,* and *protoporphyrin*). Increased levels of these compounds can be detected variably in the plasma, in the urine, or in the stools, either between or during attacks.

TABLE 3-19. DIFFERENTIAL DIAGNOSIS OF ERYTHROCYTOSIS

Primary Polycythemia
Polycythemia vera
Secondary Polycythemia
Appropriate increase in erythropoietin secondary to tissue hypoxia
  High altitude
  Chronic pulmonary disease
  Cyanotic congenital heart disease
  Low cardiac output states
  Hypoventilation syndromes (neuromuscular disease, pickwickian syndrome, sleep
    apnea)
  High-affinity hemoglobin variants
  Methemoglobin variants
  Carboxyhemoglobinemia
Inappropriate increase in erythropoietin
  Neoplasms (hypernephroma, hepatoma, uterine myoma, cerebellar hemangioblastoma,
    pheochromocytoma)
  Renal artery stenosis
  Renal transplantation
  Renal cysts
  Hydronephrosis
Relative Erythrocytosis
Dehydration and other secondary causes of volume depletion
Gaisböck's syndrome (stress erythrocytosis)

From Pittiglio, DH, and Sacher, RA: Clinical Hematology and Fundamentals of Hemostasis. FA Davis, Philadelphia, 1987, p 183, with permission.

GENETIC PORPHYRIAS

The patterns of excretion of these compounds are useful in the diagnosis of the different porphyrias, but it is the clinical expression of these syndromes that is most important in diagnosing the type of porphyria. The clinical manifestations may be neurologic (excruciating pain and other neurologic symptoms), cutaneous (particularly cutaneous blisters and solar sensitivity), or hepatic. Major clinical syndromes are called *acute intermittent porphyria (AIP), porphyria variegata (PV),* and *porphyria cutanea tarda (PCT).* The latter is an acquired porphyria, particularly seen in alcoholics (see later in this section). Other, unusual types are the *erythropoietic porphyrias* and *hereditary coproporphyria.* Table 3–20 lists these disorders and the compounds that are present in excess in asymptomatic periods and during acute attacks.

One of the many implications of diagnosing these disorders is that the clinical features can be prevented, since the acute attacks are precipitated

TABLE 3–20. CLASSIFICATION OF DISORDERS OF PORPHYRIN METABOLISM

	Erythrocyte			Urine				Feces		
	UP	CP	PP	ALA	PBG	UP	CP	UP	CP	PP
Acute intermittent porphyria (AIP)	N	N	N	LI	LI	—	I,N	N	N	N
Hereditary coproporphyria	N	N	N	—	—	N	—	N	—	N
Variegate porphyria (acute attacks)	N	N	N	—	—	I,N	I,N	N	—	LI
Congenital erythropoietic porphyria	LI	LI	—	N	N	LI	—	N	—	N
Erythropoietic protoporphyria	N	N	LI	N	N	N	N	N	—	—
Symptomatic porphyria	N	N	N	N	N	LI	—	N	I,N	I,N
Lead poisoning	N	I,N	—	I	I,N	N	—	N	N	N

UP = uroprophyrin; CP = coproporphyrin; PP = protoporphyrin; N = normal; I = increased; LI = large increase; I,N = increase or normal.

From Henry, JB: Clinical Diagnosis and Management by Laboratory Methods, ed 17. WB Saunders, Philadelphia, 1985, p 144, with permission.

by exposure to certain drugs, particularly of the barbiturate and sulfonamide classes. Individuals with a history of porphyria must not be given these drugs.

Laboratory evaluation is usually performed in patients who have unusual neurologic manifestations, particularly unexplained abdominal pain or cutaneous blisters. Often a family history warrants laboratory assessment for the presence of abnormal or excess porphyrins. Assays of these porphyrin compounds are not available in smaller laboratories and are often done by a reference laboratory. The assay systems are fairly simple, using either Ehrlich's reagent (hydrochloric acid and a benzaldehyde indicator), which turns a magenta color with porphyrins, or the fluorescent properties of these compounds. During the acute attack, the urinary concentrations of ALA and PBG increase in AIP and PV. In PV excessive amounts of coproporphyrins are present in the stools of affected patients (see Table 3–20). These porphyrins produce a characteristic reddish-brown (port wine) color to the urine when they are present in excess quantities. They also give a characteristic pinkish fluorescence in the presence of ultraviolet light. The diagnosis may be made on a 24-hour collected urine sample that shows excessive amounts of these porphyrin pigments in the urine. Reference values for urinary ALA are 1.5 to 7.5 mg/24 hours and for PBG, <1.0 mg/24 hours. Stools should contain <500 g of coproporphyrin per 24-hour collection (see also Chapter 19).

ACQUIRED PORPHYRIAS

Acquired disturbances of porphyrin metabolism may occur with lead poisoning. This has already been discussed in the section dealing with sideroblastic anemias (see also Table 3–5). Lead interferes with several enzymes in the porphyrin biosynthetic pathway, and the precursor porphyrin accumulates in excess. Typically, elevated levels of ALA occur in the plasma and are excreted in the urine. In addition, urinary coproporphyrins are also present in excess in a 24-hour collected sample. In the acquired porphyria, *porphyria cutanea tarda*, alcohol is also associated with acute exacerbations. Alcohol is believed to interfere with enzymes later on in the porphyrin biosynthetic pathway and is associated with an excessive build-up of some of the earlier porphyrins.

SYNDROMES OF IRON OVERLOAD

Hemochromatosis is an inherited disorder causing increased gastrointestinal iron absorption and systemic iron overload. Daily iron absorption increases by 100 to 300%, an extra 1 to 3 mg per day. Over many years this translates into total iron stores between 15 and 50 g, compared to normal iron stores of only 500 to 1500 mg. About 20 g of excess iron is associated with tissue damage, producing the clinical spectrum of hemochromatosis.

The basic defect in hereditary hemochromatosis is unknown, but it is the most common autosomal recessive disease in humans, with a frequency of homozygosity in about 3/1000 persons of Central and Northern European ancestry. The gene for hemochromatosis, HLA-H (HFE), appears to be closely linked to the HLA-A on the short arm of chromosome 6. The co-association with HLA-A3 is found in 74% of patients, and the association with HLA-B14 or HLA-B7 is due to the linkage with HLA-A3. It is likely that most cases of primary iron overload in Caucasian populations are due to homozygosity for HLA-H. Heterozygotes are generally asymptomatic although body iron stores may be elevated. The term *hemosiderosis* refers to a condition in which there is *secondary iron accumulation* in association with thalassemia, sideroblastic anemia, multiple blood transfusions, or excessive iron consumption (as originally described in South African blacks who drank homemade beer produced in iron kettles). Tissue iron in these conditions appears to be distributed differently. Hemochromatosis is associated with iron deposition in liver parenchymal cells, whereas in the syndromes of secondary iron overload or hemosiderosis, excess iron occurs in parenchymal cells and Kupffer cells in the portal tract.

Clinical manifestations include the classical triad of *bronze skin, diabetes,* and *cirrhosis.* Other common clinical symptoms include arthritis and sexual dysfunction. Many patients may have subclinical homozygous disease with limited clinical or laboratory abnormalities. The full manifestations of this syndrome are abbreviated in women owing to the normal physiological losses of iron in monthly menstruation and pregnancy.

The most common laboratory findings in hemochromatosis are an increased serum iron concentration, a high percentage saturation of transferrin, and an elevated serum ferritin concentration. Heterozygotes may have values that are intermediate between the normal reference ranges and the values of homozygous individuals. Affected individuals also have abnormal glucose tolerance.

The most useful screening test is the demonstration of greater than 60% saturation of transferrin on two occasions. Liver biopsy, however, is the definitive test. Patients suspected of having hemochromatosis should undergo a liver biopsy for quantitative estimation of iron overload on both examination of a Prussian blue stain as well as atomic absorption spectroscopy providing for quantitative iron analysis. From the latter value, a hepatic iron index may be calculated (Table 3–21).

The prognosis of hemochromatosis depends upon the extent of disease. Therapy simply requires frequent phlebotomy to deplete hemoglobin iron and consequently diminish excessive iron stores. The frequency of phlebotomy is titrated according to patient tolerance and the desire to expeditiously remove iron. In this manner, progressive liver disease, glucose intolerance, and cardiac function can be improved, but there

TABLE 3-21. HEMOCHROMATOSIS: DIAGNOSTIC CRITERIA

Screening Tests

Blood Tests Reflecting Iron Stores
Transferrin saturation > 60%
Elevated Serum Ferritin Concentration
>350 µg/L in men
>150 µg/L in women

Proof of Diagnosis

Liver Biopsy
Assessment of stainable hepatocellular iron (grades 3 or 4)
Hepatic iron concentration (µmols Fe/g dry wt)
Hepatic iron index: Iron concentration ÷ Age
    >2 indicative of homozygous state
    <2 heterozygote, normal, or alcoholic liver disease
Demonstration of Homozygosity for HLA-H (HFE) gene

Adapted from Powell, LW: Hemachromatosis. In Rakel, RE: Conn's Current Therapy. WB Saunders, Philadelphia, 1994, p 381.

appears to be very little reduction of the incidence of arthritis or sexual dysfunction. An increased life-long risk of hepatocellular carcinoma remains. On initial diagnosis, a baseline *serum alpha fetoprotein* should be determined, which can serve as a monitoring parameter for early liver-cancer detection.

SUGGESTED READING

Beutler, E: Glucose 6-phosphate dehydrogenase deficiency: Population genetics and clinical manifestations. Blood Rev 10:45, 1996.

Cooper, BA, and Rosenblatt, DS: Disorders of cobalamin and folic acid metabolism. In Handin, RI, Lux, SE, and Stossel, TP (eds): Basic Principles and Practice of Hematology. JB Lippincott, Philadelphia, 1995, pp 1399–1432.

Cooper, BA, Rosenblatt, DS, and Whitehead, V: Megaloblastic anemias. In Nathan, DG, and Oski, FA: Hematology of Infancy and Childhood. WB Saunders, Philadelphia, 1993, p 354.

Edwards, CO, and Kushner, JP: Screening for hemochromatosis. N Engl J Med 325:1616–1620, 1993.

Finch, CA, and Cook, JD: Iron deficiency. Am J Clin Nutr 39:471, 1985.

Green, R: Metabolite assays in cobalamin and folate deficiencies. Bailliere's Clin Hematol 8:533, 1995.

Higgs, DR, and Weatherall, DJ (eds): The haemoglobinopathies. Bailliere's Clin Haematol, ed 6. WB Saunders, London, 1993.

Hillman, RS, and Finch, CA: Red Cell Manual, ed 7. FA Davis, Philadelphia, 1996.

Kazazian, HH, Jr: The thalassemia syndromes: Molecular basis and prenatal diagnosis. Seminars Haematol 27:209, 1990.

Liu, SC, and Derrick, LH: Molecular anatomy of the red blood cell membrane skeleton: Structure-junction relationships. Semin Hematol 29:231–243, 1992.

Moore, MR, et al: Disorders of Porphyrin Metabolism. Plenum, New York, 1987.

Oski, FA: Iron deficiency in infancy and childhood. N Engl J Med 329:190, 1993.

Palek, J, and Jarolim, P: Clinical expression and laboratory detection of red cell membrane protein mutations. Semin Hematol 30:249, 1993.

Powell, LW: Hemochromatosis. In Rakel, RE (ed): Conn's Current Therapy. WB Saunders, Philadelphia, 1994, p 381.

Sassa, S, and Kappas, A: Disorders of heme production and catabolism. In Handin, RI, Lux, SE, and Stossel, TP (eds): Basic Principles and Practice of Hematology. JB Lippincott, Philadelphia, 1995.

Stabler, SP, et al: Clinical spectrum and diagnosis of cobalamin deficiency. Blood 75:871, 1990.

Stomatoyannopoulos, G, et al: The Molecular Basis of Blood Diseases, ed 2. WB Saunders, Philadelphia, 1994.

Witte, DL, et al: Practice guideline development task force for the College of American Pathologists: Hereditary hemochromatosis. Clin Chem Acta 245:139, 1996.

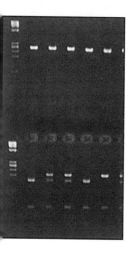

4

Diseases of White Blood Cells

CLASSIFICATION OF NONCLONAL AND CLONAL LEUKOCYTE DISEASES

An approach to the classification of leukocyte disorders is presented here. The classification is not meant to be all-inclusive but is organized to allow for an easier understanding of these complex disorders. Any classification is arranged so that the disorders are in categories that have a similar derivation, natural history, prognosis, and therapy.

Leukocytes are heterogeneous cells that have markedly different functions. Despite this, they are derived from a common stem cell that differentiates (matures) to allow these functions to be performed. The disease presentation of many of the disorders of white cells depends on which cellular precursor is involved and the degree of differentiation of the cells. There is naturally a spectrum of clinical presentations that may overlap considerably. Because common cell lines are often involved, presenting symptoms, such as failure of bone marrow function causing anemia, infection, and thrombocytopenic bleeding, may be similar. Also, because leukocytes migrate to many areas of the body, their presentations may be focal, involving specific organ systems, or reflect a more diffuse disease. An understanding of the classification of the disorders of white blood cells is made easier by referring to Color Plate 1, which outlines normal leukocyte differentiation.

White cell diseases may be classified according to whether they are clonal or nonclonal (Table 4–1). The *clonal* disorders are derived from a single precursor cell with all the affected cells (progeny) showing features of derivation from the precursor cell. The conditions included in this category are the acute and chronic myeloproliferative disorders, the acute and chronic lymphoproliferative disorders, and the myelodysplasias. Tissue macrophages, although ultimately derived from bone marrow, participate in nonhematologic conditions such as lipid and carbohydrate storage diseases, as well as participating in the lymphoreticular disorders, notably lymphomas and certain leukemias. Similarly, lymphocytes and plasma cells are intimately involved in immunologic functions, and some diseases of these cells are also clonal diseases. These conditions will be considered under the section on Immunoproliferative Disorders and Plasma Cell Dyscrasias.

TABLE 4–1. CLASSIFICATION OF DISEASES OF WHITE BLOOD CELLS

Disorders of Leukocyte Function

Neutrophils
  Chemotaxis and phagocytosis
  Chronic granulomatous disease
  Chediak-Higashi syndrome
  Myeloperoxidase deficiency
Disorders of lymphocyte-monocyte and macrophage function

Non-neoplastic (Nonclonal) Quantitative Disorders

Neutropenia
Agranulocytosis
Leukemoid reactions
Infectious mononucleosis

Clonal Neoplastic Disorders of Leukocytes

Myeloproliferative disorders
  Acute myeloproliferative disorders (acute nonlymphocytic leukemias) (see Table 4–9)
  Chronic myeloproliferative disorders (see Table 4–7)
  Myelodysplastic syndromes (see Table 4–8)
Lymphoproliferative disorders
  Acute lymphoblastic leukemia
  Leukemic chronic lymphoproliferative disorders
  Non-Hodgkin's lymphoma
  Hodgkin's lymphoma
Immunoproliferative diseases
  Waldenström's macroglobulinemia
  Multiple myeloma
  Monoclonal gammopathy of undetermined significance
  Amyloidosis primary
  Heavy chain disease

The other major category of disorders of white cells are the *nonclonal conditions*. These include **growth regulation abnormalities** (cyclic and constitutional neutropenias); **leukemoid reactions** (increased proliferative responses to various stimuli), including bone marrow aplasia and hypoplasia; and the **qualitative leukocyte disorders** (inherited or acquired), characterized by deficiencies of leukocyte function involving the differentiated cells. The functional impairment of leukocytes often can be identified by studies available only in the research setting or specialized laboratory, but the quantitative reduction of cell populations or morphologic abnormalities reflecting clonal expansion are readily appreciated by routine hematologic testing (CBC). Marker studies identifying the cells of origin and whether or not these disorders are clonal are now routine.

NONCLONAL DISEASES OF LEUKOCYTES

DISORDERS OF LEUKOCYTE FUNCTION

Neutrophils

Neutrophils are especially effective defenders against microbiologic agents, principally bacteria. Granulocytes are motile, accumulating at sites of injury in response to chemotactic stimuli (as discussed in Chapter 2). Their range of functional activities includes phagocytosis, enzymatic reactions inside the cell, and release of enzymes to the extracellular environment. Antibacterial defense requires adequate numbers of neutrophils, effective mechanisms to attract them to the site of invasion (chemotaxis), and the ability of the neutrophils to engulf (phagocytosis) and destroy the invaders. Any defects in neutrophil numbers, in chemotaxis, or in bacterial killing activity will render the host abnormally susceptible to infection. Table 4–2 lists some of the constitutional and acquired problems that affect neutrophil activity.

Defective Chemotaxis
Chemotaxis is the ability of neutrophils to be attracted to areas of infection and inflammation, where they are most needed to fight infection or remove debris. Deficient numbers of neutrophils at these sites are most commonly associated with neutropenia, which is discussed later. In some conditions, attraction fails because of deficient attractants (e.g., complement deficiencies, especially C5a), or the neutrophils may fail to respond to these attractants, as may occur with several primary or secondary disorders (see Table 4–2).

TABLE 4–2. SELECTED DEFECTS IN NEUTROPHIL FUNCTION

Defects in Migration Cascade

Congenital complement deficiencies
Decreased generation of chemotactic factors
  Congenital
  Uremia
Acquired production of chemotactic inhibitors
  Cancer
  Renal dialysis
  Chronic infection
  Idiopathic (IgG)
Congenital absence of a membrane glycoprotein
"Job's syndrome": defective chemotactic response with "boils," increased IgE,
  eosinophilia, eczema
"Lazy leukocyte" syndrome: undefined neutrophil defect, resulting in reduced release
  from the marrow associated with reduced adhesion and migration

Defects in Killing Cascade

Chronic granulomatous disease
Glucose-6-phosphate dehydrogenase (G6PD) deficiency
Myeloperoxidase deficiency (increased susceptibility to *Candida* infections)
Deficiency of H_2O_2 detoxifying enzymes

Defects with Significant Influence on Both Cascades

Congenital absence of specific granules
Congenital absence of actin polymerization
Defects in microtubule assembly
Diabetes and other causes of hyperosmolality
Alcohol intoxication

Defects in Adhesion Molecules

Leukocyte adhesion deficiency, Type I (deficiency of CD11/CD18 integrin)
Leukocyte adhesion deficiency, Type II (deficiency of ligand for L selectin)

From Winkelstein, A, et al: The White Cell Manual, ed 5. FA Davis, Philadelphia, 1998, p 61, with permission.

Tests that assess chemotaxis can be performed in vivo and in vitro. The *Rebuck skin window technique* is the in vivo method. The principle of this test is to superficially abrade an area of skin. A cover slip is then placed on the denuded area, and after a predetermined period of time the cover slip is removed and stained, and the number of neutrophils is counted. The in vitro techniques assess the ability of isolated neutrophils to be attracted through a semipermeable membrane by chemoattractants. After a set period of time, the semipermeable membrane is removed and stained, and the number of neutrophils adherent to it is quantitated. Before they can phagocytose particles, granulocytes must accumulate in the area and attach to the particles. Surface adherence requires a systematic process outlined in Figure 4–1. Initially this requires expression of a family of glycoproteins called **selectins** (see Fig. 4–1[A]) followed by up-regulation of a family of surface glycoproteins (the **integrins**). One

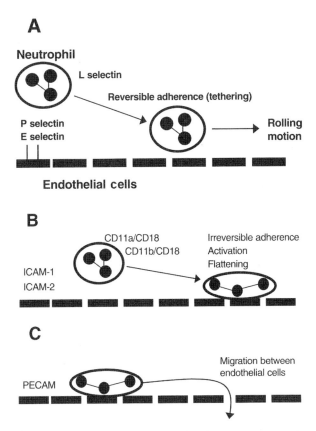

FIGURE 4–1. Stages of neutrophil adherence to vascular endothelial cells. *(A)* The initial phase consists of loose adherence (tethering), along with a rolling motion. This reversible phenomenon is mediated by the actions of the selectin molecules, L selectin on neutrophils, and P and E selectins on endothelial cells. *(B)* The second phase consists of irreversible adherence, activation, and flattening of the neutrophils. These processes are primarily due to the interactions of the integrin adhesion molecules on the neutrophil with the endothelial-cell CAM molecules. *(C)* The final phase consists of neutrophil migration between the junctions of adjacent endothelial cells. PECAM, another adhesion molecule, effects this process (see text). (From Winkelstein, A, et al: White Cell Manual, ed. 5. FA Davis, Philadelphia, 1998, p 49, with permission.)

integrin, the CD11/CD18 complex, is especially important. Neutrophils from patients with CD11/CD18 complex deficiency show poor adhesion-related functions, including a reduced capacity to exit the circulation because of an inability to adhere to vascular endothelium. Egress from the vascular system into the tissues is facilitated by adhesion molecules (e.g., PECAM—see Fig. 4–1[C]). Adhesion is enhanced if antibodies, complement proteins, or both coat the foreign particles. This process is called "opsonization." Patients with constitutional or acquired hypogamma-globulinemia lack antibodies and experience depressed neutrophilic antibacterial activity. Low complement, especially of components 3 and 5, also impairs immune adherence and response to chemotactic stimuli.

Hodgkin's disease, rheumatoid arthritis, and cirrhosis are often associated with the depressed neutrophilic function involving chemotaxis. These conditions are characterized by increased incidence of infections. Exposure to alcohol, aspirin, prednisone, and nonsteroidal anti-inflammatory agents (NSAIDs) reduces adherent properties of granulocytes. Aspirin, prednisone, and the NSAIDs are potent inhibitors of inflammation, and reduced adherence is only one of their many effects on the inflammatory process.

Defective Phagocytosis and Bacterial Killing

Phagocytosis may be assessed by exposing phagocytic cells to bacteria, fungi, latex beads, and antibody- or complement-coated particles. The engulfed particles or bacteria are then counted.

Microbial killing by phagocytic cells may be determined in the laboratory by a number of techniques, some of which were discussed in Chapter 2. Defects may initially be appreciated by examination of a peripheral blood smear, where morphologic abnormalities such as toxic granulation, Döhle bodies, intracellular organisms, vacuolization, and granule deficiency may be appreciated. The composition and functional characteristics of the granules can be assessed by a variety of cytochemical techniques and functional assays. The respiratory burst with oxidative metabolism is an important component of bacterial killing and can be assessed by the Nitroblue Tetrazolium (NBT) test. Briefly, phagocytic cells are exposed to endotoxin, which subsequently activates oxidative metabolism, stimulating the respiratory burst. A positive test is conversion of the yellow NBT dye to a black formazan pigment. Alternative tests of assessing the respiratory burst include **chemiluminescence** (light emission associated with generation of ATP). Specialized laboratories can precisely determine the amount of oxygen-free radical compounds (peroxide, superoxide) released during and after phagocytosis. The three best-characterized disorders of microbicidal function are **chronic granulomatous disease, Chediak-Higashi syndrome,** and **myeloperoxidase deficiency.**

Chronic Granulomatous Disease (CGD)   This disorder of microbicidal activity is usually an X-linked inherited disease characterized by severe recurrent infections caused particularly by staphylococci and gram-negative bacteria, in which the affected tissues show a granulomatous type of inflammatory process. The tissues contain lipid-filled macrophages and small abscesses. These patients have normal neutrophil counts, neutrophil morphology, and chemotaxis. Phagocytosis is also normal; however, bacterial killing is defective (especially against catalase-positive organisms such as *Staphylococcus aureus, Serratia marcescens, Aspergillus,* and *Candida*). The primary defect is the inability to generate superoxide and peroxide, which are essential components for bacterial killing (see Fig. 4–2). The main defect is absence of one of the *b* cytochromes (b_{558}). Consequently, organisms proliferate and grow inside the phagocytic cells, emphasizing the intracellular bactericidal defect. These patients have abnormal nitroblue tetrazolium reduction and chemiluminescence.

Chediak-Higashi Syndrome This condition, affecting all granule-containing cells, is also discussed in Chapter 2. It is associated with the

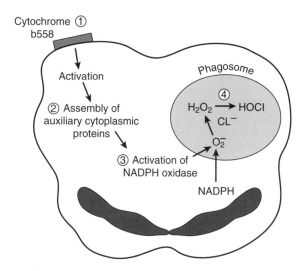

① Membrane-associated electron transporting oxidase
② Auxiliary cytoplasmic proteins: p67, p47, neutrophil cytosol factor 3
    H_2O_2 = hydrogen peroxide ⎫
    O_2^- = superoxide   ⎬ all bactericidal
    HOCl = hypochlorite ion ⎭
③ Electrons transferred from NADPH to produce superoxide
④ Myeloperoxidase

FIGURE 4–2. Polymorphonuclear function: phagocytosis and the respiratory burst.

morphologic appearance of giant lysosomal granules in cells. These abnormal cells, containing giant azurophil granules, are readily seen on peripheral blood smears. These patients have defective membrane fusion, causing decreased microbicidal activity, as well as defective chemotaxis. Patients also have partial cutaneous albinism, prolonged bleeding times (see Chapter 5) and recurrent infections.

Myeloperoxidase Deficiency   Bacterial phagocytosis requires, as a last step, interaction of hydrogen peroxide with an intracellular enzyme myeloperoxidase. Neutrophils with this disorder generate superoxide normally but have defective generation of the hypochlorite ion (see Fig. 4–2). A variant syndrome of CGD occurs if myeloperoxidase activity is congenitally absent. Acquired deficiency of myeloperoxidase occurs in granulocytic leukemia, a fact that may contribute to the increased infection rates that occur in leukemia (especially from catalase-positive microorganisms). Severe bacterial infections depress bactericidal efficiency. Laboratories equipped to perform histochemical studies in circulating white cells can stain neutrophils directly for myeloperoxidase activity.

Disorders of Lymphocyte, Monocyte, and Macrophage Function

When lymphocytes are deficient in number or function, the patient suffers from **immunodeficiency.** This may either be inherited or acquired. Table 4–3 lists some of the more common immunodeficiency disorders. See also Cellular Immunology, Chapter 7. Inherited immunodeficiency syndromes are rare but have an importance out of all proportion to their frequency because of the insight they reveal about normal immune functioning. Acquired deficiency states are increasingly common. The **acquired immunodeficiency syndrome (AIDS)** is an acquired immune deficiency state produced as a result of infection with a human immunodeficiency virus (HIV). This virus preferentially attacks helper T-lymphocytes, markedly depleting their numbers (see Chapter 8). Impairment of cellular proliferation or protein synthesis can also depress lymphocyte and plasma cell activity. Cytotoxic therapy for malignant diseases, adrenal corticosteroids, and negative protein balance are common predisposing conditions.

Blood **monocytes** and **tissue macrophages** are the same cells in different locations. The circulating monocyte is probably a young or de-differentiated form. Once in the tissues, macrophages develop organelles and enzymes that permit phagocytosis and lytic activity. The cells that line the sinusoids and spleen, liver, and lymph nodes are also derived from the same monocyte-macrophage pool. Tissue macrophages recruit new members by local cell reproduction and by repletion from bone marrow precursors. Macrophages exist as inconspicuous **histiocytes** (tissue monocytes) in most tissues, becoming obvious only when they

TABLE 4–3. IMMUNODEFICIENCY DISORDERS

Primary Immunodeficiency Diseases

T Cells
  Severe combined immunodeficiency
  Di George's syndrome
  Wiskott-Aldrich syndrome
  Chronic mucocutaneous candidiasis
B Cells
  Selective IgA deficiency in combination with various states
  X-linked agammaglobulinemia
  Common variable hypogammaglobulinemia
  Selective IgM deficiency
  IgG subclass deficiency

Secondary Immunodeficiency Diseases

Viral infections
  Acquired immunodeficiency syndrome (human
    immunodeficiency virus)
  Measles
  Cytomegalovirus
  Epstein-Barr virus
Splenectomy
Burns
Immunosuppressive drugs
  Antimetabolites
  Corticosteroids
Radiation
Prematurity
Hematologic disorders
  Lymphomas
  Leukemia
  Myeloma
  Aplastic anemia
  Sickle cell disease
Miscellaneous
Diabetes
Protein-losing states
Nephrotic syndrome
Enteropathies
Aging

engage actively in phagocytosis. When there is substantial local demand for macrophages, as in tuberculosis and other granulomatous inflammatory diseases, bone marrow and blood monocyte turnover increases, and monocytes accumulate in substantial numbers. Normal macrophages have enzyme systems capable of synthesizing and degrading sphingolipids, compounds important in biologic membranes and especially prominent in the nervous system. Several different inherited defects involve specific enzymes (acid hydrolase) necessary for lipid breakdown. In these deficiency states, lipid products accumulate in those parts of the cells that normally degrade recycled lipids. These diseases are not primarily hematologic conditions, although the macrophages of the marrow, spleen, and liver become overloaded with these metabolic precursors. The major effects of this are enlargement of the reticuloendothelial organs and numerous lipid-laden histiocytes present in the bone marrow. Some of these cells have distinctive morphologic features that characterize the disorders **Gaucher's disease** and *Niemann-Pick disease.* *Pseudo-Gaucher* cells can also be seen in the **myeloproliferative disorders.** Other morphologic curiosities include the *Sea-Blue Histiocyte Syndrome,* in which marrow histiocytes are laden with a bluish staining material on Giemsa-Wright stains. These diagnoses are often made on the basis of family history, but also on the identification of the characteristic cells, particularly in the bone marrow. The enlarged spleen often serves as reservoir for maldistribution of the peripheral blood cells and therefore leads to hypersplenism. Many patients require splenectomy for symptomatic cytopenias.

NON-NEOPLASTIC QUANTITATIVE DISORDERS

Total and differential white counts are useful, but nonspecific, diagnostic signs in many physiologic and pathologic states besides the previously covered neutropenia and immune deficiency syndromes. Changing counts may indicate that an abnormal condition exists and the body is responding; however, changes in white cell levels may also reflect conditions that directly affect blood-forming organs (see Chapter 2).

Neutropenia

Neutropenia is a decrease in the absolute neutrophil count below 2000/µL. Neutropenia may be classified as mild (a neutrophil count of between 1000 and 2000/µL), moderate (a neutrophil count of 500 to 1000/µL), or severe or agranulocytosis (a neutrophil count of less than 500/µL). This classification is useful in that it predicts the likelihood of infectious events. Individuals with severe neutrophil depletion are susceptible to bacterial infection, particularly with the organisms *Klebsiella, Escherichia, Pseudomonas,* and *Staphylococcus.* Neutropenia may occur as a result of many primary bone marrow diseases or acquired disorders (Table 4–4). Thirty percent of the black population may normally have a neutrophil count of less than 2000/µL, referred to as "constitutional neutropenia."

Evaluation of an absolute reduction in neutrophil count starts with an

TABLE 4–4. NEUTROPENIA

Definition

Neutrophil count < 2000/μL

Classification

Mild   PMN count 1000–2000/μL
Moderate PMN count 500–1000/μL
Severe   PMN count < 500/μL

Causes

Constitutional (normal in certain populations, e.g., blacks)
Deficiency in production
   Constitutional
     Familial benign neutropenia
     Cyclic neutropenia
     Infantile genetic agranulocytosis
     Many rare genetic conditions
   Acquired
     Nutritional deficiency (Vitamin B_{12}, folic acid, copper)
     Leukemia
     Aplastic anemia
     Response to infection (typhoid, hepatitis, infectious mononucleosis, tuberculosis)
     Cytotoxic drugs (cancer chemotherapy, immunosuppression)
Drug reactions (chloramphenicol, phenothiazines, propylthiouracil, phenylbutazone, phenytoins, carbamazepines)
Excessive destruction
   Immune-mediated
     Autoimmune neutropenia (idiopathic or associated with collagen-vascular diseases, lymphoproliferative diseases, or drugs)
     Acute granulocytotoxicity or leukoagglutination associated with blood transfusions
     Neonatal alloimmune granulocytopenia
     Antidrug antibodies
   Nonimmune
     Splenomegaly (portal hypertension, storage diseases, leukemias, lymphomas, rheumatoid arthritis)
     Extracorporeal circulation (heart-lung machines, renal dialysis)
     Disorders of pulmonary microcirculation
   Abnormal distribution
     Splenomegaly
     Margination shifts (see Fig. 2–3)
   Cyclic neutropenia

examination of the peripheral blood smear. A *differential count* is useful in assessing the degree of quantitative impairment as well as the percentage of immature cells present. Analogous to the reticulocyte count in anemia, the evaluation of bands in neutropenia can be helpful, and suggests increased neutrophil turnover. *Bone marrow examination* is important in categorizing the nature of the neutropenia. If the bone marrow is hypercellular and shows many normal neutrophil precursors in the presence of peripheral neutropenia, this suggests a peripheral destructive cause for the neutropenia. Normal neutrophil counts in the presence of increased bone marrow activity accompany maldistribution of the neutrophil pools—for example, change in the distribution between the marginating and the circulating pool, or in conditions associated with hypersplenism (in which a large percentage of the circulating neutrophil pool is sequestered in the spleen). Neutrophils may also be consumed in the peripheral blood by increased destruction that can be immune- or nonimmune-mediated. Unfortunately, there is no simple test like the Anti–Human Globulin Test for immune hemolytic anemia, but autoimmune neutropenia should be considered when all other conditions have been excluded and the marrow shows an increased number of normal neutrophil precursors without an enlarged spleen. Antineutrophil antibodies can be detected using immunofluorescence and other immunologic techniques. However, these tests are not readily available in routine laboratories. The *most common cause* of neutropenia, however, is bone marrow suppression or failure. This may occur with the primary marrow diseases or particularly associated with secondary suppression from drugs, medications, irradiation, and infections. Some of these conditions are listed in Table 4–4.

Another unusual disorder, in which *cyclic neutropenia* occurs, is characterized by periodic and often marked depletion of total neutrophil counts in the peripheral blood. Individuals with this disorder show an increased cyclic susceptibility to infection, characterized by cyclic fever and oral infections. These cycles may occur regularly, often at 21-day intervals. It is felt that this disorder is due to a defect in control of granulocyte differentiation, maybe related to cyclic disappearance of controlling colony-stimulating factors.

In several rare constitutional conditions, granulocytopenia occurs as part of the spectrum that may also include failure to produce neutrophils (reticular dysgenesis), defective granulocyte differentiation (infantile genetic agranulocytosis—Kostmann's syndrome), decreased gamma globulins, the presence of inhibitors to granulopoiesis, or the presence of leukoagglutinating antibodies. Moreover, the range of symptoms is wide. In familial **benign chronic neutropenia,** the condition may be discovered by chance, whereas in **infantile genetic agranulocytosis,** death from infection usually occurs before the first birthday.

Investigation of suspected constitutional neutropenia should begin with observation of the bone marrow cellularity and maturational pattern. These individuals may also have defects in leukocyte chemotaxis and bacterial killing (discussed above). A search should also be made for simultaneous abnormalities of lymphocytes, of immune activity, and of red cell and platelet development. In addition, the patient's family should be studied to detect a possible familial incidence.

Agranulocytosis

Agranulocytosis is a severe, acute neutropenia characterized by the disappearance of neutrophil precursors in the bone marrow and a severe depletion of the granulocyte count in the peripheral blood. The differential white count shows an absence or less than 500/μL of neutrophils or granulocytic cells. This may occur suddenly in an otherwise normal individual, and more especially occurs as an idiosyncratic drug reaction. It can also occur in association with autoimmune diseases and with some infections. Drugs sometimes affect the granulocyte levels without affecting the other marrow elements, but often red cells and/or platelet numbers are reduced as well. Antibodies may affect white cells only, but drug antibodies that damage cells through the "innocent bystander" effect (see Chapter 3) sometimes affect all three cell types in the blood as well.

Most of the agents and pathophysiologic conditions that cause anemia can depress granulocytes. Agranulocytosis is characterized clinically by the presence of fever and a severe throat infection, often with a white plaque-like membrane on the pharynx.

Most patients recover spontaneously following discontinuation of the offending drug. Antibiotic therapy is invariably given for those patients who are infected. The earliest signs of marrow recovery are associated with an increased number of monocytes, and subsequently bands, in the peripheral blood. In the early stages of marrow recovery, there is a predominance of promyelocytes, which can mimic the morphology of acute promyelocytic leukemia.

Some drugs produce a dose-related depression of white cells. In particular, drugs such as carbamazepine *(Tegretol)* are associated with gradually declining neutrophil counts. In some of these patients, this may herald the onset of agranulocytosis, but in many others the white cell count improves if the dosage is decreased. Periodic monitoring of WBC counts in patients taking such medications is important. Phenothiazines, phenytoins, some sulfonamides, and some antithyroid drugs also depress leukocyte production. Neutropenia persists for several weeks after therapy ceases, but granulopoiesis resumes when the drug is stopped. Chloramphenicol-induced marrow depression, however, may last for months or years.

Diagnosis depends on careful evaluation of total and differential white counts. If agranulocytosis causes necrotizing mouth infections, prostration, and fever, it may be difficult to distinguish between drug-induced agranulocytosis, acute leukemia, and the granulocyte-suppressive effects of massive infection. Evaluation must include meticulous inquiry about drugs and food additives and about exposure to materials involved in industrial, domestic, recreational, and environmental activities. It is important to evaluate red cell and platelet numbers and bone marrow cellularity. Aplastic anemia may present with features of agranulocytosis. With pure agranulocytosis, the total white count is low, and mature lymphocytes are virtually the only leukocytes in the circulating blood. Red cell and platelet levels, both in blood and in bone marrow, are normal. Pure agranulocytosis is relatively rare because many exogenous agents also tend to depress red cell and platelet production. In leukemias, the marrow usually has an increased proportion of blasts and immature cells, and the marrow is often hypercellular despite low levels of circulating cells. A list of the more common drugs associated with neutropenia is shown in Table 4–5.

Leukemoid Reactions

Reactive leukocytosis assumes florid proportions, with immature as well as mature white cells flooding the circulation. Because the blood picture resembles chronic leukemia, this event is called a "leukemoid reaction." It is not a primary marrow disorder and is usually secondary to some other condition. Granulocytes are most often involved, but striking monocytosis can occur in tuberculosis, whereas leukemoid lymphocytosis has been reported in tuberculosis, whooping cough, and infectious mononucleosis.

Granulocytosis of leukemoid proportions may accompany malignant tumors with or without metastases to the bone, severe pyogenic or tuberculous infection, heavy metal poisoning, sickle cell crises, severe metabolic disturbances involving the kidney or liver, and diabetic ketoacidosis. A patient recovering from agranulocytosis or from recent chemotherapy may have an intense white cell overproduction that suggests a leukemic proliferation, but leukopoiesis seldom continues at this rate for longer than a week.

When a leukemoid reaction is secondary to some obvious, underlying condition, distinction from leukemia is not difficult. It should be remembered, however, that leukemia can coexist with other diseases.

TABLE 4–5. MORE COMMON DRUGS PRODUCING UNEXPECTED NEUTROPENIA AND AGRANULOCYTOSIS

Anti-inflammatory	Phenylbutazone, oxyphenbutazone
Antimicrobials	Chloramphenicol, sulphonamides, trimethoprim
Anticonvulsants	Phenytoin, carbamazepine
Tranquilizers	Phenothiazine group
Antithyroid	Thiouracil group
Hypoglycemia agents	Tolbutamide
Miscellaneous	Allopurinol, chlorothiazides, cimetidine, gold, isoniazid, ibuprofen

TABLE 4–6. COMPARISON OF LEUKEMOID REACTION WITH CHRONIC MYELOGENOUS LEUKEMIA

Leukemoid Reactions	Chronic Myelogenous Leukemia
WBC usually < 50,000/μL	WBC usually > 50,000/μL
Toxic granulation and Döhle bodies	Toxic granulation ± –0
Basophilia absent	Greater basophil count (usual)
Bands particularly prominent	All stages, myelocytes
Leukocyte alkaline phosphatase (LAP) elevated (>100)	LAP < 10
Spleen usually not palpable	Spleen usually enlarged
Philadelphia chromosome not present	Philadelphia chromosome present in 90% of cases

Leukemia and tuberculosis, for example, can occur together, and each exacerbates the other. If the primary condition is not apparent, the picture alone may suggest the presence of leukemia. Features that distinguish a leukemoid reaction from chronic myelogenous leukemia are shown in Table 4–6.

Infectious Mononucleosis

Infectious mononucleosis (IM) is caused by infections with the Epstein-Barr virus (EBV), a member of the human herpes group of viruses. It is, however, not uncommonly associated with a marked elevation in the total white cell count, and in particular in the lymphocyte differential count. The EBV invades B lymphocytes by attaching to the receptor of the third component of complement (C3d, or CR2/CD21). The white count may be low when the disease begins, but by the end of the first week, leukocytosis of 10,000 to 30,000/μL is usual. There is an absolute increase in lymphocytes, many of which are large (see Color Plate 23) and atypical (Downey cells). These are **transformed T-lymphocytes.** These cells are reacting to the infected B lymphocytes. Circulating "virocytes" of this appearance are not unique to IM. In other viral diseases as well, circulating T lymphocytes manifest these reactive changes to viral infections of other cells or tissues. In IM, the atypical lymphocytes are prominent during the second to the fourth weeks of the illness. Table 2–9 lists the disorders that can cause an absolute lymphocytosis that may sometimes be mistaken for IM. Serologic tests described in Chapter 14 would confirm the diagnosis.

CLONAL LEUKOCYTE DISORDERS

MYELOPROLIFERATIVE DISORDERS

The myeloproliferative disorders are a group of clonal, neoplastic diseases that involve the pluripotent hematopoietic stem cells. In these conditions there is unregulated and uncontrolled growth and proliferation of the ancestral progeny of multipotent cells that exhibit differing degrees of differentiation. These disorders can be further divided into the acute and chronic types. The **acute myeloproliferative disorders** are the **acute nonlymphocytic leukemias** and are characterized by unregulated growth with limited or no differentiation. The **chronic myeloprolifera-tive diseases** include a group of disorders causing unregulated and excessive proliferation of cells with substantial differentiation, usually producing an excess of the mature, differentiated hematopoietic cells. Tables 4–7 and 4–8 list classifications of the acute and chronic myeloproliferative diseases.

Another variant of these clonal nonlymphocytic disorders are the **myelodysplastic syndromes,** a group of diseases in which there is unstable and unregulated growth of cells with varying degrees of differentiation. These syndromes differ from the above disorders in that they cannot be classified as acute leukemias because their clinical course is generally more benign and the cell populations are more mature. However, a substantial number of these disorders *may transform* into the leukemic stage after a variable latent period. It is because of this potential for leukemic transformation that these disorders have been called "preleukemic syndromes." They should, however, be broadly grouped together with the myeloproliferative diseases. Because of their propensity for unstable growth, they are classified in a subcategory called the **myelodysplasias.** Table 4–9 is a list of these diseases grouped together as the *myelodysplastic syndromes.*

Color Plate 1 is a comprehensive diagram showing the differentiation of marrow elements from the pluripotent stem cell. This cell is capable of proliferating and differentiating into progenitor cells that can give rise to granulocytes, erythrocytes, and platelets. Evidence supporting the clonal nature of these disorders has been derived from both cytogenetic and isoenzyme studies, using glucose-6-phosphate dehydrogenase isoenzymes, in black female heterozygotes. In these women, if a tumor is of clonal origin, only a single isoenzyme will be found in the tumor cells. Tumors with a multicentric origin would show both isoenzymes in these heterozygous women.

Despite their apparent homogeneity, in terms of specific cell types and morphology, the myeloproliferative disorders are probably extremely heterogeneous and may exhibit a markedly differing array of cell surface types, which may explain why some patients have a more aggressive

TABLE 4–7. ACUTE NONLYMPHOCYTIC LEUKEMIA (ANLL) CLASSIFICATIONS

	Features	Alternate Names	Cytogenetics	Genes
M0	Minimally differentiated		—	—
M1	Myeloblastic, without maturation (<10%)	Acute myelocytic Acute granulocytic leukemia Acute non-	—	—
M2	Myeloblastic, with maturation (>10%)	lymphocytic leukemia	t(8;21)	AML1-ETO
M3	Promyelocytic (APL)	Acute progranulocytic	t(15;17)	RARα-PML
M3V	Microgranular variant of APL			
M4	Myelomonoblastic	Naegeli-type leukemia	11q23	HRX/MLL
M4Eo	Myelomonoblastic with abnormal eosinophils		inv(16)	CBFβ-MYH11
M5A	Monoblastic, without maturation (<20%)	Schilling-type	11q23	HRX/MLL
M5B	Monoblastic, with maturation (>20%)			
M6	Erythroblastic (blasts > 30% nonerythroid cells) (Erythroleukemia)	DiGugliemo's disease Erythremic myelosis	—	—
M7	Megakaryoblastic	Acute myelofibrosis	3q27	?TPO

AML = Acute myeloid leukemia; RAR = retinoic acid receptor; PML = promyelocytic leukemia; TPO = thrombopoietin. (Other abbreviations refer to translocated oncogenes).

course than others. Studies of various oncogenes may also lead to an understanding of the pathogenesis of these disorders and their differing growth patterns.

TABLE 4–8. CLASSIFICATION OF CHRONIC MYELOPROLIFERATIVE DISORDERS

Preferred Name	Abbreviations	Common Synonyms
Chronic myelogenous leukemia	CML	Chronic myelocytic leukemia Chronic myeloid leukemia Chronic granulocytic leukemia
Polycythemia vera	P. vera	Erythrocytosis Erythremia True polycythemia
Agnogenic myeloid metaplasia	AMM	Myelofibrosis Idiopathic myelofibrosis Osteomyelosclerosis Myelosclerosis
Essential thrombocythemia	ET	Primary thrombocythemia Hemorrhagic thrombocythemia Primary thrombocytosis

TABLE 4–9. MYELODYSPLASTIC SYNDROMES

FAB: Myelodysplastic Syndromes	Other Terms
Refractory anemia (RA)	Chronic erythremic myelosis Refractory megaloblastic anemia
RA with ring sideroblasts	Acquired idiopathic sideroblastic anemia
RA with excess blasts (RAEB)	Acute myeloproliferative syndrome
RAEB in transformation	Primary acquired panmyelopathy with myeloblastosis (PAMP)
Chronic myelomonocytic leukemia	Subacute myelomonocytic leukemia

The Acute Myeloproliferative Disorders

Acute nonlymphocytic leukemia (ANLL) may be subdivided into seven main types and several subtypes on the basis of morphology. A classification system proposed by the French, American, British (FAB) Cooperative Group provides the morphologic and cytochemical standards for grouping these acute leukemias into the differing categories. As can be seen from Table 4–7, there are eight main variants of ANLL (M0 to M7) with some subvariants that may be derived from the pluripotent or multipotent stem cells, or from clonal proliferation of cells committed toward myeloid, erythroid, and megakaryocytic lines. Consequently, some of these leukemias may present with morphologic features of myeloid, monocytic, erythroblastic, or megakaryoblastic characteristics. Presumably, the predominant morphologic type depends on where the clonal neoplastic event occurs in the development of the nonlymphocytic cells.

The importance of identifying these cell types is to separate them from the acute lymphoblastic leukemias. This distinction is important since specific therapy and prognosis are different. Table 4–10 outlines some of the features that distinguish ANLL from the acute lymphoblastic leukemias (ALL). In clinical usage, the FAB classification numbers have not replaced the descriptive diagnostic terms that are routinely employed in common practice. **Acute myeloblastic leukemia** (M1 or M2) and

TABLE 4–10. FEATURES USEFUL IN DISTINGUISHING ANLL FROM ALL

Feature	AML	ALL
Morphology		
Cell size	Large	Small
Nuclear chromatin	Diffuse	Some clumping
Nucleoli	Multiple	One, often large
Cytoplasm	Moderate	Scanty
Auer rods	Sometimes present	Absent
Special Stains		
Esterases	+	−
Myeloperoxidase	+	−
PAS	− (except M6)	+
TdT	−	+
Immunophenotyping		
CD33	+	−
CD13	+	−
CD14	+ (M4, M5)	−
CD7	−	+ (T cells)
CD5	−	+ (T cells)
CD2	−	+ (T cells)
CD19	−	+ (B, pre-B cells)
CD10	−	+ (pre-B cells)
Cytoplasmic μ	−	+ (pre-B cells)
Cytoplasmic CD3	−	+ (pre-T cells)
Cytoplasmic CD22	−	+ (pre-B cells)

ALL = acute lymphoblastic leukemia; AML = acute myeloblastic leukemia
Adapted from Winkelstein, A, et al: White Cell Manual, ed 5. FA Davis, Philadelphia, 1998, p 29, with permission.

myelomonocytic leukemia (M4) are the two most common subtypes. **Acute megakaryocytic** (M7) and **acute monoblastic leukemia** (M5) are the two more unusual categories of ANLL.

Epidemiology and Clinical Presentation

ANLL tends to be a disease of adults, whereas ALL is primarily a disease of children. Only 10% of ANLL is found in children, and its incidence increases with advancing age. It represents more than 80% of adult acute leukemias. It is more common in whites than in blacks, and in men rather than women. (The male:female ratio is 3:2.)

Most of the acute myeloproliferative syndromes present with varying degrees of bone marrow failure. Consequently, clinical symptoms associated with anemia, leukopenia, and infection or thrombocytopenia predominate in varying degrees. Special presenting symptoms may occur in the **acute promyelocytic leukemias** (M3), which cause a disseminated intravascular coagulation syndrome and substantial bleeding manifestations. Acute myelomonocytic leukemia (M4) and acute monocytic leukemia (M5) in particular may present with gum hypertrophy due to monocytic invasion into the gum tissues. Fatigue and fever, however, are nearly universal. The actual white count is unpredictable. About 25% of patients have white blood cell counts above 50,000/μL. Another 25% have subnormal counts below 5,000/μL. About 15% have normal white cell counts (5,000 to 10,000/μL), but these are morphologically abnormal and immature cells. About half the patients with newly diagnosed acute leukemia have high serum uric acid levels and elevated lactate dehydrogenase (LDH) levels. The M4 and M5 FAB types may also have decreased serum potassium and serum calcium due to marked liberation of lysozyme, which passes out in the urine and may damage the renal tubules. This produces an excess urinary loss of calcium and potassium in these leukemias. The laboratory effects of therapy are discussed below. Table 4–11 outlines possible etiologic factors that have been associated with acute leukemia.

Laboratory Diagnosis of Acute Leukemia and Differentiation of Subtypes

Diagnosis of acute leukemia is made on the basis of the following:

1. Demonstration of immature cells in the peripheral blood with confirmation of immature cells in the bone marrow. Usually the bone marrow contains greater than 20% "blastic" morphology.
2. Categorizing the leukemic cells as acute nonlymphocytic leukemia or acute lymphoblastic leukemia.
3. Categorizing the cell type enables placement within the FAB classification (see Color Plates 34 to 42).

In ANLL, the blasts that overrun the marrow have finely dispersed (diffuse) or granular chromatin, several or numerous nucleoli, delicate

TABLE 4–11. ETIOLOGIC FACTORS ASSOCIATED WITH ACUTE LEUKEMIA

Inherited

Down syndrome
Fanconi's syndrome
Bloom's syndrome
Ataxia telangiectasia
Oncogenic activation

Acquired

Drugs and chemicals
  Benzene
  Alkylating drugs (nitrogen mustard, melphalan, chlorambucil, cyclophosphamide,
    procarbazine)
Radiation
Viruses
  Human T. leukemia virus type I (HTLV-I)-Jamaica, Japan
  Epstein-Barr virus (Burkitt's lymphoma-L3)
Oncogenes
  C-abl, C-sis (CML)
  C-myc (Burkitt's lymphoma-L3)
  Chromosomal instability

regular nuclear membrane, and modest amounts of cytoplasm, although the cell outline usually is regular. Although maturation is minimal, promyelocytes are present and often numerous, particularly in the M3 type. A variant of M3 is the **microgranular acute promyelocytic leukemia.** In this type the granules are inconspicuous but stain strongly for myeloperoxidase, and the nuclei have a folded morphology. Auer rods often can be seen in the cytoplasm (see Color Plates 26 and 34). In ANLL, cytochemical stains are positive for the peroxidase reaction and positive with Sudan black stains. Esterase stains are variable, as was discussed in Chapter 2.

Nucleated red cells and diffuse polychromatophilia tend to be more conspicuous in ANLL than in ALL. Platelet depression is often less extreme than in ALL; nearly half of ANLL patients present with platelet counts in the 30,000 to 100,000/µL range. Coagulation abnormalities are particularly prevalent in acute promyelocytic leukemia (M3), where the prothrombin time, partial thromboplastin time, and thrombin time are all prolonged (see Chapter 5). In addition, in this variant, fibrin degradation products are markedly elevated and fibrinogen values are decreased (see Disseminated Intravascular Coagulation, Chapter 6). In **acute myelomonocytic leukemia (M4)** and **acute monocytic leukemia (M5),** monocytic cells proliferate in addition to myeloblastic cells. A variant of M4, the M4 *Eo* subtype, contains more than 5% eosinophil precursors with prominent eosinophil granules. In the M4 type, equivalent numbers of monoblastic and myeloblastic cells may be seen, but in the M5 type, most cells are monoblastic and morphologically show twisted or indented nuclei, fine chromatin patterns, and a positive, nonspecific esterase stain. As already mentioned, urinary lysozyme levels are increased in these types, presumably reflecting an increased turnover of these cells, liberation of the enzyme into the blood, and filtration through the kidney into the urine. Color Plates 35 to 39 show some of the morphologic variants of the different cells seen in the acute nonlymphoblastic leukemias.

In **erythroleukemia** (FAB M6), the erythropoietic precursors predominate in the marrow and exceed 50% of all the marrow elements. The morphology of these erythroid cells closely resembles that of a megaloblastic type of picture, described in Chapter 2 (Color Plate 43). In addition, however, there are usually more than 30% myeloblasts and promyelocytes in the bone marrow. The disease is therefore a neoplastic, malignant, clonal proliferation of cells with capabilities of expressing erythroid and myeloid, as well as monocytic, markers. Any megakaryoblasts may also be abnormal in morphology. In the unusual variant M7 (acute megakaryoblastic leukemia), the blast cells show cytoplasmic blebs and contain platelet peroxidase rather than myeloperoxidase (Color Plate 44). The marrow may also show intensive fibrosis, which is coexistent with the blasts. The prognosis is particularly poor in this variant.

Immunophenotypic and Cytogenetic Characterization of Leukemia
The technique of **flow cytometry** allows for cell identification using specific monoclonal antibodies labeled with a fluorescent marker that will associate its corresponding surface antigen (Fig. 4–3). Each cell is then counted as a fluorescent event as it flows past an optical detector. In addition, the forward scattering of the fluorescent light determines cell volume, whereas a right-angled detector will evaluate cell granularity. In this manner the cellular phenotype, size, and cytoplasmic constitution can be determined.

This technique has defined a diversity of cellular phenotypes in leukemias and lymphomas and allows better definition of the malignant clone and prognosis. For example, in acute myeloblastic leukemia, cells usually express CD13 and CD33 (Table 4–12). Cells of monocyte lineage express CD14, cells of erythroid lineage express glycophorin, and those of megakaryocyte lineage express CD41. The finding of the "stem cell" marker CD34 on the AML cells carries a poor prognosis and may justify a more aggressive therapeutic approach. Table 4–12 shows the more common immunophenotypes found in acute nonlymphoblastic leukemia. Table 4–13 shows the corresponding immunophenotype characteristics in antilymphoblastic leukemia.

Cytogenetic abnormalities are also found in several of these leukemias (Table 4–14). The most consistent abnormality is found in acute promyelocytic leukemia (M3) in which the majority of cases exhibit a

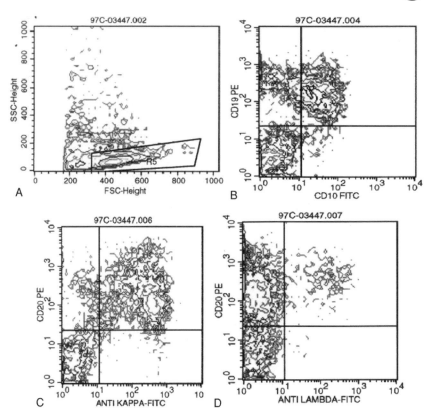

FIGURE 4–3. Flow cytometric immunophenotyping of lymphocytes obtained by fine needle aspiration of a lymph node from a patient with follicular center non-Hodgkin's lymphoma. The lymphocytes show low side scatter and variable forward scatter, suggesting *(A)* nongranular lymphocytes of different sizes with *(B)* predominantly CD19+ and CD10+, *(C)* anti-kappa and CD20+, and *(D)* low staining with anti-lambda. "Kappa" and "lambda" refer to immunoglobulin light chains; having a predominance of one chain implies clonal expansion. In this case, the kappa/lambda ratio was 12:1 (normally 2:1), confirming the abundance of kappa-positive cells. The features indicate a clonal expansion of B lymphocytes (CD19+, 20+) with kappa light chain restriction. SSC = side scatter (granulation), FSC = forward scatter (size), FITC = fluorescein isothiocyanate (a fluorescent stain), PE = phycoerythrin (a fluorescent stain).

translocation between chromosomes 15 and 17. Other abnormalities found in these leukemias include a translocation between chromosomes 8 and 21, found more particularly in ANLL (particularly M2), and the inverted chromosome 16 variant, which is found in acute myelomonocytic leukemia-*FAB-M4 Eo* (M4) (with a prominence of eosinophil precursors in this variant).

TABLE 4–12. IMMUNOPHENOTYPING IN ACUTE NONLYMPHOBLASTIC LEUKEMIA (ANLL)

Types of ANLL	Immunophenotypes
M0	CD13, 33, 34; HLA-DR
M1	CD13, 14, 15, 33, 34; HLA-DR
M2	CD13, 15, 33, 34; HLA-DR
M3	CD13, 15, 33
M4	CD13, 14, 15, 33, 34; HLA-DR
M5	CD13, 14, 33, 34; HLA-DR
M6	CD13, 33, 41, 71; HLA-DR glycophorin
M7	CD41, 61

Laboratory Effects of Treatment The aim of treatment in acute, nonlymphocytic leukemia is to eradicate the malignant clone and allow normal hematopoiesis to reestablish itself. The first objective is to induce remission with remission-induction chemotherapy. Once remission is induced, it is consolidated with further chemotherapy, and current chemotherapeutic regimens using intensification treatment with subsequent courses of mixed chemotherapy are the rule. Two drugs, cytosine arabinoside and daunomycin, are the main drugs used. Other regimens call for intensive combinations of additional drugs. In 70 to 75%, an initial remission is induced; however, the median duration of remission is between 12 and 16 months. With more intensive regimens, five-year survival figures are improving, with approximately 25% of patients alive after five years.

The intensive chemotherapy markedly suppresses total blood counts, which remain at low levels for two to three weeks. During this time patients require transfusion support with red blood cells for severe symptomatic anemia and platelet transfusions for both prophylaxis against bleeding and the treatment of thrombocytopenic bleeding. White cell transfusions are generally unhelpful. Initial chemotherapy is associated with massive destruction of leukemic cells, with liberation of chemicals from inside of the cell to the plasma. This is associated with the syndrome termed the "tumor lysis syndrome," which produces a marked elevation of uric acid, an increased serum potassium and phosphate, and a marked increase in serum LDH. Because of the propensity of uric acid crystals to precipitate in the urine, compounded by an excessive secretion of phosphate, renal function must be carefully monitored. For septic episodes during the periods of marked pancytopenia—in particular, marked neutropenia—blood cultures need to be taken, and infecting organisms identified. The usual organisms associated with infection

TABLE 4-13. IMMUNOLOGIC CLASSIFICATION OF ACUTE LYMPHOBLASTIC LEUKEMIA

Most (>95%) are TdT-positive

Very helpful to answer two questions: Is lineage B or T? What is the degree of maturation?

Pan B-cell antigens: CD19, CD20, CD22, CD24, HLA-DR

B-maturation antigens: TdT → CD10 → Cµ → Smlg

Pan T-cell antigens: CD2, CD3, CD5, CD7

T-maturation antigens: TdT → CD1a, CD4, CD8 → CD3, CD4, or CD8

Types	Morphology	Immunologic Features									
		CD15	CD2	CD3	CD5	CD19	Sig	Cig	CD10 (CALLA)	TdT	CD45R (HLA-DR)
Undifferentiated ALL	L1/L2	–	–	–	–	–	–	–	–	+	–
Common ALL	L1/L2	–	–	–	–	+	–	–	+	+	+
Pre-T-ALL	L1/L2	–	–	+	+	–	–	–	+	+	+
T-ALL	L1/L2	–	+	+	+	–	–	–	±	+	–
Pre-B-ALL	L1/L2	–	–	–	–	+	–	+	+	+	+
B-ALL	L3	–	–	+	–	+	+	–	–	–	+

ALL = acute lymphoblastic leukemia
CALLA = common ALL antigen
Cig = cytoplasmic immunoglobulin
HLA-DR = Ia-like antigen; L1, L2, L3 refer to the FAB classification
Sig = surface immunoglobulin
T = T-cell antigen
TdT = terminal deoxynucleotidyl transferase
CD15 = marker for monocytes and granulocytes
CD2 = E-rosette receptor (Pan T)
CD3 = Pan T
CD5 = Pan T
CD19 = Pan B

TABLE 4–14. CYTOGENETIC ABNORMALITIES FOUND IN LEUKEMIA

Translocations
    t9;22 (CML)
    t4;11 (ALL)
    t8;21 (AML)
    t8;14 (Burkitt's lymphoma)
Inversions
    inv 16 (AML)
Deletion
    5q- (myelodysplasia, preleukemia)
Monosomy 7

during the chemotherapy phase include gram-negative organisms and opportunistic fungal infections (see Chapter 13). The use of the antifungal agent amphotericin B is associated with potassium wasting, which also needs to be monitored during this phase.

Therapy for acute promyelocytic leukemia during the initial induction phase requires close monitoring of coagulation parameters, including the prothrombin time, partial thromboplastin time, and fibrinogen levels, and may require the use of heparin and replacement of coagulation factors (see Laboratory Monitoring of Disseminated Intravascular Coagulation in Chapter 6).

Chronic Myeloproliferative Syndromes

Table 4–8 is a list of the chronic myeloproliferative diseases and Table 4–15 shows the major features seen in these disorders. These conditions are clonal disorders of the hematopoietic stem cell that are associated with unregulated growth and proliferation of multipotent cells that are capable of differentiation to maturity. Depending on the predominant cell lines involved and the predominant cell type found in the peripheral blood, these conditions may be classified as shown in Table 4–8. These conditions comprise several disorders that have some common clinical and hematologic features. They are usually diseases of adults, and in particular elderly adults. Chronic myelogenous leukemia usually occurs in the 40- to 60-year age group, polycythemia vera in the 50- to 60-year age group, and agnogenic myeloid metaplasia and essential thrombocythemia in the 50- to 70-year age group. Patients may present with symptoms of disturbed marrow functioning, including anemia and recurrent infections, bleeding, or thrombotic tendency. On clinical examination, most patients have an enlarged spleen, often massive. Very few conditions give rise to massive splenomegaly; these are listed in Table 4–16. Common laboratory findings include a normochromic, normocytic anemia (except in polycythemia vera), diffuse polychromatophilia, teardrop poikilocytosis (especially marked in agnogenic myeloid metaplasia—myelofibrosis), high blood uric acid levels, elevated serum vitamin B_{12} levels, and usually an elevated leukocyte alkaline phosphatase, except in chronic myelogenous leukemia, where it is decreased. Specific cytogenetic abnormalities may be found in some of these disorders. The consistent chromosomal abnormality found in chronic myelogenous leukemia is the Philadelphia chromosome (translocation of chromosome 22 to 9). Marrow fibrosis (myelofibrosis) may complicate any of these myeloproliferative disorders, but it is usually more evident in agnogenic myeloid metaplasia.

Chronic Myelogenous Leukemia (CML)

Chronic myelogenous leukemia, also called **chronic granulocytic leukemia (CGL),** is characterized by unregulated growth, proliferation, and differentiation of myeloid precursors committed toward granulocytic development. As a consequence, all stages of granulocytic development

TABLE 4–15. MAJOR FEATURES OF CHRONIC MYELOPROLIFERATIVE DISEASES

Feature	CML	Polycythemia Vera	Essential Thrombo-cythemia	Agnogenic Myeloid Metaplasia
Major clinical abnormality	Leukocytosis	Erythrocytosis	Thrombo-cytosis	Extramedullary hematopoiesis, marrow fibrosis
Typical age of onset	40–60	60+	40–70	60+
HCT	Usually ↓	↑	N or ↑	↓
WBCs	↑↑↑	↑	↑	↓, N, or ↑
Platelets	N or ↑	↑	↑↑↑↑	↓, N, or ↑
Ph chromosome	+	−	−	−
LAP	↓	↑↑	↑	N or ↑
Tendency to transform into acute leukemia	++++	+	+/−	+

+ = positive, − = negative; ↓ = decrease, ↑ = increase, N = normal; CML = chronic myelogenous leukemia; HCT = hematocrit; LAP = leukocyte alkaline phosphatase; Ph = Philadelphia; WBC = white blood cells.

From Winkelstein, A, Sacher, RA, Kaplan, SS, and Roberts, GT: White Cell Manual, ed 5. FA Davis, Philadelphia, 1998, p 34, with permission.

TABLE 4–16. DISEASES PRODUCING MASSIVE SPLENOMEGALY

Chronic myelogenous leukemia
Agnogenic myeloid metaplasia
Lymphomas
Chronic lymphocytic leukemia
Visceral leishmaniasis (kala-azar)
Gaucher's disease
Schistosomiasis (bilharziasis)
Malaria

are markedly increased. Other granulocytic cells, including eosinophils and basophils, also may be abundant. Leukemia literally means "white blood," and in CML white cell counts may be so high that the blood actually assumes a grayish hue. White cell levels are characteristically between 50,000 and 250,000 per µL but can go even higher. This condition accounts for 15% of all leukemias. It is usually a disease of older adults; only occasional cases are seen in persons below 20 years of age.

CML usually begins insidiously. Patients may present with symptoms of hypermetabolism due to the numerous, dividing, metabolically active cells and complain of malaise, fatigue, abdominal fullness, or low-grade fever. The anemia is usually mild, with hematocrit between 25 and 35%. Thrombocytopenia is uncommon. Red cell and platelet levels vary independently of the white cell count. More than half of CML patients have platelet counts above 450,000 per µL. Abnormal bleeding may occur despite the elevated platelet counts because of qualitative platelet defects. The spleen is almost always enlarged, and sometimes it virtually fills the abdominal cavity. Hepatomegaly is common, but less impressive. Bone marrow tenderness is frequent, especially over the sternum. This is probably related to excessive marrow volume (marrow expansion) and activity. Serum uric acid levels are elevated, and there may be urate kidney stones or clinical gout.

Serum vitamin B_{12} and vitamin B_{12}–binding proteins usually are above normal. Values for serum potassium often are high and glucose levels low, but these are artifactual findings, the result of prolonged contact between serum and huge numbers of metabolizing white cells and platelets. If serum is separated promptly, glucose and potassium levels are normal in the clinically stable state.

The disease has three main clinical stages: the stable, chronic phase as described above; the phase of metamorphosis; and the acute leukemic phase. CML is a true preleukemia in that nearly all cases evolve into an acute blastic transformation. During this phase of evolution, the mature cells become dedifferentiated, and many more immature cells are seen. At this stage, patients may present with more profound symptoms, and thrombocytopenia may predominate and produce marked bleeding manifestations.

White Cell Findings The blood and bone marrow look much alike in CML (Color Plate 45). Vast numbers of granulocytes are present in all stages of maturation, but an interesting peculiarity is that there are more myelocytes and metamyelocytes. CML granulocytes retain bactericidal capacity, and increased susceptibility to infection is rare at the time of diagnosis. The leukocyte alkaline phosphatase (LAP) is nearly always low and can be zero (0). Occasionally, it may increase in patients who are infected or are in the metamorphosis or blast transformation stage. The pathognomonic feature of CML is the finding of the Philadelphia chromosome, which occurs in 90% of patients.

Philadelphia Chromosome The **Philadelphia chromosome** is a translocation of genetic material from the long arm of chromosome 22 to another chromosome, usually chromosome 9. Other translocations can occur but are unusual. Standard nomenclature defines the short arm of a chromosome as p and the long arm as q. The Philadelphia chromosome, then, is $t(9;22)$ $(q34;q11)$ (see Fig. 2–16). The finding of this chromosomal translocation is diagnostic of CML. The genome of the translocation has been studied intensively, and it has been found to involve two human sequences of homologous retroviral transforming genes (the proto-oncogenes c-abl and c-sis), which are located on chromosomes 9 and 22, respectively, at the sites of the breakpoint translocations. The v-abl is the viral sequence of the transforming gene that causes leukemias in mice. The molecular studies of the translocation in CML have shown that the translocation of chromosome 9, c-abl to chromosome 22, involves not only c-sis but a region called the "breakpoint cluster region (BCR)." This rearrangement produces recombinant genetic material that is capable of synthesizing marker proteins. Several marker proteins can be identified in different types of CML. The most consistent protein coded by the bcr/abl chimeric gene is a 210 kD molecule with transforming tyrosine kinase activity. A mouse model of CML has actually been generated by using a retroviral construct of the bcr/abl gene. Further analysis of proteins from the reciprocal translocation (i.e., abl/bcr) may identify heterogeneity of CML. Future advances in laboratory technology will not only facilitate understanding of the pathogenesis of this disorder but also will provide more precise diagnostic and prognostic categories of CML subtypes. In the future, recombinant DNA technology and genetic probes are very likely to refine into different subtypes the diagnosis of a disease once thought to be homogeneous.

Accelerated Phase and Acute Leukemic Phase of CML The initiating event causing the chronic, stable disease to accelerate into an acute transformation is unknown. Whether this involves activation of the proto-oncogene sequences or whether another inciting stimulus promotes the unregulated, undifferentiated growth, this event is the almost inevitable termination of CML. Apart from the apparent clinical manifestations of increasing spleen size, increasing bone pain, and symptoms of anemia or hypermetabolism, certain laboratory findings may herald the onset of the unstable phase and accelerated growth. The peripheral blood shows increasing basophilia and blasts, and the leukocyte alkaline phosphatase may rise. Cytogenetic studies performed during the accelerated phase may show multiple cytogenetic abnormalities, including double or triple Philadelphia chromosomes. Another feature is the cytochemistry staining on the blasts, which in approximately 25% of cases shows lymphoblastic markers. This may represent a dedifferentiation or imply that the primary disease is one of an immature stem cell with capabilities of exhibiting myeloid and lymphoid characteristics. The lymphoblastic marker terminal deoxynucleotidyl transferase (TdT) may be present in these blasts. Approximately 60 to 70% of patients will have a myeloblastic transformation.

The median duration of chronic, stable CML is 40 months. After this, the accelerated phase with blastic acute leukemia develops, and patients die within 1 to 6 weeks if untreated. Even with treatment, the median duration of survival is dismal, approximately 3 months. Patients with the lymphoid markers treated with vincristine and prednisone may have a higher rate of remission, but their long-term survival is only marginally better.

Philadelphia Chromosome–Negative CML   About 10% of patients with all the clinical features of CML do not demonstrate a Philadelphia chromosome on cytogenetic study. Many of these patients may be negative on cytogenetic analysis but have the bcr/abl fusion gene. This group of Ph-negative patients are generally older and have lower initial white counts and platelet counts. Their median duration of survival is only 8 months, compared with 40 months for Ph-positive CML. Ph-negative CML, then, may be an even poorer prognostic CML category.

Some laboratory findings may be interpreted as having especially poor prognostic implications. These include leukocytosis greater than 100,000/μL, a blast count greater than 1% in the peripheral smear and 5% in the marrow, a basophil count greater than 15 to 20%, a platelet count greater than 700,000/μL or less than 150,000/μL, or the presence of additional Philadelphia chromosomes or other cytogenetic abnormalities.

Polycythemia Vera

"Polycythemia" literally means "many blood cells," but usually it refers to increased red cell mass. A better term for this is **erythrocytosis** or **erythremia.** When red cells increase to meet a recognizable physiologic stimulus, the condition is called **secondary** or **reactive polycythemia.** Spontaneous or seemingly unprovoked increase in red cell production and blood volume is called **polycythemia vera (PV)** or **"true poly-cythemia."** *Secondary* polycythemia, or erythrocytosis, is discussed in Chapter 3. PV belongs to a group of myeloproliferative cell disorders characterized by unregulated growth and proliferation of hematopoietic precursors with excessive erythrocytic proliferation. Because this involves a clonal, multipotent stem cell, other marrow elements may also be present in excess (leukocytosis in 75% of cases, thrombocytosis in 50%). PV occurs in older adults, slightly more often in men than in women, and usually has an insidious onset easily confused with other causes of erythrocytosis, from which it must be excluded (see Chapter 3).

The clinical presentations of PV are those of excessive red cell proliferation. Patients may present with a ruddy complexion or symptoms of hyperviscosity such as headaches, visual disturbances, or thrombotic events. These patients have a higher incidence of peptic ulcer disease. They may also present with symptoms of increased blood histamine (released from basophils), including itching, particularly after a hot shower. They usually have a plethoric cherub face, and 75% have an enlarged spleen. The differential diagnosis involves exclusion of all the causes of secondary erythrocytosis discussed in Chapter 3.

Laboratory diagnosis of this disorder aims at the major diagnostic criteria used in establishing the clinical diagnosis of PV (Table 4–17). The first three criteria listed were originally introduced by the Polycythemia Vera Study Group for the purpose of classifying patients with PV. They have been retained by many clinicians to standardize the diagnosis. To establish a diagnosis of PV, a patient must show an increased red cell mass; an elevated hematocrit or red cell count may be due to contracted

TABLE 4–17. CRITERIA FOR ESTABLISHING DIAGNOSIS OF POLYCYTHEMIA VERA

Category A (Major Criteria)

Elevated red cell mass
Normal arterial oxygen saturation
Splenomegaly
Erythropoietin (see text)

Category B (Minor Criteria)

Leukocytosis
Thrombocytosis
Elevated leukocyte alkaline phosphatase score
Increased serum vitamin B_{12} or vitamin B_{12}–binding proteins

To establish a diagnosis of polycythemia vera, either the first three diagnostic criteria from Category A must be present, or the first two criteria from Category A and two criteria from Category B.

plasma volume. The patient also must have a normal PO_2, or blood oxygen, to exclude conditions in which the red cell mass is appropriately increased due to erythropoietin stimulation. If these two conditions are met and the spleen is enlarged, the diagnosis is established. Without enlargement of the spleen, two of the minor criteria listed on Table 4–17 also must be met to make the diagnosis. Clearly, these minor diagnostic criteria are features that are seen in many of the other myeloproliferative disorders.

An additional criterion used by many clinicians is the finding of a low serum erythropoietin, which invariably occurs in patients with PV. An increased red cell mass in the presence of a decreased or even normal erythropoietin suggests autonomous erythropoiesis, which is the hallmark of PV, but an assay of serum erythropoietin is not required for diagnosis.

The red cell count, hemoglobin concentration, and hematocrit are all elevated unless there is significant associated iron deficiency. If iron deficiency exists, examination of the peripheral smear will reveal normochromic, normocytic red cells with hypochromic, microcytic cells. Myelocytes and metamyelocytes are occasionally seen in the peripheral blood smear of patients with PV, and the basophil count may be elevated. Platelets are often morphologically abnormal, and platelet aggregation studies may reveal functional defects.

The bone marrow usually is hypercellular with an abundance of all cell lines and normal maturation. Stainable iron is often reduced or absent.

PV usually progresses in a relatively indolent fashion, and prolonged survival is common. Treatment is aimed at reducing the red cell mass by frequent, therapeutic bloodletting (phlebotomy). This usually controls thrombotic and hemorrhagic complications, but about one-third of patients will suffer from them. After a variable period (average, 10 years), the proliferative, erythrocytic phase of the disease evolves into the "spent phase" in approximately 15 to 20%. The clinical picture of this phase features progressive anemia and increasing enlargement of the spleen or liver enlargement. This syndrome resembles agnogenic myeloid metaplasia (discussed next) in many respects, with an abundance of teardrop poikilocyte red cells and nucleated red blood cells in the peripheral blood (Color Plate 46). The bone marrow biopsy shows extensive marrow fibrosis; bone marrow aspirate is usually a dry tap—that is, unobtainable. Life expectancy in this phase is less than 3 years. Among patients who have received alkylating drug therapy, PV can terminate in acute leukemia in as many as 15%, compared to fewer than 5% of patients treated only with phlebotomy.

Agnogenic Myeloid Metaplasia

Agnogenic myeloid metaplasia, also called **myelofibrosis** or **idiopathic myelofibrosis,** is a clonal disorder of the hematopoietic stem cell characterized by unregulated proliferation of hematopoietic precursors within the bone marrow and within extramedullary sites. The two major clinical components of this disorder represent expansion of reticuloendo-thelial organs, including the liver, the spleen, and, more rarely, lymph nodes, as well as replacement of the bone marrow by fibrous tissue. The clinical presentations are anemia with tiredness, fatigue, and palpitations; hypermetabolism with fever and weight loss; and massive splenomegaly producing abdominal fullness, splenic pain, and fever. The enlarged spleen may also serve as a reservoir sequestering white cells, red cells, and platelets. Many times the platelets are malfunctional, so patients may have a bleeding tendency despite the high levels that can occur.

Studies using the G-6-PD isoenzyme marker have shown that the clonal proliferation involves the hematopoietic precursors in the marrow and extramedullary sites, but the fibrosis in the marrow is nonclonal, indicating that it is not derived from the abnormal clone. It is believed that the fibroblastic proliferation occurs as a result of liberation of platelet-derived growth factor from the abnormal platelets.

Laboratory Data   Most patients develop a normochromic, normocytic anemia, but some have a macrocytic anemia. Others have a chronic bleeding tendency, with iron deficiency and hypochromic, microcytic anemia. Red cell morphology is strikingly abnormal on the peripheral smear, showing the presence of abundant teardrop poikilocytes, which are always prominent in this disorder (see Color Plate 14). Nucleated red blood cells are also evident, as are many other morphologic variations in the red cell series, including the presence of inclusion bodies such as Howell-Jolly bodies. Other features consistent with a chronic myelopro-liferative syndrome include an elevated LDH, increased uric acid, and increased vitamin B_{12} binders. The leukocyte alkaline phosphatase is usually raised. Platelets are often morphologically very abnormal on the peripheral smear, and megakaryocytic fragments may also be seen. The leukocytes may show hypersegmentation and other immature precursors also may be evident, but blasts are not a conspicuous feature. The typical blood picture is termed a "leukoerythroblastic reaction" (see Color Plate 46). The causes of a leukoerythroblastic reaction are shown in Table 4–18. Bone marrow aspiration is usually a dry tap, and biopsy shows the presence of extensive fibroblastic replacement with numerous bizarre, atypical, and dysplastic megakaryocytes. Patients may also develop osteosclerosis, which may appear on x-rays as increasing bone density. Cytogenetic abnormalities are not consistent, but their presence suggests a worse prognosis.

Clinical Course   Patients who are asymptomatic at presentation tend to remain stable for approximately 5 years. When symptoms develop, particularly increasing transfusion dependency and symptoms referable to increasing cytopenia (anemia, decreased white cell count, and decreased platelet count) or enlarging splenic size with painful symptoms of splenic infarction, these patients may require splenectomy or palliative drug or radiation therapy. In most patients, however, once the disease

---

TABLE 4–18. CAUSES OF A
          LEUKOERYTHROBLASTIC REACTION

Blood Loss

Infective Causes

Granulomatous disease
  Tuberculosis
  Syphilis
  Brucellosis
  Disseminated fungemia
  Schistosomiasis

Neoplastic Causes

Primary hematologic diseases
  Leukemia (acute and chronic)
Myeloproliferative disorders
Lymphomas
  Hodgkin's and non-Hodgkin's
Secondary solid tumors
  Breast, kidney, prostate, thyroid, lung
Autoimmune Disorders
  Hemolysis

Ischemia

Myocardial infarct
Shock

Idiopathic Myelofibrosis

---

progresses, the median duration of survival is less than a year. Some patients end with acute leukemia.

Essential Thrombocythemia (ET)

Essential thrombocythemia (ET) is a clonal disorder of the pluripotent stem cell characterized by excessive proliferation of cells of the megakaryocytic lineage with the production of excess numbers of platelets. The condition is associated with an unexplained elevation in the platelet count, usually to levels greater than 1 million per microliter. This condition, however, usually has a much more benign course than the other conditions classified as chronic myeloproliferative syndromes. The condition may occur at a younger age and often appears in otherwise asymptomatic patients. Some patients may present with thrombotic or thromboembolic symptoms, and others with bleeding tendency—despite the excessive numbers of platelets—because these platelets may be functionally abnormal. The gastrointestinal tract is the most common site of bleeding, but mucous membranes also may bleed. These patients may have more substantial bleeding with trauma or surgery. About half also have an enlarged spleen, which is usually mild. In the younger patients, the prognosis is excellent; older patients present with more hemorrhagic and thrombotic problems. Of all the myeloproliferative syndromes, ET has the lowest potential for termination in acute leukemia.

Laboratory Features The hallmark of ET is the elevated platelet count, usually greater than 1 million per microliter. The peripheral blood smear usually shows normochromic, normocytic red cells, but teardrop poikilocytes may be present. The most striking features are the abundant platelets and megakaryocytic fragments with abnormal morphology. Bone marrow aspirate may be a dry tap; usually it is cellular and shows a marked abundance of megakaryocytes and platelet debris. Bone marrow biopsy may show increased fibrous tissue. Many of the megakaryocytes display abnormal morphology. Iron is often absent in the bone marrow. In keeping with some of the other myeloproliferative disorders, the white cell count is usually elevated, in the range of 10,000 to 20,000 per microliter. Chromosomal findings are not consistent, but the Philadelphia chromosome is absent. Platelet function studies are usually abnormal, but coagulation tests (see Chapter 6) are usually normal. Table 4–19 lists the causes of thrombocytosis.

Differential Diagnosis of Thrombocytosis Elevated platelet counts may be found in a number of other acute and chronic diseases listed in Table 4–19. ET is suspected when there is a *sustained* elevation in the

---

TABLE 4–19. CAUSES OF THROMBOCYTOSIS

Primary
Chronic myeloproliferative syndromes
    Primary thrombocythemia
    Myelofibrosis
    Polycythemia vera
    Chronic myeloid leukemia
    5q syndrome

Secondary
Infections
    Acute (e.g., abscess)
    Chronic (e.g., bronchiectasis)
Injury
Malignant solid tumors
Inflammatory disorders (e.g., rheumatoid arthritis)
Acute and chronic blood loss

Idiopathic

platelet count, whereas reactive thrombocytosis (RT) usually abates after the associated disease is treated. Some patients with ET may have counts below 1 million per microliter, whereas occasional RT can have platelet values greater than 1 million. These conditions are sometimes difficult to differentiate and require a full work-up. Since elevated platelet counts in RT are often associated with malignancy, inflammation, and chronic blood loss, these conditions must be excluded. The routine evaluation of these patients should include a complete history (noting especially thrombophlebitis or bleeding) and physical examination. In RT, the peripheral blood smear may show iron deficiency, reticulocytosis, a leukoerythroblastic blood picture, or poikilocytosis. In ET, morphology is usually normal with the possible exception of large and sometimes abnormal platelets. Further laboratory work-up should be undertaken to exclude the conditions listed in Table 4–19. A bone marrow examination for morphology and cytogenetics completes the investigation.

Myelodysplastic Syndromes

These syndromes are a heterogeneous group of disorders in which there is clonal, unregulated, and unstable growth characterized by disturbed maturation, refractoriness to standard vitamin and iron therapy, and a propensity to develop acute leukemia. Because of this last feature, these conditions were previously termed the *"preleukemic syndromes,"* but only about 25 to 35% of them evolve into acute leukemia. Certain clinical and laboratory features may herald this transformation. These conditions were discussed in Refractory Anemia in Chapter 3, and the classification of these disorders in Table 4–9, gives the nomenclature of the French, American, and British (FAB) Cooperative Group. The hallmark of these conditions is ineffective hematopoiesis, which includes erythroid development, granulopoietic development, and platelet production. The unstable growth may affect any combination of these major cell lines of maturation. The ineffective growth is characterized by hypercellularity in the bone marrow, but with cytopenia of varying degrees in the peripheral blood because of intramedullary cell death. The major clinical presentations of these disorders are anemia unresponsive to standard hematinic treatment (vitamins and iron), fever, recurrent infections, or a bleeding tendency. Splenomegaly usually is not a feature of the myelodysplastic syndromes. Patients may, however, present with other clinical features of a hypermetabolic state, including fever and weight loss, as well as features of increased cellular turnover, such as gout due to hyperuricemia or bone pain due to marrow expansion.

Refractory Anemia (RA)

Refractory anemia (RA) is the most benign of the myelodysplastic syndromes and has the least likelihood of transformation into acute leukemia (<10%). It occurs more commonly in elderly people and is associated with a normochromic, normocytic anemia, or a macrocytic anemia, in the presence of a hypercellular marrow that shows megaloblastic features. Blasts are less than 5% of marrow cytology. Cytogenetic findings are unusual. Repeated marrow aspirates are often needed to follow these patients.

Refractory Anemia with Ringed Sideroblasts (RARS)

This condition, also called "acquired idiopathic sideroblastic anemia," is typically associated with an elevated serum iron and percentage iron saturation (see Chapter 2). Patients also usually present with a hypochromic, microcytic anemia, but a dimorphic blood picture, showing some cells hemoglobinized and others underhemoglobinized, is also common. The white cell count and platelet count are usually normal. A bone marrow is usually hypercellular due to erythroid hyperplasia that shows megaloblastic features. The pathognomonic finding in this condition, however, is the presence of numerous positive iron granules arranged in a ring or partial ring around the nucleus on an iron stain: **ring sideroblasts.** Finding ring sideroblasts does not necessarily imply a myelodysplastic process. Table 3–4 lists the classification of sideroblastic anemias (see Color Plate 12A). To be classified as RARS, at least 15% of developing erythroid cells must contain these ring forms. Blasts constitute less than 5% of the marrow cytology. The inability to utilize iron is felt to be due to a defect in iron incorporation from mitochondria into developing erythroid cells (see Fig. 2–3). This condition also has a relatively chronic course, but it transforms into acute leukemia in about 10% of patients.

Refractory Anemia with Excess Blasts (RAEB)

The hallmark of RAEB is a normochromic or macrocytic anemia in the presence of a hypercellular marrow that shows 5 to 20% myeloblasts and no Auer rods. This condition has also been called a "smoldering leukemia" or "subacute leukemia." Circulating peripheral mononuclear cells may show abnormal granulation, hypersegmentation, or the pseudo-Pelger-Huet anomaly. Most patients remain stable for many months or even years, but RAEB transforms into ANLL in 30%.

RAEB in Transformation

This condition represents a more advanced stage of RAEB, with a greater percentage of blasts (20 to 30%) developing in the marrow in association with a severe anemia. The features are intermediate between cells with normal differentiation and evolution into acute leukemia. This condition is more refractory to chemotherapy than ANLL presenting *de novo.*

Chronic Myelomonocytic Leukemia

This condition is characterized by an increased absolute monocyte count in the peripheral blood without a secondary stimulus such as tuberculosis or chronic inflammation. Many of the monocytes appear atypical or immature and may show nucleoli. The bone marrow may also show an abundance of cleaved and clefted cells with horseshoe-shaped nuclei characteristic of monocytic precursors, as well as dysplasia of the other hematopoietic precursors. These patients may also have an elevated lysozyme, a feature that is seen in acute monocytic leukemia. Typically, there is no gum infiltration by these abnormal cells. This condition also carries a high likelihood of transformation into acute myelomonocytic or monocytic leukemia (M4 or M5).

Chromosomal Abnormalities in the Myelodysplastic Syndromes

Cytogenetic abnormalities in patients with myelodysplastic syndromes usually impart a worse prognosis with a greater likelihood of leukemic transformation. Transformation into acute leukemia is more commonly associated in these syndromes with the 5q chromosomal abnormality, which represents a loss of the long arm of chromosome 5. The 5q abnormality appears more commonly in leukemia that follows alkylating drug therapy (so-called therapy-related myelodysplasia [t-MDS]). Other chromosomal abnormalities seen in these myelodysplasias are monosomy 7 and trisomy 8. These findings are generally thought to be associated with a poorer prognosis or a greater likelihood of leukemic transformation.

The 5q chromosomal abnormalities may sometimes be associated with a specific constellation of findings that includes macrocytic anemia and leukopenia but a normal or elevated platelet count. This **5q syndrome** paradoxically is associated with a better prognosis and less likelihood of leukemic transformation.

LYMPHOPROLIFERATIVE DISORDERS

The lymphoproliferative disorders represent unregulated growth and proliferation of cells of the lymphoid lineage. These disorders are classified into the **acute lymphoproliferative disorders,** in which there is little or no differentiation to terminal maturity, and the **chronic lymphoproliferative disorders,** in which there is an unregulated growth with differentiation and an abundance of mature cells. These conditions are also clonal in origin, representing expansion of a single clone of cells, all exhibiting the same phenotypic markers as the parental cell. These lymphoproliferative disorders may be subclassified in terms of their functional characteristics into the **T-cell disorders** (disorders of lymphocytes programmed or under the influence of the thymus) and the **B-cell disorders** (disorders programmed or influenced by the bone marrow). Finally, lymphoproliferative disorders also may be subcategorized according to their anatomic distribution into those predominantly involving the bone marrow and peripheral blood, called the **leukemias,** and those predominantly involving the reticuloendothelial organs (lymph nodes, spleen, and liver), called the **lymphomas.** On the basis of these various criteria, lymphoproliferative disorders can be grouped into distinct subtypes. This chapter will discuss the diagnosis, differentiation, functional characteristics, and distribution of each type.

Chapter 2 outlines normal lymphoid differentiation and functional classification. Because lymphoproliferative disorders involve a neoplastic clonal change somewhere in their development and maturity, excess growth and proliferation of cells frozen at a specific stage in differentiation can occur. These cells may be defined by the clinical laboratory.

Lymphoreticular cells can be either fixed or mobile. B lymphocytes and their plasma-cell derivatives constitute a mobile, or potentially mobile, population, even though at any one time most B cells reside in the lymphoid tissues. T lymphocytes are in continuous movement between tissue sites, blood, and lymph fluid. The monocyte-macrophage-histiocyte population is less conspicuous in body fluids, the cells spending most of their active life within the tissues. Since there is a continual exchange between the tissue sites, blood, and bone marrow, all of these sites may be involved in some stage of a lymphoproliferative disease.

The Acute Lymphoproliferative Disorders

The three types of acute lymphoproliferative disorders are as follows:

1. **Acute lymphoblastic leukemia (ALL),** the most common acute leukemia of childhood
2. **Undifferentiated leukemia**
3. **Lymphoblastic transformation of chronic myelogenous leukemia**

All of these disorders may present in a similar way, so they will be discussed together.

Acute Lymphoblastic Leukemia

Acute lymphoblastic leukemia is the major childhood leukemia, accounting for nearly all leukemias before age 4, and more than half of the leukemias through puberty. It is rare in patients over the age of 30. Although ALL occurs in about 15% of adult leukemias, many of these cases may be the initial presentation of an acute transformation of CML. The major distinction is the demonstration of the Philadelphia chromosome.

Clinically, ALL and acute myeloblastic leukemia (AML) have similar features, but the onset of ALL tends to be strikingly acute. It almost never has a smoldering or preleukemic phase. Lymph node enlargement and hepatosplenomegaly occur more often in ALL than in AML, as do bone pain and bone lesions. Leukemic meningitis can occur late in the disease. Because the central nervous system tends to be a sanctuary for relapse in this leukemia despite an apparent blood and bone marrow remission, all patients with ALL routinely receive prophylactic chemotherapy and radiation therapy to the CNS.

Table 4–20 shows the FAB classification of lymphoblastic leukemias. This classification includes three morphologic categories: L1, L2, and L3. The lymphoblastic leukemias are separated from the myeloblastic leukemias on the basis of morphology and cytochemical staining. The morphologic differences were listed in Table 4–10, and as shown there, these differences are confirmed by cytochemical staining patterns using myeloperoxidase, Sudan black, and nonspecific esterase stains (see Chapter 2), which stain the acute myeloblastic leukemias, and the PAS and TdT stains, which stain the acute lymphoblastic leukemias. Occasionally, cytology and cytochemistry cannot define the cell lineage. Immunophenotypic characterization of the acute leukemias is now routine and substantially enhances classification by the origin of the leukemia (see Tables 4–12 and 4–13). The FAB classification defines not only cytologic differences but also prognostic categories, L1 having the best prognosis, L2 intermediate, and L3 the worst. The nature of aggressive chemotherapy thus can be planned accordingly. LI-ALL consists of a monotonous population of uniform cells with a high nucleo-cytoplasmic ratio and very scanty cytoplasm. There are usually two or fewer nucleoli that are fairly well defined (see Color Plate 40). The nucleus is usually regular in shape.

L2-ALL is characterized by more heterogeneity, in that both small and large cells can be seen replacing the bone marrow and in the peripheral blood. The larger cells often show nuclear clefting, prominent nucleoli, and abundant cytoplasm (see Color Plate 41).

L3, or Burkitt's type, consists of a uniform population of uncleaved immature cells with both nuclear and cytoplasmic vacuolization. The cytoplasm is usually basophilic and may be abundant (see Color Plate 42).

Blood and Bone Marrow Findings Very few recognizable neutrophils circulate in ALL, and even in the bone marrow normal red and white cell elements may be hard to find. The predominant cell, both in blood and in the marrow, is a blast that may have morphologic characteristics as mentioned above under the FAB types. However, the blasts usually have scant cytoplasm, contain no Sudanophilic granules, no peroxidase-reactive granules, and no Auer rods. The few neutrophils that are present have normal leukocyte alkaline phosphatase scores. Anemia is usually pronounced, with few reticulocytes and a very low platelet count.

A marrow aspirate shows the marrow spicules to be almost totally replaced by blasts. Very few normal marrow elements are in evidence. Culturing marrow for chromosomes usually shows no distinct chromosomal abnormalities, but a translocation of chromosome 4 and 11 is sometimes seen in infantile ALL, a 9–11 translocation is occasionally seen in childhood ALL, and a Philadelphia chromosome may be detected in adults presenting with an ALL, representing *de novo* presentation of the blastic phase of CML.

TABLE 4–20. CELL CHARACTERISTICS IN ACUTE LYMPHOBLASTIC LEUKEMIA (FAB CLASSIFICATION)

Cell Characteristics	L1	L2	L3
Cell size	Predominantly small cells, homogeneous	Large, heterogeneous	Large, homogeneous
Nuclear chromatin	Homogeneous in any one case	Heterogeneous	Stippled, homogeneous
Nuclear shape	Regular, round, occasional clefting	Irregular, clefting	Regular, round to ovoid
Nucleoli	Inconspicuous	One or more, may be large	One or more, prominent
Cytoplasm	Scanty	Variable, moderately abundant	Moderately abundant, strongly basophilic
Cytoplasmic vacuolation	Variable	Variable	Prominent

From Pittiglio, DH, and Sacher, RA: Clinical Hematology and Fundamentals of Hemostasis. FA Davis, Philadelphia, 1987, p 234, with permission.

Cell Surface Markers   Acute lymphoblastic leukemia can be subdivided into different cells of origin using surface antigens as markers. This allows more vigorous evaluation of treatment regimens and epidemiologic features than is possible if all cases of ALL are considered together. These markers may subcategorize the FAB types. Most ALL (about 70%) involves cells lacking features of either B or T lymphocytes (see Chapter 2). These neoplastic cells have a distinctive surface membrane marker called the "common ALL antigen (CALLA)(CD10)"; this form of leukemia is called **common ALL.** These cells also stain positive for the marker TdT (see Chapter 2). This type of ALL, the usual FAB LI category, usually has the best prognosis. Patients present with low white cell counts. There are three other types of ALL also identified on the basis of immunologic markers:

- T-cell ALL
- B-cell ALL
- Null or undifferentiated ALL, which stains negative for B, T, and CALLA.

The prognosis appears to be worse for these three types, so these patients usually undergo more aggressive chemotherapy. The immunologic classification of ALL is shown in Table 4–13.

The next most common type (20 to 22% of ALL) is **T-cell ALL.** These cells are positive for monoclonal T-cell markers, CD2, CD3, CD7 and may be positive for CD8 or CD4. They are capable of forming rosettes with sheep red blood cells. Other characteristics are listed in Table 4–13. This form tends to affect older patients and has unfavorable clinical findings, including occurrence in males with mediastinal tumors and a white cell count of greater than 50,000/μL. The most significant adverse prognostic feature for all types of ALL is a white cell count of greater than 50,000/μL. Although T-cell ALL responds well to initial therapy, remissions tend to be shorter, and long-term prognosis is much less favorable than in common ALL. As it becomes possible to distinguish helper T cells from suppressor T cells routinely, different subsets of T-cell leukemia may emerge and enable further categorization of the more aggressive or better prognostic types. A rare type of T-cell ALL is associated with hypercalcemia and previous exposure to the retrovirus HTLV-I (human T-cell lymphotropic [leukemia] virus 1 type I). This condition has a higher prevalence in Jamaica and Japan. (See also Chapter 14.)

B-cell ALL represents 1 to 3% of ALL and tends to carry a poorer prognosis. These cells show surface immunoglobulins and receptors for F_c and complement characterizing the circulating cells, which resemble cells from the center of germinal follicles and are morphologically similar to the cells of Burkitt's lymphoma. They also type positive for B-cell antigens CD19 and CD20 with specific monoclonal antibodies, and virtually all cases have specific chromosomal translocations t(8;14), t(8;22), or t(2;8).

Still poorly characterized is a moderately large group of ALL patients in whom common ALL antigen is present but the cells also have immunoglobulin (IgM or its heavy chain) in their cytoplasm. This is considered a pre–B-cell leukemia. It has a better prognosis than the B-cell leukemia, resembling that of common ALL.

Treatment　Before 1950, 80% of children with ALL were dead 8 months after diagnosis. By 1970, 5 to 10% of children with ALL could expect long-term survival of 5 years or longer, and most had disease-free intervals of 1 to 2 years. At present, 50% of children newly diagnosed as having ALL can anticipate long-term survival and complete cessation of therapy (cure).

Certain features at diagnosis have favorable prognostic significance. The most favorable category is diagnosis between the ages of 2 and 9, peripheral white cell count no higher than 20,000/μL at diagnosis, little or no organ involvement, and normal immunoglobulin status. The L2- and L3-type morphology, male gender, black ethnicity, and the presence of CNS leukemia are relatively poor prognostic signs. Chromosomal number also influences prognosis, with hyperdiploidy having the best prognosis and normal diploid or hypodiploid karyotypes being less favorable. In addition, the finding of a positive Philadelphia chromosome t(9;22) is an adverse finding.

The strategy in treating ALL is to attempt to eradicate every malignant cell so that none remain to cause recurrent disease. Combination chemotherapy employs agents that exert different kinds of damaging effects to the multiplying cells and is directed toward damaging cell growth at different stages. The three common drugs used are vincristine, prednisone, and L-asparaginase. CNS prophylaxis is usually accomplished by the administration of methotrexate into the spinal fluid and courses of cranial irradiation. Maintenance chemotherapy is also continued for 2 to 3 years with 6-mercaptopurine and methotrexate. Patients receiving these drugs need to have regular blood counts checked for bone marrow suppression and liver function studies to evaluate liver toxicity. The principles of therapy and the requirements of transfusion support, vigorous antibacterial therapy, and microbiologic searches for causes of sepsis are the same as were discussed under the treatment of acute myelogenous leukemia. A comparison of the features of acute myelogenous leukemia and acute lymphoblastic leukemia are listed in Table 4–10.

Leukemic Chronic Lymphoproliferative Disorders

These conditions are characterized by unregulated clonal growth of differentiated cells, each expressing individual immunologic characteristics, either B subtypes, T subtypes, or undifferentiated subtypes. These disorders are broadly grouped into the leukemic chronic lymphoproliferative disorders and the lymphomas. The major diseases in the former category are *chronic lymphocytic leukemia, prolymphocytic leukemia,* and *hairy cell leukemia* (see Color Plates 47–49).

Chronic Lymphocytic Leukemia

Chronic lymphocytic leukemia (CLL) differs from the other leukemias in that it runs a typically indolent course over many years in most cases. It occurs almost exclusively in adults over the age of 40. In most CLLs, the proliferating cells are B lymphocytes, which have normal surface characteristics and no detectable immunologic activity but characteristically express the CD5 antigen. Leukemic B cells survive as long as 5 years, compared with 1–year survival for normal "long-lived" B lymphocytes. Because the lymphocyte production rate also increases as much as tenfold, the net result is massive cellular accumulation. The accumulating cells are immunologically inert, and their presence crowds out normally reactive B cells. The spleen, lymph nodes, and bone marrow are overrun by these cells, which interfere with the movement of normal granulocytes, monocytes, and erythrocytes across vascular membranes.

Clinical Findings Chronic lymphocytic leukemia always develops gradually. Often it is discovered incidentally during a blood count performed for other reasons. The white cell count runs between 10,000/µL and 100,000/µL; 95% of the circulating white cells are small lymphocytes of normal appearance (see Color Plate 47). Granulocytes, although sparse in the differential count, are present initially in normal absolute numbers. As the lymphocytes overrun the marrow, platelet counts and red cell production may decline, but intrinsic erythropoietic and thrombopoietic capabilities are normal. Since these lymphocytes are functionally inert, both humoral and cell-mediated immunity are defective, and individuals are at risk for infections with bacterial and opportunistic microbes.

Chronic lymphocytic leukemia adversely affects immune function. Half of the CLL patients have decreased immunoglobulin levels, especially IgM, at some time during their disease. One-third of patients experience autoimmune manifestations and have a positive direct antiglobulin test (Coomb's Test) (see Chapter 8). This may be associated with an autoimmune hemolytic anemia, whose effect may be profound since the marrow cannot mount an appropriate response due to the overcrowding by lymphocytes (see Autoimmune Hemolytic Anemia, Chapter 3). The clinical stages of chronic lymphocytic leukemia are listed in Table 4–21.

Some patients in stages 0 to 2 may live for 10 to 20 years, whereas for those with stages 3 and 4, the median survival is less than 5 years. Some untreated persons survive for years with a CLL. Symptomatic anemia and thrombocytopenia are indications for therapeutic intervention. If red cells and platelets remain adequate, patients may never need therapy and may succumb to other cardiovascular problems and diseases of old age. Many

TABLE 4–21. STAGING SYSTEMS FOR CHRONIC LYMPHOCYTIC LEUKEMIA

	Criteria	Median Survival (Years)
RAI Staging System		
*Stage**		
0 (low-risk)	Lymphocytes $> 15 \times 10^9$/L	>10
	Bone marrow > 40% Lymphocytes	
I and II (intermediate-risk)	Blood and bone marrow lymphocytosis, lymphadenopathy, liver or spleen enlargement	6
III and IV (high-risk)	Blood and bone marrow lymphocytosis plus anemia (hemoglobin < 11 g/dL) or thrombocytopenia (platelets < 100×10^9/L)	2
Binet Staging System		
*Group**		
A	No anemia or thrombocytopenia, less than three of the following five areas involved: axillary, inguinal, cervical (unilateral or bilateral) lymphade-nopathy; liver, spleen	9
B	No anemia or thrombocytopenia; three or more involved areas	5
C	Anemia (hemoglobin < 10 g/dL) or thrombocytopenia (platelets < 100×10^9/L)	2

*Autoimmune hemolytic anemia and thrombocytopenia are independent of stage or group.

From Foon, KA, and Gale, RP: Chronic Lymphoid Leukemias. In Handin, RI, Stossel, TP, and Lux, E (eds): Blood: Principles and Practice of Hematology. JB Lippincott, Philadelphia, 1995, p 789, with permission.

patients, however, do experience a progressively more aggressive course. As organ infiltration progresses, CLL and well-differentiated lymphocytic lymphoma become difficult to distinguish both clinically and histologi-cally. Indeed, the need to distinguish between these two disorders may be only technical because therapy would generally be the same. In the terminal phase of CLL, increasing immunologic impairment, anemia, hemorrhagic complications, and infection develop. An unexplained observation is the finding that patients with CLL have solid cancers more often than age-matched controls; skin and colon are especially common sites.

In treating CLL, it is impossible to eradicate all malignant cells because leukemic proliferation is widespread, longstanding, and massive by the time disease becomes apparent. Chlorambucil and cyclophosphamide are drugs used to control disease proliferation. Therapy seeks mainly to prevent bone marrow replacement and alleviate symptoms or bulk disease arising from splenomegaly or lymph node enlargement. Agents useful in treating acute leukemia are generally ineffective in combating the accelerated terminal phase of CLL. Newer agents such as 2-chlorodeoxyadenosine (2-CdA), fludarabine, and rituximab appear to be more successful in controlling the disease progression and in treating more advanced disease.

Prolymphocytic Leukemia

Prolymphocytic leukemia is a more aggressive and dedifferentiated form of chronic lymphocytic leukemia, in which the proliferating cells have a more rapid growth potential and more abundant cytoplasm with very prominent nucleoli (usually fewer than two), and patients usually present with high leukocyte counts and a markedly enlarged spleen. This course tends to be more aggressive, and patients may have an elevated blood calcium (note T-cell ALL and HTLV-I and hypercalcemia in the previous section).

Hairy Cell Leukemia

This condition is a clonal proliferation of morphologically distinct cells that are characterized by the presence of fine, cytoplasmic projections; a distinctive nuclear pattern (salt and pepper chromatin); and the presence within the cells of a specific tartate-resistant isoenzyme of acid phosphatase (TRAP test; see Color Plate 49). These patients also show an enlarged spleen. The disorder may present with increased numbers of these cells in the peripheral blood, and may mimic chronic lymphocytic leukemia, but *pancytopenia* is common. In contrast to CLL, these cells characteristically express the CD25 antigen (IL-2 receptor). Another distinctive differentiating feature is the fact that, in most cases, a bone marrow aspirate performed on these patients is usually a dry tap. Bone marrow biopsy shows a characteristic eosinophilic interdig-itating material that looks very much like fibrous tissue but is negative for fibrous stains. Electron microscopy of the cells characteristically shows the hairy projections and abnormal ribosomal lamellar com-plexes. The differentiation of this disorder from CLL is extremely important because therapy is distinctly different. This disorder may be well controlled or even cured using 2CdA therapy. Other active agents in this disease are interferon treatment or 2-deoxycoformycin. Another name for this disorder is "leukemic reticuloendotheliosis." Figure 4–4 shows the characteristic morphology of these cells. The patients also characteristically have a severe peripheral pancytopenia (see also Color Plate 48).

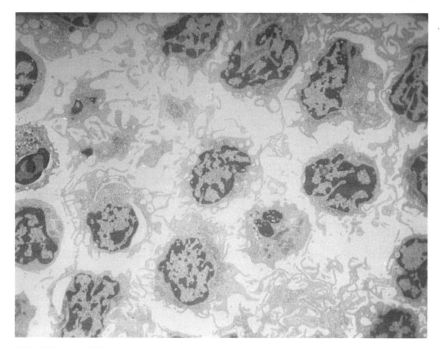

FIGURE 4–4. Electron micrograph of hairy cells from a patient with hairy cell leukemia.

The Lymphomas

Lymphomas are malignant neoplasms of the lymphoid organs character-ized by autonomous neoplastic growth of cells committed toward lymphoid differentiation. These tumors primarily affect lymphoid tissues, particularly lymph nodes and spleen but may involve other lymphoreticular sites, including the liver, gastrointestinal tract, nasopha-ryngeal tissues, and the lungs. Diagnosis is by tissue biopsy; laboratory data are suggestive or confirmatory at best. Because of the close association of lymphomas with the hematologic and immunologic diseases already considered, a brief discussion of diagnosis and classification follows.

Hodgkin's Disease

Categorized as one of the lymphoproliferative disorders, lymphomas fall into two major categories: Hodgkin's disease and the non-Hodgkin's lymphomas.

Classification **Hodgkin's disease** is classified separately because the neoplastic cell has not yet been fully determined and because the prognosis and therapy are distinctly different from those of non-Hodgkin's lymphomas. Hodgkin's disease is further subclassified into four major subtypes, all of which have the presence of the pathognomonic cell, the **Reed-Sternberg cell** (Fig. 4–5). The subtypes of Hodgkin's disease are classified according to the preponderance of lymphocytes and larger transformed cells or Reed-Sternberg cells. Table 4–22 is a breakdown of the subtypes of Hodgkin's disease. Hodgkin's disease almost invariably originates in the lymph nodes and spreads from one chain of nodes to adjacent ones in a regular progression. The diagnosis of Hodgkin's disease is made by tissue histology and the finding of Reed-Sternberg cells, which are giant cells with mirror-image nuclei and prominent nucleoli—an owl's eye nucleus. The precursor of these cells remains controversial. The lymphocytes are clearly of T-cell origin, but they may not be the distinctive neoplastic element. Controversy also surrounds the etiology of the disease; epidemiologic features suggest infection as a contributing cause, but no specific agent has been implicated, and it is obvious that other unknown considerations critically influence the development of the disease.

Clinical Features   Painless asymmetric swelling of the lymph nodes is the most common presenting feature of Hodgkin's disease. Some patients

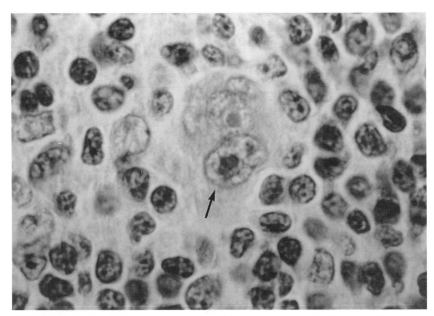

FIGURE 4–5. Reed-Sternberg cell *(arrow)* from a lymph node biopsy in Hodgkin's disease. (From Pittiglio, DH, and Sacher, RA: Clinical Hematology and Fundamentals of Hemostasis. FA Davis, Philadelphia, 1987, Fig. 204, with permission.)

TABLE 4–22. CLASSIFICATION OF HODGKIN'S DISEASE

Pattern	General Age Group	Description	Presence of Reed-Sternberg (RS) Cells	Frequency (% of Cases)	Prognosis
LP (lymphocyte predominant)	Young individuals	Characterized by a diffuse infiltrate of mature lymphocytes mixed with variable numbers of histiocytes.	Few in number	5–10	Best
NS (nodular sclerosis)	Young individuals (often females)	Represents a distinct entity with a different epidemiology and biologic significance from the other 3 patterns. Unique to this pattern are 2 characteristics: 1. biopsy specimen characterized by birefringent bands of collagen, which traverse the lymph node, enclosing nodules of normal and abnormal lymphoid tissue; and 2. presence of a Reed-Sternberg cell variant called a lacunar cell, which looks like a Langhans' giant cell that sits in a lacunal space.	RS variant (lacunar cells present)	35–60	Second best
MC (mixed cellularity)	Middle-aged (30 yr old)	Characterized by a diffuse infiltrate of lymphocytes, histiocytes, eosinophils, and plasma cells, which obliterate the underlying nodal architecture.	Usually plentiful	30–50	Third best
LD (lymphocyte depletion)	Middle-aged	Characterized by a paucity of lymphocytes and diffuse fibrosis.	Few in number	1–5	Worst

Adapted from Pittiglio, DH, and Sacher, RA: Clinical Hematology and Fundamentals of Hemostasis. FA Davis, Philadelphia, 1987, p 299.

present with constitutional symptoms that include night sweats, fever, and weight loss. These symptoms, termed "B" symptoms, are prognostically adverse. Thus the disease can be classified on the basis of the presence or absence of these symptoms into A or B types.

Laboratory Findings Table 4–23 lists the laboratory findings often associated with Hodgkin's disease. The peripheral blood may show a normochromic, normocytic anemia, and monocytosis and eosinophilia may also occur. The platelet count is often increased, with an elevated sedimentation rate reflecting increased cell turnover and inflammation. The sedimentation rate serves as a useful, nonspecific marker of the disease activity. Involvement of other organs may produce specific chemical abnormalities such as abnormal liver function.

Another feature of this disorder is decreased cell-mediated immunity, reflecting abnormal T-cell function. A common finding is the absence of skin reactivity following intradermal injections of common antigens such as *Candida,* mumps, and streptokinase. This failure to elicit a skin reaction is termed **cutaneous anergy.**

Therapeutic response and long-term prognosis correlate not only with the morphologic type but also with the extent of the disease at the time of diagnosis. Table 4–24 indicates the staging of Hodgkin's disease. In stage I disease, the least extensive at the time of diagnosis, only a single lymph node group or a single extranodal site is involved. Stage IV disease, the most widespread, involves many lymph node groups and also nonlym-

TABLE 4–23. LABORATORY FINDINGS IN HODGKIN'S DISEASE

Early in Course

Mild normochromic, normocytic anemia from depressed erythropoiesis
Moderate leukocytosis with eosinophilia to 10%
Normal or increased platelet count
Increased ESR
Decreased serum iron and iron-binding capacity, normal or increased marrow iron
Decreased cell-mediated immunity; antibody activity normal

Later in Disease

Lymphopenia
More severe anemia
Coombs'-positive hemolysis (relatively rare)
Thrombocytopenia
Mild hypoalbuminemia, hyperglobulinemia
Hypercalcemia
Hyperuricemia
Low serum zinc, high serum copper

TABLE 4–24. CLINICAL STAGING OF LYMPHOMAS (HODGKIN'S DISEASE)

Stage I	One group of lymph nodes involved with disease, either above or below the diaphragm.
Stage II	Two different groups of lymph nodes involved with disease, both being either above or below the diaphragm.
Stage III*	Two different groups of lymph nodes involved with disease, one on each side of the diaphragm.
Stage IV	Extranodal involvement in areas not contiguous with lymph nodes (includes bone marrow or liver involvement).†

*Stage IIIA is subdivided into 1 and 2.
†E classification indicates extension from a lymph node area.

phoid organs like bone marrow, liver, and spleen. At any given stage, patients without constitutional symptoms like fever, weight loss, and night sweats, do better than those with symptomatic disease. In recent times, combination chemotherapy, radiation therapy, or both have proven very successful in the management of Hodgkin's lymphoma. Complete and durable long-term remission has been achieved in more than 85% of patients. Patients are generally followed up at regular intervals by monitoring complete blood counts, a chemistry profile screen, and a sedimentation rate. The presence of cytopenias and an elevated sedimentation rate may herald the onset of relapse.

Non-Hodgkin's Lymphomas

Non-Hodgkin's lymphomas are characterized by autonomous proliferation of lymphoid cells that are classified according to their histopathologic morphology (nodular or diffuse), the cell type (small cells, large cells, lymphocytic, histiocytic, mixed), and cytologic differentiation (well differentiated, poorly differentiated). Because of the complexity of lymphocyte differentiation and lymphocyte subtypes, several classifications have been developed. A "working formulation" of the non-Hodgkin's lymphomas has been categorized by international experts into low-grade, intermediate-grade, high-grade, and other types, as listed in Table 4–25. This compromise classification reconciles some of the advantages of the various other classifications. A new Revised European American Lymphoma (REAL) Classification has been suggested because of an increasing number of unclassifiable types (see Fig. 4–3). Table 4–26 cross-references the REAL and Working Formulation Classifications. Table 4–27 also lists the differential diagnoses of small lymphocytic types.

Low-Grade Malignant Lymphoma   Low-grade malignant lymphomas include **small-cell lymphocytic, follicular small cleaved,** and **follicular**

TABLE 4–25. CLASSIFICATION OF NON-HODGKIN'S LYMPHOMAS (WORKING FORMULATION)

Low-grade Malignant Lymphoma

Small, lymphocytic
Follicular, predominantly small, cleaved
Follicular, mixed small, cleaved, and large cell

Intermediate-grade Malignant Lymphoma

Follicular, predominantly large cell
Diffuse, small, cleaved
Diffuse, mixed small and large cell
Diffuse large cell

High-grade Malignant Lymphoma

Large cell, immunoblastic
Lymphoblastic
Small, noncleaved
Miscellaneous
  Composite
  Mycosis fungoides
  Histiocytic

---

mixed. Small-cell lymphocytic lymphoma is analogous to chronic lymphocytic leukemia developing within the B lymphocytes of the lymph nodes. There is a clonal expansion of well-differentiated small lymphocytes replacing the normal architecture of the lymph nodes. This produces lymph node swelling and may spill over into the peripheral blood, producing a leukemic-like picture. The morphology of this leukemia is like CLL, and the clinical features and stages are very similar. A Coomb's-positive autoimmune hemolytic anemia and thrombocytopenia may also coexist in this disorder.

In follicular small cleaved and follicular mixed lymphomas, the follicular (or nodular) pattern prevails. The histology is further classified according to whether small cells with clefted nuclei or a mixture of these cells and larger cells coexist. The behavior of these lymphomas resembles that of the small lymphocytic type.

Intermediate-Grade Lymphomas This type may be subclassified into the *diffuse* and *follicular* types. The diffuse large-cell lymphoma is more common. It usually presents with asymmetric enlargement of lymph nodes and other clinical features of non-Hodgkin's lymphoma, such as splenomegaly. The condition was formerly called "diffuse histiocytic lymphoma" and represents an unregulated growth of transformed

TABLE 4–26. SIMPLIFIED COMPARISON OF THE REAL CLASSIFICATION WITH THE WORKING FORMULATION

Revised European American Lymphoma (REAL) Classification	Working Formulation
Precursor B-lymphoblastic lymphoma/ leukemia	Lymphoblastic
B-cell chronic lymphocytic leukemia/ prolymphocytic leukemia/small lymphocytic lymphoma	Small lymphocytic, consistent with CLL
Lymphoplasmacytoid lymphoma	Small lymphocytic, plasmacytoid
Mantle cell lymphoma	Diffuse, small cleaved cell
Follicular center lymphoma, follicular	
Grade I	Follicular, predominantly small cleaved cell
Grade II	Follicular, mixed small and large cell
Grade III	Follicular, predominantly large
Follicular center lymphoma, diffuse, small cell [provisional]	Diffuse, small cleaved cell
Extranodal marginal zone B-cell lymphoma (low-grade B-cell lymphoma of MALT type)	Small lymphocytic
Nodal marginal zone B-cell lymphoma [provisional]	Small lymphocytic
Splenic marginal zone B-cell lymphoma [provisional]	Small lymphocytic
Hairy cell leukemia	—
Plasmacytoma/myeloma	Extramedullary plasmacytoma
Diffuse large B-cell lymphoma	Diffuse, large cell
Primary mediastinal large B-cell lymphoma	Diffuse, large cell
Burkitt's lymphoma	Small noncleaved cell, Burkitt's
High-grade B-cell lymphoma. Burkitt-like [provisional]	Small noncleaved cell, non-Burkitt's
Precursor T-lymphoblastic lymphoma/ leukemia	Lymphoblastic
T-cell chronic lymphocytic leukemia/ prolymphocytic leukemia	Small lymphocytic
Large granular lymphocytic leukemia T-cell type NK-cell type	Small lymphocytic
Mycosis fungoides/Sezary syndrome	Mycosis fungoides
Peripheral T-cell lymphomas, unspecified [including provisional subtype: subcutaneous panniculitic T-cell lymphoma]	Diffuse, mixed small and large cell Large cell immunoblastic
Hepatosplenic γ-δ T-cell lymphoma [provisional]	Diffuse, mixed small and large cell Large cell immunoblastic
Angioimmunoblastic T-cell lymphoma	Diffuse, mixed small and large cell Large cell immunoblastic
Angiocentric lymphoma	Diffuse, mixed small and large cell Large cell immunoblastic

(Continued)

TABLE 4–26. SIMPLIFIED COMPARISON OF THE REAL CLASSIFICATION WITH THE WORKING FORMULATION *(Continued)*

Revised European American Lymphoma (REAL) Classification	Working Formulation
Intestinal T-cell lymphoma	Diffuse, mixed small and large cell
	Large cell immunoblastic
Adult T-cell lymphoma/leukemia	Large cell immunoblastic
Anaplastic large cell lymphoma, T- and null-cell types	—

Adapted from Harris, NL, et al: A Revised European-American Classification of Lymphoid Neoplasms: A Proposal from the International Lymphoma Study Group. Blood 84:1364, 1994.

lymphocytes, usually of the B-lymphocyte type. These "immunoblasts" are really not histiocytes at all, so the earlier Rappaport terminology is inaccurate. These cells are usually larger than those found in the small-cell lymphomas and have a vesicular nucleus and prominent nucleoli. The large cells can be arranged in a follicular pattern or may be mixed with small, non-cleaved cells in a diffuse pattern. A variant of the intermediate-grade lymphomas is a diffuse arrangement of small cleaved cells (a condition previously termed "poorly differentiated lymphocytic lymphoma"). The leukemic phase of this disorder is characterized by the appearance of cleaved or clefted lymphocytes in the peripheral blood. There may or may not be leukopenia and thrombocytopenia, depending on marrow involvement. This type of morphology has been referred to as **lymphosarcoma cell leukemia.** Surface marker studies show the B-cell origin of these cells.

High-Grade Lymphomas   These lymphomas include, among others, the aggressive lymphoproliferative neoplasms listed in Table 4–25. The major features common to these lymphomas are their rapid growth and systemic symptoms. T-cell lymphoma, for instance, is a rare lymphoma that tends to occur in young men and is associated with an enlarged thymus and often an increased number of T lymphoblasts in the peripheral blood. This condition may be considered the lymphomatous counterpart of ALL of the T-cell type.

Burkitt's Lymphoma   This is an aggressive lymphoproliferative disorder associated with an infiltration of B lymphocytes of noncleaved, uniform size, producing a diffuse sea of closely packed cells with round to oval nuclei and frequent mitotic figures. Interspersed within this background are pale-staining histiocytes that produce a starry-sky

TABLE 4-27. LOW-GRADE B-CELL LYMPHOMAS: MORPHOLOGIC FEATURES IN DIFFERENTIAL DIAGNOSIS

Lymphoma	Pattern	Small Cells	Large Cells
B-CLL/SLL	Diffuse with pseudofollicles	Round (may be cleaved)	Prolymphocytes Paraimmunoblasts
Lymphoplasmacytoid lymphoma	Diffuse	Round (may be cleaved) Plasma cells	Centroblasts Immunoblasts
Mantle cell lymphoma	Diffuse, vaguely nodular, mantle zone, rarely follicular	Cleaved (may be round or oval)	None
Follicle center lymphoma	Follicular +/– diffuse areas, rarely diffuse	Cleaved (centrocytes)	Centroblasts
Marginal zone B-cell lymphoma	Diffuse, interfollicular, marginal zone, occasionally follicular (colonization)	Heterogeneous: round (small lymphocytes), cleaved (marginal zone/monocytoid B cells), plasma cells	Centroblasts Immunoblasts

From Harris, NL, et al: A Revised European–American Classification of Lymphoid Neoplasms: A Proposal from the International Lymphoma Study Group. Blood 84:1365, 1994, with permission.

appearance. Epstein-Barr virus has been implicated in the pathogenesis of this disease. This condition may have a leukemic counterpart with "undifferentiated" lymphoblasts appearing in the peripheral blood. These cells fail to show any consistent staining characteristics, and immunologic markers are usually negative. Another feature of this disorder is a markedly elevated serum LDH and often an elevated serum calcium.

Adult T-Cell Leukemia   See section on ALL—HTLV-I.

Other T-Cell Lymphomas (Mycosis Fungoides; Sezary Syndrome)
Mycosis fungoides is a cutaneous T-cell lymphoma characterized by reddening of the skin (erythroderma) and shedding of the outer layers of the epidermis (exfoliation). The condition is the result of neoplastic T cells invading the skin, often producing a fungal-like elevated appearance (hence the name "fungoides"). The **Sezary syndrome** is the cutaneous condition associated with the finding of abnormal T lymphocytes in the peripheral blood. These T lymphocytes characteristically have a Sezary-cell morphology—one of an immature cell with a cleaved and convoluted nucleus termed "cerebriform," or brain-like. Sezary cell counts can be performed on buffy coat preparations of peripheral blood to follow the course of cutaneous disease or the effects of systemic chemotherapy. These patients may also have associated lymphadenopathy. Electron microscopy of these cells is diagnostic, showing the characteristic cerebriform convolutions.

Angio-Immunoblastic Lymphadenopathy   This is a rare disorder that mimics a lymphoma and is really a nonclonal proliferation of immuno-blasts within the lymph nodes. The condition probably represents an immunologic malfunction and occurs particularly in elderly people. Laboratory features in this disorder are often consistent and comprise a polyclonal hypergammaglobulinemia, a positive Coomb's test, and occasionally the presence of circulating immunoblasts (transformed B cells) in the peripheral blood. This condition has a high likelihood of transforming to a clonal immunoblastic lymphoma.

Malignant Histiocytosis/Hemophagocytic Syndromes   **Malignant histiocytosis** is a true neoplasm of histiocytes (tissue monocytes), the phagocytic cells of the reticuloendothelial system. These phagocytic cells may produce a severe wasting disorder characterized by spiking fevers and enlargement of the liver and spleen. The condition can also be diagnosed in the presence of the clinical syndrome and the finding of abnormal, malignant histiocytes in the bone marrow that show phagocy-tosis of other marrow elements **(hemophagocytosis).** This hemophago-cytosis is a characteristic finding in this disorder and produces peripheral blood pancytopenia. The indirect bilirubin is occasionally elevated as a result of the hemophagocytosis of the red cells. The Coomb's test is negative. This condition has a poor prognosis.

Malignant histiocytosis must be distinguished from a **viral-associated hemophagocytic syndrome (VAHS).** Again, hemophagocytosis, which may be demonstrated in the bone marrow aspirate, is the main element and is associated with peripheral blood pancytopenia. The liver and spleen are enlarged. The "reactive" histiocytes do not appear neoplastic. This condition has a poor prognosis. It is associated with viral syndromes that include infectious mononucleosis (EBV infection).

Clinical Laboratory Findings in the Lymphomas

Laboratory findings in non-Hodgkin's lymphomas are not consistent. Depending on the degree of marrow involvement, a leukoerythroblastic blood picture may be seen (see Color Plate 46). Occasionally, circulating abnormal lymphocytes are found in the peripheral blood. A bone marrow biopsy and aspirate are useful in staging of the disorder. Approximately 40% of patients with lymphoma may have bone marrow involvement at the time of diagnosis. If marrow involvement occurs, there is a greater likelihood of CNS involvement.

IMMUNOPROLIFERATIVE DISORDERS AND PLASMA CELL DYSCRASIAS

The **immunoproliferative disorders** are a heterogeneous group of diseases characterized by the unregulated growth and proliferation of B lymphocytes that may or may not be capable of immunoglobulin production. These disorders are also characterized by disturbance of immunoglobulin secretion, producing either an excess of one immuno-globulin type **(monoclonal gammopathy)** or an absent or decreased gammaglobulin production (hypogammaglobulinemia). The ability to secrete immunoglobulin and the type of immunoglobulin secreted depend on the timing of neoplastic transformation of these cells during the normal maturation sequence. Neoplastic change can occur at any stage during B-cell development and immunoglobulin production (Fig. 4–6). **Chronic lymphocytic leukemia** is a proliferation of B cells that can fail to produce immunoglobulins; it was discussed earlier. In *Waldenström's macroglobulinemia* there is unregulated production of cells that are intermediate in physiologic transformation between mature B lymphocytes and plasma cells. Characteristically, then, there is an excess of *plasmacytoid lymphocytes* (Color Plate 50) that elaborate the initial immunoglobulin in immune stimulation, namely *IgM* (see Chapter 7). As a consequence, a monoclonal IgM is produced, resulting in *macroglobulinemia.* In *multiple myeloma,* the unregulated production of cells involves the *plasma cells,* which may or may not be capable of excess immunoglobulin proliferation. These are classified according to the *type of immunoglobulin* that they produce and their ability to manufacture whole

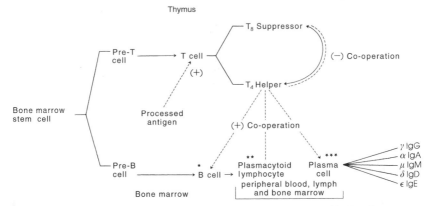

FIGURE 4–6. B-lymphocyte and plasma cell development with T-cell cooperation. Asterisks indicate the sites of immunoproliferative disorders: *chronic
lymphocytic leukemia; **Waldenström's macroglobinemia; ***multiple myeloma.
(Adapted from Pittiglio, DH, and Sacher, RA: Clinical Hematology and Fundamentals of Hemostasis. FA Davis, Philadelphia, 1987, p 268, with permission.)

immunoglobulins or components of the immunoglobulin molecules such
as *light chains* or *heavy chains* (see Chapter 7). In *heavy chain disease,*
proliferating abnormal cells cause a lymphoma-like syndrome in addition
to unbalanced production of heavy chains that are not incorporated into
the immunoglobulin molecules.

Monoclonal Gammopathies and Multiple Myeloma

The **monoclonal gammopathies** are a group of disorders that have one
common denominator: they represent excessive production of an
immunoglobulin molecule or parts of an immunoglobulin molecule
caused by the uncontrolled proliferation of cells of B-lymphocyte or
plasma-cell origin. These cells result from expansion of a single clone of
B lymphocytes, having undergone neoplastic transformation during the
normal maturation sequence. Consequently, the term "monoclonal"
refers to the cellular abnormality. The term "gammopathy" refers to the
abnormal excess of immunoglobulin proteins—**gamma globulins.** Table
4–28 is a classification of monoclonal gammopathies.

The Clinical Laboratory Evaluation of Immunoglobulin Disorders

Serum Protein Electrophoresis In serum protein electrophoresis, the
patient's serum proteins are separated by electrical charge and molecular
size when exposed to an electrical current. The serum is placed on a
support medium, most commonly agarose, suspended in an electrostatic
medium. An electrical charge is applied to the medium, and the serum

proteins are made to migrate. Separation occurs because of their different charges and molecular weights. Figure 4–7 shows the major serum protein components separated into albumin and the globulin fractions. **Immunoglobulins** separate electrophoretically as the gamma globulins. The separated protein bands are identified by staining with a protein stain, and the intensity of the stain reflects the amount of protein present. The density of the different bands is read by a densitometer, which translates the staining intensity into the amount of protein and gives a **tracing,** which is the familiar serum protein electrophoresis profile. Differing profiles are outlined in Figure 4–7. In the monoclonal gammopathies, an abnormal protein, the **monoclonal protein** or **M protein,** is identified. In this case, a single population of immunoglobulin-producing cells proliferates and secretes a single immunoglobulin type, which migrates in the same position on the serum protein electrophoresis, producing a single, dense band. The serum protein electrophoresis, therefore, differentiates a monoclonal paraprotein from polyclonal hypergammaglobulinemia, where there are several clones of immunoglobulin-producing cells, each producing different immunoglobulins migrating at different rates during protein electrophoresis. The serum protein electrophoresis *will not identify the class of immunoglobulin* but indicates the relative percentage of the separated proteins.

TABLE 4–28. CLASSIFICATION OF MONOCLONAL GAMMOPATHIES

Monoclonal Gammopathy of Uncertain Significance (MGUS)
Tumor-associated gammopathy
Biclonal gammopathy
Monoclonal gammopathy associated with miscellaneous disorders

Malignant Monoclonal Gammopathy
Multiple myeloma
   Smoldering myeloma
   Nonsecretory myeloma
   Plasma cell leukemia
Plasmacytoma
   Localized (solitary)
   Diffuse
   Extramedullary
Monoclonal gammopathy associated with:
   Lymphoproliferative disease
   Malignant lymphoma
   Waldenström's macroglobulinemia
Heavy chain disease
Primary systemic amyloidosis

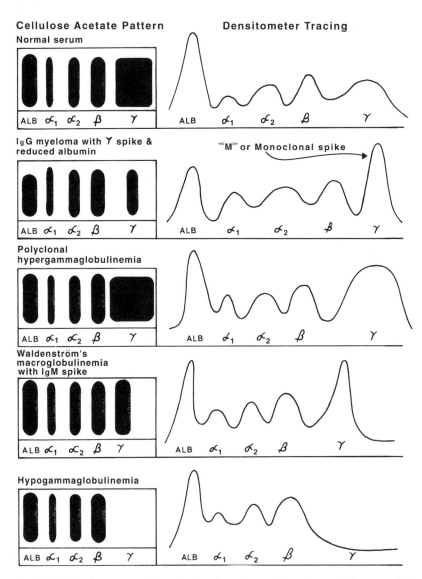

FIGURE 4–7. Serum protein electrophoretic profiles in differing medical conditions. (From Pittiglio, DH, and Sacher, RA: Clinical Hematology and Fundamentals of Hemostasis. FA Davis, Philadelphia, 1987, p 272, with permission.)

Immunoelectrophoresis **Immunoelectrophoresis** couples electrophoretic separation of the immunoglobulins with a two-dimensional immunodiffusion reaction and is used to identify the specific immunoglobulin types. A serum sample is placed in an agar gel, and electrophoresis is carried out. After the serum protein separation has occurred, the protein diffuses into the gel and then immunoprecipitates with an antibody of a known specific anti–heavy chain (gamma, alpha, mu, delta) or anti–light chain (anti-kappa or anti-lambda). If an immunoprecipitation line occurs following diffusion with the known antibody, then the protein is the specific corresponding immunoglobulin (Fig. 4–8) (see Chapter 7). This technique enables the identification of the immunoglobulin type as well as the identification of single chains. It is, therefore, mainly a qualitative test and is only semiquantitative. The urine may also be analyzed using this method if protein excretion has occurred. The urine is concentrated prior to immunoelectrophoresis in an effort to identify the presence of light or heavy chains (discussed later).

A refinement of serum protein electrophoresis and immunoprecipitation is the qualitative test of **immunofixation electrophoresis (IFE)** (Fig. 4–9). In this technique, protein electrophoresis is facilitated and then reacted with antisera that will immunoprecipitate a specific immunoglobulin if it is present.

Immunoglobulin Quantitation   The method of immunoglobulin quantitation is discussed in Chapter 7. A common technique also uses an **immunoprecipitation** reaction (but not electrophoresis) in an agar gel that is impregnated with a specific anti-immunoglobulin. The protein is allowed to diffuse into the gel in a radial fashion that will produce an immunoprecipitate in a ring around the application point. The diameter of the immunoprecipitation ring is proportional to the amount of immunoglobulin present. Immunochemical and nephelometric (turbidity-measuring) methods are now available for the quantitation of IgG, IgM, and IgA, and are faster than immunodiffusion techniques. Immunodiffusion is an overnight test, whereas the immunochemical methods give quantitative results in minutes (see also Chapters 7 and 15).

Urine—Tests for Light Chains   Urine immunoelectrophoresis is the definitive test that allows differentiation between kappa and lambda light chains in the urine.

The Sulfosalicylic Acid Test is the procedure used for quantitating the amount of protein excreted in a 24-hour period. It is a protein precipitation test.

The *Heat Precipitation Test*, or the Bence-Jones Protein Test, is based on the original test described by Bence-Jones for the detection of urine light chains. On heating a sample of urine to 56°C, Bence-Jones proteins (light chains) will precipitate but will redissolve again at about 100°C.

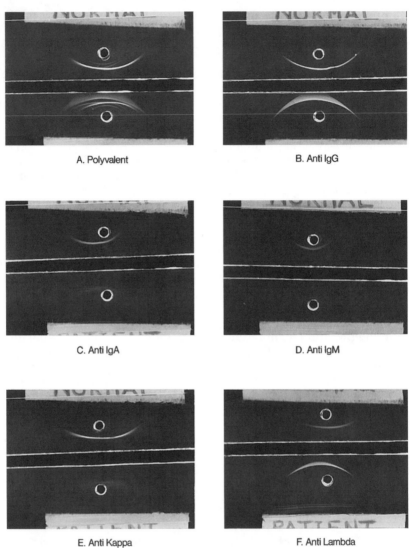

A. Polyvalent

B. Anti IgG

C. Anti IgA

D. Anti IgM

E. Anti Kappa

F. Anti Lambda

FIGURE 4–8. Immunoelectrophoretic serum patterns from a patient with IgG-lambda multiple myeloma. Each photograph shows a normal control sample *(upper well)* and patient sample *(lower well)*. The antiserum used for each analysis is specified on the lower border of each photograph. The patient's serum protein is defined by a precipitation arc in the lower part of each figure. The most intense areas are IgG *(Photo B)* and lambda *(Photo F)*.

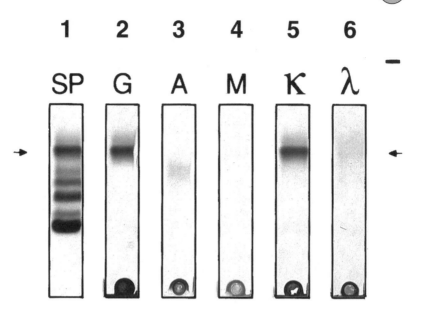

FIGURE 4–9. Immunofixation electrophoresis showing IgG Kappa monoclonal gammopathy *(Lanes 2 and 5)*. Lane 1 = polyclonal; 2 = gamma (IgG); 3 = alpha (IgA); 4 = M (IgM); 5 = K (kappa); 6 = λ (lambda).

Classification of Plasma Cell Dyscrasias

The classification of monoclonal gammopathies (see Table 4–28) uses the following criteria:

- The clinical course (benign or malignant)
- The proliferating cell type (e.g., lymphocytes in the lymphomas, plasmacytoid lymphocytes [cells intermediate between lymphocytes and plasma cells] in macroglobulinemia, and plasma cells in multiple myeloma)
- The nature of the abnormal immunoglobulin produced (IgG, IgA, IgM light chains)

Waldenström's Macroglobulinemia

As already mentioned, this condition is an immunoproliferative disorder, but its clinical features are intermediate between those of a lymphoproliferative disorder and a plasma-cell dyscrasia (see later). The clinical syndrome is one of lymph-node enlargement with enlargement of the liver and spleen and bone marrow involvement, but excess IgM immunoglobulins are also produced. The clinical features may vary—depending on whether lymphadenopathy or hepatosplenomegaly predominates—from a lymphoma-like condition to a consequence of the excess production of the IgM macromolecule. IgM is a large molecule consisting of a pentamer of immunoglobulin chains attached by disulfide bridges (see Chapter 7). It causes the hyperviscosity syndrome, characterized by increased blood viscosity with symptoms of sluggish circulation, increased blood volume, and macroglobulin (IgM) excess, impairing platelet function and hemostasis. Consequently, if it predominates, the major clinical features are neurologic impairment, congestive cardiac failure, and a bleeding diathesis characterized by nosebleeds, cutaneous bleeding, and other mucosal bleeding. Ocular effects also occur and vision impairment is common.

Laboratory Findings The peripheral blood smear shows rouleaux formation (see Color Plate 51A), and plasmacytoid lymphocytes may be seen in the differential leukocyte count (see Color Plate 50). Depending on the degree of involvement of the plasmacytoid lymphocytes and the predominance of hypersplenism, a pancytopenia may be present. The sedimentation rate is variable but may be normal or low. The serum viscosity, which is the ratio of the flow of serum in a graduated tube compared with water, is usually elevated, often above 4 (normal is 1.4 to 1.8) (see Color Plate 51C). A bone marrow aspirate may show the presence of abundant plasmacytoid lymphocytes. These cells have an eccentric nucleus with prominent basophilic cytoplasm and may have a supra-nuclear halo similar to those of plasma cells. The cytoplasm is not as abundant as in typical plasma cells. Waldenström's macroglobulinemia also can involve other organ systems, producing liver dysfunction, renal insufficiency, and nephrotic syndrome. Immune globulin quantitation usually shows an increased level of IgM macroglobulin, often associated with decreased levels of IgG and IgA. Immunoelectrophoresis confirms the presence of an IgM of monoclonal type (mu-heavy chain), and *either* kappa *or* lambda light chain (see also Chapter 7).

Multiple Myeloma

Multiple myeloma is characterized by progressive, unregulated growth and proliferation of a clone of plasma cells, leading ultimately to the death of the patient. It is a disease of the elderly, characterized by a diffuse, plasma-cell infiltration in the bone marrow and overproduction of either intact monoclonal immunoglobulins (IgG, IgA, and, rarely, IgD) or light chains only. The disorder usually presents with a diffuse involvement of the marrow, but occasionally can present as focal tumor masses **(plasmacytomas),** which may be in the marrow or at an extramedullary site (usually the nasopharynx). Variant forms of multiple myeloma include smoldering myeloma, nonsecretory myeloma, plasma cell leukemia, and plasmacytomas.

Multiple myeloma is more common in blacks than in whites and is one of the most common hematologic malignancies of the black population. It also occurs at earlier ages in black patients.

Clinical Features The clinical features and complications of multiple myeloma are shown in Figure 4–10. Patients may be asymptomatic at the time of presentation but usually present with multiple symptoms, of which bone pain, infections, anemia, and renal insufficiency predominate.

Skeletal destruction and bone pain occur as a result of the elaboration of *osteoclast-activating factor (OAF),* which stimulates bone resorption and demineralization of the bone and lytic areas. The presence of other clinical features depends on the amount and type of abnormal protein released by the malignant plasma cells. These features can include hyperviscosity syndrome and bleeding disorders due to interference with clotting factors and platelet function. Other proteins causing clinical features include **cryoglobulins** (proteins that precipitate on exposure to the cold) and abnormal plasma cells or abnormal parts of immunoglobulins *(amyloid),* which are deposited in tissues and cause organ failure.

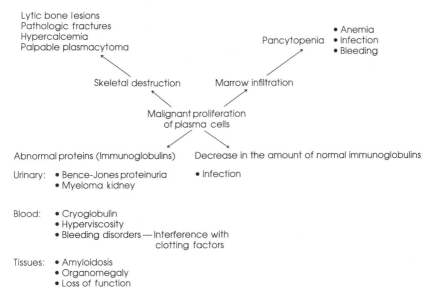

FIGURE 4–10. Diagram outlining the clinical features and complications in multiple myeloma. (From Pittiglio, DH, and Sacher, RA: Clinical Hematology and Fundamentals of Hemostasis. FA Davis, Philadelphia, 1987, p 276, with permission.)

Laboratory Features Patients usually present with a normochromic, normocytic anemia that can be macrocytic. The hemoglobin is usually below 10 g/dL, and the hematocrit is usually below 30%. Red cell morphology is usually unremarkable, with the exception of rouleaux formation as a result of protein coating the erythrocytes; this also contributes to a markedly elevated erythrocyte sedimentation rate (see Color Plate 51A). Sedimentation rates in excess of 100 mm/hour are common in multiple myeloma (see Chapter 2). Initially, the white cell count and platelet count are not decreased, but pancytopenia may develop as the disease progresses or as chemotherapy is used. Some patients may show a leukoerythroblastic blood picture, and occasionally plasma cells may be seen on the peripheral smear (if in excess of 5%, termed "plasma cell leukemia") (see Color Plate 51A).

A bone marrow aspirate usually shows a markedly hypercellular marrow with an abundance of plasma cells in all stages of maturity. Characteristically, the abnormal plasma cell has a "punched-out" nucleolus that is very prominent. Binucleate plasma cells may be seen. In multiple myeloma, the plasma cells constitute more than 20% of the marrow cell population, and the marrow may be almost entirely replaced by malignant plasma cells.

If renal insufficiency occurs, levels of blood urea nitrogen and creatinine will be elevated, in addition to uric acid, a purine nucleotide breakdown product. Serum calcium may be markedly increased because of bone resorption. If beta$_2$ microglobulin levels are increased, the prognosis is worse. Serum protein electrophoresis usually shows the monoclonal ("M") protein. Usually the M spike is greater than 2 g/dL, but the level is dependent on what type of myeloma is present. Light-chain myeloma is not associated with a serum M spike, but the monoclonal light chains are found only in the urine. Additional tests can be performed to demonstrate the presence of cryoglobulins or hyperviscosity. The frequencies of monoclonal paraproteins in multiple myeloma are as follows:

- IgG—52%
- IgA—25%
- Bence-Jones (light chain myeloma)—22%
- Others—1%

Immunoelectrophoresis is used to identify the type of protein, and immunodiffusion or nephelometry is used to determine the absolute quantity of the immunoglobulin. Protein may be identified in the urine and quantitated with a 24-hour urine specimen. Occasionally, protein levels in excess of 4 g per 24 hours may be seen, in which case one must consider the possibility of light-chain deposition in the tissues—amyloidosis—which is associated with **nephrotic syndrome.** Examination of urine sediment may reveal the presence of hyaline protein casts or uric acid crystals.

Monoclonal Gammopathy of Undetermined Significance (MGUS)

This category of disorders includes those patients who present with an *incidental finding* of a serum M spike on routine testing. The accumulation of this monoclonal protein usually occurs in the absence of any clinical disease or symptoms. In most instances, the patients are not aware of any problem, and the M spike is discovered incidentally. This condition was formerly called "benign monoclonal gammopathy," a term that is misleading because a certain percentage of these disorders go on to the malignant variety, namely multiple myeloma. The problem is that the clinical or laboratory features at initial presentation cannot allow a distinction between those cases that will become aggressive and those that will not. There is a 10% likelihood of progression to hematologic malignancy. The monoclonal protein may result in expression of a complete immunoglobulin or light chain only. Patients with MGUS usually have less than 2 g/dL of monoclonal protein in the serum and less than 5% plasma cells in the marrow. MGUS is frequent; it has been found in about 3% of persons over the age of 70 years, and in 1% over 50 years. Since it is impossible to predict which patients are likely to evolve into the more malignant presentation, periodic examination of these patients is the only definitive way of evaluating incipient myeloma. Table 4–29 is an approach to the differential diagnosis of the monoclonal gammopathies.

Amyloidosis This disorder includes a heterogeneous group of conditions characterized by the extracellular deposition of an amorphous, waxy-like material derived from different proteins by different mechanisms. The term "amyloid" was originally derived from the waxy, starch-like property of the material. The accumulation of this material within tissues and organs leads to a loss of function and organ enlargement. Diagnosis is usually made on tissue histology, but

---

TABLE 4–29. PRINCIPLES IN DIFFERENTIAL DIAGNOSIS OF MONOCLONAL GAMMOPATHIES

Establish presence of a monoclonal gammopathy by documentation of an M spike.
  Serum protein electrophoresis
  Urine protein electrophoresis
  Serum immunoelectrophoresis
Establish nature of proliferating cell type.
  Bone marrow aspirate/biopsy
  Skeletal survey
Establish presence of entire or partial protein and activity of the protein.
  Urine light chains
  Quantitative analysis of immunoglobulin
Establish the degree of organ system involvement.

patients with this disorder, particularly the type that occurs in association with multiple myeloma, may present with excess light chains in the urine and may produce excess loss of protein in the urine (nephrotic syndrome).

Heavy Chain Diseases These disorders are characterized by an uncontrolled production of the heavy chain components of immunoglobulins. These proteins are elaborated by monoclonal B lymphocytes. There are three main types, all of which are rare: gamma chain disease, alpha chain disease, and mu chain disease. The most common of these three is **alpha chain disease,** a condition that has also been referred to as "Mediterranean lymphoma." This condition more commonly afflicts younger individuals from the Middle East. The patients typically present with a malabsorption syndrome due to the deposition of plasma cells and lymphocytes in the mucous membrane of the small bowel. An excess amount of the abnormal component of immunoglobulin may be seen in the serum of any of these conditions.

SUGGESTED READING

Anger, B, et al: Polycythemia vera, a clinical study of 141 patients. Blut 59:493–500, 1989.

Bennett, JM: Classification of the myelodysplastic syndromes. Clin Haematol 15:909, 1986.

Boultwood, J, Lewis, S, and Wainscoat, JS: Review: The 5q–Syndrome. Blood 84:3253–3260, 1994.

Brunning, RB, and McKenna, RW: Tumors of the bone marrow. In Atlas of Tumor Pathology. Fascicle 9, Armed Forces Institute of Pathology, Washington, 1994.

Chan, WC, and Greiner, TC: Diagnosis of lymphomas by the polymerase chain reaction. Amer J Clin Pathol 102:273–274, 1994.

Foon, KA, and Todd, RF: Immunologic classification of leukemia and lymphoma. Blood 68:1–31, 1986.

Kantarjian, HM, et al: Chronic myelogenous leukemia: A concise update. Blood 82:691–703, 1993.

Kyle, RA: "Benign" monoclonal gammopathy: After 20 to 35 years of follow-up. Mayo Clin Proc 65:25, 1993.

Lukes, RJ, and Collin, RD: Tumors of the hematopoietic system. In Atlas of Tumor Pathology. Fascicle 28, Armed Forces Institute of Pathology, Washington, 1992.

Mitus, AJ, and Schafer, AI: Thrombocytosis and thrombocythemia. Haematol Oncol Clin North Amer 4:157–78, 1990.

O'Brien, SO, del Giglio, A, and Keating, M: Review: Advances in the biology and treatment of B-cell chronic lymphocytic leukemia. Blood 85:307–318, 1995.

Stossel, TP, and Babior, BM: Structure, function and functional disorders of the phagocyte system. In Handin, RF, Stossel, TP, and Lux, SE (eds): Blood: Principles and Practice of Hematology. JB Lippincott, Philadelphia, 1995, pp 575–619.

Wachtel, M: Cancer cytogenetics: A guide for clinical laboratories. Laboratory Medicine 25:566–572, 1994.

Weinstein, HJ, and Griffin , JD: Acute myelogenous leukemia. In Handin, RF, Stossel, TP, and Lux, SE (eds): Blood: Principles and Practice of Hematology. JB Lippincott, Philadelphia, 1995, pp 543–574.

Weinstein, IM: Idiopathic myelofibrosis: Historical review, diagnosis and management. Blood Rev 5:98–104, 1991.

Yang, KD, and Hill, HR: Neutrophil function disorders: Pathophysiology, prevention and therapy. J Pediatr 119:343–353, 1991.

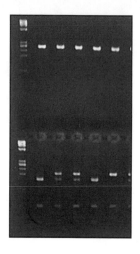

5

Hemostasis and Tests of Hemostatic Function

"Hemostasis" is the collective term for all the physiologic mechanisms the body uses to protect itself from blood loss. It is the process by which the body simultaneously stops bleeding from an injured site, yet maintains blood in the fluid state within the vascular compartment. Hemostasis involves synchronized cooperation between several interrelated physiologic systems.

Failure of hemostasis leads to **hemorrhage**; failure to maintain fluidity leads to **thrombosis.** Both hemorrhage and thrombosis are extremely common and dangerous clinical problems. Characterizing the defects that cause hemorrhage is, at present, easier than characterizing potentially treatable conditions that predispose to thrombosis.

Normal hemostatic mechanisms comprise four main systems: (1) the vascular system, (2) platelets, (3) the coagulation system, and (4) the fibrinolytic system.

Vascular System: Blood vessels have one or more layers of smooth muscle surrounding endothelial cells that cover the luminal surface. When vessels are damaged, the muscle constricts, narrowing the path through which blood flows and sometimes halting blood flow entirely. This **vascular phase** of hemostasis affects only arterioles and their dependent capillaries; large vessels cannot constrict sufficiently to prevent blood loss. Even in small vessels, vasoconstriction provides only the briefest sort of hemostasis.

Platelets: Permanent repair requires that breaks in the vessel wall be plugged; the effective hemostatic plug consists of platelets and the gel-like protein fibrin. Platelets are nonnucleated fragments of megakaryocytic cytoplasm, but they are living entities with complex structure, active metabolism, and a reactive biologic constitution. Platelets may plug small holes in blood vessels and can form an effective primary hemostatic mechanism.

Coagulation System: Coagulation is a chemical process whereby plasma proteins interact to convert the large, soluble plasma protein molecule **fibrinogen** into the stable, insoluble gel called **fibrin.** The active compound is the enzyme **thrombin,** which preferentially converts fibrinogen (soluble) into fibrin (insoluble). There is a delicate balance between coagulation and maintaining blood in a liquid state. Imbalance in one direction can lead to excessive bleeding, whereas in the other it may lead to thrombosis.

Fibrinolytic System: The **fibrinolytic system** limits coagulation to the sites of injury and wound repair and prevents coagulation from becoming more widespread and uncontrolled. The active compound of this system is the enzyme **plasmin** (derived from the plasma protein plasminogen); it is a relatively nonselective enzyme that more preferentially digests fibrin and fibrinogen.

The relative importance of the hemostatic mechanisms varies with vessel size. Capillaries may rapidly seal injured sites by the formation of hemostatic plugs with little disruption of local blood flow. Larger vessels quickly become occluded by numerous fused platelets. Failure in the formation of hemostatic plugs causes **petechiae**—small, pinpoint hemorrhages. Larger areas of bleeding into the tissues produce severe bruising and confluent hemorrhages called **ecchymoses,** which, when large, form confluent areas of **purpura.** The practical application of laboratory tests to evaluate clinical disorders of hemostasis and thrombosis requires an understanding of the organization of the coagulation and fibrinolytic systems. This may best be appreciated by considering the above four mechanisms responsible for normal hemostasis.

Tables 5–1 and 5–2 list normal values for platelet and coagulation studies.

TABLE 5–1. NORMAL VALUES FOR PLATELET STUDIES

Bleeding time	
Ivy	3–6 min
Template	6–10 min
Platelet count	150–450 × 10³/µL
Clot retraction	>40% retraction at 1 hr
Platelet aggregation	Results are compared against light-transmission of normal platelets
Von Willebrand factor	
Antigen	60–160% of normal
Activity	50–130% of normal

TABLE 5–2. COAGULATION FACTOR NOMENCLATURE AT A GLANCE

Factor	Synonym	Clotting Pathway	Molecular Weight (kd)	Site of Production
I	Fibrinogen	Intrinsic, extrinsic, common pathway	340	Liver
II	Prothrombin	Intrinsic, extrinsic, common pathway	70	Liver (vitamin-K–dependent)
III	Tissue thromboplastin (tissue factor)	*Extrinsic	44	Thromboplastic activity present in most tissues
V	Labile factor proaccelerin	Intrinsic, extrinsic, common pathway	330	Liver
VII	Stable factor proconvertin	*Extrinsic	50	Liver (vitamin-K–dependent)
VIII	Antihemophilic factor (AHF)	Intrinsic	330	Possibly, liver endo-thelial cells & megakaryocytes
vWF	von Willebrand factor	Intrinsic; also helps platelets react with endothelial cells	1000	Endothelial cells
IX	Christmas factor, plasma thrombo-plastin component (PTC)	Intrinsic	57	Liver (vitamin-K–dependent)
X	Stuart-Prower factor	Intrinsic, extrinsic, common pathway	59	Liver (vitamin-K–dependent)
XI	Plasma thromboplastin antecedent (PTA)	Intrinsic	143	Liver
XII	Hageman factor/ contact factor	Intrinsic	76	Liver
XIII	Fibrin stabilizing factor (FSF)	Intrinsic, extrinsic, common pathway	300	Liver or platelets
Prekallikrein	Fletcher factor	Intrinsic	80	Liver
High molecular weight kininogen	Fitzgerald factor	Intrinsic	120	Liver

Note: Although not a coagulation protein or factor, calcium is sometimes denoted as factor IV.

*In classical hypothesis; in combination may activate IX (see revised hypothesis in text).

Half-life Disappearance (hr)	Minimum Hemostatic Level (Concentration)	Storage Stability	Active Form	Other Characteristics (All Factors Are Present in Normal Fresh Plasma)
80	0.5–1.0 g/dL	Stable	Protein	Activity destroyed during coagulation process/present in absorbed plasma
90	40%	Stable	Serine protease	Consumed during coagulation process
			Cofactor	
25	5–10%	Labile	Cofactor	Activity destroyed during coagulation process/present in absorbed plasma
5	5–10%	Stable	Glycoprotein	Present in serum
12	30%	Labile	Cofactor	Activity destroyed during coagulation process/present in absorbed plasma
	30%	Stable		vWf transports VIII
24	30%	Stable	Serine protease	Present in serum
40	8–10%	Stable	Serine protease	Present in serum
48	20–30%	Stable	Serine protease	Present in serum and absorbed plasma
60	0%	Stable	Serine protease	Present in serum and absorbed plasma
150	1%	Stable	Transglutaminase	Actively destroyed during coagulation process/present in absorbed plasma
?	?	?Stable	Serine protease	
?	?	?Stable	Cofactor	

THE VASCULAR SYSTEM

The formation of the hemostatic plug is initiated by vascular damage, tissue damage, or both, producing a sequence of orderly events. Vascular injury is usually associated with the contraction of blood vessels **(vasoconstriction),** contact activation of platelets with subsequent platelet aggregation, and activation of the coagulation pathway. Under normal circumstances, the endothelial lining of the blood vessels is smooth and uninterrupted. Damage to this endothelial lining exposes underlying collagen, to which circulating platelets can adhere **(platelet adhesion).** This, in turn, induces the recruitment of more platelets to "plug" the injured vascular site (platelet aggregation). The vessel wall is also a source of **von Willebrand factor** (discussed later) and the platelet antiaggregant **prostacyclin.**

PLATELETS

Platelets serve two different functions: (1) they protect the vascular integrity of the endothelium, and (2) they initiate repair when blood vessel walls are damaged. This platelet–vessel wall interaction is termed **primary hemostasis.** Persons whose platelets are defective in number or function experience petechiae on skin and membrane surfaces; they are also unable to stem bleeding that occurs following accidental or induced injury to blood vessels.

PRODUCTION AND STRUCTURE

As mentioned in Chapter 2, platelets are fragments of the cytoplasm of their parent, precursor cell, the **megakaryocyte.** Platelets vary in size from approximately 1 to 4 microns and circulate for approximately 10 days as disc-shaped, anucleate cells. Regulation of platelet production is ascribed to **thrombopoietin,** analogous to erythropoietin for erythrocyte production. This substance has only recently been identified and appears to be the ligand for the receptor c-mpl. Interleukin-II also has thrombopoietic activity and is used therapeutically. Thrombopoietin has substantial homology with erythropoietin and increases not only platelet production but also megakaryocyte proliferation. With pronounced hemostatic stress or marrow stimulation, platelet production can increase seven- to eight-fold. Newly generated platelets are larger and have greater hemostatic capacity than mature, circulating platelets. Normally, one-third of the circulating platelet pool is sequestered in the spleen.

A diagrammatic representation of platelet structure is shown in Figure 5–1. The platelet membrane is rich in phospholipids, among them **platelet factor 3,** which promotes clotting during hemostasis. This membrane phospholipid serves as a surface for interaction of plasma proteins involved in blood coagulation. The membrane of the platelet also becomes sticky, allowing for other essential platelet functions of adhesion and aggregation. The cytoplasm of the platelet contains **microfilaments,** which are composed of **thrombosthenin,** a contractile protein similar to actinomyosin, the contractile protein involved in muscle tissue contrac-

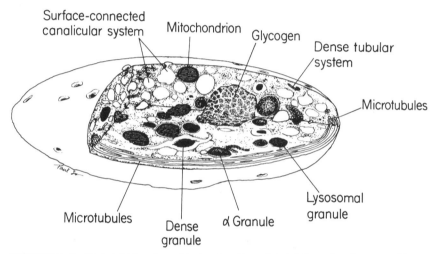

FIGURE 5–1. Platelet structure. Understanding platelet fine structure provides a morphologic basis for platelet function. The peripheral surface coat mediates the membrane contact reactions of adhesion and aggregation. Plasma membrane, which also contributes the phospholipid procoagulant activity, forms an invaginated, sponge-like open canalicular membrane system that represents an expanded reactive surface to which plasma hemostatic factors are selectively adsorbed. Submembranous filaments and other cytoplasmic microfilaments of the sol-gel zone appear to constitute the platelet's contractile actomyosin system. Residual endoplasmic reticulum, free of ribosomes, forms a calcium-binding dense tubular membrane system. Microtubules form a circumferential cytoskeleton that maintains the discoid shape. Following stimulation, the microtubules undergo a concentric central shift with an inner clustering of organelles; concurrently, cytoplasmic pseudopods form on the periphery. Constituents from the alpha-granules, dense granules, and lysosomal granules are then released into the open canalicular system in association with contraction of the actomyosin filaments, which results in a fused impermeable platelet mass. Energy for these events is derived by aerobic metabolism in the mitochondria and anaerobic glycolysis, utilizing glycogen granule stores. (From Thompson, AR, and Harker, LA: Manual of Hemostasis and Thrombosis, ed 3. FA Davis, Philadelphia, 1983, p. 10, with permission.)

tion. **Microtubules,** which form an internal skeleton, are also found in the cytoplasm. Lying beneath the platelet membrane, they comprise a circumferential band of hollow, tubular structures similar to the microtubules of other cells. The microtubules and microfilaments forming the platelet cytoskeleton are responsible for platelets maintaining the normal discoid platelet shape and allow shape changes, as well as facilitating the platelet release reactions. Also interspersed within the platelet cytoplasm are **platelet granules** of two main types: **dense granules** contain adenosine diphosphate (ADP), adenosine triphosphate (ATP), ionized calcium, and serotonin; **alpha granules** contain platelet-specific proteins, especially platelet factor 4, beta-thromboglobulin, platelet-derived growth factor, and (among others) thrombospondin. In addition, plasma proteins, in particular fibrinogen and von Willebrand factor (see factor VIII), are present in the alpha granules. The alpha granules are more numerous than the dense granules. The dense granules represent the storage pool of adenine nucleotides. Prostaglandin synthesis, which is also an integral part of normal platelet function, is believed to occur in an internal tubular system called the **dense tubular system,** which is another component of the cytoplasm of the platelet (see Fig. 5–1). **Platelet factor 4** and **beta-thromboglobulin** are substances normally present only within intact platelets. The presence of these proteins in the circulating plasma indicates excessive platelet turnover or accelerated platelet destruction. Assays for these substances are available in reference laboratories.

FORMATION OF PRIMARY HEMOSTATIC PLATELET PLUG

For normal primary hemostasis to occur, and for the platelets to fulfill their role in forming the initial platelet plug, adequate numbers of circulating platelets must be present, and they must be functioning normally. Normal function requires their participation in an orderly manner, which is important in the formation of the primary hemostatic plug (Fig. 5–2). This involves, initially, platelet adhesion, platelet aggregation, and, finally, platelet release reaction with additional recruitment of other platelets.

Platelet Adhesion

Platelets become activated by exposure to subendothelial collagen and areas of tissue injury. Platelet adhesion involves an interaction between the platelet membrane glycoproteins and exposed or injured tissue. Platelet adhesion is dependent on a plasma protein factor called the **von Willebrand factor,** which has a complex and integral relationship with

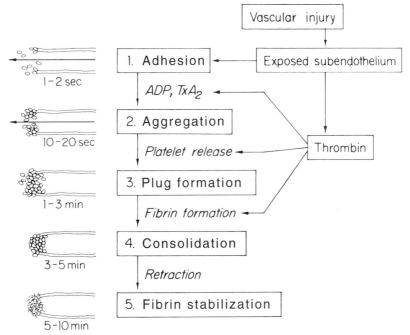

FIGURE 5–2. Hemostatic plug formation. The formation of a platelet plug proceeds through the sequence of: *(1)* platelet adhesion to exposed subendo-thelial connective tissue structures; *(2)* platelet aggregation by ADP, thromboxane A₂, and thrombin recruitment through transformation of discoid platelets into reactive spiny spheres that interact with one another through calcium-dependent fibrinogen bridges; *(3)* contribution of platelet procoagulant activity to the coagulation process, which stabilizes the plug within a fibrin mesh; and *(4)* retraction of the platelet mass to form a dense thrombus. (From Thompson, AR, and Harker, LA: Manual of Hemostasis and Thrombosis, ed 3. FA Davis, Philadelphia, 1983, p. 11, with permission.)

the plasma **antihemophilic coagulant factor VIII** and a platelet receptor called the **platelet membrane glycoprotein Ib.** Individuals lacking the von Willebrand factor have a defect in platelet adhesion called **von Willebrand's disease** (discussed later); those lacking the platelet glyco-protein Ib display the rare **Bernard-Soulier syndrome.** Platelet adhesion is associated with an increase in platelet stickiness, which allows platelets to adhere to themselves as well as to the area of damaged endothelium or tissue. Thus, an initial or primary hemostatic plug is formed. Activation of the platelet surface and the recruitment of other platelets produces a sticky platelet mass and is facilitated by the process of platelet aggregation.

Aggregation

Aggregation is the ability of platelets to stick to one another to form a plug. Initial aggregation is produced by surface contact and release of ADP from other platelets adhering to the endothelial surface. This is termed the **primary wave of aggregation.** Subsequently, as more and more platelets are involved, more and more ADP is released, producing a **secondary wave of aggregation** with recruitment of additional platelets. Aggregation is associated with platelet shape changes from discoid to spherical shape. The secondary wave of platelet aggregation is an irreversible phenomenon, whereas the initial shape change and primary aggregation are reversible. (Fig. 5–3 shows patterns of platelet aggregation as determined by a platelet aggregometer.)

Binding of ADP released from activated platelets to the platelet membrane activates the enzyme **phospholipase,** which hydrolyzes phospholipids in the platelet membrane to produce **arachidonic acid.** Arachidonic acid is the precursor of very potent chemical mediators of both aggregation and inhibition of aggregation involved in the **prostaglandin pathway.** Through this process, arachidonic acid is converted in the cytoplasm of the platelet by the enzyme cyclooxygenase to cyclic endoperoxides, PGG2 and PGH2. The potent stimulator of platelet aggregation, the compound **thromboxane A_2,** is produced by the action of the enzyme thromboxane synthetase on these cyclic endoperoxides (Fig. 5–4). Thromboxane A_2 is a very active, yet unstable, compound that degrades to its stable, inactive form thromboxane B_2. Thromboxane A_2 is also a very potent vasoconstrictor that further prevents blood loss from damaged blood vessels.

Release Reaction

During this process, platelet factor 3, a compound that is released from the internal cytoplasm of the platelet, enhances the coagulation cascade (which is the next phase of hemostasis) and the formation of the secondary, or stable, hemostatic plug. Aggregation can be induced in vitro with reagents ADP, thrombin, epinephrine, serotonin, collagen, or the antibiotic ristocetin.

In vitro aggregation also occurs in two phases: (1) primary, or reversible, aggregation and, (2) secondary, or irreversible, aggregation. Primary aggregation involves platelet shape change and is brought about by contraction of the microtubules. The secondary wave of platelet aggregation involves, predominantly, release of the chemical mediators contained within the dense granules. This, then, completes the third major function of platelets, the release reaction. Augmentation of the release reaction is facilitated by an increase in intracellular calcium, which produces further activation and release of thromboxane A_2.

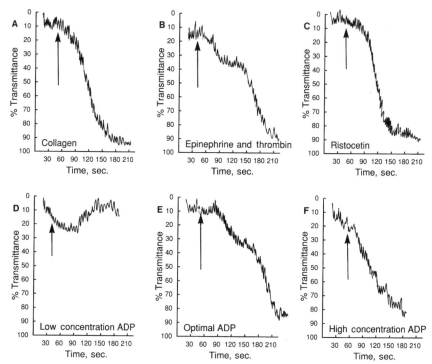

FIGURE 5–3. Patterns of platelet aggregation. Aggregation curves with various aggregating agents: *(A)* Aggregation curve induced by collagen. Note the lag time before aggregation, followed by a single wave of aggregation. *(B)* Aggregation curve induced with epinephrine and thrombin. Note the biphasic wave of aggregation. *(C)* Aggregation curve induced by ristocetin. Note the generally single wave of aggregation.

Aggregation curves with various concentrations of ADP: *(D)* Very low concentrations of ADP induce a primary wave of aggregation followed by disaggregation. *(E)* The optimal concentration of ADP induces a biphasic wave of aggregation. *(F)* High concentrations of ADP induce a broad wave of aggregation. Note: Arrow indicates point of application of aggregation inducer. (Reproduced, by permission, from Triplett, DA, et al: Platelet Function: Laboratory Evaluation and Clinical Application. © 1978 by American Society of Clinical Pathologists, Chicago.)

LABORATORY TESTS USED TO ASSESS PLATELET FUNCTION

Patients experience defects in hemostasis if they have either too few platelets **(thrombocytopenia)** or platelets that function poorly **(thrombopathy).** The clinical consequences of these platelet defects are small **petechial hemorrhages,** larger hemorrhages (ecchymoses), or bleeding from mucous membranes, the gastrointestinal tract, and also bleeding

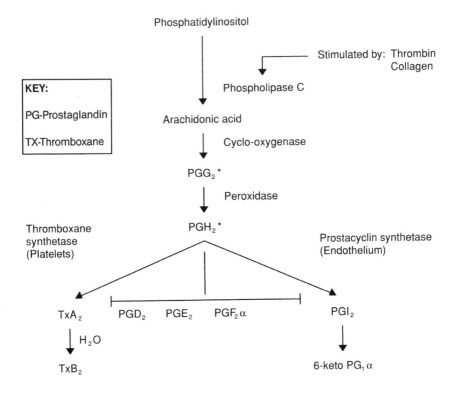

TxA$_2$ - aggregates platelets directly; enhances effect of ADP on aggregation; induces release. *Cyclic Endoperoxides*

FIGURE 5–4. Prostaglandin pathway. (From Treating Hemostatic Disorders: A Problem-Oriented Approach. American Association of Blood Banks, Arlington, Virginia, 1984, p. 15, with permission.)

from venipuncture sites. Thrombocytopenia occurs a great deal more often than the **thrombopathia.** Causes of thrombocytopenia are discussed in Chapter 6. Table 5–1 is a list of normal values for platelet studies.

Platelet Count

The quickest and simplest, but least accurate, way to assess platelet number is to examine a stained blood film. This approach has the advantage of revealing platelet size and morphology, but the disadvantage that adherence to glass or uneven distribution within the smear can produce marked differences in the apparent degree of platelet concentration. A rule of thumb is that the platelet count is adequate if the smear contains one platelet per twenty red cells, or two to three platelets per oil immersion field. Examination of the smear should always be undertaken whenever low platelet counts are obtained because platelet clumping may give rise to a spuriously low count.

Manual Platelet Count

The best manual counting method uses phase-contrast microscopy on a sample diluted 1:100 in ammonium oxalate. If the platelet count is known to be low, a lower dilution factor can be used. The major causes of error, besides technical conditions or inaccurate dilution, are inadequate mixing and the occurrence of adherence or aggregation.

Electronic Counting

Automated cell counters are able to directly measure platelet counts in addition to white cell counts and red cell values. Most of these use an ethylenediaminetetraacetic acid (EDTA) blood sample. Most electronic counters count red cells and platelets together; however, they are differentiated on the basis of size. The smaller particles are counted as platelets and the larger particles are counted as red cells. With electronic particle counting, larger numbers of platelets are examined. This technique is subject to error if the white cell count is over 100,000/µL, if there is severe red cell fragmentation, if the diluting fluid contains extraneous particles, if the plasma sample settles too long during processing, or if platelets stick to one another. As with red cell analysis, a **mean platelet volume (MPV)** is also measured and may be useful in the analysis of thrombocytopenic states. A larger MPV may suggest a peripheral destructive cause for the low platelet count.

Interpretation

Normal platelet counts are between 150,000 and 450,000/µL. The mean is about 250,000/µL. The blood must be drawn briskly through a clean, nontraumatic venipuncture, and it must be mixed promptly and adequately with anticoagulant. If the coagulation sequence is even minimally activated, platelet clumps occur and may adhere to the walls of the test tube, causing spuriously low counts. Excessive agitation should be avoided because this too causes adherence. A properly drawn specimen mixed with EDTA and kept at room temperature retains a stable platelet count for as long as 12 hours.

Platelet Aggregation

Measurement

Platelet aggregation can be measured by bringing platelet-rich plasma into contact with known aggregation inducers. Most inducers such as collagen, epinephrine, and thrombin act through the effects of ADP that the platelets themselves release. Adding exogenous ADP causes aggregation directly. Aggregation is quantitated by determining whether turbid, platelet-rich plasma becomes clear as evenly suspended platelets aggregate into larger clumps that scatter light less, thereby increasing transmission through a tube. Aggregometers are spectrophotometers adapted to record changes in light transmission while maintaining constant temperature and gentle agitation of the platelet suspension.

After a normal curve of light transmission is obtained, the test platelets can be exposed to the various agents and to various conditions. Aspirin, other anti-inflammatory agents, and many phenothiazines markedly inhibit the aggregating ability of collagen and epinephrine but do not interfere with the direct action of ADP. Constitutional disorders of platelet function differ from one another in the nature of the agents that fail to elicit aggregation. It is essential that patients suspected of these disorders abstain from all medications for at least 1 week before testing.

In performance of the tests, it is important that a clean (nontraumatic) venipuncture be obtained. The number of platelets used in the test must be standardized because aggregation responses may vary with the platelet count. Consequently, patients with thrombocytopenia are difficult to evaluate. Aggregation studies should be performed within 3 hours of the sample collection. The samples must never be refrigerated because this inhibits platelet function; consequently, the test is performed at 37°C. The anticoagulant used is sodium citrate, and the samples must never be collected in glass because this activates platelets. Hemolyzed and lipemic samples may interfere with the interpretation of optical density.

Interpretation

The most commonly induced aggregating agents are ADP in varying concentrations, collagen, epinephrine, ristocetin, thrombin, and arachidonic acid.

Low concentrations of ADP induce a biphasic aggregation containing a primary and a secondary wave (see Fig. 5–3). High concentrations of ADP induce only a single wave of aggregation. Patients with platelet release disorders fail to show a secondary wave of aggregation. Patients with **Glanzmann's thrombasthenia** fail to aggregate with ADP.

Aggregation with collagen produces a latent period followed by a single wave of aggregation (see Fig. 5–3). Decreased aggregation to collagen occurs in patients taking aspirin and anti-inflammatory drugs.

Aggregation with epinephrine is usually biphasic. Epinephrine-induced aggregation is also defective in patients taking aspirin and anti-inflammatory agents (see Fig. 5–3). Similarly, thrombin aggregation is also biphasic and may be defective in certain intrinsic platelet defects.

The aggregation response produced by the antibiotic reagent ristocetin is normally monophasic. In patients with von Willebrand's disease, the platelets respond normally to epinephrine, collagen, and ADP, but fail to respond to ristocetin. Their platelets are normal; it is the plasma that fails to contain the von Willebrand factor (vWF). As mentioned previously, this factor is essential in encouraging platelet–vessel wall interaction. In the quantitative assay for vWF activity, the patient's plasma is compared against graduated dilutions of normal plasma by measuring ristocetin-induced aggregation of formalin-fixed platelets suspended in the different concentrates. Abnormal ristocetin-induced platelet aggregation may also occur in other disorders, in particular Bernard-Soulier syndrome. Correction of abnormal ristocetin aggregation in von Willebrand's disease can be induced by the addition of normal plasma, which provides the vWF.

Although congenital defects in platelet function are rare, many acquired conditions depress the release mechanisms. Aspirin is undoubtedly the most common etiologic agent, but few patients develop severe enough bleeding that platelet testing becomes necessary. Patients with uremia, severe liver disease, or advanced alcohol-related conditions often develop a complex bleeding disorder that includes platelet dysfunction. These three conditions depress the ADP release-inducing effect of collagen, epinephrine, or exogenous ADP added directly. Myeloproliferative disorders and dysproteinemias may create a similar problem.

Other Tests of Platelet Function

Platelet Retention

The quantitative determination of the number of platelets that adhere to glass beads can be determined. Platelet retention is abnormal in von Willebrand's disease and other rare, hereditary disorders. It is also abnormal in some acquired disorders, including myeloproliferative syndromes. This test is rarely performed these days.

Beta-Thromboglobulin and Platelet Factor 4

The assay of certain products of platelet release such as beta-thromboglobulin, platelet factor 3, platelet factor 4, and prostaglandin intermediates can also be determined. These generally reflect increasing platelet sequestration and turnover and have been used as tests that are predictive of intravascular coagulation or hypercoagulability. These will be discussed in the section on hypercoagulable states.

Bleeding Time

The single best indication of functional platelet deficiency is prolonged bleeding after a controlled, superficial injury. The bleeding time is prolonged in thrombocytopenia of any cause, in von Willebrand's disease, in most dysfunctional conditions, and after aspirin ingestion. The bleeding time test is somewhat difficult to standardize and to use repeatedly for the evaluation of changing clinical conditions. Every operator performs it differently. The nature of the "standard" injury differs each time it is inflicted, and the results differ with different skin sites and external conditions. In addition, it is unpleasant for patients to be subjected to a standard skin incision time after time. Some patients may also exhibit excess scar tissue formation.

General Techniques and Interpretation Capillaries subjected to a small, clean incision bleed until the defect is plugged by aggregating platelets. If blood accumulates over the incision, coagulation occurs, and the overlying fibrin prevents additional bleeding. Welling blood must be removed, but gently so as not to disrupt the fragile platelet plug. A blood pressure cuff is inflated on the upper arm to 40 mm, and an incision is made on the forearm. Oozing blood is removed at 15-second intervals by touching filter paper to the drop of blood without touching the wound itself. As platelets accumulate, bleeding slows, and the amount of blood oozing decreases over each interval. The endpoint occurs when there is no fluid blood left to produce a spot on the filter paper. Some variation is inevitable; results of duplicate tests performed on the same individual should agree within 2 to 3 minutes at most.

The bleeding time is prolonged when platelet counts fall below 100,000/µL. Aspirin prevents platelet aggregation and prolongs the bleeding time for as long as 5 days after a single dose of 300 mg. Patients should be warned not to take aspirin or any over-the-counter pain remedies for 5 days before the test is scheduled. Congenital absence of fibrinogen and hereditary coagulation defects do not prolong the bleeding time, but acquired fibrinogen problems do. Bleeding time may be less prolonged than expected in some thrombocytopenic patients if all their circulating platelets are young because young platelets have enhanced hemostatic capabilities. Such a condition may occur in sequestrative disorders associated with increased destruction, such as **immune thrombocytopenic purpura (ITP).**

IVY and Template Techniques The bleeding time test is best done on the volar surface of the forearm, a site that is readily accessible, has a reasonably uniform superficial blood supply, is relatively insensitive to pain, and can easily be subjected to mildly increased hydrostatic pressure. The incision should be made at a cleansed site that is free of skin disease and away from obvious underlying veins. A constant pressure of 40 mm Hg should be applied throughout the test. In the **IVY technique,** incisions 3 mm deep are made freehand with the blood lancet. With the **template method,** it is possible to achieve a reproducible, precise incision every time. A normal IVY bleeding time is 3 to 6 minutes. A normal template bleeding time is 6 to 10 minutes. The Simplate II method is a standardized modification of the template procedure and employs a commercially available device. The device is disposable and makes a uniform incision in the forearm. The incision is 5 mm long and 1 mm deep. Bleeding time values of greater than 15 minutes in the absence of a low platelet count indicate a qualitative platelet disorder that needs further investigation (e.g., aggregation studies or von Willebrand factor assay).

Following the activation of platelets and the release of platelet factor 3 (platelet phospholipid), activation of the coagulation cascade with formation of thrombin occurs. This sequence involves two major pathways. **Intrinsic coagulation,** with contact activation of blood clotting factors, initiates the process of clot formation (Fig. 5–5), augmented by the platelet phospholipid factor III. **Extrinsic coagulation,** which is stimulated by tissue factors released from the damaged tissues, also leads to the development of the clot or thrombus.

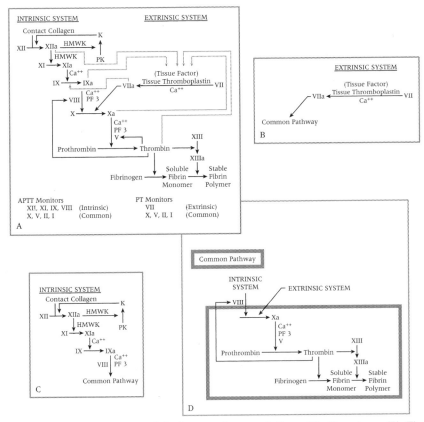

FIGURE 5–5. The "cascade" theory of coagulation. *(A)* Overview. *(B)* The extrinsic system. *(C)* The intrinsic system. *(D)* The common pathway. (From Harmening, DM, and Lemery, LD: Introduction to hemostasis: An overview of hemostatic mechanism, platelet structure and function, and extrinsic and intrinsic systems. In Harmening, DM: Clinical Hematology and Fundamentals of Hemostasis, ed 3, FA Davis, Philadelphia, 1997, p. 495, with permission.)

COAGULATION CASCADE

The purpose of the coagulation system is to generate the active serine protease enzyme thrombin, which in turn acts selectively on the soluble plasma protein fibrinogen, converting it into insoluble fibrin. Fibrin is the visible end product of coagulation and is a gelatinous protein easily identified in tissues or test tubes. Conversion of fibrinogen to fibrin is the last step in a highly complex series of protein reactions that are described schematically in Figure 5–5. Official nomenclature uses Roman numerals to identify the coagulation factors. Some have descriptive or eponymic names as well. Almost all of these factors are present in circulating blood in an inactive, precursor, or zymogen form. The activated form that participates in this sequence is designated by an "a" after the Roman numeral. Table 5–2 is a list of the coagulation factors and some of their synonyms. Fibrin, in essence, acts as the cement substance to stabilize the initial primary platelet plug. Thrombin formation can be generated by the intrinsic coagulation pathway or the extrinsic coagulation pathway.

INTRINSIC COAGULATION PATHWAY

Activation of this pathway occurs through "contact" activation of circulating plasma proteins—the **contact coagulation factors** (XII, XI), which become activated by exposure to damaged vascular endothelium, tissue, or foreign surfaces. In an orderly manner or cascade, the factors are sequentially activated to convert prothrombin into thrombin. Thrombin (IIa) preferentially converts fibrinogen (I) into fibrin through a process of enzymatic cleavage of certain **fibrinopeptides** to produce **fibrin monomer.** The fibrin monomer subsequently **polymerizes** into an **insoluble polymer,** which is then stabilized into the stable clot.

Contact Activation of Intrinsic Coagulation

An important aspect of the intrinsic coagulation sequence is the activation of the contact coagulation factors, factors XII and XI. Factor XII also serves as a key factor in linking several different physiologic pathways synchronously, as is shown in Figure 5–5. Therefore, in addition to coagulation activation, humoral factors are released from complement activation that bring neutrophils and other cells to the area to help clean the debris. In addition, kinins are activated, and these compounds have very potent effects on smooth muscles that facilitate vessel constriction or dilatation to limit bleeding or to enhance the inflammatory response. Furthermore, the fibrinolytic pathway is activated, which is a check system to ensure that coagulation is kept under control through the breakdown or lysis of more extensive clots. Intrinsic coagulation begins when the contact with appropriate surfaces or materials activates factor XII (Hageman factor). In vivo activators include collagen and other subendothelial vessel wall constituents, and such other activators as gram-negative bacterial endotoxins, cell wall products from gram-positive organisms, fatty acids, and antigen-antibody complexes. In the laboratory, factor XII is activated by contact with glass, kaolin, or ellagic acid, but not with silicon or plastic surfaces. Activated factor XII (factor XII) is assisted by a cofactor called **high-molecular-weight (HMW) kininogen (Fitzgerald factor),** which converts prekallikrein (Fletcher factor) to kallikrein, which in turn serves to activate more factor XII. This is a self-amplifying system. Factor XI is converted to its active form by factor XII_a, with HMW kininogen serving as the cofactor. As was mentioned above, contact activation of factor XII and kallikrein initiates more than just coagulation. It promotes conversion of plasminogen to the fibrin-dissolving agent plasmin (see the section on Fibrinolysis). Kallikrein activates **bradykinin,** a vasodilating agent that causes increased vascular permeability and is responsible for acute inflammation. The contact system also initiates parts of the complement sequence (see Fig. 7–2). Kallikrein may also be involved in the extrinsic coagulation system (discussed later). Because persons congenitally deficient in factor XII, Fletcher factor, or HMW kininogen suffer no apparent hemostatic abnormalities or defects in inflammation, the significance of contact activation remains mysterious. This provides additional support to the alternate hypothesis of coagulation (discussed below). Absence of factor XI, however, does cause a bleeding disorder.

Activation of Factor X by the Intrinsic Pathway

Factor XIa activates factor IX in a calcium-dependent, enzymatic cleavage. Factor IXa, along with platelet factor 3 released from stimulated platelets, reacts with factor VIII to produce factor X activator complex. Ionized calcium is required, and thrombin, if present, enhances the process. Factor IXa and phospholipid can, by themselves, activate factor X, but factor VIII enhances the process a thousandfold. Congenital deficiency of factor VIII is called **hemophilia A** and a deficiency of factor IX is called **hemophilia B.**

EXTRINSIC COAGULATION PATHWAY

Products of damaged tissue cause fluid blood to coagulate. **Tissue factor (tissue thromboplastin)** is the term used to describe the clot-promoting activity of lipoproteins present in all tissues. Tissue factor (TF) acts on factor VII, converting it to VIIa, which directly affects factor X. Factor VII can undergo activation in the presence of kallikrein, a suggestive link with the contact phase of coagulation.

In the classic cascade or waterfall hypothesis of coagulation, the extrinsic system seems to be an alternate route of the common goal of factor X activation, but in a clinical sense, the extrinsic and intrinsic pathways are not substitutes for one another. Factor VII deficiency, by itself, is very rare but can cause severe bleeding. The hemorrhagic diathesis of factor VIII and factor IX deficiency, however, is far more severe. An alternative tissue factor pathway cascade has been proposed to explain recent findings (see below).

In the laboratory, factor X can also be activated by exposure to the Russell's viper snake venom or to trypsin. This appears to be a direct proteolytic cleavage that does not require the presence of factor VII.

THE COMMON PATHWAY

Both the intrinsic and extrinsic pathways converge to form the **"common" pathway,** which ultimately activates the plasma protein prothrombin (II) into its active form, thrombin (IIa). Activation of factor X initiates the terminal phase of coagulation and, as described, can be activated by both intrinsic and extrinsic coagulation. The reaction of factor Xa with prothrombin requires calcium ions and phospholipid and is markedly enhanced by association with another plasma protein, factor V.

Thrombin is a proteolytic enzyme of tremendous potency and relatively little discrimination. The quantity of thrombin that evolves from a single milliliter of plasma, if released simultaneously throughout the circulation, could solidify the entire bloodstream. Under normal hemostatic conditions, only small amounts of thrombin develop at a time. Besides converting fibrinogen to fibrin, thrombin also enhances platelet release reactions as described above, and augments the activation of factor V and factor VIII and amplifies factor IX activation. The process is thus autocatalytic and regulatory. Under pathologic conditions, thrombin can split the peptide bonds in a wide range of other proteins.

Fibrinogen becomes fibrin when thrombin removes the tips of two pairs of peptide chains, releasing fibrinopeptides A and B. The resulting molecule, which consists of 97% of the original molecule, is fibrin monomer. Fibrin monomer polymerizes spontaneously to form a loosely adherent gel that quickly depolymerizes if exposed in the laboratory to 5M urea solution or a 1% monochloroacetic acid solution. In vivo, the fibrin monomer constitutes a bulky but fragile clot. Irreversible polymerization occurs when activated factor XIII causes the peptide bonds to cross-link. Thrombin is also responsible for activating factor XIII. Table 5–2 lists the properties of the various clotting factors.

COAGULATION CASCADE THEORY: NEW CONCEPTS—THE TISSUE FACTOR PATHWAY

Laboratory tests that evaluate the integrity of the extrinsic and intrinsic pathways of the coagulation cascade—that is, prothrombin time (PT) and partial thromboplastin time (PTT)—have proven very useful in the diagnosis and management of hemorrhagic disorders. An enigma remains, however, as to why deficiencies of the pivotal factor XII (Hageman factor) are not associated with a hemorrhagic tendency, whereas factor VII deficiencies cause bleeding.

A recently described endogenous regulator of coagulation, the tissue factor pathway inhibitor (TFPI) (see section on Natural Anticoagulants) has prompted a re-evaluation of the coagulation cascade hypothesis. This revised hypothesis of blood coagulation is shown in Figure 5–6 and in some way explains the quandary just mentioned. In this model, the "extrinsic" coagulation pathway is propagated when factor VIIa and tissue factor (TF) directly activate not only factor X, but also factor IX. This has led to a greater appreciation of tissue factor's pivotal role. Furthermore, TFPI is an extremely important natural inhibitor of the tissue factor (extrinsic) pathway, and its unregulated activity can account for a substantial bleeding diathesis. TFPI directly binds and inhibits factor Xa and factor VIIa tissue factor complex. This inhibition involves the binding of Xa-TFPI with TF-VIIa complex. This compound therefore seems to be an important natural anticoagulant, as well as a key regulator of the coagulation cascade. These properties of TFPI have led to the revised hypothesis of blood coagulation shown in Figure 5–6. Thus, coagulation is initiated following exposure of plasma proteins to damaged blood vessels and the release of tissue factor. Factor VII is converted into VIIa, binds to tissue factor, and the complex activates factor X to factor Xa. Some factor IX is also activated to IXa. The generation of Xa induces the inhibitory effect of the natural anticoagulant TFPI and prevents further production of Xa and IXa by the VIIa-TF

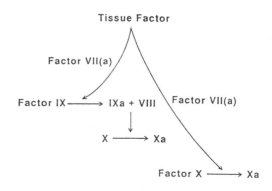

FIGURE 5–6. Revised hypothesis of coagulation: two limbs of the tissue factor pathway.

complex. As can be seen from the figure, factor Xa can only be more actively produced by the pathway involving factor IXa, factor VIII, and factor XIa. This mechanism can therefore explain the clinical need for both intrinsic and extrinsic pathways. Extrinsic activation initiates the process, whereas the contact activation process further consolidates thrombin generation intrinsically in the clot.

THE CLOTTING FACTORS

Table 5–2 shows the nomenclature of coagulation factors.

Factor I (fibrinogen) is a glycoprotein of 340 kilodaltons (kd) and is composed of three pairs of polypeptide chains. Synthesized in the liver, it has a half-life of about 3.5 to 4 days. Fibrinogen levels increase with hemostatic stress, and also with nonspecific stresses such as inflammation, pregnancy, and autoimmune diseases. Normal plasma concentration is 150 to 400 mg/dL.

Factor II (prothrombin) is a glycoprotein with a molecular weight of 70,000 daltons. It is closely related to factors VII, IX, and X; together they comprise the **vitamin K–dependent factors.** They are all manufactured in the liver and require fat-soluble vitamin K for synthesis. All four of these "liver factors" are heat-stable and retain their potency in stored blood or plasma. Prothrombin has a half-life of 0.5 to 3 days.

Factor III (tissue factor [TF] or tissue thromboplastin), and the numerical designation is never used. Tissue factor apoprotein is located in tissue adventitia and is released after vascular injury. It is a glycoprotein of 44 kd that is tightly associated with phospholipid. The gene for TF is located on chromosome 1. The most active tissues are brain, lung, and placenta, but all tissues have this clot-promoting activity.

Factor IV, or **ionized calcium,** is necessary for activation of factor IX, factor X for conversion of prothrombin to thrombin by Xa, and for polymerization of fibrin monomers. There must be at least 2.5 mg/dL of calcium before coagulation can occur in vivo or in vitro. Hypocalcemia never causes clinical bleeding difficulties because more profound neurologic and hemodynamic effects, as well as cardiac arrhythmia, occur well before clotting is disturbed. Anticoagulants such as citrate, oxalate, and ethylene diaminetetraacetic acid (EDTA) chelate calcium and anticoagulate blood by making calcium unavailable for participation in coagulation.

Factor V is a single-chain (MW 330 kd) protein that is synthesized in the liver and in megakaryocytes. The gene coding for factor V is also located on chromosome 1. The gene structure of factor V shows many similarities to factor VIII, and both are labile coagulation factors. Its activity disappears rapidly when anticoagulated blood or plasma is stored in the liquid state. It also disappears rapidly from the circulating blood and has a half-life of only 15 to 25 hours.

Factor V is also an important co-factor in activated protein C (APC)'s ability to function as a physiologic anticoagulant. Mutations affecting arginine 506 to glutamine (factor V Leiden) are thought to be responsible for up to 40% of idiopathic and hereditary thrombophilia. Thus, factor V is both an important procoagulant and anticoagulant.

The term "factor VI" is not used.

Factor VII is a single-chain glycoprotein of MW 50 kd. Factor VII has the shortest half-life of all coagulation factors (5 hours) and is one of the vitamin K–dependent liver factors. Its amino acid sequence is highly homologous with the other vitamin K–dependent factors. It is the first clotting factor to decline after administration of vitamin K antagonists such as oral anticoagulants.

Factor VIII (antihemophilic factor [AHF]) is a large molecule (MW 330 kd) that has several physiologic functions. Procoagulant activity resides on this molecule, which is organized into a heavy chain of 200 kd and a light chain of 80 kd, a low-molecular-weight fragment determined by a gene on the X chromosome. This factor is capable of normalizing the clotting time of hemophilia-A patients. Males whose single X chromosome carries a defective VIII gene suffer from hemophilia A. This factor was formerly referred to as VIII:C. Factor VIII is one of the few clotting proteins not totally synthesized by the liver, and it appears also to be synthesized by endothelial cells in all tissue. Factor VIII has a short biologic half-life of approximately 12 hours and disappears fairly rapidly from plasma stored at refrigerated temperatures. It is present in high concentrations in the cryoprecipitate fraction of plasma (see Transfusion Medicine section, Chapter 8).

Von Willebrand factor (vWF) is the factor that corrects the bleeding time defect in von Willebrand's disease. vWF and factor VIII are two distinct proteins that circulate as a complex in plasma. vWF both transports and stabilizes factor VIII. The antigenic expression of the vWF is called **vWF:Ag.** Another property of vWF that promotes aggregation of platelets in the presence of the antibiotic ristocetin is called the **ristocetin cofactor** or **vWF activity** (previously referred to as "VIIIR:RCo"). Quantitative and qualitative abnormalities of vWF as seen in von Willebrand's disease are inherited in an autosomal manner. vWF is synthesized by endothelial cells and is in fact stored in these cells in so-called Weibel-palade bodies. It circulates in plasma in multimeric configurations.

Factor IX, or **Christmas factor,** plasma thromboplastin component, and PTC, is another vitamin K–dependent liver factor. The disease hemophilia B, or Christmas disease, closely resembles factor VIII deficiency (hemophilia A) in clinical and general laboratory aspects. The factor has a physiologic half-life of about 24 hours but remains at high levels in stored liquid plasma. It is also present in serum. The molecular weight of the protein has been estimated at between 56 kd and 110 kd.

Factor X (58.8 kd), also called **Stuart factor** or **Stuart-Prower factor,** is another of the vitamin K–dependent liver factors and is the key entry protein in the common pathway. The gene for factor X is located on chromosome 13. Isolated congenital deficiency does occur, though rarely, causing moderately severe clinical bleeding. It also exists as an acquired deficiency in some cases of amyloidosis. This factor has a biologic half-life of about 40 hours.

Factor XI is a glycoprotein of 143 kd molecular weight synthesized in the liver and circulating in plasma complexed with HMW kininogen. Factor XI does not diminish in liver disease, however, and is *not* vitamin K–dependent. It is stable in stored blood or plasma and is present in serum. Isolated deficiency occurs as an autosomal recessive trait, especially in Ashkenazi Jewish people, where the gene frequency is 1 in 8. The gene for factor XI is located on chromosome 4. After factor VIII and factor IX deficiencies, it is the next most common congenital deficiency state, but the bleeding diathesis is rather mild. Biologic half-life is about 2 days.

Factor XII, commonly called **Hageman factor,** is a single-chain beta globulin that has a molecular weight of between 76 kd. It appears to be one of the links with other physiologic pathways, including contact activation of clotting, activation of the kinin pathway, activation of complement, and activation of fibrinolysis. It is activated in vitro by contact with negatively charged surfaces (e.g., glass) and in vivo by a variety of cell components such as fatty acids, cerebrosides, tissues such as skin, and endotoxin. Its ability to activate factor XI is also enhanced by two other factors, Fletcher factor and HMW kininogen. Deficiency of Hageman factor is paradoxically not associated with substantial hemostatic problems, but more usually with a thromboembolic tendency. The half-life of Hageman factor is 60 to 70 hours.

Factor XIII, also called **fibrin stabilizing factor (FSF),** stabilizes the conversion of fibrin monomer to polymerized fibrin and a stable clot. In fact, it participates in the formation of a number of stabilizing intermolecular bonds between plasma proteins and extracellular matrix proteins. It appears to be synthesized in both the liver and the megakaryocytes, and more than half of blood factor XIII exists in platelets. The rest circulates in association with fibrinogen. Factor XIII has a long biologic half-life (5 to 10 days), but disappears when plasma is converted to serum. Deficiency of factor XIII is associated with a bleeding tendency, delayed wound healing, and recurrent spontaneous abortion.

COMPARISONS BETWEEN PLASMA AND SERUM

Plasma is the liquid part of fluid blood. Outside the vascular system, blood can be kept fluid by either removing fibrinogen or adding anticoagulants, most of which prevent coagulation by chelating or removing calcium ions. Citrate, oxalate, and EDTA are anticoagulants of the chelating category. Heparin prevents coagulation by directly inhibiting thrombin; it prevents the conversion of fibrinogen to fibrin by augmenting a natural anticoagulant molecule, antithrombin III (ATIII) to neutralize thrombin. Heparin fails to influence the calcium concentration in its anticoagulant effect. Freshly drawn plasma contains all the proteins present in circulating blood; as plasma is stored, however, factor V and factor VIII activity gradually declines.

Serum is the fluid remaining after blood coagulates. Coagulation converts all fibrinogen into solid fibrin and consumes factor VIII, factor V, and prothrombin in the process. The other coagulation proteins and proteins, not related to hemostasis, remain in serum at the same levels as in plasma. Normal serum lacks fibrinogen, prothrombin, factor VIII, factor V, and factor XIII, but it contains factors XII, XI, X, IX, and VII. If the coagulation process proceeds abnormally, serum may contain residual fibrinogen and fibrinogen cleavage products or unconverted prothrombin.

FIBRINOLYSIS

Concomitant with the activation of coagulation is activation of one of the natural anticoagulant defense mechanisms, the fibrinolytic system. This system is also a multicomponent enzyme system that results in the generation of the active enzyme plasmin. Plasmin's function is to remove the fibrin clot by digesting fibrin into small fragments or degradation products (fibrin degradation products or FDPs). In this way, fibrinolysis enzymatically regulates the formation of fibrin as it is occurring in the site of fibrin deposition. It is, in this sense, an extremely integral part of normal hemostasis. Plasmin has a very high affinity for both fibrinogen and fibrin. Generation of plasmin occurs from the inactive plasma protein plasminogen, and this process is initiated by means of **plasminogen activators.** Stimulation of these activators can occur by activated Hageman factor (factor XIIa) in the coagulation system, kallikrein, and other plasminogen activators released by various tissues. A specific **tissue plasminogen activator (tPA)** released at the site of blood vessel damage is probably the most important activator, converting plasminogen to plasmin within the fibrin clot at the site of injury. This activator has an extremely high affinity for fibrin and not fibrinogen, therefore localizing the activation of fibrinolysis within the clot and not within the circulating fluid blood. Normal plasma contains 10 to 20 mg/dL of the precursor substance plasminogen. Plasminogen is converted to plasmin by other plasminogen activators, including **urokinase** and **streptokinase.** Urokinase is an activator that has full activity at the time it enters the circulation. It is an enzyme that is released from tissues of the genitourinary tract. Streptokinase is a streptococcal product that has plasminogen-activating capability. Urokinase and streptokinase have been used therapeutically to activate plasminogen to plasmin in an attempt to dissolve clots. The problem with these two compounds is that they are nonselective and their activity is widespread, producing fibrinolysis and breakdown of fibrinogen throughout the vascular system. There is much interest in the therapeutic use of tPA in dissolving thrombi because its affinity for the fibrin is more specific.

For normal hemostasis to be accomplished, a delicate and dynamic balance between the coagulation cascade and the fibrinolytic pathway needs to be maintained. Once generated, plasmin exerts rather indiscriminate proteolytic activity. Besides digesting fibrin, it also cleaves fibrinogen into peptide fragments that are incoagulable and prevent coagulation of normal fibrinogen. Plasmin also degrades factor VIII, factor V, and factor XIII. Normally, very little plasmin accumulates. Plasma contains two agents that neutralize plasmin: a rapidly acting alpha-1 antiplasmin and a slower-acting antagonist called alpha-2 macroglobulin.

tPA adsorbs to fibrin deposits and activates plasminogen in the local region of the fibrin clot, a process that under normal conditions generates just the right amount of plasmin to prevent excessive fibrin accumulation. Excessive accumulation of activated plasmin can cause proteolysis directed locally at proteins other than fibrin. Systemic activation of plasmin may also occur, or plasmin antagonists may be exhausted. The section on Disseminated Intravascular Coagulation in Chapter 6 discusses some of these consequences.

ANTITHROMBINS AND THE NATURAL ANTICOAGULANTS

Three physiologic natural anticoagulant mechanisms (Table 5–3) exist to keep blood in a fluid state and to prevent hemostatic mechanisms from

---

TABLE 5–3. THE NATURAL ANTITHROMBOTIC MECHANISMS

Antiplatelet

Prostacyclin

Anticoagulant

Antithrombin (heparin[oids])

Protein C ⎫
Protein S ⎭ Thrombomodulin

Tissue factor pathway inhibitor

Fibrinolytic

Plasminogen activator

Plasminogen/plasmin

extending beyond the local need. The checks and balances in the coagulation and fibrinolytic systems prevent unnatural activation of hemostasis, and specific inhibitors exist to limit the activated coagulation factors from proceeding in an unregulated manner. Deficiencies of these mechanisms produce a hypercoagulable state and lead to thrombosis (thrombophilia), discussed later.

ANTITHROMBIN

Antithrombin (also called antithrombin III) is a serine protease inhibitor (MW 58 kd) that preferentially binds thrombin as well as some other serine proteases (Xa, IXa, XIa) within the coagulation cascade, neutralizing their activity. The ability of antithrombin to neutralize thrombin's activity is rapidly enhanced by the presence of heparin. Antithrombin inhibits serine proteases by developing a 1:1 stoichiometric complex between the serine active center and its arginine reactive site before the protease can act on other proteins. Antithrombin abolishes activity not only of thrombin, but also of activated factors IX, X, and XI. Another name for the antithrombin is **heparin cofactor.** Heparin augments a hundredfold the affinity between ATIII and the serine protease enzymes. Patients whose blood lacks antithrombin derive no therapeutic benefit from heparin (heparin resistance). Naturally occurring heparinoid substances exist in the body that are probably released from the vascular endothelium. The heparin antithrombin complex will rapidly neutralize any thrombin that is generated by activation of the coagulation cascade. Antithrombin is formed in the liver and therefore can be depleted as a result of both liver disease and consumptive disorders such as disseminated intravascular coagulation. Inherited deficiency of antithrombin can also occur in which individuals are prone to intravenous thromboembolism (see Thrombophilia). Lysis of platelets releases platelet factor 4, which inhibits AT and heparin activity.

PROTEIN C AND PROTEIN S

These two physiologic anticoagulants, which work in unison, are also both dependent on vitamin K for their action.
Protein C, a polypeptide like the vitamin K–dependent coagulation factors, is also manufactured by the liver and circulates in its inactive (zymogen) form. Activation of coagulation, and specifically thrombin generation, facilitates protein C's conversion into its active form, protein Ca. **Thrombomodulin,** an additional substance produced by the blood vessel, is necessary for this process and may help focus the neutralization at the site of vascular injury. Protein C's action as an anticoagulant is due to its rapid neutralizing activity of factors VIIIa and Va. **Protein S** accelerates the inactivation of Va and VIIIa by protein C. A mutant factor

V (factor V Leiden), which is highly prevalent in white populations (up to 8%), is resistant to activated protein C neutralization and is responsible for a predisposition to venous thrombosis. Protein C may also activate fibrinolysis through an interrelated pathway.

One therefore can see a dynamic relationship between coagulation on one hand and fibrinolysis on the other, with numerous interconnections both augmenting and neutralizing the pathways (see Fig. 5–5). This delicate balance can be altered by deficiencies of various factors, and the clinical syndromes so produced may manifest either as hemostatic disorders or as thrombotic disorders. These will be discussed in the section dealing with disorders of hemostasis (Chapter 6).

Tissue factor pathway inhibitor (TFPI) is a 33 kd protein that circulates in the plasma bound to lipoproteins. This recently described inhibitor of the extrinsic or tissue factor pathway inhibits factor Xa and the TF/VIIa complex. The inhibitory mechanism involves the formation of a quaternary complex of TFPI/Xa/TF/VIIa in which the catalytic sites of Xa and VIIa are bound to TFPI. TFPI can also directly inhibit TF/VIIa without Xa. TFPI also increases following a heparin infusion and may be induced by natural heparins in endothelium.

TESTS OF THE COAGULATION SYSTEM

Only the tests in common use in the clinical laboratory will be discussed in this section. Many other tests of coagulation function using more sophisticated substrates are available in reference laboratories. Table 5–4 shows the normal values for common coagulation studies.

LEE-WHITE CLOTTING TIME

The oldest but least accurate test of coagulation is to measure how long it takes for blood to clot in a test tube. The Lee-White clotting time employs three tubes incubated at 37°C, each containing 1 mL of whole blood. These are gently tilted at 30-second intervals to enhance the contact between the blood and the glass surface to see when clotting occurs. Normal blood clots firmly within 4 to 8 minutes.

Interpretation

This test is extremely insensitive. It was formerly a test to monitor heparin therapy, which prolongs the clotting time. When used as a test of heparin monitoring, the clotting time should be prolonged to double its baseline.

TABLE 5–4. NORMAL VALUES FOR COAGULATION STUDIES

Clotting time, Lee-White	4–8 min
Activated coagulation time (Celite)	<100 sec
Prothrombin time (PT)	11–13 sec or within 2 sec of control
Partial thromboplastin time (PTT)	60–85 sec
Activated partial thromboplastin time (APTT)	28–40 sec or within 5 sec of control
Thrombin clotting time (TCT)	10–15 sec or within 1.3 times as long as control
Fibrinogen	150–450 mg/dL
Clot dissolution (5-M urea)	Clot intact at 1 hr, 24 hr
Euglobulin lysis	Lysis >2–6 hr
Fibrinogen degradation products	
Latex particles	<20 μg/mL
Tanned red cells	<5 μg/mL
Antithrombin III	
Coagulation assay	≥50% of normal pool
Chromogenic	85–125% of normal pool
Immunologic	22–33 mg/dL
Protein C	3–5 μg/mL
Activated protein C ratio	1.9–3.9
Protein S (total)	20–25 μg/mL
Free protein S (30–40%)	6–10 μg/mL

ACTIVATED COAGULATION TIME

Some centers have found that adding **Celite,** a finely divided clay, shortens the whole blood clotting time, reduces test variability, and allows more precise correlations between heparin dosage and laboratory results. Normal blood clots in less than 100 seconds when added to a tube containing Celite. With heparin, the goal is to achieve an **activated coagulation time (ACT)** of 300 to 600 seconds. The ACT has found greatest use in monitoring heparin therapy used during extracorporeal circulation such as cardiac bypass procedures, hemodialysis, and hemapheresis. Repeated bedside determinations can be correlated with the patient's clinical status, and heparin or its antagonist (protamine) can be given to induce desired changes in direction. The ACT is less suitable for intermittent checks of heparin dosage, partly because it must be done immediately after the blood is drawn and therefore cannot be done on specimens submitted to a central laboratory. Many laboratories have found the activated partial thromboplastin time to be the most satisfactory test for hospital-wide monitoring of heparin therapy. Monitoring of plasma heparin levels using the anti-Xa assay is also being used by some laboratories.

PARTIAL THROMBOPLASTIN TIME (PTT)

This test is performed on a specimen of citrated blood. The plasma is removed and placed in a sample tube, where it is recalcified, and a reagent containing surface-active factors such as kaolin and phospholipid is added. The kaolin enhances the speed of contact activation, the phospholipid provides a surface on which the coagulation enzyme substrate reactions can occur (see diagram), and the calcium replaces the calcium chelated by the citrate. The time taken for a clot to form represents the **partial thromboplastin time (PTT).** The normal "activated" PTT varies from 28 to 40 seconds. The test may be done manually, but it is more often evaluated using automated instruments that dispense the respective reagents. The PTT assesses the intrinsic coagulation and common coagulation pathway. This test measures the presence of factors VIII, IX, XI, and XII, which must all be present at adequate levels to have a normal PTT. Factors X and V, prothrombin, and fibrinogen must also be present. Factor VII is not required for the PTT because the test bypasses the extrinsic system. The PTT is more sensitive in detecting minor deficiencies of the common pathway than is the prothrombin time. As a general rule, factor levels below 30% of normal prolong the PTT.

PROTHROMBIN TIME (PT)

The **prothrombin time (PT)** is the most frequently performed coagulation test. Reagents for the prothrombin time are tissue thromboplastin and ionized calcium. When added to citrated plasma, these substitute for tissue factor to activate factor X in the presence of factor VII without involving platelets or the procoagulants of the intrinsic pathway (see Fig. 5–5). To get a normal PT result, plasma must have at least 100 mg/dL of fibrinogen and adequate levels of factors VII, X, V, and prothrombin.

Brain extract is the tissue most often used as the tissue thromboplastin reagent that is standardized to elicit a firm fibrin clot in the normal time of 11 to 13 seconds. Recombinant reagents are also available and have greater sensitivity. Prolongation of the PT as an isolated finding when the PTT is normal occurs only in factor VII deficiency. Prolongation of the PT and PTT can occur for a variety of reasons, including multiple coagulation factor deficiencies, oral anticoagulation therapy, liver disease, vitamin K deficiency, and deficiencies of factors in the common pathway.

The PT values are dependent on the type of reagents used and are therefore subject to wide interlaboratory variations. Prothrombin times have been standardized according to an **International Normalized Ratio (INR),** which compares the local thromboplastic reagent against an International Reagent. Thus each reagent has a relative value (International Sensitivity Index, ISI) with respect to the standard reagent, which has an ISI of 1.0. Consequently the PT value corrected for this ratio will give an INR that is "normalized" across laboratories, independent of the variability of the reagents used. The INR is most applicable in standardizing anticoagulant intensity independent of variations in the different laboratories. It is therefore only useful in prescribing oral anticoagulants and has no known significance in the patient whose prothrombin time is short or whose prothrombin time is prolonged from causes other than anticoagulant use (i.e., liver disease, malabsorption, or vitamin K deficiency). INR values recommended for Coumadin control in a variety of clinical conditions are listed in Table 5–5.

The INR is calculated from the following formula:

$$INR = \left[\frac{PT \text{ (patient)}}{PT \text{ (control mean)}} \right]^{ISI}$$

THROMBIN CLOTTING TIME

The **thrombin clotting time (TCT)** test measures the time taken for a citrated blood specimen to clot after calcium and a known amount of thrombin are added. The test consequently evaluates thrombin-fibrinogen interaction in that it bypasses both the extrinsic and intrinsic pathways and assesses the terminal steps of the common pathway. Consequently, the thrombin time may be prolonged if there is deficiency

TABLE 5–5. RECOMMENDED INR BY CONDITION

Condition	Recommended INR
Prevention of venous thrombosis (high risk)	2.0–3.0
Treatment of venous thrombosis	2.0–3.0
Treatment of pulmonary embolism	2.0–3.0
Acute MI	
Prevention of stroke	2.0–3.0
Prevention of recurrent MI	2.5–3.5
Reduction of mortality	2.5–3.5
Peripheral arterial disease	2.0–3.0
Atrial fibrillation	
Prevention of systemic embolism	2.0–3.0
Cardiac valve replacement	
Tissue valves	2.0–3.0
Mechanical prosthetic valves (high risk)	2.5–3.5

Adapted from Hirsch J, et al: Oral anticoagulants: Mechanism of action, clinical effectiveness and optimal therapeutic range. Chest (Suppl) 108(4):231–246, 1995.

of fibrinogen or if there are circulating anticoagulants that are active and interfering with thrombin's action, such as heparin. Abnormal fibrinogen or abnormalities of the fibrinogen molecule may also be evaluated using this test.

Thrombin-induced clotting is very rapid, and the test result can be standardized to any desired normal, usually 10 to 15 seconds. The TCT is prolonged if fibrinogen levels are below 100 mg/dL. In all the conditions that substantially prolong the TCT, the PT and PTT are prolonged as well. Fibrinogen deficiency can be distinguished from inhibitory conditions by adding small volumes of normal plasma to the patient's plasma and repeating the TCT.

FIBRINOGEN MEASUREMENT

Fibrinogen is unique to plasma. After clotting has occurred, serum should contain no residual fibrinogen. To measure plasma fibrinogen, it is necessary to make one of several assumptions. **Classic procedures** depend on the assumption that adding a standard amount of thrombin will convert all the available fibrinogen to fibrin. What is actually measured is the amount of protein in the resulting clot or the time it takes to generate a clot; the quantity of precursor fibrinogen is extrapolated from this value. In **immunologic techniques,** the assumption is that the plasma constituent that reacts with antifibrinogen antibodies is indeed fibrinogen. Plasma levels are determined by comparing plasma reactivity against a curve derived from known fibrinogen concentrations. **Heat precipitation tests** proceed on the comparable assumption that all the material responsive to the precipitation technique really is fibrinogen.

Immunologic techniques in which antifibrinogen antibodies are adsorbed to inert indicator particles use visible agglutination or immunoprecipitation as the endpoint, and quantitation depends on the results observed with successively diluted samples (see Chapter 7). Reliability depends on the purity of the antibody and the accuracy of the original standardization done by the manufacturer of the kit. The test is quick and easy, but the user is entirely dependent on the quality of the kit.

Depletion of fibrinogen may occur in situations in which there is decreased synthesis, as may occur in liver disease; however, this is uncommon. The other major reason for fibrinogen depletion is consumption of fibrinogen, which may occur in intravascular coagulation or in the activation of fibrinolysis.

FIBRINOPEPTIDES AND FIBRIN MONOMER

The action of thrombin on soluble fibrinogen releases two peptides, **fibrinopeptide A** (FpA) and **fibrinopeptide B** (FpB), and generates fibrin monomer as summarized by the reaction:

$$\text{Fibrinogen} \underset{\searrow \text{FpA and FpB}}{\xrightarrow{\text{Thrombin}}} \text{Fibrin (monomer)} \xrightarrow[\text{XIII}]{\text{Polymerization}} \begin{array}{c}\text{Fibrin}\\\text{(stable)}\end{array}$$

The resultant fibrin monomer polymerizes, and in the presence of factor XIII a stable crosslinked fibrin clot occurs.

Components of this reaction may be assayed and may be useful in evaluating ongoing intravascular coagulation. Sensitive immunoassays exist for FpA and FpB, although FpA is more frequently determined. As discussed later, fibrin monomer may complex with soluble fibrinogen or with fibrin degradation products. Either can be measured and may reflect active thrombin generation or fibrinolysis by plasmin (see Chapter 6, Disseminated Intravascular Coagulation).

TESTS TO IDENTIFY SPECIFIC FACTOR DEFICIENCIES

Interpretation of PT or PTT Prolongations

It is possible to infer which factors are deficient by comparing the PT with the PTT result. A normal PT with a prolonged PTT points to factors VIII, IX, XI, and XII, or to von Willebrand's disease (abnormalities of the intrinsic pathway). Fletcher factor deficiency causes a prolonged PTT that reverts to normal if plasma is incubated with kaolin for 10 minutes. A normal PTT with a prolonged PT occurs only with factor VII deficiency. Congenital isolated deficiency of factor VII is extremely rare, but the combination of a normal PTT and prolonged PT occurs fairly often in patients with liver disease or in patients who are on vitamin K–inhibitory anticoagulant factors such as warfarin. This is because factor VII has such a short half-life that it is the first of the liver factors to decline when hepatic synthesis falters. As warfarin dosage is changed or as hepatic disease is first developing, factor VII may be the only liver factor to decline significantly.

Both the PT and PTT are prolonged with severe liver disease or established warfarin therapy. Prolongation of both tests also occurs with disorders of factors V, X, or prothrombin; with acquired complex deficiencies; or inhibitors. With high heparin levels or with congenital or acquired fibrinogen defects and the resulting high levels of fibrin degradation products (FDP) (see following section), the PT and PTT are usually prolonged together. Neither test measures factor XIII activity. On a more practical level, the PTT is used to follow patients on heparin therapy, and the PT (INR) is used to follow those taking warfarin treatment.

Mixing Studies

After a tentative diagnosis has been reached by observing abnormal screening results, presumptive confirmation of deficiency or inhibitor is possible by adding different agents to the patient's plasma to see what corrects the abnormality. The usual diagnostic dilemma lies in separating factor VIII deficiency from factor IX deficiency. The clinical findings are indistinguishable: Both have prolonged PTT with normal PT, both occur in males with sex-linked inheritance pattern, and both are relatively common in the general population.

After the patient is known to have an abnormal PT or PTT, or both, the laboratory can repeat such tests on a mixture of the patient's plasma and added materials that contain clotting factors. In addition, the mixing studies can also determine whether there is a specific factor deficiency present, or whether there is a circulating inhibitor. When an inhibitor is present, mixing normal plasma with the patient's plasma fails to correct the apparent deficiency. In addition, patient's plasma may prolong the normal PT or PTT of normal plasma, indicating that inhibitor is present. Specific inhibitors can be determined by mixing studies—again using a specific plasma factor as the replacement and then mixing.

Factor Assays

Assays for specific factor levels require both a high degree of technical expertise and, often, a bank of frozen rare plasma. Factor assays are used to discriminate among mild, moderate, and severe deficiency patterns and to follow the course of a defined factor inhibitor. The factor assays are performed by evaluating the effects of dilutions of known specific factors to correct either the PT or the PTT on patients with prolonged tests. A specific percentage of the factor may be obtained from a standard curve.

Deficiency of factor XIII is an uncommon cause of severe, lifelong hemorrhagic tendency. The diagnosis should be considered in a patient with a well-documented bleeding tendency, but without abnormalities of any of the tests previously described, including PT, PTT, TCT, fibrinogen quantitation, bleeding time, or platelet count. Factor XIII promotes stable cross-linkage between individual fibrin monomers. Without factor XIII, fibrin forms, but the clot disintegrates easily.

The screening test for factor XIII deficiency is very easy. A fibrin clot is generated by adding ionized calcium to the patient's citrated plasma. Once the clot is firm, 1 mL of 5M urea solution is added to the tube, which is incubated at 37°C for 12 hours or overnight. Normally, stabilized fibrin remains firm, but a factor XIII–deficiency sample will completely reliquefy. A 1% solution of monochloroacetic acid can be used instead of urea, or both can be used in parallel tubes. Normal control plasma should always be tested simultaneously. The test is not a quantitative test and reports the result as presumptively normal or abnormal factor XIII.

TESTS OF THE FIBRINOLYTIC PATHWAY

THROMBIN TIME

Thrombin time may also be used as a test to assess fibrinolytic pathway activation (Table 5–6). Because fibrinolytic activation results in the release of plasmin, which cleaves fibrin and fibrinogen, fibrinogen may be decreased, or the fibrinogen degradation products so released may competitively inhibit thrombin/fibrinogen interaction. Consequently, if circulating fibrin degradation products are present, this competitive inhibition of thrombin/fibrinogen interaction may prolong the thrombin time.

FIBRINOGEN DEGRADATION PRODUCTS

Plasmin degrades fibrin as its physiologic substrate, but it readily cleaves fibrinogen as well if disproportion develops between plasmin, fibrin, and fibrinogen. Not only do the fragments that remain after plasmin digestion fail to clot, they also interfere with the clotting of whatever fibrinogen has escaped proteolysis. High concentrations of **fibrinogen degradation products (FDPs)** also interfere with the formation of hemostatic platelet plugs. Whenever fibrin undergoes fibrinolysis, low levels of degradation products enter the circulation, but these are normally cleared by the liver and reticuloendothelial system. With excessive plasmin activity, fibrin and FDPs—also called fibrin or fibrinogen split products—can circulate in levels high enough to cause serious hemostatic difficulty.

Tests for FDP are done on serum. Because FDPs do not coagulate, they remain in the serum after fibrinogen is removed through clotting. Their presence is documented immunologically. Antifibrinogen antibody is normally used; however, more recently antibodies against individual degradation fragments have found greater utility (see D-dimer assay).

TABLE 5–6. TESTS OF FIBRINOLYTIC SYSTEMS

Thrombin time
Fibrin degradation products
D-dimer
Euglobulin lysis time
Plasminogen activator inhibitor-1
Alpha$_2$ antiplasmin
Plasminogen

One simple and widely used procedure employs antibodies adsorbed to inert indicator particles. These fragments may be immunologically quantitated by means of a latex test in which latex particles coated with the specific antibodies are added to the patient's serum. If agglutination occurs, this may be titrated and a value recorded.

Interpretation

Because normal serum contains neither fibrinogen nor FDP, there should be nothing present to react with antifibrinogen antibodies. In patients with widespread bleeding or brisk hemostatic activity, small quantities of FDP may circulate, enough to react at a low level with reagent antibody. Very high levels of FDP are seen if the fibrinolytic system is inappropriately active, or if there is widespread intravascular coagulation. Patients with these disorders have blood that clots poorly or not at all.

D-DIMER ASSAY

The **D-dimer assay** makes use of the principle that when fibrin but not fibrinogen is cleaved by plasmin, neoantigens are released, in this case two D fragments from the gamma crosslinkage site of fibrin. The test uses a monoclonal antibody directed against the DD fragment (D-dimer). The test has no specificity for fibrinogen and therefore identifies plasmin action on cross-linked fibrin in a local or disseminated action. These fibrin-specific degradation products have been found in over 90% of patients with thrombotic or thromboembolic disorders.

EUGLOBULIN LYSIS TIME

Euglobulins are proteins that precipitate from acidified dilute plasma. The euglobulin fraction of plasma contains fibrinogen and all the plasminogen and plasminogen activators of plasma, but only traces of the antiplasmins. Thrombin added to a euglobulin solution converts fibrinogen to fibrin. In euglobulins prepared from normal blood, the initial clot undergoes dissolution in 2 to 6 hours. Even with excessive fibrinolysis, there is usually sufficient fibrinogen to form a clot when thrombin is added, but its appearance is often abnormal from the start. Lysis may take place in minutes; if the process is less severe, complete dissolution may occur in 60 to 90 minutes. The euglobulin lysis time is abnormally short in blood with normal fibrinolytic activity but reduced fibrinogen; this is because less fibrin is present to be lysed. An alternative method in this case may be **fibrin plate lysis,** in which euglobulin from a patient is applied to a standard fibrin plate and the degree of dissolution of the fibrin is determined.

Interpretation

These tests are generally not that practical because it is difficult to differentiate whether the fibrinolysis has occurred through a primary mechanism specifically activating the fibrinolytic pathway or through a secondary intravascular coagulation with secondary fibrinolytic activation. The tests are very rarely used, therefore, to differentiate between intravascular clotting or intravascular fibrinolysis.

OTHER TESTS OF FIBRINOLYTIC PATHWAYS

Other tests are also available to assess fibrinolytic pathway activation, including quantitation of plasminogen or specific fragments. These, however, are not practical and are not readily available.

Plasminogen Activator Inhibitor-1

Plasminogen activator inhibitor (PAI-1) is released from endothelial cells in response to fibrin. This naturally occurring inhibitor appears to play a key physiological role in preventing unregulated fibrinolysis. It is an inhibitor of tissue plasminogen activator, urokinase, and activated protein C. PAI-1 appears to be elevated in patients experiencing venous thrombosis and following myocardial infarction. It is assayed by determining the degree to which that plasma inhibits a known amount of tPA's action on a chromogenic substrate.

Alpha$_2$ Anti-plasmin Assay (α_2 AP)

Alpha$_2$ antiplasmin is a natural physiologic inhibitor of the fibrinolytic serine protease plasmin. Deficiency of this inhibitor can be associated with excessive fibrinolysis. Deficiencies may be inherited or may be acquired as a consequence of disseminated intravascular coagulation, therapy with tissue plasminogen activator, or liver disease. Assays are usually based on inhibition of plasmin's lytic activity on specific chromogenic substrates (functional activity) or measured by immunological methods.

Plasminogen

Plasminogen is the inactive precursor of enzyme plasmin, the active derivative of the fibrinolytic cascade. Plasminogen is synthesized in the liver and is activated by plasminogen activators such as tissue plasminogen activator (tPA), urokinase, and streptokinase. Plasminogen may be measured by immunologic assays such as radial immunodiffusion or by

TABLE 5–7. LABORATORY EVALUATION OF DISORDERS OF HEMOSTASIS

Hemostatic Defect	Cause	Platelet Count	Bleeding Time	PT	PTT	TT
Vascular	Collagen disorder Vitamin C deficiency	N	Prolonged	N	N	N
Platelet disorders						
Thrombocytopenia	All causes except immune thrombocytopenic purpura	Low	Prolonged	N	N	N
Thrombocytopathy	Von Willebrand's disease	N	Prolonged	N	Prolonged	N
	Drugs: Aspirin Anti-inflammatory (nonsteroidal)	N	Prolonged	N	N	N
	Renal failure	N	Prolonged	N	N	N
	Hematologic dyscrasias	Variable ↓	Variable	N	N	N
Coagulopathies						
Inherited	Hemophilia (VIII deficiency)	N	N	N	Prolonged	N
	Hemophilia (IX deficiency)	N	N	N	Prolonged	N
Acquired	Vitamin K deficiency	N	N	Prolonged	Prolonged	N
	Disseminated intravascular coagulation	Low	Variable (N)	Prolonged	Prolonged	Prolonged
	Liver disease	Variable (N)	Usually normal	Prolonged	Prolonged	Prolonged
	Lupus anticoagulant	N	N	Variable (N)	Prolonged	N

functional assays. The latter method often employs plasminogen activator ability to facilitate amidolytic plasmin cleavage of synthetic chromogens. Increased levels of plasminogen are found in pregnancy, oral contraceptive use, postoperative states, and obesity.

Table 5–7 summarizes the categories of hemostatic disorders and the effects on the screening coagulation tests. It must be emphasized that further work-up of the coagulation abnormalities may involve specific factor assays. The factors assayed will depend on which coagulation pathway (i.e., extrinsic, intrinsic, or fibrinolytic) is abnormal.

THROMBOPHILIA (HYPERCOAGULABLE STATES)

A **thrombus** is an insoluble mass of clot in the bloodstream or in the cardiac chambers that is produced by the action of thrombin on fibrinogen to produce fibrin or by the aggregation of platelets to form a platelet mass. Thrombosis may occur in either the venous or arterial system, and the pathogenesis of each of these thrombotic events is somewhat different. Venous thrombosis involves venous stasis, vascular damage, and hypercoagulability. The hypercoagulability in this situation more generally occurs as a result of tissue thromboplastin, producing thrombin that subsequently acts with fibrinogen to produce fibrin. In arterial thrombosis, platelet interaction is much more evident. This may involve platelet-platelet interaction or interaction of platelets with vessel walls and thrombin.

Laboratory assessment of those disorders associated with a propensity to thrombosis should involve analysis of deficiencies of the natural anticoagulant systems (see Table 5–3)—deficiencies that facilitate spontaneous thrombosis or thromboembolic disease. In addition, laboratory markers indicative of intravascular coagulation and increased platelet turnover may also represent markers of an increased propensity to thromboembolic disease. These conditions may be classified broadly as the thrombophilic disorders or hypercoagulable states.

The term thrombophilia therefore refers to an unnatural tendency to pathologic thrombosis. Such states may be subclassified into those disorders in which there are (1) laboratory abnormalities identifying a prethrombotic state or (2) clinical conditions that are associated with an increased thromboembolic risk. Factors that favor thrombotic tendency are listed in Table 5–8.

CLASSIFICATION OF THROMBOPHILIA

Thrombophilia may be classified as **inherited,** in which there is a family history; **primary,** in which there is no underlying predisposing cause; or

TABLE 5–8. FACTORS FAVORING THROMBOTIC TENDENCY

Local factors
  Blood stasis*
  Vascular damage
Coagulation-fibrinolytic imbalance
  Unimpeded activation of coagulation—DIC (intravascular thrombin generation)
  Deficiency of natural anticoagulants
    Antithrombin III
    Proteins C and S
  Qualitative abnormalities of coagulation factors
    Factor V leidein (activated protein C resistance)
    Prothrombin variant
  Defective fibrinolysis and abnormal plasmin generation
    Quantitative depletion
    Qualitative abnormalities
Increased platelet turnover†
  Prosthetic valves
  Valvular heart disease

*Usually venous thromboembolism.
†Usually arterial thromboembolism.

secondary, in which thromboembolism is associated with some preexisting clinical condition or disease. Inherited predisposition to thrombosis (hereditary thrombophilia) may be associated with depleted levels of natural anticoagulants or increased or abnormal procoagulants. These categories are listed in Tables 5–9 and 5–10.

LABORATORY TESTS OF THE PRETHROMBOTIC STATE

The clinical laboratory has the potential for a considerable impact on the diagnosis of thromboembolic disease and defining the hypercoagulable state (Table 5–11). Laboratory evaluation could be applied to (1) detection of prethrombotic changes—the truly hypercoagulable situation; (2) diagnostic enhancement (e.g., in identifying subclinical or silent forms of thromboembolism); (3) monitoring high-risk patients (patients with known risk factors such as past history of thromboembolism, cardiac disease, cancer, genetic tendency, obesity, etc.); and (4) rational therapeutic intervention and monitoring with anticoagulant, anti-platelet, and fibrinolytic drugs.

An ideal screening test should be sensitive, specific, reproducible, easy to perform, and inexpensive. Unfortunately, in the evaluation of the prethrombotic state, there are no ideal laboratory tests that can approach these standards.

Certain laboratory tests are, however, potentially useful, and these will be discussed. Laboratory assessment of platelet turnover will not be presented, since its use in defining the hypercoagulable state existing in arterial thromboembolism is still controversial. The tests include beta thromboglobulin, platelet factor 4 release assays, and platelet survival studies.

Because all of the recognizable primary thrombophilic states are associated with defects of the coagulation system and/or the fibrinolytic system (see Table 5–9), and since hypercoagulability is manifested by pathologic hemostasis, study of the hemostatic and fibrinolytic system, as mentioned above, should always be performed. This would include screening tests for extrinsic (PT), intrinsic (PTT), and thrombin-fibrinogen interaction (TCT) pathways. An appreciation of the disorders classified as hereditary or primary thrombophilic states is essential to the selection of laboratory tests for their evaluation. The conditions listed in Table 5–10 are hereditary thrombophilias. In many instances, the patient may be entirely asymptomatic until some minor challenge predisposes them to thromboembolic phenomena. In other instances, the patients may be discovered as part of a routine evaluation for family studies and work-up of a relative with thrombosis.

Expensive laboratory tests of thrombophilia should only be undertaken after a complete clinical evaluation is performed. Hereditary thrombophilia should be suspected in the following situations:

1. recurrent thromboembolic disease
2. presentation at a young age or without any predisposing factors (e.g., pregnancy or surgery)

TABLE 5–9. CLASSIFICATION OF THE HYPERCOAGULABLE STATES

Primary
Antithrombin III deficiency
Protein C & S deficiency
Resistance to activated protein C (APC resistance)
Factor V Leiden
Mutations of factor II (prothrombin) and factor VIII
Factor XII deficiency
Dysfibrinogenemia
Fibrinolytic deficiency
Plasminogen activator inhibitor-1 (PAI-1) (excess)

Secondary
Acquired disorders of coagulation and fibrinolytic impairment
Lupus anticoagulant
Antiphospholipid antibody
Acquired platelet disorders

TABLE 5–10. INHERITED THROMBOPHILIA

Mutation	Locus	Clinical Effect	Lab Association Diagnosis
Mutations of Procoagulants			
Factor V Leiden	1691 A → G Chromosome 1	Venous thrombosis	Resistance to activated protein C
Factor II	20210 (3′) A → G	Venous thrombosis	Elevated factor II levels
Factor VII	Several polymorphism R 353Q	Familial myocardial infarction or stroke	Usually elevated factor VII levels ↑ Triglycerides
Mutations Involving Natural Anticoagulants			
Antithrombin III	Chromosome 1	Venous thrombosis	Decreased ATIII activity and protein
Protein C	Chromosome 2	Venous thrombosis	Decreased protein C activity and protein
Protein S	Chromosome 3	Venous thrombosis	Decreased free protein S
Mutations Involving Fibrinolysis			
Plasminogen-1 activator inhibitor	?	Venous and ? arterial thrombosis	Elevated inhibitor ↓ Fibrinolysis
Other Mutations			
Methylene tetrahydrofolate reductase (MTHFR)		Premature arterial disease (atherosclerosis)	↑ Homocysteine ↓ Folate

3. thromboembolism at an unusual site
4. positive family history

Blood testing should preferably be performed before any anticoagulation therapy, because heparin depletes antithrombin III and Coumadin depletes the vitamin K–dependent factors, protein C and protein S.

Antithrombin III Deficiency

As was discussed earlier, antithrombin III (ATIII) has several levels of activity but primarily inhibits thrombin's ability to clot fibrinogen. Assays for AT may determine immunologically the amount of antithrombin protein present, or may use a functional assay of the ability of the protein to inhibit thrombin/fibrinogen interaction or thrombin's amidolytic action on synthetic chromogenic substrates in the presence of heparin. Deficiency of this protein allows unimpeded thrombin-mediated conversion of fibrinogen to fibrin. Consequently, most patients with this disorder manifest clinically with spontaneous thromboembolic events. Furthermore, in most cases, the thrombotic events tend to be venous thromboses. Depletion of ATIII may occur as an inherited disorder. The homozygous deficiency is probably incompatible with life, and most patients with heterozygous deficiency are asymptomatic. However,

TABLE 5–11. LABORATORY TESTS USED IN THE EVALUATION OF THROMBOPHILIA

Test	Mechanism
Prethrombotic State	
Antithrombin	Deficiency of natural anticoagulant
Protein C	Deficiency of natural anticoagulant
Protein S	Deficiency of natural anticoagulant
Lupus anticoagulant	Unknown or complex
Antiphospholipid antibody	Unknown or complex
Activated protein C resistance	Resistance to natural anticoagulants
Factor V Leiden	Resistance to natural anticoagulants
Tissue factor pathway inhibitor	Deficiency of natural anticoagulant
Fibrinogen	Elevated zymogens
Plasminogen	Deficiency of natural anticoagulant Defective fibrinolysis
Tissue plasminogen activator	Deficiency of natural anticoagulant
Plasminogen activator inhibitor-1	Defective fibrinolysis
Alpha$_2$ antiplasmin	Elevated zymogens
Lipoprotein a	Defective fibrinolysis
Thrombotic State	
Prothrombin fragment 1 & 2	Activation of coagulation
Thrombin/antithrombin complex	Activation of coagulation
Fibrinopeptide A & B	Activation of coagulation
Fibrin monomer	Activation of coagulation
D-dimer	Activation of coagulation
Activated protein C assay	Inhibition of coagulation
Beta-thromboglobulin	Activation of platelets
Platelet factor 4	Activation of platelets
Post-thrombotic State	
Fibrin degradation products	Fibrinolysis
D-dimer	Fibrinolysis
Euglobulin lysis time	Fibrinolysis
Fibrin plate lysis	Fibrinolysis

certain patients with heterozygous deficiency may present with sponta-neous thrombosis. The incidence of this disorder is estimated to be approximately 1:2000, and patients who are heterozygotes may have ATIII levels ranging between 25 and 60% of normal. Other conditions that can be associated with a depletion of antithrombin III include pregnancy, liver disease, nephrotic syndrome, widespread thrombosis, and/or disseminated intravascular coagulation, and following L-asparaginase chemotherapy.

Protein C and Protein S Deficiency

It has recently been appreciated that these two natural anticoagulants, protein C and protein S, which are vitamin K–dependent proteins, are important in the physiologic prevention of thrombosis (see Fig. 5–5). Again, these two proteins are synthesized by the liver, and their disorders are most frequently associated with congenital or hereditary deficiencies. The homozygous condition is incompatible with life, and heterozygosity is usually asymptomatic but can present with recurrent venous throm-boses. Protein C deficiency may develop in patients who take oral anticoagulants because of interference with vitamin K action. This is particularly evident in those rare patients who develop warfarin hyper-sensitivity, manifested by skin or digital necrosis. Protein S deficiency is less recognized but may be equally as common.

As can be seen from Figure 5–5, proteins C and S work together to inhibit factors Va and VIIIa. Both natural anticoagulants can be measured by immunologic assays (e.g., Laurell rocket—see Chapter 7) or functional assays using chromogenic substrates. In the functional assay, protein C is activated by thrombin (Ca) and activated protein C is assayed by its ability to release a specific chromogen from a synthetic substrate. The best test for protein S is the functional assay; next best is free protein S (since most of it is bound to C4b binding protein), and then immunologic assays.

Resistance to Activated Protein C

A new cause of hereditary thrombophilia has been described and appears to be of increasing importance. This disorder is the inherited resistance to the actions of activated protein C (APC resistance). Affected subjects may be identified by a familial thrombophilic predisposition. Under normal circumstances, when APC is added to an aPTT system, the PTT is prolonged because of the inactivation of factors VIIIa and Va. Subjects with APC resistance do not experience this prolongation and may have shorter PTT values. They may be identified by the **APC ratio,** which is expressed as a ratio of the PTT with and without added APC. (The normal ratio is greater than 2.5 to 2.9.) The explanation for this resistance has only recently been elucidated by the finding of a genetic mutation causing a single amino acid substitution on factor V (affecting one of the APC cleavage sites, Arg 506 to Gln). This mutation has been found in a high percentage of idiopathic recurrent thromboembolism—up to 60% in some studies. This resistance is likely to be more common than ATIII, protein C, and protein S deficiencies combined and is the most frequent cause of hereditary thrombophilia. Its prevalence in normal populations approaches 4 to 8%. It appears to be higher in whites, particularly of Northern European origin. It may be that individuals who inherit this genetic variation are predisposed to a greater thromboembolic risk, especially when other co-existent factors are present (e.g., surgery, pregnancy, prolonged inactivity, or birth control pills).

The mutation can be detected by molecular diagnostic techniques using the polymerase chain reaction, as is shown in Figure 5–7.

Hyperhomocysteinemia

Homocysteine is a sulphur-containing amino acid that is formed during metabolism of methionine and is an integral component of folate and cobalamin metabolism (Fig. 5–8).

Mild to moderate hyperhomocysteinemia is an independent risk factor for atherosclerotic vascular disease and may be as significant as elevated cholesterol levels. **Hyperhomocysteinemia** is caused by nutritional or genetic disturbances. The most common genetic defect occurs as a result of a mutation (a C to T substitution at base pair 677 causing alanine to be replaced by valine, on chromosome 1 p.36.3) in the enzyme methylene tetrahydrofolate reductase (MTHFR), which catalyzes conversion of 5,10 methylene tetrahydrofolate to 5-methyl THF (the major circulatory form of folate). The mutant enzyme impairs homocysteine remethylation to methionine (see Fig. 5–8).

The increased prevalence of the homozygous mutant genotype in cardiovascular disease has been confirmed by several studies from around the world. It has been estimated that for each increase in total homocysteine above 5 $\mu mol/L$ there is a 40% increase in relative risk of coronary artery disease. (Normal is <10 $\mu mol/L$ in the fasting state.)

Homocysteine levels can be determined in reference laboratories. The test is indicated in patients with premature arterial disease or those with a strong family history. Analysis for the presence of the thermolabile MTHFR mutation includes a number of genetic techniques, the most common being PCR using restriction enzymes and sequence-specific primers and probes.

The Lupus Anticoagulant

Lupus anticoagulant (LAC) is a term used for a circulating immunoglobulin factor that is responsible for inhibition of the prothrombin time, partial thromboplastin time, or both. This immunoglobulin factor inhibits

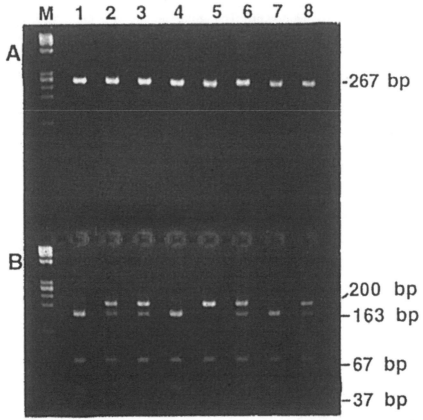

FIGURE 5–7. Detection of factor V Leiden (1691G → A, Arg 506 Gln) mutation by PCR. *(A) Undigested* with restriction enzyme. Lane M, molecular weight markers; lanes 1 to 8, PCR products amplified from genomic DNA of patients with thrombophilia. *(B)* PCR product *digested* with enzyme Mnl I. PCR samples used were same as in *A.* Patients in lanes 1, 4, and 7 are negative for F V Leiden mutation. Patients in lanes 2, 3, 6, and 8 are heterozygous. The patient in lane 5 is homozygous for F V Leiden mutation.

the phospholipid interaction with the coagulation proteins, but it is associated with a thrombotic tendency, not bleeding. LAC is most easily identified when citrated plasma from the patient is mixed with normal plasma in serial dilutions, and then a PTT is performed on the mixture. LAC prolongs the PTT—or less often, the PT—of normal plasma. Stated another way, normal plasma does not correct the prolonged PTT of the patient's plasma as it would do if there were a coagulation factor deficiency. This signifies that an inhibitor is present (see the section on Mixing Studies). Therefore, mixing studies are very helpful in identifying the LAC.

The LAC is termed "lupus" because it was first identified in patients with systemic lupus erythematosus (SLE). However, this inhibitor is only found in approximately one-third of patients with lupus, and only about one-third of patients with the LAC have lupus erythematosus. Other conditions associated with the LAC include other autoimmune diseases, lymphoproliferative disorders, AIDS, and therapy with chlorpromazine. The presence of the LAC is associated with venous and arterial thrombosis as well as recurrent fetal loss and thrombocytopenia. This syndrome is termed the **antiphospholipid syndrome.** The term "anticoagulant" really is a misnomer, because it really only applies to the prolongation of the clotting times in the test tube, and the LAC is more often associated with clinical thromboembolic disease.

The LAC has also been associated with habitual spontaneous abortions and is concomitantly associated with the presence of an anticardiolipin autoantibody in these cases. The LAC is one of a number of features that characterize these antibodies that inhibit phospholipid reactions.

The two most notable **antiphospholipid antibodies** are the LAC and the **anticardiolipin antibody (ACA).** The most recognizable phospholipid-dependent coagulation tests are the **activated partial thromboplastic time (aPTT)** and the prothrombin time (PT). The PTT is prolonged more often than the PT. Another test that is useful in

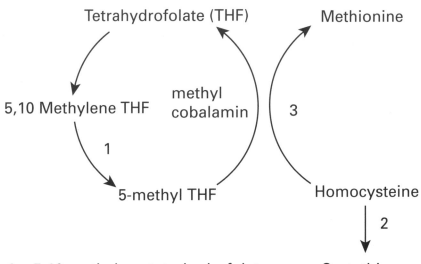

1 = 5,10 methylene tetrahydrofolate reductase
2 = cystathione synthase
3 = N_5 methyl THF homocysteine methyl transferase

FIGURE 5–8. Biochemical pathway showing formation of homocysteine by metabolism of methionine. 1, 2, 3 = enzymes involved in metabolism.

diagnosing the presence of the LAC is the **dilute Russell viper venom time (DRVVT).** (Russell's viper venom directly activates factor X which requires phospholipid Ca^{++} and factor V to activate prothrombin. An antiphospholipid antibody, the LAC prolongs this time.)

The DRVVT is performed by incubating the patient's plasma with dilute Russell's viper venom (RVV), dilute phospholipid, and calcium. Then RVV activates factor X directly and initiates the common pathway. The test is repeated with normal plasma or added phospholipid, which fails to correct the mixture, confirming the presence of an inhibitor. The presence of heparin may cause a false-positive test. A positive test occurs when the DRVVT is greater than 1.2× the normal pool.

A dilute tissue thromboplastin inhibition assay (TTI) may be used as an alternative test; however it is less sensitive than the DRVVT.

ACQUIRED THROMBOPHILIA

A tendency for thromboembolic disease may be seen in a diverse group of conditions from their adverse effects on coagulation or fibrinolytic systems. Disturbance in platelet function or impairment of blood flow may occur in many disorders. Virchow, the eminent pathologist, proposed a triad of pathologic features that are associated with the development of venous thrombosis: hypercoagulability (which has already been discussed), vascular damage, and venous stasis. Disorders included are diseases associated with impairment of venous blood flow, such as pregnancy or abdominal tumors; varicose veins; conditions producing vascular damage, such as inflammatory disorders of the vessels (vasculitis); or the hypercoagulable states previously listed. Laboratory evaluation should be directed toward excluding these secondary causes.

The acquired disturbances of hemostasis leading to thromboembolic disease are far more common than the familial thrombophilias. One such disorder, antiphospholipid syndrome in conjunction with the lupus anticoagulant, has already been discussed. Other, more common disturbances include coronary artery disease, diabetes, malignancy, nephrotic syndrome, L-asparaginase chemotherapy, postsurgery state, pregnancy, and sepsis. Some of these conditions are discussed in Chapter 6. Laboratory findings in these disturbances are complex and variable. Their general treatment is primarily directed to the underlying condition. Treatment of the hemostatic disorder is either prophylactic or supportive.

SUGGESTED READING

Adcock, DM, Fink, L, and Marlar, RA: A laboratory approach to the evaluation of hereditary hypercoagulability. Am J Clin Pathol 108:434–449, 1997.

Alving, BM, Bass, CF, and Tang, DB: Correlation between lupus anticoagulants and anti-cardiolipin antibodies in patients with prolonged activated partial thromboplastin time. Amer J Med 88:112, 1990.

Bick, R: Platelet function defects: A clinical effectiveness and optional therapeutic range. Chest (suppl) 108(4):231–246, 1995.

Boushey, C, et al: A quantitative assessment of plasma homocysteine as a risk factor for vascular disease. JAMA 274:1049–1057, 1995.

Broze, GJ: The role of tissue factor pathway inhibitor in a revised coagulation cascade. Sem Haematol 29:159–169, 1992.

Brubaker, DC, and Simpson, MB (eds): Dynamics of Hemostasis and Thrombosis. American Association of Blood Banks, Bethesda, MD, 1995.

Coleman, RW, et al (eds): Hemostasis and Thrombosis: Basic Principles and Clinical Practice, ed 3. JB Lippincott, Philadelphia, 1994.

Dahlback, B: Physiological anticoagulation—Resistance to activated protein C and venous thromboembolism. J Clin Med 94(3):923–927, 1994.

Dahlback, B, and Hildebrand B: Inherited resistance to activated protein C is corrected by anticoagulant co-factor found to be a property of factor V. Proc Natl Acad Sci (USA) 91:1396, 1994.

Frosst, B, et al: A candidate genetic risk factor for vascular disease: A common mutation in methylene tetrahydrofolate reductase. Nature Genetics 10:111–113, 1995.

Hirsch, J, et al: Oral anticoagulants: Mechanism of action, clinical effectiveness and optimal therapeutic range. Chest (Suppl) 108(4):231–246, 1995.

Hirsh, J, and Poller, L: The international normalized ratio: A guide to understanding and correcting its problems. Arch Intern Med 154:282–288, 1994.

Iacoviello, L, et al: Polymorphism of the coagulation factor VII gene and the risk of myocardial infarction. N Engl J Med 338:79–85, 1998.

Koepke, JA: Testing for hereditary hypercoagulability: Activated protein C resistance. Am J Clin Pathol 106:161–163, 1996.

Nachman, RL, and Silverstein, R: Hypercoagulable states. Ann Intern Med 119:819–827, 1993.

Roberts, HR, and Lozier, JN: New perspectives on the coagulation cascade. Hosp Prac 15:97–112, 1992.

Schafer, AI: Approach to bleeding. In Loscalzo, J, and Schafer, AI (eds): Thrombosis and Hemorrhage. Blackwell Scientific Publications, Boston, MA, 1994, pp. 407–422.

Simioni, P, et al: The risk of recurrent venous thrombus embolism in patients with an $Arg^{506} \rightarrow Gln$ mutation in the gene for factor V (factor V Leiden). N Engl J Med 336:399–403, 1997.

Svenson, P, and Dahlback, B: Resistance to activated protein C as a basis for venous thrombosis. N Engl J Med 330:517, 1994.

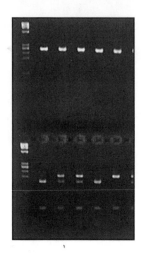

6

Disorders of Hemostasis

Patients with hemostatic disorders may present a spectrum of conditions ranging from no symptoms to severe hemorrhage. Patients may seek medical attention (1) because the patient has noticed abnormal bleeding manifestations, (2) because a responsible clinician notices abnormal physical signs or elicits a suspicious history, or (3) because the clinician specifically tests for hemostatic abnormalities before undertaking a surgical, obstetric, or dental procedure. Medical history, physical examination, and laboratory tests are all important in evaluating the significance and nature of bleeding problems.

COAGULATION FACTOR DISORDERS

MEDICAL HISTORY

Specific information obtained from the patient can be very helpful in directing the nature of laboratory tests. The medical history should include the following:

Presentation of Symptoms

It is important to find out whether the bleeding tendency is a new problem or whether the individual has noticed easy bruising since

284

childhood. The presentation of hemostatic abnormalities in a male infant at the time of circumcision may suggest a congenital or hereditary bleeding problem. Certainly a lifelong history of bleeding will suggest a congenital coagulation or platelet disorder.

Onset of Bleeding

Is the bleeding provoked by injury, or does it occur spontaneously? *Spontaneous* bleeding is more commonly seen in the hemophilia syndromes and von Willebrand's disease. Hemostatic abnormalities manifesting only with *trauma* or *surgery* may suggest a mild coagulation factor deficiency or factor XI or XIII deficiency. Factor XIII deficiency usually presents 24 to 48 hours after surgery.

Location of the Bleeding

Coagulation factor abnormalities such as hemophilia rarely present with mucous membrane bleeding, and more commonly present with spontaneous hemorrhages into the joints, in particular the knees and elbows. Platelet disorders most often present with mucous membrane bleeding or cutaneous bruising and bleeding, and are indicated by the presence of point hemorrhages (petechiae), discussed later.

Family History

Family history is important since a sex-linked preponderance may suggest hemophilia (factor VIII deficiency) or Christmas disease (factor IX deficiency). Obviously, in this situation male family members, particularly those on the maternal side, are affected. An autosomal dominant inheritance is more commonly seen with von Willebrand's disease.

Drugs and Medications

Certain drugs may be associated with impairment of platelet function, in particular aspirin and the nonsteroidal anti-inflammatory agents. Some drugs and medications, such as quinidine or quinine, are associated with rapid reduction of platelet count on an allergic basis; other drugs, such as thiazide diuretics, are notorious for suppression of bone marrow production of platelets. Many drugs may cause idiosyncratic reactions that may affect platelet function or production.

Other Systemic Diseases

Patients should always be questioned regarding the possibility of other systemic diseases that can be associated with bleeding abnormalities, such as recent infections, the presence of other hematologic diseases, nutritional deficiencies, autoimmune disease, and liver disease.

Bruising is difficult to evaluate by history since it occurs so commonly, particularly on the thighs and upper arms, especially in postmenopausal women. Duration of symptoms may determine whether the condition is congenital or acquired, and the anatomic site of hemorrhage is important in determining the nature of the hemostatic abnormality.

PHYSICAL EXAMINATION

General physical examination may reveal evidence of a bleeding abnormality. Notable categories of bleeding episodes include bleeding into joints **(hemarthroses)** and into soft tissues **(hematomas)**, especially muscles, diffuse oozing from mucosal surfaces, blood in the urine **(hematuria)**, and pinpoint or spreading hemorrhages into skin **(petechiae, ecchymoses,** or **purpura)**. Poorly healed scars may be seen in patients with connective tissue diseases and coagulation factor deficiencies or with factor XIII deficiency. Chronic bleeding into the joints may produce, in addition, joint deformities or impaired joint mobility. Bleeding disorders associated with diseases such as lymphomas or leukemias may present with anemia, bone marrow tenderness, or enlargement of the liver, spleen, or lymph nodes.

LABORATORY SCREENING TESTS

For an apparently normal patient about to undergo an operation, the prothrombin time (PT), partial thromboplastin time (PTT), and platelet count probably constitute an adequate screening profile. If the history is suggestive, the bleeding time and thrombin clotting time (TCT) should also be performed. In this manner, the extrinsic coagulation pathway (PT), intrinsic coagulation pathway (PTT), thrombin/fibrinogen interaction, and platelet count, as well as platelet function screen (bleeding time), may elucidate whether a bleeding problem exists, as well as its nature. If these screening tests are all normal despite a suggestive clinical history, it is highly unlikely that the patient has a significant bleeding problem. If an abnormality of one or the other of these tests is identified, then further characterization can be performed to elucidate the specific nature of the problem and to define a preventive measure or specific treatment. The laboratory work-up of many of the disorders of coagulation has been presented in Chapter 5. Specific disorders are discussed in this chapter, and the confirmatory laboratory tests are explained.

Clinical and Laboratory Observations

Although acquired bleeding problems are far more common than congenital disorders, characterization and treatment of congenital syndromes are far easier. Congenital deficiency syndromes attract investigators who use these isolated defects as experiments of nature that elucidate fundamental physiologic and pathologic events. Table 6–1 lists some of the inherited factor deficiencies.

Acquired disorders often accompany other diseases. Aside from treating the underlying disease, the clinician may have few options other than to treat the hemorrhagic diathesis empirically with platelets and plasma for factor replacement. Coagulation problems are probably less common than platelet disorders, but the coagulation mechanisms can be studied and manipulated more readily than can functional disorders of platelets.

Laboratory tests that are useful in evaluating hypercoagulability are generally not easy to perform and not reproducible except in some rare inherited deficiencies or in association with the lupus anticoagulant. These are discussed in Chapter 5 and mentioned briefly in this chapter.

CONGENITAL DISORDERS OF COAGULATION

Deficiencies of Factor VIII and Factor IX (Hemophilias)

Hemophilia, in general terms, refers to a severe, lifelong tendency toward excessive bleeding, occurring almost exclusively in men and following an X-linked inheritance pattern. Defects of factor VIII or factor IX produce this syndrome. Hemophilia has been recognized for thousands of years. The Talmud states that a male infant should not be circumcised if two or more of his brothers died from postcircumcision bleeding. In the United States, approximately 1 out of 10,000 boys has hemophilia of greater or lesser severity; 4 out of 5 cases are factor VIII deficiencies, and thus factor IX problems are less common. **Factor VIII deficiency** (*hemophilia A,* or *"classic hemophilia"*) and **factor IX deficiency** (*hemophilia B,* or *"Christmas disease"*) were not differentiated until 1952. Clinical findings and genetic transmission are identical. The conditions can be distinguished by cross-correctional studies (mixing studies) or specific factor assays or molecular genetic analysis (see Chapter 5).

TABLE 6–1. INHERITED FACTOR DEFICIENCIES

Factor	Deficiency	Minimum for Hemostasis	Half-Life	Laboratory	Clinical
I	Afibrinogenemia (rare) Autosomal recessive—homozygous	50–100 mg/dL	120 hr	No clot formation Abnormal PT, APTT, TCT; no fibrinogen	Umbilical stump bleeding, easy bruising, ecchymosis, gingival oozing, hematuria, poor wound healing
	Hypofibrinogenemia (rare) Autosomal recessive—heterozygous			Abnormal PT, APTT, TCT; low fibrinogen	Mild bleeding, thrombotic episodes
	Dysfibrinogenemia Variable inheritance Uncommon variants			Fibrinogen: Qualitative—abnormal Quantitative—normal	Possible hemorrhage, possible thrombosis, possible asymptomatic
II	Hypoprothrombinemia (extremely rare) Autosomal recessive	30–40%	100 hr	Abnormal PT, APTT	Postoperative bleeding, epistaxis, menorrhagia, easy bruising
V	Autosomal recessive 1/1,000,000—homozygote	10%	25 hr	Abnormal PT, APTT, BT	Epistaxis, menorrhagia, easy bruising
VII	Incomplete autosomal recessive Variable expression— 1/500,000	10%	5 hr	Abnormal PT, normal APTT	Epistaxis, menorrhagia, cerebral hemorrhage

Factor	Disorder / Inheritance	%	Half-life	Laboratory	Clinical Manifestations
VIII	Hemophilia A (classic hemophilia) Sex-linked recessive 1/10,000	30%	8–12 hr	Abnormal APTT; normal PT, BT	May be severe, moderate, mild Spontaneous hemorrhage, hemarthroses, crippling, muscle hemorrhage, post-traumatic or postoperative bleeding
	von Willebrand's syndrome Autosomal dominant variable penetrance—1/10,000 Variable inheritance, variants—1/80,000	20–40%	16–24 hr	Variable results of platelet studies, BT, APTT	Variable depending on level of VIII activity Mucous membrane bleeding, superficial wound bleeding
IX	Hemophilia B (Christmas disease) Sex-linked recessive— 1/100,000	30–50%	20 hr	Abnormal APTT, normal PT	May be severe, moderate, mild Spontaneous hemorrhage, hemarthroses, crippling, muscle hemorrhage, post-traumatic or postoperative bleeding, ecchymoses
X	Stuart-Prower defect Autosomal recessive <1/500,000—homozygous 1/500—heterozygous	10%	65 hr	Abnormal PT, APTT	Menorrhagia, ecchymoses, central nervous system bleeding, excessive bleeding after childbirth
XI	Hemophilia C Incomplete autosomal recessive pseudodominant 1/100,000	20–30%	65 hr	Abnormal APTT, normal PT	Mild bleeding, bruising, epistaxis, retinal hemorrhage, menorrhagia

(Continued)

TABLE 6-1. INHERITED FACTOR DEFICIENCIES (Continued)

Factor	Deficiency	Minimum for Hemostasis	Half-Life	Laboratory	Clinical
XII	Hageman trait (rare) Autosomal recessive	Unknown	60 hr	Abnormal APTT, normal PT	Asymptomatic Rarely bleeding, thrombosis
XIII	Factor XIII deficiency Autosomal recessive	1%	150 hr	Normal PT, APTT; clot soluble in 5 M urea	Umbilical cord bleeding, delayed wound healing, minor injuries causing prolonged bleeding, fetal wastage, excessive fibrinolysis, male sterility, intracranial hemorrhage
PK	Prekallikrein (Fletcher factor) Autosomal recessive	Unknown	35 hr	Abnormal APTT: shortening of time after prolonged incubation with activator	Asymptomatic
HMWK	Fitzgerald deficiency (rare) Autosomal recessive	Unknown	156 hr	Abnormal APTT	Asymptomatic

PT = prothrombin time, APTT = activated partial thromboplastin time, BT = bleeding time, TCT = thrombin clotting time, HMWK = high-molecular-weight kininogen.
Source: Adapted from Pittiglio, DH: Hemostasis Overview. American Association of Blood Banks, Arlington VA, 1984, pp. 28–29, with permission.

Clinical Findings

Depending on the level of available circulating factor, clinical severity of both hemophilia A and B can range from severe to mild or almost asymptomatic. As a rule, affected males in any one family tend to have comparable factor levels and comparably severe clinical disease. *Severely* affected patients have less than 1% activity, *moderately* affected patients have between 1 and 5%, and *mildly* affected patients have between 6 and 30% activity (Table 6–2).

Excessive bleeding after obvious trauma is only part of the problem, an aspect that usually can be treated successfully (Table 6–3). Of more serious, long-term consequence is bleeding into joints, which often occurs without any apparent incitement and is extremely painful. The sequelae of progressive joint deformity produce severe crippling. This more often affects the lower extremities. Before the advent of effective therapy, hemophiliac patients who survived early bleeding episodes almost invariably became severely crippled by adolescence and young adulthood. Even though therapy now controls most lethal and many disabling symptoms, hemarthroses have not been eliminated; however, their frequency, magnitude, and crippling effects have been markedly reduced.

Soft tissue bleeding, especially subcutaneous and intramuscular hemorrhage, can cause compressive damage to muscles and nerves. Hematomas into soft tissues of the head and neck may compress respiratory passages and cause death by asphyxiation. Bleeding into the urinary or alimentary tract is common but usually causes no long-term complications. Intracranial hemorrhage, on the other hand, sometimes occurs without apparent predisposing trauma and can be extremely dangerous.

Persons with hemophilia suffer not only from hemorrhage, but also from delayed wound repair. Before adequate therapy was available, dental or surgical procedures were extremely hazardous. Bleeding after an operation or tooth extraction often can be the first sign of the disease in mildly affected persons with previously unsuspected hemophilia.

TABLE 6–2. CLINICAL AND LABORATORY CLASSIFICATION OF HEMOPHILIA

Degree of Severity	Level of Factor	Frequency
Mild	6–30%	15%
Moderate	1–5%	15%
*Severe	<1%	70% of cases

*45% of these patients have an unstable inversion of Intron 22 toward the telomeric end of the long arm of chromosome.

TABLE 6-3. TREATMENT SCHEDULE FOR SEVERE HEMOPHILIA (<1% OF FACTOR PRESENT) WITHOUT AN INHIBITOR

Disorders	Degree of Hemorrhage	Initial Dose of Concentrate	Subsequent Doses	Duration
*Hemophilia A: classic hemophilia (factor VIII deficiency)	Minor Hemarthrosis Muscle hematoma Mild hematuria	18 units/kg†	10 units/kg every 8–12 hr	Until objective bleeding and pain resolve; single dose may be sufficient
	Moderate	26 units/kg†	14 units/kg every 8–12 hr	7–10 days to permit adequate healing
	Severe Life-threatening surgical procedure Major trauma Head injury	35 units/kg†	18 units/kg every 8–12 hr	7–10 days to permit adequate healing

Hemophilia B: Christmas disease (factor IX deficiency)	Minor Hemarthrosis Muscle hematoma Mild hematuria	25 units/kg‡	5 units/kg every 12–24 hr	Until objective bleeding and pain resolve; single dose may be sufficient
	Moderate	35 units/kg‡	8 units/kg every 12–24 hr	7–10 days to permit adequate healing
	Severe Life-threatening surgical procedure Major trauma Head injury	45 units/kg‡	10 units/kg every 12–24 hr	7–10 days to permit adequate healing

*Mild factor VIII deficiency is treated by the intravenous administration of Desmopressin (DDAVP) at a dose of 0.4 µg/kg.
†Factor VIII concentrates.
‡Factor IX concentrates.
From Sacher, RA. Hemophilia. In Tintinalli, UE, Rothstein, RJ, and Krome, RL (eds): Emergency Medicine: A Comprehensive Study Guide. American College of Emergency Physicians. McGraw-Hill, New York, 1988, p. 530, with permission.

Laboratory Findings

Initial diagnostic procedures have been discussed in Chapter 5. After a presumptive diagnosis has been made, it is important to determine the level of factor activity and to test whether an inhibitor exists. **Anti–factor VIII antibodies** develop in as many as 5 to 10% of treated classic hemophiliacs; it is rare to find antibodies at initial diagnosis. Factor IX antibodies are less common. When adequate replacement fails to have therapeutic effect, or if the PTT remains severely abnormal after treatment, an antibody should be suspected. The presence of inhibitor is demonstrated by incubating the patient's plasma with a known concentration of factor VIII or factor IX and measuring the coagulant activity of the resulting mixture. This can be done either by determining the PTT or by performing a *specific inhibitor assay* that determines how much factor VIII or IX is neutralized by the inhibitor.

Treatment

Factor VIII is available as a purified recombinant protein, a highly potent monoclonal antibody purified concentrate prepared from large pools of cryoprecipitated plasma, and as a moderately rich factor VIII cold precipitated plasma concentrate or *cryoprecipitate* prepared from single donor plasma. Factor VIII concentrate is dispensed with a predetermined activity noted on the vial (see Chapter 8). It can be reconstituted by adding a diluent solution. Cryoprecipitate gives good results in treating minor or uncomplicated problems but still carries the risk of any blood component and is not subjected to a viral inactivation step (see Chapter 8). The recombinant factor VIII is commercially synthesized and does not carry the risk of transfusion-transmitted infection but can still cause allergic reactions and allosensitization. All the other factor VIII and IX concentrates are treated to reduce the risk of transfusion-transmitted infections by heat and solvent detergent treatment. The latter strategy eliminates the risk of lipid-coated virus transmission. No case of HIV disease has been transmitted since the implementation of these strategies. Concentrates are ideal for treating severe hemorrhagic episodes and for elevating factor VIII levels prior to surgical procedures. Mild factor VIII deficiency is now effectively treated by the administration of desmopressin (DDAVP) (Table 6–4).

Factor IX is available as a product derived with other liver factors (prothrombin, factor VII, and factor X). The concentrate of these four "vitamin K–dependent factors" formerly carried a very high risk of hepatitis transmission. However, viral inactivation steps listed in Table 6–5 and the availability of *recombinant* factor IX have now substantially reduced this risk.

Carrier State

Women, who have two X chromosomes, almost always have one normal gene to balance the hemophilia gene. Theoretically, a woman who

TABLE 6–4. CURRENTLY AVAILABLE FACTOR VIII PRODUCTS*

	Origin	Viral Inactivation
Intermediate Purity		
Humate P†	Plasma	Pasteurization
Profilate SD†	Plasma	Solvent detergent
High Purity		
Koate HP†	Plasma	Solvent detergent
Beriate	Plasma	Pasteurization
Immunate	Plasma	Vapor heating
Hyate C	Porcine plasma	
Ultrapure‡		
Hemofil M	Plasma	Solvent detergent
Monoclate P	Plasma	Pasteurization
Recombinant		
Recombinate‡	CHO cells	
Kogenate‡	BHK cells	
Refacto** (B domain deleted)	CHO cells	

*Other concentrates available in Europe
†Contains vWF
‡Human albumin added; insignificant vWF
**Not yet available
Note: Helixate and Bioclate, marketed by Centeon, are the same as Kogenate and Recombinate respectively.

TABLE 6–5. CURRENTLY AVAILABLE FACTOR IX PRODUCTS*

	Origin	Viral Inactivation
Intermediate Purity *(Prothrombin Complex Concentrates)*		
Konyne 80	Plasma	Dry heat 80°C
Proplex T	Plasma	Dry heat 60°C
Profilnine SD	Plasma	Solvent detergent
Bebulin VH	Plasma	Vapor heating
High Purity		
Mononine	Plasma	Ultrafiltration, chemical
Alphanine	Plasma	Solvent detergent
Recombinant		
BeneFIX	CHO cells	Pasteurization

*Other FIX concentrates are available in Europe.

received an abnormal gene from her carrier mother, and another from her hemophiliac father, would have true hemophilia. Such a case is extremely rare in humans. When there is one normal and one abnormal gene, the woman often has less than the normal level of factor activity. This deficiency is highly variable and usually too mild to be detected in routine PTT. The presence of the normal gene supplies an adequate amount of activity to normalize the PTT in most cases. The carrier state, therefore, cannot be diagnosed reliably by quantitative assays of factor activity. Sufficient variation occurs that a woman can have normal or near normal assays and still be a carrier. The diagnosis of the carrier state can be determined by comparing the percentage level of coagulant factor with the percentage level of vWF antigen. As was mentioned in Chapter 5, the von Willebrand factor antigen (vWF:Ag—formerly called VIII:RAg) is invariably normal or even high in hemophiliacs, and the basic defect is a defect or deficiency of the procoagulant activity. Therefore in hemophilia carrier states the ratio of von Willebrand factor antigen to factor VIII coagulant is greater than unity. This assay system is also useful in differentiating mild classic hemophilia from mild von Willebrand's factor. In the latter disorder, procoagulant (VIII:C) is equally decreased, as is vWF:Ag. These assay systems were discussed in Chapter 5. Molecular assays can now also help in an accurate diagnosis.

Factor IX carriers have not been as substantially characterized as factor VIII carriers, and the carrier status may be difficult to diagnose without the use of molecular genetic analysis.

Fibrinogen

Plasma may contain either severely abnormal fibrinogen or no fibrinogen at all. Patients with **afibrinogenemia** are paradoxic in having totally incoagulable blood, but nevertheless bleed less often and less danger-ously than patients with procoagulant deficiencies. Bleeding episodes, bruising, and poor wound healing characterize this disorder, which is usually inherited as an autosomal recessive trait. In rare autosomal dominant conditions, the fibrinogen molecule is structurally or function-ally defective. These **dysfibrinogenemias** cause relatively mild hemor-rhagic symptoms; a few patients, indeed, have a thrombotic tendency.

Laboratory Findings

Blood that lacks fibrinogen fails to clot in the PT, the PTT, or the TCT, but the addition of afibrinogenemic plasma to normal plasma does not inhibit fibrinogen formation. All the tests that measure fibrinogen measure zero. There is no precipitate to analyze and nothing reacts with anti-fibrin/ fibrinogen antibodies.

The dysfibrinogenemias, on the other hand, show qualitative as well as quantitative abnormalities. When incubated with normal plasma, this dysfibrinogenemic plasma inhibits clotting. Discrepancy exists, often strikingly, between the amount of coagulable fibrinogen and the quantity of immunoreactive or precipitable protein. Therefore, the functional tests show discrepant values with the protein assays. Another test that is useful in diagnosing dysfibrinogenemia, which empirically gives a prolonged thrombin clotting time, is the **reptilase time.** This is a test that is very similar to the thrombin clotting time; however, it uses the snake venom reptilase to produce cleavage of the fibrinopeptide molecules from fibrinogen. Therefore, following this direct cleavage, which bypasses the clotting pathway, fibrinogen can form an insoluble fibrin monomer and a fibrin clot. If an individual has an abnormal fibrinogen molecule, the reptilase time is substantially prolonged. As was mentioned in Chapter 5, most of the tests of fibrinogen utilize a functional assay that requires the addition of thrombin to clot an unknown amount of fibrinogen. Heparin is a powerful antithrombin and is used as an anticoagulant because of this property. Reptilase can be used to assay fibrinogen in the presence of heparin.

Other Factors

Except for the hemophilias and the dysfibrinogenemias, inherited deficiencies of coagulation factors follow an autosomal recessive inheritance pattern. All are rare (less than 1:500,000) except for **factor XI deficiency,** which occurs in up to 1:10,000 in certain Jewish populations. Most cause a lifelong tendency toward severe bleeding episodes, but hemarthroses are rare. Factor XI deficiency causes much milder symptoms, often menorrhagia, epistaxis (nosebleeds), or bleeding after dental or surgical procedures. **Factor XII, Fitzgerald,** and **Fletcher factor deficiencies** do not cause any symptoms at all, and indeed, as was previously mentioned in Chapter 5, deficiency of **factor XII (Hageman factor)** may, paradoxically, be associated with a thrombotic tendency. Table 6–1 lists the clinical features of congenital deficiency syndromes for all the coagulation factors.

Von Willebrand's Disease

Von Willebrand's disease (vWD) is a hemostatic disorder that is transmitted as an autosomal dominant trait with variable penetrance. It occurs with equal frequency in both sexes. The condition and the clinical manifestations may vary, despite the inheritance patterns. Since factor VIII levels are low, von Willebrand's disease earned the name **pseudohemophilia,** creating much confusion for early workers studying hemophilia. Besides the low factor VIII:C levels, there is a prolongation of the bleeding time, a phenomenon inspiring the alternate name "vascular hemophilia" for this disease.

Pathophysiology

The interactions of Factor VIII and von Willebrand factor and vWF and platelets are important to understand in order to appreciate the complexities of von Willebrand's disease and involves the **procoagulant activity (VIII:C)**, the **antigenic activity (vWF:Ag)**, and the **von Willebrand factor activity** (**vWF:activity,** formerly called "VIII:vWF"). This third function is important in the interaction between the vascular endothelium and the platelets and prevents excessive capillary bleeding by enhancing platelet plug formation. The name "von Willebrand factor" has been applied to the protein properties with these complex results. In classic hemophilia, the procoagulant activity of factor VIII is low, but von Willebrand factor and cross-reactive antigenic factor (vWF:Ag) are normally active. In vWD, all three aspects are variably abnormal, and the degree to which these abnormalities may manifest produces the several different types of von Willebrand's disease syndromes. Variable clinical and laboratory features created much confusion in the past. Recently, a more practical classification has been adopted and is summarized in Table 6–6.

Briefly three main types have been described. *Type 1* is associated with a quantitative defect causing reduction in all vWF components in equal distribution (Fig. 6–1). *Type 2* results from qualitative abnormalities usually associated with reduced high molecular weight (MW) multimers. Several subtypes are described based on the nature of the abnormality (e.g., 2A, B, N). *Type 3* is the most severe and most uncommon variant and is associated with almost no vWF (see Fig. 6–1). The primary reason that factor VIII levels are low is that vWF is not available to transport and stabilize factor VIII. There is no defect in factor VIII synthesis in vWD. Table 6–7 compares the properties of factor VIII and vWF. Most patients have mild clinical symptoms. Small vessel bleeding (such as mucocutaneous bruising, nosebleeds, and menorrhagia) is the most common event. Aspirin enhances the bleeding tendency and exaggerates the defective interaction between the platelets, plasma factor VIII, and vessel wall that characterizes vWD.

Laboratory Findings

Routine tests of hemostatic functions are somewhat unpredictable. The classic findings are a prolonged bleeding time due to deficiency of vWF and an abnormally long PTT due to the low factor VIII levels. Bleeding time varies only moderately in most patients, but there may be a marked fluctuation in factor VIII levels. The platelet count and clot retraction are normal, but there exists a characteristic abnormality of platelet activity that provides the best single diagnostic test for vWD. When exposed to **ristocetin,** platelets from vWD patients fail to exhibit aggregation (see Chapter 5). In addition, when passed through a column of glass beads, they fail to adhere. Infusion of plasma or factor VIII–rich cryoprecipitate causes temporary improvement of ristocetin aggregation and glass bead

TABLE 6–6. CLASSIFICATION OF VON WILLEBRAND'S DISEASE

Type	Frequency	Inheritance	vWF:Ag	Factor VIII Activity	vWF Activity	Clinical Features
1	70–80%	Dominant	↓	↓	↓	**Variable** **Mild–Severe** **Hemostatic Defect**
2	15–20%	Dominant or recessive	↓ Usually (esp. high MW multimers)	↓ or N	↓	**Variable** **Mild–Severe**
2A	Commonest type 2	D/R	Absent High MW multimers	N or ↓	↓	• Variable ↓ platelet dependent functions
2B	Low prevalence	D/R	Same	N or ↓	↑	• Associated with thrombocytopenia • ↑ Affinity for gp Ib receptor • Lack of high MW forms
2N (vWD Normandy)	Rare	Dominant	N	↓		• Mild–moderate mimics hemophilia • Normal multimers • Inability to complex with F.VIII
3	Very rare	Recessive	↓↓	↓↓	↓↓	**Severe**

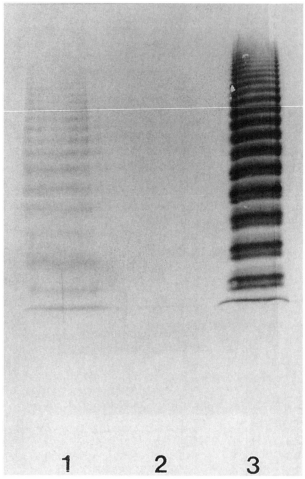

FIGURE 6–1. Von Willebrand factor multimers in cryoprecipitate and absence of multimers in cryoprecipitate-poor plasma. Lane 1: One unit of cryoprecipitated plasma showing normal, albeit reduced, multimer patterns. This pattern could also be seen in type 1 vWD. Lane 2: Absent vWF multimers from cryopoor plasma. This pattern would also be seen in type III vWD. Lane 3: Normal vWF multimers taken from normal plasma. (From Caruana, CC, and Schwartz, SL: Disorders of plasma clotting factors. In Harmening, DM (ed): Clinical Hematology and Fundamentals of Hemostasis, ed 3. FA Davis, Philadelphia, 1997, p. 540, with permission.)

TABLE 6–7. PROPERTIES OF FACTOR VIII AND VON WILLEBRAND FACTOR (vWF)

Property	Factor VIII	vWF
Clinical disorder due to deficiency	Hemophilia A	von Willebrand's disease
Production site(s)	Hepatocytes	Endothelial cells, megakaryocytes
Location of genetic information	Long arm of the X chromosome	Chromosome 12
Molecular mass (kDa)	240	270 (monomer)
Molecular dimension	Heterodimer	Multimer
Plasma concentration	1 nmol/L	50 nmol/L (monomer)
Function	Pro-cofactor for factor IXa in the intrinsic factor X–activating complex	Platelet adhesion to the injured vessel wall; carrier protein for factor VIII

From Vlot, AJ, et al: Factor VIII and von Willebrand factor. Thromb Haemostat 79:456–465, 1998, with permission.

retention tests, as well as an increase in procoagulant activity that lasts much longer than the survival of passively administered factor VIII.

In most vWD patients, there are comparably low levels of antigenic and procoagulant activity. A minority of patients have a normal quantity of protein with aberrant immunologic activity. There seem to be several different fundamental mechanisms involved. Most patients have quantitatively normal synthesis of the entire factor VIII complex, whereas others have a qualitative defect of synthesis (see Fig. 6–1). Not surprisingly, laboratory observations vary more widely among patients with qualitative or structural variants than among those with quantitative deficiency.

PLATELET DISORDERS

Disorders of platelet number or function cause prolonged bleeding time and poor clot retraction. The platelet count allows quantitation of circulating platelets. To evaluate how many platelets are being produced, it is necessary to examine the bone marrow megakaryocytes. If platelet counts are normal but clinical symptoms and screening laboratory tests suggest platelet failure, qualitative tests of platelet function are indicated, as was outlined in Chapter 5.

QUANTITATIVE PLATELET ABNORMALITIES

Platelets may be either *decreased* (**thrombocytopenia**) or *increased* (**thrombocytosis** or **thrombocythemia**).

Thrombocytopenia

The major causes of thrombocytopenia may be classified into two categories: (1) the failure of the bone marrow to produce an adequate number of platelets and (2) increased peripheral destruction or sequestration of platelets.

The diagnosis of thrombocytopenia is usually made using *automated platelet counters.* It is essential, however, that these counts be verified by examination of the *peripheral blood smear.* Corroboration with the peripheral smear may also reveal other possible causes of the apparently low platelet count such as **artifactual thrombocytopenia (pseudothrombocytopenia).** In this condition, platelet clumping occurs after collection of the blood sample, particularly in blood collected in the anticoagulant EDTA. The automated platelet counter interprets this as an apparent decrease in the platelet count due to the multiple platelets adherent in one aggregant mass. These clumps may readily be seen on a peripheral smear examination. Furthermore, the peripheral smear may also reveal clues as to the cause of the disorder. For example, fragmented red cells **(schistocytes)** would suggest a **microangiopathic hemolytic anemia** in association with thrombocytopenia, as may occur in disseminated intravascular coagulation, hemolytic uremic syndrome, and thrombotic thrombocytopenic purpura. The presence of altered red cell and white cell morphology may suggest a **megaloblastic anemia,** a **marrow failure syndrome,** or **leukemia.** In most cases, however, evaluation of a bone marrow is essential for categorizing the cause of the thrombocytopenia.

If bone marrow examination reveals abundant megakaryocytes with normal maturation of all the other cell lines, this strongly suggests a peripheral destructive process causing reduction in the platelet count. This may occur in **autoimmune thrombocytopenia** or **splenic platelet sequestration.** The bone marrow may also reveal **abnormal hematopoiesis, marrow fibrosis,** the presence of foreign cells, leukemia, or marked reduction in hemopoietic tissue, as may occur in **aplastic anemia.** It is also extremely important that any patient presenting with thrombocytopenia be thoroughly examined and have a detailed medical history, particularly with emphasis on recent viral syndromes, family history, and a drug history.

Thrombocytopenia Due to Decreased Platelet Production

Conditions that generally affect bone marrow cellular maturation often cause thrombocytopenia as one of several hematologic manifestations; therefore, anemia and leukopenia often coexist. Table 6–8 lists causes of thrombocytopenia associated with decreased platelet production.

TABLE 6–8. ACQUIRED THROMBOCYTOPENIA SECONDARY TO DECREASED PLATELET PRODUCTION

Aplastic anemia
Paroxysmal nocturnal hemoglobinuria
Leukemia (acute, chronic, hairy cell)
Myelodysplastic syndromes
Metastatic lymphoma or carcinoma
Myelofibrosis (primary or secondary)
Folate and vitamin B_{12} deficiencies
Cytotoxic and immunosuppressive chemotherapy
Viral infections*
Drugs*
Idiopathic*

*Conditions in which thrombocytopenia is often the predominant hematologic finding.

Aplastic anemia is discussed in Chapter 3 and usually occurs as a result of some undefined insult to the pleuripotent or multipotent stem cell in the bone marrow. Consequently there is failure of one or all of the major hemopoietic cell lines, producing variable degrees of anemia, leukopenia, and thrombocytopenia. Disorders in which there is abnormal growth or maturation of the pleuripotent or multipotent stem cell occur in the **clonal hematologic diseases** that are discussed in Chapter 4, and include leukemia, the **myelodysplastic syndromes,** and **paroxysmal nocturnal hemoglobinuria.** Metastatic malignancies and lymphomatous involvement of the bone marrow may produce a gross disturbance of the bone marrow architecture with the production of a **leukoerythroblastic (myelophthisic) peripheral blood picture** (see Color Plate 46). In **megaloblastic anemia,** folate and vitamin B_{12} are necessary for maturation and normal development of all rapidly dividing cells; although these conditions usually produce a more profound anemia, more often pancytopenia occurs. Cancer chemotherapeutic drugs usually produce suppression of all marrow elements; however, in some situations, more profound thrombocytopenia may exist, such as the agents **mitomycin C** and the **nitrosoureas.**

These disorders are often associated with specific findings on history and physical examination as well as laboratory examination. In most cases, examination of a bone marrow aspirate and biopsy is necessary to confirm the correct diagnosis. Some viral infections are associated with thrombocytopenia (HIV, Epstein-Barr virus, cytomegalovirus, and hepatitis B). These conditions can also be associated with immune destruction of platelets.

Relatively few drugs affect platelet production selectively. Chlorothiazide causes mild thrombocytopenia in some patients, but this rarely causes bleeding. Alcohol depresses platelet production; low platelet counts are found in most alcoholics examined during or immediately after acute or continued ingestion. Alcohol may have varied effects on the bone marrow and may produce thrombocytopenia by direct suppression of platelet production, hypersplenism secondary to cirrhosis of the liver, and folate and other nutritional deficiencies. Thrombocytopenia from direct alcoholic suppression is usually associated with recovery of the platelet count in a few days after alcohol withdrawal.

Rarely, thrombocytopenia may occur as a result of selective deficiency of megakaryocytes. This may be as a result of a primary or constitutional defect, or it may be acquired in association with myelodysplastic syndromes. Occasionally this disorder may be seen in collagen-vascular diseases and may occur as a result of autoimmune destruction of platelet precursors.

Thrombocytopenia as a Result of Platelet Sequestration

Thrombocytopenia associated with normal megakaryocytes in a bone marrow aspirate indicates that the life span of the platelets is significantly shortened. The presence of abundant megakaryocytes in association with a peripheral thrombocytopenia is the hallmark of these conditions. These disorders associated with shortened platelet survival are classified according to the mechanisms of platelet destruction. In addition to alloantibodies and immune complexes, antibodies can be directed specifically against the platelet membrane, producing an autoimmune thrombocytopenic syndrome.

The spleen, under normal conditions, contains up to one third of all circulating platelets, although relatively few platelets undergo destruction in any one passage through the spleen. Massive splenic enlargement increases the number of platelets removed from active circulation by splenic sequestration and reduces the survival time of all circulating platelets. Liver disease, portal hypertension, and the lymphomas are common causes of splenomegaly great enough to affect platelet numbers (see also Table 3–19).

Because platelets adhere to damaged endothelial surfaces, platelet counts often drop dramatically in conditions characterized by widespread endothelial damage. **Rocky mountain spotted fever** and the hemorrhagic rash of **meningococcemia** are outstanding examples. In these cases, the infection and the localized capillary damage cause hemorrhage and thrombocytopenia; it is not the thrombocytopenia that causes the hemorrhagic rash. Other causes of vascular inflammation **(vasculitis)** can be associated with thrombocytopenia (due to platelet destruction or adherence to vessel walls) and similar hemorrhagic rash.

Thrombocytopenia is one of the most common hematologic abnormalities occurring in pregnant women (Table 6–9). It may occur as an incidental finding in asymptomatic pregnant women, the so-called gestational thrombocytopenia, or may occur in association with a variety

TABLE 6–9. THROMBOCYTOPENIA SYNDROMES IN PREGNANCY

Incidental (gestational) thrombocytopenia
Immune thrombocytopenic purpura
Pregnancy-induced hypertension syndromes
    Preeclampsia
    HELLP syndrome
    Thrombotic thrombocytopenic–hemolytic uremic syndrome
Immune thrombocytopenia with antiphospholipid antibodies
Thrombocytopenia associated with DIC
    Abruptio placentae
    Amniotic fluid embolism
    Septic abortion
    Defibrination syndromes
    Severe postpartum hemorrhage

of other disorders, including ITP (as described above), preeclampsia, and the pregnancy-associated hypertensive disorders that include the HELLP syndrome. The latter disorder is an acronym for microangiopathic *h*emolysis, *e*levated *l*iver function tests (usually transaminases—see Chapter 12) and *l*ow *p*latelet counts. The mechanism of thrombocytopenia in these disorders is probably platelet consumption on damaged endothelial cells and this also contributes to the microangiopathy. These conditions are usually corrected by delivery; however these disorders may have serious consequences to the mother and/or fetus. The syndromes of TTP-HUS in pregnancy probably represent a variant spectrum of the above conditions.

Another curious syndrome not associated with DIC occurring in pregnancy is the triad of arterial or venous thrombosis, spontaneous abortions, and thrombocytopenia, with the finding of antiphospholipid antibodies. This condition has a 50 to 75% fetal loss or maternal thrombosis. Diagnosis of the hypercoagulable state with the antiphospholipid antibody is discussed in Chapter 5 and includes a prolonged PTT, prolonged dilute Russell viper venom time, and tissue thromboplastin inhibition.

Thrombocytopenia Due to Immune Destruction of Platelets

Alloantibodies. Platelets may be destroyed by **autoantibodies,** by **alloantibodies,** and by the action of antibodies directed against drugs. Alloantibodies cause problems relatively rarely, except in thrombocytopenic patients who receive multiple platelet transfusions and develop antibodies to human leukocyte antigens (HLA). Such patients are refractory to platelet transfusions from random donors and require platelets from donors of compatible HLA phenotype (see Chapter 8).

Much rarer are antibodies to specific platelet antigens; anti-HPA-1a (formerly PI^A,) is the usual offender, and pregnancy is the usual immunizing event. Occasionally, maternal anti-HPA-1 crosses the placenta and destroys fetal platelets. The newborn suffers from **neonatal alloimmune thrombocytopenia,** a disorder that is pathogenetically similar to hemolytic disease of the newborn, except in this situation thrombocytopenia is the end result (see Chapter 8). If purpura or the threat of hemorrhage makes it necessary to transfuse HPA-1a-negative platelets, the mother is usually the best donor if her clinical condition permits. Very rarely, HPA-1a-negative women become profoundly and symptomatically thrombocytopenic 6 or 7 days after receiving whole blood or red cells. In this **post-transfusion purpura** (see Chapter 8), the patient's own platelets are destroyed, but the inciting event is exposure to HPA-1-positive material in the transfusion. Immune complex formation (see Chapter 7) may be at fault. Later transfusions exacerbate the problem, which can be treated by plasma exchange.

Drugs and Immune Complex Formation. Many drugs have been implicated in acute thrombocytopenic episodes; most cases are isolated *idiosyncratic* reactions. Frequent offenders are *quinine* and its optical isomer *quinidine. Digitoxin, heparin,* and the *thiazides* occasionally cause problems.

Characteristically, the antibody is directed against the drug (such as quinidine), not against the platelets. If platelets adsorb the drug from the plasma, the antibody damages the platelet while attaching to the drug. High blood levels are often necessary before platelets become coated with the drug.

High drug doses are not necessary for the quinine antibodies and others with comparable activity. These antibodies unite with free drug to form **immune complexes,** insoluble macromolecules that settle onto the receptive surface of circulating platelets. The immune complex activates complement; because the immune complex attaches to the platelets, the activated complement sequence acts on the platelets and actively destroys them. Although neither the antibody nor the complement has specific affinity for the platelet, it is the platelet that suffers as an "innocent bystander."

Roughly 5% of all patients receiving heparin (either prophylactic or therapeutic) display a clinically significant heparin-induced thrombocytopenia (HIT) syndrome, making heparin the most common cause of drug-induced thrombocytopenia. Thrombocytopenia may occur in patients receiving either prophylactic or therapeutic heparin. The syndrome is usually characterized by (1) a decrease in platelet counts to values below 100×10^9/L or >40% decline during heparin treatment in patients who originally had normal counts, (2) normalization of platelet counts within several days of discontinuation of heparin, and (3) absence of any other cause of the thrombocytopenia.

Of patients with HIT, 20% may develop so-called white clot syndrome (the paradoxical occurrence of venous or arterial thrombosis in patients receiving heparin who develop HIT), which is associated with a 50% incidence of serious morbidity.

Patients who develop HIT have heparin-IgG complexes that bind to platelet Fc receptors and cause phagocytic removal by reticuloendothelial cells from the circulation. Patients with HIT can also produce antibodies to platelet factor 4-heparin complex, which may enhance platelet or endothelial cell activation.

Several test systems are available to aid in the diagnosis of HIT. They use either enzyme immunoassay technology or platelet aggregation detection methods. They are, however, not universally reproducible. Thus, the diagnosis is made on a clinical basis as outlined in Table 6–10. Once the diagnosis is made, heparin should be discontinued, and alternatives such as low-molecular-weight heparin, the snake venom ancrod, or thrombin inhibitors, (e.g., hirudin) should be considered.

Autoimmune Thrombocytopenia.   This condition, formerly called **idiopathic thrombocytopenic purpura (ITP),** results from the effects of an IgG antibody that coats circulating platelets and causes them to be rapidly destroyed in the reticuloendothelial system. Idiopathic thrombocytopenic purpura is a disorder in which the individual develops an autoantibody against antigens (usually IIb/IIIa glycoprotein complexes) on the platelet membrane. As a consequence of this attack, platelet survival is markedly shortened and thrombocytopenia occurs. Idiopathic thrombocytopenic purpura is a diagnosis of exclusion and may occur as a *primary* or *idiopathic* condition, or as *a secondary disorder* in association with other diseases such as collagen vascular disorders, lymphomas, carcinomas, and drugs. The clinical manifestations of this disorder may be *acute* (less than 6 months) or *chronic* (persisting for longer than 1 year). The *acute* type occurs more commonly in children and is usually transient and self-limiting in more than 80% of cases, whether treatment is administered or not. The *chronic* type is more commonly seen in adults and it usually worsens. The IgG antibody coats both the patient's own platelets and also transfused donor platelets if they are administered. In

---

TABLE 6–10. DIAGNOSTIC CRITERIA FOR HEPARIN-INDUCED THROMBOCYTOPENIA

Decrease in platelet count to <100,000/µL, or >40% reduction from pretreatment value during heparin treatment
Normalization of the counts within 3–5 days after stopping heparin
Absence of other causes of thrombocytopenia

general, platelet transfusions are not recommended and usually are unsuccessful in elevating the platelet count. The transfused platelets would also be destroyed by the underlying disease process at the same rate as the patient's platelets, which are being produced in vastly greater quantities.

Many studies have demonstrated the pathogenesis of this condition, but in the individual patient the diagnosis of ITP is not easy to make because there is no simple, reliable in vitro test for plasma antibody. Procedures to demonstrate IgG on circulating platelets are not available in most clinical laboratories; reference laboratories use antiglobulin consumption tests, radiolabeled antiglobulin tests, tests using radiolabeled staphylococcal protein A, or enzyme-linked immunosorbent antiplatelet antibody tests. All these tests are designed to detect, using different mechanisms, the presence of IgG on the platelet surface. It is important to remember that ITP is a diagnosis of exclusion, and all the secondary causes listed in Table 6–11 must be excluded. Laboratory studies, therefore, are also addressed at excluding some of the secondary causes. The spleen, although the site of major platelet destruction, is not enlarged in ITP. Splenomegaly, if present, requires investigation for other causes of thrombocytopenia.

The usual treatment is corticosteroid therapy (completely successful in only one-third of chronic cases), which if unsuccessful is often followed

TABLE 6–11. THROMBOCYTOPENIA SECONDARY TO INCREASED PERIPHERAL DESTRUCTION OF PLATELETS

Immune-Mediated Thrombocytopenia

Idiopathic thrombocytopenic purpura (ITP)
 ' Acute ITP
  Chronic ITP
  Intermittent/recurrent ITP
Secondary immune thrombocytopenias
  Viral infections
  Collagen vascular diseases
  Lymphoproliferative malignancies
  Carcinomas
  Drugs
  After blood transfusions

Non-Immune-Mediated Thrombocytopenias

Thrombotic thrombocytopenic purpura
Hemolytic uremic syndrome
Disseminated intravascular coagulation (DIC)
Complications of pregnancy
Infections

by splenectomy. Splenectomy not only removes the site of platelet destruction but also a significant site of platelet sequestration (see above). Table 6–11 gives a list of the causes of thrombocytopenia producing increased platelet destruction. As can be seen, a systematic approach to this cytopenia is similar to that discussed in Chapter 3, that is, the exclusion and diagnosis of autoimmune hemolytic anemia. Occasionally, **autoimmune hemolytic anemia** and **immune thrombocytopenia** may coexist. This condition is called **Evans's syndrome.**

Secondary Immune Thrombocytopenia. As with autoimmune hemolytic anemia (see Table 3–17), immune destruction of platelets may also occur in association with viral syndromes. In about 50% of cases of idiopathic or primary type, an antecedent viral infection may have predated ITP. Viral disorders such as HIV, EBV, CMV and hepatitis B may also be associated with ITP. In any patient presenting with ITP, serologic work-up for exposure to HIV must be performed. Lupus erythematosus and other collagen-vascular disorders may produce immune destruction of platelets or may be associated with sequestration of platelets in conjunction with vasculitis, as was described previously. Thrombocytopenia may be a presenting feature of a collagen-vascular disease such as systemic lupus erythematosus. Immune thrombocytopenic purpura may also occur secondary to hematologic malignancies such as chronic lymphocytic leukemia, Hodgkin's and non-Hodgkin's lymphomas, and other solid tumors such as adenocarcinoma of the large bowel. These conditions should also be excluded before the diagnosis of primary or idiopathic ITP is made.

Nonimmune Thrombocytopenia with Destruction of Platelets

Destruction and consumption of platelets may occur in the bloodstream in clinical syndromes not associated with immune (antibody) destruction of platelets. Two main clinical syndromes in which this occurs are themselves associated with complex hematologic problems. These are (1) disseminated intravascular coagulation and (2) syndromes of thrombotic thrombocytopenic purpura (TTP) and hemolytic-uremic syndrome (HUS). The syndrome of DIC is discussed fully in the section on Acquired Complex Bleeding Disorders later in this chapter.

Thrombotic Thrombocytopenic Purpura and the Hemolytic-Uremic Syndrome. These conditions may be part of a similar spectrum of diseases that represent the sequelae of different stimuli. **Thrombotic thrombocytopenic purpura (TTP)** is a disorder in which there is **disseminated intravascular platelet aggregation** associated with deposition of mainly platelet thrombi in the microcirculation. Many vessels in different organs are affected, and the consequence is organ circulatory insufficiency (particularly of the brain and kidneys), and microangiopathic hemolytic anemia as well as thrombocytopenia. TTP classically presents as a pentad of clinical features that include: (1) thrombocytopenia, (2) microangiopathic hemolytic anemia, (3) renal disorders, (4) neurologic impairment, and (5) fever.

DIC is generally *not a feature of TTP* since the syndrome rarely reflects localized fibrin deposition but is more an intravascular platelet consumption and aggregation. The peripheral blood smear shows a striking schistocytosis of erythrocytes and profound thrombocytopenia. The reticulocyte count is invariably elevated, and chemical analyses on the serum show variable impairment of renal function, usually including an elevated blood urea nitrogen and creatinine. A urine sediment is usually active. Since the microvasculature of many organs can be involved, including the liver and the heart, variable enzyme changes or other test parameters reflecting insufficiency of these organs may be seen.

TTP is a serious disorder that formerly was associated with a greater than 80% mortality. In recent times the mortality has decreased; however, it still carries approximately a 20 to 30% mortality. It is usually a disease of young adults who have a viral-like prodrome in many instances. The clinical features are typically those of the predominant organ failure, thrombocytopenia, and anemia. Other laboratory studies reflecting hemolysis may also be evident, including an elevated indirect bilirubin, reticulocytosis, elevated lactate dehydrogenase (LDH), and often an elevated leukocyte count reflecting panhyperplasia of the bone marrow.

The pathophysiology of this disorder is unclear, and it may be associated with collagen-vascular diseases, infections, drugs, or a postpartum state. A recent finding suggests that TTP may have an autoimmune basis with autoantibodies directed against a vWF cleaving protease. The autoantibody thus prevents breakdown of high-molecular-weight vWF multimers, which activate platelet aggregation. Treatment is directed toward removing this platelet aggregating factor or replacement of the protease by means of plasma or fresh frozen plasma infusion. Corticosteroids are also generally used.

Hemolytic-Uremic Syndrome. The **hemolytic-uremic syndrome** may represent a focal manifestation of TTP involving predominantly the kidneys. The main features are a severe microangiopathic hemolytic anemia with schistocytes in the peripheral blood and a reticulocytosis, as well as all the other clinical and laboratory features of hemolysis. However, in this condition, a major feature is the presence of renal failure. Hemolytic anemia and thrombocytopenia appear to be secondary to local renal abnormalities. Fever and neurologic impairment, which may occur in TTP, are generally absent. This condition more usually occurs in children who present with profound reduction of urine output and hematuria. Platelet consumption occurs in the microcirculation of the kidney.

Hemolytic-uremic syndrome can also occur following pregnancy **(postpartum hemolytic-uremic syndrome)** and has been reported following chemotherapy with the agent mitomycin C or associated with infections with *E. coli.*

Thrombocytosis

Thrombocytosis is the term that refers to an elevated platelet count, usually as a result of secondary stimulation. The term **thrombocytopenia** is used for unregulated, uncontrolled production of platelets, as occurs in the myeloproliferative syndromes (see Chapter 4). Elevated platelet counts are commonly encountered in the hospitalized population and may be seen in conditions such as inflammatory disorders, infections, malignancy, and following acute bleeding. Platelets may be elevated as part of an acute phase response to inflammation or infection. Table 6–12 is a list of the causes of thrombocytosis.

The laboratory determination of the platelet count by electronic counters will document the presence of an elevated platelet count. *Sustained* platelet count elevations above a million are generally *not* encountered in reactive thrombocytosis and are more commonly seen in primary thrombocythemia; however, occasionally more marked platelet counts may be seen in the reactive disorders. The peripheral smear may also show the appearance of giant or large platelets, which are usually more indicative of either abnormal production or increased platelet turnover (Fig. 6–2). Sample testing, particularly serum samples, may give

TABLE 6–12. CAUSES OF THROMBOCYTOSIS

Myeloproliferative Syndromes
Essential thrombocythemia
Polycythemia vera
Myelofibrosis with agnogenic myeloid metaplasia
Chronic myelogenous leukemia

Secondary (Reactive) Thrombocytosis
Mobilization of pooled platelets
  Postsplenectomy
  After epinephrine administration
Rebound thrombocytosis
  After blood loss (including surgery)
  Accompanying bone marrow recovery
    After cytotoxic chemotherapy
    After treatment of vitamin B_{12} or folate deficiency
Iron deficiency
Malignancy
Chronic inflammatory conditions
  Collagen vascular diseases
  Inflammatory bowel diseases
Chronic infections
  Tuberculosis
  Osteomyelitis

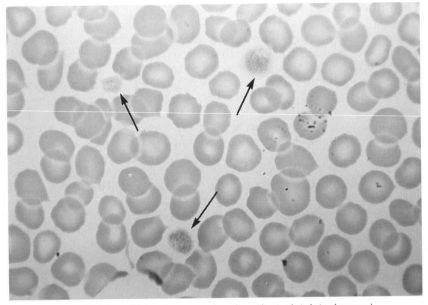

FIGURE 6–2. Peripheral blood smear showing giant platelets *(arrows).*

spurious elevation of potassium levels **(spurious hyperkalemia)** because platelets contain intracellular potassium, and as the blood clots, potassium is released. This produces a spurious hyperkalemia. A more accurate determination of blood potassium is achieved by a **plasma potassium,** which is the determination of choice in patients with elevated platelet counts. In reactive thrombocytosis, platelet function studies are usually normal, and patients are not at increased risk for thrombotic events. In thrombocythemia, platelet function studies may be quite abnormal, including abnormal aggregation studies, and patients may be at risk for either bleeding or thrombotic events.

Thrombocytosis may also occur in patients who have had a splenectomy because the normal splenic pool constitutes one-third of the total platelet mass. Splenectomy will result in an immediate increase in platelet count, but the platelet count may return to a normal or high normal value within 1 to 2 months.

QUALITATIVE PLATELET DISORDERS

Abnormal platelet function in the presence of a normal platelet count suggests a **qualitative platelet abnormality.** These defects in platelet function may be *inherited* (von Willebrand's disease) or *acquired* (drugs, infections, renal disease, or dysproteinemias). The most common qualitative platelet abnormality is that occurring in association with drugs, and in particular aspirin and the nonsteroidal anti-inflammatory agents. Alcohol may also produce qualitative platelet malfunction. Patients with qualitative platelet abnormalities usually have an abnormally prolonged bleeding time and variable disturbances of platelet aggregation. These are discussed in Chapter 5. Table 6–13 is a list of the qualitative platelet abnormalities that may occur. One of the most common inherited disorders of platelet function is von Willebrand's disease, and this is discussed earlier in this chapter. Reduction of platelet numbers is far more common than disorders of function. Most dysfunctional syndromes do occur as part of other diseases. Note: Constitutional defects of platelet function are very rare. Of these, von Willebrand's disease is the most common, but, as already mentioned, it is not primarily a platelet disorder.

TABLE 6–13. QUALITATIVE PLATELET ABNORMALITIES

Inherited Platelet Abnormalities

Intrinsic platelet defects
    Bernard-Soulier syndrome
    Glanzmann's thrombasthenia
    Storage pool disorders
Extrinsic platelet abnormalities
    von Willebrand's disease
    Congenital afibrinogenemia

Acquired Platelet Abnormalities

Intrinsic platelet abnormalities
    Preleukemic and acute nonlymphocytic leukemia
    Myeloproliferative syndromes*
    Paroxysmal nocturnal hemoglobinemia*
Drug-related platelet abnormalities
    Aspirin and other nonsteroidal anti-inflammatory agents
    Abciximab
    Sulfinpyrazone
    Dipyridamole
    Dextran
    Heparin*
    Penicillins
Extrinsic platelet abnormalities
    Uremia
    Paraproteins (multiple myeloma, Waldenström's macroglobulinemia)

---

*Associated with increased risk of thromboembolic events.

PLATELET DISORDERS SECONDARY TO OTHER DISEASES

Severe **uremia** impairs the platelet release reaction (see Chapter 5); the patient's own platelets behave abnormally, and transfused normal platelets acquire this abnormality. Oozing and mucocutaneous bleeding often complicate advanced uremia. Although dialysis often restores platelet function to normal, the bleeding problem may remain difficult to control.

Platelets also experience difficulty in functioning normally when there are high levels of abnormal serum proteins, as seen in **multiple myeloma** and other **dysproteinemias.** High-molecular-weight dextrans produce the same effect.

The presence of fibrin-fibrinogen split products seems to inhibit both aggregation and release. The normal liver clears from the circulation the low levels of degradation products that occur with everyday trauma and repair. Platelet function is diffusely abnormal in severe liver disease, and failure to clear fibrin split products may contribute to this situation.

The high platelet counts that accompany **myeloproliferative syndromes** often predispose, paradoxically, to both bleeding problems and a thrombotic tendency.

EFFECT OF DRUGS

Many drugs impair platelet function; aspirin is undoubtedly the leading offender. Once exposed to aspirin, platelets have impaired release reactions for their entire life span. Other anti-inflammatory drugs have comparable effects but may not irreversibly impair platelet function. Alcohol inhibits ADP-related aggregation; this probably does have clinical significance, at least in patients whose liver functions also have been damaged by alcohol. The use of specific anti-IIb/anti-IIIa antibody therapy (abciximab) in percutaneous coronary interventions produces impaired platelet function for intentional therapeutic purposes.

ACQUIRED COMPLEX BLEEDING DISORDERS

DISSEMINATED INTRAVASCULAR COAGULATION

The complex disorder, variously called **disseminated intravascular coagulation (DIC), consumption coagulopathy,** and **defibrination syndrome,** is a common, acquired cause of bleeding tendency. It is a complex disorder that is due to pathologic generation of thrombin in the vascular compartment. As a consequence, there is intravascular coagulation with consumption of coagulation factors, thrombin generation, and secondarily, consumption of platelets. DIC usually occurs as a complication of some other life-threatening illness; the superimposed bleeding problem is often the last event in a rapidly deteriorating situation.

Pathophysiology

The mechanisms that lead to DIC are exaggerated physiologic processes, in which the coagulation cascade is activated, leading to fibrin deposition in the small blood vessels of many tissues and organs. Several stimuli activate the coagulation cascade (Table 6–14). The result of this process is impaired oxygenation of multiple organs, consumption of coagulation proteins, consumption of platelets, and secondary activation of the fibrinolytic system in an attempt to remove the fibrin. Without the checks and balances that normally regulate thrombin and plasmin, both of these powerful proteolytic enzymes meet little resistance to their lytic attack on whatever factor VIII, factor V, fibrinogen, and platelets survive the coagulation process. The severity, chronicity, and natural history of DIC is extremely variable, and prognosis often depends on the primary disease causing the DIC rather than the syndrome itself.

Clinical Findings

A complex clinical syndrome with thrombotic and hemostatic-hemorrhagic features occurs. In the full-blown state of DIC, there is severe depletion of all coagulation proteins, especially of factors V and VIII, platelets are markedly decreased, little or no clottable fibrinogen exists, and high levels of fibrin-fibrinogen degradation products circulate and inhibit fibrin formation. The reticuloendothelial system and the liver attempt to clear these abnormal proteins and restore a semblance of normal coagulation protein synthesis. Unfortunately, DIC usually occurs in a setting of circulatory stasis, shock, hypovolemia, or increased vascular permeability. These conditions impair circulation and make it very difficult to initiate compensatory activity.

Inciting Events

The classic stimuli to DIC are infectious, surgical, obstetric, or traumatic events that allow thromboplastic material to enter the circulation. These events include amniotic fluid embolism, trauma, or large-scale operations, especially those involving the brain, lungs, or the genitourinary system, severe burns, and conditions in which blood cells undergo intravascular destruction such as hemolytic transfusion reactions, bacterial toxemia, and acute promyelocytic leukemia. Generalized sepsis and

TABLE 6–14. PROFILE OF DISSEMINATED INTRAVASCULAR COAGULATION (DIC)

Synonyms	Conditions Associated with DIC	Suggested Triggering Mechanisms	Clinical Manifestations	Clinical Laboratory Findings	Sequential Therapy
1. "Consumptive coagulopathy"	Obstetric accidents	Amniotic fluid	1. *General signs:* hemorrhaging (usually from 3 unrelated sites), fever, hypotension, acidosis, hypoxia, proteinuria, hematuria	Hypofibrinogenemia	1. Remove or treat triggering process
2. Defibrination syndrome	Intravascular hemolysis	Retained fetus		Abnormal PT	2. Stop or slow coagulation process
	Septicemia	Byproduct of red cell hemolysis		Abnormal PTT	a. Heparin
	Viremia (varicella)	Antigen/antibody complexes		Abnormal thrombin time	b. Antiplatelet drugs
	Leukemias:	Endotoxin release		Abnormal platelet count	c. AT-III concentrates
	APL	Chronic stasis		Abnormal factors V and VIII	3. Blood component replacement
	Other	Complement activation	2. *Specific signs:* petechiae, purpura, gangrene	Positive fibrin(ogen)-split products	a. Platelets
	Solid malignancy			Leukocytosis	b. Fibrinogen ⎤
	Acidosis/alkalosis			Schistocytosis	c. AHF ⎦ Cryoprecipitate
	Burns		3. *Microthrombi*	Thrombocytopenia	4. Antifibrinolytic therapy*
	Crush injury and tissue necrosis		4. *End organ dysfunction*	Reticulocytosis	a. Epsilon amino caproic acid (EACA)
	Vascular disorders				

*Sequential therapy used only after clotting is stopped. (Three percent of patients may need this therapy.) Generally used in conjunction with heparin.

AHF = antihemophilic factor (factor VIII); AT-III = antithrombin III; APL = acute promyelocytic leukemia.
Adapted from Pittiglio, DH, and Sacher, RA: Clinical Hematology and Fundamentals of Hemostasis. FA Davis, Philadelphia, 1987, p. 389.

severe liver disease can cause acute or gradually developing DIC. Other conditions that can be associated with DIC are listed in Table 6–15.

Laboratory Diagnosis of DIC

Laboratory assessment of DIC must consider:

1. Activation of coagulation with thrombin generation and fibrin formation
2. Possible consumption of coagulation factors, particularly factors VIII and V
3. Consumption of platelets
4. Secondary activation of the fibrinolytic pathway with parts of fibrin and fibrinogen digestion increasing in the bloodstream

TABLE 6–15. CLINICAL CONDITIONS ASSOCIATED WITH DIC

Thromboplastin Release—Factor VII Activation

Placental abruption
Trauma
Fat emboli syndrome
Sepsis*
Promyelocytic leukemia
Retained dead fetus syndrome
Acute intravascular hemolysis*
Amniotic fluid embolus*
Cardiopulmonary bypass surgery

Endothelial Cell Damage—Factor XII Activation

Immune complex disease
Intravascular hemolysis*
Liver disease*
Heat stroke
Sepsis*
Burns
Vasculitis
Anoxia
Acidosis

Factor X and II Activation

Snake venoms
Acute pancreatitis
Liver disease*
Fat emboli syndrome*

*More than one mechanism may be involved.

5. The inherent clinical and laboratory manifestations of clinical syndromes inciting the DIC (Table 6–14 is an outline of the laboratory tests reflecting these manifestations.)

Activation of the coagulation cascade and thrombin generation can be assayed in the clinical laboratory (see Chapter 5). Simple screening tests of thrombin/fibrinogen interaction make use of the property that thrombin cleaves two fibrinopeptides from fibrinogen called **fibrinopeptide A** and **fibrinopeptide B.** These may be assayed by radioimmunoassay techniques. Assays for fibrin monomer or the presence of thrombin/antithrombin complexes suggest intravascular thrombin formation but are performed in specialized coagulation laboratories. These tests have all been used as an index of intravascular thrombin generation.

Consumption of the coagulation factors V, VIII, and fibrinogen will obviously, by necessity, prolong the PTT and the PT to a variable degree, depending on the degree of consumption.

Platelet determination can easily be performed by electronic counters and may be verified by examination of the peripheral blood smear. In addition, large platelets may be seen reflecting increased platelet turnover (Fig. 6–2). Furthermore, microangiopathic hemolytic anemia and schistocytes may be seen and are indicative of mechanical damage to the erythrocytes (see Color Plate 16).

Fibrinolysis causes liberation of the active enzyme **plasmin,** which cleaves fibrinogen and fibrin into **degradation products** (see also Chapter 5). These are consequently increased in DIC as fibrinogen is decreased.

The primary condition inciting the DIC may, in addition, be evident on laboratory testing: for example, positive blood cultures in association with sepsis, abnormal leukocytes in association with promyelocytic leukemia, evidence of liver cell decompensation with liver disease, clinical evidence of trauma, or the postpartum state.

Management

The best therapy is to correct or reverse the initial inciting events. With massive trauma, sepsis, cardiogenic shock, and other clinical catastrophes, this tends to be difficult. The second major therapeutic thrust is to maintain blood volume and hemostatic function by means of replacement of the coagulation factors that have been consumed and attention to cardiovascular hemodynamics. Usual blood component replacement includes red cells for the anemia, platelet transfusions to correct the thrombocytopenia, and cryoprecipitate to correct factor VIII and fibrinogen deficiencies. Fresh frozen plasma is also used in an attempt to correct a complex coagulopathy. There is very little role for heparin in the treatment of DIC unless complicated by profound thrombotic events.

LIVER DISEASE

Patients with severe liver disease nearly always have abnormal results in laboratory tests of hemostatic function and may bleed significantly after liver biopsy or other surgical procedures. Spontaneous bleeding, however, is surprisingly uncommon unless there is an obvious hemorrhagic lesion such as esophageal varices or hemorrhagic gastritis. The liver manufactures so many coagulation proteins that factor deficiencies are to be expected when hepatic function fails. Platelet problems, excessive fibrinolysis, and low-grade intravascular coagulation are additional complicating events.

Liver Factors

Deficiency of the vitamin K–dependent factors (II, VII, IX, and X) is the most frequent coagulation abnormality. This deficiency affects both PT and PTT. Early in the disease, factor VII may be the only depressed factor; this leads to a *prolonged PT* with a *normal PTT.*

If liver cells are badly diseased, giving vitamin K does nothing to increase factor levels, but administering parenteral vitamin K can help to distinguish *obstructive* from *nonobstructive jaundice.* In biliary obstruction, factor levels are low because fat-soluble vitamin K is not being absorbed. The liver is capable of synthesizing the proteins, but no bile salts reach the intestine to facilitate absorption of fat, including the fat-soluble vitamin K. In cases of biliary obstruction, PT and PTT should improve within 48 hours after vitamin K is injected.

When hepatocellular failure has caused coagulation factor deficiencies, albumin production is also depressed. In addition, *antithrombin III* and *protein C* and *protein S* are decreased. It is rare to have hypoprothrombinemia without pre-existing hypoalbuminemia. A prothrombin time more than 1.5 times normal correlates with poor clinical prognosis, but it is hepatic insufficiency rather than hemorrhagic complications that causes clinical deterioration. When hemorrhage occurs, large volumes of fresh or fresh frozen plasma may correct the coagulation defect temporarily.

Other Abnormalities

Factor V levels decline unpredictably in liver disease, but it is not clear whether this contributes to clinical bleeding. Factor VIII, by contrast, may give *higher* than normal results. Recall that factor VIII is also synthesized by endothelial cells and that von Willebrand factor (vWF) is probably the only major factor *not* synthesized by the liver. Fibrinogen levels are variable, depending on whether or not fibrinolysis occurs. Even when fibrinogen levels appear normal, coagulation may be qualitatively abnormal. There is a defect in polymerization, but it is not clear whether the abnormality lies in the fibrinogen molecules or in factor XIII.

Activated products of both coagulation and fibrinolysis normally circulate in small quantities and are cleared by the liver. With hepatic failure, activated coagulation and fibrinolytic factors may persist and accumulate. These factors affect laboratory tests for disseminated intravascular coagulation and for the occurrence of fibrin-fibrinogen degradation products.

Severe liver disease impairs both platelet production and platelet function; this is especially marked in alcoholics. The transfusion of platelet concentrates gives disappointing clinical results, although it may be necessary if active bleeding is present.

INHIBITORS TO COAGULATION FACTORS

In addition to the inhibitory antibodies that develop in repeatedly transfused factor-deficient patients, antibodies have been observed to develop *spontaneously*. Antibodies to factor VIII, or rarely to factors V and VIII, occur in previously normal individuals of either sex. Usually IgG, these antibodies resemble autoimmune red-cell or platelet antibodies. They occur without discernible stimulus, they react with tissue or protein from other humans as well as from the patient, and they can cause clinically significant disease.

Spontaneous anti–factor VIII usually occurs in older people, although it has been reported in young patients with chronic immuno-inflammatory diseases such as rheumatoid arthritis, lupus erythematosus, and ulcerative colitis. There is also a puzzling association with pregnancy. Pregnancy-associated anti–factor VIII usually develops after delivery rather than during the pregnancy itself. Its management may be quite complicated.

A patient with antibody to factor VIII has bleeding symptoms very like those of constitutional hemophilia, including hemarthroses, soft tissue hematomas without apparent trauma, and excessive bleeding after minor injuries. The patient's plasma has low or absent levels of procoagulant activity and, after incubation, inhibits the coagulation of previously normal plasma ("mixing study"). Treatment is extremely difficult; non-human (usually porcine) factor VIII concentrates can be used for one-time correction of a crisis, but these products are immunogenic under the best of circumstances. Coagulation factor replacement usually consists of replenishing activated products of coagulation or excessive amounts of factor VIII concentrate. Immunosuppression has been tried with variable success. Another approach has been to administer concentrates of the "liver factors," including factors IX and X, thereby bypassing the step that involves factor VIII.

SUGGESTED READING

Ballem, PJ: Diagnosis and management of thrombocytopenia in obstetric syndromes. In Sacher, RA, and Brecher, M (eds): Obstetric Transfusion Practice. American Association of Blood Banks, 1993, pp. 49–76.

Boshkov, LK, et al: Heparin induced thrombocytopenia and thrombosis: Clinical and laboratory studies. Brit J Haematol 84:322–328, 1993.

Colman, RW, et al (eds): Hemostasis and Thrombosis: Basic Principles and Clinical Practice, ed 3. JB Lippincott, Philadelphia, 1994.

Evers, JP, Capon, SM, and Sacher, RA: The liver in coagulation disorders. In Rustgi, VK, and van Thiel, DH (eds): The Liver in Systemic Disease. Raven, New York, 1993, pp. 303–320.

George, JH, and Shattil, SJ: The clinical importance of acquired abnormalities of platelet function. N Engl J Med 324:27–39, 1991.

Lusher, JM, and Warrier, I: Hemophilia. Pediatr Rev 12:275–81, 1991.

Marder, VJ, et al: Consumptive thrombohemorrhagic disorders. In Coleman, RW, et al (eds): Hemostasis and Thrombosis. Basic Principles and Clinical Practice, ed 3. JB Lippincott, Philadelphia, 1994, pp. 1023–1063.

McCrae, KR, Samuels, P, and Schreiber, AD: Pregnancy associated thrombocytopenia: Pathogenesis and management. Blood 80:2697–2714, 1992.

Perry, JJ, and Alving, BM: von Willebrands disease. Am Fam Physician 41:219–24, 1990.

Rao, AK, and Holmsen, H: Congenital disorders of platelet function. Semin Hematol 23:102–18, 1986.

Seligsohm, U: Disseminated intravascular coagulation. In Hardin, RI, Lux, SG, and Stossel, TP (eds): Blood: Principles and Practice of Hematology. JB Lippincott, Philadelphia, 1995, pp. 1289–1318.

Triplett, DA: Laboratory diagnosis of von Willebrands disease. Mayo Clin Proc 66:832–40, 1991.

White, GC, et al: Approach to the bleeding patient. In Coleman, RW, et al (eds): Hemostasis and Thrombosis: Basic Principles and Clinical Practice, ed 3. JB Lippincott, Philadelphia, 1994, pp. 1134–1148.

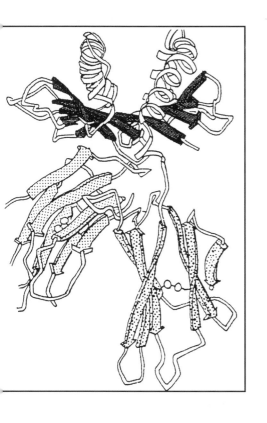

Section Three

Immunology

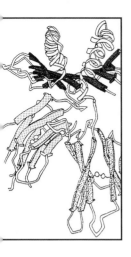

7

Principles of Immunology and Immunology Testing

This chapter details elements of the immune system, laboratory procedures that measure the activity of the immune system, and how such laboratory tests can be used effectively for diagnosis and monitoring of immune disorders.

Challenges to the body from bacteria, fungi, viruses, and parasites or from other foreign antigens such as transfused blood cells elicit various degrees of involvement of the three major divisions of the immune system:

1. humoral immunity (immunoglobulins or antibodies)
2. complement and its cascade of activation
3. cell-mediated immunity

Although these three divisions do have distinct components, they frequently, if not usually, work in concert when confronted with a foreign material such as a microorganism.

Beyond this role in infectious diseases, principles of immunology have major significance in autoimmune diseases, in allergy and hypersensitivity, in immunodeficiency states, and in modalities of therapy involving immunosuppression for organ transplantation and immunoenhancement for rejection of malignancies.

HUMORAL IMMUNITY

This portion of the immune system refers to the immunoglobulins or antibodies that circulate in the blood plasma and are also secreted at mucosal surfaces of the body. Immunoglobulin molecules are proteins composed of heavy chains (55,000 or 70,000 daltons in molecular weight) and light chains (24,000 daltons). The basic structure of an immunoglobulin molecule consists of two light chains plus two heavy chains. The light chains are attached to the heavy chains by way of disulfide (S-S) bonds between cysteine residues in the amino acid backbone of each chain. The heavy chains are also linked to one another through disulfide bonds (Fig. 7–1). This basic monomeric structure has a molecular size of approximately 160,000 daltons. Spatially, it points in three directions: two arms with identical Fab regions that can combine with a specific antigen and a third Fc portion that is constant in structure between different antibodies. The Fab region varies considerably in amino acid composition between different antibodies. This difference in Fab structure is what accounts for the extremely diverse range of different antigens to which specific antibodies can be synthesized by the immune system. Both heavy and light chains have what are called **variable (V) regions** near their amino ends in the Fab segments and also **constant regions** toward their carboxy ends in the Fc segment.

During the maturation of B cells, the genes encoding immunoglobulin heavy chains (on chromosome 14) and light chains (kappa on chromosome 2 and lambda on chromosome 22) go through a process of DNA rearrangement that commits an individual cell to synthesize a particular immunoglobulin. The gene for the heavy chain has approximately 100 variable (V) regions of which only one will be selected in the final rearrangement (Fig. 7–2). There are also 15 to 20 **diversity (D) encoding regions** and 6 **joining (J) regions.** The gene also contains 9 constant regions in the order mu, delta, gamma3, gamma1, alpha1, gamma2, gamma4, epsilon, and alpha2.

The initial step in heavy chain gene rearrangement consists of removing the extra V and D regions and some of the J regions (V-D-J rearrangement). If the resulting gene product cannot be made (e.g., due to introduction of a premature termination codon), the allele on the other chromosome 14 has an opportunity to rearrange. If rearrangement of both alleles is faulty, the cell dies. Following successful rearrangement, the mRNA transcript is spliced to remove extra J regions, and the final protein is translated. The choice of heavy chain type is also dictated by gene rearrangement in which a particular constant region is directly linked to the J region. Conversion of an immunologic response from IgM antibody to IgG antibody requires further removal of the mu constant region as well as the delta to create IgG3 (with gamma3) and so forth to yield any of the other immunoglobulin types (IgA, IgD, IgE).

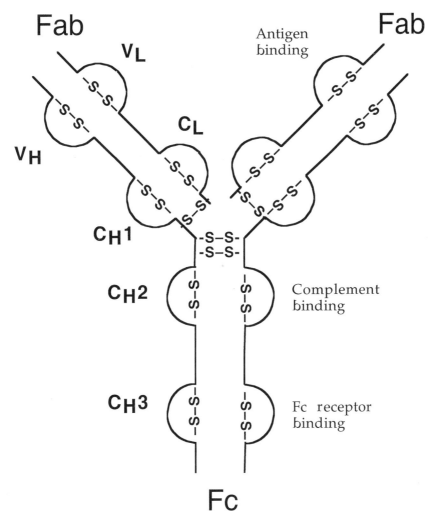

FIGURE 7–1. Molecular structure of immunoglobulin, consisting of two heavy chains (H) and two light chains (L) linked by disulfide bonds (-S-S-). Each chain has variable (V) and constant (C) regions. The Fab region of immunoglobulin binds to specific antigens; the Fc region binds complement. This structure is the basic unit of immunoglobulins. IgG consists of a single one of these units, whereas IgM is a pentamer consisting of five of these units (10 heavy chains and 10 light chains) further linked with a "joining chain" at their Fc regions. Secretory IgA occurs as a dimer of two units with a joining chain plus another peptide designated "secretory piece."

Immunoglobulin heavy chain gene

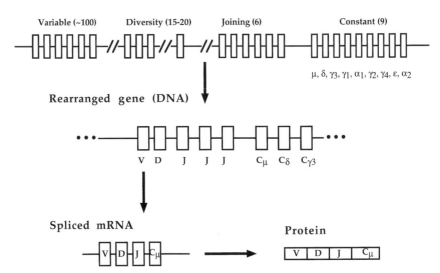

FIGURE 7–2. Immunoglobulin heavy chain gene map with a rearranged gene, the spliced mRNA, and final immunoglobulin protein molecule.

The genes for immunoglobulin light chains are similar to the heavy chain gene with the exception that they lack diversity regions. Otherwise the rearrangement process is similar. Following successful heavy chain gene rearrangement, each kappa chain gene and then each lambda chain gene has an opportunity to rearrange until a single light chain gene is successfully rearranged. For the rest of its life, that cell and its daughter cells will synthesize an immunoglobulin with only that light chain type. The choice of the particular variable regions of the heavy chain and of the light chain determines what antigens will be recognized by that immunoglobulin molecule.

The particular cells that make immunoglobulins for release into the circulation are called **plasma cells** (see also Chapter 4). They reside in the bone marrow along with precursors of the blood cells. An individual plasma cell produces only a single type of immunoglobulin molecule, which recognizes its specific antigen. As that plasma cell divides and produces a line of **descendent cells** (also termed a **clone** or **clonal line**), those resultant cells continue to synthesize the same antibody specific for that single antigenic site. Monoclonal antibodies are used extensively as diagnostic reagents for measurement of such substances as drugs and hormones and are also now finding therapeutic applications (e.g., to facilitate removal of digoxin from the circulation of digoxin-overdose cases by intravenous administration of a monoclonal antidigoxin antibody).

The class of an immunoglobulin is determined by the type of its heavy chain. IgG has gamma-heavy chains, IgM has mu-heavy chains, IgA has alpha-heavy chains, IgE has epsilon-heavy chains, and IgD has delta-heavy chains. The antibody molecules made by a single clone of plasma cells have exactly the same heavy chains and also contain only a single type of light chain. There are two general types of light chains, designated kappa and lambda. Both **kappa** and **lambda light chains** occur in all classes of antibodies. Overall, there is a slight predominance of kappa versus lambda by a ratio of roughly 3:2 in the serum of normal individuals. The major clinical use of measuring light chain type is in distinguishing whether proliferations of plasma cells or lymphoid cells are **monoclonal** (in which case there is almost complete predominance of only kappa or only lambda) or **polyclonal** (both kappa and lambda are present in major amounts) (see Chapter 4).

Immunologic responses against infections or other foreign antigens are typically polyclonal, whereas malignant proliferations of lymphoid cells are typically monoclonal. In some clinical situations, it is not always possible to characterize fully a lymphoid proliferation by assessment of the light chain protein expression (e.g., due to mixtures of normal polyclonal cells with the monoclonal tumor cells). In that case, it is possible to examine the DNA of lymphocytes, lymph nodes, or tumor biopsy for evidence of a clonal population with the same immunoglobulin gene rearrangement (see Appendix B: B- and T-Cell Gene Rearrangements; Fig. B–1). The method used for this examination is Southern blot analysis in which cellular DNA is enzymatically cut into fragments, electrophoresed in agarose gels, transferred to a membrane, and hybridized with a marker DNA probe for the gene of interest.

Subclasses of immunoglobulins occur because of minor differences between heavy chains that occur in the constant regions of some classes. There are four subclasses of IgG (IgG1, IgG2, IgG3, and IgG4), two of IgA (IgA1 and IgA2), and two of IgD. Some of these subclass differences result in altered function of an immunoglobulin. For example, IgG1, IgG2, and IgG3 molecules generally can fix complement (see below), whereas IgG4 cannot. IgG3 has a structure that allows it to remain in the circulation for a much shorter period than the other IgG subclasses before it is cleared. Maternal IgG2 does not cross the placenta to the fetal circulation, although the other IgG subclasses can. IgA1 can be cleaved and thereby inactivated by some bacterial (streptococcal and gonococcal) enzymes, whereas IgA2 is not susceptible to those proteases.

In addition to the basic monomeric immunoglobulin structure mentioned above as two heavy chains plus two light chains (H_2L_2), there are polymeric linkages in which IgM and IgA participate. Normally, IgM in the serum is a pentamer of five monomeric units as $(H_2L_2)_5$ with interconnection through the mu-heavy chains in their Fc regions. There is another small fragment designated the J chain, which is involved in joining these IgM monomers together (see Fig. 7–1). In the case of IgA, the J alpha chains join at the Fc location. One further modification of IgA occurs as it passes across epithelial cells and enters body secretions such as saliva, in which IgA is the major immunoglobulin. This modification entails the attachment to IgA of another protein segment designated **secretory piece.**

A typical immune response consists initially of a rise in IgM antibody directed against the stimulating antigen (immunogen). This phase is followed by production of IgG antibody against the antigen. Repeated stimulation with the antigen leads to greater production of the IgG antibody, but with shorter time lag after each succeeding antigenic stimulus. This ability of the immune system to remember and respond more efficiently to an antigen is called an **anamnestic response.** The time sequence of IgM followed by IgG is used extensively in the diagnosis of infectious diseases (see Fig. 15–1). In general, significant levels of IgM antibody against a virus, bacterium, or other infectious agent are interpreted as evidence for acute infection, whereas a high level of specific IgG is consistent with persistence of immunity in the convalescent phase after a previous infection. A common application of this principle is the measurement of IgM antibody against hepatitis A virus to diagnose acute or recent infection with that virus. Antibody of the IgG class against hepatitis A virus merely indicates infection in the (distant) past and is not very useful clinically for the evaluation of current hepatitis (see also Chapter 15).

ANTIGENS

The chemical nature of materials that can be recognized by antibodies is extremely wide and includes proteins, lipids, nucleic acids, and small molecules such as drugs and steroid hormones. This is due in part to the fact that any particular antibody reacts with only a small region of an antigen. This antigenic site is designated an **epitope.** Monoclonal antibodies by their very nature are very specific for a single epitope. This degree of specificity has allowed the development of different antibodies that can distinguish between such closely related antigens as thyroxine (T_4) versus triiodothyronine (T_3), hemoglobin A versus hemoglobin S, and procainamide (parent drug) versus N-acetyl procainamide (drug metabolite).

Polyclonal antibodies are typical of the immune response in a normal animal on stimulation with foreign antigens, such as by immunization or by infection. Polyclonal antibodies consist of many different clones, each with potentially different specificities for a large number of epitopes on the surface of the foreign antigen. A distinct advantage for many different antibody clones to recognize an array of epitopes on an invading microorganism is that mutation by the infectious agent will likely alter only one epitope. The microbe may then escape one clone of antibody, but the other clones can still recognize the remaining epitopes. Polyclonal immune responses to infectious agents can therefore be seen to confer significant survival advantage to an animal.

Whether or not an antigen elicits an antibody response depends on the ability of the immune system to recognize that antigen as foreign and not as a self antigen. The vast number of self antigens present on our own tissues, cells, and proteins do not trigger immune responses except in cases of autoimmune disorders.

A foreign antigen is essentially one that has not been present in the body during development or afterward until it is introduced by infection, by trauma, by injection (as with immunization), by blood transfusion with erythrocytes, or by pregnancy, with fetal cells that cross the placenta to the mother (e.g., Rh incompatibility). Even some small molecules normally present in the circulation can be made immunogenic (i.e., capable of stimulating an immune response) by coupling them to large foreign proteins. Examples of this strategy include coupling of thyroxine or steroid hormones to an enhancer called **keyhole limpet hemocyanin,** which induces an intense immune response when injected into animals. Some of those antibody clones will react with the small hormone molecule even though it was previously tolerated as a self antigen. In other instances, drugs such as penicillin or heparin on rare occasion can cause autoimmune responses when those drugs become bound to cell surfaces, thereby converting a self antigen to a foreign-appearing one.

Antigens of similar chemical structure may be able to cross-react with the same antibody. There is very likely a measurable difference in affinity or binding strength between an antibody and those different antigens, but when the antibody is present in high concentration, the reaction may be clinically significant. An example of this may be similar epitopes on the surface of a virus or bacterium and also on some protein in the body. Infection with such a microorganism could then trigger an antibody response, which has the undesired side effect of attaching to the common epitope on tissues and causing damage to the body. Examples of this type are streptococcal antigens and rheumatic fever or acute glomerulonephritis.

IMMUNE COMPLEXES

When antibodies interact with antigens, the two Fab arms of the immunoglobulin monomer can bind to separate antigen molecules, each containing the same epitope. If the antigen is large enough for another antibody to combine with another epitope on its surface, there can result a large matrix of alternating antigen and antibody molecules. This meshwork is referred to as an immune complex. It can be so large as to be physically insoluble and may actually form a visible precipitate, thereby removing both antigen and antibody from solution. If the concentration of either antigen or antibody greatly exceeds that of the other, a matrix cannot form. When the antigen is in excess, the Fab regions are saturated with individual antigens. When the antibody is in excess, available antigen is coated with antibody. The point at which concentration of antigen and antibody form an interlocking matrix is termed **equivalence.**

These different states of immune complexes have importance for laboratory test procedures that use the point of equivalence to detect assay endpoints by immunodiffusion or by nephelometry. They also can have enormous clinical significance because large immune complexes that form at equivalence in the circulation are filtered by the kidney, potentially giving rise to glomerulonephritis. In addition, any infectious disease can be separated into a stage in which there is excess antigen (early in the disease before an immune response is mounted) and another in which the antibody is in excess (convalescence). For example, human immunodeficiency virus (HIV) and its antigens are present in an infectious form in the body and blood of individuals for several weeks after initial infection before there is sufficient time to develop a detectable response to that virus.

COMPLEMENT

Once an antibody has lodged on the surface of an invading microorganism, an orderly sequence of plasma proteins called **complement** may be activated (Fig. 7–3). These complement proteins are capable of delivering a fatal blow to the invader. This process is initiated by a conformational change in the Fc region of an antibody on combining with an antigen. If that antigen were floating freely in the circulation as an individual molecule, the immune complex that formed may bind complement components to it. Complement in the complex could then help to attract phagocytic cells, which will engulf and remove the inactivated antigen from the circulation.

If the antigen is part of a bacterial cell wall, complement can fix onto the bound antibody, ultimately weakening the bacterium and killing it. The same process can occur with transfused red blood cells if they are incompatible with the recipient, thereby leading to hemolysis.

By the so-called classic pathway of complement activation, the first component C1q attaches to Fc regions of two adjacent IgG molecules that have been brought into proximity by binding onto a foreign surface. Alternatively, a single IgM molecule can attract C1q since each IgM has five Fc regions. Next, the subunits C1r and C1s bind to C1q. These subunits have enzymatic activities that cleave two other components (C4 into C4a and C4b, and C2 into C2a and C2b). C4 binds directly to the surface near where it was generated, and C2a binds to the C4b. The

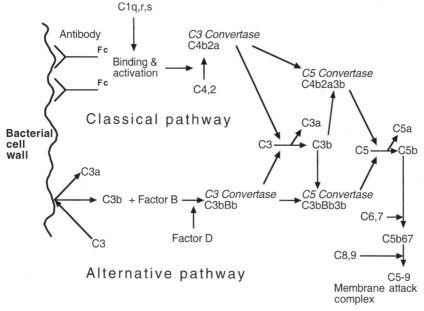

FIGURE 7–3. Schematic representation of the classical and alternative pathways for complement activation. Both pathways use the same final reactions and result in formation of the membrane attack complex.

C4b–C2a complex then cleaves C3 into C3a and C3b, which in turn binds nearby on the surface. The interaction of C2a and C3b cleaves C5, which then binds C6 and C7 and also attaches to the surface. C8 and C9 are attracted to form the final additions to this complex. At this point, the surface of the cell or bacterium is seriously damaged, leading ultimately to lysis. This sequence of complement activation is the same regardless of the specific antigens involved in the immune complex. It is the specificity of the antibody that directs and initiates the whole process (see Fig. 7–3).

The **alternative pathway** is another means by which complement can be activated. This pathway is independent of antibody. It occurs when C3 combines with factor B and binds to a substance such as a bacterial cell wall. This complex further activates more C3, which then continues the activation and attachment of C5 through C9.

Complement activation is down-regulated by individual plasma proteins that selectively inhibit C1, C4b, or C3b. Congenital deficiency of one such protein, C1 esterase inhibitor, results in a clinical syndrome called **hereditary angioedema.** In this disorder, edema occurs in the gastrointestinal and respiratory tracts when complement is activated by trauma or for frequently unrecognized reasons.

Congenital deficiencies of individual complement components may manifest themselves as increased susceptibility to infections with pyogenic bacteria (deficiency of C1, C4, C2, or C3) or *Neisseria* (C3, C5, C6, C7, C8, or C9). In addition, there is a greater frequency of rheumatic diseases (in particular systemic lupus erythematosus) with deficiencies of C1, C2, or C4, perhaps due to impaired clearance of immune complexes.

CELL-MEDIATED IMMUNITY

The recognition, uptake, and processing of foreign antigens are performed by cellular elements of the immune system. These include macrophages, which initially ingest foreign materials and then present them to T lymphocytes in a process that relies on mixed histocompatibility (MHC) antigens on the macrophage and antigen receptors on the T lymphocyte. With all these control signals acting properly, a subset of the T lymphocytes called **T-helper cells** then stimulates B lymphocytes to produce antibody against the processed antigen. These B lymphocytes are also stimulated to divide as a further means to amplify antibody production. This sequence is slowed down by other types of T lymphocytes called **T-suppressor cells,** which limit the antibody response. This on-off feature of the immune response permits a multitude of different antibodies to be made and subsequently to be turned off when the need for those particular antibodies is over. Discovery of unique antigenic markers on the surfaces of lymphocytes has led to the classification of helper T cells as **CD4 cells** (CD = cluster of differentiation) and suppressor T cells as **CD8 cells** (Table 7–1).

One other type of lymphocyte is **cytotoxic killer T cells** (positive for CD16 or CD56), which have the capacity to lyse target cells. An example is interaction of cytotoxic T cells with virally infected cells. If the infected cells have both viral antigens and major histocompatibility antigens on their membranes, they constitute targets that the cytotoxic T cells recognize and kill, thereby protecting the body from further virus production and release.

The nature of the T-cell antigen receptor genes deserves special mention as they go through rearrangements in a manner parallel to that of the immunoglobulin genes to confer antigen-recognizing specificity to any particular T cell. The T-cell antigen receptor consists of two subunits: either alpha plus beta or gamma plus delta. The alpha/beta heterodimer is present on the surfaces of most T cells in the blood and lymph nodes, whereas the gamma/delta receptor occurs predominantly on lymphocytes in the skin. The gene for the alpha chain is on chromosome 14; the gene for the delta chain is contained within the alpha gene. The beta and gamma chain genes are located in separate locations on chromosome 7. The beta and delta genes contain V, D, J, and C regions analogous to immunoglobulin heavy chain genes; the alpha and gamma genes contain

TABLE 7–1. WORLD HEALTH ORGANIZATION RECOMMENDED NOMENCLATURE FOR HUMAN LEUKOCYTE DIFFERENTIATION ANTIGENS*

Antigen	Monoclonal Antibodies	Positive Leukocytes
CD1	Leu 6, T6, OKT6	Thymocytes
CD2	Leu 5B, T11, OKT11	T and NK cells (E-rosette receptor)
CD3	Leu 4, T3, OKT3	Mature T cells
CD4	Leu 3, T4, OKT4	Helper-inducer T cells, monocytes
CD5	Leu 1, T1, T101	T cells, B-cell subset, CLL cells, PLL cells
CD6	T12	T cells
CD7	Leu 9, 3A1	T, T-ALL, and NK cells
CD8	Leu 2, T8, OKT8	Suppressor-cytotoxic T cells, NK subset
CD9	BA-2	Monocytes, pre-B cell
CD10	CALLA, J5	Granulocytes, pre-B leukemia cells
CD11	CR3/Leu 15, OKM1	(C3bi receptor) monocytes, granulocytes
	MO-1	NK cells
CD13	MY7	Neutrophils and monocytes
CD14	MY4, MO-2	Monocytes
CD15	Leu M1	Monocytes, granulocytes
CD16	Leu 11	(IgG Fc receptor) NK cells, PMNs
CD19	Leu 12, B4	Pan B cell marker
CD20	Leu 16, B1	B cells, dendritic cells
CD21	CR2, B2	(C3d receptor) Mature B cells
CD22	Leu 14	B cells
CD23	Blast-2	B cells
CD24	BA-1	B cells, most B neoplasms
CD25	TAC	(IL-2 receptor) Activated B and T cells
CD34	My10	Myeloid, lymphoid precursors (stem cells)
CD45		Leukocytes
CD56	Leu 19	NK cells
CD71	38-18	(Transferrin receptor) Proliferating cells

CLL, chronic lymphocytic leukemia; PLL, prolymphocytic leukemia; ALL, acute lymphocytic leukemia; CALLA, common ALL antigen; NK, natural killer.

*Newer antigens have been discovered since this list was formed, and more than 75 have now been described.

V, J, and C regions similar to immunoglobulin light chain genes. The maturation process of a T cell involves gene rearrangement of a particular pair of alpha/beta or gamma/delta genes that produce a unique antigen receptor inserted in the lymphocyte surface membrane.

The major clinical utility of examining the T-cell antigen receptor gene is to determine whether a proliferation of T cells consists of a monoclonal population, in which case Southern blot analysis shows predominance of a rearranged gene (see Fig. B–2). Such a finding of monoclonality of a T-cell population is strong evidence for malignancy (lymphoma). Gene rearrangement studies are generally done for both B- and T-cell genes at the same time to establish both the clonality and lineage (B vs. T) of a lymphoid proliferation.

HISTOCOMPATIBILITY ANTIGENS

The immunologic identity of human cells is determined by histocompatibility antigens on the surface membranes of all cells except for erythrocytes and trophoblasts. These tissue antigens are what account for rejection of transplanted organs. **Class I antigens** consist of two protein components: heavy chains from one of the three different genetic loci designated HLA-A, HLA-B, and HLA-C and a common light chain called beta-2-microglobulin. The large number of alleles for the heavy chain genes accounts for an almost unlimited number of different antigen combinations. For this reason, a perfect genetic cross-match between organ transplant donor and recipient is virtually impossible to achieve except in the case of identical twins.

Another set of antigens is restricted primarily to monocytes and lymphocytes. These are the **class II antigens,** which consist of two protein chains. Class II antigens include HLA-D, HLA-DP, HLA-DQ, and HLA-DR, which also has multiple alleles. The function of all these antigens appears to be at the level of cell-to-cell communication regulating the immune response.

Human leukocyte antigen typing is used clinically for cross-matching solid organ and bone marrow transplants and also for better typing of platelet transfusion products in patients who have become HLA sensitized after multiple transfusions. Human leukocyte antigen typing is also used medicolegally for paternity testing because of the relatively high degree of certainty in tracing lineages through familial inheritance of the HLA alleles or haplotypes (see Chapter 8).

The genes for both class I and class II antigens are located on chromosome 6 along with genes for some complement components. Some HLA types have been associated with diseases that have an autoimmune etiology, perhaps because of faulty immune regulation related to antigen type. In particular, HLA-B27 has an association with the rheumatic diseases, ankylosing spondylitis, and Reiter's syndrome; different HLA types are associated with narcolepsy, multiple sclerosis, diabetes mellitus, and other disorders (see Chapter 8).

DISORDERS OF THE IMMUNE SYSTEM

IMMUNE DEFICIENCIES

Deficiencies of selective parts of the immune system usually result in increased susceptibility to infection with different microorganisms. These immune deficiencies can be inherited or acquired (Table 7–2; see Table 4–3).

Congenital deficiency typically presents early in the life of a newborn as recurrent infections, sometime after maternally transferred immunity has waned (IgG immunoglobulins that cross the placenta; IgA absorbed from swallowed breast milk). There are distinct hereditary deficiencies of immunoglobulins, of lymphocyte functions, and of complement (discussed above). In general, absence of antibodies **(agammaglobulinemia)** or severely reduced levels of antibodies **(hypogammaglobulinemia)** are manifested by increased susceptibility to bacterial infections. Immunoglobulins that normally bind to bacterial cell walls **(opsonization)** promote phagocytosis and removal by leukocytes.

In contrast, impaired cellular immunity typically shows infections with viruses or fungi. This is because it requires lymphocytes to recognize and kill other cells infected with viruses and to kill the large cellular forms of the fungi. Combined immunodeficiencies involving both immunoglobulins and cell-mediated immunity are severe disorders that show multiple infections and usually result in death at an early age unless treated with heroic measures such as immune system reconstitution by bone marrow transplantation (e.g., severe combined immunodeficiency disease).

Acquired immunodeficiency may be due to replacement of normal immune cells in the bone marrow by leukemia or to loss of cells with immunosuppressive therapy. Hypogammaglobulinemia can leave a patient susceptible to pneumococcal pneumonia or other bacterial infections. Malignancy involving the immune system, such as lymphoma, can also impair cellular immunity, resulting in such infections as *herpesvirus* and *candida* species.

The disorder known as acquired immune deficiency syndrome (AIDS) is due to human immunodeficiency virus (HIV), which infects and destroys helper T lymphocytes (CD4-positive T cells). Loss of these helper cells affects the body's ability to produce functional antibodies and to induce cellular immune responses. Patients with this syndrome therefore become infected with a wide array of microorganisms, many of which are not normally pathogenic except in such disorders. These include *Pneumocystis carinii, Candida, Mycobacterium avium-intracellulare,* and many species of parasitic organisms (see Chapters 13 and 14).

TABLE 7-2. CONDITIONS ASSOCIATED WITH IMMUNOGLOBULIN DEFICIENCIES*

Condition	Population Affected	Immunoglobulin Abnormality	Other Findings
Acquired hypogammaglobulinemia	Malignancy of lymphoreticular system Autoimmune diseases Protein loss or malnutrition Immunosuppressive drugs	Unpredictable	T-cell function also depressed Findings of primary disease
Selective IgA deficiency	1 in 500–1000 persons	$\downarrow\downarrow$ IgA Other Ig normal	Sinopulmonary infections frequent Often asymptomatic May have anaphylactoid response to transfused IgA
X-linked hypogammaglobulinemia	Males, from birth	All Ig classes very low	No B lymphocytes or plasma cells T-cell function intact
Wiskott-Aldrich syndrome	X-linked	IgG, IgA normal or $\uparrow$ IgE $\uparrow$, IgM $\downarrow$	Eczema, thrombocytopenia, recurrent infections T-cell function decreased; may have $\downarrow$ number of T cells
IgG and IgA deficiency	X-linked or acquired	$\downarrow$ IgG; $\downarrow$ IgA; $\uparrow$ IgM, to 10 × normal $\downarrow$ IgA in 70%	Frequent infections Plasma cells numerous
Ataxia telangiectasia	Rare; both sexes		Neurologic symptoms prominent Cutaneous vessels abnormal Lymphoid malignancies often develop
Severe combined immunodeficiency (SCID)	Very rare	All Ig classes $\downarrow\downarrow$, except sometimes IgM present	Deficiency of progenitor lymphocyte Absent T-cell functions Lymphoreticular malignancies develop in those who do not succumb to infection

*Listed in approximate order of decreasing incidence.

IMMUNOSUPPRESSION/ENHANCEMENT

Chemotherapy with antimetabolites such as methotrexate is designed to kill rapidly dividing cancer or leukemia cells. One of the undesired side effects of chemotherapy is suppression of the bone marrow and also of the immune system, which limits the extent to which cancer treatment can be tolerated. Organ and bone marrow transplantation recipients must be treated with immunosuppressive agents and/or irradiation in order to prevent rejection of the grafted organ or cells as foreign antigens. These strategies are directed primarily at moderating cellular immunity. In addition to using antimetabolites, physicians employ steroids, cyclosporine, antithymocyte globulin, and FK-506 to control the immune response.

Some exciting new developments in cancer therapy are based on the idea that tumor cells have escaped destruction by the immune system due to a breakdown in normal immune surveillance for antigens that are present on the tumor cells. The new strategies of therapy are based on enhancing or reconstituting the body's own immune response by activating lymphocytes with one or more of the chemicals that normally modulate immune function. These substances are the lymphokines such as interleukin-2 (IL-2). By injecting IL-2 into the body or by treating lymphocytes outside the body and then returning those cells to a cancer patient, the hope is that **lymphokine-activated killer (LAK) cells** will target the tumor for destruction. Other biologic response modifiers that affect immune system and are undergoing clinical trials include alpha and gamma interferons.

AUTOIMMUNITY

When the immune system produces antibodies against (self) antigens of the body, serious damage to many organs can result. A classic example of autoimmunity is **systemic lupus erythematosus (SLE),** in which extensive damage occurs in the kidneys due to deposition of circulating immune complexes in the glomeruli followed by activation of complement that indiscriminately injures the glomeruli. A target antigen for these autoantibodies is frequently DNA as well as other nuclear antigens such as ribonuclear protein (RNP) and also many cytoplasmic antigens. Other forms of autoimmune disease include mixed connective tissue disorder (MCTD), rheumatoid arthritis, and many organ-specific diseases (e.g., thyroid-Graves disease, adrenal, skin).

ALLERGY/HYPERSENSITIVITY

Inappropriate excess activity of the immune system is sometimes an undesirable reaction on exposure to allergens such as pollens, dust, animal hairs, or foodstuffs. These reactions are mediated by IgE, which is

TABLE 7–3. IMMUNOLOGIC MECHANISMS OF TISSUE INJURY

Type	Examples	Mechanism
I	Immediate hypersensitivity Anaphylaxis Allergies Asthma	Allergens bind to IgE on mast cells/ basophils to release vasoactive amines (e.g., histamine)
II	Antibody directed against cells Autoimmune hemolytic anemia Goodpasture's disease	IgG, IgM bind to antigens on cell surfaces leading to phagocytosis or lysis (antibody-dependent cell-mediated cytotoxicity, ADCC)
III	Immune complex diseases Serum sickness Acute glomerulonephritis	Antigens and antibodies (IgG) form complexes that bind and activate complement; deposition in tissues
IV	Delayed hypersensitivity Contact dermatitis Tuberculosis Foreign Organ transplant rejection	Sensitized T lymphocytes mediate cytotoxicity

the only immunoglobulin class to bind onto mast cells or basophils (see Chapter 2). These cells contain granules of histamine and similar substances that are the direct chemical mediators of allergy. When an allergen such as ragweed pollen comes in contact with antiragweed IgE bound onto mast cells in the respiratory tract, the mast cells release their contents, causing constriction of smooth muscle around bronchioles. This action results in limited air movement, mucus secretion, and wheezing—a condition known as asthma. Other manifestations of this IgE-mediated reaction can occur in other parts of the body. These reactions can be relatively mild, in the form of hayfever and nasal congestion, or they can be extremely severe and result in sudden death from anaphylactic shock, which produces circulatory collapse (Table 7–3).

DIAGNOSTIC TEST PROCEDURES IN IMMUNOLOGY

The detection of many substances has been greatly facilitated by the use of antibodies as reagents. The principles of these immunologic assays deserve some consideration as fundamental to understanding how various analytes are measured and what interferences may be expected to occur in different conditions.

ANTIGEN-ANTIBODY EQUIVALENCE

The principle of detection using an antibody is specific recognition of an antigen at concentrations near saturation of the antibody's capacity to bind that antigen. Many of the earliest immunoassays were based on visual detection of an actual precipitation of the antigen-antibody complexes in some semisolid medium such as agarose. Precipitation of these complexes occurs when antigen and antibody are in equivalent concentrations and can form large interlocking macromolecular structures that are more turbid than either the antigen or antibody alone in solution **(antigen-antibody equivalence)** (Fig. 7–4). Under conditions in which either the antigen or antibody is in excess of the other, complexes can form, but they are generally very small, do not form a large macromolecular structure, do not scatter light, and so are not detected visually.

IMMUNODIFFUSION

Immunodiffusion takes place in a translucent semisolid medium such as agarose, through which both antigen and antibody are able to diffuse freely. In the simplest form, wells are punched into a layer of agarose on a glass slide. Into adjacent wells are placed preparations of antigen and antibody. Following diffusion over 24 to 48 hours, antigen-antibody complexes form a precipitin line between the wells. This method can be used to detect either antigens (in the presence of known reagent antibody) or antibodies (in the presence of known reagent antigen). This method is frequently referred to as **Ouchterlony** or **double diffusion** because both the antigen and antibody diffuse through the medium. By alternating placement of antigen wells around a central antibody well, it is also possible to determine from intersection of the precipitin lines whether the antigens are identical or have different recognition sites.

A common variation of this method is **radial immunodiffusion (RID),** in which reagent antibody is incorporated into the agarose in a uniform concentration. Samples containing antigen are placed into wells cut into the agarose, and the antigen is allowed to diffuse through the agarose, where it comes into contact with antibody. Initially the antigen is in excess near the well and so it continues to migrate in a circular manner until it comes into equilibrium with antibody concentration, where it forms a precipitin ring at antigen-antibody equivalence. The precipitin ring is visually detected (generally a few millimeters in diameter) and measured in comparison with the size of rings from standards applied to the same

Antigen-Antibody Complex Formation

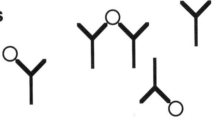

Antigen excess
Low turbidity

Equivalence
High turbidity
Precipitate

Antibody excess
Low turbidity

FIGURE 7–4. Variations in antigen-antibody complex formation with different concentrations of reactants. Methods of detection based on precipitation or scattering of light rely on the antibody and antigen being in equivalent concentrations.

agarose in other wells. The concentration of antigen is proportional to the area of the precipitin ring. RID has been used extensively in the past for quantitating a large number of serum proteins such as immunoglobulins and complement. Because of the long time required to complete RID (typically 48 hours) and the expense of labor, most laboratories today have converted these measurements to nephelometry or ELISA. However, understanding the principles of RID is useful for comprehending other immunoassays.

COUNTERIMMUNOELECTROPHORESIS AND LAURELL ROCKET IMMUNOELECTROPHORESIS

To overcome the disadvantage of waiting overnight or up to 2 days for the results of simple immunodiffusion, **electrophoresis** is used to bring the antigens and antibodies together (replacing the long diffusion step) in a period of minutes to an hour. **Counterimmunoelectrophoresis (CIE)** entails putting the antigens to be tested in a well adjacent to a paired well containing a reagent antibody. A buffer fixes the pH so that the antigens have net negative charge and the antibodies have net positive charge. When an electrical field is imposed on the pairs of wells, the antigens and antibodies are driven in opposite (counter) directions toward one another. At the completion of electrophoresis, the CIE plate is allowed to sit for an additional brief period of several minutes for precipitation of antigen-antibody complexes to occur. This procedure has been very useful in the past for expediting the detection of bacterial antigens in cerebrospinal fluid for suspected cases of bacterial meningitis and in other body fluids. CIE has largely been replaced with simple agglutination assays.

Laurell rocket immunoelectrophoresis (RIE) consists of electrophoresing samples through an agarose gel, in which is incorporated an antibody at uniform concentration. If the antigen is present in a sample, it will migrate electrophoretically into the gel and form a precipitin pattern that is an elongated parabola with an area proportional to concentration of the antigen. The precipitin is generally approximated as a triangle whose height is measured and plotted versus concentration in a standard curve. RIE has been used a great deal in the past for quantitating some plasma proteins such as von Willebrand antigen. Most applications of RIE are now being replaced with ELISA.

IMMUNOELECTROPHORESIS AND IMMUNOFIXATION ELECTROPHORESIS

Immunoelectrophoresis (IEP) and **immunofixation electrophoresis (IFE)** are reserved for use in the detection and characterization of clonal immunoglobulins (paraproteins) in disorders such as multiple myeloma. IEP is depicted in Figure 4–8. IEP requires an initial electrophoresis step followed by an overnight diffusion step after addition of reagent antibodies. IFE is a more modern method that can generally be completed in less than 4 hours. The initial step of IFE is also electrophoresis through an agarose gel. The second phase of IFE is to overlay replicate lanes of the patient's electrophoresed serum sample with the individual antihuman IgG, IgA, IgM, kappa, and lambda reagent antibodies (generally produced in rabbits or goats). Wherever in the electrophoretic lane the patient sample has immunoglobulins, the overlaying reagent antibodies react and form a precipitate. If the patient has normal polyclonal immunoglobulins, the precipitates formed are broad and diffuse and contain both light chain types. If a monoclonal protein is present, it forms a precipitate with a single type of heavy chain antibody and also with a single type of light chain. Visual inspection of an IFE easily reveals the specific type of paraprotein (Fig. 7–5).

WESTERN BLOT

This method consists of an initial step in which protein antigens are electrophoresed in a gel such as polyacrylamide that separates them according to molecular size. The antigens are then transferred to the surface of a membrane such as cellulose nitrate or nylon; the antigens remain in the same positions on the membrane as in the electrophoretic gel. The membrane is then cut into strips, and each segment is incubated with a dilution of patient serum. If the patient's serum contains an antibody against one of the antigens (e.g., proteins of the HIV or of the

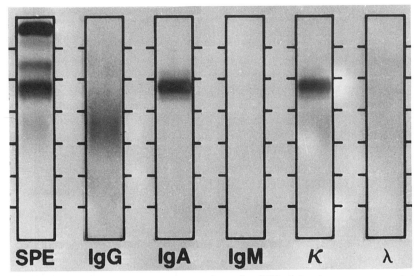

FIGURE 7–5. Immunofixation electrophoresis (IFE) following serum protein electrophoresis. The patient's serum was applied to each lane, electrophoresed, and then overlaid with precipitating acid to fix all proteins in the serum protein electrophoresis (SPE) or with reagent antibodies against the immunoglobulin heavy chains (gamma—IgG, alpha—IgA, mu—IgM) and light chains (kappa—κ, lambda—λ). This sample demonstrated a monoclonal band of IgA-kappa plus some normal polyclonal IgG.

hepatitis C virus), the antibody will bind to that antigen. The strip is then washed free of unbound serum proteins and incubated with an antibody against human immunoglobulins that is labeled with an enzyme such as alkaline phosphatase. The strip is then washed again to remove unbound enzyme, and it is soaked in a solution containing a substrate for the enzyme. The result is formation of a colored band at locations where the patient's antibody bound to antigen on the membrane. Because all the antigens remain in reproducible register from strip to strip, the molecular size of each antigen is clear on visual inspection. The Western blot has had most application as a confirmatory test for viral antibodies after a screening test such as ELISA has been found positive.

LATEX AGGLUTINATION

The development of monoclonal antibodies in large amounts has made possible the production of many basic immunoassays into a simple format in which the reagent antibody is linked to microscopic particles of latex that form a creamy suspension **(latex agglutination).** If antigen is present (e.g., bacterial antigen in CSF), the complexes formed between it and the antibody cause the latex particles to be linked together into clumps that are easily distinguished from a negative sample, in which the latex particles remain uniformly suspended. Latex agglutination tests are rendered specific by the nature of the antibody coating the individual particles. This method is fast and can be done at the point of care with the proviso that personnel performing the test should be well trained in interpreting results including borderline positive ones.

NEPHELOMETRY

For rapid and reliable quantitation of individual serum proteins, most laboratories now use instruments that are based on **nephelometry.** The principle employed relies on the turbidity that occurs when antigen and antibody approach equivalence in concentrations. To make these measurements in a brief period, the rate of formation rather than the final amount of turbidity is measured as a sample is mixed in solution with the reagent antibody in a precisely controlled sequence within the nephelometer. Nephelometry is so automated and rapid that it has almost completely replaced RID and other immunoassays that relied on visual detection steps.

ENZYME-LINKED IMMUNOSORBENT ASSAY

Enzyme-linked immunosorbent assay (ELISA) is performed with plastic microtiter plates that typically contain 96 wells, thereby facilitating simultaneous analysis of multiple specimens. A reagent antibody is coated on the bottom of each well. Patient samples are added to wells, and if the antigen is present, it will bind to the solid phase (capture) antibody in the well. A second (detector) antibody is then added, which also is capable of reacting with the antigen. The second antibody is labeled with an enzyme. After washing away any unbound second antibody, substrate for the enzyme is added to each well in a precisely timed sequence, and the resulting formation of colored product is monitored spectrophotometrically. The amount of antigen in a sample is directly proportional to the amount of colored product formed at the last step.

After many years of development, ELISAs have been exceedingly well standardized and automated. They have applications in measuring a wide variety of serum and plasma proteins that are present in quantities too small for adequate detection by nephelometry (e.g., protein C, protein S, von Willebrand antigen).

RADIOIMMUNOASSAY AND ENZYME IMMUNOASSAY

The most sensitive immunoassays, which are reserved for quantitation of very low-concentration analytes (e.g., hormones, vitamins, therapeutic drugs), are **radioimmunoassays (RIAs)** and **enzyme immunoassays (EIAs)** and also more recently, the similarly based chemiluminescent immunoassays. RIAs depend on having a radioactively labeled analyte that is displaced from reagent antibody by unlabeled analyte in the patient sample being tested. The amount of radioactivity bound to the antibody is inversely proportional to the concentration of the analyte in the test sample. In the RIA format, the bound radioactivity must be separated from the free radioactivity by a maneuver such as precipitation with a second antibody or adsorption by charcoal. Following separation, the radioactivity must be quantitated with a gamma or scintillation counter. RIAs are very labor intensive and have not been readily automated.

EIAs overcome some of the problems of RIAs by not requiring a separation step, owing to different reactivities of the labeled enzyme in bound versus free forms. Furthermore, EIA detection steps are done in a single automated instrument. Accordingly most laboratories have switched virtually all former RIA procedures to EIA whenever it has been possible to do so. In addition, EIAs generally are performed in minutes, whereas RIAs require hours for completion.

HUMAN ANTIMOUSE ANTIBODY (HAMA)

Many of today's automated immunoassays such as EIAs employ mouse monoclonal antibodies as reagents due to the ability to produce large amounts of consistent reactivities. Mouse monoclonal antibodies are also used in some therapeutic approaches in which they are administered intravenously to patients who then can develop antibodies against mouse immunoglobulins. Other individuals can also develop such antimouse antibodies for reasons not known. In either case, those **human anti-mouse antibodies (HAMAs)** can very seriously interfere with immunoassays that use monoclonal antibodies. Thus patients who have consistently abnormal assay results that do not appear clinically correct may in fact have HAMAs that invalidate those assays. One approach to rectifying this problem is to selectively preincubate the patient's serum sample with a large amount of mouse immunoglobulins to neutralize the HAMA before performing the immunoassay.

IMMUNOHISTOCHEMISTRY, DIRECT IMMUNOFLUORESCENCE, INDIRECT IMMUNOFLUORESCENCE ASSAY

Immunohistochemistry (IHC) is performed on tissue biopsies to demonstrate presence of particular antigens in a tumor or other mass. The sections of the tissue are fixed onto glass slides and then incubated with a reagent antibody labeled with an enzyme (such as peroxidase) and directed against the target antigen (e.g., a tumor antigen such as carcinoembryonic antigen). The antibody will bind to locations where the antigen is present. Unbound antibody is then washed off, and the section is incubated with enzyme substrate. Reaction product precipitates in locations where the antigen occurs, and the sections are visualized microscopically. Tumors can frequently be identified by this means; a particular example is examination of lymph node biopsies for presence of lymphoma, which is a clonal malignancy.

   Direct immunofluorescence is performed by incubating a biopsy sample with a fluorescein-labeled antihuman antibody to demonstrate the presence of immunoglobulin deposits in tissue. Examination utilizes a fluorescent microscope. Examples are biopsies of kidney or skin that may have accumulations of immunoglobulin or complement as the basis of disease (e.g., systemic lupus erythematosus). **Indirect immunofluorescence assay (IFA)** examines a patient's serum sample for presence of an antibody directed against antigens in cells or tissue sections that are mounted on glass slides. A major application of this assay is in autoantibody testing, discussed later.

SPECIFIC IMMUNOLOGIC MEASUREMENTS

SERUM IMMUNOGLOBULINS

Several methods are commonly available to evaluate the level of immunoglobulins present in serum and other body fluids. Major elevations or reductions of immunoglobulins are broadly indicated by measurement of total proteins and albumin in serum. The difference between these two values yields the value of the serum globulins, of which immunoglobulins form a major component in the gamma globulin fraction (see Chapter 9, Proteins). Since other globulin fractions can also vary, a better appreciation of the immunoglobulin quantity can be obtained from serum protein electrophoresis, which gives a direct measure of total gamma globulins. The gamma globulins can be qualitatively identified as having a monoclonal (narrow) versus polyclonal (wide) distribution by visual examination of the electrophoresis strip or of the densitometric scan (see Chapter 4 and Fig. 4–4).

The next step in qualitative evaluation of elevated gamma globulins is IEP or IFE, using as reagents (animal) antibodies directed against the heavy and light chains of human immunoglobulins. This technique gives information on whether there is a predominance of IgG, IgA, or IgM versus elevation of all three. In rare cases an otherwise unidentified protein band in the gamma region may be IgD or IgE, both of which can be detected using anti-IgD and anti-IgE antibodies. With predominance of a single immunoglobulin class, it is essential to establish whether that protein component is monoclonal or polyclonal. This determination is based on the presence of only one light chain type (i.e., kappa or lambda) indicating monoclonal gammopathy. This finding is typical of multiple myeloma and other plasma cell dyscrasias and lymphoreticular disorders (see Chapter 4 and Fig. 4–4). If, on the other hand, both kappa and lambda light chains are present in large amounts, the elevation of immunoglobulins is polyclonal. This type of response is frequently seen in states of chronic inflammation or chronic infection.

Quantitation of immunoglobulin types is useful for monitoring progress in diseases such as myeloma, where the amount of monoclonal protein in serum is related to disease activity. Serial measurements should be separated by at least a few weeks to allow for natural clearance from the circulation even after successful treatment of myeloma. In cases in which the patient's plasma is replaced by plasmapheresis to reduce high levels of a monoclonal immunoglobulin causing hyperviscosity and circulatory problems (usually an IgM), completeness of the removal can be ascertained by quantitative immunoglobulin levels soon after the procedure is completed. The methods for quantitation usually employ precipitation in solution with nephelometry on automated equipment (a few minutes for assay time) or diffusion through agarose to form precipitin rings (a 1- to 2-day procedure)—both making use of class-specific antihuman immunoglobulin antibodies.

The diagnosis of immunodeficiency states also relies heavily on quantitative immunoglobulin levels. Very low levels of IgG, IgA, and IgM near zero are characteristic of agammaglobulinemia. Selective deficiency of one immunoglobulin class is also established by quantitation, for example IgA deficiency. In this condition there is a unique risk of anaphylactic reactions from blood transfusion containing IgA into deficient individuals, owing to immune anti-IgA antibodies (see Chapter 8).

In addition to clear-cut deficiency states and gammopathies, immuno-globulins are measured to define and to monitor moderate elevations as an index of disease progression in autoimmune conditions such as systemic lupus erythematosus and rheumatoid arthritis. Documentation of below-normal levels may also be useful for explaining mild im-munodeficiencies, particularly in children. In that light, it should be well noted that immunoglobulin levels normally increase throughout child-hood until maturity. Thus, interpretation of quantitative immunoglobulin levels in children requires age-specific reference ranges.

Some patients develop a high concentration of an immunoglobulin that precipitates in the cold and can cause blockage of small capillaries in regions of the body (e.g., fingertips, ears) exposed to cold in winter weather. These cryoglobulins are measured by collecting a blood sample, keeping it warm while centrifuging, and then cooling the serum in a refrigerator to observe the formation of a precipitate in 1 to 2 days. This procedure is performed in a special graduated tube. The volume of sedimented precipitate is then read as a percentage of the whole serum sample to yield a numerical value of the **cryocrit** analogous to hematocrit. The cryoglobulin can be further washed, redissolved at warm tempera-ture, and specifically identified as to immunoglobulin class by IEP, IFE, or other immunologic analysis.

When immunoglobulins are produced in a disordered manner by myeloma and similar cells, light chains may be synthesized in excess and released into the circulation. These free kappa or lambda light chains enter the urine because of their small molecular size. Such a finding in urine is termed **Bence-Jones protein.** It can be detected by traditional heating methods that cause a precipitate that redissolves at higher temperatures. Modern methods for Bence-Jones protein are based on immunologic detection. This protein can be toxic to the tubule cells of the kidney, which become overloaded with intracellular protein while attempting to reabsorb it from the renal filtrate. In some patients, further modification of light chains by proteolytic enzymes in the body can lead to deposition of insoluble protein complexes termed **amyloidosis.** In this condition, the extracellular deposition of the protein causes pressure on normal cells (e.g., of spleen, liver, heart, gastrointestinal tract). The normal, functioning cells of those organs are gradually replaced by the acellular amyloid. Diagnosis of this disorder is established by tissue biopsy (usually rectal or gingival). Amorphous deposits that demonstrate apple-green birefringence of polarized light when stained with Congo red dye are characteristic of amyloidosis.

Tissue biopsies are sometimes stained by immunofluorescence tech-niques to demonstrate the deposition of immunoglobulins as part of a pathologic process. Kidney biopsies are commonly evaluated for deposi-tion of IgG, IgA, and IgM in the glomeruli to help make the diagnosis of glomerulonephritis. Circulating immune complexes of antigens and antibodies are normally filtered out of the circulation by the glomeruli. The presence of those complexes in glomeruli activates complement, leading to localized tissue destruction. This filtration of immune complexes performed in the circulation (e.g., in systemic lupus erythematosus) leads to an irregular or lumpy-bumpy staining pattern for immunoglobulin in the glomerulus. When the antibody is directed against the glomerulus itself (e.g., poststreptococcal glomerulonephritis), the immunoglobulin staining pattern is smooth and more homogeneous within the glomerulus. Deposition of immunoglobulin in tissues is also of diagnostic significance in other autoimmune disorders (e.g., the skin in pemphigus), although laboratory assessment of autoimmunity rests largely on the demonstration of autoantibodies in the serum.

SERUM COMPLEMENT

The integrity of the entire complement system and all its components is conveniently screened for by a hemolytic assay designated the CH50. In this assay, dilutions of human serum to be tested for complement activity are mixed with a standardized suspension of sheep erythrocytes presensitized by the adsorption of specific antibody. The complement present in the test serum leads to hemolysis, which is quantitated spectrophotometrically as the amount of hemoglobin released from lysis of the sheep erythrocytes. The CH50 should be used to screen for complement function in such conditions as suspected congenital deficiency of one component. The CH50 has been used in the past to provide quantitative information of complement activation as part of a disease process. However, modern immunoassays for individual components (discussed later) have largely supplanted the role of CH50 in disease monitoring. One reason that even excellent immunochemistry laboratories may show marked variation in the CH50 levels is that the sheep cells demonstrate a seasonal fluctuation in stability. Thus, the functional CH50 assay should be deferred in most instances in favor of more specific component assays, which are rigorously standardized over long periods of time. CH50 has a normal range of approximately 50 to 200 units. Levels just below normal range can indicate increased consumption (and hence active disease process) or decreased synthesis. The hemolytic assay has particular sensitivity to levels of the components C2, C4, and C5. A zero value of hemolytic activity indicates deficiency of one or more components and should be followed up by detailed investigation to delineate the abnormality. An elevated level of CH50 has no significance except that of other acute phase reactants.

The components of complement most frequently measured in serum are C3 (75–175 mg/dL) and C4 (15–45 mg/dL). They are normally the most abundant of the complement factors in serum and so are naturally most easily quantitated by immunologic methods (usually nephelometry or immunodiffusion). Reductions in their levels can be related to one another serially with time to provide a reasonable monitor of autoimmune disease activity. Low levels indicate depletion due to activation secondary to disease progression. Normal or high levels indicate the opposite: disease regression or response to therapy. Other more sophisticated component assays are available from specialized reference laboratories. These include determinations of C1q, C2, C3, C4, C4d, C5, C6, factor B (properdin), and C1 esterase inhibitor. These assays can be used to distinguish immunologic disorders from other inflammatory states and also to diagnose specific deficiencies.

IMMUNE COMPLEXES

The combination of antigen and antibody leads to the formation of immune complexes. When there is continuous release of antigen into the circulation plus synthesis of antibody to that antigen, immune complexes can form in the blood. **Circulating immune complexes (CICs)** are significant in many diseases such as acute glomerulonephritis, systemic lupus erythematosus, chronic viral hepatitis, and vasculitis. Immune complexes probably mediate and direct the pathologic response involving chemotaxis, infiltration of cells, and release of proteolytic enzymes at sites in the kidney, heart, lung, synovium, and so on.

Immune complexes can be grossly screened for in the form of cryoprecipitable substances extracted from serum suspended in cold temperatures (1–4°C). This approach is sensitive only to very large amounts of CIC. Two major methods are commonly used to detect and quantitate CICs down to very low levels. The first is **C1q binding,** in which radiolabeled C1q is added to serum sample. If CICs are present, some of the C1q will preferentially bind to the Fc portion of immunoglobulins engaged in that complex. Addition of polyethylene glycol differentially precipitates the CICs, which have now become labeled with radioactivity proportional to the number of Fc sites on each CIC. Radioactivity trapped in the precipitate is counted. The C1q binding is expressed as a percentage of total C1q added, which should be less than about 15% (see the laboratory report form for specific ranges).

The second method for evaluating CICs is the **Raji cell assay.** This is a lymphoblastoid B cell line that came originally from a patient with Burkitt's lymphoma. Raji cells have receptors for complement components (e.g., C3) that are participating in the CICs. They do not specifically bind immunoglobulins, but bind complement, so their specificity is for CICs that activate complement. In assay, Raji cells are mixed with test serum samples and incubated. Any CICs present bind to the Raji cells through the complement attachment. The cells are then washed and incubated with radiolabeled antihuman immunoglobulin, which binds in turn to CICs on the surface of the Raji cells. The cells are finally washed and counted for radioactivity as a measure of CICs. This assay is conveniently standardized with known amounts of aggregated human globulin to simulate various concentrations of actual CICs.

CELLULAR IMMUNITY

This branch of the immune system can be assessed both by provocative tests performed on the body and with procedures done on lymphocytes collected outside of the body. **Skin tests** utilize extracts of various infectious microorganisms such as mycobacteria, yeasts *(Candida)*, and bacteria *(Streptococcus)*, which are injected intradermally. If the individual has functioning cellular immunity, a region of redness and induration will develop around each injection site that contains antigen to which the individual has immunologic experience. If an individual shows no such positive reaction to any common antigen to which all humans are exposed, that person has a defective cellular immune response and is said to be **anergic.** This is a severe disorder that can leave a patient susceptible to infections from many opportunistic viruses, fungi, bacteria, protozoa, and parasites.

Lymphocytes can be separated from the other cells of heparinized whole blood by centrifugation in a special density-adjusted medium (e.g., Ficoll-Hypaque). Those lymphocytes can then be stimulated with materials such as phytohemagglutinin (PHA) that act as foreign antigens and cause normal lymphocytes to undergo blastic transformation. Such **lymphocyte stimulation** and transformation are measured by adding radiolabeled thymidine, which becomes incorporated into the DNA of the lymphoblasts that are stimulated to divide. Low-level incorporation indicates a poor capacity to mount an immune response.

A variation of this procedure is used for cross-matching organ donors and recipients, particularly for bone marrow transplantation. In this procedure, lymphocytes are isolated from the blood of both recipient and the potential donors and then mixed in various combinations to test the reactivity of antigens on the donor's lymphocytes with the recipient's lymphocytes and vice versa. This assay is termed the **mixed lymphocyte culture (MLC).** It is based also on lymphoblastic transformation and incorporation of radiolabeled thymidine after 10 days of co-culturing the lymphocytes. Incompatibility of cross-match is indicated by greater counts of radioactivity incorporated into the lymphocyte DNA. Very low counts indicate probability of a good match. The MLC is used as a more definitive test of compatibility after screening for HLA typing has been done to establish candidate donors.

LYMPHOCYTE SURFACE MARKERS

Lymphocyte surface markers are antigens carried on a lymphocyte's surface. These antigens are related to specific functions and subgroups of those cells and are defined by the use of antibodies against each one. Early methods employed to delineate these markers included immunofluorescent staining of cells fixed on a glass slide. Modern methods for surface marker analysis are based on **flow cytometry,** which uses labeled antibodies to stain cells. Initial categorization of cells into granulocytes, lymphocytes, monocytes, and so on, is based on size measurement (forward scatter of light) and internal complexity or granularity (side scatter). The cells exhibiting particular surface markers are then quantitated by fluorescence intensity of the bound monoclonal antibodies. Flow cytometry requires sophisticated instrumentation but has the advantages of excellent quantitation and fast analysis time. The markers commonly used include ones for total B cells, total T cells, and subsets of the T cells (see Table 7–1). The monoclonal antibodies specific for each cell type have given rise to designations such as CD3 for T cells, CD4 for helper T cells, and CD8 for suppressor T cells (as previously mentioned, "CD" indicates "cluster of differentiation"). Other markers are specific for thymocytes (CD1), early T cells (CD5), and several other antigens (see Table 7–1).

This spectrum of markers is used for clinical classification of immunodeficiency states, lymphoid leukemias, autoimmune diseases, and for monitoring their response to therapy. Multiple markers can be assayed on a single cell using different monoclonal antibodies (each labeled with a different dye) simultaneously. A basic lymphocyte enumeration panel consists of the following individual results: CD2 (T and NK cells), CD3 (T cells), CD4 (helper T cells), CD8 (suppressor T cells), CD19 (B cells), and CD56 (NK cells). This panel would yield information about lymphocyte production particularly in HIV infection; serial measurements on AIDS patients concentrate on CD4 and CD8. In AIDS, the CD4 cells are depleted by infection with HIV, whereas the CD8 cells persist. The absolute number of CD4 cells is a marker of progression of HIV infection to more overt AIDS. The result is a characteristic reduction in the ratio of CD4/CD8 cells from a normal value of roughly 2.0 to far below 1.0 (Fig. 7–6). Evaluation of acute leukemias uses other antibodies to test for presence of myeloid versus lymphoid markers on blasts in blood or bone marrow. Autoimmune diseases frequently demonstrate clonal populations positive for CD5.

TISSUE TYPING

The **histocompatibility antigens** are so named because of the role they play in the rejection of allogeneic tissue grafts and organ transplants. They are encoded by genes on the short arm of chromosome 6 in humans in a cluster called the **major histocompatibility complex (MHC)** (see Chapter 8). These antigens are present on most cell surfaces, but because they were initially discovered on human lymphocytes, they are termed **human leukocyte antigens (HLAs).** The **class I antigens** are HLA-A, HLA-B, and HLA-C, each of which consist of a unique heavy chain plus a common light chain called beta-2 microglobulin. **Class II antigens** are related to the HLA-D locus and consist of two peptide chains

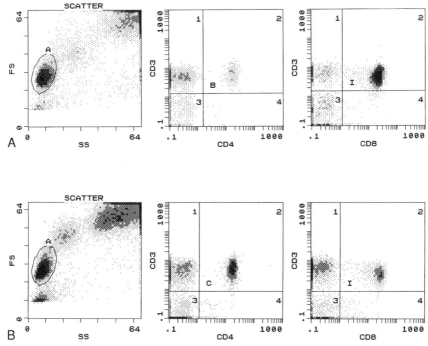

FIGURE 7–6. Scattergrams from three-color flow cytometry for lymphocyte surface markers. The left-hand panels show how lymphocytes are gated (enclosed within line A) by size (forward scatter of light, FS) versus internal granularity (side scatter of light, SS). The middle panels show lymphocytes marked for CD3 (general T-cell marker) versus CD4 (helper T cells). Events (points) in the region designated 2 represent cells with sufficient surface antigens to be categorized as true CD4-positive T cells. The right-hand panel shows lymphocytes marked for CD3 versus CD8 (suppressor T cells); events in region 2 represent true CD8-positive T cells. Row A is from an AIDS patient whose CD4 cells were markedly decreased and had a very low CD4/CD8 ratio of 0.17. Row B is from a normal individual whose ratio of CD4/CD8 cells was 1.53.

without beta-2 microglobulin. Human leukocyte antigen typing is performed with defined antisera that are specific for the individual antigens. The binding of an antibody to lymphocytes leads to cell death on addition of complement. This microcytotoxicity assay is a common means for identifying the corresponding antigen on the lymphocyte surface membrane.

Human leukocyte antigen typing is used for histocompatibility typing as in organ transplantation and in paternity testing and also for disease association or risk assessment (e.g., specific linkages of disease with HLA types: hemochromatosis, ankylosing spondylitis) (see Chapter 8).

AUTOANTIBODIES

The diagnosis, classification, prognosis, treatment, and monitoring of the progression of autoimmune diseases depend on the detection and quantitation of various autoantibodies (Table 7–4). These autoantibodies have reactivities with specific antigens frequently characteristic of distinct diseases. In general, autoantibodies are screened for by a few common methods. The first of these is indirect immunofluorescent antibody (IFA) staining of fixed cells or tissues prepared and mounted on glass slides in a standardized manner. These substrate slides contain multiple antigens (both protein and nucleic acid) for detection of whichever autoantibodies may be present in a patient's serum. The test procedure consists of incubating a dilution of the patient's serum in contact with the cells or tissue on the slide. Unbound serum immunoglobulins are then washed off along with the rest of the serum sample. A second incubation is performed with fluorescein-labeled antihuman immunoglobulin to detect the autoantibodies bound to their respective antigens. Microscopic examination is done with ultraviolet illumination to excite the fluorescein, which gives off the visible light from the cellular and subcellular locations where the autoantibodies are bound (see Color Plates 52 and 53). A titer

TABLE 7–4. ASSOCIATION OF AUTOANTIBODIES WITH RHEUMATIC DISEASES

ANA Finding	Confirmatory Test	Likely Diagnosis with Positive Antibody*
Homogeneous with drug history	Anti-DNA	SLE
	Anti-histone	Drug-induced SLE
Rim (peripheral)	Anti-DNA	SLE
PCNA	None	SLE
Speckled	Anti-Sm	SLE
	Anti-RNP	MCTD
	Anti-SS-A (Ro)	Sjögren's syndrome
	Anti-SS-B (La)	Sjögren's syndrome
	Scl-70	PSS
Nucleolar	None	PSS
Centromere	None	CREST syndrome

*Clinical suspicion and symptoms are also used as diagnostic criteria in addition to serologic findings.
SLE = systemic lupus erythematosus; MCTD = mixed connective tissue disease; PSS = progressive systemic sclerosis (scleroderma); CREST = calcinosis cutis, Raynaud's phenomenon, esophageal dysmotility, sclerodactyly, telangiectasia; a subset of PSS.

is reported as the highest dilution of patient serum that yields a strong fluorescent response under the microscope. This procedure is referred to as **antinuclear antibody (ANA)** testing because of its ability to detect antibodies against many different nuclear antigens. As detailed below, the ANA can identify antibodies to cytoplasmic antigens as well.

In general, the ANA is considered a screening test, which may be followed by confirmatory testing for specific autoantibodies (see Table 7–4). A common method for confirmatory testing of a positive ANA utilizes a soluble extract of tissue such as spleen or thymus, which is particularly rich in a variety of nuclear antigens. The preparation of **extractable nuclear antigen (ENA)** is tested for reactivity with patient samples by double diffusion in agarose gels or by counterimmunoelectrophoresis in agarose. Because the ENA is performed with a mixture of antigens, identification of any particular reactivity depends on lines of identity between precipitates formed by the patient's serum and positive prototype serum samples containing known autoantibodies. With improvements in purification of specific antigens, most of the ENAs have been converted to ELISA formats that are readily automated and have considerable advantages in standardization. ELISAs have also been used to screen for positive ANAs by using a complex cellular extract that contains all the significant antigens.

The ANA and ENA detect autoantibodies directed against antigens present in virtually all cells of the body, and so these assays are designed to study systemic autoimmune diseases. For those patients suspected of having autoantibodies that react with only selective organs (e.g., thyroid, adrenal, heart), their serum is tested by IFA, using as substrate fixed and mounted tissue slices of those organs from animals or autopsy material. By this means organ-specific autoantibodies can be detected and quantitated in serum to assist in diagnosis and to mark disease progress.

Antinuclear Antibody (ANA)

This procedure can identify autoantibodies against DNA, histones, or soluble nuclear antigens. The microscopic fluorescent staining distributions within cell nuclei assume characteristic distributions. A *homogeneous pattern* may be due to antibodies directed against either DNA or histones or a combination of both. A homogeneous stain indicates uniform staining throughout each nucleus with all nuclei staining to the same extent (see Color Plate 52A). Mitotic cells show *positive staining* corresponding to daughter chromosomes along the metaphase plate and in the newly formed nuclei just before final cell division. This finding is frequently associated with systemic lupus erythematosus (SLE). The titer of a homogeneous ANA is also a useful index for monitoring the progress of SLE. If the staining pattern is distributed more toward the nuclear membrane, where native DNA is concentrated, it is referred to as a *peripheral* or *rim staining pattern* and is usually a reliable index activity of SLE.

Further discrimination of whether these above types of positive ANAs are due to anti-DNA antibodies versus antihistone antibodies is conveniently accomplished by specific assay for the anti-DNA antibody by staining of the microorganism *Crithidia* (which has an organelle called the kinetoplast that contains DNA but is devoid of histone) or by an ELISA using purified DNA as antigen. This distinction has clinical significance because SLE associated with antihistone predominant antibodies has been associated with a drug-induced etiology that can be reversible with discontinuation of that drug (e.g., procainamide). By contrast, anti-DNA antibodies are more associated with idiopathic SLE. Antibodies against DNA can also be classified into those specific for the native or double-stranded molecule (n-DNA or ds-DNA), those specific for the denatured or single-stranded molecule (ss-DNA), and those that react with both ds-DNA and ss-DNA. Antibodies against ds-DNA are generally considered to be clinically significant (especially IgG), whereas antibodies reactive solely with ss-DNA are neither very sensitive nor specific for disease activity. SLE typically demonstrates high levels of ds-DNA antibodies; those levels are frequently correlated with a degree of glomerulonephritis most likely due to immune complex formation with DNA released from tissue destruction. Other autoimmune diseases besides SLE may sometimes have positive homogeneous ANAs that can be used as markers of those diseases' progression as well.

A staining pattern that is localized to the nucleus but consists of multiple small intersecting globules is designated as the *speckled pattern* (see Color Plate 52B). It typically shows negatively staining regions within the nucleus corresponding to the position of nucleoli. In addition, in contrast to a homogeneous pattern that stains the DNA within chromosomes of dividing cells, speckled staining shows negative regions corresponding to chromosomes in mitotic cells. Thus, speckled pattern antibodies are directed against antigens other than DNA and histones. These antigens are called the **soluble** or **extractable nuclear antigens (ENA),** which include Sm (initially designated for a patient named Smith who had SLE) and RNP (for ribonucleoprotein). High titers of anti-Sm antibody are suggestive of SLE, whereas high levels of anti-RNP antibody are characteristic of mixed connective tissue disease (MCTD) as well as SLE and some other rheumatic disorders. Because of varying sensitivities and specificities of the test procedures, it is reasonable to perform both ANA and ENA assays in order to establish the precise autoantibody present and also its titer.

A unique variant of the speckled pattern is the autoantibody against proliferating cell nuclear antigen (PCNA). The PCNA pattern shows speckled nuclear staining, but the intensity of staining varies markedly between different cells, proliferating ones staining the brightest. The PCNA antibody is highly specific for SLE, but only about 3% of SLE patients have PCNA antibody.

Another striking finding of the ANA is a *positive nucleolar pattern* (see Color Plate 53A). This pattern is complementary to a true speckled pattern in that it shows stain deposition in the precise regions that are negative in the speckled pattern. The antigen in this case is nucleolar RNA. While this autoantibody may occur in SLE (often in association with other ANAs), it is more specific for **scleroderma,** also called **progressive systemic sclerosis (PSS),** a progressive disorder involving fibrosis and degeneration of skin, blood vessels, muscles, joints, and other organs (viscera). In addition to reacting with nucleolar antigens, autoantibodies characteristic of PSS can also react with the centromeres on each of the chromosomes. The anticentromeric pattern consists of multiple small positive dots distributed uniformly throughout the nucleus of interphase cells, but aligned with the chromosomes in metaphase cells. Results of ENA testing in PSS frequently show reactivity with an antigen designated Scl-70, although this autoantibody may also occur in other rheumatic diseases.

Two other commonly noted soluble antigens are *SS-A* and *SS-B,* which have a particular association with Sjögren's syndrome, a disorder of keratoconjunctivitis, sicca, and xerostomia with other connective tissue disease. These ENA reactivities can be of great clinical help in the diagnosis of Sjögren's syndrome, which can have no positive immuno-flurescent findings. In another terminology, the SS-A antigen is the same as the *Ro* antigen and the SS-B is the same as the *La* antigen.

There are several other ENA autoantibodies identified by routine testing of large numbers of patients with rheumatic diseases. Some of these antibodies also have disease correlation (rheumatoid arthritis-associated nuclear antigen, RANA; PM-1, Jo-1, and Ku antigens in polymyositis, dermatomyositis, and overlapping syndromes).

Because antigenic reactivity and rheumatic disease classification overlap considerably, a practical clinical approach is simply to identify those autoantibodies present in a particular patient early in the stage of the disease and then to monitor the titer of those antibodies with time. Occasionally autoantibodies will be detected that have almost amazing specificities for antigens without any recognized disease correlation. Among these findings are antibodies against the spindle apparatus, centrioles, Golgi apparatus, ribosomes, and other nondescript subcellular antigens. It is important that the laboratory performing the ANA recognize these autoantibodies as well and correctly classify them so as to avoid confusion with autoantibodies of true clinical significance and so that they will be reflected as an accurate baseline against which to gauge any change in the patient's status in later years.

Two very important anticytoplasmic autoantibodies are **anti-smooth muscle (ASMA)** and **antimitochondrial (AMA),** both of which can usually be detected by ANA test procedures using fixed cells grown in monolayers (see Color Plate 53B). However, for accurate identification and for determination of antibody titer, it is necessary to test patient serum against fixed slices of tissues rich in those antigens, usually mouse stomach and kidney. The finding of a high-titer ASMA is strongly suggestive of chronic active hepatitis, whereas low titers may be found in other liver pathology, other rheumatic disease, malignancies, or in healthy persons. The AMA is a useful marker for primary biliary cirrhosis and also for other obstructive hepatic disorders.

Rheumatoid factor (RF) is an autoantibody (usually IgM) that reacts with other immunoglobulins (usually IgG) to form immune complexes. As indicated by its name, the RF has particular application to diagnosis and monitoring of rheumatoid arthritis. There are numerous methods for quantitating the RF based on its ability to induce flocculation visible to the eye. Unfortunately for purposes of diagnosis, RF is not usually positive in cases of juvenile rheumatoid arthritis. A frequently employed marker for degree of disease activity in addition to specific autoantibody titer is the quantitation of **C-reactive protein (CRP),** which shows a very good correlation with amount of tissue necrosis, as may occur with inflammatory destruction in rheumatoid arthritis (see Table 7–3; also Chapter 10, Serum Proteins). Paradoxically CRP typically remains low (normal) in SLE. The erythrocyte sedimentation rate is a universally useful test for assessing activity of most rheumatoid diseases.

Antiphospholipid Antibodies

The **antiphospholipid antibody (APA) syndrome** consists of thrombosis or recurrent spontaneous abortions in association with autoantibodies that react with a complex formed between a normally occurring serum glycoprotein and phospholipids. APA is tested for by ELISA. Cardiolipin is commonly used as a reagent in the assay, giving rise to the term **anticardiolipin antibody (ACA),** which is a synonym for APA. This autoantibody frequently is associated with the lupus anticoagulant, an antiphospholipid antibody that causes prolongation of the activated partial thromboplastin time. Despite its ability to inhibit clot formation in the test tube, the lupus anticoagulant (and phospholipid antibodies in general) paradoxically cause thrombosis, inappropriately excessive amounts of clotting, in the body. Antiphospholipid antibodies are acquired; they may occur in association with systemic autoimmune disorder or by themselves. Patients remain at risk for thrombosis as long as they have this autoantibody.

Organ-Specific Autoantibodies

Many patients with disease of a particular organ have antibodies directed against antigens unique to that organ (Table 7–5). It is often difficult to untangle cause and effect, to know whether the antibody has caused the tissue problem or whether organ damage provoked the antibody response. Patients with autoantibodies reactive against the diseased organ often have additional antibodies that react with other tissues. Thyroid and stomach are often linked in this way: many patients with

TABLE 7–5. ORGAN-SPECIFIC AUTOANTIBODIES IN HUMAN DISEASE

Disease	Associated Autoantibodies
Thyroiditis	Thyroid microsomal antigen (thyroid peroxidase), thyroglobulin
Grave's disease	Thyroid-stimulating hormone (TSH) receptors
Pernicious anemia	Gastric parietal cells, intrinsic factor
Myasthenia gravis	Acetylcholine receptors (in skeletal muscle)
Dermatositis; polymyositis	Jo-1, PM-1, Ku
Goodpasture's syndrome	Alveolar and glomerular basement membrane
Wegener's granulomatosus	Anti-neutrophil cytoplasmic antibody (ANCA)
Chronic active hepatitis	Smooth muscle (actin); liver-kidney microsomal antigen (LKM)
Primary biliary cirrhosis	Mitochrondria
Celiac disease	Gliadin (wheat protein); reticulin; endomysium
Addison's disease	Adrenocortical cells
Diabetes mellitus	Pancreatic islet cells; insulin; glutamic acid decarboxylase
Rheumatoid arthritis	IgM anti-IgG (rheumatoid factor); RANA
Chronic demyelinating neuropathies	Gangliosides; sulfatides; myelin-associated glycoprotein
Paraneoplastic neurologic syndromes	Cerebellum (Purkinje cells); anti-neuronal nuclear antibodies
Pemphigus	Epidermal cells
Bullous pemphigoid	Basement membrane zone of skin/mucosa
Autoimmune hemolytic anemia	Erythrocyte membrane proteins
Immune thrombocytopenia	Platelet membrane proteins
Rheumatic fever	Myocardium

immune thyroiditis (Hashimoto's disease) have antibodies to gastric parietal cells, and many patients with pernicious anemia have antithyroid antibodies in addition to antibodies against intrinsic factor and gastric parietal cells. Another confounding observation is that first-degree relatives of patients with autoantibody-related diseases often have the same circulating antibodies but no evidence of disease.

The role of cell-mediated immunity in diseases characterized by autoantibodies is another field of inquiry. Insulin-dependent diabetes mellitus (IDDM) is especially challenging. Although antibodies to pancreatic islet cells (detected by indirect immunofluorescence), insulin (detected by radioimmunoassay), and glutamic acid decarboxylase (detected by ELISA) are strongly associated with IDDM, they probably do not initiate islet cell damage. It may be that cell-mediated autoimmunity plays a significant etiologic role in the disease after some primary insult to the pancreas such as acute viral infection.

Kidney and Lung Diseases

Several types of renal disease result from autoimmune activity. In glomerulonephritis of lupus erythematosus and poststreptococcal states, immune complexes deposit on the glomerular membranes and induce complement-mediated damage. These antibodies damage not only the patient's kidneys but may, if persistent, damage transplanted kidneys also. A different form of glomerulonephritis occurs in patients with disease-causing antibodies directed specifically against glomerular basement membrane (anti-GMB). The anti-GBM also reacts with alveolar basement membranes in the lungs. The clinical condition of antibody-mediated hemorrhagic damage in the lungs and kidneys is called **Goodpasture's syndrome.** Rapid diagnosis of this condition is essential to initiate immunosuppressive therapy and plasmapheresis to lower the anti-GBM titer before irreversible damage occurs.

Wegener's granulomatosus (WG) is an inflammatory disorder affecting the lungs that was formerly diagnosed only by excluding all other causes until recent years, when it has been found that WG is associated with *antineutrophil cytoplasmic antibodies (ANCA)*. The specific antigen is proteinase 3 in the so-called cytoplasmic (c-ANCA) pattern; for the peripheral (p-ANCA) pattern associated with some forms of vasculitis, the antigen is myeloperoxidase.

Liver and Gastrointestinal Diseases

Chronic inflammatory states of the liver such as viral hepatitis or autoimmune hepatitis frequently are accompanied by autoantibodies. One of the most common and yet least specific of these is **anti-smooth muscle antibody (ASMA; antiactin),** which is often present along with either homogeneous or speckled ANA in autoimmune hepatitis. Liver and kidney share a microsomal antigen *(LKM)*, against which autoantibodies frequently react in chronic hepatitis. Additional autoantibodies have been described that react with specific liver antigens (e.g., asialoglycoprotein receptor, liver membrane) in hepatitis; despite much apparent clinical promise, these assays are not yet well standardized, nor are they widely available.

Primary biliary cirrhosis is marked by high titers of antimitochondrial antibodies (AMA). Both ASMA and AMA can be detected using HEp-2 cells, but they are better characterized on substrate slides using sections of mouse stomach and kidney, which also demonstrate the LKM pattern.

The intestinal disorder termed **celiac disease** derives from dietary intolerance to wheat protein (gluten, gliadin). In addition to forming antibodies against gluten, these individuals also develop autoantibodies against reticulin and endomysium.

Neuromuscular Disease

The weakness of myasthenia gravis is directly related to titer of auto-antibody against the acetylcholine receptor that blocks neuromuscular transmission. Success of treatment with plasmapheresis or other therapies can be documented by serial measurements of antibody titer. Other autoimmune muscle diseases such as dermatomyositis or polymyositis show such autoantibodies as Jo-1, PM-1, and Ku.

Recent work has demonstrated a large group of chronic demyelinating neuropathies that are caused by autoantibodies reactive with the neuronal components gangliosides, sulfatides, and myelin-associated glycoprotein. These peripheral neuropathies respond to reduction in antibody titer. Some cancers, such as breast and lung, stimulate immune responses against tumor cells that also cross-react with antigens on brain cells, giving rise to various sensory and motor disorders. These paraneoplastic syndromes are marked by antibodies against cerebellar Purkinje cells or by **antineuronal nuclear antibodies (ANNA).**

Other Organ-Specific Antibodies

Indirect immunofluorescence is used to demonstrate most organ-specific antibodies, but other procedures are used in special cases in which the antigens can be solubilized or purified. Antithyroid antibodies are measured by an immunofluorescence or agglutination procedure in which antigen is adsorbed to red cells. Intrinsic factor antibodies are measured by radioimmunoassay. Other radioassays are used to detect antibodies against the acetylcholine receptor in myasthenia gravis and against cell surface receptors in Graves' disease (TSH receptor) and also in some forms of diabetes mellitus. Many other organs or cell types can be seen to have autoantibodies directed against them. These include adrenal (Addison's disease), myocardium, skeletal muscle, various endocrine cells, skin components, colonic mucosa, salivary gland ducts, erythrocytes, platelets, and more. While most of these antibodies may simply reflect existing tissue damage rather than be the cause of it, many of them may extend the damage or stimulate cell-mediated immunity to those tissues that could cause the primary insult or contribute to it.

ALLERGY TESTING

Persons suffering from asthma can be tested for sensitivities to a wide variety of potential allergens by skin tests in which each allergen is applied separately through a scratch in the skin. The development of redness and swelling around a scratch application site indicates that the patient is allergic to that particular antigen. Because of the discomfort involved and a limited number of sites that can be used at any one sitting, other procedures involving detection of IgE have been introduced. Diagnosis of allergic disorder can be further substantiated by quantitation of total IgE levels in the blood. Allergic individuals tend also to have higher than expected concentrations of total IgE. Solid phase immunoassays also are available to detect the presence of specific IgE antibodies against a battery of individual allergens. These include different food groups, pollens, animal hairs, and other common environmental exposures. These allergens are linked to a solid bead that is incubated with the patient's serum in the test procedure to allow any IgE against that antigen to attach to it. The bead is then washed and further incubated with a labeled anti-IgE antibody. The bead is then washed one more time and the amount of bound label is quantitated (either radioactive or enzymatic label) as a direct measure of the specific IgE in the patient's serum directed against that particular antigen. These allergen-specific IgE assays are called radioallergosorbent tests (RAST). Before embarking on a blind survey of these allergens (most of which will likely show no reaction), it is extremely useful to determine by careful history what classes of allergens may be within the exposure experience of the patient. As part of allergy and allergic reaction testing, it is frequently useful to determine the absolute count of eosinophils in the blood and also to look for eosinophils in nasal secretions to confirm an allergic origin.

EVALUATION OF IMMUNODEFICIENCY STATES

Patients who experience repeated infections are candidates for evaluating immune function. HIV infection is highly prevalent and should be considered foremost in the differential diagnosis. Serologies for antibodies to HIV, detection of the viral p24 antigen in blood, or polymerase chain reaction to detect and quantitate the viral nucleic acid may all be employed at various stages of evaluation. The cellular defect of AIDS can be assessed by flow cytometry for lymphocyte enumeration, by in vitro lymphocyte stimulation tests, and by skin tests for common organisms against which healthy individuals generally demonstrate reactions. As AIDS progresses, the ability of lymphocytes to respond to stimulation diminishes, as do the responses to skin tests.

Repeated bacterial infections suggest possible immunodeficiency due to abnormalities of neutrophils (chronic granulomatous disease, especially pyogenic infections from infancy). Neutrophil function may be assessed by the **nitroblue tetrazolium blue test (NBT)** and by assays for **superoxide production.**

A complete evaluation for immune dysfunction includes quantitative measurement of immunoglobulins (IgG, IgA, IgM), CH50 to search for any component deficiency (to be confirmed with individual component measurements), lymphocyte enumeration by flow cytometry (to determine presence of B cells, T cells, and appropriate T cell subsets: CD4, CD8), specific antibody titers against common organisms or vaccines (*Haemophilus influenzae,* pneumococcus, tetanus toxin, diphtheria toxin), and skin tests against common organisms. Classification of deficiency type depends on finding specific abnormalities of the humoral or cellular immune functions or both.

SUGGESTED READING

Bellanti, JA: Immunology III. WB Saunders, Philadelphia, 1985.

Bodmer, JG, Marsh, SGE, Albert, ED, et al: Nomenclature for factors of the HLA system. Hum Immunol 41:1, 1994.

Carson, DA, Chen, PP, and Kipps, TJ: New roles for rheumatoid factor. J Clin Invest 87:379, 1991.

Cline, MJ: The molecular basis of leukemia. N Engl J Med 330:328, 1994.

Colten, HR, and Rosen, FS: Complement deficiencies. Ann Rev Immunol 10:809, 1992.

Davenport, A, Lock, RJ, Wallington, TB, et al: Clinical significance of anti-neutrophil cytoplasm antibodies detected by a standardized indirect immunofluorescence assay. Q J Med 87:291, 1994.

Engelhard, VH: How cells process antigens. Sci Am 271(2):54, 1994.

Hulett, MD, and Hogarth, PM: Molecular basis of Fc receptor function. Adv Immunol 57:1, 1994.

Kipps, TJ, Meisenholder, G, and Robbins, BA: New developments in flow cytometric analyses of lymphocyte markers. In McPherson, RA, and Nakamura, RM (eds): Laboratory immunology II. Clin Lab Med 12:237, 1992.

Lockshin, MD: Antiphospholipid antibody syndrome. JAMA 268:1451, 1992.

Manns, MP: Autoimmune diseases of the liver. In McPherson, RA, and Nakamura, RM (eds): Laboratory immunology I. Clin Lab Med 12:25, 1992.

Mills, JA: Systemic lupus erythematosus. N Engl J Med 330:1871, 1994.

Mongey, AB, and Hess, EV: Antinuclear antibodies and disease specificity. Adv Intern Med 36:151, 1991.

Nossal, GJV: Current concepts: Immunology: The basic components of the immune system. N Engl J Med 316:1320, 1987.

Reth, M: Antigen receptors on B lymphocytes. Ann Rev Immunol 10:97, 1992.

Theofilopoulos, AN, and Dixon, FJ: The biology and detection of immune complexes. Adv Immunol 28:89, 1979.

Wolfe, F, and Michaud, K: The clinical and research significance of the erythrocyte sedimentation rate. J Rheumatol 21:1227, 1994.

Zeballos, RS, and McPherson, RA: Update of autoantibodies in neurologic disease. In McPherson, RA, and Nakamura, RM (eds): Laboratory immunology I, Clin Lab Med 12:61, 1992.

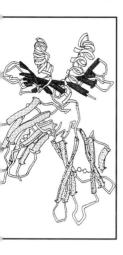

8

Transfusion Medicine

IMMUNOHEMATOLOGY OF ERYTHROCYTES

The red cell membrane contains many different proteins and carbohydrates capable of evoking antibody formation. At present there are 26 established blood group systems, consisting of 194 antigens representing the products of 27 genes (Table 8–1). For a few, the molecule's biologic role has been inferred; for a few others, the chemical composition has been characterized; for most, the structure, function, and reasons for their immunogenicity all remain mysterious. However, the genes that determine red cell antigens seem to follow the mendelian laws of inheritance. If the individual possesses a specific genetic pattern (genotype), these antigens usually express themselves on the red cell (phenotype). This inheritance pattern is called **codominant.** Chemically, red cell antigens may be proteins such as Rh, M, and N blood group substances, or carbohydrates on a lipid or protein framework such as the ABH, Lewis, Ii, and P blood group substances. The antigenicity of these various compounds is influenced by biologic and chemical properties, molecular size, and three-dimensional configuration. Some blood group substances, such as Lewis antigens, are distributed widely throughout the body tissues. Others are more restricted to red cells, such as the Rh antigens and the Kell blood group substances.

The most practical aspect of these antigens on red cells is their ability to evoke antibody formation when transfused into recipients. Evidence is emerging that some abnormalities of the red cell antigens are associated

TABLE 8–1. ESTABLISHED BLOOD GROUP ANTIGEN SYSTEMS

	Group	Chromosome	Common Antigens	Structure/Function
Carbohydrate Blood Groups	ABO (H)	9 (19)	A, B, AB (H)	?Ion transport function
	Lewis	19	Le^a, Le^b	Facilitates *H. pylori* attachment to gastric mucosa
Protein Blood Groups	P	22	pk, P_1 P_1	?Viral parvovirus B-19 receptor
	ii	2	ii	Expressed on ABH framework
	Rhesus (Rh)	1	C, D, E, c, e	?Transport protein
	MNS	4	M, N, S, s, u	Glycophorins A, B
	Kell	7	K k	?Endopeptidase
	Duffy	1	Fy^a, Fy^b	Receptor for *Plasmodium vivax*
	Kidd	7	Jk^a, Jk^b	Urea and/or water transport
	Lutheran	19	Lu^a, Lu^b	Lutheran glycoprotein
	Gerbich	2	Ge	Glycophorins C, D.
	Cromer	1	Cr	Delay accelerating factor (CDSS)
	Landsteiner-Weiner	19	LW	LW glycoprotein
	Cartwright	7	Yt^a, Yt^b	Acetylcholinesterase
	Xg	X	Xg^a, Xg	Xg glycoprotein
	Dombrook	?	Do^a, Do^b	Dombrook glycoprotein
	Chido/Rodgers	6	Ch/Rg	Complement C4
	Indian	11	In	CD44 adhesion molecule
	Wright		Wr^a, Wr^b	?
	Scianna	1	Sc^1 (Sm), Sc^2 (Bu^a)	Scianna protein
	Knops/McCoy	1	Kn/McC	CRl complement receptor
	Gregory/Holley		Cyl/Hy	?
Unknown Structure	En		En	?
	Colton	7	Co^a, Co^b	Water channel integrin protein
	Diego	17	Di^a, Di^b	Anion transport

Adapted from Vengelen-Tyler, V (ed): Technical Manual, ed 12. American Association of Blood Banks, Bethesda, MD, 1996, with permission.

with a predisposition to certain diseases. Some of the more important antigen systems will be discussed in this chapter.

BLOOD GROUPS

THE ABO BLOOD GROUP SYSTEM

Discovered in 1900 by the Austrian-born pathologist Karl Landsteiner, the ABO system is of paramount importance in blood banking and transfusion medicine. The major antigens are called A and B; the major antibodies are anti-A and anti-B. The genes that determine the presence or absence of A or B activity reside on chromosome 9. Normal persons older than 6 months of age almost always have naturally occurring antibodies that react with A or B antigens that are absent from their own cells. The occurrence of these antibodies and their specificity are not genetically determined. Instead, antibodies develop after exposure to apparently ubiquitous environmental antigens that share structure and specificity with red cell antigens. Although exposed to both A and B activity in the environment, individuals will not produce antibodies that react with their own red cell antigens.

Genes and Antigens

DNA analysis has demonstrated that the ABO system is actually a multiplicity of polymorphisms. Antigenic activity depends on specific sugar linkages located at the end of a short sugar chain that is attached to a large, complex molecule with either protein or lipid structure (Fig. 8–1). Most of the red cell antigens reside as terminal sugar chains or membrane lipids called **glycosphingolipids,** but glycoproteins also possess ABO activity. The A antigen results when N-acetylgalactosamine links to a D-galactose moiety. B activity occurs if a D-galactose is present on that terminal D-galactose moiety. The A gene characterizes the presence of a glycosyltransferase enzyme that is responsible for attaching N-acetylgalactosamine to galactose; the B gene produces a galactose transferase. These transferase enzymes encoded by the genes on chromosome 9 are capable of adding sugars to the basic precursor substance.

Figure 8–1 shows the schematic structure of the A, B, and H antigens. Before the D-galactose can accept the sugars that determine A or B activity, it must have a fucose sugar already attached. A D-galactose moiety with fucose already attached, but without A-active N-acetylgalactosamine or B-active D-galactose, has antigenic activity described as H. Cells with only

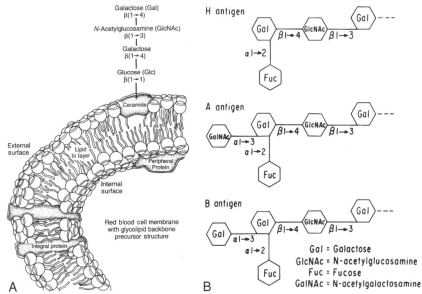

FIGURE 8–1. Schematic structure of A, B, H antigens on red blood cells. *(A)* Red blood cell membrane with the glycolipid backbone. (From Harmening, DM, and Firestone D: The ABO blood group system. In Harmening, DM: Modern Blood Banking and Transfusion Practices, ed. 4. FA Davis, Philadelphia, 1999, p 96, with permission.) *(B)* Molecular attachments to galactose, conferring A, B, or H antigenic activity. Gal added to the subterminal Gal confers B activity; GalNAc added to the subterminal Gal confers A activity to the sugar. Unless the fucose moiety that determines H activity is attached to the number 2 carbon, galactose does not accept either sugar on the 3 carbon. (From Vengelen-Tyler, V (ed): Technical Manual, ed 12. American Association of Blood Banks, Bethesda, MD, 1996, p 232, with permission.)

the H-active sugar configuration have neither A nor B activity and are called Group O.

The glycosyltransferases determined by the A and B genes depend on the presence of precursor H substance for their activity to become apparent. Attachment of fucose to D-galactose provides this precursor. Fucose attachment is mediated by another enzyme, fucose-transferase, the presence of which is determined by the H gene. The H gene is independent of the ABO locus and is found on chromosome 19. The H gene is extremely common, and nearly everyone has H substance on the red cells. A few people are homozygous for an inactive gene at that site, called *h*. Since persons with two *h* genes cannot generate the enzyme needed to attach fucose, their red cells have no H activity. In the absence of H substance, A- or B-active transferases have no substrate on which to work; therefore the red cells of these persons lack A or B activity as well.

Individuals whose red cells lack A, B, or H activity consistently have strong anti-A, anti-B, and anti-H in their serum. This constitution is called a **Bombay phenotype** because it was first discovered in that city and the very rare, inactive *h* gene seems to have its greatest concentration there (Fig. 8–2).

Many alleles exist at the ABO locus. The three most common are A, B, and O. A and B produce sugar transferases that alter H activity. The O gene has no detectable product; it is called an **amorph.** Persons with two O genes produce no enzymes capable of transforming the H substance into A or B. Their cells possess only H activity, and their serum contains anti-A and anti-B. A single A or B gene can generate enough enzyme to fully convert the H substance to A or B, respectively. The red cells of a person with the genotype A-O do not differ from those with the genotype A-A. Persons with both A and B genes attach N-acetylgalactosamine to some of their H, and D-galactose to the rest of it. These group AB individuals have both A and B activity on their cells, with very little residual H, and their serum contains neither anti-A nor anti-B. Table 8–2 shows the blood findings and the frequency of the common ABO groups.

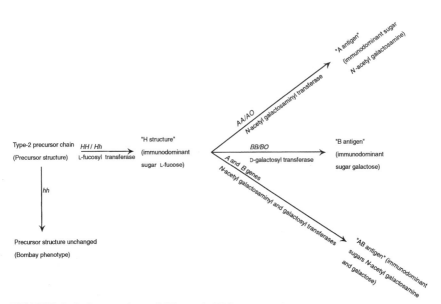

FIGURE 8–2. Interaction of Hh and ABO genes. (From Harmening, DM, and Firestone, D: The ABO blood group system. In Harmening, DM: Modern Blood Banking and Transfusion Practices, ed 4. FA Davis, Philadelphia, 1999, p 99, with permission.)

TABLE 8–2. ANTIGENS AND ANTIBODIES IN ABO BLOOD GROUP SYSTEM

Routine ABO Grouping							
Reaction of Cells Tested With		Reaction of Serum Tested Against			Interpre- tation	Frequency (%) in US Population	
		A_1	B	O	ABO		
Anti-A	*Anti-B*	*Cells*	*Cells*	*Cells*	*Group*	*Whites*	*Blacks*
0	0	+	+	0	O	45	49
+	0	0	+	0	A	40	27
0	+	+	0	0	B	11	20
+	+	0	0	0	AB	4	4

+ = agglutination; 0 = no agglutination.

From Vengelen-Tyler, V (ed): AABB Technical Manual, ed 12. American Association of Blood Banks, Bethesda, MD, 1996, p 230, with permission.

Subgroups of A

Two different A genes are common in the general population: A_1 and A_2. The A_2 transferase is less efficient than the A_1 transferase in converting H to A. A single A_1 gene produces a transferase that converts nearly all the available H to A, but A_2 produces red cells with weaker A antigenic activity and more residual H antigen. Persons with genotypes A_2-A_2 or A_2-O have red cells of the A_2 phenotype. Persons with one A_1 gene and one A_2 gene have A_1 red cells. A coexisting B gene does not alter A_1 or A_2 activity. About 20% of AB are A_2B, whereas the majority are A_1B, just as 20% of group A persons are A_2.

Still other variant A genes exist, producing progressively less active transferases. These are uncommon, but occur sufficiently often that the number of weak A subgroups has been identified and classified. Inheritance of these weak variants follows normal mendelian distribution. The reason for their "deficient" activity is unknown. Also unexplained is the fact that variant A transferases exist so often, whereas B variants are uncommon. Only a few "weak B" genes have been found.

The presence of the A_2 antigen cannot be determined in the presence of A_1 antigen. It is felt that this may merely represent a simple quantitative deficiency; however, certain qualitative changes in the A antigen may also be present in A_2 individuals. Certain A_2 and A_2B individuals can have anti-A_1 in their serum. Subgroups of A can, in this instance, give discrepant ABO grouping characteristics, as may occur when an individual's red cells type as AB, yet the serum contains anti-A. This is, in fact, an anti-A_1, and the correct blood groups are A_2 or A_2B, respectively.

Antibodies in the ABO System

Although anti-A and anti-B react strongly and specifically with the corresponding red cell antigens, the stimulus to anti-A and anti-B production is not exposure to red cells. The same linkages of galactose with N-acetylgalactosamine or galactose that characterize red cell glycosphingolipids also exist in bacterial cell walls. Continuous environmental exposure to these widely distributed antigens elicits continuous antibody production in immunocompetent persons, provided the antigen is not a "self-constituent" of the individual's own red cells. Group A subjects form only anti-B, and those in Group B have only anti-A. Persons of Group O have both anti-A and anti-B, whereas Group AB individuals have neither antibody (see Table 8–2). Infants are too young to form antibodies, and patients with defective humoral immunity will not have these antibodies.

Environmental bacteria also possess the galactose-fucose linkage that confers H activity. Anti-H, however, occurs very rarely because nearly all red cells possess H antigen in quantities ranging from slight to substantial. A_1 or A_1B persons occasionally develop weak anti-H, but the only people who form strong anti-H are those of the Bombay phenotype, whose red cells are devoid of H activity.

Anti-A and anti-B are strong agglutinins, easily demonstrated in the laboratory. In the circulation they cause rapid, complement-mediated destruction of any incompatible cells that chance to enter the bloodstream. Except for the few fetal cells that enter the mother's bloodstream during pregnancy and delivery, the only way that ABO-incompatible cells get into the circulation is by incorrectly identified transfusions. Incorrect identification of patients, blood samples, or donor blood, or incorrect clerical notations, cause the vast majority of hemolytic, ABO-incompatible transfusion reactions.

Most anti-A and anti-B activity resides in the IgM class of immunoglobulins, which produce immediate agglutination (Fig. 8–3) and/or hemolysis. Some activity, however, is IgG, and antibodies of this class attach to the cell surface without immediately affecting the viability. Anti-A or anti-B of the IgG class readily crosses the placenta and can cause hemolytic disease of the newborn (see later). Group O persons more often have IgG anti-A and anti-B than do A or B individuals. ABO hemolytic disease of the newborn affects almost exclusively the offspring of O mothers (see later in this chapter).

Secretors and Nonsecretors

A, B, and H substances can be found in body tissues in soluble forms (e.g., saliva). The ability to secrete ABH substances resides in the secretor (Se) gene also on chromosome 19. All secretors have H substance in their saliva. Group A, B, or AB secretors have the respective A substance, B

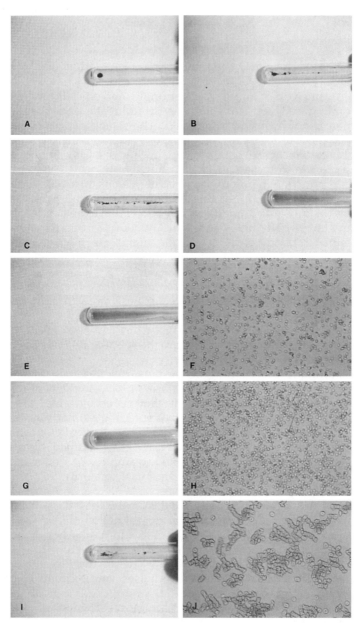

FIGURE 8–3. Agglutination reactions. *(A)* 4+: One solid aggregate of red cells. *(B)* 3+: Several large aggregates. *(C)* 2+: Medium-sized aggregates, clear background. *(D)* 1+: Small aggregates; turbid, reddish background. *(E)* +w (weak): Tiny aggregates; turbid, reddish background, or *(F)* +2: Microscopic aggregates only (original magnification × 10). *(G)* Negative: No aggregates. *(H)* Negative: No aggregates—microscopic appearance (original magnification × 10). *(I)* Pseudoagglutination or strong rouleaux (2+). *(J)* Rouleaux: Microscopic appearance (original magnification × 10). (From Harmening, DM: Modern Blood Banking and Transfusion Practices, ed 2. FA Davis, Philadelphia, 1989, Plate 2, with permission.)

substance, or both A and B substances in their saliva as well. Individuals who lack the secretor gene do not have any A, B, or H substance in their saliva, irrespective of what their ABO blood group types are. Secretor status testing can be valuable in forensic laboratories. In most whites, the incidence of the secretor gene, which manifests its activity as a dominant inheritance, is 85%.

Change in ABH Types with Various Diseases

Weakening of the A antigen may occur in some persons with acute leukemia or in chronic myeloproliferative diseases with leukemic evolution (Table 8–3). Certain cancers, particularly cancer of the colon, may be associated with the acquisition of a B antigen termed the **acquired B.** Acquired B can also occur with certain gram-negative infections and intestinal obstruction. Thus, occasionally with these diseases an individual of Group O phenotype may acquire a B and apparently type as B, or a Group-A person may acquire a B and type as AB.

THE RH SYSTEM

After the ABO system, the Rh system is the group of red cell antigens with the greatest clinical importance. Unlike anti-A and anti-B, which reliably occur in normal, unimmunized individuals, Rh antibodies do not develop without an immunizing stimulus such as pregnancy or blood transfusion. The major antigen of the Rh system (D) is more likely to provoke an antibody than any other red cell antigen if introduced into a person who lacks the antigen. The D antigen is present on the red cells of 85% of whites, and a higher percentage of blacks, American Indians, and Asians. Since 15% of whites lack the antigen, they are capable of forming the antibody if exposed to D; but only 50 to 75% of Rh-negative persons

---

TABLE 8–3. CONDITIONS CAUSING CHANGES IN ABO BLOOD GROUPS

Weakening of A
Acute leukemia
Chronic myeloproliferative diseases with leukemic transformation

Acquired B
Cancer of large intestine
Gram-negative infections
Intestinal obstructions

Transfusions of Group-Compatible But Not Group-Specific Blood
O blood to any ABO type
A, B, or O blood to AB recipients

exposed to large numbers of Rh-positive cells actively form an antibody. Nevertheless, no other blood group antigen has comparable immunizing potential.

Historically, Rh antigens and genes were described in two different terminologies, reflecting differences in experimental and theoretical approach. Current usage now tends toward simplification of the symbols, at written and spoken levels, with a numerical nomenclature available for highly technical communications.

Antigens of the Rh System

The Rh system includes many different antigens. Persons whose red cells possess D are called Rh-positive, and those whose cells lack D are called Rh-negative, no matter what other Rh antigens are present. See Table 8–4 for the frequencies of the principal Rh-positive genotypes. Besides D, there are four other Rh antigens of major clinical significance. The genes for the Rh system reside on chromosome 1. Thus, each gene controls the presence of several different Rh antigens on the red cell surface and determines a different combination of two or three major antigens, and numerous other antigens of less clinical significance.

Because it so readily provokes an identifying antibody, D was the first Rh antigen to be discovered. The other four major antigens are C, E, c, and e; antibodies to these occur less frequently but still fairly often. Many other antigens exist that are either very rare themselves or require rare antibodies to demonstrate their presence.

Rh Genes

The Rh genes common in the United States' white and black populations are given in Table 8–4. The r gene determines a product that lacks D but possesses c and e, whereas the R gene possesses the D antigen. A single group of Rh antigens defined by their alleles on one chromosome is called a **haplotype.** Rh material has a high lipid content and is a more integral part of the red cell membrane than are the ABH antigens, but its three-dimensional structure and function are unknown.

Since every person has two examples of chromosome 1, everyone has two Rh alleles. These may be either identical or different. If two examples of the same allele are present on the two chromosomes, the red cell will only have one set of antigens. If two different alleles are present, there will be two haplotypes (see Table 8–4). Of the five common Rh antigens, the minimum number that a normal person could have is two—c and e ("d" has not been identified and exists only by inference in the absence of D). This occurs in persons with the r gene on both chromosomes. A single cell tested with five major antibodies can have the maximum five different antigens—DCEce. This occurs with the genotype R^1R^2(CDe/cDE) (see Table 8–4).

TABLE 8–4. FREQUENCIES OF THE MORE COMMON GENOTYPES IN D-POSITIVE INDIVIDUALS

Phenotype	Genotype		Genotype Frequency (%)		Likelihood of Zygosity for D (%)			
					White		Blacks	
CDE	*CDE*	*Rh-hr*	*Whites*	*Blacks*	*Homo-*	*Hetero-*	*Homo-*	*Hetero-*
CcDe	CDe/ce	R^1r	31.1	8.8	10	90	59	41
	CDe/cDe	R^1R^0	3.4	15.0				
	Ce/cDe	$r'R^0$	0.2	1.8				
Cde	CDe/CDe	R^1R^1	17.6	2.9	91	9	81	19
	CDe/Cde	R^1r'	1.7	0.7				
cDEe	cDE/ce	R^2r	10.4	5.7	10	90	63	37
	cDE/cDe	R^2R^0	1.1	9.7				
cDE	cDE/cDE	R^2R^2	2.0	1.2	87	13	99	1
	cDE/ce	R^2r''	0.3	<0.1				
	CDe/cDE	R^1R^2	11.8	3.7				
CcDEe	CDe/cE	R^1r''	0.8	<0.1	89	11	90	10
	Ce/cDE	$r'R^2$	0.6	0.4				
cDe	cDe/ce	R^0r	3.0	22.9	6	94	46	54
	cDe/cDe	R^0R^0	0.2	19.4				

For the rare phenotypes and genotypes not shown in this table consult the reference books listed at the end of this chapter. cd (cde/cde) is the most common D-negative genotype, representing 15% in whites and 7% in blacks.

From Vengelen-Tyler, V (ed): Technical Manual, ed 12. American Association of Blood Banks, Bethesda, MD, 1996, p 261, with permission.

Rh-positive cells always have D as part of at least one haplotype. In routine testing, it is not feasible to distinguish cells with a single dose of D from persons who are homozygous for D (double dose). This distinction sometimes can be inferred from the presence of other antigenic factors that commonly accompany D or from gene frequency tables. Rh-negative cells, which lack D, may have c or C or both, as well as e or E or both. Most Rh-negative persons have two examples of the allele r, which determines c and e, but some Rh-negative persons have less common alleles.

Rh Antibodies

As already mentioned, not every Rh-negative person exposed to Rh-positive cells develops anti-D. Transfusion immunizes more consistently than pregnancy, largely because more cells are involved. About 20% of Rh-negative mothers develop anti-D after carrying an Rh-positive infant, whereas antibody develops in between 50 and 70% of Rh-negative persons transfused with Rh-positive blood. For this reason, every reasonable effort is made to avoid giving Rh-positive blood to Rh-negative recipients. The next most antigenic of the Rh antigens is C, followed by E. Antibodies to the other Rh antigens occur only sporadically. In routine transfusion practice, no effort is made to match the non-D antigens in donor and recipient (except in selected patients with sickle cell disease who require frequent transfusions). A few people have anti-E spontaneously (i.e., without having been exposed to blood, blood products, or pregnancy). Other Rh antibodies almost never develop spontaneously.

When Rh antibodies develop, they are predominantly IgG. Some specific IgM appears early as part of the primary immune response, but it tends to disappear soon after the immunizing event, whereas IgG can persist for a lifetime. Rh antibodies do not, as a rule, activate complement. The usual biologic effect of Rh antibodies is to **opsonize** (coat) circulating cells containing the corresponding antigen and set them up for destruction by the reticuloendothelial system. The hematologic result is hemolysis of the antibody-coated cells in the reticuloendothelial organs, predominantly the spleen or liver. Destruction may be complete within a minute or two, or proceed slowly over hours or days. In the test tube, Rh antibodies can cause a modest degree of agglutination, but surface coating usually predominates. Agglutination is enhanced by Coomb's sera (AHG), albumin, or enzyme treatment of the red cells.

Rh antibodies readily cross the placenta from mother to fetus. Historically, anti-D has been the most common cause of severe hemolytic disease of the newborn. Passive Rh antibody prophylaxis successfully prevents antibody formation when given to an unimmunized Rh-negative woman at 28 weeks antenatally and just after the birth of an Rh-positive child. Women with anti-D existing at the time pregnancy begins are very likely to have an affected infant. Other Rh antibodies can cause hemolytic disease much less frequently, and pharmacologic means of prevention are not available (see Hemolytic Disease of the Newborn, later in this chapter).

Rh Immunoprophylaxis

Anti-D formation in pregnant Rh-negative women can be prevented by giving a dose of preformed anti-D by injection at the time that Rh-positive cells enter the circulation or at periods of increased risk. The passive antibody interferes with the interaction between the antigen on the cell surface and the recipient's immune system. The cells are not destroyed, but they lose their ability to trigger the individual's own antibody production. Both the timing and the dosage must be correct. The usual dose is 300 µg at 28 weeks antenatally and at term, following delivery of an Rh-positive infant. If an Rh-incompatible blood transfusion is inadvertently given, approximately 25 µg of passive anti-D should be given for every milliliter of blood infused. The anti-D coats the circulating Rh-positive cells and apparently causes accelerated splenic destruction to the extent that the individual does not experience immunization or severe hemolytic reaction. Rh immune globulin can be given effectively at any time during the first 72 hours after Rh cells are introduced. Insufficient data exist to indicate whether this interval can be prolonged safely.

During pregnancy, if more than 50 mL of fetal cells have entered the circulation, more RhIg can be given. If an Rh-negative woman undergoes an amniocentesis, or spontaneous or induced abortion, she should similarly be protected with adequate levels of RhIg immunoprophylaxis. If a woman is administered antenatal prophylaxis, it is extremely important that this be noted in her medical history because otherwise the presence of anti-D in a postpartum blood sample might be considered evidence for preexisting immunization. Whether or not she has received RhIg during pregnancy, the unimmunized Rh-negative woman should always receive RhIg after giving birth to an Rh-positive child (discussed later).

OTHER BLOOD GROUPS

Table 8–1 outlines some of the more common red cell antigen systems of clinical importance. A blood group system is a series of antigens controlled by allelic genes inherited independently of other genes. The ABO and Rh systems dominate the blood bank scene, but many other systems exist. Blood group antigens are clinically significant if they elicit antibodies following transfusion, if they react with antibodies in such a way that in vivo hemolysis occurs, or if they are implicated in hemolytic disease of the newborn. Besides ABO and Rh, the blood group systems of greatest clinical significance are Kell, Duffy, and Kidd. Other antigens and antibodies create clinical problems in relatively few cases, but often enough that their presence must be sought and acknowledged.

RED CELL ALLOIMMUNIZATION

Alloantibody production to red cell antigens occurs when foreign erythrocytes enter the circulation of an individual whose red cells lack the antigens. Transfusion and pregnancy are the usual ways in which red cell antigens are transferred between individuals. Immunization characteristically elicits first a relatively transient IgM antibody, and then an IgG antibody that persists for years. Once an antibody is present, it will hemolyze or coat cells that possess the relevant antigen. Antibody screening and crossmatching attempt to prevent such hemolytic episodes by detecting and identifying the antibodies so that antigen-positive cells will not be transfused.

Antibodies differ in their incidence, in the frequency with which they cause clinical problems, and in the methods in which they are detected in the laboratory. Patients may have several different antibodies simultaneously; this makes it difficult to identify the weaker ones and sometimes causes more specificities to be overlooked.

Sometimes antibodies weaken as time passes so that it is difficult or impossible to demonstrate that a person has been immunized. If antigen-positive cells are transfused to such a patient, the antibody very rapidly reappears. This rapid return of antibody, called an **anamnestic response,** may destroy the transfused antigen-positive cells **(delayed hemolytic transfusion reaction)** (see section on Adverse Effects of Transfusions later in this chapter.) The Rh antibodies anti-E and anti-c are especially likely to cause delayed hemolysis, as are antibodies of the Kidd system (anti-Jk^a and anti-Jk^b). Kidd antibodies are often weak to begin with and tend to exist as one of several different antibodies in the same sensitized person.

Hemolytic reactions are rare, but antibodies are fairly frequent, occurring in 6% or more of persons with previous transfusions or pregnancies. Finding blood that lacks the one or several antigens reactive with a patient's antibodies can seriously delay transfusion, but failure to find and give compatible blood can cause even worse problems. These IgG antibodies provoked by transfusion or pregnancy can also cause hemolytic disease of the newborn (see section on Hemolytic Disease of the Newborn, later in this chapter).

ANTIBODY FORMATION WITHOUT KNOWN STIMULATION

Although anti-A and anti-B are the only antibodies regularly found in the serum of unimmunized individuals, antibodies active against other red cell antigens occasionally occur in persons who have never been exposed to human red blood cells. Such antibodies are sometimes called "naturally occurring," but a better term is **non–red cell stimulated.** The immunizing stimulus is presumably exposure to environmental material antigenically similar to red cell antigens, but the mechanism is unknown.

Antibodies that develop without red cell stimulus are usually IgM and usually react best at temperatures of 30°C or below. Because of their low thermal optimum, they seldom cause problems in a transfusion setting. Some retain activity at 37°C and must be considered to have potential clinical significance. These antibodies, being IgM, do not cross the placenta and do not cause hemolytic disease of the newborn. The most notable and most clinically important IgM antibodies of this type, of course, are anti-A and anti-B, which can cause serious hemolytic transfusion reactions when ABO-incompatible blood is given.

Other non–red-cell-stimulated (natural) antibodies (not including ABO), usually have specificity against antigens in the systems designated Lewis, Ii, P, or MNS. In cold-reactive autoimmune hemolytic anemia associated with *Mycoplasma pneumoniae* infections (see Chapter 3), anti-I is often implicated. Anti-I and anti-IH often cause laboratory problems in crossmatching because high titer examples tend to have persistent agglutinating activity even at 37°C. Lewis antibodies occur fairly commonly in the unimmunized population. In vivo hemolysis from anti-Le^a occurs only rarely. Most Lewis antibodies are clinically insignificant, but there is enough unpredictability that many blood bankers are reluctant to ignore them if they are active at 37°C.

ANTIHUMAN GLOBULIN (COOMBS') SERUM TEST

Immunoglobulins, the antibody molecules themselves, are antigenic if introduced into a nonhuman host. In 1945, Coombs, Mourant, and Race injected whole human serum into rabbits; the resulting antihuman serum antibody proved remarkably useful as a laboratory reagent. The term Coombs' serum is still applied to antibodies that react with human globulins. A panspecific antihuman globulin (polyspecific) or a monospecific antihuman globulin directed to a specific component of the antibody or complement can be preferentially used to identify antibody (or complement) either coating the red cells or floating free in the serum. Currently, newer methodology using monoclonal antibodies is defining specific globulins with more precise specificities (see Chapter 7). In blood banking, the significant test reagent specificities are against IgG and, to a lesser degree, complement, especially C3d.

Antiglobulin serum (antihuman globulin or AHG) detects the presence of antibody or complement molecules on the red cell surface in the direct

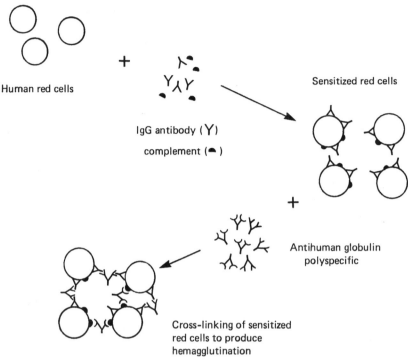

FIGURE 8–4. The antiglobulin reaction. The indirect test is employed to determine in-vitro sensitization of red cells, whereas the direct test is used to detect in-vivo sensitization. Polyspecific antihuman globulin contains anti-IgG and anticomplement activity. (From Simpson, PP, and Hall, PE: The antiglobulin test. In Harmening, DM: Modern Blood Banking and Transfusion Practices, ed 4. FA Davis, Philadelphia, 1999, p 77, with permission.)

antiglobulin test (DAT) (Fig. 8–4). Red cells can become coated with gammaglobulin either in vivo or in vitro. Most blood banks use a single antiglobulin reagent capable of detecting IgG globulin and complement (polyspecific) and then have specific reagents that react only with IgG or certain complement components (monospecific). In vivo coating is detected by the DAT (see Fig. 8–4 and Table 8–5). In vitro manipulations are used in antibody screening, in crossmatching, and in special applications of blood typing.

The principle of the test is to amplify the presence of immunoglobulin and/or complement on erythrocytes using AHG to **agglutinate** (stick red cells together) (see Fig. 8–3) the coated red cells, either directly **(direct antiglobulin test)** or following incubation with serum-containing antibodies **(indirect antiglobulin test)**.

THE DIRECT ANTIGLOBULIN TEST IN AUTOIMMUNE HEMOLYTIC ANEMIA

It is never normal for circulating red cells to be coated with immuno-globulins (IgG or IgM). In the DAT, cells are tested directly as they come from the circulation and are treated only by thorough washing to remove unbound proteins. If the polyspecific antiglobulin reagent agglutinates the cells, it is desirable to use individual reagents that can demonstrate whether the coating is IgG or complement or both.

Table 8–5 lists the uses of the DAT. An important cause of a positive DAT result is **autoimmune hemolytic anemia (AIHA)** (see Chapter 3 section on Immune-Mediated Hemolytic Anemia). In this condition, patients have antibodies that react with their own cells. These autoanti-bodies may be IgG or IgM, and nearly always react with red cells from all other persons as well as those of the patient. Red cells coated with IgG, IgM, or complement experience mechanical difficulty passing through tiny capillaries, especially in the spleen. More important, the globulin coating renders them liable to adhesion and phagocytosis by macro-phages of the reticuloendothelial system. Coated red cells undergo accelerated destruction (hemolysis), and if the bone marrow is unable to compensate for the lost red cells, the patient becomes anemic. The causes of these conditions are discussed in Chapter 3.

Autoimmune hemolytic antibody syndromes are usually classified as **cold reactive** or **warm reactive,** depending on the thermal optimum of the autoantibody. IgM autoantibodies usually react at temperatures well below 37°C; often they attach only briefly to the red cell so that few or no IgM molecules remain to coat the cell. In their brief interaction, however,

TABLE 8–5. CAUSES OF A POSITIVE DAT RESULT

Autoimmune Hemolytic Anemia

Primary immune
Collagen vascular diseases (SLE, rheumatoid arthritis, etc.)
Infections (infectious mononucleosis, *Mycoplasma pneumoniae*)
Drugs (alpha methyldopa, penicillin, quinidine)
Malignancy (lymphomas, CLL, adenocarcinoma)

Alloimmune Disorders

Hemolytic disease of newborn
Incompatible blood transfusions
Delayed hemolytic transfusion reactions

Other Causes

Nonspecific adsorption of immunoglobulin on RBC (drug)
Passive antibody therapy
Idiopathic/unknown

they may initiate the complement sequence activation, and various components of complement remain firmly attached to the circulating cells. These can be identified with monospecific AHG. In cold-reactive AIHA, the antiglobulin activity is often due solely to complement components. This form of AIHA occurs as a primary event in older people of both sexes or after such infections as *Mycoplasma pneumoniae* and infectious mononucleosis. It constitutes 20 to 25% of autoimmune hemolytic anemias.

Warm-reactive autoimmune hemolytic anemia is due to IgG autoantibodies, which remain on the red cell surface for as long as the red cell remains in the circulation. The condition is often a primary, idiopathic event that can affect any age group. Warm-reactive AIHA may also occur in conjunction with leukemias, lymphomas, disseminated carcinoma, or collagen vascular diseases, especially lupus erythematosus. Up to 70% of AIHA is the warm-reactive IgG type. Drug reactions are also a common cause of warm AIHA (see Chapter 3).

DIRECT ANTIGLOBULIN TEST WITHOUT AUTOIMMUNITY

Not every positive DAT result is due to autoantibodies. In many instances, antibody coating of the red cells may occur for some unknown reason and are not associated with any apparent anemia. It has been estimated that approximately 7% of the elderly hospital population may have a positive DAT result. In some instances, these may be related to drug reactions. Drug antibodies can cause a positive DAT result because the red cell may be coated with the drug or because an immune complex of drug and antibody attaches to the red cell surface and initiates complement activation. The antihypertensive drug alpha-methyldopa *(Aldomet)* produces a positive DAT result in up to 15% of patients taking it, although hemolysis rarely accompanies the phenomenon. In these cases, the antibody seems truly to be directed against the red cell membrane, but the manner in which the drug leads to the formation of antibody remains unclear.

Alloantibodies cause a positive DAT result in several other special circumstances. In hemolytic disease of the newborn, maternal IgG crosses the placenta and attaches to the fetal cells, which become coated with IgG. At birth, the cord cells are seen to have a positive DAT result, with monospecific AHG to IgG. If Rh immune globulin is inadvertently given to an Rh-positive individual, the DAT result will be positive, but hemolysis, if it occurs, is mild. Similarly, transfusion of antibody-containing plasma may, on rare occasions, cause the recipient's red cells with the corresponding antigen to be coated with antibody, but significant hemolysis is extremely rare.

Delayed hemolytic transfusion reactions cause a clinically significant positive DAT result. If an antigen on transfused red cells provokes anamnestic antibody production, the resulting IgG attaches to the circulating transfused cells and causes their accelerated destruction. The DAT in these cases affects only the transfused cells, not the patient's own cells, which are negative for the antigen. This type of partial activity in any agglutination reaction is called **mixed field agglutination** (see section on Delayed Consequences of Transfusions and Fig. 8–3).

ANTIBODY SCREENING TEST (INDIRECT ANTIGLOBULIN TEST)

It is important to know whether patients or donors have any antibodies in their serum other than natural anti-A and anti-B. Standard practice calls for screening every blood sample from patients for the presence of unsuspected antibodies prior to each transfusion. Routine screening for antibodies is also performed empirically during pregnancy to detect those antibodies likely to be associated with hemolytic disease of the newborn. Most donor bloods are also screened, although antibodies in donor plasma are much less significant. Table 8–6 is a list of the uses of the antibody screening test. The antibody screening test is sometimes (inaccurately) called the "indirect antiglobulin test" or "indirect Coombs' test." The antibody screening test identifies antibody in the serum and is a modified system that uses indicator red cells containing a variety of red cell antigens to define the presence of the serum antibody by agglutination. In this system, the indicator red cells become coated with antibody in vitro (in the test tube during blood banking procedures).

Antibody screening is important, not only in a transfusion setting, but also in evaluating pregnant women for the possible occurrence of hemolytic disease of the newborn. Table 8–7 lists the interpretation of antibody screening tests and crossmatching.

Type and Screen

In certain surgical procedures, blood is transfused in less than 25% of cases, and in some procedures less than 10% of the time. Blood should not

---

TABLE 8–6. USES OF THE ANTIBODY SCREENING TEST

To Detect IgG Antibody

In maternal serum during pregnancy and in association with hemolytic disease of the newborn

In recipient's serum prior to transfusion—major crossmatch

In donor serum prior to transfusion—minor crossmatch

In recipient's serum after hemolytic transfusion reaction

be crossmatched for a patient unless the chances are high that the unit will be transfused. In situations in which blood is infrequently used, yet the likelihood is possible for it to be required, a type and screen system can be set up. In this manner, the blood bank determines the ABO and Rh type and performs an antibody screen on the serum. The specimen is usually held for crossmatching of donor units if needed. If the antibody screen is positive, crossmatching will usually be performed despite the low likelihood of the blood's being needed. If no antibodies are detected, units are generally not fully crossmatched or can be matched to units in inventory by computer matching (computer crossmatch). There is always an adequate inventory of type-specific blood available in the event that the patient actually needs to be transfused. If blood is urgently needed it can be issued as "partially crossmatched" blood within 15 minutes. Issuing blood in this manner is 99.9% as safe as performing the crossmatch and vastly improves the efficiency of blood banking. Even in situations in which there is an incompatible crossmatch with a negative antibody screen, it is highly unlikely that the antibodies are going to be clinically significant. Tables for Transfusion Service blood order guidelines in elective surgical procedures should be established in each individual hospital and, in most instances, should be established with collaboration between the blood bank physician, surgeon, and anesthesiologist (Table 8–8). If a positive antibody screen is identified and is deemed to be clinically significant, blood lacking the corresponding antigens should be available and complete crossmatching should be performed using the antihuman globulin test.

TABLE 8–7. ROUTINE INTERPRETATION OF ANTIBODY SCREENING AND CROSSMATCHING (INDIRECT ANTIGLOBULIN TEST)

Result	Interpretation
Negative antibody screen	No antibody against antigens on reagent RBCs.
Crossmatch compatible	No antibody in recipient serum against donor erythrocytes.
Positive antibody screen	Irregular antibody against reagent erythrocyte antigens.
Alloantibody	Identify antibody by testing with cell panels of known
Autoantibody	antigenic specificity.
Drug antibody	
Crossmatch incompatible	Recipient antibody against donor erythrocyte antigens.
	Identify antibody by testing with cell panels of known antigenic specificity.
	Select donor who lacks corresponding antigen.
	If crossmatch is still incompatible, multiple alloantibodies, unusual antibodies, or autoantibody artifacts are responsible.

TABLE 8–8. EXAMPLE OF A MAXIMUM SURGICAL BLOOD ORDER SCHEDULE

Procedure	Units*
General Surgery	
Breast biopsy	T/S
Colon resection	2
Exploratory laparotomy	2
Gastrectomy	2
Hernia repair	T/S
Laryngectomy	2
Mastectomy, radical	T/S
Pancreatectomy	4
Splenectomy	2
Thyroidectomy	T/S
Cardiac-Thoracic	
Aneurysm resection	6
Coronary artery bypass graft, adults	4
Coronary artery bypass graft, children	2
Lobectomy	2
Lung biopsy	T/S
Vascular	
Aortic bypass with graft	4
Endarterectomy	T/S
Femoral-popliteal bypass with graft	4
Orthopedics	
Arthroscopy	T/S
Laminectomy	T/S
Spinal fusion	3
Total hip replacement	3
Total knee replacement	2
OB-GYN	
Abdominoperineal repair	T/S
Cesarean section	T/S
D & C	T/S
Hysterectomy, abdominal	T/S
Hysterectomy, radical	2
Labor/delivery, uncomplicated	(Hold)
Urology	
Bladder, transurethral resection	T/S
Nephrectomy, radical	3
Prostatectomy, perineal	2
Prostatectomy, transurethral	T/S
Renal transplant	2

*Numbers may vary with institutional practice.
T/S = type and antibody screen.
From Vengelen-Tyler, V (ed): Technical Manual, ed 12. American Association of Blood Banks, Bethesda, MD, 1996, with permission.

Crossmatching

Before blood is administered, the donor cells and the recipient's serum are tested for the presence of serologic incompatibility by crossmatching. The crossmatch is the final check that the patient does not have a circulating antibody reactive against the transfused red cells.

The crossmatch may be performed as an "immediate spin crossmatch," in which the ABO and Rh compatibility are confirmed by mixing patients' serum and donor red cells with immediate centrifugation and observance of the absence of agglutination. This is usually performed when the recipient's serum has not demonstrated any red cell autoantibodies or alloantibodies (as already described).

Alternatively, when the recipient has a positive antibody screen, the antibody is identified, and donor cells lacking the corresponding antigen are crossmatched using the indirect antiglobulin test for assessment of compatibility. The strategy of pretransfusion testing is shown in Figure 8–5.

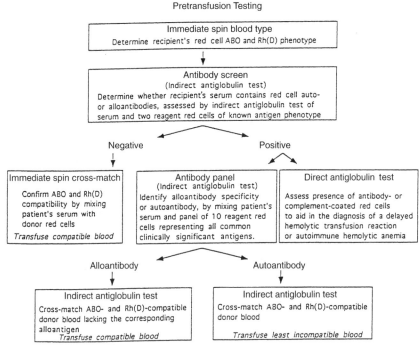

FIGURE 8–5. Laboratory algorithm for detection of red blood cell antigens and antibodies. (From Frattali, AL, Silberstein, LE, and Spitalnik, SL: Human blood group antigens and antibodies. In Rossi, G, Simon, TL, Moss, GS, and Gould, SA (eds): Principles of Transfusion Medicine, ed 2. Williams & Wilkins, Baltimore, 1986, p 84, with permission.)

Antiglobulin serum (AHG) markedly enhances the sensitivity of in vitro testing. Strong IgM antibodies usually cause grossly visible agglutination of cells possessing the relevant antigen, but weaker antibodies are difficult to detect, and many IgG antibodies do not agglutinate cells no matter how strong the antibody is. All tests for antibodies, including the crossmatch, use centrifugation of serum and cells as the first phase of testing. Agglutination indicates a positive result (see Fig. 8–3). The serum and cells are then allowed to incubate, usually for 15 to 30 minutes, to allow any antibody that is present in the serum every opportunity to attach to the donor red cells. After unbound proteins are washed away, antiglobulin serum is added. If the serum contains an antibody that reacts with and attaches to an antigen on the cell surface, adding AHG causes the antibody-coated cells to agglutinate. If there is no agglutination after the addition of AHG, it means that no antigen-antibody reaction has occurred. The serum may well contain an antibody, but if the cells do not have the relevant antigen, the reaction will be negative, and the transfused cells will be crossmatch compatible.

The crossmatch is the best available test to predict satisfactory transfusion outcome. A negative crossmatch does not, however, guarantee that the red cells will survive normally or that the patient will experience no ill effects from the transfusion.

PRETRANSFUSION TESTING

Table 8–7 outlines the interpretation of antibody screening and compatibility tests.

ON DONOR BLOOD

Blood drawn from the donor's vein must be processed for safe transfusion. Regardless of subsequent fractionation, the blood must be found to be free of hepatitis B surface antigen (HBsAg), HIV p-24 antigen and antibodies to human immunodeficiency virus (HIV) type 1 and 2, human T leukemia virus (HTLV) type I/II, hepatitis C virus, and hepatitis B core antibodies (see section on Infectious Disease Transmission by Blood Components). In addition, blood is also tested for exposure to syphilis. Blood that is positive for any of these tests is never transfused. Blood found to have unexpected red cell antibody is separated into plasma and red cells. The red cells can be used for transfusion, but the plasma is either pooled for large-scale fractionation procedures or saved for reagent purposes.

ON RECIPIENT'S BLOOD

Before a patient receives blood, his or her ABO group and Rh type must be known and the patient must be tested for unexpected red cell antibodies as described above. Every blood sample received from each patient undergoes these tests, and the results are compared against previously recorded results stored in the blood bank. A person's ABO and Rh types do not change naturally, but there is always the danger of incorrectly identified blood samples; comparing present with previous results on the "same" patient has detected many instances of mistaken identity and prevented many transfusion-associated disasters. Antibody screening tests often do change, going from negative to positive in the days, weeks, or months that follow transfusions. It is important to document whether immunization has occurred.

COMPATIBILITY TESTING FOR RED CELLS

Before blood is transfused into a patient, samples from donor and recipient should be tested for serologic compatibility. The likelihood of incompatibility is much reduced if both patient and donor have negative antibody screening test results, but no screening procedure can ensure against specific rare antibody antigen reactions. For patients with known antibodies, pretransfusion compatibility testing is crucial.

SELECTION OF BLOOD PRODUCTS

Transfused red cells must lack antigens to which the recipient has antibodies. If anti-A is present, A or AB cells cannot be given; the same applies to B or AB cells in a patient with anti-B. Although antibodies in donor plasma are far less important, occasional units of Group O blood contain potent anti-A or anti-B that can damage A, B, or AB recipient cells on transfusion. The concept of Group O as a "universal donor" applies to red cells, not to whole blood. It is good practice to give group-specific blood at all times. When this is impractical, Group A or Group B recipients can receive O red cells, and AB recipients can receive red cells of any ABO type. An O recipient can only receive Group O blood.

Because Rh antibodies are not naturally occurring, no immediate harm results from giving Rh-positive blood to an Rh-negative patient. Subsequently, however, 60 to 70% of Rh-negative recipients will develop anti-D, and the practice is considered generally undesirable. It is important to avoid giving Rh-positive blood to Rh-negative girls or women capable of childbearing because hemolytic disease of the newborn is almost certain to occur in any Rh-positive child they would subsequently bear. More flexibility is possible in selecting plasma products and platelet concentrates than in red cell selection. Ideally, all such products should be group specific. In practice, transfused anti-A and anti-B rarely cause problems except in very small children and rare cases of intensively treated hemophilia receiving intermediate-purity products. Group O plasma is more likely to be dangerous than other groups and should be the last choice for transfusing recipients of blood groups other than O.

The situation with platelet concentrates is awkward. Concentrates stored at room temperature contain at least 50 mL of plasma, which possesses antibodies that might have the potential for injuring the recipient's cells. In addition, platelets have ABH antigenic activity that can react with the recipient's antibody. Group-specific platelets are definitely the product of choice, but non–group-specific platelets are preferable to none at all.

METABOLIC CHANGES IN BLOOD DURING STORAGE

Metabolic changes occur both within the red cells and in the plasma on storage. These are listed in Table 8–9. The metabolic changes occurring with storage are termed the **storage lesion** and have some importance when large volumes of whole blood are replaced, as in massive blood transfusion (see section on Acute Transfusion Reactions). Ordinarily, metabolic changes in the red cells during surgery are not clinically important for adults. However, because of leakage of potassium from erythrocytes into the plasma during storage, as well as a drop in the erythrocyte 2,3 DPG (diphosphoglycerate responsible for oxygen delivery), especially after 1 week of storage, these changes may be important in neonatal transfusions or in massive-transfusion replacement.

BLOOD COMPONENT THERAPY

CELLULAR COMPONENTS

A unit of blood consists of cellular and noncellular elements that serve diverse functions. Transfusion therapy is directed toward replacing a component or components that are deficient in a symptomatic patient. There is always some risk associated with any product, and the risk/benefit ratio should always be ascertained. Table 8–10 summarizes the use of blood and components in transfusion therapy and also outlines some of the risks associated with each specific component.

TABLE 8–9. BIOCHEMICAL CHANGES IN STORED RED BLOOD CELLS

Variable	CPD Whole Blood	CPD Whole Blood	CPD Red Blood Cells	CPD Red Blood Cells	CPDA-1 Whole Blood	CPDA-1 Red Blood Cells	AS-1* Red Blood Cells
Days of Storage	0	21	0	0	35	35	42
% Viable cells (24 hours posttransfusion)	100	80	100	100	79	71	76 (64–85)
pH (measured at 37°C)	7.20	6.84	7.55	7.60	6.98	6.71	6.6
ATP (% of initial value)	100	86	100	100	56 (±16)	45 (±12)	60
2,3-DPG (% of initial value)	100	44	100	100	<10	<10	<5
Plasma K$^+$ (mmol/L)	3.9	21	5.10	4.20	27.30	78.50†	50
Plasma hemoglobin (mg/L)	17	191	78	82	461	658.0†	N/A
% Hemolysis	N/A	N/A	N/A	N/A	N/A	N/A	0.5

CPD = citrate phosphate dextrose; A = adenine; AS = additive solution.

*Based on information supplied by the manufacturer

†Values for plasma hemoglobin and potassium concentrations may appear somewhat high in 35-day stored RBC units. The total plasma in these units is only about 70 mL.

Adapted from Vengelen-Tyler, V (ed): Technical Manual, ed 12. American Association of Blood Banks, Bethesda, MD, 1996, p 138, with permission.

TABLE 8–10. INDICATIONS AND COMPLICATIONS OF BLOOD COMPONENT THERAPY

Cellular and Plasma Components	Content	Indications	Amount of Active Substance per Unit	Volume (mL)	Shelf Life	Dosage Effect	Precautions and Complications
RBC concentrates, PRBCs	70–80% RBCs, some plasma, WBCs, and platelets or their degradation products	Improves oxygen-carrying capacity, increases red blood cell mass for symptomatic anemia and hemorrhagic shock, preferred over whole blood to reduce complications	175–280 mL PRBC mass	250–350	ACD—21 days, CPD—21 days CPDA-1—35 days ADSOL—42 days	Increases Hct 3% per unit	Must be ABO compatible FR ++ UR ++ AR + H +++ PTP ++ INF ++
Washed RBCs	>80% erythrocytes suspended in saline	Reduces febrile reactions due to leukocyte debris in patients with preformed leukocyte antibodies	200 mL PRBC mass	200–250	Open system: 24 hours	Increases Hct 3%	ABO compatible FR 0 → +/– UR 0 AR 0 H +++ PTP 0
Leukocyte concentrates	WBCs, platelets, some erythrocytes	Granulocytopenia with sepsis (neutrophils < 500/mm³) unresponsive to appropriate antibiotics after 48 hours or positive blood culture; sepsis in premature infant with depleted WBC reserve	>1.0 × 10¹⁰ granulocytes	200–600	24 hours	Cannot be determined	FR +++ UR +++ AR ++ H 0 PTP +++ INF ++ (CMV ↑)

(Continued)

TABLE 8–10. INDICATIONS AND COMPLICATIONS OF BLOOD COMPONENT THERAPY (Continued)

Cellular and Plasma Components	Content	Indications	Amount of Active Substance per Unit	Volume (mL)	Shelf Life	Dosage Effect	Precautions and Complications
Platelet concentrates (single unit random donor; single donor—apheresis, HLA matched also available)	Platelets, some WBCs and plasma	Bleeding due to thrombocytopenia or thrombocytopathy, platelet disorders, DIC, massive transfusions (6–8 units per 10 units PRBCs transfused)	At least 5.5×10^{10} platelets	30–60 per unit	72–120 hours at RT depending on container, 48 hours at 1–6°C	Increases platelet count 5000–8000 per concentrate	Do not use microaggregate filter FR +++ UR +++ AR ++ PTP ++++ INF ++
FFP	Plasma, all coagulation factors, no platelets	Treatment of multiple coagulation disorders or in massive transfusions (2 units per 10 units PRBCs transfused)	0.7–1.0 units of factors II, V, VII, VIII, IX, X, XI, XII, XIII; 500 mg fibrinogen	200–250	Frozen—1 year, thawed—6 hours	Increase of 20–30% in coagulation factor activity per dose of 10–15 mL of plasma per kg body weight	UR +++ AR ++ INF ++ Fluid overload +

Cryoprecipitated plasma AHF (CRYO); purified AHF (factor VIII) and factor IX complex also available	Fibrinogen, factor VIII:C, factor XIII, von Willebrand factor, fibronectin	Factor VIII deficiency (hemophilia A when concentrates are not available), von Willebrand disease, factor XIII deficiency, fibrinogen deficiency, consumption of fibrinogen—DIC	10–25	80 units of factor VIII:C, 200 mg fibrinogen (usually given every 15–20 hours), 40–70% of von Willebrand factor present in initial unit	Frozen—1 year (–18°C or below); thawed—6 hours; if entered or pooled—4 hours	Increase of 50–100 units of factor VIII per unit of cryoprecipitate (about 10 mL volume)	UR ++++ AR ++++ INF ++
Albumin (5%, 25%)	96% albumin, 4% globulins (α-β)	Plasma volume expansion	50 or 250	12.5 g albumin	3 years at RT, 5 years at 2–8°C		Fluid overload ++ UR + AR 0 Very expensive

ACD = acid citrate dextrose; AHF = antihemophilic factor; AR = anaphylaxis; C = coagulant; CMV = cytomegalovirus; CPD = citrate phosphate dextrose; CPDA = citrate phosphate dextrose adenine; DIC = disseminated intravascular coagulation; FFP = fresh frozen plasma; FR = febrile reaction; H = hemolysis; Hct = hematocrit; INF = infection; PRBCs = packed red blood cells; PTP = posttransfusion purpura; RBCs = red blood cells; RT = room temperature (20–24°C); UR = urticarial reaction; WBCs = white blood cells.

Modified from American Association of Blood Banks, Blood Component Therapy: A Physician's Handbook. American Association of Blood Banks, Arlington, VA, 1981.

Red Cell Products

Red cells contain hemoglobin, which transports the oxygen that is necessary to maintain life. Red cell transfusions are given to replace or restore oxygen-carrying capacity. Red cell components can be administered in several forms.

Whole Blood

Circulating blood consists of plasma, red blood cells, white cells, and platelets. When blood is drawn from the donor, anticoagulant preservative solution is added to prevent clotting during storage. The resulting component consists of about 450 mL of blood, diluted with 63 mL of anticoagulant preservative. Since neither white cells nor platelets survive very long at refrigerated temperatures (1 to 6°C), stored whole blood consists, functionally, of red cells and plasma. Albumin and most globulins survive throughout storage, but the labile coagulation factors deteriorate unpredictably.

Metabolic changes occur both within the red cells and in the plasma on storage. These are listed in Table 8–10. The use of whole blood can really be justified only when both oxygen-carrying capacity and volume expansion are required. Transfusion reaction rates are also higher with whole blood use. Overall, whole blood use has declined with the advent of component separation and is now rare.

Patients with adequate blood volume but deficient hemoglobin derive little benefit from the plasma of transfused whole blood, and patients whose cardiac function is precarious may suffer congestive heart failure if given whole blood.

Concentrated Red Blood Cells

Red cells can be separated from the rest of the blood by centrifugation. The resulting red blood cell preparation has all the oxygen-carrying capacity of the original unit without much plasma to dilute its therapeutic effect. This is especially important for patients with chronic anemia, congestive heart failure, or other individuals who have difficulty regulating blood volume. Red cells are more effective than whole blood in supplying oxygen-carrying capacity and raising the recipient's hematocrit. Like whole blood, refrigerated red blood cells stored in CPD-A1 have a shelf life of 35 days. With the use of additive anticoagulant solutions (AS-1, Adsol, and Nutricel), the shelf life can be extended to 42 days. The amount of plasma and white cells that remain in refrigerator-stored red cells is not enough to perform any physiologically useful function but is sufficient to induce immunization or cause immune reactions in sensitized recipients. Concentrated erythrocytes are the treatment of choice in individuals who have symptomatic loss of oxygen-carrying capacity due to either acute or chronic anemia. Concentrated erythrocytes should be used only when an individual is symptomatic from the anemia and should not arbitrarily be used to raise a hematocrit value to some set level in absence of symptoms, although it can sometimes be justified prior to surgery.

Leukocyte-Reduced Red Blood Cell Concentrates

A unit of red blood cells usually has greater than 10^9 leukocytes present (see Table 8–11). Leukocytes may be removed from red cell concentrates by means of centrifugation, mechanical separation using filters, or washing procedures using saline or glycerol. Glycerol is used as a cryopreservative agent in frozen red cells but is subsequently washed and removed on thawing from storage. The efficiency of leukocyte removal varies with the different preparation. Whatever method is used, the component must retain at least 80% of the original RBCs. Leukocyte removal is indicated in individuals who have experienced febrile, nonhemolytic transfusion reactions to contaminating white cells (see Acute Transfusion Reactions, later in this chapter). Other indications include prevention of cytomegalovirus (CMV) infections or HLA alloimmunization (see Table 8–12). Centrifugation is the simplest means of removing leukocytes prior to transfusion; however, it is the most inefficient method. Microaggregate filtration is a very practical method of leukocyte removal but is also relatively inefficient. The newer leukocyte depletion filters are the most efficacious. They should be used empirically if a patient has had two **febrile nonhemolytic transfusion reactions (FNHTR).** For prevention of FNHTR the component should have less than 5×10^8 leukocytes remaining, whereas for prevention of CMV and

TABLE 8–11. APPROXIMATE LEUKOCYTE CONTENT OF BLOOD COMPONENTS (PER UNIT)

Whole blood	10^9
RBCs	10^8
Washed RBCs	10^7
RBCs, deglycerolized	10^6-10^7
RBCs, leukocyte-reduced by filtration*	$<10^7$
Platelets, apheresis	10^6-10^8
Platelets	10^7
Platelets, pheresis, leukocyte-reduced*	$<10^7$

*Leukocyte reduction with third-generation leukocyte adsorption filter.
From Vengelen-Tyler, V (ed): Technical Manual, #24. American Association of Blood Banks, Bethesda, MD, 1996, with permission.

TABLE 8–12. INDICATIONS FOR LEUKOCYTE-REDUCED BLOOD COMPONENTS

Prevention of recurrent febrile, nonhemolytic reactions due to red blood cells
Prevention of alloimmunization to HLA antigens in patients who receive multiple transfusions
Prevention of cytomegalovirus transmission by cellular components

---

HLA alloimmunization (FNHTR), fewer than 5×10^6 leukocytes should be present.

Washed red cell components are indicated in patients with IgA deficiency who have experienced anaphylactoid reactions to plasma.

Frozen Deglycerolized Red Blood Cells

This component is almost devoid of platelets and plasma and is provided usually when rare donor blood is required (e.g., from a stored rare donor registry). Red cells cannot simply be placed in a freezer for storage; there must be some cryoprotective agent to prevent damage to the cell membrane. Glycerol is the agent most often used. As red cells are exposed to the glycerol solution, all traces of plasma and nearly all the platelets and white cells are removed. Red cells can be kept in a frozen state for years; on reconstitution, at least 70% of the original cells survive normally if properly transfused. The recommended shelf life of frozen cells is 3 years, but they can be stored up to 10 years if stored at –65°C or colder. Once the cells are deglycerolized, they have a shelf expiratory time of 24 hours. Frozen, deglycerolized red cells are indicated in individuals who have had severe reactions to leukocytes and plasma components in packed red cells and, in particular, in those patients who have experienced febrile reactions or anaphylactoid reactions to washed red cells. Frozen blood can also be stored for individuals who have rare blood types and for whom it is difficult to find compatible blood. Furthermore, frozen cells may also be used for autologous transfusion, although this greatly increases the costs.

Patients severely immunized to plasma proteins or white blood cells usually tolerate transfusion with deglycerolized, thawed red cells without ill effect. Frozen storage is also useful for inventory management or in military medicine because red cells have a long shelf life stored in this manner. It also facilitates stockpiling blood of rare types needed for patients with difficult antibody problems. Many centers encourage patients with complex antibody mixtures or antibodies against high-incidence antigens to store their own blood for possible future use.

Platelet Concentrates

Random and Single Donor

Two kinds of platelet preparations are currently available: (1) Single-unit concentrates termed **platelets from whole blood** are platelets concentrated from a single whole blood donation containing greater than 5.5×10^{10} platelets suspended in a small amount of plasma. (2) **Platelet pheresis concentrates** are prepared by cytapheresis, containing a minimum of 3×10^{11} platelets (platelets, pheresis). The platelet pheresis concentrates from one single donor contain the equivalent of 6 to 8 units of platelets derived from 6 to 8 random donors of whole blood. Hemapheresis procedures make it possible to process large volumes of blood from a donor because the red cells and other elements are immediately returned to the donor. Large quantities of plasma, platelets, or white cells can also be harvested by means of this technique. Platelet-pheresis concentrates are derived from a single donor, thereby reducing the number of donor exposures compared with random pooled concentrates derived from whole blood. Consequently, the risk of transfusion-transmitted infection or immunization is reduced. However, with the substantial reduction in the risk of transfusion-transmitted infections (Table 8–13), this risk using pooled concentrates is now considered only marginally greater, whereas the cost is substantially less.

As mentioned above, one unit of random platelet concentrate consists of the platelets collected from a single whole blood unit (450 mL of blood). The platelets are separated from the whole blood after collection into a multipack and are resuspended in 50 to 75 mL of plasma. Platelets can be stored for up to 5 days at 22°C on a platelet agitator to prevent platelet clumping. Platelets have a shorter lifespan than red cells, surviving only 8 to 10 days in vivo, compared with 120 days for red cells. Survival in vitro is also much shorter. Platelets have a maximum shelf life of up to 5 days, but their postinfusion survival and effectiveness decline severely during storage.

TABLE 8–13. VIRAL DISEASES TRANSMITTED BY BLOOD TRANSFUSION: CURRENT RISKS

Human immunodeficiency virus	1 : 493,000
Human T-lymphotropic virus I/II1	1 : 641,000
Hepatitis C virus	1 : 103,000
Hepatitis B virus	1 : 63,000

Therapeutic Effects

An average single-unit platelet concentrate contains 5.5×10^{10} platelets. Although specific figures vary widely, this is a realistic mean figure when careful techniques of donor selection, phlebotomy, preparation, storage, and transportation have been employed. In a hematologically stable patient, transfusion of one unit of platelets elevates the platelet count approximately 5,000 to 10,000 per microliter per square meter of body surface area. The posttransfusion increment is usually measured at 1 hour and 24 hours after the transfusion and is expressed as the corrected count increment (CCI), corrected for the number of platelets transfused and the size of the recipient.

$$CCI = \text{Absolute platelet increment/}\mu L \text{ (posttransfusion − pretransfusion platelet count)} \times \frac{\text{Body surface area (m}^2)}{\text{Number of platelets transfused (}10^{11})}$$

(The number of platelets transfused is determined by multiplying the number of units [bags] by 0.55 expressed as 10^{11}.)

The primary indication for platelet therapy is in an individual with symptomatic thrombocytopenia. Clearly, thrombocytopenia has many mechanisms, and platelet transfusions are most effective where there is defective platelet production, such as occurs with marrow aplasia (e.g., postchemotherapy, or with marrow failure). Thrombocytopenia associated with secondary destruction or peripheral sequestration generally does not have the same response following platelet transfusion (e.g., ITP). When platelets are given to a bleeding patient, the therapeutic effect is measured by improved hemostasis and not necessarily by improved laboratory values. If platelet consumption (see Chapter 5) has caused the bleeding and a low platelet count, transfused platelets suffer the same entrapment and destruction as the patient's own platelets. Platelet transfusions cause only slight clinical improvement, if any, in such cases. Patients with large spleens or with autoimmune platelet destruction derive little benefit from transfused platelets. Infection or high fever from any cause also reduces the survival of the transfused platelets. Nevertheless, the evaluation of platelet increments following transfusions, particularly at 1 hour and 24 hours, is very valuable in determining the in vivo platelet survival. This is clinically important from the point of view of assessing whether the person receiving the platelet transfusion is alloimmunized to platelets and also in determining and defining the most effective platelet therapy (Table 8–14).

Platelet Antibodies

Transfused platelets can be destroyed rapidly by alloantibodies in the recipient's plasma. Platelets lack red cell antigens other than A, B, and H, but they share HLA antigens (primarily Class I) with white cells and other

TABLE 8–14. CAUSES OF POOR PLATELET RESPONSES FOLLOWING TRANSFUSION

Immune Causes

Alloimmunization: anti-HLA antibodies, antiplatelet-specific antibodies
Autoantibodies: immune thrombocytopenic purpura
Drug antibodies: quinidine, heparin
Immune complexes

Nonimmune Causes

Fever/septicemia
Disseminated intravascular coagulation
Splenomegaly
Veno-occlusive diseases of the liver
TTP/HUS

body tissues and have unique platelet antigens as well. Anti-A and anti-B cause much less damage to incompatible platelets than to incompatible red cells. It is desirable, but not essential, that the platelets and the patient's plasma be ABO-compatible. Antibodies to HLA antigens, elicited by past transfusions and multiple pregnancies, damage platelets far more than do ABO antibodies. Alloimmune antibodies to HLA antigens (or, much more rarely, to specific platelet antigens) rapidly destroy transfused, incompatible platelets. For the immunized patient who requires platelet transfusions, HLA-typed platelets are often desirable. Difficulties in antibody identification, the expense of HLA typing, and the tremendous range of HLA phenotypes among donors and recipients make it unlikely that routine type and crossmatch will precede uncomplicated platelet transfusions in the near future. Nevertheless, newer technologies associated with identifying platelet-associated antibodies are being developed. Rapid platelet crossmatching techniques using microtiter plates are available. There are, of course, many other reasons why platelet transfusions may not produce the expected posttransfusional increment (see Table 8–14). The dosage of platelets given should not be an empiric dose but should be evaluated on the basis of the underlying cause of the thrombocytopenia, the location of the bleed (in CNS bleeds the platelet count should be greater than 80–100,000/µL, whereas lower levels might be appropriate for nosebleeds in the thrombocytopenic patient). In general, platelet counts above 50,000/µL are sufficient for adequate hemostasis except with bleeding into the central nervous system. Values greater than 20,000/µL are usually satisfactory for prevention of spontaneous bleeding. Empiric use of platelet therapy for management of the thrombocytopenia associated with cardiopulmonary bypass or open heart surgery is not warranted.

Leukocyte Reduced Platelets

When leukocyte reduction of the platelet component is desired (indications are the same as for red cells), the white cells should be eliminated at the same efficiency as for red cells (i.e., $<5 \times 10^8$ for FNHTR and $<5 \times 10^6$ for prevention of CMV and alloimmunization) (see Table 8–12).

White Cell Concentrates

Unfortunately, the data supporting the use of white cell transfusions in septic, granulocytopenic persons are less than satisfactory in adults, but fresh buffy coat granulocytes collected from one or two units of fresh, whole blood may be useful in the management of sepsis in the newborn. These are a suspension of granulocytes in plasma prepared by cytapheresis, more appropriately termed **Granulocytes, Pheresis.** This component should contain a minimum of 1.0×10^{10} granulocytes.

Granulocytes, Pheresis provides approximately 10^{10} granulocytes in 300 to 500 mL of plasma; about 25 mL of red cells inevitably contaminate the granulocyte product, and substantial numbers of platelets are also present.

Granulocyte concentrates are indicated only for treating documented bacterial sepsis in patients with severe granulocytopenia (< 500 granulocytes/μL) who have not responded to appropriate antibiotic therapy for at least 48 hours, have a positive blood culture, or both. Repeated infusions are always necessary, imposing a high risk of transfusion-related reactions and a very high cost. Granulocyte transfusions are rarely used in treatment regimens for leukemia, but optimal use remains controversial, and they should only be used in a protocol setting.

PLASMA COMPONENTS

Plasma contains coagulation proteins, albumin, immunoglobulins, and innumerable other constituents. Commercial plasma fractionation makes it possible to separately recover albumin, gammaglobulins, and coagulation factors and some serine proteases such as alpha-1-antitrypsin and antithrombin III from large pools of donor plasma. Solutions of albumin or of less purified plasma proteins are used for volume expansion; when properly prepared, they carry virtually no risk of hepatitis because they are pasteurized. Similarly, albumin does not transmit HIV infection. Coagulation factor concentrates formerly carried a significant hepatitis and HIV risk because pooling plasma from large numbers of donors multiplies the risk contributed by just a few infective units. With the advent of better infectious disease screening of donor units and viral inactivation strategies (see Table 8–15), these risks have been substantially reduced (see also Table 8–13).

TABLE 8–15. VIRAL INACTIVATION METHODS: PLASMA COMPONENTS

Heat/pasteurization
Filtration
Ionizing irradiation
Photochemical
  Psoralens
  UVA
Solvent/detergent treatment

Fresh frozen plasma (FFP) is the liquid portion of the whole blood unit collected and frozen within 6 to 8 hours and stored at –18°C. Because fresh frozen plasma is processed so rapidly, it contains the labile coagulation factors (VIII, V), all the other coagulation factors, and plasma proteins as well. The major indication for the use of fresh frozen plasma is in coagulation factor deficiency with hemostatic defects in which the factor deficiency is not well established or is a multiple deficiency. Fresh frozen plasma should only rarely be used, if ever, for volume expansion. It can, however, be satisfactorily used to reconstitute red cells for exchange transfusion in the newborn. Indications for the therapeutic use of fresh frozen plasma are listed in Table 8–16.

Plasma frozen within 24 hours of collection and *cryoprecipitate-poor plasma* are byproducts of component preparation and are often less costly than FFP. The levels of labile coagulation factors are more variable than in FFP, but these products have the same content of stable coagulation factors, albumin, bactericidal material, opsonins, and other constituents. Cryoprecipitate-poor FFP is the preferential component used for the treatment of **thrombotic thrombocytopenic purpura (TTP)** because it lacks von Willebrand factor (vWF) multimers that are thought to be important in the pathogenesis of the consequences of TTP and provides vWF cleaving protease activity.

Cryoprecipitate and Factor VIII Concentrates

Cryoprecipitated Antihemophilic Factor

Cryoprecipitated Antihemophilic Factor (AHF) represents the cold, insoluble portion of plasma processed from FFP. Cryoprecipitate is a gelatinous residue obtained by freezing and slowly thawing freshly drawn plasma. It contains 80 to 100 IU of factor VIII, vWF, and about 250 mg of fibrinogen (minimum 150 mg) in a volume of 10 to 15 mL/unit (Table 8–17). Cryoprecipitate is useful in treating minor or moderate bleeds in patients with von Willebrand's disease. If very high vWF

TABLE 8–16. CLINICAL INDICATIONS FOR FRESH FROZEN PLASMA

Deficiencies of clotting factors for which specific factor concentrates are unavailable
Multiple coagulation factor deficiencies in a bleeding patient
Reversal of coumadin effect or coumadin overdose
Massive blood transfusion (>1 blood volume within several hours)
Antithrombin III deficiency
Treatment of thrombotic thrombocytopenic purpura

TABLE 8–17. COMPOSITION OF CRYOPRECIPITATE

Components	Amount
Factor VIII	80–100 units of factor VIII activity/concentrate
von Willebrand factor	40–70% of original FFP
Fibronectin	150–250 µg/concentrate
Fibrinogen	20–30% of original FFP (min. 150 mg)

FFP = fresh frozen plasma.

concentrations are needed, as for life-threatening hemorrhage or for surgical procedures, some commercial concentrates containing vWF are more convenient. Fresh frozen plasma and cryoprecipitate are the only transfusion products that contain fibrinogen. Cryoprecipitate is also the best available source of vWF, which is not present in many commercial concentrates of factor VIII. It is also useful in the management of hypofibrinogenemic states and in disseminated intravascular coagulation with consumption of fibrinogen. Cryoprecipitate can also be subjected to viral inactivation procedures such as heat or solvent-detergent treatment. An increasing trend is the use of cryoprecipitate to provide fibrinogen, which can then be activated to fibrin by topical thrombin on bleeding sites during surgery. This "fibrin glue" is now becoming standard practice in many vascular surgical procedures.

Factor VIII Concentrate

This component is a lyophilized concentrate of plasma derived from up to 30,000 donors, which contains predominantly Factor VIII but also small amounts of fibrinogen and other proteins. Intermediate-purity, high-purity, or very-high-purity concentrates are available and vary according to the purification method. Most monoclonal antibody (affinity) purification procedures yield very-high-purity concentrates with few contaminating proteins. The specific Factor VIII content (units of Factor VIII activity per mg of protein) varies amongst different lots and manufacturers and is labeled on each vial. Usual ranges of total Factor VIII activity are 800 to 1600 IU/mg.

The Factor VIII molecule has been cloned and is also available as a recombinant protein. This preparation is more expensive than the plasma-derived concentrates but has the advantage that it does not transmit blood-associated infectious diseases. It can still, however, be immunogenic and elicits immune responses, including alloimmunization (Factor VIII inhibitors). Table 8–18 summarizes Factor VIII concentrates in treatment or prophylaxis of hemophilia A (Factor VIII deficiency).

TABLE 8–18. FACTOR VIII CONCENTRATES

Purity	Purification Methods	Viral Inactivation	Specific Activity μ/mg*
Intermediate <10 μ/mg			
Profilate	PEG precipitation—	S/D	1–2
Humate P	alcohol fractionation	Pasteurization	6–10
High			
Alphanate	Affinity	S/D	9–22
Koate HP	Gel filtration chromatography	S/D	
Very High			
AHF-M	Monoclonal immunoaffinity	S-D	2–11
Hemophil-M	Monoclonal immmunoaffinity	S-D	2–11
Monoclate-P	Monoclonal immunoaffinity	Pasteurization	5–10
Recombinant VIII			
Recombinate	CHO cells	—	10
Kogenate	BHK cells	—	8–30
Porcine			
Hyate C	—	—	100

CHO = Chinese hamster ovary; BHK = British hamster kidney; M = monoclonal; P = pasteurized; S/D = solvent/detergent; PEG = polyethylene glycol.

*Activity per mg of protein, includes protein stabilizers, e.g., albumin (values much higher in the more purified products if protein stabilizers not considered).

Factor IX Concentrate

This component contains concentrates of the vitamin K–dependent factors II, VII, IX, and X that are derived from pools of thousands of donors. This component, therefore, has similar risks to factor VIII concentrate; however, it is prepared by plasma fractionation rather than cryoprecipitation. These products are the treatment of choice for bleeding or prophylaxis in Christmas disease patients (factor IX deficiency). Other indications are congenital deficiencies of prothrombin factors VII and X. This component is also heat treated and/or solvent-detergent treated, as is factor VIII. Some factor IX concentrates also contain small amounts of activated coagulation factors and therefore can be useful in the management of hemophilic patients with inhibitors to factor VIII. A recently approved recombinant factor IX concentrate is now also available.

Serum Globulin Preparations and Plasma Protease Inhibitors

Commercial plasma fractionation can also concentrate gammaglobulin for administration to patients with severe humoral antibody deficiency. Plasma pools containing high titers of specific gammaglobulins may be used as hyperimmune gammaglobulin serum preparations for the management of individuals who have been exposed to varicella-zoster immune globulin (VZIG) or hepatitis B immune serum globulin. Normal plasma also contains natural inhibitors to proteins that are activated during physiologic processes, such as thrombin in coagulation, trypsin in protease digestion, or C1 esterase in complement activation. Some natural inhibitors can also be concentrated during plasma fractionation for therapeutic use in congenital and acquired deficiency states (e.g., antithrombin-deficient thrombophilia, alpha-1-antitrypsin deficiency [emphysema], and C1-esterase deficiency [angioneurotic edema]).

AUTOLOGOUS TRANSFUSION

The safest transfusion uses the patient's own blood. Before an elective operation, many individuals can donate several units of blood for their own later use. With appropriate iron supplementation and clinical surveillance, it is possible to draw two or more units of blood, even as much as one unit/week, in the 35 or 42 days before the operation. Samples collected in this manner are stored in a liquid state; however, if frozen storage is available, the time between phlebotomy and autologous transfusion can be extended indefinitely. Autologous transfusion should always be indicated for any individual going for elective surgery for whom blood is likely to be used. Half-units can even be collected from smaller persons, or even adolescents going for surgery, despite the fact that they may fail to qualify as regular blood donors.

A procedure that is useful in harvesting patients' own blood is that which occurs during surgery, termed intraoperative salvage. In this manner, blood lost at surgery is filtered and washed and can be reinfused back into the patient. Another technique of autologous transfusion is using preoperative (normovolemic) hemodilution to the extent that blood lost at surgery contains fewer red cells. Autologous donations have the major advantage of eliminating the risk of transfusion-transmitted disease and alloimmunization. This type of blood product should always be offered to all qualified patients.

IRRADIATED BLOOD PRODUCTS

Graft vs. host disease (GVHD) is a rare complication of transfusion therapy that occurs predominantly in immunocompromised patients (see section on Graft vs. Host Disease, later in this chapter). In this

---

TABLE 8–19. PATIENTS WHO REQUIRE IRRADIATED BLOOD

Absolute Indications

Recipients of allogeneic or autologous bone marrow or peripheral progenitor transplants
Recipients of cord blood progenitor transplants
Congenital immunodeficiency syndrome
Fetuses receiving intrauterine transfusion
Recipients of donor units from a blood relative

Relative Indications

Neonatal exchange transfusion
Hodgkin's and non-Hodgkin's lymphoma
Acute leukemia
Chronic leukemia
Recipients of HLA-selected platelets or platelets known to be homozygous

No Definite Indications

Nonpremature neonate
Solid tumors
Acquired immunodeficiency syndrome (AIDS)
Aplastic anemia
Agammaglobulinemia
Chronic granulomatous disease (CGD)

condition, the viable transfused T-lymphocytes attack the host's cells. Exfoliative dermatitis, diarrhea, liver inflammation, and marrow aplasia are the main clinical features. Posttransfusion GVHD is almost always fatal.

GVHD can be prevented by irradiating the blood components given to persons at risk. Radiation is usually performed by placing the blood unit in a gamma radiation field with an exposure of at least 2500cGy. This dose kills lymphocytes but does no harm to erythrocytes, platelets, or granulocytes. The blood itself is not radioactive and can be given to any recipient. Table 8–19 is a list of those types of patients who require irradiated blood products.

THERAPEUTIC HEMAPHERESIS

Therapeutic hemapheresis involves the exchange of "diseased" blood or components with "healthy" blood or components. **Plasmapheresis** refers to the removal of plasma and replacement with plasma or plasma substitutes and has been reportedly successful in the diseases listed in Table 8–20. **Cytapheresis** is the term used to describe the removal of cellular components (**thrombocytapheresis**—platelets, **leukocytapheresis**—white cells, and **erythrocytapheresis**—red cells). The mechanisms of injury in certain diseases involve the presence of harmful circulating plasma or cellular factors, which may be removed by mechanical means. A notable example is the hyperviscosity syndrome, in which an excess amount of abnormal viscous plasma may induce clinical symptoms. Removal of the abnormal plasma and replacement by crystalloid or colloid substitutes can effectively reduce these symptoms. The efficiency of plasmapheresis is substantially better when the abnormal compound or substance is distributed in the intravascular fluid. In this situation, a single plasma exchange may remove up to 90% of the factor (e.g., hyperviscosity syndrome due to macroglobulinemia). However, in many conditions in which plasmapheresis has been used, pathogenesis is uncertain and the effectiveness or utility has been undefined.

Hemapheresis may be accomplished by means of continuous flow or intermittent flow cell separators. The blood volume of the patient must be estimated, and a CBC, coagulation screen, and electrolyte evaluation need to be obtained. In this manner, replacement solutions can be titrated accordingly, and electrolytes replaced to keep the patient as physiologic as possible. Specific laboratory tests may be performed in specific diseases (e.g., serum viscosity levels prepheresis and postpheresis may be monitored in patients with hyperviscosity syndrome). Similarly, in individuals with myasthenia gravis, one might monitor the titer of acetylcholine receptor antibodies.

TABLE 8–20. GUIDELINES FOR THERAPEUTIC HEMAPHERESIS: DISEASE CATEGORIES

CATEGORY I

Standard and acceptable under certain circumstances, including primary therapy
PLASMA EXCHANGE
Coagulation factor inhibitors
Cryoglobulinemia
Goodpasture's syndrome
Guillain-Barré syndrome
Homozygous familial hypercholesterolemia
Hyperviscosity syndrome
Myasthenia gravis
Posttransfusion purpura
Refsum's disease
Thrombotic thrombocytopenic purpura
CYTAPHERESIS
Leukemia with hyperleukocytosis syndromes
Sickle cell syndromes (also see Category IV)
Thrombocytosis *symptomatic*

CATEGORY II

Sufficient evidence to suggest efficacy; acceptable therapy on an adjunctive basis
PLASMA EXCHANGE
Chronic inflammatory demyelinating polyneuropathy
Cold agglutinin disease
Drug overdose and poisoning (involving protein-bound toxins)
Hemolytic uremic syndrome
Idiopathic thrombocytopenic purpura (ITP) (Protein A chromatography)
Pemphigus vulgaris
Rapidly progressive glomerulonephritis (RPGN)
Systemic vasculitis (primary, or in association with SLE and RA)
CYTAPHERESIS
Cutaneous T-cell lymphoma
Hairy cell leukemia
Rheumatoid arthritis

CATEGORY III

Insufficient evidence for efficacy; uncertain benefit/risk ratio. Conditions that may fall into this category might be an exceptional effort for an individual case or a research project for numerous cases.
PLASMA EXCHANGE
Alloantibody removal (red cell, platelets, HLA)
Maternal treatment of maternal fetal incompatibility (hemolytic disease of the newborn)
Hyperthyroidism, including thyroid storm
Multiple sclerosis
Polymyositis/dermatomyositis
Progressive systemic sclerosis
Pure red cell aplasia
Warm autoimmune hemolytic anemia

(Continued)

TABLE 8–20. GUIDELINES FOR THERAPEUTIC HEMAPHERESIS: DISEASE CATEGORIES *(Continued)*

CYTAPHERESIS
  Multiple sclerosis
  Renal transplant rejection
There are numerous other diseases for which plasmapheresis has been done from which no conclusions can be drawn.

CATEGORY IV

Lack of efficacy in controlled trials.
PLASMA EXCHANGE
  AIDS (for symptoms of immunodeficiency)
  Amyotrophic lateral sclerosis
  Aplastic anemia
  Fulminant hepatic failure
  Psoriasis
  Renal transplant rejection
  Rheumatoid arthritis
  Schizophrenia

From Sacher, RA, Brubaker, DB, Kasprisin, DO, and McCarthy, LJ (eds): Cellular and Humoral Immunotherapy and Apheresis. American Association of Blood Banks, Bethesda, MD, 1991, pp. 22–23, with permission.

ADVERSE EFFECTS OF TRANSFUSIONS

Adverse reactions to blood component transfusions are classified as **acute** or **delayed** (Table 8–21). These transfusion reactions are defined as any unexpected or unfavorable symptom or clinical sign occurring in a patient during or immediately following the administration of a blood component. Delayed reactions may occur days to many years after the transfusion. The clinical interpretation of whether a transfusion reaction has occurred must be made with the understanding of (1) the patient's condition, (2) any underlying primary disease, (3) the type of component that has been administered, (4) the volume administered, and (5) whether the patient previously had a positive antibody screen. Whenever a decision is made to transfuse a patient, the potential side effects must be weighed against the likely benefits. Reactions in common with other intravenous solutions may further complicate a blood transfusion and include: (1) pyrogens, (2) bacterial contamination, (3) circulatory overload, (4) air embolism, and (5) thrombophlebitis.

GENERAL COMPLICATIONS

Pyrogenic substances are toxins capable of evoking a fever. Following an intravenous infusion of pyrogens, fever will occur. Pyrogens were formerly a problem but are now tested for during manufacturing of intravenous solutions or intravenous administration sets.

Bacterial contamination may complicate a blood transfusion (see later) or may occur in other intravenous solutions that serve as culture mediums (e.g., high sugar solutions). Organisms may grow in the solution, and when infused into a patient, they may evoke a serious reaction mimicking a hemolytic transfusion reaction.

Circulatory overload occurs particularly in patients with chronic anemia and in the elderly or those with heart disease. The clinical features are mostly cardiopulmonary symptoms, and management is to stop or slow the infusion and administer diuretics. Circulatory overload is one of the most common complications of blood component administration.

Thrombophlebitis, or inflammation of the walls of the veins, may occur if an intravenous site has been used for extended periods or if large needles are placed in small veins. Clinical features include pain, redness, and tenderness at the infusion site. Intravenous lines should be replaced regularly, and the infusion site must be inspected frequently.

TABLE 8–21. ADVERSE REACTIONS TO BLOOD COMPONENTS

Cause of Reaction	Acute Transfusion Reactions	Delayed Transfusion Reactions
Nonimmune	Hemolytic	Infection
	Septic	Bacterial
	Circulatory	Viral
	Aggregates and pulmonary infiltrates	Parasitic
	Metabolic	Iron overload
	Coagulopathy	
	Citrate toxicity	
	Hypothermia	
	Hyperkalemia	
Immune	Nonhemolytic	Alloimmunization
	Febrile	Delayed hemolytic
	Urticarial	Graft vs. host disease
	Anaphylactoid	Posttransfusion purpura
	Transfusion-related acute lung injury (TRALI)	Platelet-refractory
	Acute hemolytic	Immunomodulation
	Incompatible transfusion	

ACUTE TRANSFUSION REACTIONS

Acute complications of transfusion of blood components may be categorized into two types: (1) **nonimmunologic,** which are not associated with preformed immune antibodies (immunoglobulins), and (2) **immunologic** (antibody-mediated), in which preformed antibodies are responsible for damaging transfused blood components (see Table 8–21).

Nonimmune Reactions

Hemolytic

Destruction of donor red cells by the patient and the release of hemoglobin from inside of the erythrocytes **(hemolysis)** usually results from patients' preformed antibodies but can occur due to mechanical destruction, such as from bypass circuits or infusion pumps. Bacterial sepsis is a rare complication and its frequency is unknown. Occasionally, bacteria may contaminate blood transfusions if strictly aseptic techniques are not followed during collection of the donated blood. It appears to be more often associated with platelet components (possibly pooled concentrates derived from whole blood rather than apheresis platelets) than with red blood cells. The risk increases with platelet storage interval and is three to five times higher if platelets are 5 days old (maximum storage time). Release of bacterial enzymes can cause hemolysis of red blood cells. Blood is a very favorable culture medium for these organisms and therefore must be refrigerated and kept between 1 and 6°C. Organisms such as *Yersinia, Serratia, Pseudomonas,* and coliforms may grow even under these temperature conditions. Prior to release from the blood bank, blood is always inspected for visible hemolysis to screen against this complication. However, if infused into a patient, this contaminated blood may evoke the clinical features of an immediate hemolytic transfusion reaction, with shock, fever, and the release of the bacterial endotoxins. In any fever associated with transfusions, particularly if severe rigors are accompanied by cardiovascular collapse or fever over 40°C within 90 minutes of the transfusion, bacterial sepsis must be considered and the transfusion stopped. Once the specimen is submitted to the blood bank, routine Gram stains and cultures are performed on the posttransfusion specimen and bags returned to the blood bank.

Aggregates

Under conditions of storage, white cell and platelet debris and minimal amounts of fibrin may develop. If transfused into a patient, these may occlude the microcirculation in the lungs and cause pulmonary distress. A routine blood filter usually removes these aggregates so that they are not transfused into the patient. Cellular components in particular must always be infused using a standard blood filter (150 µ). In situations of massive blood replacement, these filters may have to be changed after three to four units have been infused, to prevent cellular debris from entering the lungs and impeding pulmonary circulation.

Metabolic

Electrolyte and metabolic changes occur while blood is stored (see Table 8–9). Potassium leaks out of the erythrocytes, red cells continue to undergo anerobic metabolism, and the anticoagulant solutions may cause metabolic imbalances or coagulopathy. This is called the **storage lesion** and refers to the changes occurring in blood during storage. Metabolic effects of transfusion include hyperkalemia, hypocalcemia, citrate toxicity, acidosis, hypernatremia, and hypothermia. The larger the amount of blood transfused, the more clinically significant these electrolyte problems may become (see section on Whole Blood).

Antibody-Mediated Acute Transfusion Reactions

Immune antibodies may be directed against the erythrocyte (hemolytic) or nonerythrocyte, cellular, and noncellular (nonhemolytic) components.

Acute Hemolytic Transfusion Reactions

These are the most serious, but fortunately one of the least common, transfusion reactions. They arise mostly because of major ABO incompatibilities due to clerical or administrative errors. When anti-A and anti-B destroy incompatible red cells, hemolysis occurs immediately, usually in the circulation itself. This is because the isohemagglutinins, anti-A and anti-B, are IgM antibodies that efficiently bind to A and/or B antigens on the erythrocytes and rapidly activate complement. Most other antibodies attach to the surface of transfused compatible cells, coating them for removal by the extravascular reticuloendothelial cells. Pretransfusion crossmatching reduces the danger of hemolysis; however, no matter how accurate the pretransfusion testing is, if the wrong sample is tested or the wrong blood is administered to the patient, these severe hemolytic reactions may occur. No serologic subtleties are involved when group A blood is given to a group O patient. It is sheer carelessness. Occasionally, crossmatching fails to demonstrate very weak or atypical antibodies that later cause hemolysis, but hemolytic reactions on this basis are very uncommon.

Clinical Spectrum

Hemolytic transfusion reactions often begin with a rising temperature, shaking chills, and falling blood pressure. Other symptoms include palpitations, anxiety, substernal pain, flank pain, and warmth and tenderness at the site of infusion. These events are the result of widespread interaction between antibody and antigen. The major and severe clinical sequelae result from hypotension, disseminated intravascular coagulation, and renal failure.

Most fatalities occur in the anesthetized patient, since the patient cannot complain about the immediate and distressing symptoms. This situation may be recognized only by a drop in blood pressure and the presence of diffuse bleeding from the surgical wounds.

Disseminated intravascular coagulation occurs as a result of the complement activation, with subsequent activation of the coagulation cascade and intravascular thrombin generation (see Chapter 6). Fibrinogen is converted to fibrin in the vascular system. In addition, the fibrinolytic system is also activated and fibrin and fibrinogen breakdown occurs, also within the vascular system. Coagulation factors are consumed and a coagulopathy develops. Bleeding occurs because of consumption of normal coagulation factors, poor clot formation, and enhanced lysis of the weak clots. In addition, platelets may also be consumed and microangiopathic hemolytic anemia (MAHA) may develop as the red cells become scythed and chopped by the fibrin strands (see Chapter 3 and Color Plate 16).

Renal failure occurs as a result of occlusion of the renal tubules by antibody-coated red cell membranes and acute tubular necrosis (ATN). In addition, an early manifestation may be evidence of the release of hemoglobin from the damaged red cells (intravascular hemolysis). As the red cells are destroyed, hemoglobin is released into the plasma. Although a large protein, hemoglobin readily crosses the glomerular filter and hemoglobinuria commonly follows hemolysis. Free hemoglobin itself does not produce renal damage. Renal failure is a result of the combined effects of hypotension, massive antigen-antibody reaction, and intravascular coagulation. Treatment is aimed at re-establishing renal blood flow and blood pressure control, forced diuresis to flush out the occluded renal tubules, and correction of the coagulation abnormalities. In view of critical blood volume problems, strict attention to fluid control is mandatory. To prevent posthemolytic renal failure, blood pressure should be maintained and brisk diuresis established for the next several hours. This may involve the use of the osmotic diuretic mannitol or the loop diuretic furosemide *(Lasix).*

Some IgG antibodies can also produce acute hemolytic transfusion reactions (anti-Jk^a, Jk^b, anti-Duffy, Kell, etc.). IgG-coated cells are usually destroyed in the reticuloendothelial cell (extravascular hemolysis) and not in the circulation, with the exception of anti-Jk^a and Jk^b. Plasma hemoglobin levels rise only if cell destruction is so massive that it overloads the capacity of the reticuloendothelial system for hemoglobin disposal (see section on Hemolytic Anemia, Chapter 2). If extravascular destruction occurs gradually, the only sign that there has been a transfusion reaction may be a drop in hematocrit or failure to achieve the expected rise in hematocrit following the transfusion (see section on Delayed Hemolytic Reactions).

Laboratory Examination

At the first suspicion of a hemolytic transfusion reaction, the transfusion must be discontinued, but the intravenous line or catheter should be kept patent. Verification of the patient's name and blood type must be performed. Mislabeling and misidentification cause most transfusion disasters. Diagnosing this cause is easy enough; however, it may be more difficult to ascertain how and why the mistake occurred.

Laboratory investigation requires examination of the patient's posttransfusion blood. A sample of clotted blood must be sent to the laboratory, where the crossmatch and pretransfusion sample is verified. It is examined for the presence of free hemoglobin in the serum. The pretransfusion and posttransfusion samples are compared. The presence of antibody-coated cells is tested by the performance of the direct antiglobulin test (see section on The Direct Antiglobulin Test). If this result is positive, the blood bank will then verify the nature of the antibody coating the red cells. Absence of ABO incompatibility and negative test results make it unlikely that a hemolytic reaction has occurred. If the results are positive, further studies must be performed, including an administrative evaluation as to how the problem occurred.

Acute Nonhemolytic Reactions

Febrile Reactions

A febrile reaction is defined as 1°C or more rise in temperature during or immediately after the transfusion, with no precipitating cause.

Certain patients, in particular persons who have received multiple transfusions and women who have had multiple pregnancies, may become immunized to blood proteins or other cells, including platelets and white cells. If these people are given blood transfusions, they may mount an immune attack against these transfused components that elicits fever and shaking chills and is termed a **febrile (nonhemolytic) transfusion reaction (FNHTR).** The clinical features are usually headaches, general malaise, and a rapid rise in temperature of less than 24 hours' duration. The shaking chills are often the most distressing symptom. More often, these reactions are relatively mild. Since bacterial contamination and hemolytic reactions may mimic this milder cause of fever, the transfusion must be stopped and evaluated for these possibilities.

Febrile reactions are estimated to occur with a frequency of 0.5% per unit. Most often, these reactions are caused by white-cell antibodies causing release of pyrogenic cytokines (IL-1, IL-6, and TNF-alpha). These antibodies can be specific for granulocyte antigens, or may react with HLA antigens common to nearly all tissues. It is not practical to attempt matching of the recipient against the donor's white cells. Simply, this type of reaction may be prevented by using leukocyte depletion filters, particularly for red blood cell components or platelets (see Table 8–12). The leukodepletion filter for platelet components allows passage of platelets but restricts most of the leukocytes. Leukocyte or platelet antibodies do not account for all FNHTR, and it appears that in some cases cytokines are released into the plasma during storage. This is particularly evident in platelet preparations stored for 5 days. Prestorage filtration of these components blocks cytokine release and decreases FNHTR. These mediators obviously are not removed by leukodepletion filters, so reactions during infusion must be treated by antipyretics, hydrocortisone, or both.

Urticaria

Itching, hives, and urticaria are also commonly seen in patients who have received multiple blood products (up to 3% of all transfusions). They occur as a result of allergies in the recipient to proteins in the donor blood. The mechanism is an immediate hypersensitivity to transfused blood proteins affected by IgE (histamine-releasing) antibodies. Therefore, this reaction often can be premedicated or treated by means of antihistamines. In most instances, if the patient's vital signs are stable, the transfusion may simply be slowed and antihistamines administered. If the patient has a more severe reaction, including bronchospasm, the transfusion may have to be stopped. Stopping of a transfusion is a clinical decision. If patients have severe cutaneous reactions to blood components with hypotension, a more severe immunologic reaction must be suspected, such as an anaphylactoid reaction.

Anaphylactoid Reactions

Approximately 1 in 4000 people have low or deficient IgA levels. These people may develop naturally occurring IgA antibodies. Deficiency of IgA is often associated clinically with recurrent infections of the body tracts, since this antibody is the prime humoral antibody lining body cavities. Recipients of blood products should always be questioned regarding recurrent respiratory or gastrointestinal infections or a history of hypogammaglobulinemia. These patients may also develop immune anti-IgA antibodies that avidly bind to IgA in transfused blood. Under these circumstances, an immune complex activation of complement cascade occurs and the patient manifests a severe anaphylaxis (see Immunology section). These patients must either receive blood that is deficient in IgA from rare donor registries or must receive blood that has been treated to remove plasma by extensive washing or following freezing and deglycerolization.

Transfusion-Related Acute Lung Injury

Transfusion-related acute lung injury (TRALI), also called transfusion-related noncardiogenic pulmonary edema, is the consequence of acute respiratory distress and cyanosis occurring within 4 hours of the transfusion, often requiring ventilatory assistance. Although this condition can be fatal, if it is recognized and immediately treated, more than 80% of patients survive. The cause may be unclear, but it can be the result of passive antileukocyte (HLA- or neutrophil-specific) in the transfused blood. The resulting antibody-leukocyte reaction induces leukoaggluti-nation and trapping in the pulmonary vasculature. Cytokines and inflammatory mediators are then released, increasing vascular permeabil-ity and producing alveolar edema. Investigation of suspected TRALI involves screening of both the donor and recipient's plasma for anti-HLA or antileukocyte antibodies.

DELAYED CONSEQUENCES OF TRANSFUSIONS

These may be defined as any side effect of blood component administra-tion occurring 24 hours or more following infusion. Again, this group may be classified according to whether they are antibody mediated or not. The most publicized delayed effect of transfusion is infectious disease transmission. Immune antibodies may produce delayed ef-fects, including delayed hemolytic reactions, GVHD, and posttransfusion purpura (see Table 8–21).

Delayed Hemolytic Reactions

These occur when an immune antibody previously undetectable in pretransfusion testing is reinduced by exposure to the same antigens in the transfused blood. The recipient has immune memory that, following exposure to the transfused cells containing the antigen, evokes an amplified immune response **(anamnestic response)**. A **delayed hemo-lytic reaction** is diagnosed by failure to achieve a sustained increment in hemoglobin or hematocrit following the transfusion. Other effects of the hemolysis (which is usually extravascular) may occur, including the demonstration of the antibody by screening, coating of transfused red cells several days after the transfusion by the antibody (positive DAT), and elevated bilirubin, LDH, and even reversible renal failure. The antibodies mostly involved in this type of reaction include anti-Rh antibodies (c and E) and anti-Duffy and anti-Kidd. A recipient who has had such a reaction should be given the information. This should always be written down and carried with the person, and future transfusions must be negative for these specific antigens.

Graft vs. Host Disease

Graft vs. host disease is a rare complication that may occur in patients with the indications listed in Table 8–20. It is avoided by the use of irradiated blood (see section on Irradiated Blood Products).

Posttransfusion Purpura

Posttransfusion purpura is a rare delayed consequence of transfusion associated with a thrombocytopenia developing 1 week following transfusion. It is seen in persons who lack the platelet antigen HPA-1A (Pl^{A1}) and have anti–HPA-1A preformed antibodies from prior pregnancies or transfusions. Exposure to HPA-1A–positive platelets causes immune adherence of antibody/antigen complexes to their own platelets and subsequent sequestration and thrombocytopenia. These recipients must always receive HPA-1A–negative blood components.

Transfusion Hemosiderosis

A unit of concentrated red blood cells contains 250 mg of iron. Since the body stores of iron are only 500 to 1500 mg, six transfusions may saturate these stores. Once this occurs, iron is deposited in other parenchymal cells in various organs (e.g., liver, pancreas, skin, and heart). Iron overload syndromes occur particularly in persons who have received over 100 units of red cell transfusions. Individuals receiving so many transfusions include patients who are critically dependent on transfusion support for life (e.g., thalassemia, sickle cell anemia, myelofibrosis [see section on Iron Overload Syndromes in Chapter 2]). These patients usually die from cardiac failure due to iron deposition in the cardiac tissues. Iron overload from transfusions may be retarded by the use of iron chelation therapy.

INFECTIOUS DISEASE TRANSMISSION BY BLOOD COMPONENTS

Table 8–13 is a list of the viral diseases transmitted by blood transfusion and their current risks. Table 8–22 lists the infectious diseases that can be transmitted by blood transfusion, indicating those where testing is obligatory versus those where testing is not routine. Although in recent times AIDS has preoccupied concerns about transfusion-transmitted diseases, hepatitis transmission continues to be the most frequent serious infectious complication of transfusion therapy. Several viral diseases can be transmitted by blood transfusion. Prevention of transfusion-transmitted infections is one of the main thrusts of modern blood banking and pretransfusion testing. Because of improved screening methods, all transfusion-transmitted viral disease has dramatically decreased and now bacteria and other organisms are increasing in significance.

TABLE 8–22. BLOOD BANK SCREENING TESTS

Routine Tests

Human immunodeficiency virus (HIV) I/II
Anti-HCV
Hepatitis B surface antigen (HB$_s$Ag)
Anti-HBc (hepatitis B core)
Serological test for syphilis (STS)
P-24 antigen
Human T lymphotrophic virus (HTLV) I/II

No Routine Tests

Trypanosoma cruzi (Chagas' disease)
Cytomegalovirus
Yersinia enterocolitica (sepsis)
Parvovirus B-19 (aplasia)
Borrelia burgdorferi (Lyme disease)
Babesia microti (babesiosis)
Plasmodia (malaria)
Leishmania tropica (leishmaniasis)

Human Immunodeficiency Virus (HIV-1, HIV-2)

The transmission of the HIV virus by blood products to produce the acquired immunodeficiency syndrome (AIDS) is still a worldwide concern. Recipients of blood products collected in the United States from 1978 to early 1985, before the advent of serologic screening, were particularly at risk.

Blood components collected in the United States have been screened for the presence of antibody to the HIV type 1 since April 1985, and for HIV type 2 (HIV-2) since March 1992. Donors are screened using a serologic test that detects the presence of anti-HIV-1 and HIV-2 using an enzyme-linked immunosorbent assay (ELISA) system. This test is very sensitive. The diagnosis of posttransfusion HIV is made by obtaining a positive test identifying antibody to HIV in the recipient. Seroconversion is thought to occur 6 to 8 weeks after infection. Since the screening test identifies only antibody, there exists a window period in which a potential donor can still be infectious (Fig. 8–6).

Several tests for HIV antibody measure IgG or total antibody. The ELISA is the most common test. The source of the antigen is either inactivated virus that has been grown in a human lymphoid cell line but also contains other antigens in the cell line (HLA antigens) or recombinant viral sequences. The ELISA antibody test is the initially performed test, and donors who are positive with this test are excluded

The Family of HIV Seroconversion Windows

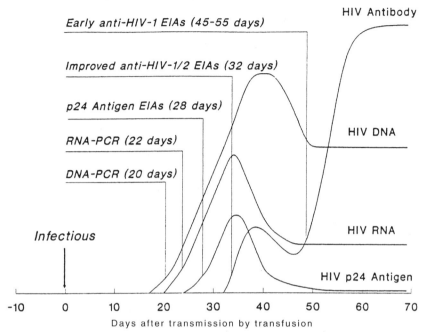

FIGURE 8–6. Current concept of HIV seroconversion window. Infection window is defined as beginning (day 0) when a seronegative person becomes infectious by transfusion of a unit of his or her blood into a transfusion recipient. Estimated days (after becoming infectious) to positivity by polymerase chain reaction (PCR), p24 antigen enzyme immunoassays (EIAs), and progressively improved anti-HIV EIAs of the seronegative donor are shown. (From Busch, MP: Retroviruses and blood transfusions. In Nance, SJ (ed): Blood Safety: Current Challenges. American Association of Blood Banks, Bethesda, MD, 1992, p 29, with permission.)

from future donations. The test is usually performed in duplicate. If one of the results is positive, an additional ELISA test is performed. If again positive, the donor is termed repeatedly reactive and the sample is sent to be confirmed by another test called the Western blot test. If the Western blot sample is negative, or if two of the three initial ELISA tests are negative, the test is considered to be a negative test. The confirmatory Western blot test utilizes the principle of immunoblotting and separation of the viral antigens so that specific antiviral antibodies can be identified. It is used to confirm all positive ELISA tests since the ELISA has a high false-positive rate. Approximately 1 in every 1000 donors is positive (repeatedly reactive) initially, of which 2 in 10,000 is Western blot positive (confirmed positive).

The method uses the electrophoretic separation of viral proteins and glycoproteins, followed by nitrocellulose blotting and fixation of the antibody. Patient sera are applied and incubated either with peroxidase-conjugated goat antihuman IgG followed by staining, or with radioimmunoprecipitation. Seropositivity is considered in the presence of a specific envelope protein for the virus termed gp-41 band, or gp-120 in its absence and in the presence of antibody to the viral core proteins p24 and p55. More sensitive and specific assays for both IgG and IgM antibodies are also available using recombinant DNA protein methods.

Transfusion-transmitted HIV infection has effectively been eliminated from the blood supply by means of these testing methods. Donor education and specific predonation questions regarding high-risk groups are still used as additional safeguards. There is a theoretical possibility that a viremic, seronegative donor (window of seronegativity) who does not consider himself to be part of a high-risk group may donate a unit of blood that is eventually transfused (see Fig. 8–6). To further decrease this window, a test for the presence of the HIV p24 antigen has also been added to the screening profile. This has now decreased the risk of TT-HIV to less than 1 in 493,000 transfusions. Nucleotide amplification testing (NAT) will soon be used and will further reduce this risk. Pooled plasma products used in the treatment of hemophilia are now additionally heat treated, pasteurized, or refined by monoclonal antibody to prevent transfusion-transmitted HIV, and recombinant factors VIII and IX are not associated with any HIV risk (see also Plasma Components).

Transfusion-Transmitted Hepatitis

Hepatitis C Virus (HCV, Non-A, Non-B Hepatitis)

Since the introduction of screening assays for HCV there has been a marked reduction in the incidence of transfusion-associated hepatitis (TAH). The organism responsible for most cases of what was previously called non-A, non-B hepatitis is hepatitis C. Before the HCV antibody assays were implemented, two surrogate tests were used: the antibody to the hepatitis B core antigen (anti-HBc) and the liver enzyme alanine aminotransferase (ALT; serum glutamic-pyruvic transaminase [SGPT]), both of which reduced the likelihood of non-A, non-B hepatitis by 40%. Since HCV antibody screening, TAH has declined to between 1 in 5000 and 1 in 50,000 and with newer assays is estimated at 1 in 103,000 (see Table 8–13). ALT testing has since been abandoned because of its lack of specificity. ALT levels may also be increased nonspecifically in obesity, following exercise, and with certain medications. The major clinical features of HCV hepatitis are subclinical, and jaundice is infrequent. Raised serum enzymes are typically fluctuant and may be missed. The major significance is the tendency to develop progressive liver disease. One of the major complications of HCV hepatitis is the development of chronic active hepatitis and, subsequently, postnecrotic cirrhosis. Formerly, a diagnosis of non-A, non-B hepatitis could only be made after serologic studies had excluded hepatitis A, B, CMV, EBV, and HIV. The introduction of the HCV antibody test has been a major breakthrough in infectious disease screening prior to blood transfusion. Of the patients with HCV hepatitis, 15 to 20% may develop cirrhosis and 5% to 10% may develop hepatocellular carcinoma.

Hepatitis B Virus

Jaundice with raised enzymes occurring 6 to 12 weeks after transfusion is more commonly produced by hepatitis B transmission by blood products. Screening of blood donors for the presence of hepatitis B virus has effectively reduced this likelihood to 1 in 63,000 transfusions. This virus may produce a spectrum of liver disease ranging from a fulminant hepatitis to a mild, subclinical infection. The incidence has greatly decreased since the abolition of paid donors and the institution of screening procedures for hepatitis B virus (see Hepatitis; Virology section).

Cytomegalovirus and Epstein-Barr Virus

These viruses reside within granulocytes and mononuclear cells and cause a viral illness with hepatitis and other visceral inflammatory manifestations. Individuals at risk for transfusion-transmitted CMV infections are persons who lack antibody to the cytomegalovirus (CMV seronegative) and who are immunocompromised, such as neonates and bone marrow transplant recipients. The use of CMV seronegative blood products is the most effective means of preventing this complication. Indications for use of CMV seronegative cellular blood components are shown in Table 8–23. The prevalence and the likelihood of transfusion-transmitted CMV infection vary across geographic regions. It is still uncertain whether transfusion-transmitted CMV infection occurs because of reactivation of dormant virus in the transfused cells or the transfusion of active virus from the donor. An alternative source of cellular components with reduced likelihood of transmitting CMV is leukodepleted preparations.

TABLE 8–23. INDICATIONS FOR USE OF CMV-SERONEGATIVE CELLULAR BLOOD COMPONENTS

CMV-seronegative recipients of CMV-seronegative bone marrow transplants
CMV-seronegative patients with AIDS
Premature infants less than 1200 g born to CMV-seronegative mothers
CMV-seronegative pregnant women

Hepatitis A Virus (HAV)

Posttransfusion hepatitis A is a rare event. The incubation period is 28 days, which is shorter than for both hepatitis C and hepatitis B. It has been reported using pooled fractionated plasma components (IvIg and Factor VIII concentrates) despite the use of solvent and detergent viral inactivation. This is because HAV is not a lipid-enveloped virus and is not inactivated by the S/D process. Another virus that can be transmitted by blood transfusion, parvovirus B-19, is also unaffected by S/D treatment.

Table 8–22 lists other infectious agents that can be transmitted by blood transfusion.

HEMOLYTIC DISEASE OF THE NEWBORN

DEFINITION AND PATHOPHYSIOLOGY

Hemolytic disease of the newborn (HDN), also termed **erythroblastosis fetalis,** is a syndrome of hemolytic anemia and jaundice occurring as a result of the destruction of antibody-coated (sensitized) erythrocytes in the infant. In this syndrome, the mother develops immune (IgG) antibodies from a **transplacental hemorrhage (TPH)** of incompatible fetal cells. These antibodies are harmless to the maternal cells, but cross the placenta into the fetal circulation and attack antigens present on the fetal erythrocytes. Depending on the severity of red cell destruction in the fetus or newborn, a spectrum of disease ranging from hydrops fetalis (fetal congestive cardiac failure) to a milder jaundice in the newborn period may develop.

When any fetal blood group factor inherited from the father is not possessed by the mother, there is the possibility of a maternal alloimmune reaction. Depending on the degree of antigenicity involved, this transplacental passage may lead to HDN. Blood group incompatibility for the Rhesus D antigen was formerly the major cause of HDN. The overall incidence of HDN due to anti-Rh_o (D) (18% in untreated mothers) has dramatically changed (<0.1%), and deaths from Rh-HDN are now uncommon. There has been, concomitant with this decrease, a relative rise in the frequency of mothers with other antibodies to Rhesus antigens and to antigens of the non-Rhesus systems. The immunologic conditions for ABO HDN occur most commonly, and group A or B infants born to group O mothers often have maternal IgG antibody on their cells. However, ABO HDN is rarely serious, although infants may have mild disease.

All pregnancies are associated with the passage of some fetal blood cells into the mother. This is particularly evident at 28 weeks, and occurs more especially at birth. This passage is termed transplacental hemorrhage (TPH) and may especially be seen to occur with antenatal procedures such as amniocentesis (sampling the amniotic fluid of the fetus), or manually changing the position of the baby from a breech position. TPH may also occur with spontaneous or induced abortions. Fetal cells comprise surface antigens from both parents. If the mother lacks erythrocyte antigens possessed by the father and transferred to the fetus, and if TPH occurs, the mother is likely to become immunized to these cells. The mother then develops, initially, IgM antibodies and, subsequently, IgG antibodies to these foreign antigens. Since IgG antibodies are capable of being transported across the placenta, if the antibodies are directed to erythrocyte antigens on the fetal cells, they may undergo immune adherence to the erythrocytes of the fetus. These cells are now coated with antibody (opsonized) and are then capable of being removed by the reticuloendothelial system of the fetus, where they are destroyed. Extravascular hemolysis then occurs. There are two main effects:

1. As the increased numbers of red cells are destroyed, hemoglobin is liberated and undergoes conversion to bilirubin and other bile pigments that diffuse across the placenta back into the mother's circulation. The mother's liver readily conjugates and excretes the fetal bilirubin. Some bile pigments leak back into the amniotic fluid and are not directly excreted. Sampling of the amniotic fluid may therefore give an index of the severity of hemolysis.
2. If the fetal bone marrow cannot compensate for the shortened red cell survival, progressive anemia develops. As the hemoglobin drops, tissue oxygenation declines and a severely anemic fetus may go into congestive heart failure and develop systemic edema. The fetus with severe HDN may die of congestive cardiac failure around the time of delivery. This disorder is called **hydrops fetalis,** which emphasizes the edematous appearance of these stillborn infants. The fetal bone marrow responds to the hemolytic process by increasing red cell production in an attempt to maintain adequate erythrocyte levels and avoid anemia. The marked increased in erythropoiesis causes many immature nucleated red cells to circulate prematurely. Erythroblasts may then be seen in the fetus's circulation and sometimes the term **erythroblastosis fetalis** is used to describe this situation.

RH HEMOLYTIC DISEASE OF THE NEWBORN

In Rh hemolytic disease of the newborn (Rh-HDN), the development of anti-D antibodies by the mother occurs following exposure to the Rh-positive (D cells) of the fetus. Pregnancy and childbirth are the immunizing events, since Rh-positive blood almost never is given to an Rh-negative woman of childbearing age. In regard to other antibody specificities, either transfusion or prior pregnancies may be the immunizing stimuli. Rh-HDN was formerly the most common cause of HDN, and at one time was responsible for close to 50% of all perinatal deaths. In Rh-HDN, laboratory testing for the detection of such antibodies is used to determine the clinical strategy: intrauterine transfusion, premature delivery, or term delivery. Exchange transfusions may be needed after birth, as determined by the bilirubin and/or degree of anemia.

Anti-D, in practical terms, is the only antibody for which HDN is severe and creates serious risk to the fetus. When anti-D is present, it is important to perform all available procedures to evaluate the fetus's condition. Titering the antibody may be useful in indicating the timing for amniocentesis, to assess fetal risk, and to determine a strategy for management during pregnancy.

Prevention of Rh Hemolytic Disease of the Newborn

One of the major accomplishments of the last 25 years has been the almost total conquest of Rh-HDN. This success has occurred because of recognition of the Rhesus-D antigen in the pathogenesis of the disease, and widespread use of passive antenatal and postnatal anti-RhIgG immunotherapy. Table 8–24 lists the indications for RhIg.

All $Rh_o(D)$-negative mothers who are nonimmunized (negative irregular antibody screen), who are pregnant, or who have any procedure associated with an increased likelihood of transplacental bleeding should receive RhIg prophylaxis. If the blood group of the father is known to be $Rh_o(D)$-negative, RhIg immunoprophylaxis can be avoided. The appreciation that antenatal TPH can occur has prompted the administration of RhIg at 28 weeks of pregnancy in women who are unimmunized. This has allowed a reduction in the incidence of Rh sensitization in pregnancy from 1.8% (the level associated with only postpartum RhIg therapy) to less than 0.07% of all Rh-negative women. Administration of antenatal RhIg is not associated with any significant adverse clinical effects on the infants. Infants may, however, have weakly positive direct antiglobulin tests. More transplacental bleeding occurs during delivery and is sufficiently covered by routine administration of postpartum RhIg. The usual dose of 300 µg is sufficient to cover a 15 mL TPH of fetal erythrocytes.

Diagnosis of Transplacental Hemorrhage

Usually less than 1 mL of fetal erythrocytes cross the placenta during delivery, and even less during pregnancy. However, occasionally a large TPH may occur. This can be detected by the rosette screening test, and then quantitated by the acid-resistant hemoglobin test **(Kleihauer-Betke test)**.

TABLE 8–24. INDICATIONS FOR Rh IMMUNE GLOBULIN IN THE NONSENSITIZED Rh-NEGATIVE PREGNANT PATIENT

Routine
  28 weeks gestation
  Within 72 hours postpartum if neonate is Rh positive
After invasive prenatal diagnostic procedures
  Chorionic villus biopsy
  Amniocentesis
  Percutaneous umbilical blood sampling
Ectopic pregnancy
Spontaneous or therapeutic abortion
External cephalic version
Antepartum bleeding
  Threatened abortion
  Suspected placental abruption
  Placenta previa
  Blunt trauma to the abdomen
  Motor vehicle accident
Hydatidiform mole

From Sacher, RA, and Brecher, ME (eds): Obstetric Transfusion Practice. American Association of Blood Banks, Bethesda, MD, 1993, p 24, with permission.

Rosette Test

The rosette test uses the principle that if fetal D-positive cells cross the placenta into the maternal circulation, a sample of blood taken from a D-negative mother will have a minor population of D-positive cells. If reagent anti-D is added to the blood specimen, coating of the D-positive cells occurs and microscopic agglutination may be seen. To amplify the test, further reagent D-positive cells are then added and appear as a rosette of agglutinated cells when examined microscopically. The finding of rosettes is evidence that a TPH of D-positive cells has occurred. This test is a qualitative test, and does not quantitate the amount of TPH.

Acid-Resistant Hemoglobin Test for Fetal Hemoglobin (Kleihauer-Betke Test)

This test uses the principle that fetal hemoglobin is more resistant to acid pH than adult hemoglobin. If a sample of blood is taken from a mother who has had a TPH, a small population of fetal cells will be present in her circulation. If this blood is placed in an acidic solution and a stained blood smear is made, fetal cells will show preservation of hemoglobin staining, whereas adult cells will appear as ghosts (see Color Plate 30). The relative percentage of stained to unstained cells is determined. This percentage ratio is multiplied by the correction factor (50) for maternal blood volume (using an arbitrary maternal blood volume of 5000 mL), then the amount of fetomaternal hemorrhage (FMH) in milliliters is quantitated. This test is used to evaluate a large TPH, and to accurately calculate the dosage of RhIg needed. An alternative strategy is to divide the volume of FMH by 30, then round to the next whole number to determine the number of 300-µg vials to be administered. It is imperative that every nonimmunized $Rh_o(D)$ woman is identified and given Rh immune prophylaxis. At the initial visit to the obstetrician, an ABO and Rh type and the presence or absence of irregular antibodies must be determined. Rh immune prophylaxis is then given at 28 weeks and again at delivery. At the time of delivery, if the infant is Rh positive, a rosette test for the detection of TPH should be performed. If the test is negative, routine administration of RhIg should be given. If the test is positive, the degree of FMH is quantitated by means of the acid-resistant fetal hemoglobin test. Other tests such as the enzyme-linked antiglobulin test or flow cytometry also are being used in some centers.

Laboratory Management of the Immunized Rh-Negative Pregnancy

Antibody Screen

Immunization, as detected by a positive antibody screen with the identification of the anti-D antibody, represents a challenge of management of a high-risk pregnancy. Once an anti-D is identified, the antibody titer needs to be evaluated. The titration is performed by consecutively diluting the antibody in the maternal serum and letting it react with the known antigen-positive cells. The titer represents the greatest dilution with which reactivity occurs. Titer is important in this situation, since it determines the need for fetal amniotic fluid sampling.

Amniotic Fluid Analysis

Amniotic fluid, in which the fetus is suspended in the uterus, is usually straw colored. Analysis of the amniotic fluid for bilirubin concentration can give an indication of the degree of HDN. A specific test called the **delta OD 450** is usually performed in this situation. This represents the optical density difference (observed vs. expected) at the wavelength of light at which bilirubin exhibits maximal light absorption. This difference quantitates to the degree of bilirubin concentration. When this value is plotted on a graph and related to gestational age, a strategy of management can be appreciated. Three zones are identified (Fig. 8–7), called the low, moderate, and severe risk zones. A value in the severe risk zone means that fetal death is imminent. These values can be used to determine whether intrauterine transfusions, premature delivery, or term

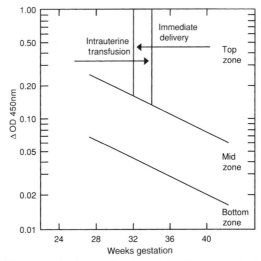

FIGURE 8–7. Liley graph for collecting data from amniotic fluid studies, identifying zones of fetal risk in hemolytic disease of the newborn (HDN). Intrauterine transfusion should be done if the OD value is in the top zone prior to 32 weeks' gestation. After 34 weeks, top zone values indicate immediate delivery. Either intrauterine transfusion or immediate delivery may be indicated for a top-zone OD between 32 and 35 weeks, depending on studies of fetal maturity. (From Vengelen-Tyler, V (ed): Technical Manual, ed 12. American Association of Blood Banks, Bethesda, MD, 1996, p 435, with permission.)

delivery is appropriate. In addition, analysis of the amniotic fluid can provide information on the fetal lung maturity. Measurement of the ratio of the phospholipids lecithin and sphingomyelin (L:S) gives an accurate reflection of fetal lung maturation that can determine a strategy for premature delivery or intrauterine transfusion (see Chapter 17).

Intrauterine Transfusions

Intrauterine transfusions are the mainstay of therapy for infants who are too premature to deliver and who have severe erythroblastosis fetalis. Blood used for this procedure is usually packed Group O Rh_o(D)-negative blood that is irradiated. The blood is irradiated to prevent the rare complication of GVHD, since these ill premature infants have an immature immune system (see section on Irradiated Blood Products). Intrauterine transfusions can be given either through the intraperitoneal route or by percutaneous intraumbilical exchange transfusion (PUBS). All these procedures are performed under direct ultrasound guidance.

The major questions that the laboratory can answer in the management of Rh sensitization are:

1. Does the pregnant woman have an antibody capable of producing HDN?
2. What is the likelihood that an intrauterine transfusion is needed?
3. What is the likelihood that premature delivery may be indicated?
4. What is the likelihood that exchange transfusions might be needed after birth?

Laboratory Management of the Neonate with HDN

General Laboratory Testing

At delivery, the infant severs connections with the mother's circulation and becomes an independent individual. This removes the source of incoming antibody but deprives the infant of an important route for bilirubin disposal. Anemia may also be a significant clinical problem in these infants. Since the infant's antibody-coated cells continue to be destroyed, excessive amounts of bilirubin continue to be produced. Before it can be excreted by the liver, bilirubin must be conjugated within the liver cells by the addition of glucuronic acid (see Chapter 12). Unconjugated bilirubin is soluble only in fat solvents and not in aqueous solution. Conjugation requires an enzyme, glucuronyl transferase, which develops slowly as the liver matures. Premature infants have a less efficient liver capacity and have very little enzyme; full-term infants, only a limited amount of enzyme. When excessive quantities of bilirubin are produced, the infant's liver cannot conjugate it rapidly enough to excrete it. The result is that unconjugated bilirubin accumulates in the infant's bloodstream.

Unconjugated bilirubin is highly lipid soluble and tends to be deposited in cells of the developing nervous system. The mature nervous system is not damaged by unconjugated bilirubin, but the infant's neurons can undergo severe, permanent damage. "Kernicterus" is the name given to localized bilirubin deposits in the brain. In severe untreated HDN, accumulation of bilirubin may deposit widely throughout the brain tissue, leading to permanent damage and even death. The immediate goal for treating an increasing bilirubin from HDN is to remove the source of bilirubin (i.e., antibody-coated red cells) and subsequently to remove excessive accumulation of unconjugated bilirubin.

Exchange Transfusion

Exchange transfusion refers to the replacement of most or all of the neonate's erythrocytes and plasma with compatible erythrocytes and plasma (or plasma components) from donor sources. Listed in Table 8–25 are the indications for exchange transfusions. The procedure of exchange transfusion is accomplished usually through the umbilical vein, and replaces the infant's blood volume with 85 to 100 mL/kg of whole blood. Aliquots of 15 mL of blood are removed and infused successively until

TABLE 8–25. INDICATIONS FOR EXCHANGE TRANSFUSIONS IN NEONATES

Hemolytic disease of the newborn
  Rh hemolytic disease
  ABO hemolytic disease
  Other antibodies
Hyperbilirubinemia
Respiratory distress syndrome
Neonatal sepsis
Disseminated intravascular coagulation

the total volume is exchanged. It is critically important that the clinical and laboratory parameters are monitored during this procedure. These include fluid volume infused and removed, serum, electrolytes, hemoglobin, and bilirubin levels. Usually Group O $Rh_o(D)$-negative blood is used and is irradiated. The blood must be compatible with both the infant and the maternal serum. Blood should be as fresh as possible, and preferably less than 5 days old (maximum, 7 days). Potassium values should be determined in the blood used for exchange, and if higher than normal, the red cells should be washed and reconstituted with fresh frozen plasma. When performed by experienced personnel, complications are infrequent, usually less than 1%.

HEMOLYTIC DISEASE OF THE NEWBORN DUE TO OTHER MATERNAL ANTIBODIES

The most common cause of mild HDN is anti-A or anti-B. The reasons for this are that most natural anti-A and anti-B antibodies are IgM class and therefore incapable of crossing the placenta; however, Group O individuals often may have anti-A or anti-B antibodies of the IgG class as well. Why these IgG antibodies occur in some Group O people and not in others is unknown. Neither pregnancy nor blood transfusion is needed as an immunizing event. It is also unclear why Group A people do not have IgG anti-B and vice versa. A fetus whose erythrocytes are Group A, B, or AB, and whose mother is Group O with IgG anti-A or B antibodies, may suffer red cell hemolysis. However, in view of the relatively low likelihood of severe HDN in these patients, neither immune prophylaxis nor antibody titering and screening is warranted unless determined by a previously severe obstetrical history.

Many other immune antibodies have been implicated in HDN, some causing severe disease in the infant; more recently, because of the declining incidence of Rh HDN, these antibodies are relatively more important. Anti-c and anti-K are next most frequent. Evaluation for ABO HDN is appropriately made after delivery when an infant manifests symptoms of clinical jaundice. Laboratory testing entails establishing neonatal-maternal incompatibility. The presence of anti-A, anti-B, or other antibodies in the serum or in red cell eluates from cord blood samples is considered diagnostic. It is extremely unlikely that intrauterine transfusions or premature delivery will be needed for antibodies other than anti-D.

ROUTINE ANTENATAL LABORATORY TESTING

Antibody screening tests in the early or middle part of pregnancy detect antibodies likely to cause HDN, but do not identify IgG, anti-A, or anti-B in Group O women. Any woman whose earlier pregnancies were affected by HDN must be carefully observed in subsequent pregnancies. For each specific antibody capable of inducing hemolytic disease of the newborn, a critical titer can be developed at each hospital. This represents the value of the diluted serum above which no cases of hemolytic disease of the newborn have occurred. For example, a titer of 1:32 of anti-D will react with D-positive cells when diluted 32 times. Maternal titers have some correlation with severity of disease in the infant, but this is not consistent.

HUMAN LEUKOCYTE ANTIGENS AND ANTIBODIES

Human leukocyte antigens (HLA) are a complex system of polymorphic glycoproteins that are important in immune regulation, transplantation (histocompatibility), and transfusion. They are the products of genes located on the short arm of chromosome 6. The different antigen groups belonging to the HLA system are closely linked in this region, which also contains genes for several enzymes and serum proteins, including components of complement (Fig. 8–8). Because of its complexity, the term "locus" is inappropriate for this chromosomal segment; it is usually described as the HLA region or major histocompatibility complex (MHC). The antigens constituting the HLA system are designated A, B, C, D, and DR DQ and DP (see Fig. 8–8). There are 27 distinct antigens in the A group, at least 57 in the B, 10 in C, and 26 in D, as well as 24 in DR, 9 in DQ, and 6 in DP. Each chromosome includes genes that define a single antigen in each of the groups; the assortment of HLA genes present on a single chromosome and transmitted as a single unit is called haplotype. Since every cell except the erythrocyte possesses two examples of chromosome 6, each person has two haplotypes, one from each parent.

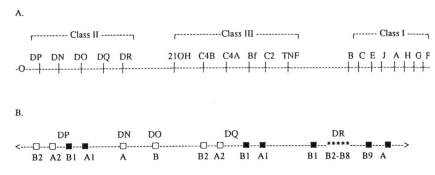

FIGURE 8–8. *(A)* The major histocompatibility complex located on the short arm of chromosome 6. The centromere is to the left. The key Class I, II, and III genetic loci are shown. The Class III region contains complement system genes (C2, Bf, C4A, C4B), the 21-hydroxylase gene (21OH) and the gene for tumor necrosis factor (TNF). *(B)* Greater detail of the Class II region. (From Vengelen-Tyler, V (ed): Technical Manual, ed 12. American Association of Blood Banks, Bethesda, MD, 1996, p 310, with permission.)

Within a single sibship (family of siblings), there can be only two maternal haplotypes and two paternal haplotypes, making a maximum of four different genotypes that the offspring can possess (see example in Fig. 8–9). The variety of haplotypes in the general population, however, is extremely variable and very diverse.

The HLA antigens consist of two main classes and a lesser third class. **Class I HLA antigens** consist of the A, B, and C antigens, which are present on the surface membranes of virtually all cells (including platelets) except mature red blood cells. The D and DR, DP, and DQ antigens seem to reside only on B-lymphocytes and early hematopoietic cells, antigen presenting cells, and endothelial cells. They are called **class II HLA antigens.**

The class I antigens consist of two chains—an alpha chain, which is glycosylated and subdivided into three regions termed alpha$_1$, alpha$_2$, and alpha$_3$, and a beta chain, which consists of the beta$_2$ microglobulin (a plasma globulin). The alpha chain is a transmembrane chain, whereas the beta$_2$ microglobulin is situated on the cell surface. The alpha$_3$ portion of the alpha chain seems to have a close homology with the F$_c$ portion of the immunoglobulin G. There is obviously, therefore, a very close and as yet ill-defined relationship between these class I antigens and the immune response or synthesis of specific antibodies (Figs. 8–10 and 8–11).

The class II antigens are also heterodimers and consist of an alpha chain and a beta chain, each of which is transmembrane and is divided up into two sections: alpha$_1$ and alpha$_2$ and beta$_1$ and beta$_2$, correspondingly.

These antigens are on the surface of all B-lymphocytes, and their role is to augment the sensitization limb of the immune system. They bind processed foreign antigens in the receptor-like cleft formed by the variable domains of the alpha and beta chains. The T-cell receptor of helper cells recognizes the processed antigen. T cells then release IL-2, and undergo clonal proliferation leading to expansion of the helper T-cell (CD4) population. The sensitized helper T cells augment clonal matura-tion of the sensitized B cells to plasma cells. This requires recognition by the T-cell receptor of the helper T lymphocyte by surface immunoglobulin and class II self-antigens or the B cell. The class II antigens also have a close homology with some of the serum complement components. There is, therefore, a complex interrelationship between the immunoglobulins, the surface antigens on these reactive cells, and complement. It is not surprising that these antigens are involved in tissue rejection or recognition of foreign tissue, and are therefore important in transplanta-tion biology. Haplo-identical grafts, in particular bone marrow trans-

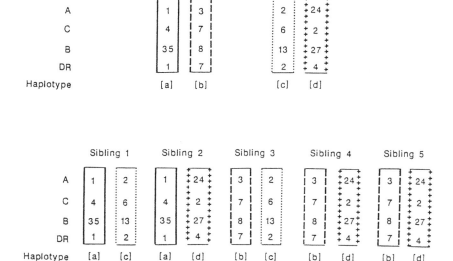

HLA Identical; MLR-Negative

FIGURE 8–9. The linked genes on each chromosome constitute a haplotype. The figure represents a family of seven persons all typed for HLA-A, B, C, and DR antigens. The data reflect the genotypes of each family member, as well as the parental haplotypes. (From Vengelen-Tyler, V (ed): Technical Manual, ed 12, American Association of Blood Banks, Bethesda, MD, 1996, p 311, with permission.)

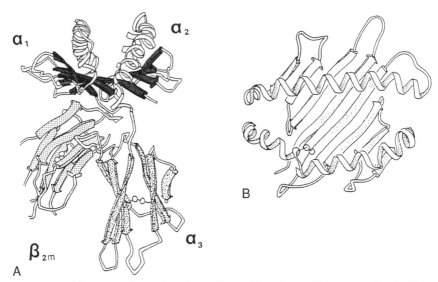

FIGURE 8–10. Three-dimensional structure of the Class I HLA molecule. *(A)* Side view of a Class I antigen molecule. *(B)* View of the antigen-binding pocket looking down toward the cell membrane. (Modified from Bjorkman, PJ, et al: The foreign antigen binding site and T-cell recognition regions of class I histocompatibility antigens. Nature 329:508, 509, 1987.)

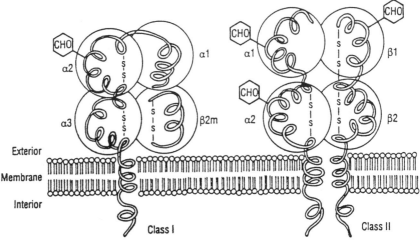

FIGURE 8–11. Stylized diagram of class I and class II MHC molecules showing alpha and beta polypeptide chains, their structural domains, and attached carbohydrate units. (From Vengelen-Tyler, V (ed): Technical Manual, ed 12. American Association of Blood Banks, Bethesda, MD, 1996, p 313, with permission.)

plants, have a much lower likelihood of graft rejection or GVHD. The D antigens appear to be very important in this regard.

HLA TESTING

HLA typing is much more complicated than testing for red cell antigens. Testing strategies are defined in three categories: *serologic assays, cellular assays,* and *DNA assays.*

Serologic Assays

Most reagent antibodies come from persons immunized through transfusions or pregnancies, but monoclonal antibody methodology is supplying specific commercial monoclonal antibodies to define specific HLA types. The number of antigens that must be studied on each lymphocyte is greater than that for red cells, and different examples of single antigens exhibit different levels of reactivity. Each cell sample must be examined against a battery of antisera so all relevant antigens are excluded. The overall reactivity determines antigenic interpretation, not just the results of one or a few individual reactions.

HLA testing usually uses agglutination or cytotoxicity as endpoints. Agglutination procedures are easier, but less sensitive, less specific, and more susceptible to false-positive results. The class I antigens are identified by their reactivity with specific antibodies, and cytotoxicity is the usual endpoint for these serologic tests. Cytotoxicity testing uses complement-binding antibodies that are allowed to attach to the cells during incubation in a complement-free system. Adding active complement to the surface-bound antibody initiates complement fixation that causes lethal damage to the cell. Cell death is most easily demonstrated by adding a macromolecular dye to the medium. Viable cells are able to exclude the large dye molecules. Because a dead cell loses this barrier function, the dye enters and stains the entire dead cell. As the reaction between antibody and cell-surface antigen increases in strength and specificity, the number of stained cells in the suspension increases. This permits a degree of qualitative comparison between serum samples that contain different combinations of antibodies. An example of such a technique is the "trypan blue dye exclusion technique." The technique has been miniaturized: HLA sera of known antibody specificities are placed in the wells of a microdroplet test plate. The test lymphocytes are added to the wells and observed for microcytotoxicity. Lymphocytes containing the corresponding antigen take up the dye. HLA-D and DR are found on B lymphocytes; thus the target lymphocytes are enriched for these cells by differential absorption using monoclonal antibody through such techniques as the use of magnetic beads. Patient serum samples can also be screened using the microlymphotoxicity test to detect HLA alloimmunization. In this case, lymphocytes of known specificity are used as the target panel (often 30 to 60 cell specificities) and are mixed with patients' sera. Reactivity is defined by microlymphocytoxicity (again using indicator dyes). In this way panel reactive antibodies (PRA) can be identified. The results are reported as percent PRA, depending on the number of lymphocytes with which the patient's serum reacts. This test is also routinely performed in histocompatibility crossmatching prior to transplantation, in which patient's serum is reacted with donor lymphocytes.

Cellular Assays

Mixed lymphocyte culture (mixed lymphocyte reaction) can detect HLA differences not evident in serologic assays. The HLA-D antigens are identified by induction of DNA synthesis assessed by the incorporation of the pyrimidine base thymidine, following reactivity of lymphocytes from the recipient and the donor. This test is used in selection of bone marrow and kidney donors. Radioactive thymidine incorporation is determined by measuring the counts of radioactivity per minute, with the higher values indicating mismatches. The corollary is that when unknown lymphocytes are reacted with known lymphocytes and low reactivity is determined, the HLA-D type can be inferred. The HLA-D locus antigens are very complex and include HLA-DR, DP, and DQ. There are many cross-reactive specificities. The functions of these antigen systems are as yet unknown. They do, however, allow closer tissue typing and presumably better transplantation-graft matches. Serological testing for Type I antigens (in particular, HLA-A and HLA-B), as well as type II (DR), are generally easily measured and available in many laboratories. Mixed lymphocyte testing for HLA-D antigens is not readily available in most laboratories; neither are antibodies for detection of the C antigens.

DNA-Based Assays

The application of DNA-based methodologies to HLA testing has greatly improved sensitivity, specificity, turnaround time, and knowledge of the molecular complexity of the MHC. For example, serologic methods identify 15 different DR antigens, but DNA-based methods identify more than 100 DR1 alleles. Several molecular testing techniques are used for the detection of HLA antigens. These include restriction fragment length polymorphism (RFLP) (see Fig. 8–12), allele-specific PCR, PCR with sequence-specific oligonucleotide primers, and PCR sequencing of HLA-RNA sequences. These techniques have varying degrees of resolution. PCR sequencing yields specific allele information and high-resolution typing. PCR allows for the generation of amplified target DNA sequences, which lend themselves to further analysis using dot blot hybridization or sequencing techniques.

Interpretation

HLA phenotype is the notation of the surface markers detected in histocompatibility testing of a single individual. The HLA genotype represents a precise determination of the antigens represented by the MHC genetic DNA on chromosome 6, determined by family studies. The term **haplotype** refers to an antigenic makeup of a single chromosome 6–MCH complex (see Fig. 8–9).

LINKAGE DISEQUILIBRIUM AND ANTIGEN DISTRIBUTION

Certain combinations of HLA antigens are more common than others. Some antigens are far more common or far rarer in one population or race than in others, and some combinations of antigens have strikingly high prevalence in specific populations.

The most common HLA-B antigens in American whites, for example, are B7, B8, and B12, with frequencies of 0.23, 0.20, and 0.24, respectively. In American blacks, the most common of the B series are Bw17 (0.26), Bw35 (0.32), and a specificity characterized as 1AG (0.34). This contrasts with African blacks, whose most common B antigens are B7 (0.18), Bw17 (0.33), and 1AG (0.31).

In American whites, association often exists between HLA-A1 and B8, A3 and B7, and Aw25 and B18. American blacks also have frequent associations of A1 and B8, but in African blacks, Aw30 and Bw42 are also frequent. This genetic characteristic of the MHC, in which two alleles of different loci are co-associated with a higher frequency than the predicted frequencies, is called **linkage disequilibrium.** Linkage disequilibrium can extend to more than two loci—for example, HLA-A1-B8-DR3. The occurrence of these genetic frequencies is therefore greater than that which might be expected with random frequency expression.

Adding further to the complexity is the observation that locus recombination can occur with a possible frequency of 1%. When crossing over occurs, the C, B, and D loci remain together but separate themselves from the A locus. The portion of the region responsible for extent and intensity of immune responsiveness lies between B and D, most closely linked to D (see Fig. 8–9).

CLINICAL APPLICATIONS OF HLA TESTING

There are four main areas of clinical medicine where HLA testing is important: (1) organ transplantation, (2) transfusion medicine, (3) disease associations, and (4) paternity testing and parentage assignment.

Organ Transplantation

HLA typing is only one aspect of donor selection for organ transplantation. The donor's ABO group should be compatible with that of the recipient, and the recipient should be free from serum antibodies that react in vitro with the prospective donor's red or white cells. If there is sufficient time, and viable cells are available from prospective donor and recipient, mixed lymphocyte cultures (MLC) are useful in ruling out cell-mediated sensitization between donor and recipient. The use of immunofluorescent flow cytometry is further streamlining the cross-matching procedure.

When donor and recipient are blood relatives, HLA matching improves the chances of graft survival. Monozygotic (identical) twins, of course, share not only HLA antigens but all their genetic material. Nontwin siblings have only a limited genetic pool from which to receive phenotypic profiles. The more alike the tissues are with regard to HLA matching, the more likely the graft is to survive. In siblings, two-haplotype matches give better results than one-haplotype matches, all other things being equal. One-haplotype matches are better than complete HLA disparity.

When donor and recipient are unrelated, HLA matching provides much less predictive information. Graft survival is not much improved by using tissue from donors who share one or several A and B antigens with the recipient. However, in patients with preformed HLA antibodies, it is important to use tissue negative for the relevant antigen in selecting the donor.

The enormous polymorphism of the HLA system has many important implications in marrow transplantation. For about 1 in 10 transplants, a parent is homozygous for a specific haplotype, and the phenotypic identity should always be confirmed by family segregation studies. In unrelated donor-recipient transplants, it must be appreciated that mutants or variants can exist that cannot be detected by serology, but only by cellular techniques. DNA-based testing has substantially increased matching precision. Splits or subgroups of different HLA alleles also exist. Each HLA molecule may carry an unknown number of different epitopes.

The evaluation of recipient serum for antibodies to donor leukocytes by PRA is important before transplantation and transfusion, because evidence indicates that presensitization to HLA antigens may cause rapid rejection of transplanted tissues. In a family, there is a one in four chance that two haplotypes segregate in the same way, and therefore a one in four probability that two siblings will have identical HLA haplotypes. Similarly, there is also a one in four probability that no haplotype will be shared between two siblings. It is apparent that a parent and a child can share only one haplotype because the child must have received the other haplotype from the other parent. Therefore the possibility of an identical match between a child and a parent is remote. Similarly, other parental relatives are unlikely to have identical haplotypes with any given child.

Bone marrow transplantation is used to treat patients with severe aplastic anemia, various types of leukemia, and immunodeficiency syndromes; it is being more widely used in salvage management of various types of lymphomas and other cancers as well. Two major problems that are referrable to HLA incompatibility are graft rejection and GVHD. In the former, the foreign identity of the HLA types is recognized by the host, who rejects the graft. This is more of a problem in solid organ transplantation than in bone marrow transplantation because bone marrow recipients are conditioned by intensive radiation therapy and chemotherapy to ablate their immune systems. This creates another problem, however, in which histocompatibility is not optimal: GVHD. In this situation, the viable transplanted cells attack the host's cells by virtue of incompatibility between antigens. GVHD produces a severe immune attack against particularly rapidly dividing cell populations, particularly the gastrointestinal tract, skin, and bone marrow. The incidence of both graft rejection and GVHD is much lower in HLA-identical transplants. Rejection of marrow is unlikely if the patient is identical for HLA-A, B, C, DR, and DQ determinants and has low reactivity with the mixed lymphocyte reaction (MLR). ABO compatibility is also important, since ABO-incompatible marrow transplants may require more blood component support and have delayed engraftment.

In renal transplantation, it appears that careful matching for HLA-B and DR and DQ alleles can provide a much greater likelihood of renal transplant survival. The HLA-B alleles are highly associated in linkage disequilibrium with DR alleles.

Transfusions

Blood transfusions are a common cause of alloimmunization to HLA antigens because even concentrated red cell transfusions contain many contaminating platelets, granulocytes, and lymphocytes. Leukocyte-depleted blood contains far fewer leukocytes, and is therefore less likely to produce alloimmunization. Platelet concentrates, however, are highly immunogenic. Immunocompetent recipients of multiple platelet transfusions frequently develop antibodies to either HLA class I antigens, specific platelet antigens, or both. The incidence of HLA alloimmunization in patients receiving multiple platelet transfusion is between 30 and 60%. Once antibodies develop, platelets that contain the relevant antigens are rapidly destroyed.

Intensive chemotherapy for malignant disease and in preparation for bone marrow transplantation has caused a massive increase in the usage of platelet transfusions. Most of these patients require multiple platelet transfusions to prevent and treat thrombocytopenic bleeding. These patients may be exposed to many different donors with many HLA phenotypes, so alloimmunization is frequent. The clinical effect, of course, is that there is little or no response to platelet transfusions, and methods are suggested to reduce the degree of alloimmunization. One such method is platelet crossmatching (see section on Blood Component Therapy). This is a technically difficult procedure and is not routinely used in most laboratories. Matching for HLA antigens between the platelet donor and the recipient is used in individuals who are alloimmunized and who fail to get appropriate responses to platelet transfusions. Clearly, this limits the number of donors available, and although HLA-matched platelets are the most desirable product, they are logistically extremely difficult to obtain. Much current practice is aimed at reducing the number of donors to whom the patient is exposed, in an attempt to reduce alloimmunization. Similarly, depleting blood of contaminating leukocytes may also facilitate a reduction of alloimmunization. A complicating factor is that non-HLA platelet-derived antigens are not well understood. They may also be contributing to the degree of sensitization and lack of platelet response. It does appear, however, that platelets are less immunogenic if one or several HLA antigens are common to donor and recipient. When blood relatives are available as donors, complete HLA matching may be possible. In this case, reduction of donor exposure may allow decreased immunogenicity and sensitization. Even the use of unrelated donors with matching antigens is often better than completely random transfusion. Practical considerations do, however, complicate this provision. Technology and reagents exist for typing platelet donors, but the process is expensive and time consuming.

Antibody development becomes obvious when a patient no longer shows hemostatic improvement or when there is a reduced increment in the platelet count after platelet transfusion. At that point, the antibody must be identified and compatible donors found if further transfusions are to be effective. Screening for HLA antibodies and definition of HLA phenotypes is the most appropriate next step.

The kinds of white-cell antibodies that cause febrile transfusion reactions are not necessarily the same as those that destroy platelets. If a patient who repeatedly has febrile reactions is given platelet transfusions, the posttransfusion platelet response should be observed carefully. If platelet survival and therapeutic benefit are poor, the antibody must be identified and compatible platelets given.

HLA and Disease Association

Determining associations between diseases and HLA antigens is difficult because of the variety of phenotypes and disease presentations. Two major approaches are possible: (1) to compare the frequency of a specific antigen in a group of unrelated patients exhibiting the disease with its frequency in a control population (of the more than 150 HLA specificities, only about 20 are associated with diseases), and (2) to study families with known haplotypes to see whether a particular disease reliably occurs in individuals with a particular haplotype. In this way genetic factors coded within or near HLA complex antigens may be evaluated to confer susceptibility to the development of the disease. This susceptibility may be related to altered immunologic responsiveness.

The strongest associations between disease and HLA involve those between rheumatologic disorders and the antigen HLA-B27 and between narcolepsy and HLA-DR-2. Ankylosing spondylitis, a clearly defined subcategory of arthritis, is very closely tied to HLA-B27. This antigen occurs only in populations native to the northern hemisphere. World-wide, more than 90% of patients with ankylosing spondylitis are positive for B27, compared with 2.8% of control populations. Ankylosing spondylitis is virtually nonexistent in populations that lack B27. In populations possessing the antigen, the *relative risk* that a person having the antigen will also have the disease ranges from 49 in American blacks to more than 300 in Japan. Other arthritic syndromes, notably Reiter's syndrome (urethritis, arthritis, and conjunctivitis), juvenile rheumatoid arthritis, and arthritic complications of psoriasis, also show positivity with HLA-B27 (in descending order).

Associations have emerged between diseases of possible autoimmune etiology and antigens at the B and D loci. Myasthenia gravis, Addison's disease, and chronic active hepatitis are modestly associated with Dw3, and Sjögren's syndrome has a fairly strong association with this allele. Insulin-dependent diabetes mellitus has been linked with B8 and Bw15, as well as with Dw3 and Dw4. The nature of these associations suggests that one or two diabetogenic genes reside somewhere around or between the B and D loci, but their effect does not become apparent unless external influences also coincide.

Research is continuing in the associations of HLA typing and disease, and in particular in the understanding of the pathogenesis and immune relationships.

Paternity Testing and Parentage Assignment

HLA typing is well suited for parentage studies because the antigens are fully developed at birth, they are transmitted in simple codominant mendelian fashion, and great phenotypic diversity exists among unrelated individuals (see Fig. 8–9). Used in conjunction with red cell phenotyping, and even independently, HLA testing provides a precise means of parentage exclusion as well as probability inclusion. If the HLA phenotypes of a child and one parent are known, it becomes possible to assess fairly accurately whether or not a given individual is the other parent. In jurisdictions that allow HLA testing results as evidence, up to 75% of falsely accused men have been excluded from paternity with HLA testing alone. Strong (but by no means absolute) statistical support also can be presented that a given man is the father if the haplotype matches that of the putative father (Fig. 8–12). This is especially true if the haplotype is uncommon in the population under study.

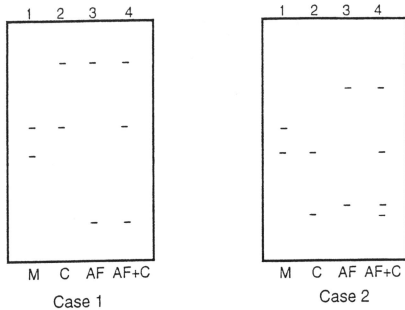

FIGURE 8–12. Diagrammatic example of DNA-RFLP analysis for paternity testing. In the two cases, two different sets of trios, mother (M), child (C), and alleged father (AF), are shown. Cut DNA fragments migrate to different positions based on their molecular weight. In lane 4, AF and C are mixed together in order to differentiate between two different bands that migrate to a similar position. In case 1, the alleged father cannot be excluded as the biologic father. Case 2 demonstrates a trio in which the alleged father can be excluded because, although the alleged father and child appear to have a similar band, the two bands are clearly separate in lane 4. (From Vengelen-Tyler, V (ed): Technical Manual, ed 12. American Association of Blood Banks, Bethesda, MD, 1996, p 324, with permission.)

SUGGESTED READING

Capon, SM, and Goldfinger, D: Acute hemolytic transfusion reaction, a paradigm of the systemic inflammatory response: New insights into pathophysiology and treatment. Transfusion 35:513–520, 1995.

Furie, B, Limentani, SA, and Rosenfield, CG: A practical guide to the evaluation and treatment of hemophilia. Blood 84:3–9, 1994.

Lublin, DM: Functional roles of blood group antigens. In Silverstein, LE (ed): Molecular and Functional Aspects of Blood Group Antigens. American Association of Blood Banks, Bethesda, MD, 1995, p. 163.

Mollison, PL, Englefriet, CP, and Contreras, M: Blood Transfusion in Clinical Medicine, ed 10. Blackwell Science, Oxford, 1997.

NIH Consensus Conference: Infectious disease testing for blood transfusions. JAMA 274:1374–1379, 1995.

Sacher, RA, and Brecher, ME (eds): Obstetric Transfusion Practice. American Association of Blood Banks, Bethesda, MD, 1993.

Vengelen-Tyler, V (ed): AABB Technical Manual, ed 12. American Association of Blood Banks, Bethesda, MD, 1996.

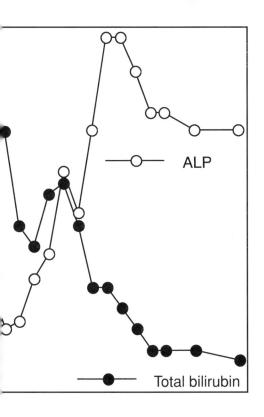

ALP

Total bilirubin

Section Four

Clinical Chemistry

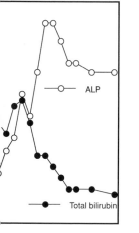

General Chemistry

SERUM CHEMISTRY ANALYSIS

The blood transports a large number of chemical substances throughout the body between organs and into the tissues. These substances reflect metabolic processes and disease states. Alterations in their concentrations are frequently useful in diagnosis and the planning and monitoring of therapy.

Those substances typically measured in serum fall generally into the following categories:

1. *Substances normally present with a function in the circulation:* glucose, sodium, potassium, chloride, bicarbonate, total proteins, albumin, calcium, magnesium, phosphorus, triglycerides, cholesterol, hormones (thyroxine, cortisol), vitamins (folate, B_{12}), individual proteins (haptoglobin, transferrin, immunoglobulins)
2. *Metabolites* (nonfunctioning waste products in the process of being cleared): urea, creatinine, uric acid, ammonia, bilirubin
3. *Substances released from cells as a result of cell damage and abnormal permeability or abnormal cellular proliferation* (usually enzymes/proteins): lactate dehydrogenase, alanine aminotransferase, aspartate aminotransferase, creatine kinase, amylase, gamma-glutamyltransferase, alkaline phosphatase, acid phosphatase, ferritin
4. *Drugs and toxic substances:* antibiotics (aminoglycosides), cardiac

445

(antiarrhythmics, digoxin), antiasthmatic (theophylline), anticonvulsants, salicylates, alcohol, and other substances of abuse

This chapter deals with several of the analytes most commonly
measured in serum. Other special chemical tests performed on serum or
plasma are described in separate chapters: Chapter 5, coagulation
proteins; Chapter 10, acid-base balance and electrolytes; Chapter 11,
enzymes; Chapter 12, liver functions; Chapters 16 and 17, hormones and
other endocrine markers; Chapter 18, drugs and toxic substances.

A special word should be said about *sample type.* The portion of the
blood that is in equilibrium with tissues and that contains substances
emanating from tissues is the **plasma.** Therefore, almost all blood
chemistry measurements are performed on plasma or more typically
on serum that is obtained after a blood sample has been clotted and
the clot separated by centrifugation. Serum is equivalent to plasma
with the prothrombin, factor VIII, factor V, and fibrinogen removed
(see Chapter 5). The use of serum instead of plasma also precludes
contamination of the specimen with an anticoagulant that may
interfere with one or more tests. Some substances do localize in
erythrocytes and therefore are usually measured in whole blood. These
include such determinations as blood gases (oxygen), the metal lead,
and the drug cyclosporin. However, the vast majority of chemical
substances in the plasma either are excluded from erythrocytes and the
other blood cells or are at much different concentrations intracellularly
than extracellularly. Thus precautions should always be taken to prevent
or minimize hemolysis in the collection of serum. Hemolysis can falsely
elevate serum levels of *potassium* and *lactate dehydrogenase* in particular
and may also cause methodologic interference in other tests due to release
of the pigment hemoglobin.

Serum has become the almost universally employed sample for
chemistry testing. To facilitate its collection and preparation, most
commercial blood drawing tubes have a vacuum sealed with a red rubber
stopper (i.e., red-topped tube). These tubes may contain a fine powder or
other nondissolving material that enhances clot formation at the contact
phase of coagulation. Some of these tubes also have at the bottom a gel
that settles out between the clot and the serum (serum separator tubes) on
centrifugation, thereby protecting the integrity of the serum sample
separate from cells in the clot. (These tubes cannot be used for blood bank
serology; see Chapter 8.)

Ever greater demands for faster turnaround times in critical care
situations and for simplified sample preparation in satellite sites and
physician office laboratories have led to new strategies for using whole
blood directly from a fingerstick drop or venipuncture samples anticoagulated with heparin. Future developments in blood chemistry testing will
most likely emerge in the fields of sample collection and analysis,
whereas the actual tests and their interpretation should remain very

much as detailed in this text. Emphasis is given to those substances most commonly measured.

CARBOHYDRATE METABOLISM

Oxidative metabolism of **glucose** provides most of the energy used in the body. Glucose is a simple six-carbon sugar. Glucose in the diet is largely present as **disaccharides** (i.e., chemically bonded to another sugar molecule: **sucrose** is glucose plus fructose; **lactose** is glucose plus galactose; **maltose** is two glucose molecules) and as the complex polysaccharide starch. The disaccharides are broken down into their constituent monosaccharides by enzymes called **disaccharidases** in the mucosa of the small intestine. These enzymes (**lactase, sucrase,** and **maltase**) are entirely specific for a single disaccharide. The starch is broken down by **amylase** secreted from the pancreas and also by the salivary glands. Sugars are absorbed by the intestine in the form of monosaccharides.

Glucose metabolism generates pyruvic acid, lactic acid, and acetylcoenzyme A (acetyl-CoA) as intermediary compounds. The complete oxidation of glucose yields carbon dioxide, water, and energy that is stored as the high-energy phosphate compound **adenosine triphosphate (ATP).**

If not immediately metabolized to produce energy, glucose can be stored in liver or muscle as **glycogen,** a polymer consisting of numerous glucose residues in a form available for subsequent release and metabolism of glucose. The liver can also convert glucose through other metabolic pathways into fatty acids, which are stored as triglycerides, or into amino acids for use in protein synthesis. Because of its large volume and its content of enzymes for multiple metabolic conversions, the liver plays a pivotal role in distributing glucose for immediate energy need or for storage and structural purposes as well. If glycogen becomes depleted and available glucose is insufficient for energy needs, the liver can synthesize glucose from fatty acids, and also from amino acids (gluconeogenesis).

The energy for most cellular and tissue functions derives from glucose. Alternative energy generation can derive from metabolism of fatty acids, but this pathway is less efficient than burning glucose and creates acid metabolites that can be harmful if allowed to accumulate. Therefore glucose in the blood is controlled by several homeostatic mechanisms that in health maintain levels in the range 70 to 110 mg/dL in the fasting state. Following ingestion of a meal with a heavy glucose load, blood glucose normally does not exceed about 170 mg/dL. Many hormones participate in maintaining adequate blood glucose levels in steady-state conditions or in response to stress (Table 9–1). Measurement of blood glucose is frequently performed to monitor the overall success of these regulatory

TABLE 9-1. HORMONES THAT INFLUENCE BLOOD GLUCOSE LEVEL

Hormone	Tissue of Origin	Metabolic Effect	Effect on Blood Glucose
Insulin	Pancreatic β cells	1. Enhances entry of glucose into cells 2. Enhances storage of glucose as glycogen, or conversion to fatty acids 3. Enhances synthesis of proteins and fatty acids 4. Suppresses breakdown of protein into amino acids, of adipose tissue into free fatty acids	Lowers
Somatostatin	Pancreatic D cells	1. Suppresses glucagon release from α cells (acts locally) 2. Suppresses release of insulin, pituitary tropic hormones, gastrin, and secretin	Raises
Glucagon	Pancreatic α cells	1. Enhances release of glucose from glycogen 2. Enhances synthesis of glucose from amino acids or fatty acids	Raises
Epinephrine	Adrenal medulla	1. Enhances release of glucose from glycogen 2. Enhances release of fatty acids from adipose tissue	Raises
Cortisol	Adrenal cortex	1. Enhances synthesis of glucose from amino acids or fatty acids 2. Antagonizes insulin	Raises
ACTH	Anterior pituitary	1. Enhances release of cortisol 2. Enhances release of fatty acids from adipose tissue	Raises
Growth hormone	Anterior pituitary	1. Antagonizes insulin	Raises
Thyroxine	Thyroid	1. Enhances release of glucose from glycogen 2. Enhances absorption of sugars from intestine	Raises

Adapted from Howanitz, PJ, and Howanitz JH: Carbohydrates. In Henry, JB (ed): Clinical Diagnosis and Management by Laboratory Methods, ed 17. WB Saunders, Philadelphia, 1984, p 165, and Guyton, AC: Textbook of Medical Physiology, ed 7. WB Saunders, Philadelphia, 1986.

mechanisms. Pronounced deviation from normal, either too high or too low, indicates faulty homeostasis and should initiate a search for the etiology.

GLUCOSE MEASUREMENT

Sample Type

Historically, blood glucose values were given in terms of whole blood, but most laboratories now measure the serum glucose level. Because erythrocytes have a higher concentration of protein (i.e., hemoglobin) than serum, serum has a higher water content and consequently more dissolved glucose than does whole blood. To convert from whole-blood glucose, multiply the value by 1.15 to give the serum or plasma level.

Collection of blood in clot (red-top) tubes for serum chemistry analysis permits the metabolism of glucose in the sample by blood cells until separated by centrifugation. Very high white cell counts can lead to excessive glycolysis in the sample with substantial reduction in glucose level. Ambient temperature at which the blood sample is kept prior to separation also affects the rate of glycolysis. At refrigerator temperatures, glucose remains relatively stable for several hours in blood. At room temperature, a loss of 1 to 2% of glucose/hour should be expected. This loss is not significant for hospital laboratories that process blood samples soon after they are drawn. However, if blood samples are sent a long distance to reference laboratories, there may be opportunity for substantial loss of glucose to glycolysis by the blood cells. This problem can be circumvented by using fluoride-containing (gray-top) tubes that inhibit glycolysis, thereby preserving the glucose level even at room temperature. Gray-top tubes are generally employed when glucose levels are to be used for diagnostic purposes (e.g., in the initial diagnosis of diabetes). Red-top serum separator tubes also preserve glucose in samples once they have been centrifuged to isolate the serum from the cells. Serum separator tubes are generally used for the majority of glucose determinations (e.g., both outpatient screening and inpatient monitoring of intravenous [IV] fluid therapy), since other analytes can be measured on the same serum samples. Particular care should be given to drawing blood samples from the arm opposite the one in which an intravenous line is inserted, to prevent contamination of the sample with intravenous fluids. Alternatively blood can be drawn from the same arm with an IV if the IV is first turned off for at least 5 minutes and the arm is elevated to drain the infused fluids away from the vein. As little as 10% contamination with 5% dextrose (D5W) will elevate glucose in a sample by 500 mg/dL or more. Arterial, capillary, and venous blood have comparable glucose levels in a fasting individual, whereas after meals venous levels are lower than those in arterial or capillary blood.

Methodology

There are two different major methodologies that have been used to measure glucose. The older one is a chemical method that exploits the nonspecific *reducing property of glucose* in a reaction with an indicator substance that acquires or changes color on its reduction. Since other compounds also present in blood are reducing substances (e.g., urea, which can build up to appreciable levels in uremia), glucose measurement can be 5 to 15 mg/dL erroneously higher by reducing methods than by more accurate *enzymatic methods* that are highly specific for glucose. These enzymatic methods generally employ the enzymes **glucose oxidase** or **hexokinase,** which act on glucose but not on other sugars and not on other reducing substances. The enzymatic conversion of glucose to product is now quantitated on automated chemistry analyzers by a color change reaction as the last of a series of coupled chemical reactions or by the consumption of oxygen on an oxygen-sensing electrode. By making several measurements over a period of minutes, modern chemistry analyzers can calculate the rate of the reaction, which is proportional to concentration of glucose. This kinetic analysis is technically preferable to endpoint analysis, by which only the final amount of product is measured. In general, kinetic analysis is superior to endpoint for many common chemical measurements due to the shorter time period required for each assay and also because interferences in endpoint assays can frequently be nullified in measuring reaction rates.

Outside of the clinical laboratory, there are presently available several brands of personal glucose monitors that diabetic patients can use for measuring their own glucose levels in a drop of blood from a fingerstick. These glucose meters are extremely useful for providing fast and frequent feedback to the patient for changing medication and therapy. Many personal glucose meters have the disadvantage that low hematocrit falsely elevates the glucose result and conversely, high hematocrit falsely lowers the result. This hematocrit effect (and a similar one for high or low protein in serum) is probable cause for many discrepancies noted between glucose values measured in blood samples sent to a hospital laboratory and simultaneously performed by a patient on a personal glucose meter. Consequently patients who use personal glucose meters should periodically (e.g., every few weeks) check them against clinical laboratory glucose measurements (the gold standard) on their own blood to account for possible physiologic interferences as well as fluctuations in meter function.

Whereas the measurement of blood glucose concentration provides information about immediate glucose homeostasis, evaluation of long-term glucose control (e.g., over the previous few weeks) is available from measurement of **glycosylated hemoglobin** in erythrocytes. Hemoglobin is glycosylated spontaneously in the circulation with larger amounts formed when blood glucose levels are high. Glycosylated hemoglobin is measured by electrophoretic or affinity chromatographic methods on a lysate of washed erythrocytes (see Chapter 16).

Clinical Correlation

The **fasting blood glucose** level gives the best indication of overall glucose homeostasis, and most routine determinations should be done on fasting samples. Conditions that affect glucose levels are shown in Table 9–2. They reflect abnormalities in the multiple control mechanisms of glucose regulation.

The metabolic response to a carbohydrate challenge is conveniently assessed by the postprandial glucose level drawn 2 hours after a meal

---

TABLE 9–2. CAUSES OF ABNORMAL GLUCOSE LEVELS

Reference Range, Fasting Serum Glucose: 70–110 mg/dL

Persistent Hyperglycemia:

Diabetes mellitus
Adrenal cortical hyperactivity (Cushing's syndrome)
Hyperthyroidism
Acromegaly
Obesity

Transient Hyperglycemia:

Pheochromocytoma
Severe liver disease
Acute stress reaction (physical or emotional)
Shock
Convulsions

Persistent Hypoglycemia:

Insulinoma
Adrenal cortical insufficiency (Addison's disease)
Hypopituitarism
Galactosemia
Ectopic insulin production from tumors

Transient Hypoglycemia:

Acute alcohol ingestion
Drugs: salicylates, antituberculosis agents
Severe liver disease
Several glycogen storage diseases
"Functional" hypoglycemia
Hereditary fructose intolerance

or a glucose load. In addition, the glucose tolerance test, consisting of serial timed measurements after a standardized amount of oral glucose intake, is used to aid in the diagnosis of diabetes. These applications are given more detailed consideration in the section on the pancreas (see Chapter 16).

OTHER SUGARS

High blood and urine **fructose** levels occur in patients with any of several relatively uncommon enzyme deficiencies **(essential fructosuria).** When reducing methods were used for glucose determinations, **fructosemia** was readily detected as an unexpectedly high blood sugar level. Now that most tests use glucose-specific enzyme techniques, fructosemia will be diagnosed only if specifically sought. Patients with hereditary fructose intolerance (deficiency of fructose-1-phosphate aldolase) experience severe hypoglycemia and hypophosphatemia after exposure to fructose or to table sugar (sucrose), which consists of one glucose and one fructose moiety. Lack of a different fructose-related enzyme impairs the ability to synthesize glucose from other sugars; hypoglycemia develops if there is no glycogen available as a reserve source of glucose.

Galactosemia results from deficiency of any of several galactose-metabolizing enzymes. Because severe mental and physical changes accompany prolonged galactosemia in infancy, it is important to test newborn infants for the presence of excess galactose. Screening tests are done on urine, but galactose will be detected only if the test is done after the infant begins to ingest milk. More definitive blood tests are indicated if screening results are abnormal.

The deposition and retrieval of glucose into and out of glycogen involve myriad enzymes; congenital deficiency states have been identified for a great many of these. Collectively designated **glycogen storage diseases,** they have an overall incidence of 1 in 40,000, with diverse clinical signs and population distribution. Definitive diagnosis requires enzyme analysis, but screening procedures include measuring fasting blood glucose and observing responses to glucose load, to glucagon infusion, to muscular exertion, and to other stimuli.

For additional discussion of carbohydrate abnormalities, see Chapter 16.

NONPROTEIN NITROGENOUS COMPOUNDS

This group of chemical substances refers to low-molecular-weight compounds that contain nitrogen and are distinguished from proteins. **Nonprotein nitrogen (NPN)** includes urea, creatinine, uric acid, ammonia, and amino acids. These compounds are by-products of protein or nucleic acid metabolism. They are present in concentrations of milligrams/deciliter or less because of ready clearance into the urine. In the past, before specific analyses were available, NPN measurement was used as an index of renal function. However, modern assays for the individual compounds has made NPN determination obsolete.

UREA

Metabolism

Amino groups are exchanged between amino acids as catalyzed by **aminotransferases** in many tissues of the body. In addition, amino groups are removed from amino acids in the transformation and recycling of the amino acid pool. The liberated amino groups are converted to ammonia that travels to the liver where it is incorporated into *urea* in a metabolic pathway referred to as the urea cycle. Urea is a small molecule with the following chemical structure:

$$\underset{H_2N-C-NH_2}{\overset{\overset{\textstyle O}{\|}}{}} \qquad \begin{array}{l} \text{Urea} \\ \text{molecular weight } = 60 \text{ daltons} \end{array}$$

Urea diffuses freely into both intracellular and extracellular fluid. It is concentrated in the urine for excretion. In stable nitrogen balance, about 25 g urea is excreted daily. Levels in the blood reflect the balance between production and excretion of urea.

Measurement

Chemical methods for determining urea have been largely replaced by enzymatic methods utilizing **urease** and therefore are highly specific for urea. By convention in the United States, urea assays are calibrated and values expressed as the nitrogen content of the molecule, also referred to as **blood urea nitrogen (BUN).** Normal serum concentration of BUN is roughly 5 to 20 mg/dL. In other countries, values are expressed as total weight of urea instead of nitrogen content. Nitrogen contributes 28/60 to the total weight of urea; the concentration of urea can be calculated by multiplying BUN concentration by 60/28, or 2.14.

Clinical Considerations

Blood urea nitrogen derives from breakdown of protein, primarily dietary in origin. Men have slightly higher mean values than do women. Blood

TABLE 9–3. COMMON CAUSES OF UREMIA

Prerenal:
Reduced blood flow to kidney
  Shock, blood loss, dehydration
Increased protein catabolism
  Crush injuries, burns, fever, hemorrhage into soft tissues or body cavities, hemolysis
Renal:
Acute renal failure
  Glomerulonephritis, malignant hypertension, nephrotoxic drugs or metals, renal cortical
    necrosis
Chronic renal disease
  Glomerulonephritis, pyelonephritis, diabetes mellitus, arteriosclerosis, amyloidosis,
    renal tubular disease, collagen-vascular diseases
Postrenal:
Ureteral obstruction by stones, tumor, inflammation, surgical misadventure; obstruction of
  bladder neck or urethra by prostate, stones, tumor, inflammation

urea nitrogen is usually on the high side of the normal range in otherwise healthy individuals whose diet is heavy in protein on a long-term basis. Low levels of BUN are not generally considered abnormal. They may be due to low protein in the diet or to expansion of plasma volume. A very low level of BUN is an important finding in severe hepatic disease, signifying that the liver is not able to synthesize urea from ammonia in the circulation.

The condition of high urea levels is called **uremia** (although in common parlance uremia is often used to refer to elevations of all nitrogenous wastes). Its most common cause is renal failure resulting in impaired excretion. **Azotemia** refers to elevation of all the low molecular weight nitrogenous compounds in renal failure. **Prerenal uremia** means an elevation of BUN due to some mechanism acting prior to filtration of the blood by the glomeruli. These causes include markedly reduced blood flow to the kidney as in shock, dehydration, or increased catabolism of protein such as massive bleeding into the gastrointestinal tract with digestion of the hemoglobin and its absorption as protein in the diet. **Postrenal uremia** occurs when there is obstruction of the lower urinary tract in the ureters, bladder, or urethra that prevents excretion of urine. The urea in the backed-up urine can diffuse back into the bloodstream. **Renal** causes of uremia include diseases or toxicities that affect either the glomeruli and renal microvasculature or the renal tubules. Causes of elevated BUN are listed in Table 9–3.

CREATININE

Metabolism

Creatinine is the endproduct of creatine metabolism. Creatine is present mostly in skeletal muscle, where it is involved in energy storage as **creatine phosphate (CP).** Creatine phosphate is converted to creatine in the synthesis of ATP from ADP catalyzed by the enzyme creatine kinase (CK).

This reaction continues as energy is utilized and CP is regenerated. In the process, small amounts of creatine are irreversibly converted to creatinine, which is removed from the circulation by the kidneys. The amount of creatinine generated in an individual is proportional to the mass of skeletal muscle present. Reference values for creatinine are 0.6 to 1.3 mg/dL for men and 0.5 to 1.0 mg/dL for women.

The daily generation of creatinine remains fairly constant, with the exceptions of crushing injury or degenerative disease that causes massive damage to muscle. The kidneys excrete creatinine very efficiently. Levels of blood flow and urine production affect creatinine excretion much less than they affect urea excretion because temporary alterations in blood flow and glomerular activity are compensated by increased tubular secretion of creatinine into urine. Blood concentration and daily urinary excretion of creatinine in an individual fluctuate very little. Consequently, serial measurements of creatinine excretion are useful in determining whether 24-hour urine specimens for other analyses (e.g., steroids) have been completely and accurately collected.

Clinical Considerations

Blood creatinine becomes elevated when renal function declines. If slow loss of renal function occurs simultaneously with slow loss of muscle mass, the concentration of creatinine in serum may remain stable, but 24-hour excretion (or clearance) rates would be lower than normal. This pattern may happen in aging patients. Thus a better index of renal function is **creatinine clearance,** which takes into account both serum creatinine and the quantity excreted in a day (see Chapter 19).

BUN and creatinine are almost always ordered together on the same blood sample to assess renal function. The ratio of BUN (expressed as mg of urea nitrogen/dL) to creatinine (expressed as mg of creatinine/dL) is a convenient index to distinguish between possible causes of uremia (Table 9–4). The BUN/creatinine ratio is usually in the range of 12 to 20. Elevated levels of BUN in a patient with normal creatinine indicate a nonrenal cause for the uremia (usually prerenal). Blood urea nitrogen rises more steeply than creatinine with declining renal function. With dialysis or successful renal transplantation, the urea falls more rapidly than creatinine. With severe long-term renal impairment, urea levels continue to climb, whereas creatinine levels tend to plateau, perhaps due to excretion across the alimentary tract.

TABLE 9–4. CONDITIONS AFFECTING BUN/CREATININE RATIO

Reference Range: 12 to 20

Low: <12
Hepatic disease or failure
Low protein diet/starvation
Acute tubular necrosis

High: >20
With normal creatinine values
Prerenal uremia
High protein diet
Gastrointestinal hemorrhage
Catabolic states
With high creatinine values
Prerenal azotemia with renal disease
Renal failure
Postrenal azotemia

Uric Acid

URIC ACID

Metabolism

Uric acid is produced as the endproduct of purine metabolism in humans. Purines (adenine and guanine) are constituents of nucleic acids. Purine turnover occurs continuously in the body with RNA and DNA synthesis and degradation, so that substantial amounts of uric acid are produced even in the absence of dietary purine intake. Uric acid is synthesized primarily in the liver, a reaction catalyzed by the enzyme xanthine oxidase. Uric acid then travels through the blood to the kidneys, where it is filtered, partially reabsorbed, and partially further secreted before final excretion in the urine. On a low-purine diet, daily excretion is about 0.5 g; on a normal diet, excretion is about 1 g daily. Organ meats, legumes, and yeast are especially high in purines.

Hyperuricemia

Uric acid is poorly soluble in water, and urate crystals readily precipitate from urine with high concentrations of urate to produce urate kidney stones. Similarly, patients with high blood uric acid levels often deposit urate crystals in soft tissues, especially joints. This clinical syndrome is **gout.** The crystals in tissues cause an inflammatory response, with release of enzymes from leukocytes and local tissue damage that leads to an acid environment favorable to formation of more urate crystals, and so forth, in a renewed cycle. The result is painful swollen and inflamed joints. Urate stones sometimes occur in patients with gout, but normouricemic persons (i.e., those with normal uric acid levels in the blood) may have urate stones if urinary levels of uric acid are excessive. The reference range of uric acid in serum is higher in healthy men than in healthy women (see Fig. 1–7), leading to a greater propensity for men to develop gout.

Both the amount of uric acid produced and the efficiency of renal excretion affect serum urate levels. Uric acid production is increased by idiopathic mechanisms associated with gout. It is also increased in proportion to cell turnover due to the degradation of nucleic acids, as with leukemia or other malignancies with a large cell mass. Cytolytic therapy of malignances should be expected to result in extremely high levels of uric acid for periods of days. In such instances it is necessary to take special precautions to prevent acute renal failure due to precipitation of urates in the kidneys. Renal failure, of course, causes uric acid and also urea and creatinine to accumulate. Thiazide diuretics and low doses of aspirin diminish urate excretion. Allopurinol, probenecid, corticosteroids, and large doses of aspirin increase urate excretion.

Although symptoms of gout occur during periods when blood urates are high, many people have hyperuricemia without gouty symptoms or urinary problems, indicating that multiple factors probably modulate urate precipitation. **Primary gout** occurs due to overproduction of uric acid or impaired renal tubular excretion. **Secondary gout** results from excessive urate production following massive nucleic acid turnover or from acquired renal disorders that diminish urate excretion. These conditions affecting serum urate levels are shown in Table 9–5.

Treatment

Uric acid production can be reduced by administering the drug, allopurinol, which inhibits xanthine oxidase activity, thereby lowering serum urate level without imposing an increased excretory load on the kidneys. The uricosuric agents probenecid and sulfinpyrazone lower serum urates by increasing the uric acid content of urine, which could lead to stone formation. Patients taking these agents must maintain a high volume of alkaline urine to keep the urates in solution. Colchicine, a drug long used to treat gouty arthritis, affects neither production nor excretion of urate, but rather alters the phagocytic response of leukocytes to urate crystals in tissue.

OTHER NPN COMPOUNDS

Ammonia and **amino acids** constitute most of the remaining low-molecular-weight nitrogenous compounds. Ammonia is discussed under liver functions tests (see Chapter 12). It is not measured as a screening test but rather for special instances such as hepatic failure causing encephalopathy. The 20 different amino acids are likewise not usually measured except in special circumstances for the evaluation of some congenital or acquired abnormalities in the metabolism of specific amino acids or in the evaluation of some causes of liver failure.

TABLE 9–5. FACTORS AFFECTING SERUM URIC ACID LEVELS

Reference Range: 4–8.5 mg/dL for Men; 2.7–7.3 mg/dL for Women

---

Increased Production, Raised Serum Levels:
Idiopathic mechanisms associated with primary gout
Excessive dietary purines (organ meats, legumes, anchovies, etc.)
Cytolytic treatment of malignancies, especially leukemias and lymphomas
Polycythemia
Myeloid metaplasia
Psoriasis
Sickle cell anemia

Decreased Excretion, Raised Serum Levels:
Alcohol ingestion
Thiazide diuretics
Lactic acidosis
Aspirin doses < 2 g/day
Ketoacidosis, especially diabetes or starvation
Renal failure, any cause

Increased Excretion, Lowered Serum Levels:
Probenecid, sulfinpyrazone, aspirin doses above 4 g/day
Corticosteroids and ACTH
Coumarin anticoagulants
Estrogens

Decreased Production, Lowered Serum Levels:
Allopurinol

From Woo, J, and Cannon, DC: Metabolic intermediates and inorganic ions. In Henry, JB (ed): Clinical Diagnosis and Management by Laboratory Methods, ed 17. WB Saunders, Philadelphia, 1984, p 133, with permission.

BILIRUBIN

METABOLISM

The normal metabolic processing of hemoglobin after its release from aging erythrocytes leads to production of the small molecule heme (see Chapter 2). Breakdown of muscle also results in the production of heme in a lesser amount as myoglobin is degraded. Heme in turn loses its iron atom and is oxidized to form the yellow pigment **bilirubin,** which is highly insoluble in water. Bilirubin does bind to albumin, enabling it to be transported throughout the body. In this form, the molecular species is termed "unconjugated bilirubin." As it circulates through the liver, hepatocytes perform the following functions:

1. uptake of bilirubin from the circulation
2. enzymatic conjugation as bilirubin glucuronides
3. transport and excretion of conjugated bilirubin into the bile for elimination from the body.

Congenital defects in each of these metabolic steps are recognized clinically:

1. defect in uptake: **Gilbert syndrome**
2. defect in hepatic glucuronyl transferase: **Crigler-Najjar syndrome**
3. defect in transport extracellularly: **Dubin-Johnson syndrome**

The intracellular conjugation of glucuronic acid onto two sites of the bilirubin molecule confers negative charge to it, thereby making "conjugated bilirubin" soluble in aqueous phase. If there is obstruction or other failure to excrete this conjugated bilirubin, it will re-enter the circulation, where it can accumulate. Functioning hepatocytes will attempt to take up conjugated bilirubin as they do the unconjugated form in step 1. A further chemical change can occur when conjugated bilirubin remains in the circulation at high levels for a prolonged time. In that instance, there is spontaneous formation of a covalent bond between conjugated bilirubin and albumin. This chemical species will not be taken up by the liver and has a long half-life in the circulation.

Once bile enters the intestine, colonic bacteria convert bilirubin to **urobilinogen,** a collective term for several colorless compounds that subsequently undergo oxidation to the brown pigment **urobilin.** Urobilin is excreted in the feces, but urobilinogen is in part reabsorbed through the intestine, and through the portal circulation is picked up by the liver and re-excreted in bile. Since urobilinogen is freely water soluble, it can also pass out through the urine if it reaches the kidneys.

MEASUREMENT

Although bilirubin is normally only a minor constituent of bile (outweighed 20 to 1 by the bile salts), measurement of bilirubin in serum is relatively simple to perform in the laboratory, and is frequently used as a sensitive indicator of hepatic functions. For clinical purposes, bilirubin is expressed as two components. These are the unconjugated insoluble form referred to as "indirect" or "prehepatic" and the conjugated soluble form described as "direct" or "posthepatic." Direct bilirubin is measured by a specific chemical reaction (diazotization) without any modification since it is water soluble. Indirect bilirubin is not quantitated separately, but instead is calculated as the difference between *total bilirubin* and the direct fraction. Measurement of total bilirubin involves solubilization of the unconjugated form before chemical quantitation. For health screening examinations, total bilirubin measurement usually suffices, since a major increase in direct bilirubin would also be reflected in the total. Most clinical laboratories report only direct and total bilirubin (which are the actual measurements), leaving calculation of the indirect fraction to the physician.

A variation on this measurement strategy is offered by slide chemistry methods (*Vitros* from Johnson and Johnson, formerly *Ektachem* from Kodak) in which both unconjugated and conjugated fractions are directly quantitated.

Optimal serum specimens for bilirubin determination should be free from hemolysis, lipemia, or other sources of abnormal pigment or turbidity that could interfere with the optical detection of the colored product in some methods of bilirubin analysis. Exposure of a specimen to light can reduce serum bilirubin concentrations. This effect is particularly important in monitoring neonatal jaundice, where the actual level is very important but the specimens are usually small (e.g., microcollections from heel sticks) thereby allowing incident light to penetrate further and denature bilirubin throughout a stored sample. Phototherapy of infants is also used clinically to lower bilirubin levels in the patient.

CLINICAL CONSIDERATIONS

Jaundice is the visible yellow discoloration of skin and sclerae that arises when serum total bilirubin levels exceed 2.0 or 2.5 mg/dL. Table 9–6 lists clinically significant causes of hyperbilirubinemia. In the serum of adults, the expected range of direct bilirubin is up to 0.3 mg/dL, and that of total

---

TABLE 9–6. CAUSES OF HYPERBILIRUBINEMIA

Reference Range: 0.3–1.1 mg/dL Total; 0.1–0.4 mg/dL Direct

Increased Indirect (Unconjugated) Bilirubin:

Hemolysis; hemoglobinopathies; spherocytosis; G-6-PD deficiency; autoimmunity; hemolytic transfusion reaction

Red cell degradation: hemorrhage into soft tissues or body cavities; inefficient erythropoiesis; pernicious anemia

Defective hepatocellular uptake or conjugation: viral hepatitis; hereditary enzyme deficiencies (Gilbert, Crigler-Najjar syndromes); hepatic immaturity, in newborns

Increased Direct (Conjugated) Bilirubin:

Intrahepatic disruption: viral hepatitis; alcoholic hepatitis; chlorpromazine; cirrhosis

Bile duct disease: biliary cirrhosis; cholangitis (idiopathic, infectious); biliary atresia

Extrahepatic bile duct obstruction: gallstones; carcinoma of gallbladder, bile ducts, or head of pancreas; bile duct stricture, from inflammation or surgical misadventure

bilirubin is 0.1 to 1.2 mg/dL. Occasionally, healthy adults have normal direct bilirubin with a total of 2.0 mg/dL or greater. Such individuals may have a mild defect in the uptake of bilirubin by the liver, a variation of **Gilbert's syndrome** (see Chapter 12). This degree of unconjugated hyperbilirubinemia may be exacerbated in Gilbert's syndrome by the fasting state.

Neonatal "physiologic" jaundice reflects both increased loads of hemoglobin breakdown and immaturity of the liver in its ability to conjugate bilirubin. Any hemolytic abnormality can be expected to increase the flow of bilirubin through its metabolic intermediates (prehepatic jaundice). In patients with normal hepatic function, an increased load of bilirubin from hemoglobin will result in a mild increase of indirect bilirubin typically not above 5 mg/dL, but the direct bilirubin will likely remain normal if the liver's excretory capacity is intact. As a consequence of more conjugated bilirubin in the intestines, there will be greater amounts of urobilinogen in the gut with reabsorption and excretion into the urine.

Hepatic testing is discussed further in Chapter 12. Generally, the direct and indirect fractions are used to determine whether liver disease primarily involves hepatocellular function (hepatic jaundice) (e.g., high total bilirubin, low direct) or a posthepatic block (e.g., high total bilirubin, high direct) (posthepatic jaundice). Frequently a patient with liver disease can go through different stages in which hepatic or posthepatic jaundice predominates.

Elevation of direct bilirubin in serum for whatever reason permits this water-soluble species to pass into the urine, where it appears as bright yellow and can be detected on dipstick analysis as "bile" (see Chapter 19).

Biliary obstruction with prolonged elevation of conjugated bilirubin in serum leads to the formation of **delta bilirubin.** This species of bilirubin molecule has only recently been recognized. Its significance comes in monitoring the timely descent of serum bilirubin after surgical correction of biliary obstruction (e.g., gallstones). Instead of leaving the circulation once biliary excretion is re-established, delta bilirubin can remain elevated (reacting as direct bilirubin) for weeks despite normal hepatic function. Thus delta bilirubin must be recognized as a possible cause of persistent direct hyperbilirubinemia that has no pathologic repercussion.

CALCIUM, MAGNESIUM, AND PHOSPHORUS

Calcium and magnesium both occur as divalent cations (Ca^{2+} and Mg^{2+}) in aqueous solution. The reference range for serum calcium is 9 to 11 mg/dL (4.5 to 5.5 mEq/L). For serum magnesium, the reference range is 1.8 to 3.0 mg/dL (1.3 to 2.1 mEq/L). Roughly one half of the total calcium and magnesium circulates as free ions in plasma, while the remaining amount is bound by charge interaction to negatively charged proteins (predominantly albumin) or complexed with small anions (Fig. 9–1).

The free (or ionized) fraction of calcium is physiologically active. The bound fraction is not active and does not play an immediate role in the endocrine control of calcium. Calcium participates in blood coagulation

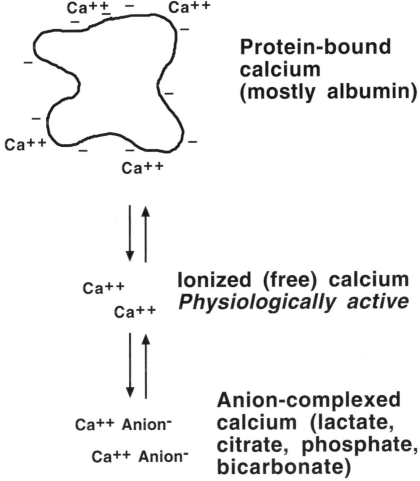

Protein-bound calcium (mostly albumin)

Ionized (free) calcium *Physiologically active*

Anion-complexed calcium (lactate, citrate, phosphate, bicarbonate)

FIGURE 9–1. Calcium in plasma can be in one of three forms that are in equilibrium with one another: (1) bound to negatively charged proteins, (2) free or ionized, and (3) complexed with small anionic species. Total calcium measurements quantitate all three forms together; ionized calcium measurements are done with ion-selective electrodes. Ionized calcium is the physiologically active form.

and also in skeletal and cardiac muscle contractility and in multiple membrane and cellular functions. Both calcium and magnesium are important in neuromuscular conduction and activation.

Phosphates, along with sugar moieties, form the backbone of both nucleic acids RNA and DNA. Phosphates are also essential for intracellular storage and conversion of energy (ATP, creatine phosphate), for the intermediary compounds of carbohydrate metabolism, and in regulatory compounds such as 2,3-diphosphoglycerate, which modulates the dissociation of oxygen from hemoglobin.

METABOLISM

Calcium and phosphorus are generally considered together in routine clinical evaluations. These ions are in a continuous flux that is controlled by action of **parathyroid hormone (PTH), vitamin D,** and **calcitonin.** The amount present in serum at any one time is small compared with the major reservoir within bone. Serum levels do reflect overall mineral metabolism and, hence, the activity of the parathyroid glands. Parathyroid hormone secretion into the blood is stimulated by lowering the calcium concentration (actually the free or "ionized" fraction of calcium). Parathyroid hormone acts to elevate calcium levels by increasing the resorption of calcium from bone and suppressing loss of calcium into the urine. Vitamin D promotes absorption of calcium and phosphorus by the intestine and accelerates turnover of the minerals in bone.

Calcium phosphate has a solubility limit that restricts how high each can rise before the other is suppressed in a reciprocal relationship. This effect is strikingly important in renal disease that causes chronically elevated serum phosphate levels. In that situation, the serum calcium level (in particular the ionized calcium) will fall. However, the resulting hypocalcemia in turn stimulates PTH secretion that mobilizes calcium from deposits in bone. Long-term consequences include serious demineralization of the skeleton and secondary hyperparathyroidism with hyperplasia of that gland.

Magnesium levels usually parallel those of calcium when abnormalities occur. However, there is no large body reservoir from which to mobilize magnesium in order to replenish it as there is for calcium. Thus deficiency states of magnesium can arise and may require dietary supplementation to correct.

CLINICAL CONSIDERATIONS

Disorders of Calcium Homeostasis

Parathyroid disease, metabolic bone diseases, and disorders of **vitamin D metabolism** are usual causes of serum calcium abnormalities (see

Chapter 16). **Hypercalcemia** is a common problem in some **malignancies** with and without bone involvement, in **multiple myeloma** (lytic lesions of bone), and in the granulomatous disease **sarcoidosis.** Hypercalcemia can produce startling changes in the mental abilities of patients, leading to confusion and inability to communicate. Hypercalcemia is sometimes present in hyperthyroidism.

Hypocalcemia, as measured in the laboratory, can be a consequence of **reduced albumin** levels. In this situation, the fraction of bound calcium is reduced independently of the ionized fraction, which should remain normal. **True hypocalcemia** frequently develops as a serious medical emergency in **pancreatitis** due to sequestration of ionized calcium in the damaged tissue and surrounding fluid. Hypocalcemia produces neurologic irritability, commonly manifesting with tetany (muscular spasm and twitching, especially evident in the hands and facial muscles). This severe form of hypocalcemia requires immediate correction with intravenous calcium infusion. Patients suffering from chronic renal disease usually must take calcium supplements in the diet. Surgical removal of the parathyroids (as with complete thyroidectomy) also results in lifelong hypocalcemia requiring continuous replacement therapy. Various causes of calcium abnormalities are listed in Table 9–7. Functional hypocalcemia with reduction in ionized calcium but normal total calcium can also occur following massive transfusion due to large amounts of citrate in the blood products that complex with free calcium in the patient.

TABLE 9–7. CONDITIONS THAT AFFECT SERUM CALCIUM

Reference Range: 9–11 mg/dL, 4.5–5.5 mEq/L

Causes of Hypercalcemia:
Hyperparathyroidism, primary
Hyperparathyroidism, secondary to renal disease
Ectopic production of PTH-like material
Malignant tumors, mechanisms various or unknown
Sarcoidosis, mechanism unknown
Skeletal immobilization
Vitamin D intoxication
Hyperthyroidism
Excessive calcium intake (milk-alkali syndrome)

Causes of Hypocalcemia:
Hypoparathyroidism, usually due to operation
Unresponsiveness to PTH (pseudohypoparathyroidism)
Vitamin D deficiency
Unresponsiveness to vitamin D (vitamin D–resistant rickets)
Malabsorption syndromes: calcium, phosphate, vitamin D, or combination
Acute pancreatitis

Disorders of Phosphate Homeostasis

The equilibrium between serum phosphates and intracellular phosphate stores is determined largely by carbohydrate metabolism and blood pH. Phosphate is essential for the insulin-mediated entry of glucose into cells by a process involving phosphorylation of the glucose plus the co-entry of potassium. Acidotic diabetic patients who have lost phosphates and water by solute diuresis may experience a sudden drop in serum phosphate levels when treated with insulin and fluid expansion. Even normal individuals will show a slight reduction of the serum phosphate levels after a meal of carbohydrates.

Disorders of Magnesium Homeostasis

Magnesium levels usually fall in parallel with reduction in calcium due to their similar binding onto albumin. Malabsorption and starvation can lead to magnesium deficiency with serum levels reflecting depletion of body stores only late in the course. Chronic diarrhea and use of potent diuretic agents can also lead to hypomagnesemia. Chemical correction of calcium loss sometimes may not produce the expected clinical improvement of neurologic or cardiac status of a patient until a coexisting deficiency of magnesium is recognized and treated. Disorders of magnesium can also exacerbate the effect of potassium abnormalities (both hyperkalemia and hypokalemia).

MEASUREMENT

Measurement of calcium usually consists of total calcium: ionized, protein-bound, and complexed together. Measurement of ionized calcium may be done with ion-selective electrodes on whole blood or serum samples.

Phosphorus is measured in body fluids as a mixture of the phosphates HPO_4^{-2} and $H_2PO_4^{-1}$, which change in relative concentrations as one of the buffering systems in the blood (see Chapter 10). Results are reported in milligrams/deciliter (reference range, 2.4 to 4.7 mg/dL) or mmol/liter (reference range 0.81 to 1.45 mmol/L), but not as milliequivalents because phosphate species with different valences are usually present together in serum.

Calcium, magnesium, and phosphorus measurements must be done on serum to avoid interferences from anticoagulants used to collect plasma. Clot formation in those samples is prevented by agents that chelate calcium. Calcium can be measured by atomic absorption spectroscopy, by dye-binding with color change, or by ion-selective electrodes. Whole blood or plasma samples collected into heparin, which does not chelate calcium significantly, can be used for ionized calcium measurements that reflect the physiologically active calcium. Such determinations are useful in evaluating parathyroid function and also for the acute monitoring of patients undergoing cardiac surgery or other high-risk procedures. Many blood gas analyzers now also conveniently provide ionized calcium measurements.

Special consideration must be given to obtaining high-quality, fresh specimens for ionized calcium measurements. Alkaline conditions cause ionized calcium to bind to proteins due to more negative charge on the protein molecules. Conversely, acidosis causes an elevation of hydrogen ions, which displace calcium from proteins, thereby increasing the ionized fraction. For accurate measurement, the sample should be drawn without prolonged venous stasis, which can cause local acidosis. Atmospheric contact will allow carbon dioxide to escape from both whole blood and serum specimens on even brief storage, resulting in rising pH of the sample (alkalosis). Thus ionized calcium determinations should either be done quickly (e.g., on whole blood) or will require re-equilibration of a sample to physiologic pH.

Both phosphorus and magnesium are measured with dye-binding methods, although magnesium can also be measured with atomic absorption spectroscopy.

It has become more widely recognized recently that total body deficiency of magnesium can develop despite normal levels of magnesium in serum. This is because magnesium is predominantly an intracellular ion. Such a deficiency state is best diagnosed by administering a test load of magnesium and then measuring the percentage that is retained in the body versus excretion in urine. Normal individuals should have retentions below 20%, whereas whole body deficiency will lead to magnesium retentions substantially greater than 20%.

LIPIDS

Lipids are carbon- and hydrogen-containing compounds that are mostly hydrophobic: insoluble in water but soluble in organic solvents. Biologically important groups are the **neutral fats,** the **conjugated lipids,** and the **sterols.** Neutral fats consist of fatty acids (primarily oleic, linoleic, stearic, arachidonic, and palmitic) in the form of **triglycerides** (i.e., three fatty acid molecules esterified to a single glycerol molecule). Adipose tissue has stores of triglycerides that serve as a pool of readily available lipids. The conjugated lipids result from the joining of phosphate or sugar groups to lipid molecules. These phospholipids and glycolipids are integral constituents of the cell wall structure. Sterols also serve as structural building blocks in cells and membranes and as constituents of hormones and other metabolites. **Cholesterol** is the sterol of major biologic significance.

Because of their insolubility in water, lipids require special transport mechanisms for circulation in the blood. Free fatty acids occur in only small amounts in the blood and generally bind in a loose complex with albumin. The major lipid components found in plasma are triglycerides, cholesterol, and phospholipids. They exist and are transported in blood as **lipoproteins,** very large macromolecular complexes of those lipids with specialized proteins **(apolipoproteins)** that help in their packaging, solubility, and metabolism.

METABOLISM

Body stores of energy are primarily in the form of **fatty acids.** As they enter and leave triglyceride molecules of adipose tissue, fatty acids provide the substance for conversion to glucose **(gluconeogenesis)** as well as for direct combustion to generate energy. Fatty acids can originate in the diet but also derive from excess glucose that the liver and adipose tissue can convert into storable energy.

Cholesterol has two sources: dietary and that endogenously synthesized in the body. Cholesterol is an important constituent in the assembly of cell membranes. Much cholesterol also goes toward synthesis of bile acids and the steroid hormones (e.g., cortisol, estrogens, androgens). In the normal biologic process, cholesterol undergoes synthesis, degradation, and recycling. Consequently, the dietary component of cholesterol is probably not necessary for essential metabolic reactions.

The **phospholipids, lecithin, sphingomyelin,** and **cephalin** are major components of cell membranes and also act in solution to alter fluid surface tension (e.g., surfactant activity of the fluid in the lungs). The circulating phospholipids originate in liver and intestine with widespread synthesis in lesser amounts. The circulating phospholipids can participate in cellular metabolism and also in blood coagulation.

Lipids in the circulation are organized into large lipoprotein particles with apolipoproteins characteristic of different classes. These apolipoproteins aid in the solubilization of the lipids and also in their transfer from the gastrointestinal tract to the liver, which contains specific receptors for apolipoproteins. Thus the metabolism and clearance of lipids is directly regulated by the apolipoproteins.

Lipoproteins in the circulation consist of different sized particles that also contain different amounts of cholesterol, triglycerides, phospholipids, and protein, resulting in different densities characteristic of each lipoprotein type. The largest and least dense of lipoproteins are **chylomicrons,** followed by **very-low-density lipoproteins (VLDL), low-density lipoprotein (LDL), intermediate-density lipoproteins (IDL),** and **high-density lipoproteins (HDL).** Most of the triglycerides of nonfasting plasma reside in the chylomicrons, whereas in fasting plasma samples, the triglycerides are mostly in the VLDL. The majority of plasma cholesterol is contained in LDL. A smaller fraction (15 to 25%) of cholesterol is in the HDL.

Exogenous (Dietary) Lipid Pathway

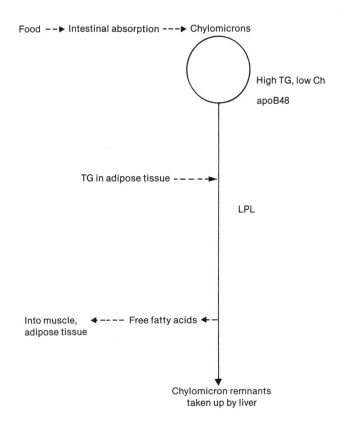

Food – –▶ Intestinal absorption – – –▶ Chylomicrons

High TG, low Ch

apoB48

TG in adipose tissue – – – –▶

LPL

Into muscle, ◀– – – – Free fatty acids ◀–
adipose tissue

Chylomicron remnants
taken up by liver

The **dietary** or **exogenous pathway of lipid transport** involves absorption of triglycerides (TG) and cholesterol (Ch) through the intestine, with formation and release of chylomicrons into the lymph and subsequently into the blood by way of the thoracic duct. The chylomicrons release triglycerides to adipose tissue as they circulate. In addition, the apoliprotein B48 on the surface of chylomicrons activates **lipoprotein lipase (LPL)** found in the vascular endothelial cells. Lipoprotein lipase cleaves free fatty acids from the triglycerides, thereby reducing chylomicrons in size to remnants ultimately taken up by the liver. The free fatty acids so liberated are in turn taken up by muscle and adipose cells.

In the endogenous pathway, there is synthesis of triglycerides from fatty acids by the liver with secretion of VLDL particles that contain apolipoproteins B100 (which is commonly referred to as apoB in clinical measurements) and E. These VLDL particles are also modified by LPL as they circulate, leading to production of IDL that can either be removed by the liver through apoE (as remnants) or can lose the apoE in that process to become LDL. The cholesterol-rich LDL particles can be taken up by the liver (70%) or into other tissues (30%) where the cholesterol goes into membranes, steroid synthesis, or deposits (atheromas).

This pathway of synthesis, transport, and deposition is modulated by HDL particles that can mobilize cholesterol from tissues and reintroduce it for continued metabolism or excretion. **Nascent HDL particles** containing phospholipid, apoA 1, and other apolipoproteins are synthesized and released by the liver. As these particles circulate, they pick up cholesterol from tissues, thereby becoming the HDL_3 fraction. **Lecithin cholesterol acyl transferase (LCAT)** catalyzes the esterification of this cholesterol in HDL_3, converting these particles to HDL_2. This fraction of cholesterol can be transferred to VLDL to participate in the metabolism of membrane and steroid synthesis. It can also be taken up by the liver and then excreted into bile.

Endogenous Lipid Pathway (Synthesis)

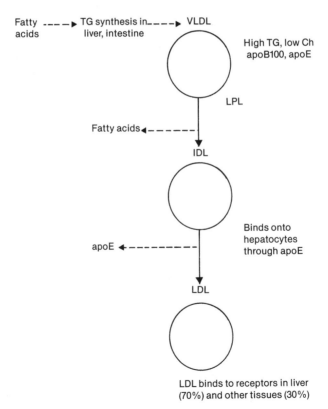

LDL binds to receptors in liver
(70%) and other tissues (30%)

HDL Pathway

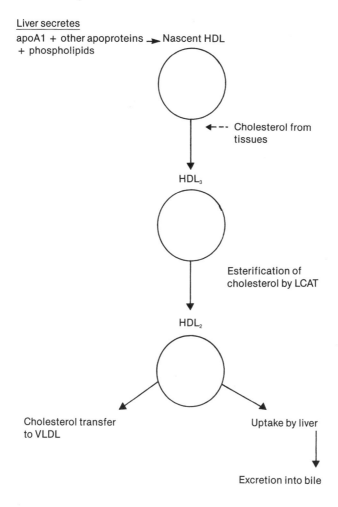

Liver secretes
apoA1 + other apoproteins → Nascent HDL
+ phospholipids

◄ -- Cholesterol from
tissues

HDL$_3$

Esterification of
cholesterol by LCAT

HDL$_2$

Cholesterol transfer
to VLDL

Uptake by liver

Excretion into bile

The efficiency of these pathways for lipid transport and clearance depends on concentrations of available apolipoproteins and also on the lipid load presented to the body by diet. The importance of HDL as a means of clearing cholesterol from tissues is emphasized by the deficiency state of HDL **(Tangier disease),** in which cholesterol forms extensive deposits in tissues. Conversely, high levels of HDL serve to protect against development of atherosclerosis due to cholesterol deposits.

Another lipoprotein fraction is Lp(a), which has densities overlapping the range between LDL and HDL and has a prebeta electrophoretic mobility. Although it is a relatively minor fraction in most individuals, genetic elevations of Lp(a) have been associated with increased risk for developing coronary artery disease, perhaps due to an amino acid sequence homology shared by apo(a) and plasminogen, which presumably interferes with naturally occurring low levels of fibrinolysis initiated by circulating tissue plasminogen activator (TPA). The Lp(a) is thought to block endogenous TPA, thereby promoting minor clot formation that proceeds to atherosclerosis.

MEASUREMENT AND FRACTIONATION

The most relevant measurements of serum lipids are total cholesterol, triglycerides, and cholesterol fractionation into the HDL fraction with calculation of the LDL fraction of cholesterol. In addition, clinical laboratories now have the capacity to quantitate **apolipoprotein AI (apoAI)** and **apolipoprotein B (apoB)** in serum samples. Free fatty acids (FFA, also called nonesterified fatty acids, NEFA) and phospholipids are not usually quantitated in serum except in cases of specific metabolic diseases.

Measurement of total cholesterol has been done in the past by colorimetric chemical methods that demonstrate interferences from other substances. Today most cholesterol methods use the enzyme cholesterol oxidase and are much more specific. The major technical problem in assuring standardization between different cholesterol assays is the relative insolubility of cholesterol, which limits its availability to the enzymatic reagents during the period of analysis. There is presently a major emphasis nationally to establish cholesterol standards to bring all laboratories into agreement on this assay.

Triglycerides are measured by hydrolytic removal of the fatty acids and then quantitation of the liberated glycerol. Since triglycerides can contain a variety of different fatty acids in unpredictable mixtures (probably dependent on diet), triglyceride determination must be standardized against a defined material that can differ in average composition from the samples being analyzed. Comparability is then based on the glycerol content.

Cholesterol fractionation originally was based on the separation of individual lipoproteins according to density by ultracentrifugation. Pure fat is less dense than water; lipids are less dense than proteins; and triglycerides are less dense than phospholipids and cholesterol. The least dense lipoproteins are those with the highest triglyceride content. Chylomicrons are lipoproteins with very high triglyceride content and a specific gravity less than that of plasma. Chylomicrons will rise to the top of a volume of plasma under conditions favorable to separation of fat from water (e.g., refrigeration overnight). The next most dense lipoprotein class is VLDL, followed by LDL and HDL. The composition of the major lipoprotein categories is given in Table 9–8.

The appearance of serum after 12 to 16 hours of refrigeration gives

TABLE 9-8. LIPOPROTEIN COMPOSITION

	Triglyceride (%)	Cholesterol (%)	Phospholipid (%)	Protein (%)	Electrophoretic Mobility
Chylomicrons	85–95	3–5	5–10	1–2	Remain at origin
Very-low-density lipoproteins	60–70	10–15	10–15	10	α_2-lipoprotein Pre-β-lipoprotein
Low-density lipoproteins	5–10	45	20–30	15–25	β-lipoprotein
High-density lipoproteins	Very little	20	30	50	α_1-lipoprotein

Adapted from Weidman, SW, and Schonfeld, G: Lipids and lipoproteins. In Sonnewirth, AC, and Jarrett, L (eds): Gradwohl's Clinical Laboratory Methods and Diagnosis, ed 8. CV Mosby, St. Louis, 1980, p 272, and Segal, P, et al: Lipids and dyslipoproteinemia. In Henry, JB (ed): Clinical Diagnosis and Management by Laboratory Methods, ed 17. WB Saunders, Philadelphia, 1984, p 133.

quick, useful information about chylomicron and VLDL content of serum with excessive triglycerides. This is summarized in the last column of Table 9–9. Freshly separated hyperlipemic serum is uniformly milky or opalescent. In chilled serum, excessive chylomicrons float to the top, appearing like a layer of cream. Uniform turbidity in the refrigerated serum indicates elevated VLDL content. Several different patterns may be seen: uniform turbidity means elevated VLDL without significant chylomicrons; "cream" atop a turbid specimen means elevation of both chylomicrons and VLDL; and "cream" atop a clear specimen means chylomicronemia without excess VLDL.

Because ultracentrifugation is not a practical method for clinical laboratory use, alternative techniques have been developed to study cholesterol fractionation. One such technique is electrophoresis, which separates as follows: chylomicrons at origin, LDL as beta, VLDL as prebeta, and HDL as alpha (Fig. 9–2). Frederickson, Goldstein, and Brown have classified six distinct lipoprotein distribution phenotypic patterns by this means (Table 9–9). These phenotypes have been correlated with genetically determined abnormalities (familial hyperlipoproteinemia) and with a variety of acquired conditions (secondary hyperlipoprotein-emias) outlined in Table 9–10. Phenotype descriptions have proven useful in classifying diagnoses and in evaluating treatment and preventive regimens. However, most hyperlipemic (elevated cholesterol and/or triglycerides) individuals can be categorized into phenotypes without electrophoresis if total cholesterol, HDL cholesterol, triglyceride level, and chylomicron status are known. Furthermore, phenotyping in itself does not provide the best measure of relative risk for developing coronary artery disease.

Present protocols for serum cholesterol fractionation involve precipitation of all the lipoproteins other than HDL, followed by direct measurement of the HDL cholesterol remaining in solution. In fasting samples, VLDL cholesterol content has been found empirically to be approximately equal to one-fifth of the serum triglyceride concentration. Thus LDL cholesterol can be calculated from measurements of total cholesterol, triglycerides, and HDL cholesterol by the Friedewald approximation:

$$LDL\text{-}C = (Total\ cholesterol) - (HDL\text{-}C) - (triglycerides)/5$$

This calculation is valid for triglyceride concentrations up to approximately 400 mg/dL. It may also need correction to account for IDL and Lp(a) cholesterol content whenever they are elevated.

Very recently, direct measurement of LDL-C has been made possible by a method involving selective immunoprecipitation of the other lipoprotein fractions. Direct measurement of LDL-C is not restricted by elevated triglycerides and is valid on nonfasting samples. Elevations of Lp(a) may falsely increase direct measurement of LDL-C.

ApoAI and apoB are proteins present predominantly on HDL and LDL lipoprotein fractions, respectively. Accordingly, measurement of these

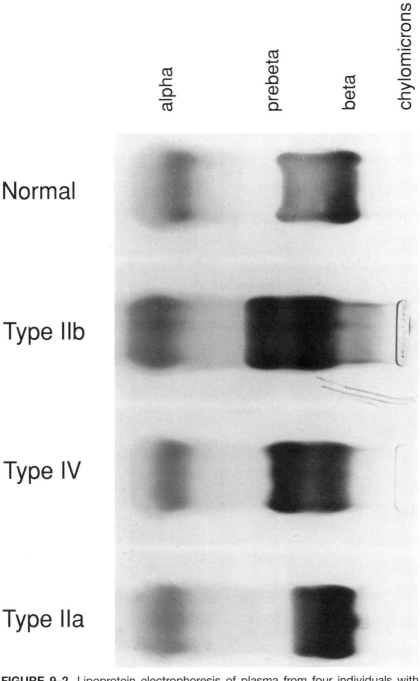

FIGURE 9–2. Lipoprotein electrophoresis of plasma from four individuals with the following patterns: (a) normal, (b) type IIb, (c) type IV, and (d) type IIa hyperlipoproteinemias. The individual fractions (alpha, prebeta, and beta) demonstrate variation in migration between patients who have different cholesterol and triglyceride concentrations. Chylomicrons remain at the origin.

TABLE 9-9. LIPOPROTEIN PHENOTYPES

Phenotype	Frequency	Chylomicrons	Pre-β-Lipoproteins (Approximates VLDL)	β-Lipoproteins (Approximates LDL)	α₁-Lipoproteins (Approximates HDL)	Total Cholesterol	Total Triglycerides	Refrigerated Serum or Plasma
I	Very rare	↑↑↑	↑	↓	↓	nl or ↑	↑↑↑	"Cream"/clear or turbid
IIa	Common	nl	nl	↑↑	nl	↑↑	nl	Clear
IIb	Common	nl	↑↑	↑↑	nl	↑↑	↑	+ or ++ turbid
III	Uncommon	nl or ↑	These two bands merge		nl	↑↑	↑↑ or ↑↑↑	+++ turbid
IV	Very common	nl	↑↑↑	nl or ↑	nl or ↓	nl or ↑	↑↑ or ↑↑↑	++ turbid
V	Rare	↑↑	↑↑	nl or ↓	nl or ↓	↑↑	↑↑↑	"Cream"/++ turbid

Adapted from Frederickson, DS, Goldstein, JL, and Brown, JS: The familial hyperlipoproteinemias. In Stanbury, JB, Wyngaarden, JB, and Frederickson, DS (eds): The Metabolic Basis of Inherited Disease, ed 4. McGraw-Hill, New York, 1978, p 604.
nl = normal.

TABLE 9–10. CLINICOPATHOLOGIC SIGNIFICANCE OF LIPOPROTEIN PHENOTYPES

Phenotype	Familial Syndrome	May Occur Secondary to	Remarks
I	Abdominal pain Eruptive xanthomas Lipemia retinalis Early vascular disease absent	Insulin-dependent diabetes Lupus erythematosus Dysglobulinemias Pancreatitis	Lipoprotein lipase is deficient
II	Early, severe vascular disease Prominent xanthomas	High-cholesterol diet Nephrotic syndrome Porphyria Hypothyroidism Dysglobulinemias Obstructive liver diseases	Familial trait is autosomal- dominant; homozygotes are especially severely affected
III	Accelerated vascular disease, onset in adulthood Xanthomas, palmar yellowing Abnormal glucose tolerance Hyperuricemia	Hypothyroidism Dysglobulinemias Uncontrolled diabetes	Diet, lipid-lowering drugs very effective
IV	Accelerated vascular disease, onset in adulthood Abnormal glucose tolerance Hyperuricemia	Obesity High alcohol intake Oral contraceptives Diabetes Nephrotic syndrome Glycogen storage disease	Weight loss lowers VLDL High-fat diet may convert to type V
V	Abdominal pain Pancreatitis Eruptive xanthomas Abnormal glucose tolerance Vascular disease not associated	High alcohol intake Diabetes Nephrotic syndrome Pancreatitis Hypercalcemia	Weight loss does not lower VLDL

two apolipoproteins gives additional clinically useful information for estimating the distribution of lipoproteins in a patient's serum. Both of these apolipoproteins can now be quantitated by immunoassays, although they have not yet found widespread acceptance for cardiac risk assessment.

CLINICAL CONSIDERATIONS

Lipid measurements have gained popularity among both medical and nonmedical personnel for assessing an individual's risk of having coronary artery disease. It is probably useful for all persons to have knowledge of their cholesterol levels in order to decide what changes in lifestyle would be helpful in reducing their risk of myocardial infarction and other atherosclerotic disease.

Effects of Diet

Dietary cholesterol and total caloric intake are the major determinants of blood lipid concentrations. People with low caloric intake have relatively low triglyceride levels on a populationwide basis. In addition, vegetarians who get very low cholesterol in their diets have relatively low blood cholesterol levels.

Fats absorbed from the diet are transported to the liver as chylomicrons rich in triglycerides. Chylomicrons should disappear from circulating blood several hours after eating, and it is abnormal to find chylomicrons in fasting serum. Prolonged consumption of a diet high in calories, specifically in fats, produces a sustained increase in triglycerides, located largely in the VLDL particles. High carbohydrate intake causes a prompt rise in triglycerides and VLDL. Dietary cholesterol increases the LDL cholesterol content, as does dietary intake of saturated fatty acids; consumption of unsaturated fatty acids may decrease total cholesterol. Alcohol increases triglyceride concentration, affecting largely VLDL and sometimes chylomicrons.

Risk Factors

Most people in the United States and other industrialized and developed nations have diets high in both calories and cholesterol. Consequently, a large proportion of those individuals have high blood lipid levels. Coupled with other risk factors (e.g., male, family history of myocardial disease, cigarette smoking, overweight, hypertension), elevated cholesterol poses a major health threat leading to coronary artery disease (CAD). The epidemiologic significance of elevated cholesterol has been established after decades of measurements correlated with clinical outcome. Efforts to deliberately lower cholesterol in hypercholesterolemic men have proven effective in alleviating CAD.

The problems inherent in guiding this form of preventive medicine include deciding what parameters of cholesterol measurement to monitor, establishing reference limits, and then standardizing the assays both nationwide and worldwide. It is now well understood that total cholesterol is generally a bad risk factor. Among the subfractions, high levels of cholesterol in the HDL fraction are negatively associated with cardiovascular disease, whereas high levels of cholesterol in the LDL fraction are positively associated with it. Thus high LDL cholesterol and low HDL cholesterol are risk factors for atherosclerotic disease, and conversely, high HDL cholesterol and low LDL cholesterol lower the risk of CAD.

To establish reference ranges for cholesterol based on observed population distributions would be erroneous because it would include many people who have or will develop CAD. To address this issue, the National Cholesterol Education Program sponsored by the National Heart, Lung, and Blood Institute has established guidelines for testing everyone over the age of 20 years, with the initial classification based on total cholesterol. For those with cholesterol less than 200 mg/dL, testing should be repeated every 5 years. Those with cholesterol between 200 and 239 mg/dL are considered borderline. Levels of 240 mg/dL or greater are considered high. Further fractionation is recommended for persons with high levels or with borderline levels plus two other risk factors. The classification according to *LDL cholesterol* is as follows:

<130 mg/dL = desirable
130-159 mg/dL = borderline
>160 mg/dL = high risk

Treatment is recommended for all high-risk persons and for those who are borderline and have at least two other risk factors.

At present, there is no national recommendation for specific desirable levels of HDL or of apoAI and apoB. However, it is clear from existing epidemiologic studies that high levels of HDL cholesterol, high levels of apoA1, and low levels of apoB are desirable because patients with these findings tend to have a lower incidence of CAD. Conversely, those individuals with low HDL cholesterol (<35 mg/dL), low apoAI, and high apoB tend to develop atheromatous disease from cholesterol deposits in vessels and are at a relatively high risk for CAD and myocardial infarction at an early age. In addition, the ratio of HDL cholesterol to LDL cholesterol and the ratio of apoAI to apoB can also be useful in assessing the combined risks of CAD from the two lipoproteins together. It should also be noted that HDL cholesterol can be further fractionated into two predominant subclasses based on density: HDL_2 and HDL_3, although the vast majority of clinical laboratories measure them together as HDL. HDL_2 goes up with exercise and estrogen, and HDL_3 goes up with consumption of alcohol.

Treatment

Specific therapies for cholesterol reduction include dietary modification, resin taken orally to sequester bile acids in the intestine to prevent absorption of cholesterol, and drugs that block intracellular synthesis of cholesterol.

Monitoring for efficacy of therapy in reducing cholesterol should be timed soon enough to produce positive feedback in patients after embarking on therapy, but long enough afterward to detect a change in cholesterol, which should take 4 to 6 weeks to occur. All such measurements should be preceded by 3 days of routine diet and fasting of 12 to 14 hours before blood draw. Patients in the hospital usually have major changes in diet plus intravenous fluid therapy, both of which can alter cholesterol levels very significantly over a few days, thereby negating their value in cardiac risk assessment.

PROTEINS OF SERUM AND PLASMA

METHODS OF ANALYSIS

Several methods are commonly employed for the routine clinical measurement of proteins in serum, urine, and other body fluids. The simplest technique is by hand-held refractometer, which quantitates proteins in solution from the change in **refractive index** caused by protein molecules in aqueous solution. The refractive index is easy to perform and requires no other reagents, but suffers from interferences due to hyperlipidemia, elevated bilirubin, or hemolysis (i.e., turbid or pigmented specimens).

Most automated methods for protein measurement today use dyes that bind to protein molecules, thereby altering the absorbance pattern of the dye molecule. **Total protein** is typically quantitated with the biuret reagent and alkaline copper sulfate. Absorbance is monitored at 545 nm. Most proteins can be expected to react equivalently with this reagent on a weight basis. Severely lipemic specimens should be ultracentrifuged to decrease potential interference from turbidity. In addition to total protein, **albumin** is also routinely quantitated on automated chemistry analyzers. Albumin reversibly binds many small molecules, including dyes that do not interact with the other serum proteins. This selective binding is usually done with dyes such as bromcresol green or bromcresol purple. The calculated difference between measured total protein and measured albumin is the **globulin fraction**. This nomenclature has been retained from the past when serum proteins were fractionated by salting out the globulins before measuring protein content. Those methods led to the use of the **albumin to globulin (A/G) ratio** as an index of disease state. The

A/G ratio can be decreased in response to low albumin or to elevated globulins. Thus the A/G ratio is not a specific marker for disease because it does not indicate which specific proteins are altered.

Modern methods of protein fractionation use **electrophoresis** on a solid support medium such as agarose or cellulose acetate. Electrophoresis separates proteins into six zones: *prealbumin, albumin, alpha-1-globulins, alpha-2-globulins, beta globulins,* and *gamma globulins* (Fig. 9–3). Each of

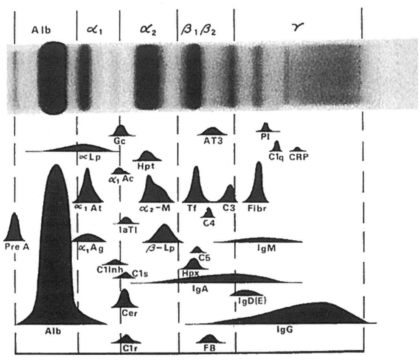

FIGURE 9–3. Plasma protein electrophoresis pattern in agarose gel is composed of five fractions, each composed of many individual species. Some of the major proteins are shown here in an artist's rendition for clarity.

α1Ac = Alpha-1-antichymotrypsin; α1Ag = Alpha-1-acid glycoprotein; α1At = Alpha-1-antitrypsin; α2-M = Alpha-2-macroglobulin; αLp = Alpha lipoprotein; Alb = Albumin; AT3 = Antithrombin III; β-Lp = Beta lipoprotein; C1q, C1r, C1s, C3, C4, C5 = Complement components as designated; C1Inh = C1 esterase inhibitor; Cer = Ceruloplasmin; CRP = C-reactive protein; FB = Factor B; Fibr = Fibrinogen; Gc = Gc-globulin, group-specific component, vitamin D–binding protein; Hpt = Haptoglobin; Hpx = Hemopexin; IαTI = Interalphathrombin inhibitor; IgA, IgD, IgE, IgG, IgM = Immuno-globulins as designated; Pl = Plasminogen; Pre A = Prealbumin; Tf = Transferrin.

(From McPherson, RA: Specific proteins. In Henry, JB (ed): Clinical Diagnosis and Management by Laboratory Methods, ed 17. WB Saunders, Philadelphia, 1984, p 204, with permission.)

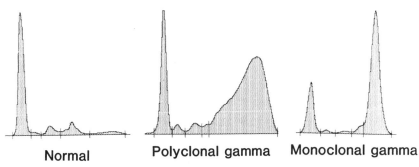

FIGURE 9–4. Electrophoretic tracings of serum proteins.

these zones is then quantitated by staining and scanning the electrophoretic strip with a densitometer that produces a tracing with peak height and area under the tracing proportional to protein concentration in each fraction (Fig. 9–4; Table 9–11). The proteins making up these fractions (Table 9–12) can be quantitated by reacting serum samples with specific antibodies raised against the individual human proteins (e.g., in rabbits or goats). The resulting antigen-antibody complex causes slight turbidity, which is used to quantitate the amount of a serum protein on an instrument called a **nephelometer.** The nephelometric measurement of some serum proteins (e.g., immunoglobulins, complement, haptoglobin, C-reactive protein) is commonly used to monitor disease progression or response to therapy. Much diagnostic information can also be gleaned from a rigorous inspection of serum protein electrophoretic patterns (Table 9–13). (See also Immunoglobulins—Chapter 4 and Fig. 4–7.)

TABLE 9–11. REFERENCE RANGES FOR SERUM PROTEIN ELECTROPHORESIS

Constituent	% of Total Protein
Albumin	52–68
α_1-globulin	2.4–5.3
α_2-globulin	6.6–13.5
β-globulin	8.5–14.5
γ-globulin	10.7–21.0

From Henry, RJ, Golub, OJ, and Soleb, C: Some of the variables involved in the fractionation of serum proteins by paper electrophoresis. Clin Chem 3:49, 1957, with permission.

TABLE 9–12. SERUM PROTEINS OF DIAGNOSTIC SIGNIFICANCE

Protein	Function	Clinical Observations
Prealbumin	Transports vitamin A	Decreased after relatively brief hepatocellular dysfunction
	Transports thyroxine	Decreased with widespread tissue damage
Transferrin	Transports iron	Increased when iron stores are low (except decreased when protein malnutrition coexists)
		Increased in pregnancy and oral contraceptive use
		Decreased with protein-losing states
		Congenital deficiency exists
Haptoglobin	Binds free hemoglobin	Disappears when hemoglobin escapes from red cells (hemolysis)
		Increased with infection, malignancy, burns
		Decreased with severe liver disease
		Genetically determined structural variants are numerous
α_1-Antitrypsin	Inhibits naturally occurring proteases	Genetically determined absence or diminution exists fairly frequently
		Levels increase with pregnancy, oral contraceptive use
		Increased with acute inflammatory conditions
Ceruloplasmin	Transports copper	Increased with chronic inflammation, tissue necrosis
		Increased with pregnancy, oral contraceptive use
		Decreased with severe liver disease, with protein-losing states
		Absent in Wilson's disease, an uncommon genetically determined disease
Antithrombin III	Enhances antithrombin effect of heparin	Decreased with hepatocellular dysfunction, protein-losing states
		Decreased with pregnancy, oral contraceptive use
		Genetically determined deficiency occurs in 1:2000

TABLE 9–13. CONDITIONS CAUSING ABNORMAL SERUM PROTEIN ELECTROPHORESIS*

Condition	Change in Electrophoretic Pattern
Hypoalbuminemia	Low spike for albumin
Chronic liver disease	Diffuse but large elevation of γ-globulins
Chronic inflammatory disease	Diffuse but small elevation of γ-globulins
Dysproteinemia (monoclonal immunoglobulin)	Sharply elevated spike in γ-globulins (occasionally β-globulins)
Hypogammaglobulinemia	Flat curve where γ-globulins should be
Nephrotic syndrome	Low albumin spike, very high α_2-globulins
Protein-losing enteropathy	Low albumin spike, moderate α_2-globulin elevation
α_1-Antitrypsin deficiency	Flat curve where α_1-globulin should be

*See also Figure 4–7.

High-resolution protein electrophoresis is generally standard practice for the detection of oligoclonal banding of immunoglobulins in cerebrospinal fluid. Still more exacting procedures such as **isoelectric focusing** offer great potential for identifying genetic variants of proteins such as alpha-1-antitrypsin with high reliability.

PREALBUMIN

The zone of protein that migrates electrophoretically most anodally (i.e., toward the positive pole) beyond albumin consists primarily of a single protein that is present in serum and also in cerebrospinal fluid (CSF). The absolute concentrations of **prealbumin** are similar in serum and CSF, but because of the low levels of other proteins in CSF, prealbumin composes a larger percentage of CSF protein. Thus, prealbumin can be used as a marker for CSF when evaluating whether, for example, fluid draining from the nose is CSF released by skull fracture versus simple nasal secretions.

Prealbumin binds thyroxine, although at physiologic levels, most thyroxine is bound to thyroxine-binding globulin (TBG). Prealbumin is sometimes referred to as **thyroxine-binding prealbumin (TBPA),** although it probably does not play a major role in thyroid hormone function.

Prealbumin also binds **retinol-binding protein (RBP),** which in turn binds vitamin A. This protein-vitamin complex formation is essential to transport the oil-soluble vitamin A throughout the body.

Prealbumin is synthesized in the liver. Its level in serum has been suggested to be useful for assessing the nutritional status of patients (see Appendix A).

A genetic variant of prealbumin is susceptible to proteolytic cleavage resulting in protein fragments that form amyloid deposits in peripheral nerves.

ALBUMIN

Normal circulating levels of albumin account in large part for the **oncotic pressure** of blood plasma. Consequently, reduction of circulating albumin concentration results in a shift of fluid from intravascular to extravascular spaces. Several different mechanisms can cause a fall in albumin levels or **hypoalbuminemia** (Table 9–14). Probably the most common one is a decrease in the production of albumin that is synthesized in the liver.

In severe liver disease such as cirrhosis, which may be due to alcohol abuse, iron storage disorder, chronic hepatitis, or drug reactions, the protein-synthesizing capacity of hepatic parenchymal cells can be drastically limited. In such instances, a major diagnostic and prognostic test is measurement of serum albumin concentration. Often in liver disease, severe hypoalbuminemia is offset by increased concentrations of the immunoglobulins, with the result that the total concentration of serum proteins may be only moderately low (see Fig. 9–4). Hepatic portal hypertension as occurs in cirrhosis (intrahepatic), but also with prehepatic and posthepatic etiologies, allows **ascites fluid** to accumulate in the peritoneal cavity. This fluid derives as a transudate that weeps from the peritoneal surface and particularly from the hepatic capsule due to blockage of hepatic lymphatics by the fibrous intrahepatic scarring of cirrhosis. Ascites fluid can accumulate in volumes up to liters, with its primary protein being albumin. This process is a major drain on the body stores of albumin, thereby further exacerbating pre-existing hypoalbuminemia (see Chapter 19).

In order for there to be abundant synthesis and release of albumin by normal liver cells, there must be adequate dietary intake of protein as well as other essential nutrients. Beyond the physiologic function of supplying oncotic pressure, albumin also serves as a circulating reservoir of amino acids, which would clear rapidly into the urine if not incorporated into a higher molecular weight protein. In this capacity as a store of amino acids, albumin is an indicator of nutritional status. Thus, decreases in dietary protein are reflected in serum albumin levels, and very low concentrations occur with malnutrition due to starvation or malabsorption. Self-induced starvation or **anorexia nervosa** produces hypoalbuminemia in addition to elevations in the serum enzymes reflecting damage to liver and muscle also secondary to starvation. Anorexia due to other medical and physical reasons over long periods likewise results in **cachexia.** The body wasting that accompanies malignancy or chronic inflammatory states is caused by a combination of anorexia plus the

TABLE 9-14. CONDITIONS CAUSING HYPOALBUMINEMIA

Condition	Relative Frequency	Mechanism
Reduced Synthesis:		
Malnutrition	Common	Deficient amino acid intake
Malabsorption syndromes	Common	Deficient amino acid intake
Chronic inflammatory diseases	Somewhat common	Depressed hepatocellular function
Acute hepatitis (lasting 14 days or more)	Common	Depressed hepatocellular function
Chronic liver disease	Very common	Inadequate volume of liver cells
Genetic abnormalities	Rare	Synthesis of defective albumin molecules
Increased Loss*:		
Nephrotic syndrome	Common	Massive albuminuria
Massive burns	Common	Escape from damaged vessels
Protein-losing enteropathy	Uncommon	Escape across intestinal mucosa
Increased Catabolism*:		
Massive burns	Common	Destruction of tissue protein
Widespread malignancy	Common	Increased energy expenditure and protein turnover; decreased intake
Multifactorial:		
Cirrhosis	Very common	Inadequate hepatocellular volume; escape into ascitic fluid; malabsorption because of portal hypertension; protein loss from GI bleeding
Congestive heart failure	Very common	Expanded plasma volume
		Depressed hepatocellular function
Pregnancy	Uncommon complication of common condition	Expanded plasma volume
		Increased metabolic turnover
		Depressed hepatocellular function

*Serum levels decline if there is insufficient hepatic function and/or available amino acids to make good the loss.

increased metabolic needs of tumor cells, thereby starving the rest of the body. Malabsorption leads to malnutrition by failure of the intestinal absorptive surface (e.g., sprue, celiac disease, lactose deficiency, or inflammatory bowel disease) or by failure to secrete pancreatic enzymes, as in cystic fibrosis. Serum albumin in particular has been used as a sensitive and highly prognostic marker in cases of cystic fibrosis.

Hypoalbuminemia as a consequence of increased loss of albumin occurs in renal disease with proteinuria, in burns with protein loss through denuded body surfaces, and in gastrointestinal disease with protein-losing enteropathy. In cases of **nephrotic syndrome,** amazingly rapid losses of protein may lead to the development of extensive body edema seemingly overnight. The mechanism for loss of albumin into the urine is increased permeability at the glomerular level resulting in passage of protein into the glomerular filtrate. This concentration of protein exceeds the capacity of renal tubular cells to reabsorb and process it. The pattern of protein electrophoresis in nephrotic syndrome is highly characteristic: low albumin, elevated alpha-2-macroglobulin, and elevated betalipoprotein. The other protein fractions are also usually diminished in serum. The pattern of proteins in the urine is complementary to that in the patient's serum, with albumin being most abundant in the urine. Traditionally, the level of proteinuria is thought of as carrying significance for assessing severity of renal disease. This is usually evaluated by some semiquantitative method as a dipstick on a spot urine read as negative, 1+, . . . , 4+. A better method for strict quantitation is measurement of the protein in a 24-hour collection of urine. In addition, this sample collection is convenient for performing a creatinine clearance study in conjunction with serum creatinine measurement. Total urine protein loss is then expressed in terms of grams per day. In severe nephrotic syndrome, proteinuria can range up to 20 or 30 g/day. In early disease, it may be only 1 or 2 g/day. In the more severe cases, other proteins besides albumin are lost, whereas in cases of only 1 g/day, predominantly albumin is lost. **Diabetic nephropathy** frequently results in losses of about 1 g/day. Early stages of renal damage in diabetes mellitus may not have levels of albumin in urine readily detected by electrophoretic methods. This problem has been addressed recently by the application of radioimmunoassay for the quantitation of **microalbuminuria** (i.e., sensitivity down to 10 mg/24 hours), which appears to carry significant diagnostic power in early diabetic nephropathy.

An apparently benign disorder called **orthostatic proteinuria** is sometimes seen in adolescents. This proteinuria is glomerular in origin with losses of albumin that cease at night when the individual is recumbent.

The loss of protein across burns of the skin is easily understood in terms of the huge surface areas that are unprotected after extensive body burns.

A much more cryptic loss of protein and predominantly albumin is that through the gastrointestinal tract. The mechanism can be exudation across an inflamed or eroded mucosal surface analogous to the loss through burns of the skin. In such instances, there is likely to be mixed causes with coexisting malabsorption. A much less obvious mechanism may operate in cases of intestinal lymphatic obstruction or congestive heart failure with elevated venous pressures. In those instances, protein can be lost directly into the digestive tract by weeping of fluids from the mucosal surfaces of the intestine.

Hereditary absence of albumin is a rare disorder termed **analbuminemia** deriving from the inability to synthesize albumin. Individuals with analbuminemia have normal concentrations of the other serum proteins and therefore have total serum protein levels markedly below the range of persons who have normal albumin. Clinically, the condition is not apparent, probably because of lifelong homeostatic mechanisms of fluid balance that compensate for the absence of albumin's oncotic pressure in the circulation.

Increases in the serum concentration of albumin result from severe dehydration in which plasma water leaves the circulation but the albumin remains due to its larger molecular size. The same effect pertains after prolonged application of a tourniquet before venipuncture, resulting in **artifactual hyperalbuminemia.**

Hereditary and Acquired Variants

Occasionally, as an incidental finding, individuals demonstrate two distinct bands of albumin on serum protein electrophoresis. This pattern is termed **bisalbuminemia** because of the distribution of albumin in two approximately equal peaks of protein. These individuals are heterozygous for the variant albumin and the normal albumin (designated albumin A), which are both expressed in a genetic codominant manner. Their other serum proteins are unaffected by the split in albumin. There are more than 20 such electrophoretic variants of albumin, all presumably due to single amino acid substitutions with resulting change in molecular charge. Despite the dramatic appearance of bisalbuminemia on serum protein electrophoresis, it appears to be a completely benign state with no physiologic consequence. As such it should be recognized for proper interpretation when it is discovered.

One variant of albumin does have markedly increased affinity for thyroxine and thereby causes substantial elevations of thyroxine in the serum of individuals with the variant. These individuals are clinically euthyroid.

Acquired bisalbuminemia is a transient phenomenon in which a small charged molecule such as a drug binds to albumin, thereby altering its electrophoretic mobility and producing two bands of albumin. As the concentration of the drug increases, the relative abundance of the abnormal albumin band increases until saturation, when it replaces the normal albumin band. The effect is reversible as the drug clears from the circulation and dissociates from the albumin molecules. Penicillin and its derivatives commonly cause acquired bisalbuminemia. However, instead of appearing as a distinct band in some electrophoretic systems, the drug-albumin complex merely broadens the normal albumin band. In addition, prolonged conjugated **hyperbilirubinemia,** such as in obstructive jaundice, results in a covalent coupling of conjugated bilirubin (which has negative charge from glucuronic acid) to albumin. This species of bilirubin is delta-bilirubin, which migrates faster than normal albumin and so broadens the albumin band toward the anode. Delta-bilirubin has a longer plasma half-life than other conjugated bilirubin because it is retained in the circulation through its covalent linkage to albumin.

The binding capacity of albumin for unconjugated bilirubin is the basic defense for prevention of **kernicterus** in hemolytic disease of the newborn or in infantile jaundice prior to maturation of the conjugating mechanism in the liver. The reserve binding capacity of albumin for bilirubin is an index of how much more the serum bilirubin concentration can rise before the albumin is fully saturated. At that point there is free bilirubin that may deposit in the brain of newborns. Thus, albumin buffers directly against shifts in free bilirubin in the face of increasing total bilirubin levels. It is revealing to consider albumin and bilirubin in molar concentrations. An albumin concentration of 3.4 g/dL corresponds to 0.5 mmol/L, whereas a typical "panic value" for bilirubin of 16 mg/dL corresponds to 0.27 mmol/L. With this conversion, it is easy to appreciate how further increases in bilirubin might saturate the reserve binding capacity. Other molecular species such as fatty acids also bind to albumin in such a way as to displace bilirubin. Therefore, nutritional and metabolic status can strongly modulate binding of bilirubin to albumin so that the reserve binding capacity cannot be reliably calculated simply from albumin and bilirubin levels alone.

Other small molecules such as hormones and drugs bind to albumin as well as do the positively charged ions calcium, magnesium, sodium, and potassium. The attraction for cations is on a charge basis, and they can be displaced by other charged species such as the antineoplastic drug cisplatin. For that reason, intravenous administration of cisplatin usually requires monitoring of serum electrolytes and supplemental administration of electrolytes, particularly Mg^{2+}, because there is no body pool of Mg^{2+} accessible for the rebound phase during drug clearance, whereas Ca^{2+} is replenished by action of parathyroid hormone.

The amino acid sequence is known for human albumin and for that of several animal species. Human albumin has 35 cysteine residues out of a total of 585 amino acids. Disulfide bond formation between the half-cystine residues results in a secondary structure in which there are nine loops arranged in three major regions, each containing three subloops, suggesting that albumin has arisen on an evolutionary basis by gene duplication and fusion. Albumin also shares regions of amino acid homology with the molecule of alpha-fetoprotein, indicating common molecular ancestry between those two proteins.

In addition to forming covalent linkage with bilirubin, albumin also becomes glucosylated by a nonenzymatic means in the circulation. Patients with chronically high levels of blood glucose in diabetes mellitus have concentrations of glucosylated albumin severalfold higher than normal individuals in a manner similar to that for the glycosylated hemoglobins. Correlation between glucosylated albumin levels and glycosylated hemoglobin levels is not good, perhaps due to different half-lives of the two proteins or to the particular molecular environment inside versus outside cells. Glucosylated albumin (also referred to as fructosamine) can be used clinically to indicate diabetic control over an intermediate period (i.e., longer than blood glucose alone and shorter than glycosylated hemoglobin).

Albumin is one of the smallest plasma proteins. Because it is generally the most abundant one too, albumin is the major serum protein found in other body fluids such as CSF, pleural fluid, and peritoneal fluid, by virtue of concentration gradient effects and molecular size. Consequently, electrophoretic analysis of the proteins in those body fluids is generally noninformative, with the exceptions of oligoclonal banding in CSF or a possible rare monoclonal spike in another fluid due to localized plasmacytoma.

As a transfusion product, albumin has the advantage that during preparation it is heated and so is not infectious. In plasmapheresis, replacement of the body plasma with 5% albumin results in a unique serum protein electrophoresis pattern that shows predominantly an albumin band. Another variation results from long-term storage of plasma prior to transfusion, allowing formation of albumin dimers between free cysteine residues that can also appear as an extra-electrophoretic band.

ALPHA-1-ANTITRYPSIN

The alpha-1-globulin fraction consists mainly of the single glycoprotein **alpha-1-antitrypsin (AAT),** which has the ability to combine with and inactivate trypsin and other proteolytic enzymes. During the normal course of inflammation, there is release of proteolytic enzymes from leukocytes in the tissues of the body. Left unchecked, those enzymes would do extensive damage to the protein structure of the tissue. Alpha-1-antitrypsin is one of the major naturally occurring inhibitors of protease activity.

Congenital deficiency of AAT can result in premature emphysema. Cigarette smoke and other volatile irritants stimulate the release of enzymes from leukocytes in the lungs. Without AAT to inhibit them, those proteases cause considerable destruction of the lung parenchyma, leading to severe and often fatal emphysema in the third or fourth decade of life. Recently, there have been experimental attempts to prevent further damage in affected individuals by the intravenous infusion of AAT concentrates.

A second clinical syndrome associated with congenital deficiency of AAT in children is **cirrhosis of the liver,** the organ where AAT is normally synthesized. This disorder may be so severe as to require liver transplantation.

Alpha-1-antitrypsin can be measured both functionally (as trypsin-inhibiting capacity) and antigenically. Deficiency of AAT can be suspected if there is no distinct band in the alpha-1 region of serum protein electrophoresis. The tracing then is flat in the alpha-1 region. The congenital deficiencies of AAT also show an aberrant electrophoretic mobility of the small quantity of AAT present (usually less than 5% of normal values). The different phenotypes of AAT are classified according to the **PI (protease inhibitor) system.** The normal variant is designated M and the severe variant is Z. There is another electrophoretic variant called S that is usually present in moderate amounts sufficient to prevent the clinical syndrome of AAT deficiency. The individuals with emphysema or cirrhosis due to AAT deficiency are homozygous ZZ. Persons with the heterozygous form MZ are clinically normal but can be detected by special electrophoretic procedures that separate the AAT variants. This procedure may be useful in screening for carriers of AAT deficiency in kindreds with afflicted family members.

Genetic studies have shown at least 75 different mutations in the AAT gene, with many alleles producing AAT molecules that fail to be secreted into the circulation and so form inclusion granules within hepatocytes.

Alpha-1-antitrypsin is an acute phase reactant that can become elevated in the serum of normal individuals undergoing the physical stress of trauma, surgery, inflammation, or other acute disease.

Alpha-1-antitrypsin is relatively specific as to the particular proteolytic enzymes with which it can combine. There are several other minor serum proteins that also inhibit selective enzymes. These include alpha-1 antichymotrypsin, antithrombin III, antiplasmin, and interalpha trypsin inhibitor (migrates between alpha-1– and alpha-2–globulins). Abnormalities of these minor protease inhibitors are below the level of detection by standard clinical protein electrophoresis.

ALPHA-2-MACROGLOBULIN

In contrast to the specific protease inhibitors, **alpha-2-macroglobulin (AMG)** combines with and inactivates a variety of different proteases. In addition, AMG is present in serum in large amounts, thereby providing considerable capacity to inhibit enzymes released during the inflammatory response or tissue injury. Without AMG, those enzymes would likely continue to autodigest body tissues inappropriately. In fact, in AAT deficiency, AMG probably is the primary protease inhibitor that inactivates those enzymes left otherwise unchecked.

The nephrotic syndrome entails loss of serum proteins into the glomerular filtrate and subsequently into the urine. The individual serum proteins are lost according to molecular size, with the smallest ones emerging most readily. Alpha-2-macroglobulin has a molecular weight of almost 800,000, making it the largest of the serum proteins (except for IgM) and allowing it to be retained in the circulation even in the face of profound proteinuria. In severe cases, the concentration of AMG in serum may approach or even exceed that of albumin. This is one of the classic abnormal patterns of serum protein electrophoresis.

HAPTOGLOBIN

The other major protein in the alpha-2 zone is **haptoglobin,** which functions by binding to hemoglobin released into the plasma from lysed erythrocytes. The haptoglobin-hemoglobin complex is rapidly taken up from the circulation by the cells of the reticuloendothelial system, thereby conserving the iron contained in the hemoglobin. In extensive hemolysis, haptoglobin in the serum is depleted. Thus, haptoglobin measurement is useful for clinical assessment of hemolysis. The binding between haptoglobin and hemoglobin is highly specific. Myoglobin, which is similar to hemoglobin monomers and contains a heme group, does not bind to haptoglobin. Both hemoglobin and myoglobin give positive reactions for occult blood in the urine due to the activity of the heme group as pseudoperoxidase. Serum haptoglobin levels will fall dramatically with hemolysis and hemoglobinuria; however, serum haptoglobin remains essentially unchanged even in severe rhabdomyolysis and heavy myoglobinuria.

The binding between haptoglobin and hemoglobin is analogous to that between an antibody and an antigen. Haptoglobin **(type 1-1)** has two heavy chains and two light chains interlinked by disulfide bonds. An allele with gene duplication yields a doubled light chain with a free sulfhydryl group that bonds to an additional light chain, leading to a series of haptoglobin polymers of different molecular sizes. An individual homozygous for the variant light chain is termed **type 2-2.** A person heterozygous for the two light chains is termed **type 1-2** and also has a series of haptoglobin polymers, but with different molecular sizes from type 2-2 polymers. Haptoglobin types 1-1, 1-2, and 2-2 are readily distinguished by high-resolution electrophoresis. Both haptoglobin light chain gene types are present at sufficiently high frequency in the human population that haptoglobin phenotyping is feasible for paternity testing in addition to blood grouping and tissue typing.

Quantitation of haptoglobin levels was formerly done as hemoglobin-binding capacity but today is more conveniently performed nephelometrically with antihaptoglobin antibodies. Both methods may underestimate the contribution of haptoglobin polymers to the total amount due to stearic hindrance of binding at the molecular level. For this reason, quantitation of haptoglobin may not be equivalent for individuals of different phenotypes. However, serial determinations in the same person should be entirely comparable and may be the best way to monitor suspected hemolysis.

Haptoglobin levels should be expected to drop slightly after transfusion of banked blood because of some small amount of obligate hemolysis, even though the transfusion is compatible. This effect is even more pronounced after several transfusions in a short period.

Haptoglobin is an acute phase reactant and is frequently elevated in medically stressful situations.

BETA LIPOPROTEIN

The lipids in serum—consisting of cholesterol, cholesterol esters, triglycerides, and phospholipids—do not circulate freely. Rather they are joined with proteins (or apolipoproteins) that keep them suspended as small globules or micelles in the aqueous environment of serum. Predominant among these forms is beta lipoprotein, which is generally appreciated as a faint band on electrophoresis when stained for protein. When stained for lipid (see Fig. 9–2), there emerge the **alpha lipoprotein** (corresponds to high-density lipids by ultracentrifugation—HDL), **prebeta lipoprotein** (very-low-density lipid—VLDL), **beta lipoprotein** (low-density lipid—LDL), and **chylomicrons** (large lipid particles rich in triglycerides that float to the top of a refrigerated sample). Administration of heparin before drawing a specimen for protein electrophoresis will alter or abolish the band of beta lipoprotein due to the action of postheparin lipoprotein lipase.

TRANSFERRIN

The transport of iron in the plasma is accomplished by transferrin, which migrates in the beta globulin region. Dietary iron is absorbed by the intestine as Fe^{2+} and bound as Fe^{3+} to ferritin in cells of the intestinal mucosa. It is then taken up by transferrin as Fe^{2+} for transport to sites of storage and utilization (primarily bone marrow and muscle). One molecule of transferrin can bind two ions of iron. The mechanism by which iron enters immature erythrocytes for incorporation into hemoglobin (as Fe^{2+}) involves receptors for transferrin on the surface of those cells. Other cells such as lymphocytes also have transferrin receptors on their cell membranes to facilitate uptake of iron. In storage cells, iron is bound as Fe^{3+} to ferritin.

The whole balance of iron metabolism is highly regulated by this exchange of iron with alternating oxidation-reduction states of the ion.

This process is described more fully under iron deficiency anemia (see Chapter 3). Relevant to patterns of serum protein electrophoresis is the finding that, in iron deficiency states, transferrin becomes elevated, giving rise to a small spike in the beta region. It is important to recognize that this phenomenon is a consequence of increased transferrin or iron-binding capacity as part of a physiologic response by the body to hold onto iron. It should not be confused with a monoclonal spike of immunoglobulin, despite a somewhat similar electrophoretic appearance.

Transferrin can be lost into the urine with severe proteinuria, thereby draining away some body supply of iron. This loss into the urine is a consequence of transferrin's relatively small molecular size (77,000 daltons). Mild proteinuria consists mainly of albumin (68,000 daltons). It is more severe renal disease that permits loss of proteins larger than albumin.

Cerebrospinal fluid (CSF) also normally contains transferrin in a small quantity. There are two electrophoretic bands of transferrin normally found in CSF. One corresponds to the band of transferrin found in serum; the other migrates more cathodally due to the loss of negatively charged sialic acid residues. This latter variant of transferrin appears to be found only in CSF and differs only in terms of posttranslational modification of that protein. Its function in CSF is not known, but it can be used as a specific marker for the presence of CSF (e.g., in questions of CSF leakage).

COMPLEMENT C3

The complement system is discussed in Chapter 7. In terms of protein electrophoresis patterns, only the C3 component is present in sufficiently high amounts to be detectable on serum samples. It migrates in the slow beta globulin region. Elevations of C3 may be appreciated in some patients but are not useful in diagnosis. Absence of C3 is significant in that it may indicate activation of the complement system and consumption of the complement factors, as in immune complex disease or systemic lupus erythematosus. For monitoring the status of autoimmune disorders, C3 (or C4) is best quantified by nephelometry.

FIBRINOGEN

The sole coagulation factor present in plasma in sufficient concentrations to be detected by standard protein electrophoresis is **fibrinogen,** which migrates between the beta and gamma globulins. In the process of clotting, all the fibrinogen in plasma is normally converted to fibrin, leaving serum devoid of fibrinogen. Incomplete clotting of a specimen, as occurs when a patient is anticoagulated with heparin, can leave a sizeable amount of fibrinogen in the serum. If not correctly recognized, this situation may lead to the suspicion of a monoclonal immunoglobulin spike.

Fibrinogen is elevated with other acute phase reactants in response to acute illness. Fibrinogen has a major impact on the erythrocyte sedimentation rate (ESR) by coating the cells and allowing them to sediment faster in clumps. Thus, elevations of fibrinogen are reflected by faster ESR.

Fibrinogen is synthesized in the liver. Hepatic failure leads to aberrant forms of the fibrinogen molecule with abnormal glycosylation that show abnormal kinetics of clotting.

Disseminated intravascular coagulation causes depletion of circulating fibrinogen, and concurrent fibrinolysis results in release of fragments of fibrin called **fibrin split products (FSP).** Fibrinolytic therapy with streptokinase or tissue plasminogen activator for treatment of acute coronary thrombosis shows a similar picture of fibrinogen depletion and elevation of circulating FSP. Rattlesnake venom contains an enzyme that clots fibrinogen, and rattlesnake bite also results in systemic depletion of fibrinogen.

Rare individuals have congenital deficiency of fibrinogen termed **afibrinogenemia,** and others have fibrinogen molecules with mutations that impair clotting, termed **dysfibrinogenemia.** Both conditions result in hemorrhagic disorders.

IMMUNOGLOBULINS

The structure and function of immunoglobulins are described in Chapter 7. All the classes of immunoglobulins (IgG, IgA, IgM, IgD, and IgE) collectively migrate electrophoretically in the gamma region. There is some minor variation in overall migration between the different immunoglobulin classes, most notably with IgA migrating into the beta globulins. However, there is so much overlap in the positions of the different classes that individual myeloma proteins cannot be identified as to heavy chain type by electrophoretic positions alone.

The single most significant clinical application of serum protein electrophoresis is for the detection of monoclonal spikes of immunoglobulins and in distinguishing them from polyclonal hypergammaglobulinemia (Figs. 9–5 and 9–6.) Uniformly migrating bands of monoclonal immunoglobulin are characteristic of multiple myeloma, Waldenström's macroglobulinemia, plasmacytoma, and monoclonal gammopathy of undetermined significance (see Chapter 4). Myeloma typically shows no normal polyclonal immunoglobulins, but a major single spike. Occasionally more than one spike of protein is observed, and in particular the urine may show a distinctly different band of free light chains that migrate away from the main band of myeloma protein (see Fig. 9–6).

The presence of a few separate bands of different immunoglobulins is called **oligoclonal banding.** While its occurrence in serum is generally without major significance, oligoclonal banding in cerebrospinal fluid (CSF) is an indication of antibody production within the central nervous system. This process is strongly associated with demyelinating disorders

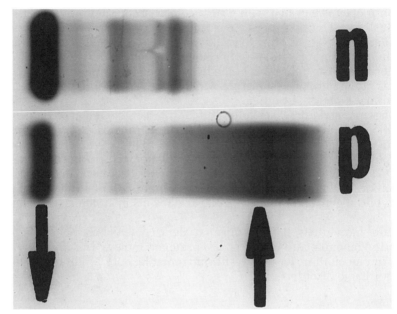

FIGURE 9–5. *Hypoalbuminemia* (downward arrow) and *polyclonal hypergam-maglobulinemia* (upward arrow) in the serum of a patient *(p)* with liver disease. Compared to normal serum *(n)*, the albumin to globulin (A/G) ratio has been markedly lowered.

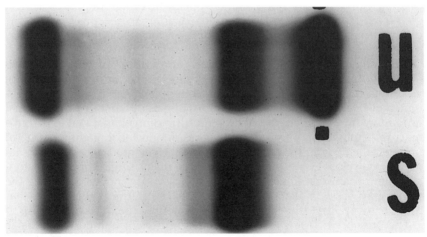

FIGURE 9–6. Myeloma proteins present in serum *(s)* and urine *(u)* of the same patient. The serum and urine both contain the intact *monoclonal immunoglobulin* (heavy and light chains) migrating in the gamma region. In addition, the urine has a major band (above mark) of *free light chains* missing from the serum.

such as multiple sclerosis, for which oligoclonal banding in CSF is a commonly used diagnostic examination.

CARRIER PROTEINS

The most abundant plasma protein albumin also has the capacity to bind a wide variety of small ions and molecules such as drugs, hormones, and metabolites. Other proteins in much lower concentrations have great specificity and high affinity of binding for individual small molecules of physiologic importance. **Alpha-1-acid glycoprotein,** or *orosomucoid*, has a great affinity for progesterone and also binds drugs such as quinidine. **Thyroxine-binding globulin** is the major serum protein involved in the transport of thyroxine (T_4) and triiodothyronine (T_3). **Hemopexin** binds heme (and in so doing preserves iron) when haptoglobin has been depleted by the release of hemoglobin. The **group-specific component (gc) globulin** binds vitamin D, thereby enabling that oil-soluble vitamin to be transported through the blood. **Retinol-binding protein (RBP)** similarly binds vitamin A. Retinol-binding protein in turn is complexed to prealbumin, which also has a moderate affinity for T_4. **Transferrin** is responsible for iron transport and uptake into cells where it is incorporated into heme groups. **Ceruloplasmin** transports copper, which is essential for life in very low levels. Ceruloplasmin concentrations are severely decreased in Wilson's disease (see Chapter 12).

ACUTE PHASE REACTANTS

As previously described in part, many plasma proteins become elevated acutely in response to illness, infection, trauma, and tissue necrosis. These proteins include alpha-1-acid glycoprotein, alpha-1-antitrypsin, ceruloplasmin, haptoglobin, fibrinogen, and C-reactive protein (CRP). The most

---

TABLE 9–15. CONDITIONS THAT ELICIT C-REACTIVE PROTEIN

Almost Always Present:
Rheumatic fever; rheumatoid arthritis; acute bacterial infections; viral hepatitis

Frequently Present:
Active tuberculosis; gout; advanced malignant tumors; leprosy; active cirrhosis; widespread burns; peritonitis

Sometimes Present:
Multiple sclerosis; Guillain-Barré syndrome; scarlet fever; varicella; postsurgical state; use of intrauterine contraceptive device

---

useful of all these species is CRP, based on its rapid rise in response to acute disease and rapid clearance once that stimulus has abated (Table 9–15). C-reactive protein is readily quantitated by immunologic methods such as nephelometry.

SUGGESTED READING

Deftos, LJ: The thyroid gland in calcium and skeletal metabolism. In Avioli, LV, and Krane, SM (eds): Metabolic Bone Disease, ed 2. WB Saunders, Philadelphia, 1990, p 702.

The Expert Panel: Report of the national cholesterol education program expert panel on detection, evaluation, and treatment of high blood cholesterol in adults. Arch Intern Med 148:36, 1988.

Frederickson, DS, Goldstein, JL, and Brown, JS: The familial hyperlipoproteinemias. In Stanbury, JB, Wyngaarden, JB, and Frederickson, DS (eds): The Metabolic Basis of Inherited Disease, ed 4. McGraw-Hill, New York, 1978, p 604.

Guyton, AC: Textbook of Medical Physiology, ed 7. WB Saunders, Philadelphia, 1986.

Henry, RJ, Golub, OJ, and Soleb, C: Some of the variables involved in the fractionation of serum proteins by paper electrophoresis. Clin Chem 3:49, 1957.

Howanitz, PJ, and Howanitz, JH: Carbohydrates. In Henry, JB (ed): Clinical Diagnosis and Management by Laboratory Methods, ed 17. WB Saunders, Philadelphia, 1984, p 165.

Jialal, I: A practical approach to the laboratory diagnosis of dyslipidemia. Am J Clin Path 106:128, 1996.

The Kroc Collaborative Study Group: Blood glucose control and the evolution of diabetic retinopathy and albuminuria. N Engl J Med 311:365, 1984.

Maciejko, JJ, Holmes, DR, Kottle, BA, et al: Apolipoprotein A-I as a marker of angiographically assessed coronary artery disease. N Engl J Med 309:385, 1983.

McPherson, RA: Specific proteins. In Henry, JB (ed): Clinical Diagnosis and Management by Laboratory Methods, ed 19. WB Saunders, Philadelphia, 1996, p 237.

Ryan, MF: The role of magnesium in clinical biochemistry: An overview. Ann Clin Biochem 28:19, 1991.

Segal, P, et al: Lipids and dyslipoproteinemia. In Henry, JB (ed): Clinical Diagnosis and Management by Laboratory Methods, ed 17. WB Saunders, Philadelphia, 1984, p 180.

Weidman, SW, and Schonfeld, G: Lipids and lipoproteins. In Sonnewirth, AC, and Jarett, L (eds): Gradwohl's Clinical Laboratory Methods and Diagnosis, ed 8. Mosby, St Louis, 1980, p 272.

Whelton, A, Watson, AJ, Rock, RC: Nitrogen metabolites and renal function. In Burtis, CA, and Ashwood, ER (eds): Tietz Textbook of Clinical Chemistry, ed 2. WB Saunders, Philadelphia, 1994, p 1513.

Woo, J, and Cannon, DC: Metabolic intermediates and inorganic ions. In Henry, JB (ed): Clinical Diagnosis and Management by Laboratory Methods, ed 17. WB Saunders, Philadelphia, 1984, p 133.

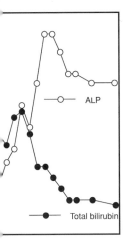

10

Acid-Base and
Electrolyte Regulation

BASIC PHYSIOLOGY

Electrolytes, blood gases, and acid-base regulators are crucial substances in the blood because of the serious consequences that can result from even modest disturbances of any one. Electrolytes are extremely important for the maintenance of electrochemical potentials across cell membranes, which in turn affect neurologic and muscular functions, as well as cellular activities such as secretion, contraction, and a vast array of other metabolic processes. Cells of the body expend a tremendous amount of energy to maintain concentrations of these simple chemical substances within narrow ranges, both intracellularly and extracellularly. Fluctuations in these levels can lead to serious malfunction of critical organs, in particular the heart, whose contractions, along with other muscle and nervous system activities, absolutely depend on correct concentrations of ions and correct pH. Rapid changes in ion concentrations can cause sudden death.

Maintaining physiologically appropriate levels of total-body water, fluid distribution, electrolyte concentration, and acid-base equilibrium requires many reactions and involves many organ systems. Water constitutes 60 to 70% of body weight (depending on body fat content), of which approximately two-thirds is intracellular water. Most of the remaining third is spread out between cells as interstitial fluid, and 3 to 4 liters of extracellular fluid circulates as blood plasma (intravascular fluid). The plasma phase contains many dissolved solutes. Some solutes (e.g., glucose and urea) do not dissociate. They do not contribute to electrical activity of fluids and membranes, and contribute only moderately to plasma osmolality. Substances that dissociate into positively and negatively charged ions strongly affect the electrical and also the osmolal functioning of the body.

IONS AND DISSOCIATION

The most abundant ions of body fluid are sodium (Na^+), potassium (K^+), chloride (Cl^-), and bicarbonate (HCO_3^-). There are also smaller amounts of other ions such as calcium (Ca^{2+}), magnesium (Mg^{2+}), and phosphates, which contribute to the total ionic content of body fluids and also play individual roles in cell functions beyond those of the more abundant ions. Fluid always contains equal numbers of positive **(cation)** and negative **(anion)** charges; this balance of charges is referred to as **electroneutrality.** The nature of the ions, the number of charges present on a single molecule, and the nature and mobility of charged molecules differ enormously among body fluid compartments. Large protein molecules that do not readily cross cell membranes have a net negative charge from all the side groups of their constituent amino acids. To achieve electroneutrality, fluids that contain protein also have accompanying cations (generally Na^+ and K^+).

Dissociation of solutes into charged particles **(ions)** depends on the chemical composition of the compound and on the concentration of other charged particles in the medium. For example, a gram molecular weight (one mole) of sodium chloride dissociates completely into one mole of Na^+ and one mole of Cl^- independent of the presence of other ions. Urea dissolves freely in water but does not dissociate further into ions. Carbonic acid (H_2CO_3) dissociates into H^+ and HCO_3^- only in media that contain few other H^+ ions.

Definitions

In order to discuss regulation of fluid and electrolyte homeostasis, a number of standard terms must be defined:

Cation. An ionized particle with a net positive charge; travels in an electrical field toward the negative pole (cathode).

Anion. An ionized particle with a net negative charge; travels in an electrical field toward the positive pole (anode).

Acid. A substance that on dissociation releases hydrogen ion (H^+) into a solution.

Fixed Acid. An acid that, when excreted through the urine, must be in salt form accompanied by a cation.

Volatile Acid. An acid that can be excreted as a gas without requiring a cation for its excretion. An example is carbonic acid.

Base. A dissociable substance capable of combining with a hydrogen ion in solution.

Hydroxyl Ion. The anion OH^-, capable of combining with H^+ to form uncharged water (H_2O).

Salt. The compound formed by the combination of an acid and a base. The H^+ of the acid is replaced by a cation that does not affect the pH. For example, NaCl is the salt formed when H^+ of HCl is replaced by Na^+ from a dissociable compound (like NaOH) in which the anion is capable of combining with H^+.

pH. A quantitative measure of the acidity or alkalinity of a solution with reference to pure water. It is expressed mathematically as the negative logarithm of the hydrogen ion concentration in a solution. A neutral solution has a pH of 7; its hydrogen ion concentration is 10^{-7} molar or 100 nEq/liter. Solutions with pH values lower than 7 are said to be acidic and have hydrogen ion concentrations greater than 100 nEq/liter. A pH of 6 corresponds to (H^+) of 1000 nEq/liter. Solutions with pH values higher than 7 are called basic (or alkaline) and have hydrogen ion concentrations less than 100 nEq/liter. A pH of 8 corresponds to (H^+) of 10 nEq/liter.

Strong Acid. A dissociable compound that separates into H^+ and an anion in solutions with low pH in which many other H^+ ions are already present (e.g., pH of 1 or less).

Weak Acid. A dissociable compound that separates to yield H^+ ions only when few other H^+ ions are present, that is, at a fairly high pH (e.g., 3 or 4).

Buffer Pair. A solution containing a weak acid and the salt of the same acid. If H^+ is added to this combination, the salt of the acid unites with H^+ to form an acid that does not dissociate at strongly acid pH. Formation of the undissociated weak acid removes free H^+ from the solution, and the pH of the solution changes relatively little. This action, called **buffering,** is extremely important for acid-base regulation in biologic fluids.

Osmolality. A measure of the number of particles dissolved in a fluid. A 1-osmolal solution contains the number of particles present in a gram molecular weight (mole) of a nonelectrolyte substance dissolved in 1 kg of pure water. The nature of the particles does not affect osmolality. One mole of an undissociated substance contributes 6.023×10^{23} particles (Avogadro's number) when dissolved. One mole of a substance like NaCl that dissociates into two ions contributes twice as many particles; $CaCl_2$, which dissociates into one Ca^{2+} and two Cl^- ions, contributes three times as many particles.

Osmotic Pressure. The tendency for solvent water to move from a solution with a lower concentration of solute particles, across a membrane (permeable to water but not to larger molecules), into a solution with a higher concentration of solute. The more dissolved particles a solution contains, the greater its osmotic pressure. Water moves from one side of a membrane to the other if one side contains particles that cannot equalize the solute concentration by entering the less concentrated compartment. In order to equalize the proportions of particles and solvent when some particles cannot equilibrate across the membrane, there must be net movement of solvent into the more concentrated compartment until particle concentration is equal on both sides. A solution with high particle concentration has high osmotic pressure because it exerts a strong attraction for water to enter.

pK. A term indicating the pH at which the associated and dissociated forms of an acid will exist in equal concentrations. Sometimes loosely referred to as **dissociation constant,** it is actually the negative logarithm of that constant.

Henderson-Hasselbalch Equation. This formula relates the pH of a solution to the dissociation properties of the weak acid, comprising the buffer pair (the pK), the concentration of the salt present $[A^-]$, and the concentration of the undissociated acid present $[HA]$. The equation is:

$$pH = pK + \log([A^-]/[HA])$$

The ratio between salt and acid is the variable that changes, and the pH depends on the proportion between salt and acid in the solution. In clinical acid-base calculations, the critical buffer pair is carbonic acid (H_2CO_3) and its salt, the bicarbonate ion (HCO_3^-). Carbonic acid has a pK of 6.1; at physiologic pH of 7.4, most of the acid is dissociated, and the ratio of HCO_3^- to H_2CO_3 is approximately 20:1.

For the bicarbonate buffering system, the Henderson-Hasselbalch equation becomes:

$$pH = 6.1 + \log \frac{[HCO_3^-]}{H_2CO_3}$$

and at normal physiologic conditions,

$$pH = 6.1 + \log ([20]/[1]) = 6.1 + 1.3 = 7.4$$

BUFFERING ACID SOLUTIONS

The normal range of pH in extracellular fluids, as reflected in circulating blood, is 7.36 (corresponds to 44 nEq/liter of H^+) to 7.44 (36 nEq/liter of H^+). These are very small quantities of dissociated H^+ ions present at any one time, despite the fact that metabolic processes generate approximately 50 to 100 mEq of fixed acid and 13,000 to 20,000 millimoles of carbon dioxide every day. To preserve pH within the narrow physiologic range, short-term buffering capacity must neutralize acids as they are generated, and long-term corrective measures must eliminate the acid permanently, but on a continuous basis.

The Bicarbonate System

The major extracellular buffer in blood is the **bicarbonate/carbonic acid system,** HCO_3^-/H_2CO_3. This buffer pair has some unique properties that are extremely important to biological functions. As long as the ratio of plasma bicarbonate to dissolved CO_2 (H_2CO_3) remains at 20:1, the blood pH remains at 7.4, even if the absolute concentrations of HCO_3^- and H_2CO_3 change. In a closed system with no additional input, buffering ceases once the salt or the acid is consumed, and generation of further H^+ causes major pH changes. However, bicarbonate and carbonic acid are renewable; even before renal mechanisms restore the constituents, the lung alters the ratio of numerator (HCO_3^-) to denominator (H_2CO_3) by blowing off CO_2. By regulating the rate of CO_2 excretion, the lungs can maintain the ratio at or near 20:1, thereby minimizing pH changes.

Proteins and Hemoglobin

Plasma proteins also exert a buffering effect for fixed acids through the charges on their surfaces. Although located exclusively within red cells, hemoglobin is uniquely effective in buffering the CO_2 generated by aerobic glycolysis because hemoglobin can off-load its oxygen and combine with CO_2 that has diffused across gradients from tissues into capillaries. In the lung, gradients of those gases reverse so that hemoglobin releases CO_2 into the expired air and acquires O_2 from inspired air.

Respiratory Control of CO_2

Blood levels of CO_2 very rapidly affect the denominator of the Henderson-Hasselbalch ratio. Additional CO_2 increases the denominator, reduces the ratio below 20:1, and causes increased acidity (falling pH); loss of CO_2 depresses the denominator, increases the proportion, and causes pH to rise. Thus respiratory control of CO_2 excretion allows rapid and very sensitive adjustments in blood pH. If excess H^+ is generated, circulating bicarbonate combines with it to form H_2CO_3, preventing H^+ accumulation from affecting blood pH. This process consumes HCO_3^- and generates H_2CO_3, changes that would affect the ratio and thus the pH were it not for the ability to control H_2CO_3 levels by increased respiratory excretion of CO_2.

As the lungs eliminate excess CO_2 to resist accumulating H^+, the proportion between HCO_3^- and H_2CO_3 readjusts to 20:1, although the absolute concentrations of each can fall below normal. Conversely, rising HCO_3^- concentration can be compensated by reducing ventilation, retaining CO_2, and allowing the 20:1 ratio to re-equilibrate at higher absolute concentrations. The lungs control the denominator of the equation, but adjustments are necessarily limited by the mechanics of respiration and the body's need for oxygen.

Renal Control of HCO_3^-

Bicarbonate concentration is under renal control, in that the kidneys regulate both the generation of HCO_3^- ions and their rate of urinary excretion. H^+ ions are excreted by the kidney, both by direct excretion as H^+ and through indirect disposal in the form of ammonium ion (NH_4^+). Water and solute regulation occur in the proximal convoluted tubule, where Na^+ is actively reabsorbed for restoration to the blood, and water and Cl^- are passively reabsorbed. Bicarbonate is also reabsorbed, a process requiring the zinc-containing enzyme carbonic anhydrase that catalyzes the following reaction:

$$CO_2 + H_2O \rightleftarrows H_2CO_3$$

The carbonic acid so produced is able to dissociate into hydrogen ion and bicarbonate. The result is salvage of bicarbonate and excretion of hydrogen ion. (Carbonic anhydrase is also present in erythrocytes, where it is the second most abundant protein after hemoglobin. It functions there to promote uptake of H^+ by hemoglobin. It also functions in the secretion of gastric acid into the stomach and in the secretion of bicarbonate into pancreatic juice.) If blood bicarbonate is below 25 mEq/liter or if blood CO_2 rises above normal, the tubule can reabsorb all the bicarbonate in the glomerular filtrate, leaving none for excretion in urine. As HCO_3^- is salvaged and actively generated, H^+ excretion increases. By this process, the whole-body acid load is reduced, and the bicarbonate numerator returns to normal.

CONTROL OVER CATIONS

Cation excretion is regulated in the distal tubules of the kidney, where H^+ is reabsorbed and Na^+ and K^+ are excreted, if necessary; or H^+ excretion is increased to the limit of permissible urinary acidity. If urine pH falls to 4.5, additional H^+ may be excreted as NH_4^+, an ion that does not affect pH but does require a balancing anion. The degree to which H^+, Na^+, K^+, or NH_4^+ will be conserved or excreted is modulated in the distal nephron in response to various stimuli. Changes in extracellular fluid (ECF) volume affect Na^+ excretion. When ECF expands, more Na^+ is excreted, whereas volume deficits cause Na^+ to be retained. If potassium levels are low, K^+ ions will be retained, and NH_4^+ will be secreted if balancing cations are needed; potassium excess causes reduced NH_4^+ excretion and increased urinary K^+.

Antidiuretic Hormone and Solute Concentration

Control over water resorption and excretion resides in the renal collecting ducts. Solute reabsorption affects water reabsorption because reabsorbed electrolytes remain concentrated in the interstitial fluid of the renal medulla through which the collecting tubules pass. The epithelium lining the collecting tubules is thus in contact with hyperosmolal interstitial fluid. **Antidiuretic hormone (ADH)** causes the epithelium to become permeable to water, and the hyperosmolal medullary environment pulls water out of the tubular fluid, leaving a concentrated urine. Without ADH, large volumes of dilute urine are excreted.

High Solute Loads

The need to excrete large amounts of fixed acids (organic acids, sulfates, phosphates, etc.) affects urinary make-up. If tubular urine contains large amounts of anions for excretion, an equal number of cations must also be excreted. Urinary H^+ concentration cannot fall below a pH of 4.5, and potential quantities of NH_4^+ are limited. To eliminate fixed acid loads, the kidneys must excrete Na^+ and K^+, regardless of the whole-body levels of these cations. In addition, high osmotic activity develops in urine with a high concentration of acid metabolites (or of any other solute, such as glucose, urea, or other nonionized and nonreabsorbable compounds). Highly concentrated tubular fluid moves rapidly past the medullary zone where fluid normally is reabsorbed. The result is excretion of large urinary volumes with loss of water as well as solutes.

Thus renal function and electrolyte regulation strongly influence acid-base metabolism. The following considerations of individual laboratory tests must be viewed in the light of these complex interrelationships. In addition, diseases that affect acid-base and electrolyte metabolism will frequently also affect the results of other laboratory tests, which can be used for confirmation of diagnosis or for extension of disease monitoring.

LABORATORY TESTS

BICARBONATE AND BLOOD GASES

Present-day instrumentation conveniently makes highly reliable measurements that can be used to assess a patient's acid-base status. As an index of **bicarbonate ion concentration,** it is customary to measure total carbon dioxide in serum. Over 90% of blood carbon dioxide exists in the ionized bicarbonate form, which is converted to CO_2 when a standard amount of acid is added to the serum. This CO_2 is then measured by one of several possible indicator techniques. Of course, this methodology is highly sensitive to variations in temperature and acidification, but these sources of error are minimized by the application of automated analyzers that operate very reproducibly. Since arterial blood has a lower total CO_2 than venous blood, measurements of bicarbonate are usually performed on serum obtained from venous samples for uniformity of comparison (normal range, 19 to 25 mEq/liter).

The amount of H_2CO_3 in blood cannot easily be measured; instead, the gaseous CO_2 dissolved is determined by measuring the partial pressure of CO_2 in an atmosphere in equilibrium with the solution. This measurement is the **partial pressure of CO_2 (Pco_2)** expressed in millimeters of mercury (mmHg) or torr. The concentration of H_2CO_3 then in mEq/liter is equal to 0.03 times Pco_2 in mmHg due to the solubility properties of the gas CO_2 in aqueous solution (normal range of Pco_2 is 38 to 42 mmHg).

Modern blood gas instruments routinely contain three electrodes that give very rapid and accurate results for direct measurement of pH, Pco_2, and Po_2 (the partial pressure of oxygen). By using these results of pH plus the modification of $0.03 \times Pco_2$ for H_2CO_3 in the Henderson-Hasselbalch equation, the bicarbonate can be calculated. This manipulation can be done manually with nomograms designed for the calculation. It is also generally performed automatically by computer-assisted reporting on blood gas instruments. In addition to these three direct measurements, blood gas analyzers now also print out calculated bicarbonate, oxygen saturation (based on the Po_2, temperature, and assumed hemoglobin value), and base excess. The calculation of base excess uses pH and Pco_2 measurements to estimate the amount of titratable base needed to normalize extracellular fluid pH to 7.4 and Pco_2 to 40 mmHg. The base excess is particularly useful when a base deficit exists to let the physician know how much base should be administered to a patient. These calculated values do not have the same accuracy and validity as direct measurements of those quantities, but they do have the advantage of being quick, being done on the same single sample as the rest of the blood gas analysis. They are close enough to true values to allow the physician to act immediately on any acute trends in the care of a patient.

As a general rule of thumb, deviations from normal in the blood gases are thought of as reflecting *acidosis* versus *alkalosis*, with the cause being either *metabolic* or *respiratory* (discussed later). It should be obvious that any change in the pulmonary or cardiac status of a patient can have marked influence on the delivery of blood to the lungs *(perfusion)*, and once there, on its oxygenation and loss of carbon dioxide *(ventilation)*.

Elevation of Pco_2 is considered a direct reflection of alveolar hypoventilation and, of course, alveolar hyperventilation leads to a lowering of Pco_2. Relatively little change of Pco_2 with a marked fall in Po_2 reflects a defect in the ability to perfuse ventilated regions of the lungs with blood. For instance, there may be pneumonia, pulmonary edema, or collapse of the lung that prevents sections of the lung from being ventilated while blood is still going through those regions. Normal values of P_{O_2} in arterial blood should be *85 to 100 mmHg*. Values down to 80 mmHg may be acceptable in healthy individuals, and down to 70 mmHg in older persons. Healthy individuals living at higher altitudes (a few thousand feet) will also show lower normal ranges of arterial P_{O_2} because of the naturally lower partial pressure of oxygen in the atmosphere and so in the inspired air.

Therapy should be designed to keep P_{O_2} above at least 50 mmHg, although the specific level of hypoxemia that will cause death varies between individuals. In addition to the medical problems related to ischemia and organ damage, patients will demonstrate a spectrum of mental changes, from mild confusion with slight hypoxemia to coma with profound hypoxemia. One of the most basic and essential reflexes of the human body is termed the **hypoxic drive,** that is, the stimulus to respiration through the central nervous system when the oxygen content of blood is reduced.

The transfer of oxygen from hemoglobin in the red cells to tissues where it is needed for metabolism is dictated by the oxygen-hemoglobin dissociation curve (Fig. 10–1). This sigmoidal (S-shaped) curve indicates what percent of the hemoglobin is oxygenated (**oxyhemoglobin;** also referred to as **percent saturation**) at different partial pressures of oxygen (**O₂ tension**). A standard reference point on this curve is the P_{50}, the partial pressure of oxygen at which 50% saturation occurs. The P_{50} and the whole curve can be shifted to the right (i.e., the hemoglobin gives up oxygen more readily to the tissues) by acidosis, fever, or increased red cell content of 2,3-diphosphoglycerate (2,3,-DPG). Alkalosis, hypothermia, and decreased amounts of 2,3-DPG shift the curve to the left, which

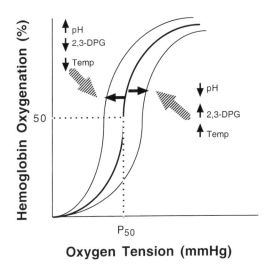

FIGURE 10–1. Normal oxygen-hemoglobin dissociation curve (bold) and the effects on oxygen affinity from changes in pH, temperature, and red cell 2,3-DPG level.

impairs release of oxygen to tissues. Concentrations of 2,3-DPG increase in red cells as a physiologic adaptation to chronic hypoxia. Hemoglobin F (fetal) normally has a curve displaced to the left of that for hemoglobin A (adult), which gives the fetus an advantage in taking up oxygen from the maternal circulation.

Normal values for blood gas measurements are given in Table 10–1.

TECHNICAL CONSIDERATIONS AND ARTIFACTS

Blood gas and pH results change rapidly, not only in the intact patient but also in the blood specimen. If the blood is exposed to ambient atmosphere (even an air bubble in the syringe), gas pressures equilibrate with the air, artifactually altering the results from true levels in the patient. This process may be accelerated if a blood specimen containing an air bubble is transported through devices such as pneumatic tube delivery systems, which can agitate the contents in transit. Continuing cellular metabolism in the sample may consume oxygen, generate CO_2, and alter the pH. Gas pressures and pH also vary with the temperature of the specimen, the temperature of the patient, and the temperature at which measurement is made.

Care of the Specimen

Arterial and venous blood differ in pH, P_{CO_2}, and P_{O_2}. The most desirable specimen is arterial blood (because it most directly reflects the status of

TABLE 10–1. NORMAL REFERENCE VALUES FOR SERUM ELECTROLYTES AND BLOOD GAS ANALYTES

	Arterial	Venous
pH	7.36–7.44	7.31–7.41
[H$^+$]	44–36 nmol/liter	41–31 nmol/liter
Total CO_2	19–25 mmol/liter	23–30 nmol/liter
P_{CO_2}	38–42 mmHg	35–40 mmHg
P_{O_2}	85–100 mmHg	35–40 mmHg
O_2 saturation	≥95% of P_{O_2}	70–75% of P_{O_2}
Sodium		135–148 mEq/liter
Potassium		3.5–5.3 mEq/liter
Chloride		98–106 mEq/liter
Bicarbonate		19–25 mEq/liter
Anion gap		12–18 mEq/liter
Serum osmolality		285–310 mOsm/kg H_2O

gas exchange at its peak in the lungs), drawn into an airtight syringe. The needle is removed and discarded, and the syringe is capped to avoid contact with air. Heparin is used for anticoagulation by drawing up into the syringe to wet its interior (no more than 0.5 mL of 1000-U/mL solution for 5 mL blood). Excess heparin should be expelled before blood collection since it can depress the Pco_2 by 12 to 25%. The specimen should then be placed immediately on ice for transport to the laboratory. It should be analyzed as soon as possible but is probably reasonably stable for up to 30 minutes on ice. The Po_2 changes more rapidly than Pco_2 or pH.

Arterial blood is the only specimen suitable for measuring Po_2, but "arterialized" capillary blood can be used for pH and Pco_2 if necessary because of sample volume constraints (e.g., heelstick draws from infants). The capillary bed should be dilated by warming the area to 45 to 47°C for 10 minutes before collecting the specimen. After a deep, free-flowing puncture, blood should be collected into heparinized capillary tubes, which are immediately sealed at both ends. Capillary "arterialization" should not be done if arterial blood pressure is below 95 mmHg or if the area has a poor blood supply.

Condition of the Patient

Blood gas results are affected by the gas mixture the patient is breathing and by the patient's temperature. Measurements are routinely made at 37°C. For each degree of fever in the patient, Po_2 will fall 7% and Pco_2 will rise 3%. If a patient is on a respirator, it is important to inform the laboratory of gas volumes and pressures. For example, a patient breathing room air (oxygen partial pressure in air is roughly 160 mmHg) may have an arterial Po_2 of 90 mmHg, which is quite acceptable. If, however, the patient were breathing a gas mixture with twice that oxygen content (40% oxygen), an arterial Po_2 of 90 mmHg would be far less than expected and should lead to medical corrective action. Respiratory adjustments can be in terms of percent inspired oxygen, depth of respiration, and frequency of respirations. After adjustments, breathing should equilibrate for at least 15 minutes before a new specimen is drawn.

Blood gas determinations may be performed on outpatients to help in the assessment of chronic pulmonary or cardiac disease or the investigation of polycythemia. They are more frequently performed on acutely ill patients—particularly those undergoing cardiac surgery, those recovering from cardiac or pulmonary events, and premature infants whose lungs are immature. Blood gas results should be back to the physician within about 10 minutes after draw in order to obtain maximum benefit from them. This immediacy of the requirement for blood gas results in order to modify life-support therapies has led to development of special equipment for the bedside monitoring of those gases. Much still needs to be done in this area in order to ensure the quality of results because these substances are highly sensitive to analytic variations. Nevertheless, it is clear that blood gas analysis is one field that will advance rapidly in the future as technology permits. These developments will include **in situ (in vivo)** monitoring of Po_2 and Pco_2, particularly in premature neonates under intensive care and in surgical and postoperative care of all ages.

Present-day blood gas analyzers generally measure pH, Pco_2, and Po_2 directly; many are also adapted to measure K^+ and Ca^{2+}. Some have a separate channel for lactate.

ELECTROLYTES

Only a few tests are necessary to delineate fluid and electrolyte status, which are physiologically related to blood gases and acid-base status. The most frequently requested of all laboratory measurements include the electrolytes sodium (Na^+), potassium (K^+), chloride (Cl^-), and bicarbonate (HCO_3^-). Modern multichannel chemistry analyzers routinely provide these four primary analyses as well as those of the other electrolytes: Ca^{2+}, inorganic phosphorus (in the form of phosphates), and Mg^{2+} (discussed in Chapter 9). The four primary electrolytes are usually sufficient to evaluate fluid and acid-base status in combination with blood gas determinations as necessary.

Historically, postsurgical patients had greatest need for electrolyte determinations because of the derangements induced by surgical intervention, replacement of blood and body fluids intravenously, and the inability of surgical patients to take fluids normally by mouth. Almost all hospitalized patients require intravenous lines for delivery of fluids when those individuals are not able to take adequate fluids by mouth. Thus, hospitalized patients in critical or unstable conditions frequently have electrolytes measured every day, along with glucose, BUN, and creatinine, to keep the physician apprised of any changes that may have occurred owing to the delivery of large amounts of IV fluids, and also how the kidneys are able to handle the load. Glucose is often present in IV fluids; thus its monitoring is also of use for assessing the response of the patient to those fluids. Outpatients may also have their electrolytes monitored periodically if they are receiving diuretics chronically. The other ions are important in critical care situations and also in the diagnosis of some endocrine abnormalities (see Chapter 16). Table 10–1 gives a list of the normal serum electrolyte reference ranges.

Specimens and Measurements

The electrolytes of physiologic importance that we can monitor are located in the plasma water phase of blood. The intracellular levels of electrolytes are of course very important, but they are not conveniently measured by methods available to clinical laboratories. It is very important to remember that potassium tends to be very high intracellularly (roughly 150 mEq/liter) and low extracellularly (about 5 mEq/liter), whereas sodium is low intracellularly and high extracellularly. These differences in ion concentrations give rise to an electrical voltage difference across membranes that, in the case of nerve and muscle cells, accounts for conduction of action potentials and initiation of muscular contraction. Other cellular functions are also affected by these levels of electrolytes and by the levels of calcium and magnesium within the cells, but we are able to measure only the extracellular levels routinely.

Of tremendous importance for the validity of electrolyte results is the quality of the specimen. In the normal course of drawing blood samples, the red cells are exposed to shear forces (narrow needles) and turbulence (flow rate too high), both of which can damage and rupture the cell membranes, leading to release of red cell contents into the plasma. This process introduces significant amounts of potassium into plasma, which then may be measured as a spurious elevation of potassium. Because potassium is the single most important chemical analyte in terms of an abnormality being immediately life-threatening, errors in its measurement can have serious consequences if therapy is based on inaccurate results. Fortunately, it is possible to recognize when this process of hemolysis has occurred by the red color of hemoglobin also released into the serum once it has been separated from the cells by centrifugation. Potassium values may be artifactually high if the patient clenches and unclenches the hand vigorously while the tourniquet is on for venipuncture.

Collected correctly, nonhemolyzed serum is an excellent specimen for electrolyte determinations. However, platelets contain potassium that is normally released into serum on clot formation. Thus serum should be expected to have slightly higher values of potassium than plasma from the same individual (increases generally less than 0.5 mEq/L). This difference becomes quite accentuated when the platelet count is elevated (e.g., thrombocythemia, in which platelet counts can be greater than a million per microliter; see Chapters 2 and 4). In fact, patients with thrombocytosis frequently exhibit serum potassium values well above the normal range. This situation can be rectified by obtaining plasma potassium values on a heparinized sample in which the platelets do not activate and do not give up their intracellular potassium.

Many laboratories standardly use heparin tubes (green top) to collect blood for stat measurements of electrolytes, glucose, BUN, and creatinine. Heparinized blood can be centrifuged to yield plasma faster than clotted samples; serum tubes (red top) also require an additional waiting period for the blood to clot before centrifugation. New-generation analyzers can also perform electrolyte measurements on whole blood samples collected with heparin. Other anticoagulants have large amounts of cations that exceed the levels circulating in the blood and so cannot be used for electrolyte quantitation. (Lavender-topped tubes for hematology tests have potassium EDTA; blue-topped tubes for coagulation tests have sodium citrate.)

The methods of analysis for sodium and potassium for many years consisted of flame photometry, on which those cations were quantitated by their atomic emission spectral line intensities when excited in a controlled flame. Flame photometry methods have been replaced almost entirely by ion-selective electrodes. These ion-selective electrodes are based on (1) glass that is permeable selectively to sodium and (2) a membrane impregnated with the antibiotic valinomycin, whose molecule has a charged cavity just the right size to admit potassium but exclude all other cations. These advances in electrode technology have not only made the job of measuring electrolytes easier for clinical laboratories, but have also made it possible to measure sodium and potassium at satellite locations such as physicians' offices and at the bedside with special monitors.

Methods for chloride are based on specific electrodes or titration techniques. Bicarbonate is measured by acidification of the sample to release the HCO_3^- as CO_2, which then diffuses across a membrane to react in a pH indicator system or to be detected by a pCO_2 electrode. An enzymatic method for bicarbonate utilizes coupled carboxylase and dehydrogenase reactions, in which bicarbonate is quantitatively consumed and NADH is converted to NAD^+ with loss of absorbance at 340 nm. This enzymatic method has gained wide acceptance on automated chemistry systems due to the ability to use absorbance at 340 nm as the indicator for multiple different chemical assays.

Spuriously low levels of electrolytes are seen in patients whose serum contains abnormal constituents that displace a quantity of the water in serum. These abnormalities are primarily (1) the paraproteins found in myeloma, which can reach concentrations of several grams per deciliter, and (2) extreme elevations of triglycerides that reside in chylomicrons. Because the electrolytes are dissolved in the aqueous portion of blood, their ionic activities in the fluids that immediately bathe cells (i.e., the levels of equilibrium with interstitial fluid) and influence physiologic functions can be perfectly normal at the same time that the laboratory measurements based on ion contents in a specific volume of serum are strikingly aberrant. Thus, in a given aliquot, the concentration of sodium in water may be perfectly normal, but if there is less water than normal in the volume examined, the amount of sodium present for measurement **(absolute content)** will be low. This effect is most striking numerically for sodium because it is in highest concentration, but the effect is proportional for all the other electrolytes too. Such plasma or serum has normal osmolality, but the problem can easily be recognized as **pseudohyponatremia** by observing milky or opalescent serum (high lipid content) or by noting excessively high serum protein values (sometimes manifested by very dense or very viscous serum). Questions of pseudohyponatremia can generally be resolved by using a method based on measuring sodium ion activity in undiluted serum, plasma, or whole blood.

Sodium Levels

Depletion of body sodium **(hyponatremia)** on an acute basis leads to symptoms of hypovolemia with hypotension, shock, and the associated cardiac abnormalities such as tachycardia. On a more chronic basis, significant hyponatremia leads to abnormalities of the central nervous system (confusion and mental aberrations). Sodium depletion can arise as the result of several different abnormalities. There may be a salt-losing renal disorder or other renal disease that impairs renal regulation of electrolytes. A not uncommon disorder is the result of chronic diuretic use in patients who are also on salt-restricted diets. On an endocrine basis, failure of the pituitary to secrete ACTH or of its target organ, the adrenal cortex, to secrete aldosterone can lead to salt loss. Inappropriate secretion of antidiuretic hormone (ADH) from the posterior pituitary causes water retention, thereby diluting out the sodium in the body. Sodium can also be lost across body surfaces such as through the gastrointestinal tract (vomiting, nasogastric suctioning, bowel fistulas, chronic diarrhea) or skin (sweating on normal skin; loss at burn sites). Hyponatremia may be treated acutely with intravenous administration of saline solutions, taking care not to volume-overload patients who may have marginal abilities to excrete urine.

Sodium retention may occur with renal or cardiac disease, but there is usually concurrent retention of water so that elevated serum sodium levels do not result. **Hypernatremia** is usually a consequence of severe dehydration, which can occur after extreme heat exposure without adequate water intake. It may also arise in debilitated patients (e.g., in nursing homes) who stop oral intake of fluids and become dehydrated. This condition is usually amenable to treatment with rehydration with hypotonic intravenous fluids.

Potassium

The vast quantity of intracellular fluid provides a large storage capacity for potassium in the body and so protects against potassium loss. In addition, excess potassium in the plasma can be taken up into this cellular storage capacity whenever it may become elevated. Serum potassium changes with alteration in blood pH. Acidosis allows H^+ to enter cells in exchange for K^+. In this situation, serum K^+ levels clearly may not be representative of total body potassium. In addition, persistent alkalosis is linked to potassium depletion (as with diuretic therapy, vomiting, laxative abuse, or hyperadrenocorticism) because of the creation of extracellular alkalosis when H^+ enters cells in place of diminished amounts of K^+, which is progressively lost.

Potassium deficit can result from decreased dietary intake over long periods. In addition, it can be caused by loss into the urine (hyperaldosteronism, diuretic therapy, prolonged osmotic diuresis as in diabetes, or with alkalosis) and into the gastrointestinal tract (vomiting, diarrhea, fistula, villous adenoma of intestine). Insulin acts to drive potassium into cells along with glucose. Therefore, in the treatment of diabetic hyperglycemia with insulin, hypokalemia will probably result unless potassium is administered intravenously along with the insulin.

Hyperkalemia can occur with tissue destruction as in massive crush injuries. In addition, patients with renal failure and impaired excretion of potassium can develop potassium excess by unrestricted dietary potassium intake.

Clinical manifestations of potassium abnormalities are potentially the most life-threatening of all disorders. Symptoms are related to the nervous system and to cardiac, skeletal, and smooth muscle. All these tissues utilize potassium to regulate cellular excitability. Both hypokalemia and hyperkalemia result in weakness and loss of deep tendon reflexes, disturbances of gastrointestinal motility, and also mental aberrations. Lethal consequences are paralysis of respiratory muscles and cardiac arrest. Because of the inability to diagnose potassium excess or depletion unequivocally from clinical examination alone, treatment should be based on accurate measurements of potassium in the serum.

Hypokalemia can be treated with oral or intravenous administration of potassium. Hyperkalemia can be treated by one of three basic approaches. The first is to drive potassium from extracellular to intracellular fluid spaces by such means as intravenous administration of glucose plus insulin, sodium, bicarbonate, or beta-adrenergic agents. The second is to remove potassium from the body by diuretics or dialysis or by the use of ion exchange resins in the gastrointestinal tract (by mouth or by rectum). The third is intravenous administration of calcium, which is an antagonist to the cardiac excitability induced by potassium. Clearly each of these methods is sensitive to fluctuations in fluid and electrolyte balance and requires frequent monitoring of serum electrolytes to ensure that desired target values are achieved and maintained.

Anion Gap

The term "unmeasured ions" refers to electrolytes in serum other than Na^+, K^+, Cl^-, and HCO_3^-. Unmeasured *anions* include the negative charges contributed by serum proteins and those of phosphates, sulfates, and other metabolites, totaling about 24 mEq/liter. *Cations* not routinely measured are Ca^{2+} and Mg^{2+}, accounting for about 7 mEq/liter. There are more unmeasured anions than cations, creating a discrepancy, or "anion gap," of 12 to 18 mEq/liter in healthy persons.

Pathologic conditions that increase cations are often easy to detect, usually by measuring Ca^{2+} or Mg^{2+}. Abnormalities that cause anionic accumulation, however, are more common and more complex to analyze. They have in common the fact that bicarbonate anions are depressed compensatorily. Chloride levels may or may not be altered, but electrical

TABLE 10–2. ALTERATIONS IN ANION GAP

Increased Anion Gap Acidosis

Chloride normal; normal or low bicarbonate (increased anions)
  Diabetic ketoacidosis (ketoacids)
  Uremic acidosis (sulfates, phosphates, fixed acids)
  Starvation (ketoacids)
  Alcoholic ketosis (ethanol metabolites; lactate)
  Lactic acidosis (lactate)
    Hypoxia/hypoperfusion
  Exogenous poisons (ketones, lactate, salicylates, alcohols)

Normal Anion Gap Acidosis

Hyperchloremic acidosis
  Diarrhea
  Renal tubular acidosis
  Hyperalimentation
  Early renal failure

Decreased Anion Gap (<6 mEq/L)

  Cationic myeloma proteins
  Hyperlipidemia with decreased plasma content of water and all electrolytes
  Erroneous report

Normal anion gap = $Na - [HCO_3^- + Cl^-] = 12–18$ mEq/L.

neutrality of the blood demands that anions of some sort be present to balance the cations (see Metabolic Acidosis). Table 10–2 is a list of conditions that cause alterations in the anion gap.

The anion gap is the difference between the sum of Na^+ and K^+ cations and the sum of Cl^- and HCO_3^- anions. The value for K^+ contributes so little, proportionately, that anion gap is often calculated with Na^+ as the only cation; the sum of Cl^- and HCO_3^- concentrations is subtracted from the figure for Na^+ concentration. The concept of anion gap allows consideration of metabolic derangements without having to measure those specific metabolites directly. Rather, their presence is effectively inferred by use of the calculated anion gap.

OSMOLALITY

Solute concentration in plasma or serum determines osmolality and affects the movement of fluid across body membranes. Osmolality of body fluids is most easily measured in the laboratory by use of the **freezing point depression** induced in water by osmotically active solute particles. Normal serum osmolality ranges from 285 to 310 milliosmoles per kilogram (mOsm/kg) of plasma water. In health, osmolality is determined largely by sodium, chloride, bicarbonate, glucose, and urea.

Calculating Serum Osmolality

It is particle number and not the nature or weight of a solute that determines osmolality. A mole of an ionized compound like NaCl contributes twice as many particles as a mole of a nondissociated substance like glucose. To use glucose or urea in osmolality calculations, concentrations must be converted from milligram units to molar units. Sodium and chloride ions have a single charge; milliequivalent concentration is the same as millimolar concentration for them, so Na^+ and Cl^- results can be used directly in calculating osmolality. The number of sodium ions in serum is just a little more than the total number of anions; for simplicity, only the figure for sodium concentration is used for determining the osmolal contribution of charged particles. A simple but reasonably accurate formula for calculating serum osmolality (based on the molecular weights of glucose and urea plus a weighted contribution from sodium and its circulating anions) is:

$$\text{osmolality} = 1.86 \times [Na^+] + \frac{\text{glucose}}{18} + \frac{\text{BUN}}{2.8}$$

A still simpler form, useful for rule-of-thumb calculations, is

$$\text{osmolality} = 2 \times [Na^+] + \frac{\text{glucose}}{20} + \frac{\text{BUN}}{3}$$

Major alterations of glucose or BUN concentration affect serum osmolality and are easily detected. If measured osmolality departs significantly from the value calculated with this formula, the problem is usually accumulation of abnormal substances like drugs, ethanol, or radiologic contrast materials. Unmeasured anions, which betray themselves by expanding the anion gap, rarely reach proportions that markedly affect serum osmolality.

Urine Osmolality

The traditional way to measure solute concentration in urine is specific gravity determination. Specific gravity compares the weight of a fluid with that of distilled water at a reference temperature. A frequently used alternative method is to measure the refractive index of the urine on a hand-held refractometer. The refractive index of an aqueous solution is related to the concentration of dissolved solutes, and refractometers are calibrated in terms of specific gravity units. Urine dipsticks now also have a pad with a colorimetric reaction for specific gravity.

In healthy persons, the kidneys can concentrate or dilute urine to cover a specific gravity range from 1.001 to 1.035, depending on the relative quantities of water and solute available for excretion. The ability of the kidney to concentrate urine is best gauged by specific gravity determination on early morning voided samples because a patient is normally water deprived when asleep. The specific gravity of plasma in health is 1.010 to 1.012.

Measuring specific gravity of urine is a relatively insensitive technique, but it adequately detects major alterations in renal capability or body fluid homeostasis. However, measuring osmolality encompasses a wider range of variation and allows more sensitive detection of urine abnormalities or altered fluid regulation. The normal range for urine osmolality is from 300 to 900 mOsm/kg; physiologically possible extremes range from 50 to 1400 mOsm/kg (see also Chapter 19).

Urine : Serum Ratio

Except in states of fluid overload, urine is more concentrated than plasma. The ratio of urine osmolality to serum osmolality ranges from 1:1 to 3:1. If renal concentrating ability is lost, the ratio of urine to serum osmolality cannot rise above 1.2:1. Ratios below 1:1 occur with water overload or diabetes insipidus.

ACID-BASE DISTURBANCES

Hydrogen ion and electrolyte disturbances may be modest or severe, acute or chronic, simple or mixed. The presence of normal blood pH does not necessarily mean absence of disease, as the body's buffering and other compensatory mechanisms often keep the pH constant despite marked variations in blood composition.

DEFINITIONS

A condition that would, if uncorrected or unmodified, lead to accumulation of excess H^+ ion and fall in pH is called **acidosis.** Conversely, the term **alkalosis** is applied to a process that would, if left to itself, cause deficiency of H^+ ions with a rise in pH. Several different processes may occur simultaneously, so it is possible to have coexisting tendencies to acidosis and alkalosis, or several different kinds of acidosis. However, blood pH can have only one measured value at any one time, so patients can display only the net condition of alkalosis, acidosis, or neutrality.

It is customary to divide these derangements into **respiratory conditions** (i.e., those that originate in pulmonary or ventilatory abnormalities) and **metabolic conditions** (those that include disturbances of renal or cellular function as well as abnormalities of intake or output). This format leads to four major categories of acid-base disturbance, which are outlined in Table 10–3.

TABLE 10–3. CATEGORIES OF ACID-BASE ABNORMALITIES

Acid-Base Disturbance	Clinical Observations	pH (nl = 7.37–7.43)	P_{CO_2} (nl = 38–42 mmHg)	HCO_3^- (nl = 19–25 mEq/L)	Limits of Expected Compensation in Uncomplicated Condition
Metabolic acidosis	Kussmaul respirations Shock, coma, moderate hypokalemia	<7.37	<30	<15; may approach 0	P_{CO_2} ↓ 1–1.3 mmHg for each mEq/liter ↓ in HCO_3^- P_{CO_2} should be 1.5 (HCO_3^-) +8 P_{CO_2} value should equal last 2 digits of pH; e.g., for pH 7.19, P_{CO_2} should be 19 Last 2 digits of pH should equal HCO_3^- concentration +15; e.g., for HCO_3^- = 15, pH should be 7.30
Metabolic alkalosis	Paresthesias, tetany, hypokalemia, and weakness	>7.45	45–55	>27	P_{CO_2} ↑ 6 mmHg for each 10 mEq/liter ↓ in HCO_3^- Last 2 digits of pH should equal HCO_3^- concentration +15

		pH	PCO2	HCO3−	Compensation
Respiratory acidosis					
Acute	Air hunger, disorientation	<7.35	50–100	>27	HCO_3^- ↑ 1 mEq/liter for each 10 mmHg ↑ in P_{CO_2} pH disturbance is more pronounced than change in HCO_3^-
Chronic	Hypoventilation, hypoxemia, cyanosis	<7.35	50–100	>35	HCO_3^- ↑ 3.5 mEq/liter for each 10 mmHg ↑ in P_{CO_2}
Respiratory alkalosis					
Acute	Hyperventilation paresthesias, light-headedness	>7.45	<30	15–20	HCO_3^- ↓ 2 mEq/liter each 10 mmHg ↓ in P_{CO_2}
Chronic	Hyperventilation, latent tetany	>7.45	<30	<15	HCO_3^- ↓ 5 mEq/liter for each 10 mmHg ↓ in P_{CO_2}

From Narins, RG, and Gardner, LB: Simple acid-base disturbances. Med Clin North Am 65:323, 1981, with permission.

METABOLIC ACIDOSIS

In metabolic acidosis of any etiology, the initial compensatory change is to convert bicarbonate to CO_2. This action buffers excess H^+ as the CO_2 is blown off through the lungs. The hallmark event is reduction in both bicarbonate and P_{CO_2}. The degree of P_{CO_2} decline should parallel the fall in HCO_3^-, but respiratory problems may also exist in the patient with metabolic abnormalities. If P_{CO_2} does not decline commensurately, faulty ventilation exists. A pragmatic approach to this expected relationship is the following formula for expected P_{CO_2} drop:

$$P_{CO_2} = 1.5 \times [HCO_3^-] + 8$$

A patient whose P_{CO_2} has not dropped to this level may need respiratory assistance in addition to metabolic therapy.

If bicarbonate levels fall and serum chloride concentration remains relatively normal, the gap between measured cations and measured anions increases. These conditions are often called **anion gap acidoses.** If there is a compensatory rise in chloride levels, the anion gap remains normal, and the condition is sometimes described as **hyperchloremic acidosis.** This condition is also referred to as **renal tubular acidosis (RTA),** which is most frequently encountered in infants and children due to inherited disease. It may also be seen in adults as an acquired disorder secondary to multiple myeloma, amyloidosis, autoimmune disease, or drug effects on the kidney (gentamicin, amphotericin B). RTA may be due to a defect in the distal renal tubules (DRTA, type I) or in the proximal renal tubules (PRTA, type II). Other variants of RTA are type 3 (combination of types 1 and 2) and type 4 (moderate renal deficiency, acidosis with hyperchloremia, and hyperkalemia). Treatment is geared to correct acidosis and electrolyte imbalance by oral administration of alkaline salts and potassium.

Diagnosis of PRTA can be made by simultaneous measurements of blood and urine pH and P_{CO_2} while the patient is maintained with steady blood HCO_3^- concentrations by intravenous infusion. Normally bicarbonate does not appear in urine until serum bicarbonate rises above 24 to 26 mmol/L. In PRTA, bicarbonate excretion into the urine occurs at a much lower serum bicarbonate level. DRTA is confirmed by examining pCO_2 in urine and blood. CO_2 is normally present in alkaline urine, but in DRTA there is failure to excrete CO_2 even in heavily alkalinized urine.

Serum potassium is usually low in hyperchloremic acidosis, although in the acidotic states that follow the use of acidifying drugs or result from inadequate aldosterone secretion, K^+ levels may be elevated. Treatment of RTA is long-term oral administration of bicarbonate and other affected constituents such as potassium or calcium. The major categories of hyperchloremic acidosis are listed in Table 10–4.

TABLE 10–4. HYPERCHLOREMIC ACIDOSES

Renal Tubular Failure:
Defective exchange of H^+ for Na^+ causes increased urinary excretion of HCO_3^-
Urine often inappropriately alkaline
Urine: Na^+ increased, K^+ increased, Cl^- decreased
Ca^{2+} excretion and bone demineralization, if prolonged
Gastrointestinal Loss of HCO_3^-:
Na^+ and K^+ loss in intestinal fluid
Fluid and electrolyte loss → hypovolemia
Increased BUN and creatinine, from dehydration and ↓ GFR
Urine Na^+ and Cl^- very low

GFR = glomerular filtration rate.

Anion Gap Acidosis

Anion gap acidosis occurs if endogenous metabolism produces excessive amounts of fixed acids like ketone bodies or lactic acid, if the kidneys fail to excrete fixed acids, or if exogenous acids or acid-producing materials are ingested. Major conditions causing anion gap acidoses are listed in Table 10–2. **Ketoacidosis** occurs with excessive (but incomplete) metabolism of fatty acids, which occurs with insulin deficiency and in states of starvation; malabsorption; or defective glucose mobilization. Stored fatty acids are burned in these conditions as an energy source substituting for glucose. Diabetic ketoacidosis is a result of this type of metabolic shift, although it should be kept in mind that diabetic coma can also be nonketotic but hyperosmolar.

The major ketone bodies produced in ketosis are **acetone** (2% of the total), **acetoacetic acid** (20%), and **beta-hydroxybutyric acid** (BOHB, 78%). Of these constituents, only the minor ones (acetone and acetoacetic acid) give a positive color reaction with the usual methods employed to detect ketones by **nitroprusside testing** (**dipstick** or **Acetest tablets**). Clearly it would be desirable to quantitate the major ketone BOHB to give a more sensitive indicator of metabolic status. An enzymatic assay for BOHB is available under special circumstances for the most sensitive indicator of ketosis (see Chapter 16).

Lactic Acidosis

Lactic acid accumulates when there is massive **anaerobic metabolism**. It is customary to divide states of lactic acidosis into *type A*, which results from tissue hypoxia due to circulatory collapse, systemic hypoxemia, or local circulatory obstruction; and *type B,* which reflects a primary defect in renal or hepatic metabolism, enzymatic defects in gluconeogenesis, or the presence of drugs (streptozotocin, biguanides) or toxins (ethanol, methanol).

In **type A lactic acidosis,** (associated with tissue hypoxia) arterial hypotension and/or hypoxemia usually exists, and the anion gap reflects fairly closely the magnitude of the acidosis. Impending shock, especially due to cardiac failure or sepsis, sometimes provokes lactic acidosis earlier than clinically apparent circulatory failure. In **type B lactic acidosis** (associated with systems disorders), the anion gap is often very large because drug anions or pathologic metabolites accentuate the electrolyte imbalance.

Blood lactate concentration is routinely measured by enzymatic assay and more recently by ion-selective electrodes. To add blood lactate concentrations into the formula for calculating anion gap, divide the measured lactate value in mg/dL by 9 to give the number of anionic milliequivalents that lactate contributes. Adding this number to the values for other anions shows whether additional unmeasured anions are present.

Effects of Alcohol

Ethyl alcohol abuse causes acidosis through accumulation of ketones and lactate and also through direct generation of H^+ ions as alcohol is oxidized. Ethanol itself also adds to the osmolality of blood. As alcohol is metabolized and H^+ accumulates, more pyruvate is converted to lactate, and gluconeogenesis is depressed. With less glucose available, fatty acids are metabolized, ketones accumulate, and the oxidation-reduction equilibrium favors generation of BOHB rather than acetoacetic acid. The nitroprusside test for ketones may be seriously misleading in this setting (false-negative due to low levels of the reactive ketones). Alcohols other than ethanol, notably methanol and ethylene glycol, produce severe metabolic derangement; the anion gap and serum osmolality both rise sharply when these materials are present.

METABOLIC ALKALOSIS

Volume Changes

Excess generation or retention of bicarbonate increases the numerator of the Henderson-Hasselbalch proportion, producing an increased pH, or alkalosis. Loss of hydrogen ions causes alkalosis by depressing the denominator. Bicarbonate concentration increases when there is stimulus to renal retention of sodium. Diminished blood volume or inappropriate reactivity to blood-volume stimuli causes the kidneys to increase return of sodium and bicarbonate to the bloodstream. Vomiting commonly causes metabolic alkalosis because massive loss of gastric fluid depletes whole-body supplies of H^+ and Cl^-, as well as body water supplies.

Effects of Sodium and Potassium

Aldosterone stimulates the kidneys to retain Na^+ and to excrete K^+ and H^+. If there is insufficient K^+ for excretion, renal generation of NH_4^+ increases, causing an associated increase in HCO_3^- generation. **Hyper-aldosteronism** or other inappropriate regulation of mineralocorticoids can thus cause an alkalosis that may produce and in turn be accentuated by hypokalemia. Blood volume and sodium stores contract, and bicarbonate concentration increases with use of diuretics that promote excretion of sodium and chloride along with water. If body fluid and sodium stores contract, tubular epithelium will conserve sodium ions by excreting H^+ or NH_4^+ as the necessary cation; this H^+ loss accentuates the alkalosis. Potassium excretion may also increase, producing hypokalemia that in turn accentuates the alkalotic state.

Decreased blood levels of Na^+, K^+, and Cl^-, and increased HCO_3^- characterize metabolic alkalosis of most etiologies. It is seldom possible to depress ventilation enough to increase Pco_2 and restore the buffer proportion to normal because of the counter need for ventilation to maintain Po_2. Each 10-mEq/liter rise in HCO_3^- should theoretically provoke a rise in Pco_2 of 6 mmHg, but this compensation is rarely complete or rapidly effective.

RESPIRATORY ACIDOSIS

With respiratory failure, carbon dioxide accumulates, a condition called **hypercapnia.** This state raises the Pco_2 and causes the pH to drop. To compensate, HCO_3^- will rise, but in respiratory acidosis, bicarbonate retention is never sufficient to restore the pH completely to normal. The longer the CO_2 retention persists, the more steeply the bicarbonate rises; total CO_2 may rise to very high levels in chronic respiratory acidosis.

Acute Conditions

Acute respiratory acidosis occurs with sudden obstruction to airways, chest trauma that damages the muscles of respiration, or acute paralysis or depression of CNS respiratory centers. The immediate treatment goal is to correct the usually obvious primary problem or render ventilatory assistance; complex laboratory evaluation is rarely necessary or feasible. Acute severe CO_2 retention first activates the buffering capacity of intracellular and extracellular proteins; the bicarbonate buffering system responds only after these buffers are exhausted. Within 10 to 15 minutes after acute respiratory failure, HCO_3^- begins to rise modestly; in acute respiratory acidosis, bicarbonate increases about 1 mEq/liter for each 10-mmHg rise in P_{CO_2}.

Chronic Respiratory Failure

Chronic respiratory acidosis occurs far more often and is far more difficult to treat than acute respiratory acidosis. Chronic obstructive pulmonary diseases (bronchitis, emphysema, pulmonary fibrosis, or scarring) impair CO_2 excretion more severely than they affect oxygenation. Accumulation of CO_2 lasting days, weeks, or months provokes a sustained increase in bicarbonate generation and leads to enhanced renal excretion of H^+. With chronic CO_2 retention, bicarbonate rises 3.5 mEq/liter for each 10-mmHg rise in P_{CO_2}. Rising bicarbonate levels cause compensatory decline in Cl^- levels. Serum levels of Na^+ and K^+ may be normal or mildly elevated.

Stimulation of Respiratory Center

Acute hypercapnia is a potent stimulus to respiration; acute respiratory acidosis produces conspicuous air hunger and ventilatory effort. Acute CO_2 retention provokes increased respiratory effort before the effects of impaired oxygen exchange influence the respiratory centers (hypoxic drive). In normal persons, frank hypoxemia is not necessary to stimulate respiratory drive. However, with prolonged CO_2 retention, respiratory drive diminishes. The respiratory center accommodates to prolonged exposure to high P_{CO_2} by achieving a new equilibrium that reflects reduced respiratory efficiency. With severe chronic hypercapnia, the respiratory center no longer responds to P_{CO_2}; only changes in P_{O_2} affect respiratory drive. Under these conditions, injudicious administration of oxygen and the consequent rise in arterial P_{O_2} may entirely remove the stimulus to respiration, and the patient simply stops breathing.

Complex Conditions

Acute respiratory acidosis can complicate chronic respiratory acidosis if infection, CNS disruption, or chest wall abnormalities compromise the usual level of respiratory activity. Treating this complication is difficult. Giving oxygen may correct the hypoxemia but depress respiration; giving sodium bicarbonate to raise the pH may overload an already precariously compensated cardiovascular system; rapidly increasing pH to normal may upset the hemoglobin-oxygen dissociation equilibrium established during chronic acidemia.

Rapid correction of longstanding hypercapnia can precipitate metabolic alkalosis in patients with severely elevated bicarbonate levels. If the ventilatory problem is corrected and P_{CO_2} drops rapidly to normal levels, more circulating bicarbonate will remain than the kidneys can handle. If P_{CO_2} is normal and bicarbonate high, the pH can rise to an acutely symptomatic alkalosis. Ultimately, equilibrium will be re-established, but it may be necessary to administer oxygen until the bicarbonate excess is eliminated.

RESPIRATORY ALKALOSIS

Overbreathing causes excessive CO_2 excretion, reducing the denominator of the fraction and causing the blood pH to rise. As with respiratory acidosis, acute respiratory alkalosis interacts with intracellular and protein buffers before affecting the bicarbonate system. When adjustment occurs, blood bicarbonate drops 5 mEq/liter for every 10-mmHg decline in P_{CO_2}. When hyperexcretion is prolonged, bicarbonate can decline to levels that completely compensate for CO_2 loss and restore pH to normal values.

Alkalosis causes plasma proteins to have greater negative charge that in turn binds more ionized calcium. This change toward hypocalcemia increases neuromuscular excitability, provoking a condition called **tetany.** In acute respiratory alkalosis, neuromuscular dysfunction first becomes apparent as tingling around the mouth and in the fingers and toes (circumoral and peripheral paresthesias). Lightheadedness and weakness may occur and progress to actual unconsciousness, which reverses itself as the CNS depression slows respiration and allows CO_2 to reaccumulate. Acute respiratory alkalosis becomes dangerous only when caused by excessive mechanical ventilation, such that the respiratory rate cannot automatically correct itself. Hyperventilation occurs in acute anxiety states and after stimulation of CNS centers by drugs or by hepatic or neurologic disease.

MIXED DISORDERS

Table 10–3 summarizes salient findings in the four major acid-base disturbances; Table 10–5 summarizes the physiologic mechanisms that compensate for these disturbances. It is important to remember that several different processes may occur simultaneously. The primary indicators are pH and P_{CO_2}. When these are abnormal, evaluating the magnitude of the changes, the associated HCO_3^-, and the existence of other derangements helps determine whether the results can be explained by a single abnormality or whether the laboratory findings reflect the summation of several different processes. Significant abnormality of P_{CO_2} or HCO_3^- in the face of normal pH suggests that a mixed disorder of

TABLE 10–5. COMPENSATION FOR SIMPLE ACID-BASE DISTURBANCES

Event	Physiologic Changes
Metabolic Acidosis	HCO_3^- consumed in order to buffer organic acids
	P_{CO_2} drops as respiration increases
Expected compensation:	P_{CO_2} drops 1–1.3 mmHg per mEq/liter fall in HCO_3^-
	15 + HCO_3^- value should give last 2 digits of pH
Metabolic Alkalosis	Excess HCO_3^- is generated
	P_{CO_2} rises as respiration is suppressed, a limited mechanism
Expected compensation	P_{CO_2} rises 6 mmHg for each 10 mEq/liter rise in HCO_3^-
	15 + HCO_3^- value should give last 2 digits of pH
Respiratory Acidosis	CO_2 is retained because ventilation is impaired
	HCO_3^- rises; acute changes are buffered by hemoglobin and other proteins; bicarbonate changes occur after some minutes. Later, kidney excretes H^+ and retains Na^+ and HCO_3^-
Expected compensation	HCO_3^- rises 1 mEq/liter for each 10 mmHg rise in P_{CO_2} (acute)
	HCO_3^- rises 3.5 mEq/liter for each 10 mmHg rise in P_{CO_2} (chronic)
Respiratory Alkalosis	Too much CO_2 is blown off during hyperventilation
	HCO_3^- falls initially as intracellular buffers remove HCO_3^-; later sustained fall occurs with renal H^+ retention and HCO_3^- excretion
Expected compensation	HCO_3^- falls 2 mEq/liter for each 10 mmHg fall in P_{CO_2} (acute)
	HCO_3^- falls 5 mEq/liter for each 10 mmHg fall in P_{CO_2} (chronic)

Adapted from Nairns, RG, and Gardner, LB: Simple acid-base disturbances. Med Clin North Am 65:321, 1981.

acidosis and alkalosis is present, with the two opposite influences canceling out the numerical change in pH, but compounding the patient's clinical problems.

WATER AND ELECTROLYTE METABOLISM

Water metabolism, electrolyte homeostasis, and acid-base regulation affect one another so closely that they should be considered together. Metabolic acidosis and alkalosis are inevitably accompanied by clinically significant electrolyte changes and often by fluid shifts, but disordered electrolyte and fluid metabolism does not always affect acid-base regulation. The information derived from measuring electrolyte concentrations can often be augmented by considering serum and urine osmolality and such other indicators as BUN, hematocrit, and urine electrolyte excretion.

It is not clinically feasible to measure body water or the magnitude of water loss. History, observation of daily fluid intake, and measurement of output in urine, vomiting, diarrhea, and gastrointestinal fistulas often provide sufficient explanation for disturbances in body fluid. Fluid can also be lost to the "third compartment" as ascites or massive gastric or colonic dilatation. Fluid balance calculations must include insensible water loss through respiration and across the skin. Patients with extensive burns also lose considerable water and electrolytes through the denuded skin. Febrile patients or those who are hyperventilating may lose substantial water through these routes without concomitant changes in electrolyte pools.

The concentration of sodium in serum accurately reflects whole-body sodium stores because this ion is predominantly extracellular. Sodium and its accompanying chloride and bicarbonate anions normally account for 92% of serum osmolality. If the value for serum osmolality is more than 2.1 to 2.3 times the value for serum sodium, diagnostic attention should be turned to the presence of hyperglycemia, uremia, or anion gap acidosis, or to the presence of osmotic diuretics (e.g., mannitol). Because sodium is so intimately involved in volume regulation, serum sodium concentration should always be considered in the light of total fluid metabolism. Table 10–6 categorizes the major conditions affecting sodium levels according to overall metabolic derangement.

Serum potassium values must be evaluated according to the source and the disposition of this highly changeable ion, as shown in Table 10–7.

In considerations of water metabolism, it is worth remembering that body water makes up about 60% of total body weight. This quantity is distributed as about 40% cell water, 15% interstitial water, and 5% plasma water. In the normal individual, there is about 15 liters of extracellular water and about 30 liters of intracellular water. The average intake of water is about 3 liters per day from all sources, and this amount also equals the output. Sources of water intake are as fluids, as water in the foods ingested, and as water of oxidation. Water losses are primarily urine, gastrointestinal (feces), and the insensible losses through the skin and lungs.

Physiologic regulation of water metabolism is primarily modulated by release of ADH from the posterior pituitary gland in response to changes in serum osmolality. Osmolar changes also stimulate thirst and the resultant drinking of more fluids. An increase in plasma/serum osmolality causes ADH to be released into the circulation. That ADH then causes a decrease in urine flow due to the reabsorption of more water from the glomerular filtrate as it passes through the tubules. The osmolality increase also causes greater thirst and consequent increased

TABLE 10–6. ABNORMALITIES OF SODIUM AND EXTRACELLULAR FLUID (ECF)

Hyponatremia (Serum Sodium Concentration Lower than Normal):
Total-body sodium and ECF volume low
    Gastrointestinal fluid loss
    Burns
    "Third compartment" accumulation (ascites, ileus)
    Salt-losing renal disorders
    Diuretic overuse
Total-body sodium and ECF volume normal
    Acute water intoxication, usually iatrogenic
    Syndrome of inappropriate ADH secretion
    Glucocorticoid deficiency
    Severe whole-body potassium depletion
Total-body sodium and ECF volume increased
    Acute renal failure with superimposed water load
    Congestive heart failure
    Cirrhosis
    Nephrotic syndrome

Hypernatremia (Serum Sodium Concentration Higher than Normal):
Total-body sodium normal, ECF volume low
    Excessive insensible loss: fever, thyrotoxicosis
    Diabetes insipidus
Total-body sodium and ECF volume low
    Gastroenteritis
    Osmotic diuresis
    Pronounced sweating
Total-body sodium increased proportionately more than increased ECF volume
    Salt ingestion, deliberate or accidental
    Inappropriate intravenous therapy

Hyperosmolality, Without Sodium Alterations:
High blood ethanol (measured osmolality increases but plasma is not hypertonic)
Hyperglycemia
Radiographic contrast media

Adapted from Goldberg, M: Hyponatremia. Med Clin North Am 65:251, 1981, and Walker, WG, and Whelton, A: Sodium metabolism. In Harvey, AM, et al (eds): The Principles and Practice of Medicine, ed 20. Appleton-Century-Crofts, New York, 1980, p 59.

intake of fluid. Both increased reabsorption of water and increased intake have the same result of lowering the plasma osmolality. When there is a decrease of serum osmolality, the converse happens: ADH secretion is suppressed, allowing more water excretion through the urine. A decrease in thirst leads to diminished intake of fluids. Both of these effects result in raising of the serum osmolality (see also Chapters 16 and 19).

TABLE 10–7. ABNORMALITIES OF SERUM AND WHOLE-BODY POTASSIUM

Hyperkalemia (Serum Potassium Concentration Higher than Normal):
Inappropriate cellular metabolism
  Insulin deficiency
  Acidemia
  Hypoaldosteronism
  Cell necrosis (burns, crush, hemolysis, antileukemia therapy)
Decreased renal excretion
  Acute renal failure
  Chronic interstitial nephritis
  Tubular unresponsiveness to aldosterone
  Hypoaldosteronism
Increased potassium intake
  Inappropriate use of salt substitutes or K^+ replacement
Potassium salts of antibiotics

Hypokalemia (Serum Potassium Concentration Lower than Normal):
Inappropriate cellular metabolism
  Alkalemia
  Familial periodic paralysis
  Very rapid generation of cells (leukemia, treated megaloblastic anemia)
Increased excretion
  Vomiting and/or diarrhea
  Diuretic overuse
  Hyperaldosteronism
  Renal tubular acidosis
Decreased potassium intake
  Anorexia nervosa
  Diet deficient in vegetables, meat
  Clay eating (binds potassium and prevents absorption)

Adapted from Cox, M: Potassium homeostasis. Med Clin North Am 65:363, 1981, and Walker, WG, and Sapir, DG: Disorders of potassium metabolism. In Harvey, AM, et al (eds): The Principles and Practice of Medicine, ed 20. Appleton-Century-Crofts, New York, 1980, p 66.

Normally, serum osmolality varies only about 1% at most. A water deficit of 1 to 2% leads to a severe thirst. In clinical situations, water deficits may go to 5% with findings in the patient of disorientation progressing to poor skin turgor, dry mucous membranes, stupor, and coma. Since this sequence can occur in persons not able to communicate with the physician, it may be necessary to resort to quantitative data in order to make the diagnosis of water deficit. Probably the most reliable indicator for change in body water on an acute basis is obtained from daily monitoring of body weight performed early in the morning after voiding and defecating and before eating. In addition, recording of intake and output is an invaluable aid in establishing a pattern of fluid flux and for suggesting how to limit or expand intake to achieve stated goals of hydration. Measurements of *serum osmolality* or *serum sodium* are particularly useful for assessing water deficit or excess. *Azotemia* from renal failure and *hyperglycemia* from diabetes mellitus out of control can add to the osmotic activity of serum, but their contributions must be subtracted out in order to assess level of water deficit. Therefore, the serum sodium is generally more convenient to use. As a general guide, serum sodium levels in the range of 150 to 160 mEq/liter indicate a moderate deficit of water, levels of 160 to 165 mEq/liter indicate severe deficit, and levels greater than 165 mEq/liter are associated with very severe deficits.

Causes of water deficit are indicated in Table 10–8. They generally result from impaired mechanisms of thirst or water removal through the kidneys and frequently also involve debilitated patients. Water deficits can be treated by replacement with intravenous administration of 5% dextrose in water for mild deficits. If it is necessary to replace the water more rapidly, lower concentrations of dextrose in water can be used, but

---

TABLE 10–8. DISORDERS OF WATER METABOLISM

Water Deficit

Reduced intake/water deprivation
   Infancy
   Elderly
   Enfeebled
   (Hot weather complicates the above.)
Defective thirst
   Head injuries
   Postneurosurgery
Excess solute intake
   Formula feeding to supplement nutrition
   Nasogastric tube feeding of heavy solute for total nutrition
Sweating (can also lose Na^+)
Renal loss of water
   Primary due to loss of renal concentrating ability in
     nephropathy
   Secondary due to diabetes mellitus
   Osmotic diuresis

Water Excess

Compulsive water drinking
Increased intake with inappropriate secretion of ADH
Renal abnormality that limits or prevents water excretion
Congestive heart failure (underperfusion of kidneys)
Cirrhosis of liver with ascites

water alone cannot be used because of the danger of inducing hemolysis intravascularly. The dextrose in solution maintains osmotic strength to prevent hemolysis but is removed by cells leaving the water to mix into body fluid spaces.

Water excess can manifest itself as an intoxication with headache, blurring of vision, and muscle cramps leading to disorientation, stupor, and convulsions. The serum sodium is used to diagnose water excess. Sodium levels between 125 and 130 mEq/liter indicate moderate water excess; levels between 118 and 125 mEq/liter are severe; and those below 118 mEq/liter represent very severe water excess. Water excess is almost never simply due to increased intake alone because of the rapid reflex responses of the body to regulate water loads. However, increased intake does play a role in exacerbating other causes of water excess such as the syndrome of inappropriate ADH secretion (see Chapter 16) or renal abnormalities that limit water elimination (see Table 10–8). Treatment of water excess is accomplished by fluid restriction, which usually takes several days to achieve normal levels. If quicker resolution is necessary because of seizures or other neurologic manifestations, hypertonic saline can be administered intravenously with monitoring of the serum sodium levels.

SUGGESTED READING

Bia, M, and Thier, SO: Mixed acid-base disturbances: A clinical approach. Med Clin North Am 65:347, 1981.

Brewer, ED: Disorders of acid-base balance. Pediatr Clin North Am 37:429, 1990.

Cox, M: Potassium homeostasis. Med Clin North Am 65:363, 1981.

Goldberg, M: Hyponatremia. Med Clin North Am 65:251, 1981.

Nairns, RG, and Gardner, LB: Simple acid-base disturbances. Med Clin North Am 65:321, 1981.

Pruden, EL, Siggaard-Andersen, O, and Tietz, NW: Blood gases and pH. In Burtis, CA, and Ashwood, ER (eds): Tietz Textbook of Clinical Chemistry, ed 2. WB Saunders, Philadelphia, 1994, p 1375.

Rutherford, EJ, et al: Base deficit stratifies mortality and determines therapy. J Trauma 33:417, 1992.

Taylor, L, and Stephens, D: Arterial blood gases: Clinical application. J Post Anesth Nurs 5:264, 1990.

Tietz, NW, Pruden, EL, and Siggaard-Andersen, O: Electrolytes. In Burtis, CA, and Ashwood, ER (eds): Tietz Textbook of Clinical Chemistry, ed 2. WB Saunders, Philadelphia, 1994, p 1354.

Tietz, NW, Siggaard-Andersen, O, and Pruden, EL: Acid-base balance and acid-base disorders. In Burtis, CA, and Ashwood, ER (eds): Tietz Textbook of Clinical Chemistry, ed 2. WB Saunders, Philadelphia, 1994, p 1412.

Waldau, T, et al: Lactate, pH, and blood gas analysis in critically ill patients. Acta Anaesthesiol Scand Suppl 107:267, 1995.

Walker, WG, and Sapir, DG: Disorders of potassium metabolism. In Harvey, AM, et al (eds): The Principles and Practice of Medicine, ed 20. Appleton-Century-Crofts, New York, 1980, p 66.

Walker, WG, and Whelton, A: Sodium metabolism. In Harvey, AM, et al (eds): The Principles and Practice of Medicine, ed 20. Appleton-Century-Crofts, New York, 1980, p 59.

Wrenn, KD, et al: The syndrome of alcoholic ketoacidosis. Am J Med 91:119, 1991.

Zelikovic, I: Renal tubular acidosis. Pediatr Ann 24:48, 1995.

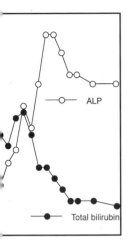

ALP

Total bilirubin

11

Enzymes and Other Markers of Tissue Dysfunction

GENERAL PRINCIPLES

Enzymes are protein molecules that catalyze chemical reactions without themselves being altered chemically. They regulate metabolism by participating in virtually every function in cells. Each enzyme is specific for a substrate that it converts to a defined product. There are literally thousands of different enzymes, but only a few are routinely studied for clinical diagnosis.

Because enzymes are contained primarily within cells, the presence of increased amounts of an enzyme in serum or plasma generally is a consequence of cell injury that permits the escape of intracellular molecules. Abnormally large amounts of enzymes in serum are therefore used clinically as evidence of organ damage. Cellular enzymes released into the circulation have no physiologic function there and are gradually cleared by normal routes of excretion.

The key to diagnostic enzymology is the association of particular enzymes with organs containing specialized cells that are rich in those

533

enzymes. Examples of such organ associations are amylase with the pancreas and ALT (SGPT) with the liver. While these enzymes are not completely restricted to those organs, they can be extremely helpful in making a diagnosis, with the background of a patient's clinical presentation.

Many essential enzymes are present in virtually all organs but have slightly different forms in different locations. These different forms are called **isoenzymes.** When dealing with enzymes such as lactate dehydrogenase, creatine kinase, or alkaline phosphatase, usefulness of total enzyme activity measurements is enhanced by fractionating or separating the isoenzymes as well. When an enzyme level is elevated in the serum and isoenzyme determinations are not feasible, the pattern of other enzyme or biochemical abnormalities is frequently used to diagnose the site of organ damage. In addition to establishing diagnosis, enzyme measurements are applied serially to monitor the progress of a disease state over time.

The terminology of naming enzymes is established by the Commission on Enzymes of the International Union of Biochemistry. Enzymes are classified according to their biochemical functions, indicating substrate and class of reaction catalyzed, and are designated by individual identification numbers. Although this precise scientific terminology is necessary to deal with the myriad enzymes, descriptive or practical names and their abbreviations are commonly used in clinical communications. For example, the enzyme that catalyzes the reversible reaction

$$\text{creatine} + \text{ATP} \rightleftarrows \text{creatine phosphate} + \text{ADP}$$

has the formal designation ATP: creatine phosphotransferase; its EC (enzyme commission) number is 2.7.3.2; its popular name is creatine phosphokinase (CPK), more recently referred to as creatine kinase (CK).

An extremely important aspect of enzymology is the standardization of the units of enzyme activity by which measurements are made. International Units (IU) have been implemented to standardize measurements between laboratories and between countries. One IU of an enzyme is the amount that will catalyze transformation of 1 μmol of substrate per minute. In Système International (SI) nomenclature, the basic unit of enzyme activity is the **katal,** corresponding to conversion of 1 mol of substrate per second. Because differences in assay conditions such as temperature can alter measurement of enzyme activities, the medical users of such measurements should refer to the reference range specified by each laboratory. Although there is not perfect agreement between methodologies in different locations, the use of IU has achieved a marked improvement in the widespread standardization of clinical enzyme measurements.

INDICATORS OF CARDIAC INJURY

CREATINE KINASE

Biochemistry and Tissue Distribution

Creatine kinase (CK), also known as **creatine phosphokinase (CPK),** catalyzes the transfer of a phosphate group between **creatine phosphate** (a storage molecule for high-energy phosphate in muscle) and **adenosine diphosphate (ADP).** The products of this reaction are **creatine,** which can be reused in the cell, and **adenosine triphosphate (ATP),** which is available for directly driving energy-requiring reactions in the cell.

Creatine kinase is a dimeric molecule consisting of a pair of two different monomers called M and B, giving rise to three possible isoenzymes of CK: CK1 (BB), CK2 (MB), and CK3 (MM). These isoenzymes are easily resolved by electrophoresis, with CK1 being the most anodal and CK3 the most cathodal. Other routine methods for CK isoenzyme separation include ion-exchange chromatography and immunochemical precipitation.

The M and B subunits are antigenically distinct proteins encoded by different genes. Tissues that contain CK can express only the B gene, only the M gene, or both genes, giving rise to relatively specific organ distribution of CK isoenzymes.

The primary tissue sources of CK are brain and smooth muscle (BB), cardiac muscle (MB and MM), and skeletal muscle (MM; normal skeletal muscle also contains a small amount of MB, less than 1%). The dimeric molecule of CK has a relatively small molecular size (60,000 daltons) that allows it to leak out of ischemic muscle or brain cells. High-resolution electrophoresis reveals subtypes or isoforms of CK isoenzymes in serum, with three isoforms of MM and two of MB. They are due to the progressive removal of a charged amino acid from one end of the M subunit after a CK molecule is released into the circulation. The relative amounts of CK isoforms indicate how long elevated CK has been in the circulation after release from an acute tissue injury (n.b., the isoform pattern continues to change in vitro before analysis). Present methodologies include electrophoresis to quantitate the isoenzymes MM, MB, and BB or the isoforms and immunoassays to quantitate CK-MB separately as a measurement of molecular mass.

The **creatine kinase relative index** is a calculation based on the mass measurement of CK-MB (in ng/mL) divided by the total CK activity (in units/mL). This index is used to account for possible release of CK-MB from noncardiac tissues when the total CK is very high (e.g., following a crush injury to skeletal muscle). Values of the index above a fixed threshold indicate probable myocardial origin of the CK-MB.

Diagnostic Applications

The constellation of substances released from damaged muscle includes CK, AST, LD, and myoglobin. Due to its small molecular size, myoglobin is released first, followed by CK. Later in the course of acute muscle injury, AST and then LD appear in serum. CK is released into the circulation in the face of virtually any ischemia, injury, or inflammation of muscle (Table 11–1). Injury to the brain releases CK into serum less regularly because of relatively poor perfusion of swollen brain tissue. Baseline CK activity in serum of normal healthy individuals depends strongly on body muscle mass and also on exercise. Thus, thin, sedentary individuals may have serum CK activities in the range of 30 to 50 U/liter, whereas muscular individuals who exercise a great deal may routinely have levels in the range of 500 to 1000 U/liter. Marathon runners generally have levels above 1000, up to 2000 U/liter as resting values. This wide range of expected values for serum CK creates a dilemma in establishing reference ranges that will identify persons with acute myocardial infarction (AMI) who have acute elevations of CK from heart, while excluding persons who normally have high CK levels from skeletal muscle.

The primary clinical use of CK is in the detection of AMI. Most laboratories choose a relatively low upper limit for total CK activity such as 180 or 200 U/liter, so as not to miss acute mild elevations in the majority of patients.

A second necessary step to demonstrate cardiac origin of CK in serum is the measurement of CK isoenzymes. The distribution of CK in myocardium is about 80% MM and 20% MB, whereas in skeletal muscle it is normally almost completely MM, with only a trace of MB (less than 1%).

TABLE 11–1. CONDITIONS AFFECTING CREATINE KINASE

Pronounced Elevation (5 or More Times Normal)
Duchenne's muscular dystrophy
Polymyositis
Dermatomyositis
Myocardial infarction

Mild or Moderate Elevation (2–4 Times Normal)
Severe exercise, trauma, surgical procedures, intramuscular
    injections
Delirium tremens, alcoholic myopathy
Myocardial infarction, severe ischemic injury
Pulmonary infarction
Pulmonary edema (some patients)
Hypothyroidism
Acute agitated psychoses

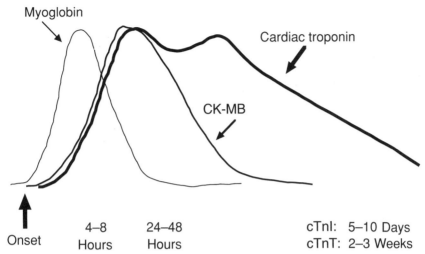

FIGURE 11–1. Idealized time course for appearance of myocardial injury markers in the circulation following onset of acute myocardial infarction. cTnI = cardiac troponin I; cTnT = cardiac troponin T.

Thus, the sudden appearance of CK-MB in serum suggests myocardial release, particularly in clinical settings of chest pain and changes in the electrocardiogram. The level of CK-MB in serum after AMI depends both on the amount (volume) of infarcted tissue as the source for extracellular release of CK-MB and on diffusion of the enzyme into adjacent unin-farcted myocardium, where it is absorbed through the vasculature and taken up into the circulation. CK-MB appears in serum within 6 hours after AMI and clears from the circulation within 24 to 36 hours (Fig. 11–1). Persistence of CK-MB in serum after that period may indicate extension of infarction into other regions of the heart or reinfarction.

New thrombolytic therapies designed to remove coronary artery obstruction soon after onset of AMI give rise to kinetics of appearance and clearance of serum CK-MB that are much more rapid than in the natural course of AMI. After reperfusion of an ischemic region of myocardium is achieved, there is sudden washout of accumulated extracellular CK-MB from the tissue with very rapid appearance in serum. In this therapy, the goal is to prevent necrosis of heart muscle by reestablishing perfusion of ischemic regions, thereby salvaging tissue that would otherwise necrose. Success of coronary artery reperfusion can be assessed by monitoring serum CK-MB values serially during the first 2 to 4 days, during which time CK-MB should fall exponentially without secondary rises, unless there is further infarction or ischemia.

Total serum CK activity is markedly elevated after trauma to skeletal muscle from electrocution, crush injury, convulsions, tetany, surgical incision, or intramuscular injections. Athletic individuals have high CK levels due to increased muscle mass and increased release during strenuous activity. Muscular dystrophy, chronic inflammation of muscle (dermatomyositis or polymyositis), and muscle hypertrophy from intense exercise all give rise to major elevations of CK from skeletal muscle. In these cases, skeletal muscle begins to synthesize more B subunit and actually contains 10% or more of CK-MB, which also appears in serum at similar concentrations. These patients may be mistakenly diagnosed as having AMI based on high CK-MB levels in serum, which actually derive from their chronically inflamed or hypertrophied skeletal muscle. In later stages, muscular dystrophy shows low CK in serum due to diminished muscle mass. It is significant that neurogenic muscle diseases (e.g., myasthenia gravis, multiple sclerosis) are not associated with increased CK levels in serum.

CK can also be elevated in hyperthermia or hypothermia, in hypothyroidism, after normal vaginal delivery (BB from myometrial contractions), and in Reye's syndrome. CK-BB is typically present in serum after brain trauma or brain surgery and occasionally after cardiopulmonary resuscitation accompanied by some period of cerebral ischemia. Some tumors of the lung, intestine, prostate, and bladder synthesize B subunits, which give rise to fairly constant levels of CK-BB in serum, thus distinguishing a tumor source from CK released after acute injury.

Atypical isoenzymes are defined as forms that migrate electrophoretically in positions different from the standard ones. Atypical CK variants are of three general types:

1. **Adenylate kinase** catalyzes the formation of ATP and AMP from ADP, which is in the reaction mixture for measuring CK. Any adenylate kinase in a sample (e.g., release from erythrocytes) may be misread as CK.
2. **Macro CK type 1** is a complex of CK with antibody giving rise to altered electrophoretic migration that can be mistaken for CK-MB. This finding has no known clinical significance.
3. **Macro CK type 2** is an oligomeric variant of CK released from mitochondria. It too can cause ambiguous isoenzyme analysis. Mitochondrial CK in serum is a poor prognostic sign, probably because its release requires severe injury to tissue.

Although rare, atypical variants should be recognized when they do occur to ensure proper interpretation of the isoenzyme pattern.

Specimen Requirements

Serum samples for CK activity or isoenzyme analysis should be free from hemolysis (to prevent contamination with adenylate kinase) and stored frozen if not assayed immediately. Serum or plasma can be used for immunoassay of CK-MB; the antigen is stable at room temperature for several hours to days, although analysis should be done without significant delay to provide clinically useful information.

LACTATE DEHYDROGENASE

Biochemistry and Tissue Sources

Lactate dehydrogenase (LD, LDH) catalyzes the reversible conversion of lactate to pyruvate using NAD^+ as a cofactor.

$$\underset{\text{Lactate}}{\overset{\text{CH}_3}{\underset{\text{COOH}}{|\ \text{HCOH}\ |}}} + NAD^+ \rightleftharpoons \underset{\text{Pyruvate}}{\overset{\text{CH}_3}{\underset{\text{COOH}}{|\ \text{C=O}\ |}}} + NADH + H^+$$

LD is present in virtually all tissues. It is a tetrameric molecule containing four subunits of two possible forms (H and M). The result is five individual isoenzymes designated LD1 (H_4) through LD5 (M_4). The isoenzymes have tissue specificities that are very useful in determining organ source (Table 11–2). LD1 and LD2 are high in heart muscle and also in erythrocytes, whereas LD5 is high in skeletal muscle and in liver.

Many techniques have been used to measure individual isoenzymes of LD. These include heating (LD5 breaks down and LD1 is stable), substrate specificity (hydroxybutyrate dehydrogenase activity is actually LD1),

TABLE 11–2. ISOENZYMES OF LACTATE DEHYDROGENASE (LD)

Isoenzyme	Chain Composition	Approximate % of Total Normally Present in Serum	Tissues Rich in the Isoenzyme
LD1	HHHH	29–37	Heart, brain, erythrocytes
LD2	HHHM	42–48	Heart, brain, erythrocytes
LD3	HHMM	16–20	Brain, kidney, lung
LD4	HMMM	2–4	Liver, skeletal muscle, kidney
LD5	MMMM	0.5–1.5	Liver, skeletal muscle, ileum

From Dietz, AA, Lubrano, T, and Rubinstein, H: LDH isoenzymes. Standard Methods in Clinical Chemistry 7:49, 1972.

electrophoresis, and immunoinhibition of selective subunits. The most commonly used method is electrophoresis, with LD1 migrating most anodally and LD5 most cathodally due to different charges on the H and M subunits (Fig. 11–2). The normal pattern of LD isoenzymes in serum shows major components LD2 greater than LD1 plus smaller amounts of LD3, 4, and 5. LD1 shows preference for the reaction lactate to pyruvate (called LD-L reaction for lactate as substrate). LD5 shows preference for pyruvate as substrate, converting it to lactate (LD-P reaction). Total LD activity in serum may be measured with either lactate or pyruvate as substrate, which leads to differences in standardization between laboratories. The LD-L reaction is now most widely used. LD activity in serum is stable at room temperature for periods of days.

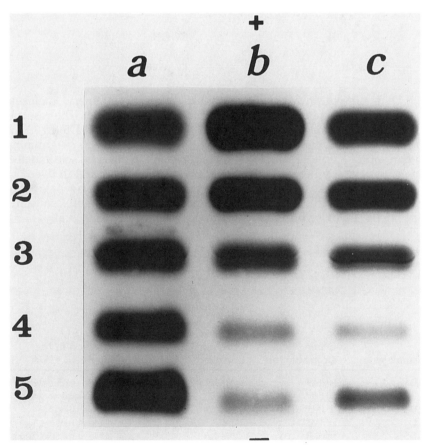

FIGURE 11–2. Lactate dehydrogenase isoenzymes 1, 2, 3, 4, and 5 separated by electrophoresis. Serum samples are from (a) liver disease (elevated LD5), (b) myocardial infarction (elevated LD1), and (c) normal individual.

**TABLE 11–3. CONDITIONS AFFECTING TOTAL
LACTATE DEHYDROGENASE ACTIVITY**

Pronounced Elevation (5 or More Times Normal)
Megaloblastic anemia
Widespread carcinomatosis, especially hepatic metastases
Septic shock and hypoxia
Hepatitis
Renal infarction
Thrombotic thrombocytopenic purpura

Moderate Elevation (3–5 Times Normal)
Myocardial infarction
Pulmonary infarction
Hemolytic conditions
Leukemias
Infectious mononucleosis
Delirium tremens
Muscular dystrophy

Slight Elevation (Up to 3 Times Normal)
Most liver diseases
Nephrotic syndrome
Hypothyroidism
Cholangitis

Diagnostic Applications

Total LD activity in serum can be expected to be elevated in virtually any disease state in which there is cell damage or destruction (Table 11–3). Although this lack of specificity of total LD activity can be a disadvantage for establishing organ source, it is also a relatively sensitive indicator that some pathologic process is going on.

The association of LD1 and LD2 with heart muscle is useful in confirming diagnosis of myocardial infarction, particularly in situations in which CK isoenzyme analysis proves equivocal or after CK and CK-MB release has returned to normal. Myocardium contains more LD1 than LD2, leading to an inversion or flip of the LD1/LD2 ratio to a value greater than 1.0 in serum after myocardial infarction. After release from damaged myocardium, the ratio of LD1/LD2 will stay flipped for several days, and total LD will also remain elevated. A similar ratio of LD1/LD2 also occurs in erythrocytes. Since erythrocytes have an extremely high content of LD, even a small amount of hemolysis in a blood sample will result in a ratio falsely suggesting myocardial release.

In vivo hemolysis due to such conditions as hemolytic anemia (e.g., sickle cell disease), megaloblastic anemia, microangiopathic hemolytic anemias such as TTP, and mechanical damage to erythrocytes from prosthetic heart valves will lead to increased values of LD, with LD1 greater than LD2.

LD emerges from skeletal muscle after the same injuries that also release CK: tetanus, convulsion, crush, electrocution, and so on. LD5 likewise is released from liver in many different hepatic pathologies: hepatitis, cirrhosis, passive congestion, etc. To distinguish liver versus skeletal muscle as the source of elevated LD5, patterns of other enzymes are very useful (e.g., CK, aminotransferases, ALP, GGT).

The LD isoenzymes 2, 3, and 4 are frequently elevated in patients with malignancy and large tumor burden due to the metabolism and turnover of tumor cells. Germ line tumors of testis and ovary tend, however, to cause elevations of LD1 or LD2. Oncologists frequently rely on total LD values to estimate tumor mass including metastases initially and also after treatment. Isolated elevations of LD detected on screening examinations may prompt search for occult malignancy. In this regard, it is worth remembering that mechanical heart valves cause elevations of LD due to repeated trauma to erythrocytes upon each passage through the heart; mild elevations of LD in such patients should be disregarded.

Multisystem disease can give rise to elevated total LD activity with "normal distribution" into the isoenzymes. LD activity in pleural fluids is useful for distinguishing transudates (hydrostatic imbalance with low LD) from exudates (inflammatory origin with many cells and high LD) (see Chapter 19).

Specimen Requirements

Serum or other body fluid should be free of hemolysis and separated from clot, which may release intracellular LD on storage. Total LD and LD isoenzymes are stable in samples at room temperature but deteriorate on freezing.

MYOGLOBIN

Myoglobin is a small protein (molecular size 17,200 daltons) that is present in muscle, where it functions in the storage and transfer of oxygen from hemoglobin in the circulation to intracellular respiratory enzymes of contractile cells. Myoglobin has a higher affinity for oxygen than does hemoglobin, thus favoring muscle stores of oxygen. Because it is a small molecule, myoglobin is one of the first protein markers to diffuse out of ischemic muscle cells, even before CK. Myoglobin is encoded by a single gene that gives rise to only one molecular form of protein, which is common to all muscle types. Consequently myoglobin of skeletal muscle is indistinguishable from myoglobin of myocardium. Myoglobin exhibits pseudoperoxidase enzymatic activity from its heme group, as does hemoglobin, but it is generally measured in serum by immunoassay. Myoglobin is cleared from the circulation by the kidneys. At high concentrations in urine, it produces a positive dipstick reaction for occult blood due to the pseudoperoxidase activity. Metmyoglobin (heme iron oxidized from ferrous +2 to ferric +3 state) does not have this activity.

Despite its relative lack of specificity for myocardium, measurement of myoglobin in serum has high sensitivity for muscle injury, including AMI. Thus serum myoglobin quantitation is effective for ruling out AMI when concentrations are low and remain low. Elevations of myoglobin may derive from myocardium or from skeletal muscle (e.g., intramuscular injection or other trauma); however, in the clinical context of acute chest pain, myoglobin elevations suggest AMI and allow treatment for that presumptive diagnosis until confirmed with more specific analyses or with evolution of symptoms and other analytes over a period of several hours.

Specimen Requirements

Myoglobin is measured in serum by immunoassay. Myoglobin is stable in whole blood or in serum kept refrigerated for several hours to days.

TROPONINS

Muscle contraction occurs upon the movement of myosin molecules along actin filaments intracellularly. This molecular interaction is mediated by tropomyosin and the troponin complex, consisting of three polypeptides:

1. **troponin C** (TnC, molecular size 18,000 daltons; binds and thereby senses calcium ions that regulate contraction)
2. **troponin I** (TnI, 24,000 daltons; inhibitory component, binds to actin)
3. **troponin T** (TnT, 37,000 daltons; binds to tropomyosin).

Fortuitously, both troponin I and troponin T (which are different proteins encoded by different genes) have unique forms that are expressed in myocardial cells, but not in other muscle types. The cardiac forms of troponin I (cTnI) and troponin T (cTnT) are released into the circulation following myocardial injury. They can be quantitated by immunoassays that have recently become widely available on automated immunochemistry analyzers. The presence of cTnI or cTnT in serum has been found to be very highly specific for myocardial injury. Skeletal muscle cells synthesize antigenically different troponin molecules that do not interfere with measurement of the cardiac troponins.

Cardiac troponin is released from injured myocardium in two phases. Upon initial damage, some cardiac troponin rapidly leaves myocardial cells and enters the circulation at about the same time that CK-MB does, peaking at 4 to 8 hours. Thus fresh appearance of cardiac troponin in serum suggests AMI. Cardiac troponin is also released from the intracellular contractile apparatus to which it is normally tightly bound. This sustained release of cardiac troponin provides information comparable to that of lactate dehydrogenase isoenzymes for late or retrospective (confirmatory) diagnosis of myocardial infarction up to days after the acute event.

The time course at which cardiac troponins first appear in the circulation following myocardial injury is slightly later than when myoglobin enters the blood. Consequently it is very useful to couple measurements of serum myoglobin (very sensitive but not wholly specific for myocardial injury) with quantitation of serum cardiac troponin (either cTnI or cTnT, both very specific for myocardial injury).

Use of CK-MB for diagnosing AMI is a widely accepted practice that generally provides correct diagnostic information, but occasionally false-positive cases with elevated CK-MB arise who in fact do not have myocardial injury. These include persons such as marathon runners or patients with muscular dystrophy who produce CK-MB in skeletal muscle or individuals with renal failure who have impaired clearance of normally released CK-MB and myoglobin. The cardiac troponins appear to remain low in such cases. Thus although CK-MB and cardiac troponins have comparable sensitivities for detecting AMI initially, the cardiac troponins have greater specificity and can also be used to document myocardial damage days later, after CK-MB has returned to normal. Cardiac troponins are sometimes persistently elevated in patients with myocardial disease who demonstrate no elevations of myoglobin, CK-MB, or LD isoenzyme 1. These patients typically have unstable angina; cardiac troponin measurements may provide a new vehicle for quantitatively monitoring clinical progression in that disease.

Specimen Requirements

Cardiac troponins are measured in serum by immunoassays. They are relatively unstable in whole blood or serum, and so specimens should be processed and analyzed quickly. If the serum must be stored for later analysis, it should be kept frozen.

CHOICE OF CARDIAC INJURY MARKERS

Laboratories providing services to acute care hospitals with busy emergency rooms now face the question of which cardiac injury markers to offer. Until recently, practice has uniformly consisted of CK and LD isoenzymes; methods have included electrophoresis and various immunoassays (especially for CK-MB). Cardiac troponin measurements have largely replaced LD isoenzymes, which are often seriously interfered with by hemolysis and other noncardiac abnormalities because of the presence of LD in essentially all tissues. With myoglobin now often used for earliest detection of AMI, laboratories must choose between the widely accepted and understood CK-MB and the less known but diagnostically superior cardiac troponins. At this time, immunoassays for cardiac troponins are substantially more expensive than those for CK-MB; this difference in cost will delay introduction of the newer assays. Nevertheless, it now seems that CK-MB measurements are likely to be completely replaced by cardiac troponins within a decade. Myoglobin may also be replaced by another analyte with similar high sensitivity but much greater specificity within the immediate post-AMI period.

OTHER ENZYMES USEFUL IN CLINICAL DIAGNOSIS

ACID PHOSPHATASE

Biochemistry and Tissue Sources

Phosphatases are enzymes that act on compounds containing single phosphate groups, thereby cleaving off the phosphate moiety (an activity designated orthophosphate ester monohydrolase). Individual phosphatases have preferential catalytic activities for different substrates. In the past, this property has led to several different assays for phosphatases based on the use of different substrate reagents.

Another characteristic of phosphatases is that they exhibit optimal activities in different pH ranges. Those optimally active at pH 5 are termed **acid phosphatases (ACP),** and those most active at pH 9 are termed **alkaline phosphatases (ALP).** Measurement of activity at these different pH levels has become a standard method for distinguishing phosphatases and their potential organ sources. Acid phosphatase is common to many tissues, but is especially rich in the prostate. There are small amounts in erythrocytes, platelets, liver, and spleen. Acid phosphatase is also found in human milk, and it is very concentrated in seminal fluid.

During the collection of blood samples, some erythrocytes can lyse, thereby releasing acid phosphatase into the serum artifactually. In addition, platelets also release acid phosphatase during clot formation. To distinguish between prostatic ACP and the others, methods have been developed to inhibit or enhance the different forms selectively. Tartrate in the assay mixture inhibits the prostatic form. Thus, [total ACP activity] – [ACP activity in the presence of tartrate] = [prostatic ACP activity]. A more recent method employs the substrate thymolphthalein monophosphate, which is highly specific for prostatic ACP alone, thereby making further fractionation unnecessary. By the thymolphthalein monophosphate method, total ACP activity measured is equivalent to prostatic ACP activity, thereby requiring only a single measurement for prostatic ACP quantitation.

Diagnostic Applications

Only the prostatic form of ACP is used extensively for clinical diagnosis. Its major application is in the evaluation of prostatic carcinoma for both metastatic and local growth of the tumor. Acid phosphatase is less useful in detecting prostatic carcinoma that has not gone beyond the capsule. Benign hypertrophy, inflammation, or ischemia of the prostate is not generally associated with elevated ACP in serum. Radioimmunoassay (RIA) of prostatic ACP antigen in serum has also been used for diagnosis. Radioimmunoassay has a higher sensitivity than enzyme activity measurement, thus leading to more false-positives when screening large populations of men for prostatic carcinoma. Prostatic ACP by RIA or enzyme activity can be used to monitor cancer patients for recurrence after prostatectomy. Immunoassays for **prostate-specific antigen (PSA)** (see Appendix B, Tumor Markers) have largely replaced ACP for evaluating prostatic carcinoma.

The other major use of ACP has been in the medicolegal evaluation of rape. Acid phosphatase activity in vaginal swab specimens taken during pelvic examination after alleged rape is substantiating evidence for sexual intercourse, since the vagina normally has little or no ACP. This medicolegal use has largely been replaced by DNA testing, which is much more powerful for uniquely identifying an assailant.

Specimen Requirements

Blood should be drawn without hemolysis and promptly removed from the clot. Because of its extremely labile nature, ACP should be measured within a few hours or the serum frozen for assay later. Acidification of the serum with citric acid will also stabilize ACP activity. Timing of sample collection with respect to the physical examination may also be important, since digital examination of the prostate gland in cases of benign hypertrophy may lead to a transient rise in serum ACP.

ALKALINE PHOSPHATASE

Biochemistry and Tissue Sources

Alkaline phosphatase is widely distributed along the surface membranes of metabolically active cells. Tissues very high in ALP activity are bone, liver, intestine, kidney, leukocytes, and placenta. ALP from these different organs has some different chemical and physical properties, allowing the organ sources to be distinguished by special assays. Four different genes encode for alkaline phosphatase expressed in different tissues: (1) placenta, (2) intestine, (3) germ cell and lung, and (4) tissues including bone, liver, kidney, granulocytes, and others. The protein products of the last group are posttranslationally modified, giving rise to isoenzymes with different stabilities, electrophoretic mobilities, and so on, despite a common gene origin.

The easiest and most common method for distinguishing ALP isoenzymes is **heat fractionation,** whereby a serum sample is heated at 56°C for 15 minutes and then assayed for remaining ALP activity. This value is compared with ALP activity in the same sample unheated. Bone ALP is extremely labile (mnemonic is "bone burns" or "bone breaks") and after heating may retain only 10 to 20% of original activity, whereas liver ALP is relatively stable and should retain 30 to 50% of its activity. Placental ALP is extremely heat stable and can retain virtually all its activity on heating. Serum normally contains ALP activities from multiple tissues, so heat fractionation results can be ambiguous. Chemical inhibition by urea (blocks placental fraction) or phenylalanine (blocks liver and bone fractions) also allows some discrimination of the ALP isoenzymes.

Recent advances in electrophoresis of ALP isoenzymes have made possible the resolution of many more forms that have much better organ specificity. Up to 16 different ALP isoenzymes can be resolved by isoelectric focusing. Despite this complexity, the most commonly encountered clinical situation with elevated serum alkaline phosphatase is simply to distinguish bone from liver as the source. This distinction can usually be accomplished by measuring other parameters of liver function such as bilirubin and gamma-glutamyltransferase. ALP isoenzyme analysis (by electrophoresis) should be reserved for definitive diagnosis in cases in which the organ source remains ambiguous despite review of these other analytes.

Diagnostic Applications

Elevation of alkaline phosphatase may occur in many conditions, listed in Table 11–4.

Liver

The hepatic isoenzyme of ALP is derived from epithelial cells of the biliary tract. The normal route of elimination of hepatic ALP is by excretion of bile into the intestine. Obstruction of the biliary tract leads to back-up of ALP and leakage into interstitial fluid and consequently to absorption of ALP into the circulation. Biliary obstruction also causes reabsorption of bilirubin. Thus, ALP is frequently used for establishing the diagnosis in jaundice (see Chapter 12).

TABLE 11–4. CONDITIONS AFFECTING ALKALINE PHOSPHATASE

Pronounced Elevation (5 or More Times Normal)
Bile duct obstruction (intrahepatic or extrahepatic)
Biliary cirrhosis
Paget's disease
Osteogenic sarcoma
Hyperparathyroidism

Moderate Elevation (3–5 Times Normal)
Granulomatous or infiltrative diseases of liver
Infectious mononucleosis
Metastatic tumors in bone
Metabolic bone diseases (rickets, osteomalacia)

Slight Elevation (Up to 3 Times Normal)
Viral hepatitis
Cirrhosis (intestinal isoenzyme often present)
Healing fractures
Pregnancy (placental isoenzyme conspicuous)
Normal growth patterns in children

Electrophoretic separation of ALP isoenzymes in serum reveals a normal band released from sinusoidal surfaces in the liver. Another fraction, termed "fast liver" because it migrates more anodally than the normal liver fraction (or even fails to enter polyacrylamide gels because of its high molecular weight), has been observed in the serum of patients with various hepatobiliary diseases including cancer. The fast liver fraction consists of molecular complexes in which the ALP protein molecule is anchored to lipid, presumably in the same form in which it was released from biliary membrane surfaces in the pathologic process.

Bone

Elevations of bone ALP in serum occur as part of osteoblastic growth responses. Children whose bones are growing have high levels of bone ALP. Similarly, adults with healing bone fractures have elevated bone ALP. Paget's disease of bone leads to very high ALP levels, as high as 10 times or more the upper limit of normal. Other pathologic conditions with elevated ALP from bone include carcinoma metastatic to bone, myeloma (with pathologic fractures), and metabolic bone disease (rickets, hyperparathyroidism, and osteomalacia). Very low levels of bone ALP occur in the metabolic disorder hypophosphatasia.

A recently released immunoassay is designed to quantitate bone-derived ALP in serum as a monitor for osteoporosis and other bone disorders. The immunoassay is not entirely specific for the bone fraction, as it also cross-reacts with the liver fraction that derives from the same gene.

Placenta

Normal pregnancy usually shows some placental ALP in the maternal circulation. This observation carries no diagnostic significance in itself, but the same gene that makes this ALP is sometimes turned on and expressed by tumor cells in adults. This oncofetal form of placental ALP is referred to as the Regan isoenzyme after the patient in whom it was first described.

Intestine

Intestinal ALP may be elevated in inflammatory bowel disease such as ulcerative colitis and regional enteritis. Of more general significance is the finding that persons with blood types O or B and blood group secretory status can also secrete intestinal ALP into the circulation after a meal. This tendency may result in elevating an otherwise normal total ALP value to the abnormal range on nonfasting specimens.

Other

Renal tubular cells have ALP activity that is normally excreted into the urine. It does not reach the serum in pathologic states. Renal ALP on sloughed tubular cells may cause artifactual positive results on some new immunoassay screening procedures such as urine pregnancy tests, which incorporate an antibody linked to ALP as indicator. This interference can be eliminated by centrifuging urine samples to remove cells and bacteria before performing a pregnancy test.

The ALP found in granulocytes does not lead to elevations in serum. It can be used as a marker of granulocyte maturity in leukocytosis by special enzymatic staining of leukocyte preparations (see Chapter 2). Lymphocytes infected with the human immunodeficiency virus (HIV) have also been found to release a specific fraction of ALP (band-10), which may be useful as a surrogate marker for HIV infection in children whose serologic results are ambiguous due to residual maternal antibodies.

Specimen Requirements

Fasting blood samples should be drawn into clot tubes to obtain serum for ALP measurement. Plasma samples collected into a chelating anticoagulant are unsatisfactory due to the need for zinc ion (Zn^{2+}) to assess ALP activity. ALP is relatively stable over time, although serum stored at room temperature shows a slight (few percent) increase in ALP activity over 1 to 4 days. Refrigerated serum shows a similar but slower rise in ALP activity.

ALDOLASE

Aldolase is a glycolytic enzyme that splits fructose-1, 6-diphosphate into two triose phosphate molecules in the metabolism of glucose. It is distributed in all tissues and becomes elevated in serum following skeletal muscle disease or injury, metastatic carcinoma (particularly to liver), granulocytic leukemia, megaloblastic anemia, hemolytic anemia, or tissue infarction in general. With such a wide range of disorders causing elevations, aldolase measurement in serum is not very specific for diagnosis.

Aldolase has found application in inflammatory disease of muscle (e.g., dermatomyositis), in which high serum levels are reflective of disease severity. In addition, aldolase may be elevated early in the serum of patients who later develop muscular dystrophy and subsequently in the course of that disease as well. CK measurements convey essentially the same information about muscle damage. Because CK assays are widely available on automated instruments, aldolase measurements are generally no longer requested to evaluate muscle diseases.

AMINOTRANSFERASES (TRANSAMINASES)

Biochemistry and Tissue Sources

Enzymes that catalyze the reversible transfer of an amino group between an amino acid and an alpha-keto acid are called **aminotransferases,** or **transaminases** by older nomenclature, which is still popular.

$$
\begin{array}{ccccccc}
\text{R} & & \text{R}' & & \text{R} & & \text{R}' \\
| & & | & & | & & | \\
\text{HCNH}_2 & + & \text{C}=0 & \rightleftharpoons & \text{C}=0 & + & \text{HCNH}_2 \\
| & & | & & | & & | \\
\text{COOH} & & \text{COOH} & & \text{COOH} & & \text{COOH} \\
\textbf{Amino acid} & & \textbf{Alpha-keto acid} & & & &
\end{array}
$$

The two aminotransferases most often measured are **alanine aminotransferase (ALT),** formerly called "glutamate-pyruvate transaminase (GPT)," and **aspartate aminotransferase (AST),** formerly called "glutamate-oxalacetate transaminase (GOT)." Both ALT and AST require pyridoxal phosphate (vitamin B_6) as a cofactor. This substance is frequently added to the assay reagents to enhance the measurement of these enzymes in cases of B_6 deficiency (e.g., hemodialysis, malnutrition).

Aminotransferases are widely distributed in the body but are particularly rich in the liver, owing to the pivotal role that organ plays in protein synthesis and in rechanneling amino acids into other biochemical pathways. Hepatocytes are virtually the only cells with high ALT content, although kidney, heart, and skeletal muscle contain moderate amounts. Lesser quantities of ALT are present in pancreas, spleen, lung, and erythrocytes. Accordingly, serum ALT has a relatively high specificity for liver damage. Large quantities of AST exist in liver, myocardium, and skeletal muscle; erythrocytes also have moderate amounts of AST. Hepatocytes contain three to four times more AST than ALT.

Diagnostic Applications

The aminotransferases are excellent indicators of damage to the liver when both are elevated. Acute injury to the liver, such as in hepatitis, can result in elevation of both AST and ALT into the thousands of IU/liter. Measuring the aminotransferases on a weekly basis may be very useful for monitoring progression and recovery in hepatitis or other hepatic injuries. Modern assays of aminotransferases are so precise that minor elevations can be used to detect the affect of acute alcohol ingestion on the liver (e.g., for alcohol rehabilitation programs). Chapter 12 details more uses of serum enzymes for diagnosis of hepatic disorders.

Elevations of AST occur in many conditions (Table 11–5), reflecting its relatively wider organ distribution compared with ALT. ALT rises in serum following AMI as soon as 6 hours after the event, peaks at 24 to

---

TABLE 11–5. CONDITIONS AFFECTING ASPARTATE AMINOTRANSFERASE

Pronounced Elevation (5 or More Times Normal)
Acute hepatocellular damage
Myocardial infarction
Circulatory collapse (shock)
Acute pancreatitis
Infectious mononucleosis

Moderate Elevation (3–5 Times Normal)
Biliary tract obstruction
Cardiac arrhythmias
Congestive heart failure
Metastatic or primary tumor in liver
Muscular dystrophy

Slight Elevation (Up to 3 Times Normal)
Pericarditis
Cirrhosis
Pulmonary infarction
Delirium tremens
Cerebrovascular accident

48 hours, and returns to normal in 3 to 4 days. Although these values can be readily obtained, they are not as useful clinically as CK levels, which rise and fall more quickly and thus provide more timely information regarding onset and evolution of an AMI. In addition, lactate dehydrogenase stays in the circulation longer than AST for late diagnosis of AMI. Notably, AST can rise in several conditions that may be confused with AMI or that may also complicate or coexist with AMI:

- Serum AST rises with shock or circulatory collapse from any cause, owing to secondary liver damage.
- Acute pancreatitis leads to very high AST levels.
- Moderate AST elevations can occur with cardiac arrhythmias or ischemic insult that does not progress to infarction.

Skeletal muscle injury from infection, inflammation, seizure, crush, or electrocution results in the release of several muscle enzymes, including AST.

Specimen Requirements

Serum free of hemolysis is optimal for aminotransferase assays, to avoid interference by hemoglobin with optical absorbance measurements and to avoid artifactual elevations of AST due to release from erythrocytes. Samples can be refrigerated or frozen if not assayed immediately.

AMYLASE

Biochemistry and Tissue Sources

Amylase (synonymous with **diastase**) is a digestive enzyme that normally acts extracellularly to cleave starch into smaller carbohydrate groups and finally to monosaccharides. The major organ sources of amylase are the salivary glands and the pancreas. Salivary amylase normally enters the mouth by secretion through the salivary ducts.

Exocrine pancreatic secretions include digestive enzymes such as amylase, lipase, trypsin, chymotrypsin, carboxypeptidases, deoxyribonuclease, and ribonuclease. These secretions leave the pancreas via the pancreatic duct on stimulation by the hormone pancreozymin (cholecystokinin) and enter the duodenum at the ampulla of Vater through the sphincter of Oddi. Low levels of amylase are also found in fallopian tubes, adipose tissue, small intestine, and skeletal muscle. Salivary and pancreatic amylases form distinct isoenzymes that can be separated by electrophoresis. As many as three subtypes of pancreatic amylase and three types of salivary amylase are distinguishable with high-resolution electrophoresis. Normal serum contains both salivary and pancreatic forms of amylase, although the salivary form usually predominates.

Diagnostic Applications

Inflammation of the pancreas causes release of amylase and other pancreatic enzymes into the circulation, most likely by direct absorption across peritoneal surfaces. In acute pancreatitis, serum amylase levels rise within 6 to 24 hours, remain high for only a few days, and return to normal in 2 to 7 days. Because of its low molecular size (50,000 daltons), amylase is readily cleared into the urine, where it can remain elevated for several days due to prolonged clearance, even when serum levels have become normal.

Conventional strategies for diagnosing acute pancreatitis in patients with abdominal pain have started with measuring serum amylase initially (because of its relative ease of measurement on automated chemistry instruments); if the serum amylase is normal, pancreatitis could still be present, but elevations of amylase in the serum presumably cleared from the circulation before the blood sample was collected. The next step may be to perform amylase measurement on a 24-hour urine collection or to measure serum lipase, which is highly specific for the pancreas. The reasoning is that lipase is a larger molecule and so remains in the circulation longer than amylase does following an acute episode of pancreatitis. Lipase measurement has traditionally been reserved as a second-step procedure because of technical difficulties with conventional methodologies. In fact, modern chemistry analyzers generally have the capacity to perform stat automated measurements of both enzymes. Interestingly, receiver operating characteristic (ROC) curve analysis (see Chapter 1) has recently demonstrated that serum amylase and lipase measurements have essentially the same power to diagnose acute pancreatitis.

Elevations of amylase in the serum are almost always pancreatic in origin, although there are some other clinically significant sources (Table 11–6). Salivary gland inflammation (parotitis) due to mumps or other causes can release amylase into the circulation. Recently it has been found that salivary amylase rises in serum following high-level exposure to ionizing radiation (e.g., nuclear reactor accidents, bone marrow ablation before transplantation). In ambiguous cases of elevated serum amylase without clear-cut pancreatitis or parotitis, measurement of serum lipase can help in the diagnosis because lipase is also released from the pancreas but not from the other organ sources of amylase. Pancreatic amylase can rise sharply in serum after administration of drugs that constrict the pancreatic duct sphincter (e.g., morphine), thereby preventing normal excretion into the intestine and allowing increased absorption of amylase into the circulation. Other abdominal pathology, including biliary tract disease, ruptured viscus, and strangulated or necrotic bowel, can raise

TABLE 11–6. CONDITIONS AFFECTING SERUM AMYLASE

Pronounced Elevation (5 or More Times Normal)
Acute pancreatitis
Pancreatic pseudocyst
Morphine administration

Moderate Elevation (3–5 Times Normal)
Pancreatic carcinoma affecting head of pancreas (late manifestation)
Mumps
Salivary gland inflammation
Perforated peptic ulcer
Ionizing radiation

serum amylase. Pleural fluid can also contain amylase that has crossed the diaphragm from accumulated peritoneal fluid in pancreatitis. Thus, measurement of amylase in pleural fluid may be of use in determining whether a pleural effusion is due primarily to pulmonary or to pancreatic abnormality (especially left-sided effusions, above the pancreas).

Patients with renal failure are not able to clear normally released amylase from the circulation and thus can demonstrate mild elevations of amylase that have no further diagnostic significance. Occasionally patients have circulating complexes of amylase with a high molecular weight compound such as immunoglobulins, thereby preventing renal clearance of the amylase, which can rise to several times normal values and persist without elevation of urinary amylase. This condition is termed **macroamylasemia.** It has been observed in malabsorption and in liver disease. It does not appear to have any diagnostic significance but must be recognized to rule out more serious pancreatic disease.

At least two types of tumors can in some instances produce amylase. Serous ovarian tumors have epithelium similar to that of the fallopian tubes and produce a cyst fluid that contains amylase. This amylase can appear in both serum and urine. In addition, carcinoma of the lung has been associated with ectopic production of amylase.

Allogeneic pancreatic transplantation for treatment of diabetes mellitus entails connecting the vasculature of the donor pancreas to the circulation of the recipient to allow the new pancreas to sense glucose levels in the blood and to perform the endocrine function of secreting insulin. Exocrine secretions of the pancreas (e.g., digestive enzymes) continue to form and are usually excreted from the body by surgical attachment of the pancreatic duct to the urinary bladder. Function of the transplant can be judged in part from the concentration of amylase in the urine: high levels indicate intact and functioning pancreas; falling or low levels suggest graft failure or rejection.

Specimen Requirements

Amylase measurements are readily performed on serum or urine collections. Because of the extremely high levels of amylase in saliva, any contamination with saliva (e.g., into a urine specimen) will lead to striking but fictitious elevations. Amylase activity is also readily quantitated in other body fluids such as pleural fluid or peritoneal (ascites) fluid.

ANGIOTENSIN-CONVERTING ENZYME

Angiotensin-converting enzyme (ACE) converts the decapeptide angiotensin 1 to the vasoconstricting octapeptide compound angiotensin 2. This conversion occurs primarily within the lung. The main tissue sources of ACE are macrophages and epithelioid cells.

The primarily diagnostic use of ACE is for active sarcoidosis, in which levels are high. Other granulomatous diseases (e.g., tuberculosis) and inactive sarcoidosis tend to have low levels of serum ACE. Disorders with macrophage involvement, such as Gaucher's disease and leprosy, can also present with high serum ACE levels. In addition, 5% of normal adults and a large proportion of normal persons under the age of 20 can have high ACE levels. Thus this measurement should be considered a special procedure to be performed only when the clinical context allows proper interpretation (e.g., evaluation of active granulomatous pulmonary disease). ACE measurements are generally available only from reference laboratories because of the complex nature of the assays and the few requests for them; serum samples should be frozen for transport.

CHOLINESTERASE

Biochemistry and Tissue Sources

Cholinesterase activity in serum is often called **pseudocholinesterase (CHS),** to distinguish it from "true" **acetylcholinesterase (AcCHS),** which is found in erythrocytes and at nerve endings. Acetylcholine is the transmitter substance that is released at a motor neuron endplate by an electrical impulse traveling down the nerve toward a muscle. Acetylcholine diffuses from the nerve ending to the muscle and causes electrical depolarization of muscle cells, followed by muscular contraction. The acetylcholine is then rapidly broken down into acetate and choline by

AcCHS locally at postsynaptic sites to terminate the process. Failure to inactivate acetylcholine results in muscular paralysis.

Pseudocholinesterase in serum (CHS) is synthesized in hepatocytes. AcCHS and CHS are different enzymes, which can be identified in the laboratory by their catalytic properties. AcCHS has a narrow range of specificity for substrate, whereas CHS is able to act on a wider variety of choline esters. In addition, AcCHS is optimally active at low concentrations of acetylcholine and is inhibited at higher ones, whereas CHS is active at both high and low substrate concentrations. Both AcCHS and CHS are inhibited by organophosphorus compounds such as common insecticides used in agriculture.

Diagnostic Applications

Serum CHS activity is severely depressed in organophosphorus insecticide poisoning, thereby serving as a sensitive index of exposure to those insecticides. Serum CHS falls early after exposure and rises soon after the exposure ceases. In contrast, erythrocyte AcCHS is inhibited less rapidly, due to the time required for the insecticide to pass from plasma into the cells. Erythrocyte AcCHS activity remains depressed even after serum CHS has returned to normal. Thus, erythrocyte AcCHS can be used to document prior exposure to organophosphorus insecticide while serum ACS is used to document acute toxicity.

Serum CHS is often depressed in hepatocellular disease, but conveys no more information about hepatic dysfunction than other more conveniently measured enzymes and serum proteins (e.g., aminotransferases and albumin).

The medication succinylcholine is a muscle relaxant that is administered intravenously by anesthesiologists to achieve rapid paralysis to facilitate tracheal intubation early in the induction of general anesthesia. AcCHS at nerve-muscle endplates does not act efficiently on succinylcholine, but succinylcholine is usually completely inactivated by CHS in the circulation over a short interval (several seconds). The remaining succinylcholine then diffuses away from postsynaptic sites, leading to reversal of the paralysis. Some patients who are homozygous for a genetic variant of CHS have an abnormal enzyme that does not inactivate succinylcholine. When treated with succinylcholine, these individuals will experience prolonged generalized muscular paralysis and apnea due to paralysis of the diaphragm and other respiratory muscles. Heterozygous carriers of the variant CHS have sufficient normal CHS from the normal gene to metabolize succinylcholine successfully.

Functionally abnormal variants of serum CHS can be elucidated by testing the response to dibucaine in the laboratory. Normal CHS activity is inhibited by dibucaine, but the abnormal CHS is resistant to dibucaine and shows normal catalytic activity on substrate even in the presence of dibucaine. The **dibucaine number** is the percentage to which CHS activity in serum is inhibited by dibucaine under standard conditions. A high dibucaine number indicates inhibition characteristic of normal enzyme; a low number suggests homozygous variant CHS.

Specimen Requirements

ACS is stable for weeks in refrigerated serum specimens. Evaluation of a patient who has experienced prolonged apnea following administration of succinylcholine may be complicated by the presence of drug metabolites until the drug has fully cleared and the patient is no longer paralyzed, at which point a fresh specimen should be obtained for analysis.

GAMMA-GLUTAMYLTRANSFERASE

Gamma-glutamyltransferase (GGT, formerly called "gamma glutamyl transpeptidase") catalyzes the transfer of glutamyl groups between peptides or amino acids through linkage at a gamma carboxyl group. This function is probably important in the transfer or movement of amino acids across membranes. Large amounts are present in renal tubular epithelium and in liver, locations where alkaline phosphatase also occurs. Other tissue sources of alkaline phosphatase (e.g., bone) do not have a correspondingly high content of GGT. Therefore, serum GGT is very useful as a marker for liver pathology, such as obstructive jaundice, cancer metastatic to liver, or intrahepatic cholestasis, in which it reaches its highest levels. Because of its specificity for liver, GGT can be used to determine whether an elevation of serum alkaline phosphate is from bone or liver.

Hepatocellular damage can release GGT in moderate amounts. Hepatotoxicity (e.g., acetaminophen poisoning) causes elevations of GGT. Chemotherapy can cause release of GGT from liver, thereby obscuring the role of metastatic disease in leading to elevations. Inducers of hepatic enzyme synthesis (alcohol, barbiturates, phenytoin) have the secondary effect of elevating serum GGT, which apparently leaks out of hepatic cells in proportion to higher intracellular levels. GGT is particularly sensitive to alcohol ingestion; it shows a sustained rise at high alcohol intake and moderate elevations at lower intake. GGT can therefore be quite useful in determining compliance in alcohol rehabilitation and withdrawal programs. Levels return to normal after 2 to 3 weeks of abstention from alcohol. Use of GGT in evaluating liver disorders is discussed further in Chapter 12.

Although renal GGT does not reach the serum, measurement of GGT in urine can be used for assessing specific renal tubular damage due to renal toxic substances.

LIPASE

Alimentary Source

Cleavage of dietary triglycerides into free fatty acids and glycerol is catalyzed by enzymes collectively referred to as **lipases (LIP),** which are secreted from the pancreas into the duodenum along with the other pancreatic digestive enzymes.

$$
\begin{array}{lcl}
\text{H}_2\text{CO-FA} & & \text{H}_2\text{COH} \\
| & \text{3 steps} & | \\
\text{HCO-FA}' & \longrightarrow & \text{HCOH} \quad + \quad \text{3 free fatty acids} \\
| & & | \\
\text{H}_2\text{CO-FA}'' & & \text{H}_2\text{COH}
\end{array}
$$

Since lipase is found almost exclusively in the pancreas, elevation of lipase in serum is highly specific for pancreatic disease. In contrast, amylase, the other major marker for pancreatic disease, has other organ sources. Until recently, lipase has been technically more difficult to measure because its substrate is lipid and therefore inherently insoluble in aqueous reaction mixtures; modern chemistry analyzers have made lipase measurements much more feasible for standard use. Although amylase is more frequently used to screen for pancreatic disease, the advantage of lipase is that it is not cleared into the urine and thus may remain elevated even after parallel release of amylase from the pancreas has returned to normal. The highest levels of lipase occur in acute pancreatitis. Administration of morphine or cholinergic drugs that cause constriction of the sphincter of Oddi results in elevations of lipase and amylase. Carcinoma of the pancreas may show a moderate increase of lipase.

Postheparin Lipoprotein Lipase

In addition to lipase from the pancreas released into the alimentary tract, a separate lipase activity in the blood cleaves fatty acids from lipoproteins and clears chylomicrons from the circulation. This lipolytic activity is bound to vascular endothelial membranes, where it has access to lipids in the blood after absorption from the intestine. Administration of the anticoagulant heparin releases these membrane-bound lipases into plasma, where they can be measured as **postheparin lipolytic activity (PHLA).** The release occurs within minutes of intravenous heparin dose. This increased lipolytic activity after heparin could be confused with pancreatic lipase if the timing of blood draw is not taken into account.

Persons who have type I hyperlipoproteinemia have enormously increased levels of circulating chylomicrons and very high triglycerides even in the fasting state, due to markedly low levels of PHLA. This deficiency can be demonstrated by special studies of the lipoprotein composition (e.g., lipoprotein electrophoresis) and lipolytic activities after the diagnostic administration of heparin. Laboratory procedures interfered with by free fatty acids can be strongly affected by administration of heparin and release of PHLA. These procedures include T_3 uptake and binding of bilirubin to albumin (reserve bilirubin-binding capacity).

LYSOZYME

Lysozyme (muramidase) is a low molecular weight hydrolytic enzyme that catalyzes the breakdown of bacterial cell walls. It is found in tears, saliva, and sputum and also in granulocytes and monocytes. Lysozyme in serum and urine is markedly elevated in acute monocytic and acute myelomonocytic leukemias owing to release from increased numbers of those leukemic cells. Levels are low in lymphocytic leukemias and generally also low in chronic granulocytic leukemias. Serial levels may be of use in detecting relapse in acute leukemia (see Chapters 2, 4).

TABLE 11–7. ENZYME–ORGAN ASSOCIATIONS

Organ	Enzyme
Liver	Aminotransferases (AST, ALT)
	Lactate dehydrogenase (LD5)
	Gamma-glutamyltransferase
	Alkaline phosphatase
Heart	Creatine kinase (MB)
	Lactate dehydrogenase (LD1 > LD2)
	Myoglobin*
	Troponins I and T*
Skeletal muscle	Creatine kinase (MM)
	Lactate dehydrogenase (LD5)
	Aldolase
	Myoglobin*
Bone	Alkaline phosphatase (heat labile)
Prostate	Acid phosphatase
	Prostate specific antigen (PSA)*
Pancreas	Amylase
	Lipase
Brain	Creatine kinase (BB)

*Other protein markers measured immunologically.

Lysozyme is readily cleared into urine. It migrates as a single tight band on protein electrophoresis and may falsely suggest a monoclonal gammopathy. This finding may be confused with the electrophoretic pattern of immunoglobulin light chains, which are also cleared into the urine.

Lysozyme is usually quantitated by its ability to lyse the bacterium *Micrococcus lysodeikticus,* converting a turbid suspension of the organism into a clear one. Lysozyme activity can be quantitated in serum or urine specimens.

A summary of enzyme-organ associations is presented in Table 11–7.

SUGGESTED READING

Adams, JE, et al: Cardiac troponin I: A marker with high specificity for cardiac injury. Circulation 88:101, 1993.

Allen, RK: A review of angiotensin converting enzyme in health and disease. Sarcoidosis 8:95, 1991.

Bhayana, V, and Henderson, AR: Biochemical markers of myocardial damage. Clin Biochem 28:1, 1995.

Bohlmeyer, TJ, Wu, AH, and Perryman, MB: Evaluation of laboratory tests as a guide to diagnosis and therapy of myositis. Rheum Dis Clin North Am 20:845, 1994.

Cogbill, TH, et al: Hepatic enzyme response and hyperpyrexia after severe liver injury. Am Surg 58:395, 1992.

Davis, L, Britten, JJ, and Morgan, M: Cholinesterase: Its significance in anaesthetic practice. Anaesthesia 52:244, 1997.

Enzyme Nomenclature. Recommendations (1984) of Nomenclature Committee of the International Union of Biochemistry on the Nomenclature and Classification of Enzyme-Catalysed Reactions. Academic Press, Orlando, 1984.

Gitlin, N: The serum glutamic-oxaloacetic transaminase/serum glutamic pyruvic transaminase ratio as a prognostic index in severe acute viral hepatitis. Am J Gastroenterol 77:2, 1982.

Gittes, RF: Carcinoma of the prostate. N Engl J Med 324:236, 1991.

Griffiths, J: Alkaline phosphatases: Newer concepts in isoenzymes and clinical applications. Clin Lab Med 9:717, 1989.

Gumaste, VV: Diagnostic tests for acute pancreatitis. Gastroenterologist 2:119, 1994.

Helander, A, and Carlsson, S: Carbohydrate-deficient transferrin and gamma-glutamyl transferase levels during disulfiram therapy. Alcohol Clin Exp Res 20:1202, 1996.

Jaffe, AS, et al: Comparative sensitivity of cardiac troponin I and lactate dehydrogenase isoenzymes for diagnosing acute myocardial infarction. Clin Chem 42:1770, 1996.

Lantz, RK, and Eisenberg, RB: Preservation of acid phosphatase activity in medico-legal specimens. Clin Chem 24:486, 1978.

Light, RW: Diagnostic principles in pleural disease. Eur Respir J 10:476, 1997.

Murthy, VV, et al: Alkaline phosphatase band-10 fraction as a possible surrogate marker for human immunodeficiency virus type 1 infection in children. Arch Pathol Lab Med 118:873, 1994.

Ohman, EM, et al: Cardiac troponin T levels for risk stratification in acute myocardial infarction. N Engl J Med 335:1333, 1996.

O'Malley, M: Clinical evaluation of pesticide exposure and poisonings. Lancet 349:1161, 1997.

Puleo, PR, et al: Use of a rapid assay of subforms of creatine kinase MB to diagnose or rule out myocardial infarction. N Engl J Med 331:561, 1994.

Puryear, DW, and Fowler, AA: Sarcoidosis: A clinical overview. Compr Ther 22:649, 1996.

Robinson, D, and Whitehead, TP: Effect of body mass and other factors on serum liver enzyme levels in men attending for well population screening. Ann Clin Biochem 26:393, 1989.

Saxena, S, et al: Higher serum alanine aminotransferase levels among Hispanics in a reference population. Lab Med 20:264, 1989.

Tietz, NW: Support of the diagnosis of pancreatitis by enzyme tests—old problems, new techniques. Clin Chem Acta 257:85, 1997.

Werner, M, Steinberg, WM, and Pauley, C: Strategic use of individual and combined enzyme indicators for acute pancreatitis analyzed by receiver-operator characteristics. Clin Chem 35:967, 1989.

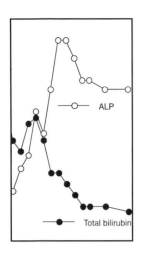

ALP

Total bilirubin

12

Tests of Liver Function

The liver is the central organ of metabolism in the body. Although it constitutes only 2% of total body weight, the liver receives 1500 mL of blood per minute, about 28% of cardiac output, in order to accomplish its functions. The liver performs multiple metabolic operations on blood constituents that come to it as waste products or nutrients, and in turn many hepatic activities are directly reflected in several of the substances circulating in the blood and also present in other body fluids. Although hepatic functions affect many metabolites, certain tests and manipulations correlate particularly well with the structural and functional integrity of the liver; these determinations are conventionally considered liver function tests (LFTs). To gain an understanding of how these tests are interpreted, it is necessary to review the functions of the liver and the ways that structure and function are related.

STRUCTURE AND FUNCTION

The liver is composed of two principal types of cells: the metabolically active **hepatocytes,** which derive from epithelium, and the phagocytic **Kupfer cells,** which are part of the reticuloendothelial system. These cells are arranged microscopically into an anatomic unit of the liver called the **lobule,** which consists of cords of hepatocytes supported by a reticulin framework around vascular channels called **sinusoids.** The entire liver is

562

made up of thousands of lobules. Vascular connections in the liver are arranged so that blood enters each lobule at its periphery, percolates inward to the center of the lobule through the sinusoids, and then exits through a small central vein. Sinusoidal blood and the liver cells lining the sinusoids have intimate contact that facilitates extensive exchange of materials between blood and the hepatocytes. The actual microscopic region between sinusoids and plates of hepatocytes is termed the **space of Disse;** it contains interstitial fluid (but not erythrocytes), through which nutrients and waste products must diffuse to transfer between circulating blood and the liver.

BLOOD SUPPLY

Blood enters the liver from two sources: arterial and venous. The hepatic artery brings arterial blood directly from the aorta. This blood supply is oxygenated; it also carries metabolic waste products from throughout the body that have previously returned through the venous circulation, to the vena cava, and thence to the heart. The portal vein introduces blood that has already drained through the capillary beds of the spleen and from the alimentary tract.

The portal blood supply is rich in nutrients absorbed from food by the intestines, materials that must undergo a vast series of metabolic changes to be utilized as carbohydrates, proteins, and lipids of the body. The connections constituting the portal venous system allow the liver to act on those materials absorbed directly from the digestive organs before they circulate to the heart and to other organs. Branches of the hepatic artery and of the portal vein reach the periphery of each lobule through special conduits called portal triads in order to achieve maximal distribution of the nutrients to hepatocytes. Sinusoidal blood consequently is a mixture of arterial and portal venous contributions. The central veins collect all the blood and return it to the systemic circulation through the large hepatic vein, which empties into the inferior vena cava.

Two-thirds of the blood circulating through the liver is from the portal vein, and only one-third comes directly from the aorta. Consequently, sinusoidal blood has less oxygen than the blood that enters most organs. Because they are performing energy-demanding activities and are operating on a rather narrow margin of oxygenation, hepatocytes are particularly vulnerable to changes in blood pressure (shock), blood flow, and oxygen content (hypoxia).

Following injury due to virtually any cause (impaired blood flow, biliary obstruction, toxic exposure, resection, or transplantation of a liver segment), the liver has a remarkable capacity to regenerate by cell division and hypertrophy of the remaining tissue. Actively regenerating liver is supplied more by the arterial blood than by the portal circulation and so is more susceptible to loss of systemic blood pressure than was the original liver tissue.

BILIARY SYSTEM

The biliary tract constitutes a system of fluid circulating through the liver separate from the blood. **Bile,** the direct secretory product of the liver, is secreted by hepatocytes into tiny tubules, called **biliary canaliculi,** situated between the cells. Approximately 1 to 1.5 liters of bile are produced daily. At the microscopic level, the biliary and circulatory systems are separated by a single layer of hepatocytes bathed on one side by blood, from which they extract nutrients, and on the other side by bile, into which they excrete metabolic products. The biliary canaliculi formed between pairs of hepatocytes coalesce into ductules, which occupy the same framework of connective tissue at the periphery of each lobule that supports portal vein and hepatic artery branches **(portal triad).** Bile ductules join into increasingly larger intrahepatic bile channels, which ultimately form the extrahepatic ducts that carry bile from liver to gallbladder. The gallbladder stores bile and releases it into the duodenum as needed for digestive processes. In the intestine, bile enhances the breakdown and absorption of fat-soluble nutrients by emulsifying lipids into small particles, thus allowing more efficient digestion by lipase and absorption by the mucosal surface of the intestine. The gallbladder is a pouch off the main bile duct; even after removal of the gallbladder, bile flow is readily established directly between liver and duodenum without impairing hepatic or digestive functions.

METABOLIC PROCESSES

There are three major categories of hepatic activity: synthesis, excretory processes, and storage functions. Energy and nutrients obtained from the diet must be processed and then stored, distributed, or transformed by hepatic action. The liver degrades, detoxifies, or otherwise alters many primary and intermediary metabolites, readying them for excretion, storage, or recycling.

The hepatocytes manufacture a great number of molecules that circulate in the blood at levels influenced by overall hepatic function. Aside from the immunoglobulins, which are produced by plasma cells of the bone marrow, the proteins circulating in blood plasma are all essentially synthesized from amino acids by the liver and then either released immediately or stored and held in reserve in the liver and released when they are needed (see Chapter 9). Regulation of this process allows complex proteins to be made available at much shorter notice than if they were synthesized from scratch. The liver also serves as a primary storage depot for glycogen and for fat-soluble vitamins A, D, and K; vitamin E is stored in the liver and also in body fat and muscle. Adipose tissue is the permanent storage site for fats, but the liver retains and reshuffles fatty acids and triglycerides; the reticuloendothelial cells of the liver store iron, copper, and other minerals that they have scavenged from the blood.

CLASSIFICATION OF TESTS

The diseases that affect the liver include secondary conditions with systemic ramifications and primary diseases more specific for the liver itself. One useful classification of liver disorders is according to the anatomic system affected—the circulation, the biliary system, or the liver cells themselves. Laboratory tests of liver function similarly can be classified according to the aspects of the disease for which they are most reflective and hence most informative. Unfortunately, the clinical effects of many conditions vary more with the number of functioning hepatic units damaged than with the location or the nature of the injury. Most liver function tests provide quantitative information about broadly defined abnormalities and cannot further discriminate the causes; however, patterns or abnormalities in several different liver function tests can be helpful in better delineating some hepatic disorders.

Circulatory Disorders

Fibrosis of the liver (as occurs in cirrhosis) and other diseases can lead to profound disturbances of the pressures and flow of the hepatic blood circulation. Measurement of these circulatory changes generally requires some form of invasive procedure such as catheterization or the introduction of radiographic contrast material into the hepatic vasculature. These procedures are beyond the scope of this chapter, which deals primarily with the biochemical abnormalities in blood that reflect liver disease. Clinical observations can suggest altered flow patterns and pressure relationships. The anatomic findings of esophageal varices, hemorrhoids, or dilated abdominal vessels indicate shunting from portal to systemic circulation caused by functional obstruction of (and high pressure in) the portal system. These vascular abnormalities occur in the venous vessels in response to increased intravascular pressures, which cause distortions in the walls of veins due to their relative weakness compared with the more muscular walls of arterial vessels. With progression of these disturbances, ascites (see Chapter 19) can present in the abdomen as a consequence of the increased pressure and excessive permeability in capillaries of the portal venous bed. Right-sided heart failure causes blood to back up in the inferior vena cava, thereby slowing central venous drainage and increasing portal venous pressure. The formation of ascites includes loss of albumin from the vascular compartment into that fluid. In addition, increased pressure on the right side of the heart may be transmitted backward to result in loss of protein from the circulation into the alimentary tract. Consequently, the primary laboratory measurement to use in monitoring these abnormalities of pressure is serum albumin because its concentration reflects the shift of protein and fluid into ascites and because of its important contribution to the oncotic pressure of plasma.

Disorders of Hepatocytes and Biliary System

Tests of the biliary system include measuring concentrations of bilirubin and its metabolites in serum and urine, evaluating secretory activity of hepatic cells, and measuring products that reflect abnormal ductal activity. Hepatocellular integrity can be studied by several approaches: measuring the concentration of normally synthesized products (e.g., plasma proteins, including coagulation factors), quantitating the substances that are normally metabolized and cleared from the circulation by the liver (generally small molecules such as organic acids), demonstrating the presence of hepatocyte breakdown products in serum (e.g., enzymes of hepatocellular origin), or quantifying activities known to require intact hepatic pathways (vitamin K–dependent coagulation factor activities). Table 12–1 indicates many of the tests that are clinically useful in assessing liver function.

BILIRUBIN AND THE BILIARY SYSTEM

PHYSIOLOGY

Bilirubin is a degradation product of heme; most (85 to 90%) results from breakdown of hemoglobin and a smaller portion (10 to 15%) from other compounds such as myoglobin (see Chapter 9). The reticuloendothelial cells take up complexes of haptoglobin with hemoglobin that has been released from red cells (see also Chapter 2). They then remove the iron from heme to conserve it for later synthesis and cleave the heme ring to produce the tetrapyrrole bilirubin, which is secreted in a form not soluble in water **(unconjugated, indirect bilirubin).** Because of this insolubility, bilirubin in plasma is bound to albumin for transport in aqueous medium. As this material circulates in the body and through the hepatic lobules, the hepatocytes detach bilirubin from the albumin and render it water soluble through conjugation with glucuronic acid **(conjugated, direct bilirubin).**

In the form of the conjugated glucuronide, soluble bilirubin enters the biliary system for excretion in the bile. When it enters the intestines, bilirubin is further degraded by colonic bacteria into urobilinogen, a colorless, water-soluble material that is easily oxidized to the pigmented compound urobilin. The urobilinogen can be converted to stercobilin and

TABLE 12-1. TESTS OF LIVER AND BILIARY FUNCTION

Test	Information Conveyed
Biliary System:	
Serum bilirubin level	Overall capacity to transport bile
Ratio of direct and total bilirubin	Patency of biliary ducts, hepatocellular metabolism of bilirubin
Serum bile acids (salts)	Overall patency of biliary ducts
Fecal color and fat content	Patency of biliary ducts
Fecal urobilinogen	Patency of biliary ducts; quantity of bilirubin processed
Urine urobilinogen	Patency of biliary ducts; quantity of bilirubin processed; hepatocellular excretory capacity
Serum alkaline phosphatase, other "obstructive" enzymes	Abnormality of bile-duct epithelium
Excretion of BSP (rarely used)	Hepatocellular function and patency of bile ducts
Urine bilirubin	Patency of biliary ducts; hepatocellular bilirubin metabolism
Hepatocellular Function:	
Serum bilirubin level	Capacity to conjugate bilirubin and secrete bile
Ratio of direct and total bilirubin	Capacity to conjugate bilirubin; quantity of hemoglobin turnover
Serum albumin level	Capacity to synthesize protein
Serum globulin level	Abnormal processing of exogenous and/or autologous antigens
Prothrombin time and response to vitamin K	Capacity to synthesize coagulation factors and/or biliary obstruction
Serum aminotransferase levels	Hepatocellular damage and necrosis
BSP excretion	Hepatocellular uptake, conjugating, and secretory capacity; patency of biliary ducts
Fasting blood glucose	Very rough indication of glycogen storage and capacity to synthesize glucose
Blood urea	If low, rough estimate of lost detoxifying capacity
Blood ammonia	Hepatocellular detoxifying reactions; integrity of portal circulation; quantity of colonic bacteria
Specific Determinations:	
Hepatitis A and B antigens and antibodies/hepatitis C antibody	Viral hepatitis
Alpha-fetoprotein	Hepatocellular multiplication: tumor or regeneration
Alpha-antitrypsin	Early developing cirrhosis; association with emphysema (inherited deficiency)
Ceruloplasmin	Low in Wilson's disease
Serum iron, ferritin	High in hemochromatosis

excreted in feces, where it imparts a dark brown color. Some of the urobilinogen is reabsorbed from the intestine in the enterohepatic pathway, and the portal blood carries it back to the liver. This recycled urobilinogen is largely excreted into the bile for passage into the intestines again, but some is carried by the systemic circulation to the kidneys, where it is excreted as a water-soluble compound into the urine (Fig. 12–1). The urine dipstick test is calibrated to yield negative results for the amounts of urobilinogen normally excreted in urine in a state of health.

Direct and Indirect Bilirubin

Most bilirubin in normal blood is the albumin-bound, insoluble form released from the reticuloendothelial cells before it is removed by the liver. There are also generally small amounts of water-soluble conjugated

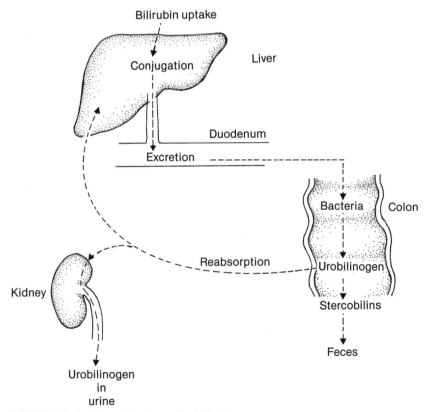

FIGURE 12–1. Normal pathway for bilirubin.

bilirubin in plasma that get into the blood because of minor leakiness of the hepatocytes in directions away from the formation and excretion of bile. Both the total amount and the relative proportions of the conjugated and unconjugated bilirubin fractions are of immense utility in the diagnosis of jaundice and liver disease. Conjugated posthepatic bilirubin reacts rapidly in commonly used tests because of its inherent solubility and is therefore described as **direct-reacting;** unconjugated bilirubin must be mixed with alcohol or other solubilizing agents before it efficiently reacts in the assay for its measurement and accordingly is termed **indirect-reacting** (see Chapter 9). Traditionally, total bilirubin and direct bilirubin have been measured separately and the difference calculated to yield the indirect fraction. Some modern methods (e.g., Kodak slide chemistry) measure conjugated and unconjugated fractions separately as distinct analytes.

PATHOPHYSIOLOGIC CHANGES

Increased Hemoglobin Turnover

In the instance of increased release of hemoglobin from red cells, as with any hemolytic disorder, serum bilirubin levels rise in response to the increased load of heme presented for degradation. If conjugation and excretion are normal, the rise in bilirubin will be due primarily to elevation of the unconjugated fraction because the liver is able to excrete large amounts of conjugated bilirubin but may have difficulty in actually conjugating greater amounts than normal. This phenomenon is termed **prehepatic jaundice,** although the peak levels of bilirubin achieved may not be more than a few milligrams per deciliter. With normal liver function, this increased amount of conjugated bilirubin entering the gut leads to greater formation of urobilinogen. Fecal and urinary concentrations of urobilinogen rise with hemolysis or after hemorrhage into soft tissues followed by resorption and degradation of hemoglobin. It is generally difficult for a patient to gauge an increase in color of feces beyond the normal dark brown color, but the levels of urobilinogen in urine can be appreciated by standard dipstick analysis or even by visual inspection.

Conjugation and Excretion Abnormalities

If the liver has difficulty in taking up bilirubin from the circulation or in conjugating it, the indirect fraction rises in serum, and the amount of bilirubin entering the gut diminishes. In that case, there may be pale-colored stools and a relative absence of urobilinogen in urine. If conjugation occurs normally but biliary excretion is obstructed, the conjugated (direct) bilirubin backs up into the circulation, and intestinal bilirubin and urobilinogen also decline. Since the conjugated bilirubin is water soluble, it also passes easily into the urine, imparting a bright yellow color that is also confirmed by the urine dipstick test designated "bile" (actually a measurement of direct bilirubin; see Chapter 19) (Fig. 12–2). Thus, an increase in circulating indirect bilirubin indicates either excessive hemoglobin breakdown or impaired hepatocellular functioning, whereas increased direct bilirubin suggests obstruction to biliary excretion (**obstructive jaundice**).

In clinical practice, this clear-cut distinction is often blurred because both disease components are frequently present simultaneously. Direct bilirubin levels may rise with hepatocellular dysfunction, although not as high as with extrahepatic biliary obstruction. Hepatocellular disease also seems to interfere with intrahepatic bile flow, and patients with severe hepatocellular disease usually have elevations of both direct and indirect bilirubin. With complete biliary tract obstruction (which may be due to gallstones, tumor, or intrahepatic cholestasis), feces become clay colored because they contain no bilirubin-based pigments; urine urobilinogen levels decline; and products of abnormal biliary tract epithelial activity enter the blood (see section on Obstructive Disease Enzymes). With partial biliary tract obstruction, those enzymes can also be released into the blood from locally obstructed regions, but conjugated bilirubin that may have been released into the blood is rapidly taken up by nonobstructed regions of the liver and excreted by those functioning hepatocytes that compensate for the obstructed hepatocytes (see Fig. 12–2).

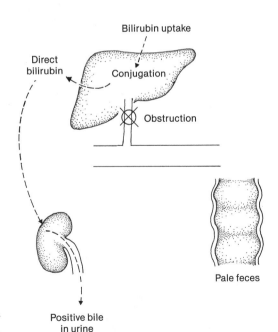

FIGURE 12–2. Model of bilirubin in obstructive jaundice.

Gilbert's Syndrome

Bilirubin is converted from a lipophilic substance to a water-soluble one through conjugation with glucuronic acid by UDP-glucuronosyltransferases (a family of 10 different enzymes derived from a single gene on chromosome 2). The different forms result from variations in the splicing of mRNA. In addition there is a transcription promoter sequence at the 5′-end of the gene that has recently been found to occur in different lengths. The longer promoter sequence binds RNA polymerase less well, leading to less transcription, and ultimately to less enzyme in hepatocytes. The gene for this variation is quite common: about two-thirds of people have the gene and 15% are homozygous. This gene defect explains the well-known phenomenon of mild unconjugated bilirubinemia (usually less than 3 mg/dL) that occurs in about 5% of the population in the United States (Fig. 12–3). This elevation of unconjugated bilirubin is an isolated finding in these asymptomatic individuals, whose other liver function tests are normal. This phenomenon should be remembered in the differential diagnosis of jaundice, as it may cause the clinician to suspect liver disease or hemolysis when in fact no more evaluation is necessary.

BILE SALTS

Bile acids exist as bile salts in the watery medium of bile or (under abnormal conditions) in plasma. The primary bile acids are cholic and chenodeoxycholic acid, as well as cholylglycine and sulfolithocholylglycine, which are synthesized by hepatocytes from cholesterol and constitute 65 to 90% of bile. They function by solubilizing cholesterol and other lipids in the bile and in intestinal contents. When concentrations of bile salts are low in the bile, cholesterol may precipitate to form gallstones. In the intestine, the bile salts are necessary to emulsify the fats for absorption. The bile salts are normally reabsorbed through the enterohepatic circulation, as is urobilinogen, and then taken back up by the liver for recycling.

Pathophysiologic Significance

Biliary obstruction prevents bile salts from entering the duodenum and leads to their accumulation in the blood. Serum bile salt levels may rise even without obstruction if there is damage to the liver cells that normally extract reabsorbed bile salts from portal blood. Salts that are not removed from the enterohepatic cycle enter the systemic circulation, where they constitute a sensitive index of hepatocellular dysfunction. It is significant that the intense itching that accompanies many forms of jaundice is caused by bile salts in the circulating blood, where they do not normally

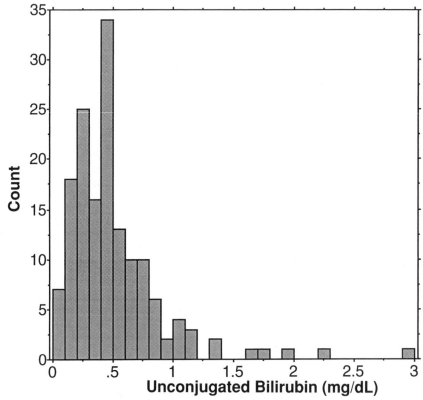

FIGURE 12–3. Unconjugated bilirubin concentrations in the serum of healthy medical students. Most of the values fall below 1.5 mg/dL. Individuals with values above 1.5 mg/dL had normal results of other liver function tests, suggesting that these persons may have a mild form of Gilbert's syndrome.

occur in high concentration. Intestinal shunting operations sometimes used to treat obesity may cause a tremendous loss of bile salts by interrupting the enterohepatic circulation. A complication of this procedure is pathologic fibrosis of the liver, suggesting that bile salts are required for the normal physiology of the liver.

Congenital abnormalities of bilirubin conjugation and excretion do not affect bile salt concentrations in serum. However, in structural liver diseases such as cirrhosis of any cause, hepatitis (acute or chronic), or drug reactions (e.g., cholestasis), the serum concentration of bile salts may be elevated even when other biochemical markers have normalized, making this assay potentially very sensitive for documenting injury or predicting disease exacerbation ahead of other liver function tests.

Laboratory Analysis

Bile salts can be quantified by spectrophotometry, chromatography, or radioimmunoassay, although such determinations are usually beyond the ability of most clinical laboratories. Since the clinical value of this measurement depends on a highly reliable assay, it is prudent to ensure that it is performed by a reference laboratory with background and experience in bile salts analysis. Testing a postprandial sample allows a more sensitive distinction between normal and abnormal values than testing a fasting sample, because of the usual increase in secretion stimulated by eating.

OBSTRUCTIVE DISEASE ENZYMES

Several enzymes appear in the circulation when bile duct epithelium is damaged, particularly with biliary tract obstruction that prevents normal clearance of those substances through biliary excretion. The increased pressure in an obstructed biliary tract pushes these enzymes backward into the circulation. In addition, there also appears to be increased synthesis of biliary tract–associated enzymes in the regenerative phase immediately after any injury to that system, with concomitant elevations in the blood.

Many of these enzymes also exist in other cell types, but relatively few extrahepatic diseases cause characteristic changes in most of them. Enzymes are very large molecules; they are normally confined within cells unless increased membrane permeability allows them to enter the blood. Enzymes enter the bloodstream with cell necrosis or sublethal cellular injury, as well as in states of rapid cellular multiplication or regeneration, when there are greater amounts of freshly synthesized enzymes and greater opportunities for cellular contents to spill out during cell division. Serum enzyme levels are diagnostically helpful in obstructive disorders of extrahepatic or intrahepatic biliary ducts, in infiltrative disorders involving the periductal tissue, and in inflammatory or regenerative conditions of small bile ducts.

Alkaline Phosphatase

The enzyme most often measured to indicate bile duct obstruction is **alkaline phosphatase (ALP)** (see Chapter 11). This enzyme functions to remove phosphate groups from proteins and from other molecules. This action is important because the degree of phosphorylation of biologic compounds frequently is responsible for their own inherent activities (as enzymes) or structural interactions with other molecules (as in membranes). High levels of ALP exist in cells that are rapidly dividing or are otherwise metabolically active. These include epithelium of biliary tract and liver, osteoblasts laying down new bone, granulocytes of circulating blood, intestinal epithelium, proximal tubules of the kidney, placenta, and lactating mammary glands. ALP levels should be expected to rise in conditions with active bone formation, in pregnancy (placental enzyme that crosses from fetal to maternal circulation), in some intestinal disorders, and rarely in renal infarcts.

In all the above conditions, the total activity of ALP can rise in serum. If it is necessary to trace the origin of an ALP elevation not evident from other laboratory or clinical findings, it is possible to partition ALP into organ- or tissue-specific isoenzymes by electrophoresis or by exploiting differences in physical properties or optimum substrates. A simple method of resolving ALP isoenzymes is heat fractionation (see Chapter 11), in which the ALP from bone is almost entirely degraded, roughly two-thirds of ALP from liver is preserved, and that from placenta is left entirely intact. If the clinical picture does not provide enough discrimination, it is often possible to demonstrate the hepatic origin of ALP by measuring associated enzymes not affected by bone growth or pregnancy. These corroborative enzymes are **5′-nucleotidase (5′-NT), leucine aminopeptidase (LAP),** and **gamma-glutamyltransferase (GGT).** Both 5′-NT and LAP determinations have largely fallen out of favor because of the hazard of their measurements, which utilize potentially carcinogenic substrates. GGT, however, is very conveniently quantitated on virtually all modern, large, multichannel chemistry analyzers and has achieved a position of great clinical utility for detecting and monitoring biliary obstruction, particularly that due to metastatic disease invading the liver. Serum GGT levels are also affected by alcohol ingestion, which induces more synthesis of GGT, some of which is normally absorbed into the circulation even without obstruction. Serum GGT is now frequently used to evaluate alcohol-induced hepatic changes because of this amplification effect from induction of new enzyme synthesis.

ALP levels reach spectacular heights (up to 20 times normal values) in primary biliary cirrhosis, in conditions of disorganized and fibrotic hepatic architecture (cirrhosis), and in diseases characterized by inflammation, regeneration, and obstruction of intrahepatic bile ductules. Obstruction of extrahepatic bile ducts causes up to tenfold elevations, even if obstruction is incomplete. Hepatocellular disease (e.g., hepatitis) often causes modest elevations of ALP and GGT. Diagnostic associations of ALP are reviewed in Table 12–2. It should be especially noted that ALP and GGT of hepatobiliary origin are very sensitive markers for metastatic cancer to the liver, and rival the sensitivity and efficiency of far more expensive, inconvenient, and invasive radiographic and other imaging procedures for the detection of small metastases. Marked elevation of both enzymes but with disproportionate increase of GGT over ALP suggests drug-induced cholestasis (with induction of increased GGT synthesis).

TABLE 12–2. CONDITIONS ASSOCIATED WITH INCREASED ALKALINE PHOSPHATASE

Disease	Other Clues
Very High Values (10 or More × Normal):	
Primary biliary cirrhosis	Antimitochondrial antibodies; high IgM; pruritus
Extrahepatic bile duct obstruction by tumor	Unremitting jaundice
Granulomatous or neoplastic infiltration of portal areas	Bilirubin may be disproportionately low
Congenital atresia of intrahepatic bile ducts	Unremitting conjugated bilirubinemia in newborn
High or Moderate Values (3–10 × Normal):	
Extrahepatic bile duct obstruction by stone	Levels of alkaline phosphatase, bilirubin may fluctuate
Incomplete occlusion, intrahepatic or extrahepatic ducts	Bilirubin may be disproportionately low
Mild or No Elevation (1–3 × Normal):	
Alcoholic liver disease	Depressed synthetic functions; increased GGT
Chronic active hepatitis	Aminotransferases higher than alkaline phosphatase
Viral hepatitis	Viral antigens and antibodies

HEPATOCELLULAR FUNCTION

Because the liver has such substantial reserve capacity, hepatocellular loss must be far advanced before it becomes clinically apparent. It is possible to detect ongoing hepatocellular damage by measuring functional indices and by observing in the circulation the products of damaged or necrotic hepatocytes. Enzyme tests are often the only indication of cell injury in early or localized liver disease because subtle changes in excretory capacity may be unapparent due to the compensation from other regions of the liver that remain functional.

Serum bilirubin rises with moderate or severe dysfunction. For patients with mild or moderate disease, waxing and waning damage is best monitored by serially testing bilirubin and serum enzyme levels. With severe loss of hepatocyte function, there may be diagnostic changes in synthetic capacities and in the functions of excretion, detoxification, and metabolic reactivity that are reflected in multiple standard and specialized tests available in most clinical laboratories.

AMINOTRANSFERASES

The two enzymes most often associated with hepatocellular damage are the aminotransferases that catalyze the reversible transfer of an amino group between an amino acid and an alpha-keto acid. This function is essential for the production of the correct amino acids needed to synthesize proteins in the liver. **Aspartate aminotransferase (AST)** mediates this reaction between aspartic and alpha-ketoglutamic acids; it was formerly called "glutamic-oxaloacetic transaminase (GOT)" and is still referred to as "serum (S)GOT." **Alanine aminotransferase (ALT)** transfers an amino group between alanine and alpha-ketoglutamic acid and was formerly called "(serum) glutamic-pyruvic transaminase (SGPT)." Although both AST and ALT are commonly thought of as liver enzymes because of their high concentrations in hepatocytes, only ALT is specific for liver; AST is widely present in myocardium, skeletal muscle, brain, and kidney. Characteristics of these aminotransferases are given in Table 12–3. Both AST and ALT require pyridoxal phosphate (vitamin B_6) as a cofactor for full enzymatic activity. For that reason, coexisting renal disease that causes deficiency of pyridoxal phosphate may give falsely low measurements of the aminotransferases unless the assay reagents are supplemented with that cofactor.

The numerical result obtained when AST activity is divided by ALT

TABLE 12–3. CHARACTERISTICS OF LIVER-ASSOCIATED AMINOTRANSFERASES

Characteristic	Aspartate Aminotransferase (AST)	Alanine Aminotransferase (ALT)
Present in tissues other than liver	More in heart than in liver; also in skeletal muscle, kidney, brain	Relatively low concentrations in other tissues
Location in hepatocyte	Mitochondria and cytoplasm	Cytoplasm only
Reference range in adult blood	10–40 IU/liter	5–35 IU/liter
Half-life in blood	12–22 hr	37–57 hr
Change with acute inflammatory damage	Moderately sensitive	Extremely sensitive
Change with primary or secondary neoplasm	Substantial rise	Moderate or no rise
Change with cirrhosis	Moderate rise	Mild or moderate rise
Change with myocardial infarct	Substantial rise	Mild or moderate rise

activity in the same serum sample is termed the **de Ritis ratio.** It is used to distinguish various clinical conditions in which both AST and ALT can be elevated to different degrees. In general, ALT is released from hepatocytes into the blood more readily in acute conditions, whereas AST is released to a greater degree in more chronic disorders with progressive damage.

Vascular Changes

With liver disease, serum levels of AST and ALT generally rise and fall in parallel. When hepatocytes are injured, these normally intracellular enzymes enter the bloodstream. Nonhepatic diseases—especially circulatory collapse, congestive heart failure, and myocardial infarction—may also cause hepatic release of aminotransferases. This sensitivity results because the hepatocytes nearest the central vein of each lobule normally have a low oxygen tension and are extremely vulnerable to hypoxic damage. Centrilobular hepatocytes are injured if arterial hypotension causes less blood to enter the liver or if increased back pressure from right heart failure slows the exit of blood out of the central veins; with this hypoxic damage, aminotransferase levels rise to a modest degree. In addition, myocardial infarction directly causes substantial increases in AST (usually a few days after the event), because this enzyme is abundantly present in heart muscle. Hemolysis also releases AST directly into the circulation.

Hepatocellular Disease

Aminotransferases rise to levels that roughly parallel the extent of hepatocellular damage. Severe viral or toxic hepatitis may produce elevations up to 20 times the normal range. A sudden drop of these enzyme levels during the course of hepatitis without corresponding clinical improvement is an ominous indication that so many cells have been damaged that only few or no viable hepatocytes remain as a source for release of enzymes. With low levels of inflammatory damage in acute hepatitis, ALT levels rise earlier and more impressively than those of AST (de Ritis ratio < 1.0). ALT measurement is a more sensitive and specific screening test for posttransfusion hepatitis or occupational toxic exposure. ALT quantitation was formerly required on blood donors to exclude individuals contagious for hepatitis viruses not then identified. The introduction of hepatitis C virus antibody has made the need for such screening less critical. ALT measurement on blood donors is no longer mandatory in the United States but is still performed in some countries to rule out other as-yet-unidentified hepatitis viruses.

In chronic active hepatitis, changing enzyme levels often (but not always) reflect the degree of ongoing cell destruction. Alcoholic hepatitis often causes functional derangement more than actual cell necrosis, so enzyme levels are often only modestly elevated. In both acute and chronic alcoholic liver damage, the elevation of AST tends to be somewhat greater than that of ALT (de Ritis ratio >1.0, often >5.0) because of its higher content in tissue. Because skeletal muscle contains AST, nonhepatic AST may be conspicuously elevated above ALT in acute alcohol-related illness like delirium tremens, trauma, or stupor with prolonged immobility, owing to release from the injured muscle. In cholestasis, extrahepatic obstruction is typically an acute process (e.g., gallstone), which elevates ALT more than AST (de Ritis ratio <1.5). In contrast, intrahepatic cholestasis is a more chronic process with greater release of AST (de Ritis ratio >1.5). The characteristic findings of various diseases are detailed in Table 12–4.

TABLE 12–4. CONDITIONS ASSOCIATED WITH ELEVATED AMINOTRANSFERASES*

Disease	Other Clues
Very High Values (20 or More × Normal):	
Viral hepatitis	Viral antigens and antibodies
Toxic hepatitis	History of drugs, occupational exposure, anesthetics
Moderately High Values (Usually 3–10 × Normal):	
Infectious mononucleosis	Heterophile antibodies; EBV antibodies
Chronic active hepatitis	Levels may fluctuate, decline with steroids
Extrahepatic bile duct obstruction	ALP very high; ratio of direct to indirect bilirubin is reversed
Reye's syndrome	Serum ammonia high; neurologic signs
Intrahepatic cholestasis	ALT often higher than AST; ALP very high
Myocardial infarction	AST much higher than ALT
Mild or No Elevation (1–3 × Normal):	
Pancreatitis	Lipase, amylase high
Alcoholic fatty liver	GGT usually high
Laënnec's cirrhosis	Decreased synthetic functions; portal hypertension
Granulomatous or neoplastic infiltration	AST usually higher than ALT
Biliary cirrhosis	ALP very high; antimitochondrial antibodies

*Aspartate aminotransferase (AST) and alanine aminotransferase (ALT).
ALP = alkaline phosphatase; GGT = gamma-glutamyltranspeptidase.

GAMMA-GLUTAMYLTRANSFERASE

Obstructive Disease

Large amounts of **gamma-glutamyltransferase (GGT;** also called **gamma-glutamyl transpeptidase)** exist in hepatobiliary cells. It appears that epithelium of pancreas and kidney has some GGT activity because modest serum elevation occurs with pancreatic or renal cell damage or neoplasia. In addition, GGT activity occurs in urine in association with renal tubule damage. Most hepatocellular and hepatobiliary diseases elevate serum GGT. Elevated GGT correlates better with obstruction and cholestasis than with pure hepatocellular damage, and GGT is considered one of the "obstructive" enzymes. Normal activity of GGT essentially rules out even very small hepatic metastases that result in segmental obstruction. In the general diagnosis of liver disease, measurement of GGT is not especially useful because it provides little information beyond that obtained from quantitating the aminotransferases, ALP, and bilirubin fractions.

Alcohol and Enzyme Induction

The other major clinical significance of GGT measurement is its developing role as an indicator of alcohol use. GGT is one of the microsomal enzymes whose activity increases in persons taking alcohol, barbiturates, phenytoin, and certain drugs because of induction of new enzyme synthesis as the physiologic response to those drug exposures. Alcohol not only induces microsomal activity but also causes hepatocellular damage, even in otherwise well-nourished alcoholic drinkers. The combination of increased GGT activity in the hepatocytes plus increased hepatocellular damage amplifies the elevation of serum GGT levels in persons with substantial alcohol intake. About 60 to 80% of patients considered to have alcohol-abuse problems demonstrate elevated serum GGT levels, whether or not they have other physical or laboratory signs of liver damage. Because of the combined new synthesis and potential cell damage, levels of GGT return to normal after as long as 3 to 6 weeks of abstention from alcohol, making it a useful test for compliance in alcohol-reduction programs and potentially also in other drug abuse treatment protocols. It should be realized that elevated GGT is not pathognomonic for alcohol-related disease because GGT can be high in 90% of patients with liver disease of any sort. Yet up to 10 to 15% of all adult hospital patients may have hidden alcohol-abuse problems, and measurement of GGT can be used by the physician to obtain concrete physical evidence of their existence in order to assist patients in recognizing the significance of that abuse.

LACTATE DEHYDROGENASE

All cells contain **lactate dehydrogenase (LD)** as an essential metabolic enzyme for the interconversion of lactate and pyruvate. As discussed in Chapter 11, LD has a tetrameric molecule composed of two possible subunits, H and M, which form a total of five possible combinations (see Table 11–2). These isoenzymes of LD have characteristic distributions in different tissues according roughly to whether an organ is more or less aerobic or anaerobic in its metabolism. Accordingly, myocardium and erythrocytes are rich in LD isoenzyme 1 (high content of the H-subunit); liver and skeletal muscle are rich in LD isoenzyme 5 (predominantly the M-subunit) (see also Fig. 11–2).

Pathophysiologic Association

The diagnostic significance of these organ associations of the LD isoenzymes is that elevations of LD due to hemolysis or myocardial infarction can easily be distinguished from elevations due to liver or skeletal muscle damage by routine LD isoenzyme analysis (usually performed by electrophoresis). In turn, liver and skeletal muscle injury can generally be distinguished on clinical evaluation or on the basis of associated biochemical markers specific for those organs.

As with the aminotransferases, elevations of LD from the liver occur in association with circulatory changes (e.g., shock) and with other hepatocellular damage (hepatitis, cirrhosis, inflammation, or infiltrative disorders).

Contemporary strategies for diagnosis of myocardial infarction no longer routinely include LD total activity or isoenzymes but instead utilize cardiac troponin I. In addition, LD provides essentially no more information about liver disease than is provided by AST, ALT, ALP, and bilirubin. Consequently LD quantitation and isoenzyme fractionation are now requested much less frequently than in former years.

SYNTHETIC FUNCTION

PROTEIN METABOLISM

Most of the blood plasma proteins, except for von Willebrand factor (from endothelial cells) and the immunoglobulins (from plasma cells), are made in the liver. In addition to synthesizing proteins from available amino acids, hepatocytes regulate amino acid conversions, breaking down endogenous or exogenous proteins and transforming worn-out protein metabolites like ammonia into urea for excretion. This action also helps to buffer the body against changes in acid-base balance due to the organic acids and ammonia produced by metabolism. More than 90% of overall hepatic function must be lost before urea production or amino acid regulation is measurably affected.

With very severe acute or chronic liver damage, generalized aminoaciduria may occur. Amino acids enter the blood and the urine because of massive protein breakdown in degenerating liver cells and loss of the regulatory mechanisms for retaining those free amino acids by incorporation into new protein synthesis. Aminoaciduria can manifest itself with unusual crystals of leucine or tyrosine that never appear in normal urine samples. In starvation or other severe systemic illnesses, normal hepatic synthetic and ·recycling mechanisms may fail to operate, even though there is no primary liver disease. In such instances of nonhepatic disease impacting on hepatic function, aminoaciduria may also arise, but it is reversible with correction of the primary disorder. Consequently, the finding of aminoaciduria is diagnostically significant only in primary liver disease.

Urea and Ammonia

Blood urea nitrogen (BUN; actually serum urea) levels drop in severe hepatic disease, largely because of a decline in the capacity of the liver to form urea from ammonia. Characteristic of severe cellular and circulatory disorders of the liver is impaired sodium and water metabolism, partly because of failure to inactivate the steroid hormones that regulate electrolyte balance. Consequently, plasma volume expands, producing dilutional changes in many circulating metabolites, including the electrolytes, urea, and creatinine. With established liver failure, inability to form urea from the amino groups of degraded proteins causes low overall urea levels and excess aminoaciduria; ammonia metabolism is also diminished. As intestinal bacteria degrade protein in food, they generate ammonia, which readily enters the portal circulation and is normally transformed into urea. In liver failure, or when the circulatory changes accommodating increased pressures from cirrhosis divert the portal blood to collateral vessels, there is bypass of the usual circulation through hepatic lobules where ammonia and other substances are removed by hepatocytes. Then the systemic ammonia levels rise and the urea levels fall. This clinical problem is best approached by reducing alimentary proteins and by eliminating colon bacteria through use of nonabsorbable antibiotics by mouth or rectum to decrease production of ammonia in the gastrointestinal tract. Another treatment is to administer the sugar lactulose, which is not metabolized by the human intestine but is metabolized by bacteria in the lower intestines. This bacterial action links ammonia to lactulose, thereby further reducing overall ammonia load. Monitoring of the success of these measures is accomplished by quantitation of plasma ammonia levels.

The blood specimen must be collected very carefully into heparin and kept on ice to prevent spontaneous formation of ammonia in the specimen itself. Serial ammonia determinations are frequently useful in following the progress of hepatic encephalopathy in such conditions as Reye's syndrome (acute postviral fatty degeneration of the liver with encephalopathy).

Protein Manufacture

When hepatocellular dysfunction is longstanding, circulating plasma protein levels drop. Serum albumin and the vitamin K–dependent coagulation factors provide the most useful indices for assessing severity of disease.

The normal liver manufactures about 12 g of albumin daily, maintaining a whole-body content of about 500 g. Albumin has a half-life of 14 to 20 days; even if albumin synthesis stops completely, it takes some time for serum levels to decline appreciably. Acute hepatocellular failure is more immediately apparent from measurement of the protein designated **prealbumin** (transthyretin). With a half-life of only 2 days, prealbumin levels decline rapidly when hepatic synthesis falters. In such acute settings as viral or toxic hepatitis, prealbumin levels sensitively reflect the intensity of liver damage. In addition, states of malnutrition, whether due to starvation or cachexia or cancer, are also occasioned by reductions in serum prealbumin.

Albumin

Serum albumin levels regularly decline when severe hepatocellular disease lasts more than 3 weeks, after which the circulating albumin has substantially cleared from the body. In rapidly developing illnesses, declining serum albumin indicates massively impaired function and has ominous prognostic significance. With gradually progressive diseases, especially cirrhosis or carcinomas, low albumin levels are almost universal and probably contribute to the edema and ascites formation often seen in these conditions by reducing plasma oncotic pressure.

Not all hypoalbuminemia comes from liver disease. Serum albumin levels are low in malnutrition, in protein-losing alimentary tract disease (enteropathy), in protein-losing renal diseases, in prolonged severe catabolic conditions like burns (which also lose albumin by exudation through the skin), and in conditions of expanded blood volume (using intravenous solutions). Liver disease may accompany any of these other problems, making it difficult to assess the relative significance of the single laboratory finding without associated tests, whose values may form diagnostic patterns of abnormalities.

Immunoglobulins

Immunoglobulins constitute much of the increased globulin fraction in chronic liver disease. The stimulus to the formation of these antibodies has generally been unclear, but they are typically polyclonal antibodies with broad distribution throughout the gamma region of protein electrophoresis and with IgA extending into the beta region (see Fig. 9–2). It has been suggested that alterations of the portal circulation allow antigenic material from food or bacteria in the gut to escape hepatic denaturation and to enter the systemic circulation as massive direct immune stimulation. If there were such specific antigenic stimuli, we should expect to find individual clones of antibodies in an oligoclonal distribution. Instead, the typical increase of immunoglobulins in liver disease is polyclonal and therefore almost certainly not due to antigenic stimulation of the immune system. A more likely explanation is that in liver disease, B-cell growth factors (such as interleukin 6 and other cytokines that are normally removed from blood by the liver) remain in the circulation, thus permitting continuous production of polyclonal immunoglobulins in a nonspecific manner independent of antigenic stimulation. Polyclonal hypergammaglobulinemia is a frequent finding in liver disease, but it is not very useful for monitoring disease progression, as it is merely an indirect indicator of liver malfunction. Chronic liver disease such as cirrhosis can be better monitored with serum albumin measurements that directly reflect hepatic synthetic capacity.

Other Globulins

The alpha globulins provide little diagnostic information in liver disease except for specific levels of alpha-1-antitrypsin. Deficiency of that protein can result in cirrhosis and associated pulmonary emphysema.

The beta fraction includes beta lipoprotein, which carries the majority of cholesterol in the plasma. This fraction is elevated in viral hepatitis, in biliary cirrhosis, and in extrahepatic biliary tract obstruction in association with high concentrations of serum cholesterol. The effect of liver disease on serum protein electrophoretic patterns is outlined in Table 12–5.

LIPID AND CARBOHYDRATE METABOLISM

The liver is very important in several steps of lipid metabolism and in particular is responsible for the synthesis of the apolipoproteins that go into the construction of the lipoprotein fractions that the liver also helps to assemble and to reabsorb in the various phases of their transport and clearance (see Chapter 9). The liver is also responsible for converting free fatty acids to triglycerides and for esterifying cholesterol. Abnormalities of lipid metabolism in the liver are manifested by fatty deposits there. In

TABLE 12–5. SERUM PROTEIN CHANGES IN SELECTED LIVER DISEASES

	Albumin	α-Globulin	β-Globulin	γ-Globulin
Acute hepatitis	nl or sl ↓	nl or sl ↑	sl ↑	↑ (IgG and IgM)
Laënnec's cirrhosis	↓↓	nl	sl ↑	↑↑ (IgM and IgA)
Chronic active hepatitis	↓↓	nl	↑	↑↑ (IgG)
Biliary cirrhosis	↓	↑	↑↑	↑ (IgM)
Extrahepatic biliary obstruction	nl	nl or sl ↑	↑	nl

nl = normal; sl = slightly; ↓ = moderately depressed; ↓↓ = severely depressed; ↑ = moderately elevated; ↑↑ = markedly elevated.

obstruction of the biliary tract, normal excretion of cholesterol in bile is prevented, leading to high total cholesterol levels in the circulation. The fat-soluble vitamins (A, D, E, and K) are also stored in the liver after being absorbed by digestive processes that depend on adequate amounts of bile salts from the liver.

Carbohydrate metabolism is also significantly controlled by the liver. The hepatic stores of glycogen are a source of glucose to go into the blood when needed to maintain normal glucose levels. In addition, gluconeogenesis occurs in the liver, as glycogen is formed from noncarbohydrate sources such as amino acids or fatty acids. This happens under such conditions as low carbohydrate intake, diabetes mellitus, or starvation. In cases of severe liver damage, hypoglycemia can occur because of the inability of remaining liver tissue to generate glucose.

COAGULATION FACTORS

The liver synthesizes most coagulation proteins of plasma, but only a few factors are routinely tested as evidence of hepatocellular disease. Levels of fibrinogen and factor V do fall with severe liver failure, but by the time these changes affect coagulation, other complicating conditions have usually developed. More straightforward is the relationship between hepatocellular disease and the so-called "liver factors," or vitamin K–dependent factors: factors II (prothrombin), VII (proconvertin), IX (Christmas factor), and X (Stuart-Prower factor) (see Chapter 6).

The normal liver synthesizes these four coagulation proteins in two stages. First there is construction of the proper primary amino acid sequence encoded in the gene and transcribed in the mRNA. The coagulation proteins at this stage are antigenically complete but functionally inactive in the coagulation cascade. If there is no vitamin K present in the liver, these incomplete proteins will be released into the circulation where they can actually interfere with the function of normal coagulation factors. However, most people have adequate stores of vitamin K, a fat-soluble vitamin, which allows the second stage of synthesis to occur. Vitamin K then catalyzes the transfer of carboxyl groups onto selective glutamic acid residues already incorporated into those four coagulation factors. This process allows the vitamin K–dependent factors to interact correctly with the other coagulation proteins and with calcium to achieve clot formation. Manufacture of these coagulation factors declines with either hepatocellular dysfunction or insufficient vitamin K in the liver. Vitamin K absorption is disturbed if bile duct obstruction prevents bile salts from entering the duodenum, or if enzymatic (e.g., lack of pancreatic lipase) or mucosal abnormalities cause malabsorption of fats. Vitamin K deficiency is infrequent but can be seen in hospitalized patients who have been chronically ill and usually have the triad of poor diet, oral antibiotics (which can deplete the intestinal bacteria that make some vitamin K), and abdominal surgery or other abnormality that limits intestinal absorption.

Prothrombin Time and Partial Thromboplastin Time

Deficiencies of the vitamin K–dependent factors prolong both the prothrombin time (PT) and the partial thromboplastin time (PTT). Factors II, VII, and X affect the PT; factors II, IX, and X affect the PTT. Of the four vitamin K–dependent proteins, factor VII has the shortest half-life, so that factor VII levels fall first as hepatic function begins to decline. For that reason, the PT will be prolonged earlier than will be the PTT. A prolonged PTT usually accompanies a prolonged PT in cases of longstanding liver disease, and both tests are available routinely.

Effect of Vitamin K

When a prolonged PT suggests deficiency of vitamin K–dependent coagulation factors, deficiency of vitamin K must be distinguished from defective hepatocellular capacity. After the baseline PT has been established, vitamin K is administered by intramuscular injection, usually 10 mg daily for 1 to 3 days. If malabsorption and deficiency of vitamin K were the problem, a PT performed 72 hours after beginning therapy should give normal results. In fact, simple deficiency of vitamin K with frank hemorrhage can show improvement and nearly normal clotting times within 6 to 12 hours after the vitamin K is replaced. Persistent prolongation of the PT despite vitamin K administration indicates loss of hepatic capacity to manufacture the proteins in the first stage of synthesis. Coagulation factor synthesis is usually defective in patients with liver disease severe enough to cause hypoalbuminemia. These patients should not receive prophylactic administration of clotting factor concentrates unless they are bleeding because those preparations contain some activated factors that may precipitate consumption of more coagulation proteins in the absence of adequate liver function to regulate their inactivation. In the instance of hemorrhage in liver failure, the administration of vitamin K and of fresh frozen plasma should be tried. In acute viral or toxic hepatitis, prolongation of the PT signifies massive cellular damage. In jaundice caused by extrahepatic biliary obstruction, administering vitamin K nearly always corrects the PT abnormality. Newborns are routinely given a dose of vitamin K in order to prevent hemorrhage due to occasional deficiency of the vitamin after full-term pregnancy (hemorrhagic disease of the newborn).

SPECIAL TESTS IN EVALUATION OF LIVER DISEASE

Cirrhosis is a chronic, diffuse disease in which there is necrosis of hepatocytes, fibrosis of the liver, and regeneration of hepatic nodules with derangement of liver architecture. It has many different causes including alcohol, other drug and toxic exposures, viral hepatitis, biliary obstruction, cardiac failure (congestion), and the genetic disorders of copper and iron metabolism. The most common cause in this country is alcohol, which causes fatty liver, acute nonviral hepatitis, and cirrhosis.

To manage patients with cirrhosis, the physician should establish diagnosis and etiology, assess the extent of the disease, and determine what complications are present. To assist in this diagnostic process, several special tests are commonly employed. Many of these are directed at detecting hepatocellular carcinoma, which often arises from cirrhosis.

LIVER BIOPSY

Because different liver disorders can have overlapping biochemical profiles and clinical appearances, diagnosis may require histologic examination of tissue obtained by liver biopsy. The main reason for doing this invasive procedure should be to evaluate patients who are not improving as expected and may have more complicated disease that requires additional therapies. The morphologic classification of the different forms of cirrhosis relies on specific histopathologic patterns. Special stains are regularly employed to indicate the extent of iron deposits, fibrosis, inflammation, and other immunologic features. Unusual features of necrosis and healing are easily revealed on biopsy, which is performed as a cored-out sample of liver through a hollow needle. The specimen must be sufficiently large to preserve a local region of hepatic architecture and keep the organization of several lobules and their component elements intact for microscopic analysis. It is easy to appreciate from microscopic examination how the grossly disordered cellular architecture encountered in cirrhosis could interfere with the normal flow of blood and bile through fine channels of the liver.

ALPHA-FETOPROTEIN

During the first 10 weeks of fetal life, the major serum protein is not albumin but **alpha-fetoprotein (AFP),** a glycoprotein that migrates more slowly on electrophoresis than albumin but more rapidly than most globulins. AFP shares amino acid sequence homologies with albumin, indicating that both probably derived from a common ancestral gene. Fetal liver synthesizes huge quantities of AFP until about the 32nd week of gestation, at which time synthesis declines sharply, although the AFP concentration in cord blood is 20,000 times that in adult blood. By 1 year of age, normal individuals have serum AFP levels of no more than 30 ng/mL.

During pregnancy, AFP levels in amniotic fluid are higher than normal if the developing fetus has a neural tube defect (see also Chapter 17). This amniotic fluid AFP is also transferred to the maternal circulation. Thus, levels of AFP in the serum of the mother are routinely used to screen for neural tube defects before birth. There is a sliding scale of normal values, depending on the exact month of the pregnancy; multiple fetuses in the same pregnancy also cause elevations compared with a single fetus. On obtaining an elevated serum AFP in a pregnant woman, confirmation is sought by performing AFP analysis on amniotic fluid collected by amniocentesis.

In the adult, the capacity to manufacture AFP is repressed in normal, resting hepatocytes, but rapidly multiplying hepatocytes resume the synthesis of AFP. If rapid hepatocyte multiplication occurs in postuterine life (regrowth of the liver following damage, lobular resection, liver transplantation, etc.), serum AFP levels also rise, although never to levels approaching those in fetal life. If there is unbridled multiplication, as in hepatocellular carcinoma, AFP levels may rise to several thousand nanograms per milliliter. More restrained regenerative activity, characteristic of active cirrhosis, chronic active hepatitis, or the recovery phase of viral or toxic hepatitis, produces AFP elevations to about 500 ng/mL.

Hepatocellular carcinoma cannot be diagnosed solely by AFP determination but also requires a tissue diagnosis from biopsied material of the tumor. However, demonstration of very high AFP levels can direct the clinical differential diagnosis toward carcinoma in cases of hepatomegaly, jaundice, and hepatocellular dysfunction when etiology is uncertain or degree of illness is more severe than anticipated. As many as 30 to 50% of American patients with liver cancer have no detectable AFP in their circulations, perhaps because of variation in tumor type that produces no

AFP or that produces AFP antigenically nonreactive with the antibodies used in a particular immunoassay. More consistent elevations are seen in those Asian and African populations with very high incidence of hepatocellular carcinoma in association with chronic infection with hepatitis B virus.

Measurement of AFP has its greatest usefulness as an index of disease recurrence. In a patient treated for hepatocellular carcinoma, disappearance of AFP indicates elimination of malignant cells, and rising levels reflect recurrence of the cancer. After therapeutic intervention, the AFP measurement should be repeated each month or so, allowing enough time for existing AFP to be cleared from the circulation. Persistence of AFP after that interval suggests continued synthesis by tumor. Because serum levels of AFP are proportional to tumor mass, however, normal levels can be interpreted as merely indicating that any residual tumor is below a certain mass, not that complete removal of all tumor cells has been accomplished. AFP is also produced by some germ cell tumors (testicular, ovarian).

CARCINOEMBRYONIC ANTIGEN

Carcinoembryonic antigen (CEA) is another commonly used tumor marker that circulates in blood when there is rapid multiplication of epithelial cells, especially those of the digestive system. Elevations of CEA occur in many cancers, and the association of CEA with liver cancer is far less specific than that of AFP. As with AFP, CEA is useful in monitoring the recurrence of tumors, particularly metastases after surgical or other ablative therapy if those tumors initially elaborated CEA. There are now several different assays available for CEA using different antibodies, some polyclonal and others monoclonal. The assays therefore can have slightly different specificities, and occasionally a cancer patient has an elevated CEA by one assay but not by another assay. In such a case, the positive result should be used for determining therapy, and the same assay must be adhered to for future determinations to make correct comparisons of serial CEA levels.

ALPHA-1-ANTITRYPSIN

Alpha-1-antitrypsin (AAT) is a normally occurring glycoprotein that migrates as an alpha-1-globulin and inhibits the proteolytic action of several enzymes, notably trypsin and plasmin. Like many other proteins, the AAT molecule has several structural variations (see Chapter 9). Allelic genes at the controlling locus result in different forms, which are synthesized at different rates. The most common form is designated MM; variant molecules have different electrophoretic mobilities and reduced capacities to inhibit proteases because of their lower concentrations in serum. The most common abnormal allele that causes disease is designated **Z;** it occurs in about 1% of the population.

The physiologic role of AAT has to do with preventing self-destruction of tissues whenever proteolytic enzymes are released, as in an inflammatory response against a foreign material or irritant (e.g., cigarette smoke). Patients whose AAT activity is defective frequently develop lung and liver conditions in which functioning units are destroyed and excessive connective tissue is generated as scarring over the damaged cells. With AAT deficiency, emphysema and cirrhosis may develop very early in life, without the usual predisposing factors. The hepatocytes that manufacture the variant AAT acquire characteristic inclusion bodies that are accumulations of abnormal AAT molecules that apparently cannot be secreted normally into the blood. These inclusions can be stained histochemically with PAS, or immunohistochemically with specific antibody to AAT on liver biopsy specimens.

Deficiency of AAT activity is appreciated on serum protein electrophoresis as a flat region where the normal alpha-1-globulin band should be. More detailed analysis by high-resolution electrophoresis and immunofixation can confirm the particular variant form that is present. Young patients with unexplained cirrhosis or cholestatic jaundice should be evaluated for AAT deficiency. Although no specific therapy has been possible until now, new experimental protocols involve the prophylactic administration intravenously or by aerosol of recombinant AAT. Liver transplantation cures the deficiency.

Asymptomatic relatives of patients who are homozygous for AAT deficiency are not considered to be at greater risk for developing lung or liver disease. However, they can be analyzed to determine whether they are carriers of the hereditary deficiency, which does have a greater likelihood among relatives of known homozygous persons. If a known carrier marries another carrier, the chance that any one of their children will have AAT deficiency is one out of four, as determined by simple mendelian inheritance.

CERULOPLASMIN

An unusual cause of hepatic dysfunction is **Wilson's disease,** or **hepatolenticular degeneration,** a genetic abnormality in which excessive copper accumulates in liver, eye, brain, and other organs. A pigmented ring around the iris (the Kayser-Fleischer ring) is pathognomonic for this condition. The most conspicuous biochemical abnormality in most cases is deficiency in serum of the copper-transport protein ceruloplasmin. When a young person presents with signs suggesting chronic active hepatitis, or when a patient with liver disease has neurologic changes of basal ganglia origin that affect motor control, ceruloplasmin should be measured. Levels below 20 mg/dL are abnormal and can be followed up with further analysis of copper metabolism.

The gene for Wilson's disease has very recently been identified as a result of masterful molecular detective work utilizing DNA clones of a related gene responsible for diminished copper absorption in **Menkes disease** (copper deficiency). The Wilson's disease gene maps to chromosome 13, and the disorder follows an autosomal recessive pattern of inheritance. The product made from the Wilson's disease gene is a transmembrane protein that transports copper across lysosomal membranes. Normally, hepatic copper is transported by this protein into the bile for excretion from the body. Mutated forms of this protein apparently permit copper to accumulate to toxic levels in hepatic lysosomes, leading to cell necrosis. The clinical presentation can include acute hepatitis due to this toxicity and may also extend to hemolysis.

The low serum concentration of ceruloplasmin in Wilson's disease is probably due to a combination of generalized hepatic toxicity with secondary impairment of all protein synthesis plus selective inhibition due to inadequate intracellular transport of copper for ceruloplasmin synthesis. About 10% of patients with Wilson's disease have normal serum ceruloplasmin concentrations. It has been hypothesized that they may have an altered Wilson's disease protein that is capable of conveying copper to the cellular site of ceruloplasmin synthesis but cannot transport copper into bile for excretion.

Chelating agents such as penicillamine have provided moderately effective treatment and have been successfully used in children to prevent manifestation of Wilson's disease. This kind of treatment works by mobilizing body stores of copper for excretion into the urine. Liver transplantation is also effective in curing Wilson's disease. Gene therapy is a possibility now that the exact gene is known, but it will be complicated by the need to introduce the correct gene into each cell. Otherwise the uncorrected cells will likely continue to accumulate copper.

SERUM IRON AND TRANSFERRIN SATURATION

The serum iron level is an important screening test in patients suspected of having **hemochromatosis.** The primary defect is at the intestinal level, resulting in unregulated absorption of dietary iron. In the normal state, iron absorption falls with increasing body iron stores, but in hemochromatosis, it remains high regardless of iron stores. In this genetic disorder, inherited in an autosomal recessive manner, excessive iron is absorbed inappropriately through the intestinal mucosa and accumulates in tissues (especially in liver, pancreas, and heart), where it is toxic. Skin pigmentation increases because of the stimulation of melanin production there. Involvement of pancreatic islet cells leads to diabetes mellitus. (This combination of skin pigmentation and diabetes mellitus in hemochromatosis is referred to as "bronze diabetes.") The liver develops fibrosis secondary to the toxic effect of iron deposits. Since iron accumulates progressively, symptoms rarely develop until early middle age in men. Because of the loss of iron in menstrual blood, women with the abnormal gene have no untoward effects while menstruation continues and seldom become symptomatic even in late adulthood.

Hemochromatosis is actually quite common; the prevalence of homozygotes in the United States is about 1 in 400, and that of heterozygous carriers has been calculated to be roughly 1 in 10. Thus an accurate and inexpensive screening test for hemochromatosis would be extraordinarily beneficial. Secondary causes of hemochromatosis are discussed in Chapter 3.

Cirrhosis develops over decades as the liver accumulates more and more iron and may proceed to hepatocellular carcinoma. Pancreatic dysfunction occurs fairly commonly, and cardiac failure from dilated cardiomyopathy or arrhythmias due to iron deposition in the conduction system often cause death. Impotence in men and amenorrhea in women result from gonadal involvement. Arthropathy is also common.

Diagnosis is made by the demonstration of high serum levels of iron to the point of nearly complete saturation of the iron-binding capacity (transferrin). Thresholds in screening for hemochromatosis by transferrin saturation are >60% in men and >50% in women after fasting overnight. In addition, there are very high levels of ferritin (normally the tissue storage molecule of iron) in serum, generally proportional to tissue concentrations of iron (see also Iron Metabolism, Chapter 2). Tissue iron levels may be so high as to set off an airport metal detector as the patient passes through. Definitive diagnosis is achieved by evaluation of iron content in a liver biopsy specimen, either by iron stain and visual examination or by specific quantitation of tissue iron content by atomic absorption spectroscopy. Liver transplantation may be used to replace an irreversibly cirrhotic liver, but it does not cure hemochromatosis, as the hepatic manifestations are secondary to the intestinal iron absorption problem. Treatment consists of decreasing iron intake, phlebotomy to remove iron in red cells, and intravenous chelation therapy to liberate iron stores into the urine (also used in acute iron toxicity).

Treatment is generally quite successful if begun prior to irreversible changes such as cirrhosis. Phlebotomy protocols are designed to remove large amounts of iron in early stages, followed by long-term maintenance removal. Monitoring of therapy for decreasing total body iron stores can be done with serum ferritin measurements, but with very high iron stores, ferritin levels may not reflect actual removal. Thus some clinicians prefer to gauge therapeutic response by quantitation of tissue iron content in serial liver biopsies.

Hemochromatosis is so readily treated and so severe if left untreated that screening programs have been widely advocated, especially by patient support groups. Family members of hemochromatosis patients should be tested for transferrin saturation to determine whether they are also homozygous; the carrier state cannot be determined by serum iron measurements. Recently the gene responsible for hemochromatosis was discovered on chromosome 6 in the vicinity of HLA genes, which have long been known to show genetic linkage with that disease. Two mutations have been described in the hemochromatosis gene (HLA-H): a cysteine to tyrosine substitution at amino acid 282 and a histidine to aspartic acid substitution at position 63. Knowledge of this gene and its mutations now makes it possible to perform definitive diagnosis and carrier studies for hemochromatosis by DNA analysis.

TISSUE AUTOANTIBODIES

Autoimmune liver diseases are mediated predominantly by a cellular response with infiltrations of T lymphocytes. There are three primary forms of autoimmune liver diseases:

1. **autoimmune chronic active hepatitis (AICAH),** which affects hepatocytes
2. **primary biliary cirrhosis (PBC),** which destroys small intrahepatic bile ducts
3. **primary sclerosing cholangitis (PSC),** which affects large bile ducts (both intrahepatic and extrahepatic)

A major tool for diagnosing these disorders is histologic examination of liver biopsy, which reveals the specific pattern of lymphocytic infiltration corresponding to each. In addition, circulating autoantibodies directed against specific tissue antigens also characterize these disorders. To detect these autoantibodies, a patient's serum sample is placed over a tissue slice mounted on a glass slide; after incubation and washing, a second antibody of fluorescein-labeled antihuman immunoglobulin is added to detect the microscopic structures to which the patient's own antibodies bind by indirect immunofluorescent assay.

AICAH probably consists of at least four subgroups:

1. Lupoid hepatitis (type 1) is marked by antinuclear antibodies (ANA) that are also common in rheumatologic diseases. In addition, anti–smooth muscle antibody (ASMA) is a frequent finding.
2. Type 2 is negative for ANA and ASMA, but shows a unique autoantibody directed against liver-kidney microsomal (LKM) antigens.
3. Type 3 is characterized by autoantibody against "soluble liver antigen" (SLA); unfortunately this assay is not yet well standardized.
4. Type 4 shows high-titer ASMA with specificity for F-actin.

These autoantibodies can be very useful in establishing diagnosis because the biopsy findings of AICAH are largely indistinguishable from those of viral hepatitis.

PBC demonstrates elevations of serum bilirubin and alkaline phosphatase even early in the disease. In addition it is characterized by antimitochondrial antibody (AMA). The antigen for AMA has recently been shown to be the mitochondrial membrane protein pyruvate dehydrogenase. AMA is a sensitive and specific marker for PBC in high titer. PBC is also associated with other extrahepatic autoimmune disorders such as the sicca syndrome and other overlap states.

Diagnosis of PSC requires radiologic examination with contrast media to demonstrate stricture of the larger bile ducts. About 50% of PSC cases also have inflammatory bowel disease, and many of those have antineutrophil cytoplasmic antibody (ANCA) in a perinuclear pattern, which reacts with some atypical antigen other than the proteinase 3 or myeloperoxidase, the usual targets of ANCAs.

Treatment for AICAH is immunosuppression. For PBC and PSC, immunosuppression is ineffective; administration of bile salts is helpful for replacement in the digestive tract. Liver transplantation is frequently done for PBC and PSC in advanced stages.

VIRAL HEPATITIS

Many infectious agents damage the liver. In systemic infection by the herpes family viruses Epstein-Barr (EBV) and cytomegalovirus (CMV), liver damage often occurs, although the liver is not the primary target of infection with these two agents. There are several clearly defined viruses whose sole or primary target is the liver. These include **hepatitis A (HAV),** a 27-nm particle that localizes to the cytoplasm of infected hepatocytes, and **hepatitis B (HBV),** a 42-nm particle consisting of a DNA core surrounded by surface protein. Viral hepatitis not caused by HAV or HBV, and not caused by EBV, CMV, or other known agents, had been given the name **non-A, non-B (NANB) hepatitis.** Most of these cases are caused by **hepatitis C (HCV,** an RNA virus), for which diagnostic tests are now standard. **Hepatitis D virus** (HDV; delta agent; RNA genome) can only replicate when the patient is also infected with HBV. **Hepatitis E virus** (RNA genome) is enterically transmitted. Attempts are continuing to be made to isolate other significant hepatitis viruses, which epidemiologic data indicate do exist.

Hepatitis A Virus

The disease formerly called **infectious hepatitis,** or **short-incubation hepatitis,** almost always results from oral ingestion of the hepatitis A virus (HAV). Infected patients shed virus in feces for several weeks before clinical illness appears and for 1 to 2 weeks thereafter. During the prodromal and early jaundiced period, there may be a viremia at low and unpredictable levels, but chronic viremia (chronic carrier state) does not occur. Epidemic spread often occurs in outbreaks related to fecally contaminated water supplies or uncooked shellfish harvested from contaminated beds. Interpersonal spread, especially between children in institutions or in close family settings, allows widespread exposure and is undoubtedly responsible for much subclinical illness. Many of the cases of hepatitis A in the United States come from acutely infected restaurant workers who accidentally contaminate food they handle.

Laboratory Testing

Diagnosis of hepatitis A depends on clinical and laboratory observations. The patient experiences malaise, anorexia, fever, and nausea. Elevated aminotransferases and bilirubinuria are almost universal; alkaline phosphatase and serum bilirubin are often high. Definitive diagnosis rests on serologic demonstration of viral exposure (see also Chapter 15). Tests for viremia are not clinically feasible, and immunoelectron microscopy (a cumbersome and expensive technique) is the only way to demonstrate virus in the feces. Anti-HAV antibodies, however, are easily demonstrated by immunoassay. An acute illness is considered to be hepatitis A if at least one of the following factors exist:

- Anti-HAV antibody titers rise between acute and convalescent serum samples.
- Postillness serum contains antibody in a person whose preillness serum was known to lack antibody.
- There is a high level of IgM anti-HAV relative to the level of IgG antibody. IgG antibody to HAV indicates infection at some time in the past, whereas IgM antibody indicates acute (present or recent) HAV infection.

Epidemiology

Hepatitis A is usually a fairly mild, self-limited illness that rarely causes prolonged debility or persisting liver damage. Many persons who have never knowingly had hepatitis have anti-HAV IgG, indicating subclinical occurrence. Worldwide, the incidence of anti-HAV positivity increases with declining socioeconomic levels and standards of sanitation. A vaccine for HAV has been successful in preventing infection and is being considered for routine childhood immunization.

Hepatitis B Virus

The disease formerly called "serum hepatitis," or "long-incubation hepatitis," is now called **hepatitis B.** Infective HB virions circulate in the blood for prolonged periods and can at times be found in feces, urine, semen, saliva, and virtually any other body fluid. Spread can occur by blood transfusion, parenteral exposure to materials containing blood, instruments contaminated with body fluids, and by person-to-person contact, including sexual activity. Vertical transmission from mother to child may occur, producing a persistent state of viral infection in the infant. Prenatal screening of mothers now includes routine testing for hepatitis B surface antigen (HBsAg). Although mild and subclinical hepatitis B infections do occur, the disease is usually more severe than hepatitis A and may be fatal, especially in the very old or persons with other illnesses. Chronic active hepatitis may follow the acute illness. A chronic carrier state can exist in some patients with minimal or no evidence of continuing liver damage; viral material may remain in the circulation for months or years, or for life. Immunization against HBV is now standard in health care workers who are at risk of exposure and in childhood, to prevent viral propagation in a whole generation and perhaps completely eliminate HBV.

Laboratory Testing

Intense laboratory scrutiny of HBV has uncovered numerous aspects susceptible to clinical or research testing. Table 12–6 lists the more commonly measured variables. Highly sensitive tests for hepatitis B antigen (HBsAg) are widely available. Testing for HBsAg allows specific diagnosis of hepatitis B even in mild, subclinical, or persistent cases. All blood destined for transfusion must be tested and found negative for HBsAg because HBs antigenemia carries a strong, almost absolute, association with infectivity. Tests for anti-HBs are also widely available and are useful for retrospective diagnosis, for epidemiologic studies, and more recently for assessing the efficacy of vaccination against HB. Tests for anti-HBc, HBeAg, and anti-HBe are also very useful for establishing the diagnosis of HBV infection if the testing has missed periods of HBs antigenemia or when the anti-HBs titer has yet to rise (see also Chapter 15).

Quantitation of HBV DNA in serum can be useful for establishing infectivity and also acute response to interferon therapy, although long-term follow-up of patients treated that way shows disappearance of HBeAg from serum to be the most reliable predictor of recovery.

Hepatitis C Virus

This virus has recently been discovered as a major cause of parenterally acquired non-A, non-B hepatitis (especially by blood transfusion). Antibody against hepatitis C rises slowly, as late as 6 months after onset of acute infection. It is also highly prevalent in intravenous drug abusers. Diagnoses and screening of blood products for hepatitis C are performed by serum antibody testing using an ELISA followed by recombinant immunoblot assay (RIBA) for confirmation (see also Chapters 8 and 15). HCV infection has a high rate of chronicity and, with chronic HBV infection, may lead to hepatocellular carcinoma. HCV infection is now recognized as a frequent cause of cryoglobulinemia, which improves with antiviral interferon therapy.

TABLE 12–6. HEPATITIS VIRUS TERMINOLOGY

Anti-HAV	Antibody to hepatitis A virus coat protein; IgM is initial immune response indicating recent acute HAV infection; IgG indicates previous infection with HAV.
HBcAg	The core protein of hepatitis B virus that binds directly to HBV DNA. HBcAg is normally covered by the outer membrane layer of HBV. It does not circulate freely in blood, and so it is not directly measured in laboratory assays.
HBeAg	The e antigen of HBV is a degradation product of pre-HBcAg. HBeAg does not associate with the virus but instead circulates freely in the blood. HBeAg is present in active HBV infection.
HBsAg	The surface antigen of HBV is embedded in a membrane layer (derived from hepatocyte endoplasmic reticulum) that coats the HBV complex of HBV DNA and HBcAg. HBsAg is measured in serum as a marker of HBV infectivity in both acute infections and chronic carrier states. Recombinant HBsAg is the basis of the HBV vaccine.
Anti-HBc	Antibody to HBV core antigen; develops before anti-HBs in acute infection. IgM anti-HBc indicates acute infection; IgG indicates previous infection and may persist for many years.
Anti-HBe	Antibody to HBeAg that develops as acute infection resolves; may persist for months to years.
Anti-HBs	Antibody to HBsAg that develops in response to acute HBV infection and persists lifelong. This antibody is also elicited by the HBV vaccine. High concentrations of HBsAg and anti-HBs in blood can form circulating immune complexes leading to extrahepatic manifestations of HBV infection such as glomerulonephritis, arthritis, or neuropathy.
HBV DNA	The DNA of HBV is complexed with HBcAg and covered with HBsAg in a membrane layer; this structure is the infectious HB virion called the Dane particle. Measurement of HBV DNA in serum is useful for assessing infectivity and also for monitoring response to antiviral therapy (e.g., interferon) in chronic HBV infection.
Anti-HCV	Antibody to hepatitis C virus; typically determined by ELISA as a screening test using a mixture of different HCV antigens.
RIBA	Recombinant immunoblot assay: supplemental test to confirm a positive anti-HCV test by ELISA.
Anti-HDV	Antibody against hepatitis D virus (delta agent). Infection with HDV requires coinfection with HBV and should also exhibit positive HBsAg. HDV serology should be reserved for evaluating cases of fulminant hepatitis.
Anti-HEV	Antibody against hepatitis E virus. No commercial assays are now available for diagnosing HEV, which occurs almost exclusively in third-world nations.

Hepatitis D Virus

HDV is a very simple virus that cannot replicate without coinfection with HBV to supply virus synthetic functions. HDV has an inner protein complex with its RNA genome; this complex is surrounded by the same membrane coated with HBsAg that also surrounds HBV. The immune system can make antibodies against the HDV protein, but it does not reach through the membrane to inactivate HDV. However, anti-HDV antibody is used for diagnosing HDV infection, which is characterized as fulminant hepatitis B, much worse than HBV infection without HDV. Thus anti-HDV measurement should be requested only in cases of confirmed HBV infection, in which worsening clinical course cannot otherwise be explained.

Hepatitis E Virus

Hepatitis E virus (HEV) is found in third-world countries and has an enteric means of transmission. Hepatitis E is an acute infection without a chronic carrier state. Pregnant women have a 20% mortality from HEV infection, but it is much more benign in others. Cases in the United States are related to travel abroad. There is no commercially available assay for HEV, but research laboratories have set up ELISAs for anti-HEV using recombinant proteins from cloned HEV.

Hepatitis G Virus

The hepatitis G virus (HGV) has recently been discovered in patients with severe hepatitis caused by the other viruses and also in persons without clinically apparent hepatitis who have had extensive exposure to blood products, such as in dialysis. Consequently, although HGV is frequently present in patients, it is not considered a significant human pathogen, and serologic methods for its detection have not yet been commercialized.

LIVER TRANSPLANTATION

Transplantation of cadaveric livers and, more recently, segmental transplants from living donors have been used for a variety of end-stage liver disorders including autoimmune, infectious, toxic, malignant, and hereditary. Key to successful transplantation is appropriate preservation of the liver from time of harvest from the donor until placing into the recipient. The actual surgical procedure entails removing the recipient's own liver and joining the circulatory and biliary systems of the donor liver to the recipient's vessels and bile ducts. The clinical laboratories are essential to liver transplantation for providing blood transfusion products (sometimes in large numbers due to excess bleeding intraoperatively) and laboratory tests of hepatic function.

The procedure for monoethyl-glycine-xylidide (MegX) is used to predict hepatic function in the donor before removal of the liver. MegX is a metabolite of lidocaine that is made in the liver following intravenous administration of lidocaine. Serum samples are obtained at 0 and 15 minutes following injection. High levels of MegX indicate functioning liver with an adequate blood supply.

Most of the tests used to monitor liver transplants are standard procedures: AST, ALT, bilirubin fractions, ALP, GGT, and coagulation times. The immediate post-transplant period is marked by clearance of

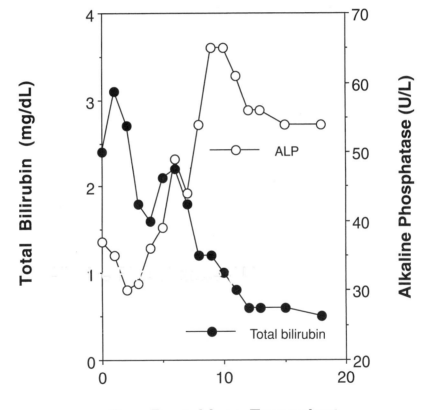

Day Post Liver Transplant

FIGURE 12–4. Serial changes in total bilirubin and alkaline phosphatase (ALP) following liver transplantation. Successful transplantation results in clearance of bilirubin. The progressive rise of ALP (remaining in the reference range) may be due to liver regeneration or to a mild degree of rejection that is expected in virtually all allogeneic transplants.

bilirubin and enzymes if the transplant is successful (Figure 12–4). Immunosuppression is standard for preventing rejection; laboratory monitoring includes blood levels of cyclosporine and lymphocyte enumeration by flow cytometry. Rejection is marked by events involving the biliary system with elevations of bilirubin, ALP, and GGT. Viral infection (especially with cytomegalovirus) is often in response to immunosuppression and is characterized by elevations of AST and ALT due to inflammation affecting hepatocytes.

SUGGESTED READINGS

Bartolo, C, et al: Differential diagnosis of hereditary hemochromatosis from other liver disorders by genetic analysis. Gene mutation of patients previously diagnosed with hemochromatosis by liver biopsy. Arch Pathol Lab Med 122:633, 1998.

Bosma, PJ, et al: The genetic basis of the reduced expression of bilirubin UDP-glucuronosyltransferase 1 in Gilbert's syndrome. N Engl J Med 333:1171, 1995.

Edwards, CQ, et al: Prevalence of hemochromatosis among 11,065 presumably healthy blood donors. N Engl J Med 318:1355, 1988.

Hoofnagle, JH, and DiBisceglie, AM: Serologic diagnosis of acute and chronic viral hepatitis. Semin Liver Dis 11:73, 1991.

Manns, MP: Autoimmune diseases of the liver. In McPherson, RA, Nakamura, RM (eds): Laboratory Immunology I, Clin Lab Med 12:3, 1992.

Markin, RS, and McPherson, RA: Laboratory support for organ transplantation: part II. Lab Med 22:319, 1991.

McPherson, RA: Laboratory diagnosis of human hepatitis viruses. J Clin Lab Anal 8:369, 1994.

McPherson, RA: Specific proteins. In Henry, JB (ed): Clinical Diagnosis and Management by Laboratory Methods, ed 19. WB Saunders, Philadelphia, 1996, p 237.

Misani, R, et al: Interferon alpha-2a therapy in cryoglobulinemia associated with hepatitis C virus. N Engl J Med 330:751, 1994.

Niederau, C, et al: Long-term follow-up of HBeAg-positive patients treated with interferon alfa for chronic hepatitis B. N Engl J Med 334:1422, 1996.

Pincus, MR, and Schaffner, JA: Assessment of liver function. In Henry JB (ed): Clinical Diagnosis and Management by Laboratory Methods, ed 19. WB Saunders, Philadelphia, 1996, p 253.

Schilsky, ML: Identification of the Wilson's disease gene: Clues for disease pathogenesis and the potential for molecular diagnosis. Hepatology 20:529, 1994.

Wulfsberg, EA, Hoffmann, DE, and Cohen, MM: α1-antitrypsin deficiency: Impact of genetic discovery on medicine and society. JAMA 271:217, 1994.

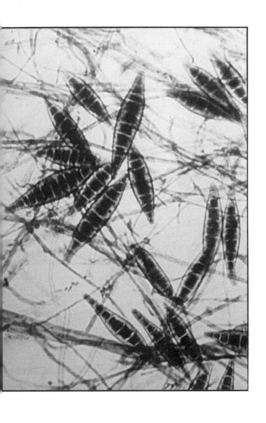

Section
Five

Clinical
Microbiology

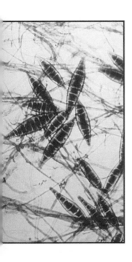

13

Principles of Clinical Microbiology

INTERACTION OF THE HOST WITH INFECTIOUS AGENTS

Microbial agents that are infectious for humans are present just about everywhere in the human environment, including soil, water, foods, and other animals. Perhaps the most significant reservoir, however, is human—both other humans' and the individual's flora. In fact, many agents that cause infection are members of the host's indigenous flora. These microorganisms ordinarily reside harmlessly in the host in a mutualistic or symbiotic relationship. However, host circumstances can arise that lead to the relationship becoming parasitic, and the same microorganisms cause morbidity and/or mortality in the host.

ENTRY OF INFECTIOUS AGENTS INTO THE HOST

Whether pathogenic microorganisms are derived from an indigenous or exogenous source, the initial step of infection is evasion of the barrier defense mechanisms of the host. **Exogenous infectious agents** enter the host through several portals, including the respiratory tract, the gastrointestinal tract, the genitourinary tract, or via breaks in the skin following trauma. **Endogenous infectious agents,** as they transition from harmless to harmful microorganisms, are already present in the host and must cope with deeper layers of the host defense system, which will be discussed later in this chapter.

Via the Respiratory Tract

Entrance of exogenous infectious agents via the respiratory tract occurs by either *inhalation* or *direct contact.* Inhaled agents are usually found within tiny fluid droplets—for example, respiratory secretion droplets produced during coughing or sneezing (e.g., influenza virus) or water droplets produced by aerosolizing machinery (e.g., *Legionella* spp). Infectious agents that enter the respiratory tract by direct contact are present in respiratory secretions found on environmental surfaces. They are usually introduced into the host's mouth, nose, or eyes via the fingers (e.g., respiratory syncytial virus).

Having entered the respiratory tract, infectious agents must cope with *secretory antibodies of the IgA class* and the trapping effect of *mucus.* Microorganism-laden mucus is ultimately swept out of the respiratory system by the **ciliated epithelial cells** lining the respiratory tract. Infectious agents also must confront microorganisms already colonizing the upper respiratory tract. Such microorganisms may produce *toxins* and/or **bacteriocins** that are damaging to the new agent. Normal microflora may already be occupying adherence sites necessary for the new agent to initiate infection. In the lower respiratory tract, infectious agents may activate the host's *cellular immune system,* resulting in an inflammatory response and increased phagocytic activity by **macrophages** and **neutrophils.** Because of the host defense and microbial factors described above, only a small fraction of infectious agents that gain entrance to the respiratory tract cause infection.

Via the Gastrointestinal Tract

Most infectious agents enter the gastrointestinal tract via *ingestion,* and assuming they survive exposure to gastric acidity, they eventually reach the more hospitable environments of the small and large intestines. Within the intestines, however, additional factors may come into play. *Competition from endogenous microflora* for adherence sites may be stiff, and infectious agents unsuccessful in finding a suitable niche are eventually eliminated from the gastrointestinal tract with the solid waste. *Secretory IgA, microbial toxins, bacteriocins* and the host's *cellular immune system* may also interfere with establishment of infection within the gastrointestinal tract (see previous section).

Infectious agents may also enter the gastrointestinal tract by *direct contact.* Anal sexual intercourse can be an efficient means of transmitting certain gastrointestinal tract pathogens (e.g., intestinal parasites, human immunodeficiency virus, and hepatitis B virus).

Via the Genitourinary Tract

The infectious agents that cause urinary tract infection and certain sexually transmitted diseases usually enter the host via the *genitourinary tract.* Most urinary tract pathogens gain access to the bladder via the urethra and typically originate from colonized periurethral sites. Access of agents to the genital tract follows direct contact with infectious material (e.g., semen, vaginal/cervical secretions, chancre fluid). Once in the genitourinary tract, infectious agents must evade the host's *humoral and cellular immune system.* In the vagina, the *acidic environment* established by the fermentative products of lactobacilli and other saprophytic anaerobes is not conducive to survival of some infectious agents.

Via Penetration Through the Skin

Infectious organisms that enter the host through the skin do so in a variety of manners. Some (e.g., *Plasmodium* spp, *Borrelia* spp, *Rickettsia* spp) require the aid of **arthropod vectors** (e.g., mosquitoes, ticks). Others (e.g., *Necator americanus, Ancylostoma duodenale,* and *Schistosoma* spp) depend upon larvae to mechanically bore through the skin and initiate infection. Most commonly, exogenous and endogenous agents pass through the skin during or soon after trauma—before the host can repair skin damage.

The most effective host defense mechanism in preventing or containing post-traumatic wound infection is the *inflammatory response,* resulting in **phagocytosis** of infectious agents and, if necessary, *walling off the infection site.* **Plasma proteins,** in the form of opsonizing **humoral antibodies, fibronectin,** and **complement,** play an important host defense role in the latter case.

HOST RESPONSE TO THE PRESENCE OF INFECTIOUS AGENTS

Once the presence of an infectious agent has been detected, additional mechanisms of the host defense system become active. More detailed information concerning these mechanisms may be found in Chapter 7.

Cellular Immune Response

The *inflammatory response* is initiated by detection and processing of infectious agents by *macrophages.* The macrophages are stimulated, triggering their migratory and phagocytic activities. The stimulated macrophages interact with and activate antigen-specific **T lymphocytes.** Signals (**lymphokines**) are released that attract phagocytic cells (initially neutrophils and later monocytes) to the infection site. *Phagocytosis* and killing of infectious agents ensue. In some situations, monocytes convert to a more active macrophage state. Opsonizing *humoral antibodies, fibronectin,* and *complement* may eventually participate in the immune response to enhance phagocytosis and killing.

Humoral Immune Response

Activated macrophages also present processed infectious agent antigens to specific **memory B lymphocytes** that, in the presence of **helper T lymphocytes,** transform to antibody-producing *plasma cells.* Plasma cells multiply and produce *antibodies* directed against specific antigens. Because many different infectious agent antigens may be recognized as foreign, the complete antibody response is polyclonal in nature, although each plasma cell produces individual (monoclonal) antibodies.

Decavalent, less avid, **immunoglobulin class M (IgM)** antibodies are the first to be produced by plasma cells. Eventually, plasma cells discontinue IgM production and switch to manufacturing more avid, divalent **immunoglobulin class G (IgG)** antibodies.

INFECTIOUS AGENT VIRULENCE FACTORS

Not all microorganisms with pathogenic properties that enter the host cause infection. Many potentially pathogenic microorganisms merely pass through the host or are rapidly killed by host defense mechanisms. Other pathogenic microorganisms transiently colonize the host but inflict no damage. The presence of colonizing saprophytic microorganisms is usually beneficial to the host in that potentially pathogenic microorganisms are intolerant of the microbial environment or unable to locate adherence sites. Furthermore, some colonizing gastrointestinal tract microorganisms produce materials essential for human nutrition (e.g., vitamin K), which pass into the bloodstream from the gut. Three of the factors that distinguish pathogenic from nonpathogenic microorganisms are discussed below.

Adherence Factors

Before a microorganism can cause infection at a particular site, mechanisms for recognizing and adhering to host cells are generally necessary. **Adherence factors** enable microorganisms to attach to specific cells within the host. Both pathogenic and nonpathogenic microorganisms found in humans produce adherence factors. What separates pathogenic and nonpathogenic microorganisms from one another are the activities that commence after adherence and the reaction of the host to those activities.

Toxin Production

Quite a few infectious agents, because of their routine metabolism, produce byproducts that are toxic to the host. The *toxins* may be produced at the site of infection (e.g., *Corynebacterium diphtheriae, Clostridium tetani, Vibrio cholerae*) or produced outside the host and later ingested (e.g., *Clostridium botulinum, Staphylococcus aureus, Bacillus cereus*).

The mechanisms of toxin action are quite varied (e.g., inhibition of host cell protein synthesis by *C. diphtheriae* toxin and interference with acetylcholine release by *C. botulinum* toxin). Some toxins act locally at the site of toxin production (e.g., toxin A of *Clostridium difficile*), and others act systemically (e.g., tetanus toxin of *Clostridium tetani*).

Resistance to Host Killing

Microorganisms that reach body sites that are ordinarily free of microorganisms generally are eradicated rapidly by various host defense mechanisms. The most effective of these mechanisms are *phagocytosis* and killing by *monocytes, macrophages,* and *neutrophils.*

Some infectious agents manufacture products that enable organisms to *inhibit phagocytosis* (e.g., *Cryptococcus neoformans*) or *prevent killing* (e.g., *Salmonella typhi*). Quite a few microorganisms produce an extracellular polysaccharide *capsule* that prevents phagocyte recognition of surface antigen markers and thus inhibits phagocytosis. The manner in which other microorganisms resist the killing effects of lysosomal enzymes and other factors after phagocytosis has occurred is not well understood, but clearly is germane to their virulence.

LABORATORY DETECTION OF INFECTIOUS AGENTS IN THE HOST

NONSPECIFIC EVIDENCE OF INFECTION

Very often, clinical suspicion of infection is first raised when the patient complains of constitutional symptoms, such as fever, chills, headache, or myalgia. If it is not possible to localize the site of infection from the patient's history and physical examination, the next step usually is to begin a laboratory test workup, initially to confirm the suspicion of infection and then to identify the specific cause of infection. Laboratory tests that provide only nonspecific evidence of infection will be discussed briefly, since they frequently are not performed in the microbiology area of the laboratory. Laboratory tests that confirm the existence of infection and/or identify the etiologic agent will be the subject for most of the remainder of this chapter.

Leukocyte Count and Differential

The existence of an *elevated leukocyte count* in the peripheral circulation or in body fluids is evidence of infection. A differential count of the leukocytes that reveals a *"shift to the left"* (i.e., abnormally high percentages of segmented neutrophils and band cells) is suggestive of bacterial infection. Elevated leukocyte counts not displaying a "shift to the left" are suggestive of viral infection (see Chapter 2).

Sedimentation Rate

One of several causes of an elevated sedimentation rate is acute inflammation. If chronic infection is on the list of possible diagnoses for a patient, an elevated sedimentation rate suggests that further workup of an infectious etiology is warranted. However, the test is not very specific; there are many causes of elevated sedimentation rates, and the clinician is cautioned not to overinterpret such test results (see Chapter 2).

C-Reactive Protein

C-reactive protein is an acute phase reactant whose concentration increases in serum or body fluids during local or systemic infection. However, many conditions besides infection also result in elevated C-reactive protein levels, and such test results should also be interpreted with caution.

Interleukins and Tumor Necrosis Factor

Cytokines are a group of low-molecular-weight proteins that regulate the amplitude and duration of the immune and inflammatory responses. Within the group are proteins known as **lymphokines, monokines, interleukins,** and **interferons,** which are produced by a variety of cells within the human body. **Interleukin-6 (IL-6),** in particular, is a particularly important mediator of the inflammatory response. It is produced in response to release of **interleukin 1** and **tumor necrosis factor** and (1) serves as a signal for *T-cell activation,* (2) stimulates *B-cell production of antibodies,* and (3) triggers *differentiation of cytotoxic T-cells.* IL-6 is also the major inducer of C-reactive protein synthesis by the liver. Several investigators have reported the presence of IL-6 in serum and CSF to be a more sensitive marker of acute infection than C-reactive protein. Similar findings have been reported by others regarding detection of interleukin-1, interleukin-8, and tumor necrosis factor in serum and CSF.

SPECIMEN COLLECTION AND TRANSPORT

The success of the microbiology laboratory in identifying the cause of infection is critically dependent upon proper collection and transport of patient specimens to the laboratory. First and foremost, the site of specimen collection must be chosen carefully to afford the greatest yield of infecting organisms, toxins, or antibodies generated by the host. The collection of the specimen itself must be conducted in a manner that minimizes contamination with endogenous host flora. Delivery of specimens to the laboratory must be performed under conditions that maintain the viability of infectious agents or the integrity of their products. The time in transit to the laboratory must be short enough to limit overgrowth by contaminating flora. Many laboratories provide reference material for hospital staff or instructions in the laboratory information system that outline specimen requirements and special conditions for specimen transport.

Blood

The importance of *aseptic technique* in the collection of blood cultures cannot be overemphasized. A single contaminating microorganism from the patient's or phlebotomist's skin can confuse, and possibly jeopardize, the correct interpretation of a blood culture result. Contaminated blood cultures lead to unnecessary expenditure of limited financial and personnel resources. The venipuncture site, as well as the rubber stoppers on the collection tubes or bottles, should be disinfected with a rapidly acting agent such as tincture of iodine or povidone iodine. The blood culture contamination rate should be less than 4% in children and 2% in adults. Many laboratories furnish broth-containing bottles for blood cultures. Venting or introduction of oxygen into bottles intended for aerobic incubation should be performed solely by laboratory personnel. Other blood culture collection containers in current use include tubes containing sodium polyanethole sulfonate (SPS) anticoagulant, or tubes containing a saponin-based lysis reagent plus SPS. When these tubes are used, laboratory personnel are responsible for inoculation of blood specimens onto agar and/or into broth culture media. Special blood culture measures for detection of anaerobic bacteria; fungi, and acid-fast bacilli are generally offered by laboratories as well.

Current recommendations call for collection of 20 to 30 mL of blood from adults and 1 to 5 mL of blood from children per blood culture. Less blood than these amounts jeopardizes the sensitivity of culture. A decreasing incidence of anaerobic bacteremia and an increasing incidence of fungemia during the past 15 years have prompted many laboratories to discontinue routine inoculation of anaerobic blood cultures and recommend allocation of that blood to aerobic or fungal blood cultures. Another laboratory practice gaining in use is requiring two blood cultures collected from separate venipuncture sites, in order to facilitate understanding of the significance of positive results. Whichever inoculation protocol is used, the consensus is that no more than three blood cultures per 24-hour period are necessary to identify uncomplicated bacteremia.

Body Fluids

Cerebrospinal fluid, synovial fluid, pleural fluid, peritoneal fluid, pericardial fluid, and fluids from other closed spaces should be collected in sterile, leak-proof containers and delivered promptly to the laboratory. The aseptic technique recommended above for collection of blood samples also applies to collection of body fluids.

Urine

The ideal time to obtain urine for laboratory workup of infection is in the morning, prior or simultaneous to the day's first voiding. At this time infecting microorganisms are present in their highest numbers, and discrimination between clinically significant and insignificant findings is easiest. *"Clean catch," catheterized,* or *suprapubically aspirated* specimens may be collected. *"Bagged"* specimens from young children should only be used as a last resort. "Clean catch" or catheterized specimens from females and uncircumcised males require disinfection of the periurethral area prior to collection. The "clean catch" specimen should be collected in midstream to avoid contamination by transient periurethral flora. Despite the utmost of precautions, "clean catch" and catheterized specimens inevitably are contaminated with small numbers of microorganisms, and care must be taken during transport to the laboratory to prevent excessive multiplication of contaminants. Storage of specimens at 4°C after collection and during transport is effective. Commercially available urine preservative tubes containing boric acid stabilize colony counts of pathogens and contaminants alike and are useful when long delays at room temperature are likely. Agar dipslide culture devices that are inoculated immediately after specimen collection can also be helpful in minimizing the problems associated with delayed specimen transport. Suprapubically aspirated urine, in effect, is a body fluid and should be handled in the manner described above.

Stool

Some pathogens that cause gastrointestinal tract infection are harmed by changes that occur in stool after defecation. One example is the drop in stool pH that occurs as fermentative waste products resulting from anaerobic microbial metabolism accumulate. To reduce the loss of pathogen viability (a problem especially relevant for *Shigella*), transport medium (e.g., buffered glycerolized saline) should be used if specimens cannot be cultured immediately. Unfortunately, *Campylobacter* spp do not survive well in buffered glycerolized saline; thus Cary-Blair transport medium is recommended for this organism. Stool for ova and parasite examination should be delivered to the laboratory promptly after collection. If this is not possible, specimens should be maintained at refrigerator temperature or placed in a formalin-based or polyvinyl alcohol-based (PVA) preservative. Stool for microbial toxin studies (e.g., those produced by *Clostridium difficile, C. botulinum,* or *Escherichia coli*) should be brought to the laboratory immediately or frozen to prevent loss of heat-labile activity.

Respiratory Tract Secretions

The diagnosis of lower respiratory tract infection is sometimes dependent upon examination of *sputum,* or in children too young to produce sputum, examination of **endotracheal** or **gastric aspirates.** These specimens are unavoidably contaminated with upper respiratory tract microflora, which can seriously hamper clinicians in determining the etiology of infection. Furthermore, what is labeled as sputum all too often is merely saliva. If a patient is unable to expectorate genuine sputum from the lower respiratory tract, an alternative means of specimen collection should be considered. Other options include techniques such as aspiration during bronchoscopy **(bronchoalveolar lavage),** using a suction apparatus that is protected from upper respiratory flora contamination during insertion, **percutaneous needle aspiration** of an abscess or empyema cavity, or **open lung biopsy.** Gastric aspirates are often relied on as an alternative procedure for diagnosis of pulmonary tuberculosis in children. The purpose here is to detect and recover mycobacteria in swallowed lower respiratory tract secretions. In any event, respiratory tract specimens, especially those contaminated with upper respiratory organisms, should be transported to the laboratory promptly or refrigerated until transport is possible.

Genital Tract Specimens

The genital tracts of humans harbor a wide assortment of nonpathogenic microorganisms. To obtain the highest diagnostic yield, specimens should be collected in a manner that maximizes the number of pathogens and minimizes the quantity of endogenous microorganisms. Careful selection of the sampling site is important. In women with gonococcal or chlamydial cervicitis, for example, a swab of the vaginal vault or collection of vaginal discharge is inferior to direct sampling of the endocervical canal. In some infections, simultaneous testing of specimens from the urethra and rectum enhances the likelihood of correct diagnosis.

Certain sexually transmitted pathogens are killed by abrupt changes in their environment. The temperature, atmosphere, and chemical characteristics of the surroundings all affect the viability of *Neisseria gonorrhoeae.* If culture is being used for detection, many laboratories furnish physicians with selective agar media warmed to ambient temperature for inoculation immediately after specimen collection. Provision can even be made for transport of such cultures in an atmosphere enriched for carbon dioxide, in case immediate delivery to the laboratory is not possible. The viability of *Chlamydia trachomatis* is maintained by placing specimens in a buffered transport medium such as sucrose phosphate broth.

Tissue/Biopsy Material

Biopsy is strongly recommended for establishing the etiology of tissue or bone infection. A single pea-sized specimen delivered to the laboratory in a timely fashion can be homogenized in sterile saline or broth and used to prepare smears and inoculate cultures for aerobic and anaerobic bacteria, acid-fast bacteria, and fungi. The primary concerns during transport are drying of the specimen, and, if anaerobic infection is suspected, extended exposure of the specimen to oxygen. Placement of the specimen in a small quantity of sterile, nonbacteriostatic saline and delivery to the laboratory in an appropriate anaerobic transport device can allay these concerns.

Swab Specimens

Culture yields from swab specimens are usually lower than those achieved by culture of the corresponding aspirate, exudate, pus, body fluid, or tissue biopsy specimen. The yield is always lower when a single swab is submitted for multiple cultures. In fact, most microbiology laboratories insist that separate swabs be submitted when multiple cultures of the same specimen site are requested. Swabs should be reserved for collection of specimens that cannot be better obtained by other means.

Their convenience and simplicity of use have misled too many practitioners to rely upon them routinely for collection of specimens.

Sterile rayon, dacron, cotton, and calcium alginate swabs are commercially available. Because cotton is a natural fiber containing oils that may be toxic to some microorganisms, synthetic fiber swabs are generally preferred for specimen collection. For the same reason, swabs with plastic shafts are superior to swabs with wooden shafts. Liquid or semisolid transport medium often is included in the swab container and is intended to maintain the viability of microorganisms during transport. Individuals collecting specimens must make certain that swabs are moistened or immersed in transport media.

Specimens for Anaerobic Culture

Oxygen is a metabolic poison for obligate anaerobes, resulting in intracellular accumulation of toxic metabolites. Detection of these organisms by culture depends on their survival during the processes of collection, inoculation, and incubation. Anaerobic specimen transport devices that include mechanisms to chemically eliminate oxygen from specimens and specimen environments are available. Most microbiology laboratories will not accept specimens for anaerobic culture unless steps have been taken to promote the survival of anaerobes.

Obligate anaerobes constitute the majority of the resident flora of the respiratory tract, the gastrointestinal tract, and the female genital tract. Even human skin itself is heavily colonized with anaerobes. Requests for anaerobic cultures on specimens collected from sites colonized with anaerobic organisms are inappropriate and will not be accepted by most microbiology laboratories. The laboratory work required is tedious, time consuming, and expensive because anaerobic infections are frequently polymicrobial in nature and often caused by mixtures of obligately aerobic, facultatively anaerobic, and obligately anaerobic microorganisms. It is in the best interests of patients, caregivers, and the laboratory for physicians to request anaerobic cultures only on appropriately collected and transported specimens from patients likely to have anaerobic infection.

DIRECT VISUALIZATION OF INFECTIOUS AGENTS

Despite the much-ballyhooed recent advances in immunodiagnostic and nucleic acid probe-based assays for infectious agents, the light microscope still occupies the central role in early diagnosis of infectious diseases. Microscopic examination of specimens provides the quickest direct evidence of infection and influences decision-making by physicians during the initial stages of patient management. The remainder of this section will be concerned with the variety of microscopic analyses available from the microbiology laboratory.

Wet Mount Preparation

Cover-slipped wet mounts of freshly collected specimens are primarily used for detection of parasitic agents. Heavy infestations of intestinal parasites can be identified by examining small portions of stool mixed with saline or, in the case of watery specimens, direct examination of the specimens themselves. Similarly, genital tract trichomoniasis is often diagnosed by seeing motile trophozoites in saline suspensions of vaginal and urethral discharges. The main advantages of wet mounts are the rapidity with which results are available, the ease of detection of motile, live organisms, and the low cost of testing.

Gram Stain

Examination of **Gram-stained smears** is still the most frequently ordered microscopic procedure in the clinical microbiology laboratory. The Gram stain procedure, first described more than a century ago, has withstood the test of time. The reasons for its success are that stained microorganisms are more easily recognized than unstained microorganisms, and bacteria are differentially stained based on structural differences of their cell walls. Purple-stained **gram-positive bacteria** possess thick cell walls, and red-stained **gram-negative bacteria** possess relatively thin cell walls bounded by a lipopolysaccharide-containing outer membrane. More important, knowledge of a bacterium's Gram reaction aids physicians in selecting suitable empirical antimicrobial therapy because many antimicrobial agents have predictable activity against gram-positive and gram-negative bacteria.

The *Gram stain procedure* is easily performed (Table 13–1). Thin smears

TABLE 13-1. THE GRAM STAIN PROCEDURE

1. Prepare a thin smear, air-dry, and fix with gentle heat or methanol.
2. Flood the smear with crystal (Gentian) violet for 10 seconds. Rinse with tap water.
3. Flood the smear with Gram's iodine for 10 seconds. Rinse with tap water.
4. Decolorize the smear with ethanol, acetone, or an ethanol and acetone mixture until no more crystal violet leaches from the smear (1 to 5 seconds). Rinse with tap water.
5. Flood the smear with safranin for 10 seconds. Rinse with tap water. Gently blot-dry or air-dry the smear.

of specimens are prepared, air-dried, and fixed with gentle heat or methanol. Smears are first stained with crystal violet; treated with Gram's iodine; decolorized with ethanol, acetone, or an ethanol/acetone mixture; and finally counterstained with safranin (a red dye). The crucial step in the procedure is the **decolorization step,** in which over- or under-decolorization is possible. It is essential to know the composition of the decolorizing agent because ethanol is a much slower decolorizer than acetone. A 1:1 ratio of ethanol and acetone yields a moderate rate of decolorization. Simultaneous staining of **quality control smears** containing both gram-positive and gram-negative bacteria is recommended to ensure that proper staining technique is being followed. One other problem to avoid is excessive heat fixation, which may disrupt the structural integrity of bacterial and inflammatory cell morphology. Use of a temperature-controlled slide warmer or use of methanol fixation eliminates this problem.

Clinician interpretation of Gram stain reports can have a major bearing on patient care. Reports should be clear, concise, and informative. They should note the presence and quantity of microorganisms, inflammatory cells, and epithelial cells. Separation of inflammatory cells into mononuclear and polymorphonuclear categories is possible, but furnishing an accurate cellular differential analysis is not. Differential analysis should be left to individuals examining **Wright-** or **Giemsa-stained smears.**

Observation of more than one microorganism per 960–1000X oil immersion field suggests the presence of at least 100,000 colony-forming units per mL (cfu/mL) of specimen—a relationship that is especially useful when examining smears of urine. Many laboratories routinely stain sputa to determine which contain material from the lower respiratory tract and which are primarily saliva. If epithelial cells outnumber inflammatory cells in the smear, then the specimen is deemed inadequate for laboratory analysis. These laboratories utilize acceptance criteria for culture of sputa based upon the inflammatory cell/epithelial cell ratio. Representative Gram-stained smears are shown in Color Plates 54 to 61.

Acridine Orange Stain

One of the shortcomings of the Gram stain technique is the minimal contrast between gram-negative microorganisms and gram-negative cellular debris and proteinaceous strands present in some specimens. The **acridine orange** staining method does not suffer from this problem: all microorganisms stand out in sharp contrast to the background. Acridine orange dye is taken up by microorganisms and intact cells, with the dye molecules intercalating within the double helix of DNA. Upon irradiation with ultraviolet light, the dye emits bright orange fluorescence that is easily visible under the microscope at 100× to 500× magnification.

Because of the stronger contrast between stained microorganisms and background material, the acridine orange stain is a more sensitive technique than the Gram stain. Five- to ten-fold fewer organisms per mL of specimen are detectable in acridine orange–stained smears. Another advantage of the acridine orange stain is that positive smears may be restained with Gram stain reagents. In this way, clinicians can be informed of the Gram reactions of bacteria detected.

Acid-Fast Stain

Mycobacterium spp, *Nocardia* spp, *Legionella micdadei,* and the oocysts of *Cryptosporidium* and *Isospora* are detectable with **acid-fast** staining reagents (Color Plates 62 and 63). Several acid-fast staining methods are used in laboratories today. All are based on the same principle, with important differences in the details of their staining protocols. In general, all of the methods call for preparing a thin smear of the specimen, allowing it to air-dry, and following that with heat fixation. The smear is flooded with a penetrative primary stain, decolorized with a strong mineral acid–containing reagent, and counterstained with a contrasting second stain. The essential differences between the staining methods are described below.

Ziehl-Neelsen Stain

The oldest of the acid-fast staining procedures, the **Ziehl-Neelsen stain** requires that the primary carbol-fuchsin stain be heated to the point of steaming during staining. The decolorizer is a mixture of concentrated hydrochloric acid and 95% alcohol, and the counterstain is usually methylene blue.

Kinyoun Stain

The **Kinyoun stain** differs from the Ziehl-Neelsen in that no heating of the primary stain is necessary. A more concentrated carbol-fuchsin reagent enables penetration of the dye and eliminates the need for heat. The Kinyoun method has replaced the Ziehl-Neelsen method in many laboratories because of the easier staining protocol.

Fluorochrome Stain

The **fluorochrome stain** requires a microscope equipped either for ultraviolet illumination or quartz-halogen illumination. In either case, appropriate excitation and barrier filters must be in the light path to promote the observation of fluorescence. The fluorochrome staining method is not a fluorescent antibody procedure. The primary stain is a mixture of auramine O and rhodamine B dyes in a carbol-glycerol base. The hydrochloric acid/ethanol decolorizer is not as strong as in the Ziehl-Neelsen and Kinyoun procedures, and the counterstain is a potassium permanganate solution that quenches background fluorescence. The advantage of the fluorochrome stain over the other stains is its higher sensitivity. Fewer acid-fast microorganisms need to be present to yield a positive result because of the striking contrast between acid-fast organisms and the background. The contrast is so great that smears may be scanned at lower magnifications, permitting examination of wider expanses of specimen in the same time. The fluorochrome and other similar fluorescent acid-fast stains are the methods of choice for screening smears for mycobacteria.

Modified Acid-fast Stain

Procedures using **modified acid-fast stain** have been developed for detection of *Nocardia, Legionella micdadei,* and the oocysts of *Cryptosporidium* and *Isospora.* These organisms are partially acid-fast and may be decolorized when stained by Ziehl-Neelsen, Kinyoun, or fluorochrome methods. In the modified procedures, a gentler decolorizer, such as aqueous 2% sulfuric acid, is used. Otherwise, the staining method and examination procedure are similar to those described above.

Potassium Hydroxide Preparation

When present in high numbers, most fungi are detected without difficulty in Gram-stained smears of clinical specimens. However, specimens like hair, skin, and nail scrapings from patients with dermatophyte fungal infections are not suitable for Gram staining. These specimens can be "clarified" by using 10 or 20% **potassium hydroxide (KOH)**, without affecting fungal morphology. The specimen is placed in a drop of KOH on a microscope slide, coverslipped, and after 5 minutes, examined microscopically under low light conditions. Gentle heating of the preparation or extended KOH treatment allows more thorough "clarification" of difficult specimens. Care must be taken during examination of KOH-treated skin scrapings to avoid confusing fungal elements with cellular division planes (Color Plate 64). Some mycologists add dyes like calcofluor white (see next section) or indelible ink to KOH to sharpen the contrast between fungal elements and background material.

Calcofluor White Stain

Laundry brighteners like calcofluor white M2R and Tinopal CBS-X are added to detergents by manufacturers to increase the "whiteness" of clothing. The added "whiteness" is due to dye fluorescence emitted when clothing is exposed to the ultraviolet light in sunlight and artificial light. Fortuitously, these dyes also bind well to the polysaccharides in fungal cell walls. Specimen smears can be stained with one of these dyes for 1 minute and examined microscopically under ultraviolet illumination. Fungi exhibit a bright, bluish-white fluorescence that stands out vividly against an unstained background. As mentioned above, these dyes may be added to 10 to 20% KOH to enhance detection of fungal elements in hair, skin, and nail specimens.

A similar fluorescent dye known as **Uvitex 2B** has been described recently for staining the chitinous inner layer of microsporidial spores in the stool of HIV-1 infected patients. The organisms exhibit a bright white fluorescence against a dark background. Calcofluor white has also been tried for visualizing microsporidia in stool but suffers from a higher degree of background fluorescence.

India Ink Preparation

The **India ink preparation** is a negative staining technique for rapid, presumptive identification of *Cryptococcus neoformans* in body fluid specimens. A tiny drop of India ink is placed next to a drop of the specimen on a microscope slide. A coverslip is placed over both drops, causing the drops to mingle. In a positive specimen, the tiny carbon particles of India ink are unable to penetrate the thick polysaccharide capsule of *C. neoformans,* resulting in the formation of a halo around the organism (Color Plate 65). Because of the clinical ramification of a positive result, extreme care must be taken to differentiate encapsulated yeast cells from inflammatory cells, which may be surrounded by the semblance of a thin capsule. It is advisable to first observe encapsulated budding yeast cells in the wet mount before deciding that a test is positive.

As is the case with all of the other microscopic wet mount procedures, the India ink preparation is likely to be negative when there are fewer than 10,000 *C. neoformans* per mL of specimen. A much more sensitive test, and almost as rapid, is the **latex particle agglutination** assay for cryptococcal antigen. This test will be discussed later in this chapter.

Toluidine Blue O Stain

The clinical importance of identifying *Pneumocystis carinii* pulmonary infection in patients with acquired immunodeficiency syndrome (AIDS) has led many microbiology laboratories to begin testing for this pathogen. Historically, detection of *P. carinii* has been the responsibility of the pathology laboratory, using Giemsa, Wright, Gram-Weigert, or methenamine silver nitrate staining methods. The **toluidine blue O stain** is simpler to perform and easier to read than the above methods, and results are available in approximately 1 hour (Color Plate 66).

The organism burden in untreated, infected AIDS patients is generally very high. Bronchoalveolar lavage specimens are easily obtained and quite adequate for testing. However, in treated AIDS patients or in untreated non-AIDS patients, fewer organisms may be present and a toluidine blue O-negative specimen may require confirmation by examining lung biopsy material.

Trichrome Stain

Laboratory confirmation of many intestinal protozoan infections requires microscopic examination of stool. Wet mounts of concentrated or unconcentrated specimens can be helpful in detecting the presence of protozoa. However, they may not provide enough morphologic detail to enable specific identification of the agent. Because many intestinal protozoa found in specimens from humans are harmless, it is mandatory that laboratories be able to differentiate pathogens from nonpathogens. The three dyes in the **Wheatley trichrome stain** (chromotrope 2R, light-green SF, and fast-green FCF) differentially stain the nuclear and cytoplasmic material of protozoa, highlighting the features essential for accurate identification (Color Plates 67 and 68). The **iron-hematoxylin stain** is similar in principle and useful for staining intestinal protozoa. Neither stain is of value for detection or identification of *Cryptosporidium, Isospora,* and intestinal helminths.

The **modified trichrome stain** has been used successfully for recognition of microsporidia in stool specimens from HIV-1 infected patients. Although the method is laborious and time consuming, it is better able than the Giemsa stain (discussed next) to differentiate between the small (1–3 μ) microsporidial spores and the background.

Giemsa Stain

Microscopic examination of Giemsa-stained blood smears is the method of choice for identifying patients with blood-borne parasitic infections, including malaria, babesiosis, trypanosomiasis, and filariasis. Examination of Wright-stained smears may be substituted in certain situations. Both thick and thin smears from fresh (preferred) or EDTA-anticoagulated blood should be prepared (Table 13–2). Prior to staining, the thick smear is not fixed and the thin smear is fixed with methanol. The thick smear should be stained with Giemsa reagents, since Wright stain reagents contain an alcohol fixative that will prevent erythrocyte lysis. Examination of the thick smear (Color Plate 69, *left*) enables the microscopist to survey a larger volume of blood because all of the piled-on erythrocytes in the dried blood drop are lysed during staining. In effect, the thick smear examination serves as a screen for the presence of infection. Any blood parasites present are left intact on the surface of the slide, but with a morphology that can be difficult to identify at the species level. Examination of the thin smear (Color Plate 69, *right*) yields

---

TABLE 13–2. METHOD FOR PREPARATION OF THICK AND THIN BLOOD SMEARS

---

1. Place one drop of blood at the end of a glass microscope slide and spread to form a circle 1.5 cm in diameter.
2. Place the end of a second glass slide along the edge of the drop nearest the center of the slide, so that a linear pool of blood forms along the end of the second slide. Tilt the second slide to form a 30 to 45° angle with the first slide, and push the second slide along the length of the first slide, leaving a broad smear of blood one erythrocyte thick. The distal end of the smear should display a "feathered edge."
3. Dry the thick smear for at least 1 hour (preferably overnight) before staining.
4. Do not fix the thick smear. The thin smear is fixed with methanol for 1 minute.

---

improved parasitic and erythrocyte morphology, features that are often required for precise identification of blood parasites. The thin smear may be stained with Giemsa (preferred) or Wright staining reagents.

IMMUNOASSAYS FOR DETECTION OF MICROBIAL ANTIGENS

Recent decades have witnessed the development of numerous immunoassays for direct detection of microbial antigens in patient specimens. The primary attraction of these immunoassays is the rapidity of results when compared to classic culture methods. For community-acquired infections like streptococcal pharyngitis and sexually transmitted diseases, patients may be diagnosed and treated during the same visit to a health care facility. A public health advantage conferred by rapid diagnosis is the assurance that noncompliant patients will be appropriately treated, assuming that single-dose antimicrobial therapy is available. Prompt contact tracing and administration of antimicrobial prophylaxis may also be initiated in the case of sexually transmitted infections.

There also are disadvantages to antigen detection testing:

- The sensitivity and/or specificity of these assays is generally inferior to those of the traditional diagnostic methods (e.g., direct visualization and culture). If the difference in sensitivity or specificity is clinically significant, negative or positive immunoassay results require confirmation.
- Antigen detection assays tend to be more expensive to perform than conventional diagnostic tests. The expense of testing is an important consideration in the current era of health care cost containment, especially if a large percentage of specimens screened for antigen need confirmatory testing.

- Antigen detection assays provide no direct information concerning the antimicrobial susceptibility of agents detected. If the detected organism's antimicrobial susceptibility is not predictable, specimens still need to be cultured and isolates tested to obtain these results.

An even larger concern over readily obtainable antigen detection results is the temptation to test patients who would not have been tested if only conventional methods were available. Rates of testing in the laboratory with rapid assays or in the clinic with point-of-care test devices have increased tremendously in recent years. These rates will continue their upward trend as assays become even easier and faster to perform. Aside from the questionable medical necessity of such practices, another problem is the decline in predictive value of positive results. If testing is carried to an extreme, the majority of positive test results could become falsely positive. Consequently, all positive results would require confirmation by more specific methods—at the cost of considerable delay and additional expense.

Most antigen detection in laboratories today is performed by direct or indirect immunofluorescence, particle agglutination, color-endpoint enzyme immunoassays (EIAs), immunochromatography, and optical immunoassay.

Immunofluorescence

There are two categories of immunofluorescence-based antigen detection assays performed in the microbiology laboratory. **Direct immunofluorescence assay (DFA),** in which antigen and antibody conjugated with a fluorescent dye react, is used exclusively for antigen detection. **Indirect immunofluorescence assay (IFA),** in which antigen and antibody react, followed by reaction with an antibody conjugate directed against the first antibody, is used both for antigen and antibody detection. IFAs will be discussed in more detail in Chapter 15.

Numerous DFAs for detection of microbial antigens are in use. Among the more popular are assays for *Chlamydia trachomatis, Legionella* spp, *Bordetella pertussis, Pneumocystis carinii, Cryptosporidium* spp, *Giardia lamblia,* herpes simplex virus, varicella zoster virus, respiratory syncytial virus, influenza virus, parainfluenza virus, and adenovirus. The assay procedure consists of preparing acetone- or methanol-fixed smears of specimens, flooding the smears with antibody conjugate, carefully rinsing the smears to remove unbound conjugate, and examining them microscopically under ultraviolet illumination (Table 13–3).

The major advantages of DFA are the rapidity of test results and the ability to examine the smear for antigen and simultaneously assess the adequacy of the specimen submitted for testing.

TABLE 13–3. DIRECT IMMUNOFLUORESCENCE ASSAY PROCEDURE

---

1. Prepare a smear of the specimen on a glass microscope slide.
2. Fix the smear for 1 minute with methanol or acetone.
3. Flood the smear with antibody conjugate. Rinse thoroughly in FA buffer.
4. Microscopically examine the smear under ultraviolet illumination for antigen-specific fluorescence.

Particle Agglutination

Another popular method for rapid detection of bacterial and fungal antigens in specimens is **particle agglutination (PA).** Microscopic particles (e.g., latex, charcoal, erythrocytes, *Staphylococcus aureus* cells) are coated (sensitized) with antibodies directed against the antigens of interest. In the presence of antigen, the particles agglutinate to form visible clumps.

Commercial products in kit form are available for assays of Groups A and B *Streptococcus, Haemophilus influenzae* type b, *Streptococcus pneumoniae, Neisseria meningitidis, Escherichia coli* K1, and *Cryptococcus neoformans* antigens, among others. PA kits for detection of viral antigens, such as rotavirus, have also been developed. PA assays for qualitative and quantitative detection of antibodies will be discussed in Chapter 15.

The standard PA antigen detection assay requires two suspensions of microscopic particles. One suspension (the **test suspension**) is sensitized with specific antibodies to the antigens being sought, and the other (the **control suspension**) is sensitized with nonspecific immunoglobulin of the same class used to prepare the test suspension. When *S. aureus* cells are used, strains with cell walls rich in protein A (e.g., the Cowan strain) nonspecifically bind most subclasses of IgG at the end of the molecule (Fc region), which does not bind to antigen. Accordingly, the antigen-reactive sites of the IgG molecules (Fab region) are all oriented so that they are available to bind antigen. In contrast, the antibody molecules clinging to other particles are bound in random orientation so that only a fraction of the antigen recognition sites are free to react with antigen.

The PA assay is performed by mixing a drop (approximately 50 µL) of specimen with 10 to 25 µL of each reagent on a cardboard or glass slide. The slide is rotated manually or mechanically for 3 to 10 minutes and observed for macroscopic agglutination of the particles (Table 13–4). A positive result is indicated by agglutination of the test suspension only (Fig. 13–1).

Specimens that are amenable to PA testing include urine, nonviscous body fluids, and liquid specimen extracts (e.g., nitrous acid extracts of pharyngeal swabs for Group A streptococcal antigen detection). Testing of

TABLE 13–4. PARTICLE AGGLUTINATION PROCEDURE

1. Mix 50 µL of specimen with 10 to 25 µL of antibody-coated test particles and antibody-coated control particles on a glass or cardboard slide.
2. Rotate the slide mechanically or manually.
3. Examine each mixture for agglutination (clumping) of the particles. A positive result is indicated by agglutination of the test particles and no agglutination of the control particles.

viscous specimens is not possible because of nonspecific agglutination of latex suspensions.

The advantages of PA assays are the rapidity of their results, improved sensitivity over immunofluorescence, and their relatively low cost.

Enzyme Immunoassay

Enzyme immunoassays (EIAs) can be configured to detect either antigen or antibody. Assays for antibody will be discussed in Chapter 15. Antigen detection EIAs currently available include kits for hepatitis B virus surface and *e* antigens, HIV-1 p24 antigen, and capsid/envelope antigens of respiratory syncytial virus, influenza A virus, rotavirus, herpes simplex virus, and varicella zoster virus. Kits for detection of *Chlamydia trachomatis, Neisseria gonorrhoeae,* Group A *Streptococcus, Giardia lamblia,*

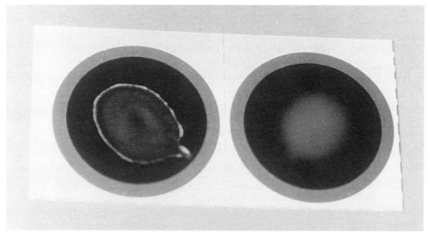

FIGURE 13–1. Photograph of positive and negative latex particle agglutination results. (Reprinted with permission of Gower Medical Publishing, Ltd., London.)

and *Cryptosporidium parvum* antigens are obtainable. Kits for detection of microbial toxins (e.g., *Clostridium difficile* toxin A and *Escherichia coli* Shiga-like toxins) also may be purchased.

Establishing an EIA for detection of microbial antigens begins with attachment of specific antibody to a solid phase, such as nitrocellulose membrane, a plastic dipstick, a plastic bead, or the inner wall of a plastic tube or microtiter tray well. The antigen-containing specimen (which may require a pretreatment step to release or expose antigen) is added to the antibody-sensitized solid phase and incubated. A careful wash step follows to remove unbound material, and a second antigen-specific antibody conjugated with an enzyme (e.g., horseradish peroxidase, alkaline phosphatase) is added to the solid phase–antibody-antigen complex. After another incubation period, the solid phase is once again carefully washed to remove unbound antibody-enzyme conjugate. The final step is the addition of enzyme substrate to the solid phase followed by incubation (Table 13–5). The positive assay endpoint usually is conversion of a colorless substrate to a colored endproduct that is detected with the unaided eye or with a spectrophotometer.

A modification of the EIA procedure described above has been used by assay developers to further enhance test sensitivity and specificity. The second antibody, instead of being conjugated to an enzyme, is **biotinylated** (chemical attachment of biotin to the antibody). Binding of the biotinylated antibody to the existing antigen-antibody complex is detected by reaction with an **avidin-enzyme** (e.g., horseradish peroxidase) conjugate followed by enzyme substrate addition and color development.

The advantages of EIAs are several. They may be more sensitive than particle agglutination by an order of magnitude or more because of the signal amplification enabled by the antibody-conjugated enzyme. A single antigen-antibody conjugate complex has the potential to produce continuous conversion of colorless substrate to colored endproduct. If the enzyme substrate is present in excess, the time allotted for color development becomes the limiting factor for signal generation. Another advantage of EIAs is their ease of reading. Most experienced observers feel that detection of a colored endpoint can be accomplished with greater

---

TABLE 13–5. ENZYME IMMUNOASSAY PROCEDURE

1. Apply the specimen to the solid phase containing the antigen capture antibody. Rinse thoroughly.
2. Flood the solid phase with the antibody-enzyme conjugate. Rinse thoroughly.
3. Flood the solid phase with the enzyme substrate. Rinse thoroughly.
4. Examine the solid phase for color development.

Immunochromatography

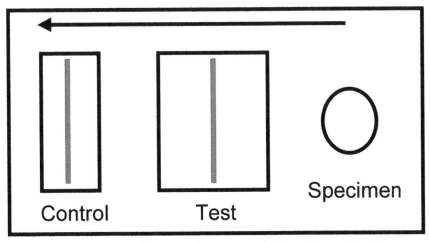

FIGURE 13–2. Diagram of immunochromatography for antigen detection.

confidence and accuracy and less training than can detection of a particle agglutination or immunofluorescence endpoint. Finally, the rapidity of EIAs (less than 10 minutes) lends itself to testing in nonlaboratory settings. Reagents are stable, minimal training is required to perform the assays, and expensive, cumbersome apparatus is not necessary for reading test results.

Immunochromatography

One of the newer antigen detection assay formats is known as **immunochromatography** (Fig. 13–2). The principle of this method involves reaction of microbial antigens with antibodies conjugated to colored particles. The resultant immune complexes then flow (chromatograph) through a membrane reaction region coated with capture antibodies to the same microbial antigens. A positive signal is indicated by visible retention of the colored particles in the reaction region of the test device. The chromatography continues until the advancing "front" encounters a second set of capture antibodies directed against nonmicrobial antigenic components of the migrating particles. The completion of the assay is indicated by retention of the non-immune-complexed particles in the quality control region of the test device. Assays for

Optical Immunoassay

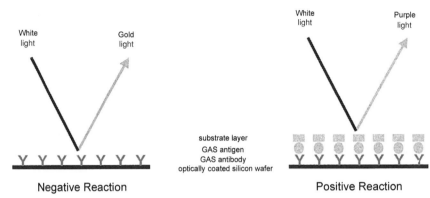

FIGURE 13–3. Diagram of optical immunoassay for Group A streptococcal (GAS) antigen detection.

detection of Group A streptococcal antigen and Group B streptococcal antigen are available in this format.

The chief advantage of the immunochromatographic method is the simplicity of the assay. One need only mix the specimen with the antibody-complexed particles, apply the mixture to the chromatography membrane, and wait the few minutes needed for chromatography to occur.

Optical Immunoassay

The newest antigen detection assay format is termed the **optical immunoassay (OIA)** by the manufacturer (Fig. 13–3). This assay technique uses an optically coated silicon wafer to which are attached capture antibodies directed against the microbial antigens of interest. The specimen is applied to the surface of the silicon wafer, washed off, and the silicon wafer is examined under bright light. The presence of a purple reaction zone superimposed on a gold background is evidence of a positive reaction. OIAs for detection of antigens of Group A streptococci, Group B streptococci, and *Chlamydia trachomatis* are commercially available.

As for immunochromatography, the major advantage of OIA is the simplicity of the assay. Moreover, the OIA method appears able to detect smaller quantities of antigen than any of the other rapid assays described.

PROBES FOR INFECTIOUS AGENT NUCLEIC ACIDS

One of the more impressive advances in diagnostic microbiology has been the development of **nucleic acid probes** for detection of microorganism-specific DNA or RNA sequences in specimens. Probe-based assays can identify specific microorganisms, and it is likely that similar assays to detect frequently occurring antimicrobial resistance genes will soon become available. Commercially available assays licensed by the Food and Drug Administration of the United States can detect *Chlamydia trachomatis, Neisseria gonorrhoeae, Mycobacterium tuberculosis,* and Group A *Streptococcus.* Several other assays for detection of infectious agents are available for investigational use only. In addition, an assay for quantitation of human immunodeficiency virus type 1 (HIV-1) viral load is available in a licensed format; other assays for qualitative detection of HIV-1 and determination of hepatitis C viral load are available for investigational use only.

Several of the licensed, commercially available assays for bacterial detection utilize a short-sequence, single-stranded DNA probe that is homologous to organism-specific ribosomal RNA (Fig. 13–4 demonstrates the hybridization protection assay). During a typical assay, microorganisms in the specimen are lysed and added to a reaction tube containing the probe. After 60 minutes incubation at a hybridization-permissive temperature, the chemiluminescent signal-generating molecule attached

Hybridization Protection Assay

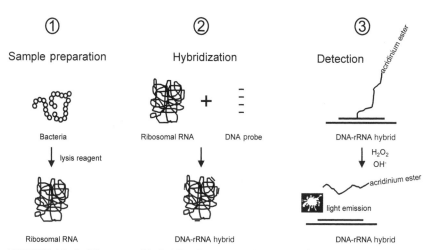

FIGURE 13–4. Diagram of hybridization protection assay for molecular detection of ribosomal RNA.

to unbound probe is removed and inactivated by the addition of separation reagent. Later, hybridized chemiluminescent probe is detected by the addition of alkaline H_2O_2, which results in a burst of light.

The main advantage of the assays described is the rapidity of test results compared to culture. These assays yield results in less than 2 hours, compared to the several days required by culture. Moreover, these assays are more sensitive than antigen detection methods, with concomitant improvement of the negative predictive value of assay results.

Despite their overall improvement in sensitivity over antigen detection, one of the theoretical disadvantages of DNA probe assays remains their lack of sensitivity compared to culture. Conventional DNA probe assays for ribosomal RNA have difficulty detecting fewer than 100 to 1000 organisms in test samples. The clinical significance of specimens harboring such low numbers of "pathogens," however, is not always clear. Another disadvantage of these assays is their higher cost compared to culture.

A solution to the problem of lack of sensitivity of these assays is the use of target or signal amplification techniques to improve their lower limits of detection by several orders of magnitude. **Target amplification techniques** like the polymerase chain reaction (PCR), ligase chain reaction (LCR), transcription-mediated amplification (TMA), and nucleic acid sequence based amplification (NASBA) increase the sensitivity of nucleic acid probe–based assays to the point that they equal or supersede that of culture. **Signal amplification techniques** like branched chain DNA (bDNA) also greatly enhance the sensitivity of nucleic acid probe–based assays.

Unquestionably, the future is bright for the use of these assays in the diagnosis of infectious diseases. Important advances in probe technology and assay development occur frequently in this rapidly evolving area. Soon it will be possible to detect a wider variety of organisms in a shorter period of time, with much-improved accuracy.

DETECTION OF INFECTIOUS AGENT TOXINS

Many infectious agents are pathogenic to humans because of elaboration of harmful toxins. These organisms do not have to invade tissues or body systems of the host to effect damage. Instead, the host ingests toxins already produced by these organisms in the environment (e.g., *Staphylococcus aureus*, *Clostridium botulinum*, or *Aspergillus flavus* food poisoning), or these organisms colonize the host and release toxins in situ that can have local or distant effects throughout the body (e.g., *Staphylococcus aureus*, Group A *Streptococcus*, *Corynebacterium diphtheriae*, *Clostridium tetani*, *Clostridium difficile*, *Vibrio cholerae*, *Shigella dysenteriae*, enterotoxigenic and enterohaemorrhagic *Escherichia coli*). In some instances, the laboratory test of choice for diagnosis of these infections is an assay for the toxin rather than for the organism producing it.

Cytotoxicity Toxin Assay

The presence of certain toxins can be demonstrated in specimens by inoculation of cell cultures. The toxins produced by serotypes of *Escherichia coli* that cause hemorrhagic colitis (verotoxin or Shiga-like toxin) are readily demonstrable by inoculation of stool extracts to African Green Monkey kidney cell culture. Similarly, a cytotoxin (toxin B) produced by *Clostridium difficile*, which correlates highly with production of an enterotoxin (toxin A) causing antimicrobial agent-associated enterocolitis, can be detected in stool extracts inoculated to a variety of cell culture lines.

For example, the set-up of the *C. difficile* cytotoxin assay requires a bacteria-free extract of a stool specimen, an appropriate cell culture line (WI-38 human diploid lung fibroblasts is recommended), and *C. difficile, C. sordellii,* or gas gangrene polyvalent antitoxin so that the necessary negative control can be included. The specimen extract with and without antitoxin is inoculated to individual cell culture tubes, incubated at 35°C, and the cells examined microscopically for cytopathic effect after 4, 24, and 48 hours of incubation (Table 13–6). A positive result is indicated by rounding of the cells in the tube lacking antitoxin, with no effect on the cells in the tube with antitoxin.

The performance of the verotoxin or Shiga-like toxin assay for diagnosis of *E. coli*–induced hemorrhagic colitis is similar in principle to the *C. difficile* cytotoxin assay.

Enzyme Immunoassay

Several FDA-licensed EIAs for detection of *C. difficile* toxin A and *E. coli* verotoxin/Shiga-like toxin are presently available from commercial sources. The assays, like those described earlier for detection of microbial antigens, yield positive color endpoints that can be read with a spectrophotometer, or in some cases with the unaided human eye. Results are available within 2 hours.

TABLE 13–6. ASSAY FOR *CLOSTRIDIUM DIFFICILE* CYTOTOXIN IN STOOL

1. Suspend the stool in pH 7 buffer and centrifuge to pellet all particulate matter. Retain and filter; sterilize the supernatant.
2. Inoculate the supernatant ± cytotoxin neutralizing antibody to a cell culture monolayer.
3. Compare the cell culture monolayers for cytotoxicity after 4, 24, and 48 hours of incubation at 35°C.

Animal Model Toxin Assay

Very few laboratories today maintain animal colonies for the purpose of detecting microbial toxins in specimens. Testing in which toxin studies in animals are necessary are usually performed by reference or research laboratories. Definitive diagnosis of food-borne, wound, and infant botulism does require demonstration of neutralizable botulinal toxin in serum, stool, or gastric contents. The use of a suckling mouse assay is the method of choice.

CULTURE OF INFECTIOUS AGENTS

For most infections, culture is still the mainstay for definitive diagnosis. Liquid and solid growth media have been developed to make growth of most bacteria and fungi possible in the laboratory. Cell culture lines for propagation of viruses and chlamydiae are available. Chicken eggs or live animals, on some occasions, may still be inoculated to demonstrate the presence of microorganisms.

Three categories of growth media are in common use: nonselective, selective, and differential. **Nonselective media** (e.g., 5% sheep blood agar, chocolate agar) support the growth of a wide variety of organisms at relatively rapid growth rates. **Selective media** (e.g., modified Thayer-Martin agar) contain additives to inhibit growth of all but a specific group of organisms. **Differential media** (e.g., MacConkey agar) display growth characteristics of organisms that aid in their presumptive identification. Growth media frequently belong to more than one category (e.g., MacConkey agar is also a selective medium).

Numerous cell culture lines are available to laboratories intent on culturing viruses and chlamydiae. Some cell culture lines are derived from human tissue, some from tissues of other mammals, and others from tissues of lower animals. Not all cell culture lines support the growth of all agents, so knowledge of which agents are being sought by the clinician is critical to success.

Rarely, chicken eggs or live animals are used as hosts for growth of infectious organisms. Again, because very few hospital laboratories these days possess adequate staffing or facilities to maintain animal colonies, such testing is referred to either reference or research laboratories.

Bacterial Culture

Bacteria can be assigned to groups that facilitate their ultimate identification by the laboratory. Knowledge of an organism's oxygen requirement, colonial and Gram stain morphology, and catalase and oxidase test reactions greatly limit the possible identifications. All of these characteristics are either apparent immediately or ascertained quickly after detection of bacterial growth. With this information at hand, focused testing can be performed to determine the definitive identification of the organism. See the algorithm in Table 13–7 for further information.

Bacterial Oxygen Requirements

All bacteria fall into one of five categories of oxygen requirement: obligate aerobes, microaerophilic aerobes, facultative anaerobes, aerotolerant anaerobes, and obligate anaerobes. **Obligate aerobes** derive energy exclusively from oxygen-dependent metabolism (aerobic respiration). **Microaerophilic aerobes** likewise require oxygen for growth, but at concentrations lower than that found in the earth's atmosphere. **Facultative anaerobes** generate energy from either oxygen-dependent or oxygen-independent (fermentation) metabolism. Because considerably more energy is generated per mole of substrate during aerobic respiration, this group of bacteria, given the choice, always prefers that mode of metabolism. **Aerotolerant anaerobes** depend exclusively on fermentation as an energy source, yet are tolerant of atmospheric levels of oxygen. **Obligate anaerobes** also derive energy from fermentation but are inhibited or killed by atmospheric levels of oxygen.

Bacterial Gram Stain Morpholoqy

The Gram stain morphology of a bacterium includes its *Gram reaction (Gram positive or negative)* and its *shape* (e.g., *coccus* or *bacillus*). Further information regarding the arrangement of the organisms (e.g., pairs, chains, clusters) can be helpful but is sometimes misleading. Gram-stained smears prepared from broth cultures more likely reflect the true arrangement of organisms than do smears prepared from agar plate colonies. The physical appearance of well-isolated colonies and the surrounding growth medium can be extremely helpful to the knowledgeable microbiologist during organism identification. The size, shape, opacity, and even the odor of colonies are characteristics that contribute to presumptive identification of isolates.

Bacterial Catalase and Oxidase Reactions

For the most part, bacteria that engage in aerobic respiration produce the hemeprotein **catalase,** which is at least partly responsible for decomposing intracellular hydrogen peroxide, a toxic byproduct of aerobic metabolism. The aerotolerant anaerobes are usually catalase negative. The results of the slide catalase test, which requires no more than 30 seconds to perform, are frequently used to differentiate staphylococci (catalase positive) from streptococci (catalase negative).

Another enzyme synthesized by certain aerobic bacteria is **cytochrome oxidase,** which catalyzes the terminal reaction of the electron transport chain, reduction of molecular oxygen to water. The results of the oxidase test, which likewise takes no more than 30 seconds, are useful in distinguishing *Neisseria/Moraxella,* most *Pseudomonas* species, and members of the *Vibrionaceae* family from other gram-negative bacteria.

TABLE 13–7. SCHEME FOR PRELIMINARY IDENTIFICATION OF BACTERIA BASED ON OXYGEN REQUIREMENT: MORPHOLOGY AND GRAM STAINING

Obligate Aerobe
  Gram-Negative Rod
    Oxidase-Positive
      Achromobacter spp
      Acidovorax spp
      Agrobacterium spp
      Alcaligenes spp
      Allomonas spp
      Bergeyella spp
      Bordetella spp
      Brevundimonas spp
      Brucella spp (except *ovis* and *neotomae*)
      Burkholderia spp
      CDC Groups EF-4a, EF-4b, EO-2, EO-3, IVc-2
      Chryseobacterium spp
      Comamonas spp
      Empedobacter spp
      Flavobacterium spp
      Legionella (some species)
      Methylobacterium spp
      Moraxella spp
      Myroides spp
      Ochrobactrum spp
      Oligella spp
      Pseudomonas spp
      Psychrobacter spp (some strains)
      Ralstonia spp
      Roseomonas spp
      Shewanella spp
      Sphingobacterium spp
      Sphingomonas spp
      Weeksella spp
    Oxidase-Negative
      Acinetobacter spp
      Afipia spp
      Bartonella spp
      Brucella ovis and *neotomae*
      Chryseomonas spp
      Flavimonas spp
      Franciscella spp
      Legionella (some species)
      Psychrobacter spp (some strains)
      Stenotrophomonas spp

(Continued)

TABLE 13–7. SCHEME FOR PRELIMINARY IDENTIFICATION OF BACTERIA BASED ON OXYGEN REQUIREMENT: MORPHOLOGY AND GRAM STAINING *(Continued)*

Gram-Negative Coccus
  Oxidase-Positive
    Moraxella catarrhalis
    Neisseria spp
Gram-Positive Rod
  Catalase-Positive
    Actinomadura spp
    Arthrobacter spp
    Aureobacterium spp
    Bacillus spp (some species)
    Brevibacterium spp
    Corynebacterium spp
    Gordona spp
    Kurthia spp
    Mycobacterium spp (almost all strains)
    Nocardia spp
    Nocardiopsis spp
    Rhodococcus spp
    Streptomyces spp
    Tsukamurella spp
    Turicella spp
  Catalase-Negative
    Mycobacterium spp (some isoniazid resistant strains)
Gram-Positive Coccus
  Catalase-Positive
    Alloiococcus spp
    Micrococcus spp
Microaerophilic Aerobe
  Gram-Negative Rod
    Oxidase- and Catalase-Positive
      Arcobacter spp
      Campylobacter spp (some strains)
      Helicobacter spp
Facultative Anaerobe
  Gram-Negative Rod
    Oxidase-Positive
      Actinobacillus spp (some strains)
      Aeromonas spp
      Cardiobacterium spp
      Chromobacterium spp (some strains)
      Eikenella spp
      Haemophilus spp
      Kingella spp
      Pasteurella spp

(Continued)

TABLE 13–7. SCHEME FOR PRELIMINARY IDENTIFICATION OF BACTERIA BASED ON OXYGEN REQUIREMENT: MORPHOLOGY AND GRAM STAINING *(Continued)*

Photobacterium spp
Plesiomonas spp
Vibrio spp
Oxidase-Negative
Actinobacillus spp (some strains)
Budvicia spp
Buttiauxella spp
Capnocytophaga spp
Cedecea spp
Chromobacterium spp (some strains)
Citrobacter spp
Edwardsiella spp
Enteric Groups 58, 60, 63, 64, 68, 69
Enterobacter spp
Erwinia spp
Escherichia spp
Ewingella spp
Hafnia spp
Klebsiella spp
Kluyvera spp
Koserella spp
Leclercia spp
Leminorella spp
Moellerella spp
Morganella spp
Obesumbacterium spp
Pantoea spp
Photorhabdus spp
Pragia spp
Proteus spp
Providencia spp
Rahnella spp
Salmonella spp
Serratia spp
Shigella spp
Streptobacillus spp
Suttonella spp
Tatumella spp
Trabulsiella spp
Xenorhabdus spp
Yersinia spp
Yokenella spp

(Continued)

Gram-Positive Rod
  Catalase-Positive
    Bacillus spp (some species)
    Callatomonas spp
    Corynebacterium spp (some species)
    Dermabacter spp
    Dermatophilus spp
    Listeria spp
    Microbacterium spp
    Oerskovia spp
    Rothia spp
  Catalase-Negative
    Arcanobacterium spp
    Erysipelothrix spp
    Gardnerella spp
Gram-Positive Coccus
  Catalase-Positive
    Staphylococcus spp
    Stomatococcus spp (some strains)
  Catalase-Negative
    Stomatococcus spp (some strains)
Aerotolerant Anaerobe
  Gram-Positive Rod
    Catalase-Positive
      Propionibacterium spp (some strains)
    Catalase-Negative
      Actinomyces spp (some strains)
      Clostridium histolyticum
      Clostridium tertium
      Lactobacillus spp (some strains)
  Gram-Positive Coccus
    Catalase-Negative
      Abiotrophia spp
      Aerococcus spp
      Dolosigranulum spp
      Enterococcus spp
      Gemella spp
      Globicatella spp
      Helcococcus spp
      Lactococcus spp
      Leuconostoc spp
      Oenococcus spp
      Pediococcus spp
      Streptococcus spp
      Vagococcus spp
      Weissella spp

(Continued)

Obligate Anaerobe
  Gram-Negative Rod
    Catalase-Positive
      Bacteroides spp (some strains)
      Bilophila spp
    Catalase-Negative
      Bacteroides spp (some strains)
      Campylobacter spp (some strains)
      Centipeda spp
      Desulfomonas spp
      Desulfovibrio spp
      Dichelobacter spp
      Fusobacterium spp
      Leptotrichia spp
      Mitsuokella spp
      Porphyromonas spp
      Prevotella spp
      Selenomonas spp
      Tissierella spp
      Wolinella spp
  Gram-Negative Coccus
    Catalase-Positive
      Veillonella spp (some strains)
    Catalase-Negative
      Acidaminococcus spp
      Megasphaera spp
      Veillonella spp (some strains)
  Gram-Positive Rod
    Catalase-Positive
      Propionibacterium spp (some strains)
    Catalase-Negative
      Actinomyces spp (some strains)
      Atopobium spp
      Bifidobacterium spp
      Clostridium spp (some species)
      Eubacterium spp
      Lactobacillus spp
      Mobiluncus spp
      Pseudoramibacter spp
  Gram-Positive Coccus
    Catalase-Negative
      Peptostreptococcus spp (some strains)
      Ruminococcus spp
    Catalase-Positive
      Peptococcus niger
      Peptostreptococcus spp (some strains)
      Staphylococcus saccharolyticus

Staphylococcal Coagulase Reaction

One additional widely performed assay for differentiation of *Staphylococcus aureus* from many other species of staphylococci is the coagulase test. The assay detects production of bound (cell wall–associated) coagulase or free coagulase. This test can be performed using any of three methods:

- the **tube coagulase test,** which detects both bound and free forms of the enzyme
- the **slide coagulase test,** which detects only bound enzyme
- the **particle clumping test,** which also detects only bound enzyme

The first of these methods is still acknowledged as the reference method and yields results after 4 to 24 hours of incubation. The other two methods are much more rapid, requiring less than 1 minute to perform, but both can produce occasional false-positive or false-negative results.

Tube Coagulase Test   The tube test is set up by inoculating a staphylococcal isolate to a small quantity of coagulase reagent (e.g., rabbit plasma) within a test tube. The test is incubated at 35 to 37°C for 4 hours and the coagulase reagent examined for evidence of clotting (gel formation). A positive result indicates the isolate is *S. aureus.* Negative tests are reincubated at room temperature for an additional 20 hours and re-examined. Isolates negative after 4 and positive after 24 hours may be *S. aureus* or members of the veterinary species *S. intermedius, S. delphini,* or *S. hyicus.* Isolates negative after both 4 and 24 hours are considered coagulase negative.

Slide Coagulase Test   The slide test is performed by emulsifying staphylococcal growth in a drop of coagulase reagent on a microscope slide. If the growth forms "clumps," the isolate is either *S. aureus, S. lugdunensis, S. schleiferi,* or *S. intermedius.* If the suspended growth is homogeneous, the isolate should be confirmed as tube coagulase negative before ruling out *S. aureus* as a possible identification.

Particle Clumping Test   Several versions of this test detect the same bound coagulase responsible for a positive slide coagulase result. In some versions of this test, particles are coated with both fibrinogen (for detection of bound coagulase) and IgG (for detection of staphylococcal protein A). Protein A is a cell wall component unique to *S. aureus* that nonspecifically binds to the Fc region of IgG molecules. The resultant *S. aureus* cell/particle lattice formation gives rise to visible clumping of the latex particles. Interpretation of positive and negative results is the same as for the slide coagulase test. Some strains of methicillin-resistant *S. aureus* (MRSA) have been shown to yield falsely negative particle clumping test results.

Aerobic Culture

There are literally dozens of growth media from which to choose when inoculating aerobic cultures. Most laboratories select media according to the nature of the specimen or the site of specimen collection. The pathogens most likely to be encountered dictate the combination of nonselective, selective, and differential media to be inoculated. Thus, it is mandatory that care providers inform the laboratory of the source of the specimen and notify the laboratory of unusual suspected pathogens in order to ensure that appropriate media are inoculated.

Most specimens are streaked for isolation to agar media using the **four-quadrant streaking method** (Color Plate 70). When quantitative culture results are desired (e.g., urine cultures), the **colony-count streaking method** can be used (Color Plate 71). Agar media in tubes are inoculated by streaking the specimen onto the slanted agar surface and/or stabbing the inoculum into the agar itself. Liquid culture media in tubes or bottles are inoculated by introducing the specimen directly into the broth.

The standard incubation temperature for aerobic bacterial cultures is 35 to 37°C. Other incubation temperatures can be used when circumstances warrant. The incubation atmosphere should be supplemented with 5 to 10% CO_2 during primary incubation of blood-containing or chocolatized blood-containing agar media. Growth of many aerobic bacteria is stimulated by added CO_2, and growth of a few important pathogens actually requires added CO_2. Differential agar media dependent on pH change (e.g., MacConkey agar) should be incubated in a non–CO_2-enriched atmosphere to prevent acidification of the medium. A reduced-oxygen atmosphere is necessary for growth of microaerophilic bacteria like *Campylobacter jejuni*.

The length of incubation for cultures varies with the pathogens being sought. As a routine, agar media in plates are held for 48 to 72 hours. Enrichment broth media, if inoculated, are incubated for 1 to 14 days. When informed that slow growing, fastidious pathogens are suspected, the laboratory should extend the culture incubation time.

Anaerobic Culture

The minimum requirements of specimens submitted for anaerobic culture were discussed earlier in this chapter. Two points deserve emphasis:

- Specimens must not have been collected from a body site ordinarily colonized with anaerobes.
- Specimens must have been transported to the laboratory in a manner consistent with survival of anaerobes.

If the above requirements are not met, it is the responsibility of the laboratory to reject requests for anaerobic culture.

Although not essential to success, *prereduction* of culture media by overnight storage in an anaerobic environment before inoculation has been suggested. The purpose is to remove oxygen dissolved in the media, thus eliminating exposure of strict anaerobes to potentially lethal levels of oxygen early in incubation. Specimens don't have to be inoculated to media in oxygen-free surroundings, but after inoculation, cultures should be placed in an anaerobic environment without undue delay.

Media should be supplemented with vitamin K and hemin to satisfy the growth requirements of nutritionally fastidious organisms. In addition, a medium further supplemented with kanamycin, vancomycin, and perhaps bile salts (sodium desoxycholate) should be included to improve recovery of the *Bacteroides fragilis* group. Measures designed to enhance detection of the *B. fragilis* group are stressed because they are the anaerobes most likely to exhibit antimicrobial resistance. Because anaerobic infections are frequently mixed with facultative anaerobes, colonies of the *B. fragilis* group may be difficult to recognize on nonselective media. Identification of pigmented *Prevotella* spp and *Porphyromonas* spp (formerly the *Bacteroides melaninogenicus* group), another anaerobic gram-negative rod group that is occasionally antimicrobial resistant, can be facilitated by inoculation of laked blood (blood lysed by repeated freeze-thaw cycles) containing media. Young colonies of these species on laked blood agar may exhibit brick red fluorescence under long-wave ultraviolet light, whereas older colonies produce a visible brownish-black melanin pigment. Finally, a companion set of aerobically incubated growth media should be inoculated from the same specimens used to inoculate anaerobic media, to enable comparison of culture results. Facultative and oxygen-tolerant anaerobes will grow on both sets of media, but obligate anaerobes will form colonies only on the anaerobically incubated media.

Provision of an anaerobic atmosphere can be accomplished in various ways: (1) use of an anaerobic chamber (glove box) complete with a self-contained incubator or (2) placement of cultures in a gas-tight container, followed by mechanical replacement of the oxygen-rich atmosphere with an oxygen-free gas mixture, or catalytic removal of the oxygen. Commercially available air-tight jars and heat-sealable plastic bags make the latter approach very popular with laboratories today.

Anaerobic cultures should be incubated at 35 to 37°C. Because anaerobes usually grow at slower rates than obligate aerobes and facultative anaerobes, culture plates should be incubated for at least 5 days. Broth cultures, if inoculated, should be incubated for at least 7 days.

Mycobacterial Culture

The **mycobacteria** are obligate aerobes that differ from other bacteria in that they are acid-fast and, for the most part, grow very slowly. Except for a small group of "rapidly growing" species (colonies form within 7 days), the pathogenic mycobacteria form visible colonies only after 3 to 8 weeks of incubation.

Mycobacteria were originally classified as "typical" or "atypical." The term *typical mycobacteria* referred to *Mycobacterium tuberculosis* (see Color Plate 62) and *M. bovis. Atypical mycobacteria* referred to members of all other species. Today, the preferred term for the "atypical" group is **nontuberculous mycobacteria** or **MOTT** (mycobacteria other than *tuberculosis*).

A convenient scheme for classification of nontuberculous mycobacteria that is still in use today was developed by Runyon in 1959. Four **Runyon groups** were designated:

1. the **photochromogens,** which produce a golden yellow pigment only after exposure to bright light (e.g., *M. kansasii, M. marinum*)
2. the **scotochromogens,** which produce a golden yellow pigment regardless of light exposure (e.g., *M. scrofulaceum*)
3. the **nonchromogens,** which don't produce yellow pigment at all (e.g., *M. avium* complex)
4. the **rapid growers,** which form visible colonies in less than 7 days (e.g., *M. fortuitum, M. chelonei*)

The Runyon group classification is handy for laboratories that don't identify nontuberculous mycobacteria to the species level, but it should be remembered that some species have members belonging to more than one Runyon group (e.g., pigmented and nonpigmented *M. avium-intracellulare*).

The slow growth rate of most mycobacteria places the laboratory at a distinct disadvantage when attempting to culture mycobacteria from contaminated specimens like sputum. To prevent cultures from ruin by overgrowth with faster species during incubation, specimens should be chemically treated (e.g., with sodium hydroxide or Zephiran-trisodium phosphate) to selectively kill contaminants. Aseptically collected body fluids that are ordinarily sterile do not require decontamination prior to culture.

The number of mycobacteria present in specimens collected from infected patients is often very low. To enhance detection rates, concentration of specimens by centrifugation is a standard practice. Viscous, tenacious specimens like sputum must be liquefied first if centrifugation is to have any benefit. The decontamination agents described above also aid in specimen digestion. Other successfully used digestants are N-acetyl-L-cysteine (NALC) and dithiothreitol *(Sputalysin).* Either of these agents, in combination with 2% NaOH, effectively decontaminates and digests sputum. Centrifugation of specimens must be thorough if concentration of mycobacteria is to be successful. Thirty minutes of centrifugation at 3000g are necessary to sediment mycobacteria effectively.

The recent resurgence of tuberculosis in the U. S., the increasing incidence of multidrug-resistant strains, and rising rates of patient-to-caregiver transmission have led to recommendations that laboratories reduce the time to detection of *M. tuberculosis* as much as possible.

Consequently, laboratories providing services to institutions with high rates of tuberculosis should use liquid culture methods to hasten detection of *M. tuberculosis.* Specimens can be inoculated to bottles containing selective broth for mycobacteria. Cultures are incubated and monitored on a regular basis for evidence of growth. Depending on the broth culture system used, the evidence of growth may be release of $^{14}CO_2$ into the bottle atmosphere, fluorescence of the medium when illuminated by ultraviolet light, or detection of growth with a continuously monitoring instrument. Average times to detection of *M. tuberculosis* are 1 to 2 weeks shorter in broth culture than on solid medium.

Conventional culture techniques call for inoculation of specimens to selective solid media. Commonly used media include an opaque **inspissated egg-based medium** (e.g., Lowenstein-Jensen medium) that does not contain agar (see Color Plate 72) and **clear agar-based media** (e.g., Middlebrook-Cohn 7H10 or 7H11 agar). Agar-based media yield earlier positive results, but egg-based media yield more positive results. Specimens should be inoculated to both types of media. Care should be taken to prevent exposure of 7H10 and 7H11 agars to light, since formaldehyde may be generated that could kill mycobacteria.

Broth cultures should be incubated at 35 to 37°C and monitored for growth as previously described. Solid media cultures should be incubated at 35 to 37°C in an atmosphere enriched with 5 to 10% carbon dioxide. Wound and skin specimens should have a second set of media incubated at 30°C to permit growth of *M. marinum, M. ulcerans,* and *M. haemophilum,* which do not grow at the higher temperature. Liquid media cultures should be incubated for at least 5 weeks, and solid media cultures for at least 8 weeks before negative results are reported.

Fungal Culture

The medically important fungi are a diverse group of organisms that cause an even more diverse group of infections. They can be divided into three groups: the **yeasts,** the **molds,** and the **dimorphic fungi.** The latter group can exhibit either a yeast or a mold phase of growth, depending on incubation conditions. Fungi can also be classified based on the infections they cause. **Dermatophyte** fungi infect hair, nails, and the superficial layers of the skin. The organisms that cause chromomycosis, phaeohyphomycosis, and mycetoma infect the subcutaneous layers of the skin. Finally, agents that cause infections that disseminate to multiple organs and body sites are termed the **deep fungi.**

In most laboratories, most clinically significant fungal isolates are yeasts. Yeasts grow equally well on bacterial culture media and fungal media (Color Plate 73A). Likewise, many of the clinically significant molds, especially those that cause opportunistic infections in immunocompromised patients, grow readily and rapidly on bacterial culture media (Color Plate 74).

One reason for inoculating fungal cultures is to enable detection of slower growing fungi in specimens containing large numbers of rapidly growing bacteria. Bacterial growth on nonselective media can easily mask the presence of fungi. Fungal growth media can be made inhibitory to bacteria by using a low pH (e.g., Sabouraud's dextrose agar), or by adding antibacterial agents (e.g., chloramphenicol in inhibitory mold agar). Thus, the yield of positive fungal cultures is greater on fungal growth media than on bacterial media. Perhaps an even more important reason for performing fungal cultures is found in the incubation conditions. Several clinically important fungi either do not grow at 35 to 37°C or take longer than 72 hours to form visible colonies. Cultures incubated under routine conditions for growth of bacteria would fail to detect such isolates. The incubation conditions described in this section result in increased numbers of positive fungal cultures.

Generally speaking, fungal cultures should be inoculated to a medium lacking antimicrobial agents (e.g., Sabouraud's dextrose agar); a medium containing antibacterial agents only (e.g., inhibitory mold agar); and a medium containing blood, antibacterial agents, and the antifungal agent cycloheximide (e.g., brain heart infusion agar with sheep blood, chloramphenicol, gentamicin, and cycloheximide). Cycloheximide prevents the growth of many saprophytic fungi that occasionally contaminate nonselective media, making detection of slower growing pathogens impossible. The media assortment just described would support the growth of almost all cultivable fungi on at least one of the media. The occasions in which more specialized media are required (e.g., cultures for *Malassezia furfur*) must be communicated to the mycology laboratory. One should also remember that a few important fungal pathogens (e.g., *Cryptococcus neoformans, Pseudallescheria boydii*) do not grow on cycloheximide-containing media. Thus, it is essential that at least one cycloheximide-free medium be included with all fungal cultures. Fungal cultures should be incubated at 25 to 30°C to allow growth of dermatophytes and other fungi unable to propagate at higher temperatures. If desired, a second set of inoculated media may be incubated at a higher temperature to hasten the growth of thermotolerant fungi. Cultures should be incubated for at least 3 weeks because many fungi that cause dermatophyte, subcutaneous, or deep infections are slow growers. When only rapidly growing yeasts or molds are being sought (e.g., *Candida* sp and *Aspergillus* sp), 5 days of incubation are sufficient. Preliminary identification of fungi can be achieved by microscopy. Yeast isolates can be examined for germ tube formation in serum or plasma after incubation at 35 to 37°C for 2 to 3 hours (see Color Plate 74B). Only *Candida albicans* and *C. stellatoidea* are germ tube–positive. Another rapid method for identification of *C. albicans* is based on detection of L-proline aminopeptidase and beta-galactosaminidase enzymatic activities. Complete identification of commonly encountered yeasts requires microscopic examination of hyphal, pseudohyphal, and conidial structures, as well as biochemical testing (e.g., sugar assimilation, urease and nitrate reduction tests). Filamentous fungi should be examined in lactophenol cotton blue wet mounts for characteristic conidial or sporangial structures (Figs. 13–5, 13–6). **Tease preparations** from primary isolation media often are unsatisfactory, and the laboratory needs to set up **coverslipped slide cultures** on starvation media such as potato dextrose or cornmeal agar.

Viral and Chlamydial Culture

The viruses and chlamydiae are **obligate intracellular parasites,** which are unable to grow on artificial media. Cultures for these pathogens must be inoculated to a source of living host cells—either a monolayer of growing cells derived from a human or other animal, or an animal itself, such as an embryonated egg or suckling mouse.

Medically important viruses are the smallest known agents capable of infection, ranging in diameter from 25 to 300 nm. Structurally, they are composed of nucleic acid surrounded by a **proteinaceous coat** (capsid), which may or may not be surrounded by a **lipid-containing envelope.** The nucleic acid may be **DNA** or **RNA,** either **single-stranded** or **double-stranded.** Most human viruses are icosahedral or spherical in shape, but brick-shaped, bullet-shaped, and filamentous morphologies

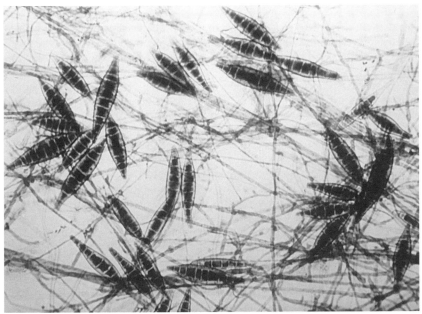

FIGURE 13–5. Macroconidia produced by *Microsporum canis.* (Reprinted with permission of Gower Medical Publishing, Ltd., London.)

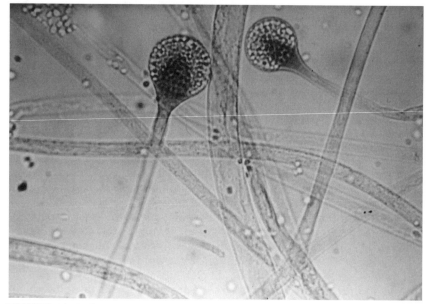

FIGURE 13–6. Sporangia produced by *Absidia* species. (Reprinted with permission of Gower Medical Publishing, Ltd., London.)

are known. Viral envelopes contain host cell lipids and proteins and become a component of viral ultrastructure when viruses emerge from infected host cells by a process known as "budding." Viruses that are released by lysis of the host cell are usually not enveloped.

Cell culture passage refers to continued growth of a cell line following transfer of a small number of cells to fresh culture medium. Not all cell lines are amenable to repeated passage during in vitro culture; some are unable to adapt to growth in an artificial environment and die. Others adapt well to atypical growth conditions and can be passaged indefinitely. Cell lines for propagation of viruses may be **primary** (passageable 1 or 2 times [e.g., primary monkey kidney]), **diploid** (passageable 20 to 50 times [e.g., WI-38 and MRC-5]), or **continuous** (passageable an infinite number of times [e.g., HeLa and HEp-2]).

Cell culture monolayers may be grown on coverslips, in test tubes, in wells of microtiter trays, or in flat-sided bottles, when large quantities of virus are desired. Monolayers are prepared by cutting the source tissue into small pieces, treating with trypsin to obtain a single-cell suspension, and allowing the cells to settle and adhere to a flat plastic or glass surface. The cells are bathed in growth medium (e.g., Eagle's medium plus fetal calf serum) containing antimicrobial agents to inhibit bacterial growth. Cells divide approximately once per day until a continuous monolayer is formed. At this point, the cell culture is ready for virus inoculation.

If a specific virus is being sought, inoculation of one or more cell lines known to support growth of the virus is all that is necessary. If an unknown virus or group of viruses is causing infection, cell lines capable of supporting the growth of a variety of candidate viruses should be inoculated. Cells are inoculated by pouring off the old growth medium, adding the specimen suspended in transport medium, and allowing the viruses to adsorb to the cells during incubation for 30 to 60 minutes at 35°C. The last step is to add maintenance medium to the cell cultures, return them to the 35°C incubator, and store any remaining specimen at −70°C in case cultures need to be reinoculated.

Cultures should be incubated and observed for **cytopathic effect (CPE)** (Fig. 13–7) for 2 to 3 weeks. Care must be taken to preserve the cell monolayer in a healthy state by periodically replacing the maintenance medium. CPE is best monitored by examination of the cell monolayer through an **inverted microscope.** CPE assumes many forms, including rounding of the cells, formation of syncytia (cell fusion), or cell destruction. Some viruses (e.g., influenza and parainfluenza viruses) cause hemadsorbing proteins to appear in the membranes of infected cells, and even though CPE may not be evident, areas of viral growth can still be identified. To detect hemadsorbing areas, the cell monolayer is flooded with an erythrocyte suspension, gently washed, and examined for erythrocyte adherence. Other methods for recognizing viral growth in

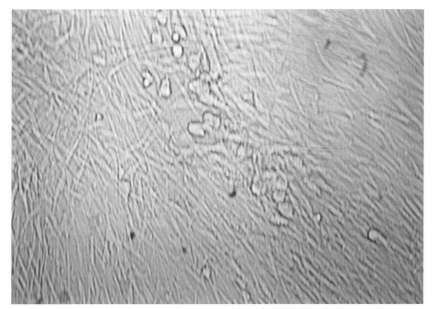

FIGURE 13–7. Cytopathic effect (CPE) due to replication of cytomegalovirus (CMV) in cell culture.

cell culture include staining for inclusion bodies, direct immunofluorescence or immunochemical staining for cell-associated viral antigens, and detection of hemagglutinating viruses in cell culture supernatants.

Some laboratories blindly passage negative cell cultures at least once to increase the yield of positive results. Cell monolayers are disrupted by agitation in the presence of tiny glass beads and then used to inoculate fresh cell cultures. The second set of cultures are incubated and examined in the manner described in the preceding paragraph.

For some viruses (e.g., cytomegalovirus, herpes simplex virus, the respiratory virus group), detection of positive cultures can be accelerated by use of the **shell vial technique.** Cell cultures are inoculated via high-speed centrifugation of the specimen onto a cell culture monolayer, usually growing on the surface of a small coverslip. The coverslip cultures are placed into small shell vials and incubated as described above. Shell vial cultures are examined after 24 to 120 hours of incubation for evidence of viral antigen production, usually via direct immunofluorescence.

The use of embryonated eggs and laboratory animals for diagnosis of viral infections is uncommon today, now that cell culture techniques are available for most viruses. Use of these hosts for propagation of large quantities of virus is still practiced in research laboratories and during the manufacture of vaccine immunogens.

Chlamydiae structurally resemble gram-negative bacteria but are unable to propagate extracellularly. They lack the ability to generate energy and depend on the host cell as a source for **adenosine triphosphate (ATP).** The life cycle of chlamydia is shown in Figure 13–8. The infectious stage is the **elementary body,** a small (0.25–0.35 μm in diameter) particle that preferentially adheres to and is taken up by mucosal columnar epithelial cells. A phagocytosed elementary body reorganizes into a metabolically active **reticulate body,** which undergoes several cycles of division to form multiple elementary bodies. The elementary bodies then leave the host cell and infect neighboring cells or susceptible cells in a new host.

Three species of chlamydia (*C. trachomatis, C. pneumoniae,* and *C.*

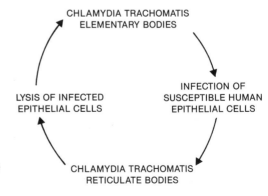

FIGURE 13–8. *Chlamydia* life cycle.

psittaci) are pathogenic for humans. A large number of serovarieties of *C. trachomatis* exist. The serovarieties that cause genital infections in sexually active individuals and ocular or respiratory infections in neonates are ubiquitous. Other serovarieties cause lymphogranuloma venereum and trachoma, a major cause of blindness in underdeveloped countries. *C. pneumoniae,* formerly known as the TWAR strain of *C. psittaci,* was recently recognized as a major cause of upper and lower respiratory tract infection in older children, young adults, and adults. Zoonotic *C. psittaci* is an important cause of infection in animals, particularly in birds, and is an occasional cause of severe lower respiratory tract infection in humans.

Only cultures for *C. trachomatis* are routinely available in clinical microbiology laboratories. *C. pneumoniae* can also be grown in culture, but very few laboratories offer this service yet on a routine basis. Most infections are identified either clinically or retrospectively via serodiagnosis. *C. psittaci* is extremely difficult to grow in the laboratory and diagnosis of infection is usually based on serologic evidence.

Specimens for *C. trachomatis* culture should be placed in *Chlamydia* transport medium (e.g., 2-sucrose phosphate broth) immediately after collection. Once in the laboratory, specimens are inoculated to cycloheximide-treated McCoy cell cultures by centrifugation of specimens onto the cells. After 48 to 72 hours of incubation at 35°C, cultures are examined for evidence of inclusion bodies by staining with Giemsa, iodine, or immunofluorescence reagents. Cultures negative at 72 hours may be blindly passaged by vortexing in the presence of tiny glass beads and reinoculating the supernatant to fresh cell cultures. The yield of positive cultures can be increased by as much as 10% by blind passage.

ANTIMICROBIAL SUSCEPTIBILITY TESTING

The global use of broad-spectrum antimicrobial agents during the previous two decades has in part led to the appearance of worrisome antimicrobial resistance (e.g., vancomycin-resistant staphylococci/ enterococci, third-generation cephalosporin-resistant gram-negative bacilli, penicillin/cephalosporin-resistant pneumococci). One of the essential functions of the microbiology laboratory is provision of antimicrobial susceptibility data for clinically significant microorganisms that do not have predictable responses to antimicrobial agents. These results guide clinicians in selecting appropriate specific antimicrobial therapy for eradication of infection. The agents suggested by laboratory data frequently replace expensive, broad-spectrum agents that were selected empirically. Aside from their high cost, the broad-spectrum agents often cause undesirable side effects when administered for extended periods of time.

There are two features of antimicrobial susceptibility testing to keep in mind:

1. The published standards that exist for antimicrobial susceptibility testing apply only to rapidly growing aerobic and anaerobic bacteria. Methods for testing fungi, parasites, and viruses have not been approved in final form by the agency responsible for overseeing such testing in the United States, the National Committee for Clinical Laboratory Standards (NCCLS). Therefore, the reproducibility of results from the same laboratory or the comparability of results from different laboratories for these types of organisms cannot be assured.
2. Antimicrobial susceptibility test results are obtained in a laboratory environment, which is different in many respects from the host environment. Thus, the laboratory results can only be assumed to predict the clinical efficacy of therapy, an assumption that clearly does not always hold.

BROTH DILUTION

The **broth dilution** method is considered the reference method for antimicrobial susceptibility testing. Its advantages are that it is quantitative rather than qualitative, both inhibitory and bactericidal antimicrobial activities can be measured, and the method is adaptable to miniaturization and automation. The latter advantage has led to development of a number of instrument-based systems capable of furnishing antimicrobial susceptibility data in as little as 4 hours.

Minimum Inhibitory Concentration Determination

The **minimum inhibitory concentration (MIC)** of an antimicrobial agent is the lowest concentration of the agent tested that inhibits visible growth of the organism (visible either by eye or instrumentation). Knowledge of the antimicrobial agent MIC, the route of administration, and the clinically achievable levels of the antimicrobial agent at the site of infection enables one to classify the organism as **susceptible (S)**, **intermediate (I)**, or **resistant (R)** to the antimicrobial agent in question.

The MIC of an antimicrobial agent may be determined in a series of test tubes, each containing growth medium plus stepwise concentrations of the antimicrobial agent. Alternatively, the MIC may be determined using the same principle in a miniaturized format (e.g., the wells of a microtiter tray or the tiny chambers within a clear plastic card). An exponentially growing broth culture or freshly prepared suspension from an overnight agar culture is used as the source of the inoculum. The inoculum is prepared by diluting the suspension sufficiently to yield a final density of 3 to 7×10^5 cfu/mL. The NCCLS-recommended media and incubation conditions follow:

- Nonfastidious bacteria are inoculated to cation-adjusted Mueller-Hinton broth and incubated aerobically for 16 to 20 hours at 35°C.
- *Staphylococcus* sp isolates being tested for methicillin/oxacillin/nafcillin resistance are inoculated from suspensions prepared from overnight agar cultures only. Suspensions are inoculated to cation-adjusted Mueller-Hinton broth supplemented with 2% NaCl. Oxacillin is the preferred agent for in vitro testing; results with oxacillin apply to all three agents. Tests are incubated aerobically for a full 24 hours at 30 to 35°C.
- *Enterococcus* isolates being tested for vancomycin resistance are inoculated to cation-adjusted Mueller-Hinton broth and incubated aerobically for a full 24 hours at 35°C.
- *Haemophilus influenzae* isolates are inoculated from suspensions prepared from overnight agar cultures only. Suspensions are inoculated to Haemophilus Test Medium and incubated aerobically for 20 to 24 hours at 35°C.
- *Streptococcus pneumoniae* and other *Streptococcus* sp isolates are inoculated from suspensions prepared from overnight agar cultures only. Suspensions are inoculated to cation-adjusted Mueller-Hinton broth supplemented with 2 to 5% lysed horse blood and incubated aerobically for 20 to 24 hours at 35°C.
- *Neisseria meningitidis* isolates are inoculated from suspensions prepared from overnight agar cultures only. Suspensions are inoculated to cation-adjusted Mueller-Hinton broth supplemented with 2 to 5% lysed horse blood and incubated for 24 hours at 35°C in an aerobic atmosphere containing 5% CO_2.
- *Listeria* sp isolates are inoculated from suspensions prepared from overnight agar cultures only. Suspensions are inoculated to cation-adjusted Mueller-Hinton broth supplemented with 2 to 5% lysed horse blood and incubated aerobically for 18 hours at 35°C.
- *Mycobacterium fortuitum* and *Mycobacterium chelonei* are inoculated to cation-adjusted Mueller-Hinton broth and incubated aerobically for 72 hours at 30°C.

The MIC is determined by visual or instrument-assisted examination of the test cultures for turbidity (Color Plate 75).

The reliability of antimicrobial susceptibility results from some instrument-based systems using rapid broth microdilution has become an issue in recent years. In fact, some manufacturers have issued warnings concerning the accuracy of their systems in determining the susceptibility of enterococci to ampicillin and vancomycin and pneumococci to beta-lactam agents. Users of these systems should maintain contact with manufacturers regarding these limitations. In addition, users must be vigilant in recognizing problems with other combinations of organisms and antimicrobial agents.

Minimum Bactericidal Concentration Determination

The **minimum bactericidal concentration (MBC)** of an antimicrobial agent is the lowest concentration of the agent that kills at least 99.9% of the original organism inoculum. Tubes or wells displaying no visible growth during an MIC determination are subcultured to determine their viable counts. If the ratio of the number of survivors to the number in the original inoculum is less than or equal to 0.001, killing has occurred; if the ratio is greater than 0.001, killing has not occurred.

In managing the antimicrobial therapy of bacterial infections, it is not necessary for clinicians to request antimicrobial MBCs routinely. Because the bactericidal properties of most antimicrobial agents are well known, qualitative disk diffusion or quantitative MIC results are usually sufficient to select appropriate antimicrobial therapy.

The bactericidal properties of beta-lactam and glycopeptide antimicrobial agents versus staphylococci, streptococci, and enterococci, however, are not always predictable, owing to the phenomenon known as **antimicrobial tolerance.** The physiologic basis for tolerance is attributed to the lack of autolytic enzyme activity in organisms whose cell wall synthesis has been inhibited. Ordinarily, it is the weakening and eventual rupturing of existing cell wall by autolytic enzymes that is responsible for the killing of affected organisms.

The most frequently used definition of antimicrobial tolerance is an MBC:MIC ratio greater than 32. When organisms are clinically tolerant to an antimicrobial agent, the MIC would suggest susceptibility and the MBC would predict resistance. The correlation between laboratory detection of antimicrobial tolerance and poor therapeutic outcome is strong enough for most clinicians to alter their choice of antimicrobial therapy when tolerance is reported.

AGAR DILUTION

The **agar dilution** method is another means of determining antimicrobial agent MICs. This method is well suited for testing large groups of isolates versus identical ranges of antimicrobial agent concentrations. One disadvantage of the method is the inability to determine antimicrobial MBCs following MIC determinations.

The agar dilution method requires the availability of agar test media with each plate containing antimicrobial agents at different concentrations. Preparation of these plates in-house is labor intensive and feasible only for larger, well-staffed laboratories. Manufactured plates are available from commercial sources at even higher cost.

An exponentially growing broth culture or freshly prepared suspension from an overnight agar culture is used as the source of the inoculum. Suspensions of test organisms are prepared and adjusted to a turbidity standard. The inoculum is prepared from dilutions of standardized suspensions so that approximately 1×10^4 colony forming units of each organism are transferred to agar plates. Transfer of test isolates may be accomplished one-by-one using a calibrated loop or may proceed simultaneously in groups of 32 to 36 isolates, using a multipronged device like the Steers replicator. The inoculum spot should contain 1 to 2 μL of organism suspension spread over an area 5 to 8 mm in diameter.

- Nonfastidious bacteria are inoculated to Mueller-Hinton agar and incubated aerobically for 16 to 20 hours at 35°C.
- *Staphylococcus* sp isolates being tested for methicillin/oxacillin/nafcillin resistance are inoculated from suspensions prepared from overnight agar cultures only. Suspensions are inoculated to Mueller-Hinton agar supplemented with 2% NaCl. Oxacillin is the preferred agent for in vitro testing; results with oxacillin apply to all three agents. Tests are incubated aerobically for a full 24 hours at 30 to 35°C.
- *Enterococcus* isolates being tested for vancomycin resistance are inoculated to Mueller-Hinton agar and incubated aerobically for a full 24 hours at 35°C.
- *Haemophilus influenzae* isolates are inoculated from suspensions prepared from overnight agar cultures only. Suspensions are inoculated to Haemophilus Test Medium and incubated aerobically for 20 to 24 hours at 35°C.
- *Streptococcus pneumoniae* and other *Streptococcus* sp isolates are inoculated from suspensions prepared from overnight agar cultures only. Suspensions are inoculated to Mueller-Hinton agar supplemented with 5% defibrinated sheep blood and incubated aerobically (+5% CO_2 if needed for growth) for 20 to 24 hours at 35°C.
- *Neisseria gonorrhoeae* isolates are inoculated from suspensions prepared from overnight agar cultures only. Suspensions are inoculated to GC agar containing 1% defined supplement and incubated for 20 to 24 hours at 35°C in an aerobic atmosphere containing 5% CO_2 (a cysteine-free supplement is necessary for testing with carbapenems and clavulanate).
- *Neisseria meningitidis* isolates are inoculated from suspensions prepared from overnight agar cultures only. Suspensions are inoculated to Mueller-Hinton agar supplemented with 5% defibrinated sheep blood and incubated for 24 hours at 35°C in an aerobic atmosphere containing 5% CO_2 (2 to 5% lysed horse blood is necessary for testing with sulfonamides).

The MIC is the lowest antimicrobial concentration that inhibits visible growth on the agar surface. A barely visible haze or growth of a single colony should be ignored.

AGAR DIFFUSION

The advantages of the **agar disk diffusion test** (Kirby-Bauer method) include a greater flexibility in selecting agents to be tested, the ease with which mixed cultures can be recognized, and its relatively low cost.

In this method, an exponentially growing broth culture or freshly prepared suspension from an overnight agar culture of a clinically significant isolate is used as the inoculum. The density of the organisms in the inoculum is adjusted to match that of a turbidity standard (McFarland 0.5). The suspension is inoculated to an agar plate with an inoculum-moistened swab. Filter paper disks 6 millimeters in diameter, impregnated with antimicrobial agents, are applied to the agar surface. The NCCLS-recommended media and incubation conditions follow:

- Nonfastidious bacteria are inoculated to Mueller-Hinton agar and incubated aerobically for 16 to 18 hours at 35°C.
- *Staphylococcus* sp isolates being tested for methicillin/oxacillin/nafcillin resistance are inoculated from suspensions prepared from overnight agar cultures only. Suspensions are inoculated to Mueller-Hinton agar with application of an oxacillin disk (serves as a class disk for all three agents) and incubated aerobically for a full 24 hours at 35°C.
- *Enterococcus* isolates being tested for vancomycin resistance are inoculated to Mueller-Hinton agar and incubated aerobically for a full 24 hours at 35°C.
- *Haemophilus influenzae* isolates are inoculated from suspensions prepared from overnight agar cultures only. Suspensions are inoculated to Haemophilus Test Medium and incubated for 16 to 18 hours at 35°C in an aerobic atmosphere containing 5% CO_2.
- *Streptococcus pneumoniae* isolates are inoculated from suspensions prepared from overnight agar cultures only. Suspensions are inoculated to Mueller-Hinton agar supplemented with 5% defibrinated sheep blood and incubated for 20 to 24 hours at 35°C in an aerobic atmosphere containing 5% CO_2.
- *Neisseria gonorrhoeae* isolates are inoculated from suspensions prepared from overnight agar cultures only. Suspensions are inoculated to GC agar with a 1% defined growth supplement and incubated for 20 to 24 hours at 35°C in an aerobic atmosphere containing 5% CO_2.

Other than the exceptions specified above, the use of a CO_2-enriched atmosphere is contraindicated for most bacteria because of the effect that a lower pH has on the activities of certain antimicrobial agents.

During test incubation, the antimicrobial agents diffuse into the agar in a radial fashion, so that a concentration gradient is established. Within the first few hours of incubation, the interaction that occurs between the changing antimicrobial agent concentration and the increasing numbers of bacteria on the agar surface determines the ultimate size of the zone of inhibition around each disk (Color Plate 76). After incubation, the diameters of the zones of inhibition are measured and compared to a reference chart. The reference chart lists zone diameter breakpoints that translate antimicrobial activity to susceptible (S), intermediately susceptible (I), or resistant (R) categories.

A variant of the agar disk diffusion method that is growing in popularity is the **E test** method, which uses a calibrated rectangular plastic strip impregnated with an antimicrobial agent concentration gradient. The test is performed in the same manner as the agar disk diffusion method with resultant formation of an elliptical rather than circular zone of growth inhibition. The intersection of the zone with the strip indicates the antimicrobial MIC by referring to the calibrated value at that strip location. The E test can be used for testing the same spectrum of bacteria as the agar disk diffusion method. In addition, E test methods for anaerobic bacteria, yeasts, and mycobacteria have been described. None of the E test methods have yet been sanctioned by the NCCLS.

BETA-LACTAMASE TEST

The beta-lactam class of antimicrobial agents includes the penicillins and cephalosporins. The most common mechanism of resistance to this class is bacterial production of an enzyme that inactivates the antimicrobial agent by breaking the beta-lactam ring.

The **beta-lactamase test** is a rapid means of determining whether an isolate produces beta-lactamase. However, it should be remembered that bacteria may be resistant to beta-lactam agents by mechanisms completely unrelated to beta-lactamase production. Thus, a positive result indicates resistance, but a negative result does not guarantee susceptibility.

The test is performed by exposing a beta-lactam substrate to the organism. The assay in general use today is the **chromogenic cephalosporin test.** The substrates used in this test (usually nitrocefin or PADAC) change color when their beta-lactam rings are broken. The test is performed by adding a heavy suspension of the test isolate to buffered chromogenic substrate (liquid or impregnated in filter paper), incubating for up to 10 minutes at room temperature, and observing for a color change.

SPECIAL TESTS

Occasional clinical situations warrant requests for nonroutine tests involving antimicrobial agents. The laboratory's ability to accommodate such requests varies with the difficulty of the test procedure and the level of staffing and sophistication of the laboratory. Generally, laboratories unable to perform requested testing in-house forward isolates or specimens to reference laboratories for testing. Following are some of the more common nonroutine test requests.

Anaerobic Susceptibility Testing

In most situations, testing of anaerobic gram-negative rods for beta-lactamase production is all that is necessary to guide antimicrobial management of anaerobic infections. However, in regions with high endemic rates of antimicrobial resistance or when individual patients fail seemingly appropriate antimicrobial therapy, it may be necessary to provide more comprehensive data.

The NCCLS-standardized method for anaerobic susceptibility testing is the agar dilution method described earlier in this chapter. Broth dilution MIC methods performed in test tubes or in microtiter trays and the E test method may also be performed.

An easier method that was widely performed by laboratories that do not perform large numbers of anaerobic susceptibility tests was the *broth-disk elution procedure.* However, this method is no longer endorsed by the NCCLS as providing accurate, reproducible results and will not be described here.

Mycobacterial Susceptibility Testing

The reference susceptibility test method is the **agar disk elution assay** (elution of antimicrobial agents from disks immersed in agar). Suspensions of mycobacteria at known cell densities are inoculated to media containing antimycobacterial agents at clinically relevant concentrations. After suitable incubation, the number of colonies growing on antimycobacterial agent–containing agar is determined. If the count is less than 1% of the number observed on growth control agar, then the isolate is considered susceptible. Colony numbers greater than 1% of the control indicate resistance.

A more rapid method for mycobacterial susceptibility testing that has become more popular than the agar disk elution technique involves the use of **radiometry.** Isolates are inoculated to antimycobacterial agent–containing broth media supplemented with ^{14}C-labeled growth substrates. The quantitative release of $^{14}CO_2$ during growth is compared radiometrically to that occurring in a control antimycobacterial agent–free broth. The advantage of the radiometric method is that results can be obtained in a matter of days rather than weeks.

Fungal Susceptibility Testing

Although broth dilution, agar dilution, disk diffusion, and E test procedures for susceptibility testing of fungi have been described, none have yet been designated by the NCCLS as an approved reference method. At the time of this writing, provisional status has been granted by the NCCLS to a broth macrodilution method for testing of yeasts.

Clinicians should be aware that the predictive value of antifungal susceptibility test results may be low because of problems inherent in the test methods themselves.

Antimicrobial Agent Synergy Testing

When two or more antimicrobial agents are administered simultaneously to a patient, the effect of the combination may be additive, antagonistic, or synergistic. An **additive effect** is noted when the antimicrobial activity of the combination equals the sum of the activities exhibited by the agents individually. An **antagonistic effect** is observed when the activity of the combination is markedly less than the sum of the individual activities. A **synergistic effect** is observed when the activity of the combination is markedly greater than the sum of the individual activities. Under most circumstances, clinicians administering antimicrobial agents in combination rely on their own experience or the experience of others in the medical literature to guide patient management. On rare occasions, however, it may be necessary to test a patient's isolate versus an antimicrobial agent combination. Such testing is difficult, time consuming, and expensive, and should be performed only when results are medically necessary.

The **checkerboard titration method** of antimicrobial agent synergy testing is usually performed in microtiter trays. The MICs and MBCs of two antimicrobial agents are determined individually and in combination by testing the isolate versus stepwise concentrations of the agents alone and versus the stepwise concentration combinations of the agents together. Synergy is observed when the MIC/MBC of one or both of the agents is reduced by at least four-fold in the presence of a subinhibitory or subbactericidal concentration of the other agent (Fig. 13–9).

The **killing curve method** of antimicrobial agent synergy testing is performed in broth culture. The viability of the test organism following exposure to each antimicrobial agent is compared to its viability following exposure to the antimicrobial agents in combination. The killing curve is constructed by plotting the number of surviving bacteria in each culture versus time. Antimicrobial agent synergy is defined as observing at least ten-fold fewer survivors in the culture containing the agents in combination than in either of the cultures containing the agents individually (Fig. 13–10).

Body Fluid Bactericidal Activity Determination

Data correlating the bactericidal activity of serum with the outcome of antimicrobial therapy exist for patients with endocarditis, osteomyelitis, bacteremia (immunocompromised patients), and meningitis. Clinical correlative data do not exist for patients with other infectious diseases;

SYNERGY, ADDITIVITY AND ANTAGONISM
DEPICTION BY ISOBOLOGRAM

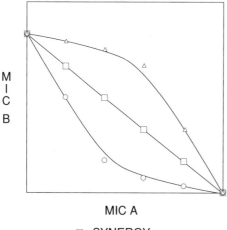

MIC A

□ SYNERGY
○ ADDITIVITY
△ ANTAGONISM

MICB

FIGURE 13–9. Antimicrobial synergy, additivity, and antagonism as determined by checkerboard titration. The MIC or MBC of antimicrobial B in the presence of varying concentrations of antimicrobial A is plotted. The resultant graph is termed *isobologram.* If the isobologram bows inward toward the origin, synergy of the two antimicrobial agents is indicated. If the isobologram bows outward, away from the origin, antagonism is indicated. If the isobologram is a straight line, additivity is indicated.

therefore the test should not be performed in those situations. If the purpose is to determine that an antimicrobial agent is achieving therapeutic levels in a fluid at the site of infection (e.g., cerebrospinal fluid in a patient with a neurosurgical shunt-associated infection), determination of a **body fluid bactericidal titer** may be helpful.

The **serum bactericidal test** is performed on sera collected just prior to antimicrobial agent administration **(trough specimen)** and 30 to 90 minutes after administration (depending on the route of administration and the antimicrobial agent) **(peak specimen).** In the laboratory, the sera are serially diluted in two-fold steps using sterile, antimicrobial-free, pooled human serum as the diluent. Pooled human serum is used to maintain a stable concentration of antimicrobial agent–binding serum proteins in each tube. Next, a turbidity-adjusted suspension of the patient's isolate is added to each dilution tube and to a growth control tube containing no antimicrobial activity. The density of organisms in each tube should approximate 5×10^5 cfu/mL, and a viable count of the inoculum suspension should be performed to determine the actual density. The tubes are incubated at 35°C for 20 hours in an organism-appropriate atmosphere. The tubes are then shaken by hand to suspend organisms that may have escaped exposure to antimicrobial activity by adhering to the walls of the tube; next, it is reincubated for 4 additional hours. At this point, the **serum inhibitory titer** is obtained by

SYNERGISM, ADDITIVITY AND ANTAGONISM
DEPICTION BY KILLING CURVES

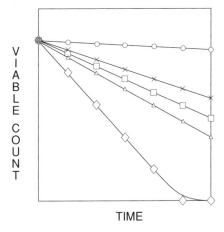

TIME

× ANTIBIOTIC B ALONE
□ ANTIBIOTIC A ALONE
○ A + B (ANTAGONISM)
△ A + B (ADDITIVITY)
◇ A + B (SYNERGY)

FIGURE 13–10. Antimicrobial synergy, additivity, and antagonism as determined by killing curve analysis. The viable count of the test organism is determined serially with time in the presence of antimicrobial agent A alone, antimicrobial agent B alone, and antimicrobial agents A + B. If the viable count in the presence of antimicrobial agents A + B is more than one log (90%) less than the viable counts in the presence of antimicrobial agents A and B alone, the combination is considered synergistic. If the viable count in the presence of antimicrobial agents A + B is more than one log (ten-fold) greater than the viable counts in the presence of antimicrobial agents A and B alone, the combination is considered antagonistic. If the viable count in the presence of antimicrobial agents A + B is within ±1 log of the viable counts in the presence of antimicrobial agents A or B alone, the combination is considered additive.

determining the highest dilution of serum that inhibited visible growth of the organism. Tubes exhibiting no visible growth are subcultured (0.1 mL) to blood or chocolate agar and incubated for 24 hours. Finally, the number of colonies present in each subculture is counted, and the **serum bactericidal titer** is reported as the highest dilution of serum that killed at least 99.9% of the original inoculum.

Studies correlating serum bactericidal test results with clinical outcome in patients with endocarditis revealed that peak serum bactericidal titers greater than or equal to 1:64 and trough titers greater than or equal to 1:32 predicted bacteriologic cure. Peak and trough titers as low as 1:8

usually predicted a successful outcome, but bacteriologic failures also occurred. The test results could not be used to predict bacteriologic failure.

In patients with acute osteomyelitis, studies indicated that the peak serum bactericidal titer had no predictive value, but the trough titer predicted bacteriologic cure at titers greater than or equal to 1:2. Trough titers less than 1:2 predicted bacteriologic failure. The interpretation of results was very different in patients with chronic osteomyelitis. Peak serum bactericidal titers greater than or equal to 1:16 and trough titers greater than or equal to 1:4 accurately predicted bacteriologic cure, and peak titers less than 1:16 and trough titers less than 1:4 predicted failure. In summary, acute osteomyelitis patients should have serum bactericidal titers greater than or equal to 1:2, and chronic osteomyelitis patients should have serum bactericidal titers greater than or equal to 1:4 throughout the course of their therapy.

For patients with other infections, studies correlating serum bactericidal titers with clinical outcome are incomplete. In general, peak titers greater than or equal to 1:32 and trough titers greater than or equal to 1:8 are considered satisfactory.

Measurement of Antimicrobial Agent Levels

Some antimicrobial agents (e.g., the aminoglycosides, chloramphenicol, vancomycin, 5-fluorocytosine) have narrow therapeutic- to toxic-level ratios, or rapidly accumulate to toxic levels in patients with renal or hepatic dysfunction. It is essential to monitor the levels of these antimicrobial agents during therapy so that necessary dose adjustments can be made before the patient is harmed.

The levels of most of these antimicrobial agents can be monitored with rapid, very accurate **instrument-based immunoassays.** The physical location of the test instrument may not be in the microbiology laboratory because the levels of other serum analytes often can be measured with the same instrument. See Chapter 18, dealing with therapeutic drug monitoring, for more information about the assays themselves.

For antimicrobial agents that cannot be measured with automated immunoassays, **bioassays** or **high-pressure liquid chromatography** assays can be devised.

The key component of the bioassay is the indicator organism, which must be susceptible to the agent being measured, yet resistant to other antimicrobial agents in the specimen that cannot be inactivated or neutralized beforehand. To perform the bioassay, the indicator organism is added to molten agar that has been allowed to cool to 45 to 50°C, and the mixture poured into a Petri plate. After the agar has hardened, the patient's serum and a series of antimicrobial standards are added to the agar, either in cylindrical wells cut into the agar or adsorbed in filter paper disks applied to the surface of the agar. The plates are incubated at 35°C in an aerobic atmosphere for as long a period as is necessary to visualize measurable zones of growth inhibition around the wells or filter paper disks. The diameters of the zones around the antimicrobial standards are used to construct a linear regression equation or a linear standard curve on semilogarithmic graph paper. The antimicrobial concentration in the patient's specimen can then be calculated by use of the equation or by plotting values on the standard curve.

The use of high-pressure liquid chromatography to measure antimicrobial agent concentrations in serum is similar to use of the same method to measure other drugs. See Chapter 18 for further information.

SUGGESTED READING

Baron, EJ, et al: Classification and identification of bacteria. In Murray, PR, et al (eds): Manual of Clinical Microbiology, ed 6. American Society for Microbiology, Washington DC, 1995, pp 249–266.

Baron, EJ, Peterson, LR, and Finegold, SM: Bailey and Scott's Diagnostic Microbiology, ed 9. Mosby, St Louis, 1994.

Doern, GV: Susceptibility tests of fastidious bacteria. In Murray, PR, et al (eds): Manual of Clinical Microbiology, ed 6. American Society for Microbiology, Washington DC, 1995, pp 1342–1349.

Espinel-Ingroff, A, and Pfaller, MA: Antifungal agents and susceptibility testing. In Murray, PR, et al (eds): Manual of Clinical Microbiology, ed 6. American Society for Microbiology, Washington DC, 1995, pp 1405–1414.

Forbes, BA, and Granato, PA: Processing specimens for bacteria. In Murray, PR, et al (eds): Manual of Clinical Microbiology, ed 6. American Society for Microbiology, Washington DC, 1995, pp 265–281.

Garcia, LS, and Bruckner, DA: Diagnostic Medical Parasitology, ed 2. American Society for Microbiology, Washington DC, 1993.

Garcia, LS, et al: Diagnosis of parasitic infections: Collection, processing, and examination of specimens. In Murray, PR, et al (eds): Manual of Clinical Microbiology, ed 6. American Society for Microbiology, Washington DC, 1995, pp 1145–1158.

Herrmann, JE: Immunoassays for diagnosis of infectious diseases. In Murray, PR, et al (eds): Manual of Clinical Microbiology, ed 6. American Society for Microbiology, Washington DC, 1995, pp 110–122.

Howard, BJ (ed): Clinical and Pathogenic Microbiology, ed 2. Mosby, St Louis, 1994.

Inderlied, CB, and Salfinger, M: Antimicrobial agents and susceptibility tests: Mycobacteria. In Murray, PR, et al (eds): Manual of Clinical Microbiology, ed 6. American Society for Microbiology, Washington DC, 1995, pp 1385–1404.

Isenberg, HD, and D'Amato, RF: Indigenous and pathogenic microorganisms of humans. In Murray, PR, et al (eds): Manual of Clinical Microbiology, ed 6. American Society for Microbiology, Washington DC, 1995, pp 5–18.

Lennette, DA: Collection and preparation of specimens for virological examination. In Murray, PR, et al (eds): Manual of Clinical Microbiology, ed 6. American Society for Microbiology, Washington DC, 1995, pp 868–875.

Merz, WG, and Roberts, GD: Detection and recovery of fungi from clinical specimens. In Murray, PR, et al (eds): Manual of Clinical Microbiology, ed 6. American Society for Microbiology, Washington DC, 1995, pp 709–722.

Miller, JM, and Holmes, HH: Specimen collection, transport, and storage. In Murray, PR, et al (eds): Manual of Clinical Microbiology, ed 6. American Society for Microbiology, Washington DC, 1995, pp 19–32.

Podzorski, RP, and Persing, DH: Molecular detection and identification of microorganisms. In Murray, PR, et al (eds): Manual of Clinical Microbiology, ed 6. American Society for Microbiology, Washington DC, 1995, pp 130–157.

Quintiliani, R, and Courvalin, P: Mechanisms of resistance to antimicrobial agents. In Murray, PR, et al (eds): Manual of Clinical Microbiology, ed 6. American Society for Microbiology, Washington, DC, 1995, pp 1308–1326.

Rippon, JW: Medical Mycology: The Pathogenic Fungi and the Pathogenic Actinomycetes, ed 3. W.B. Saunders, Philadelphia, 1988.

Sherris, JC (ed): Medical Microbiology: An Introduction to Infectious Diseases, ed 2. Elsevier Science, New York, 1990.

Specter, S, and Lancz, GJ: Clinical Virology Manual. Elsevier Science, New York, 1986.

Summanen, P, et al: Wadsworth Anaerobic Bacteriology Manual, ed 5. Star, Belmont, CA, 1993.

Wexler, HM, and Doern, GV: Susceptibility testing of anaerobic bacteria. In Murray, PR, et al (eds): Manual of Clinical Microbiology, ed 6. American Society for Microbiology, Washington DC, 1995, pp 1350–1355.

Woods, GL, and Washington, JA: Antibacterial susceptibility tests: Dilution and disk diffusion methods. In Murray, PR, et al (eds): Manual of Clinical Microbiology, ed 6. American Society for Microbiology, Washington DC, 1995, pp 1327–1341.

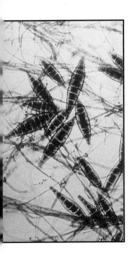

14

Systematic Clinical Microbiology

Laboratory options exist for diagnosis of infection by body site. The nine specimen types received with the highest frequency by most microbiology laboratories are shown in Table 14–1.

BLOODSTREAM SPECIMENS

Almost all clinically important bacteria and fungi are able to access the bloodstream and, in some circumstances, produce life-endangering infection. Although hospital-based microbiology laboratories are usually able to detect these agents, the cost of using optimal methods for recovery of all pathogen groups is prohibitive. For these reasons, it is vital that effective channels of communication exist between clinicians and the laboratory when uncommonly encountered organisms with unique growth requirements are suspected. Similarly, the laboratory must be notified when departures from standard blood culture techniques are necessary (e.g., extended incubation or use of specialized growth media).

The age of the patient is an essential consideration. The list of microorganisms that commonly cause bloodstream infections in children overlaps greatly with that of adults, but there are some important differences. For example, the incidence of *Streptococcus pneumoniae*, Group

661

TABLE 14–1. CATEGORIES OF SPECIMENS MOST OFTEN PROCESSED BY THE CLINICAL MICROBIOLOGY LABORATORY

1. Bloodstream specimens
2. Body fluids
3. Urine
4. Respiratory tract specimens
5. Genital tract specimens
6. Gastrointestinal tract specimens
7. Cutaneous specimens
8. Wound, tissue/biopsy specimens
9. Eye/ear specimens

B *Streptococcus,* and *Salmonella* bacteremia is distinctly higher in children, while the frequency of anaerobic bacteremia and polymicrobial bacteremia is higher in adults. Knowledge of the patient's age helps the laboratory recognize age group–associated pathogens.

The underlying medical problems of patients are a major factor. Immunodeficient patients, as a group, are susceptible to bloodstream infections with microorganisms that rarely invade the normal host. Fungal infections due to *Aspergillus fumigatus, A. flavus, Candida albicans, C. tropicalis, C. krusei, Cryptococcus neoformans,* and *Pseudallescheria boydii* are not uncommon in such patients. *Mycobacterium tuberculosis* and *M. avium* complex organisms are recovered from the blood of acquired immunodeficiency syndrome (AIDS) patients much more often than from other patients. Asplenic patients of all ages are more susceptible to infection by encapsulated bacteria like *Haemophilus influenzae* type b, *S. pneumoniae, N. meningitidis,* and *Klebsiella pneumoniae.* Patients with sickle-cell disease experience higher rates of invasive *Salmonella* infections.

Patients with intravenous lines in place for more than 48 hours are at risk of catheter-associated sepsis caused by microorganisms colonizing the skin. In such individuals, recovery of coagulase-negative staphylococci from blood should not be dismissed automatically as a skin contaminant. Nonfermentative gram-negative bacilli (e.g., *Acinetobacter* spp) and *Candida* spp (e.g., *C. parapsilosis*) are occasional causes of catheter-associated sepsis. Among neonates receiving intravenous lipid nutritional supplements, the fatty-acid-requiring yeast, *Malassezia furfur,* is a well-known nosocomial pathogen.

MICROSCOPY

Because of the low numbers of microorganisms present in the blood of most infected patients, microscopic examination of smears plays little, if any, role in diagnosis. Microorganisms occasionally can be seen in buffy coat (white blood cell fraction) or white blood cell differential smears. The likelihood of finding microorganisms, however, is low, and the probability of misleading results is high. Therefore, the predictive value of positive or negative smears is low, and microscopy cannot be recommended as a routine procedure.

The test of choice for diagnosis of blood-borne parasitic infections is examination of Giemsa- or Wright-stained blood films. Both thick and thin blood smears should be examined before ruling out the diagnosis (see Chapter 13).

ANTIGEN DETECTION

Confirmation of bloodstream infection by antigen detection methods has been unsatisfactory. First, the list of microorganisms for which commercially available reagents exist is very short. Second, of those microorganisms for which reagents do exist, the concentration of antigen in blood is frequently below the lower limit of assay sensitivity. Last, detection of antigen in blood offers little benefit to patient care. Therapeutic decisions usually await antimicrobial susceptibility test results from culture isolates.

CULTURE

Identification of bloodstream pathogens is accomplished chiefly by culture. Several blood culture methods are in current use, each with its advantages and disadvantages. Selection of a method is influenced by several factors, notably the age of the patient population, availability of funds for capital equipment, and laboratory staffing levels during the evening, night, and weekend/holiday work shifts. In some laboratories, the decision has been to use a combination of methods to maximize the advantages of each.

Conventional broth culture was the most convenient blood culture method for many years and was used by nearly all laboratories. New techniques developed over the last 25 years have convinced most users to replace or at least supplement conventional broth culture methods. Several of the methods are described below.

Conventional Broth Culture

Conventional broth culture methods call for inoculating blood to liquid media contained in bottles or tubes. There are many different media from which to choose, and most are available commercially. Cultures are incubated aerobically or anaerobically for 7 to 14 days at 35°C.

They are examined visually every day for evidence of growth (e.g., turbidity, gas production, and adherent colonies on the walls of the vessel) (Color Plate 77). In addition, blind subcultures to agar media or blind smears for Gram or acridine orange staining are prepared at scheduled intervals.

Conventional broth culture has features that are ideal for some laboratories. The methods are not solely relics of the past. Its advantages include the thoroughness with which the methods have been investigated and the flexibility afforded by the variety of media available. Virtually all parameters of these methods have been investigated. These include comparative yields from growth media prepared by different manufacturers, the optimal ratio of blood to broth, the effect of different anticoagulants on culture results, and the ideal times for performing blind subcultures.

The disadvantages of conventional broth culture are that the method is labor intensive, cultures are examined only 1 or 2 times per day, and subcultures to agar media are necessary to perform definitive identification and antimicrobial susceptibility testing. Some laboratories inoculate identification and antimicrobial susceptibility tests directly from suspensions of centrifuged broth sediments to obtain preliminary results. Results of these tests should be considered tentative until they are confirmed by standardized procedures.

Infrared Spectroscopic Broth Culture

The first inroad of automation into blood culturing occurred with development of the radiometric broth culture method. Blood was inoculated to broth culture media containing ^{14}C-labeled growth substrates. Evolution of $^{14}CO_2$ occurred during microbial growth, which was detected in bottles by instrument sampling of the atmosphere. Heeding the reluctance of customers to deal with radioactive media, the manufacturer developed a series of instruments that detect CO_2 by infrared spectroscopy. Cultures are incubated 5 to 7 days at 35°C.

The advantages of this approach are the same as for the radiometric system without the concern over disposal of radioactive waste. One advantage is that the method lends itself to instrumentation and automation. Instrument-assisted sampling of bottles for CO_2 relieves laboratory workers of having to prepare blind subcultures or smears. Positive cultures are identified by the instrument, confirmed by Gram- or acridine orange–stained smear, and subcultured to agar media. A second advantage is that instrument-detected positive cultures are usually recognized several hours before conventional broth cultures. Thus, clinicians can be notified earlier, and necessary clinical interventions can occur more rapidly. The instruments can be interfaced to laboratory information systems for electronic transfer of patient data.

The disadvantages of these systems include the cost of the instruments and the infrequency of blood culture monitoring compared to continuously monitored broth culture systems.

Continuously Monitored Broth Culture

The state of the art today is the continuously monitored blood culture instrument. These instruments enable automatic assessment of blood cultures for evidence of growth. Since cultures are checked several times per hour, clinicians can be notified of positive blood cultures within minutes of detectable growth. Systems are available from several manufacturers and identify microbial growth by detecting CO_2 production (via pH sensors or fluorescence detection) and/or gas consumption from the atmosphere of the bottle. Cultures routinely are incubated for 5 to 7 days at 35°C.

These systems have many advantages, including all of those cited for the radiometric and infrared spectroscopic systems. Each bottle location within the incubator cabinet contains a monitoring sensor, so bottles need not be manipulated during incubation. Bottles are untouched until they show evidence of growth or are ready for discarding. The continuous monitoring facilitates more rapid detection of positive cultures than with the other techniques. Management decisions regarding antimicrobial therapy can be made earlier.

Perhaps the only disadvantages of these systems are the higher costs of both the monitoring system and the proprietary sensor-compatible blood culture bottles.

Biphasic Agar/Broth Culture

The **biphasic agar/broth culture** method (Castenada bottle) has long been recommended for detection of *Brucella* and filamentous fungi in blood. The method also works well for detection of routine pathogens. It was never widely used because the bottles were difficult to prepare and were not commercially available at an affordable price. A modification of the Castenada bottle approach has been available for a number of years. The product features an agar-coated plastic paddle enclosed in a cylindrical container. The paddle is screwed onto a blood culture bottle after the bottle has been inoculated. The bottle is inverted at periodic intervals to inoculate the paddle and then reincubated. Positive cultures are identified by seeing growth of colonies on the agar surface.

The main attraction of the biphasic agar/broth culture is the ease with which subcultures can be made. Technologist time ordinarily spent on subculturing blood culture bottles can be used elsewhere in the laboratory. Furthermore, the method is superior to the broth culture methods for recovery of filamentous fungi from patients with disseminated infection.

A significant disadvantage of the biphasic agar/broth system is the risk of contamination when agar paddles are attached. Oxygen also enters the bottles during the process, lessening the likelihood of recovering anaerobes. A separate, anaerobically incubated culture must be set up to rule out the presence of strict anaerobes. The combined expense of a biphasic agar/broth culture and an anaerobic culture is too high for many laboratories to bear.

Lysis Centrifugation/Direct Plating

Two related blood culture techniques are the lysis centrifugation and lysis direct plating methods. In **lysis centrifugation,** 10 mL of blood is collected in a tube containing a proprietary detergent-like reagent **(saponin).** The saponin spontaneously lyses erythrocytes and leukocytes without affecting microorganisms. The tube is centrifuged and the resultant sediment is inoculated to agar media. The **lysis direct plating** method is intended for processing blood specimens from children. In this method, 1.5 mL of blood is added to a small tube containing saponin. The entire specimen lysate is inoculated to agar media, bypassing the need for centrifugation.

The lysis methods have several advantages:

- There is complete freedom in selecting the agar media for inoculation. This feature is helpful when pathogens with unusual growth requirements are being sought.
- The methods are effective for detecting filamentous fungi more rapidly and more comprehensively than broth culture.
- When cultures are positive (Color Plate 78), the laboratory usually has isolated colonies for inoculation of identification and susceptibility tests. This reduces the time necessary for issuing final results.
- If known amounts of lysate are inoculated to agar media, quantitative results can be reported with positive cultures. Quantitative results aid clinicians in distinguishing skin contaminants from clinically significant isolates. In some situations (e.g., *Streptococcus pneumoniae* bacteremia in children), colony counts help determine whether patients have occult bacteremia or a focal infection seeding organisms into the bloodstream.

The lysis methods also have disadvantages. They require more labor than broth culture during culture setup. This poses a problem to laboratories with limited evening, night, and weekend or holiday staffing, where specimen processing delays may negate the advantage of issuing final results more rapidly. Another problem is the higher likelihood of culture contamination during setup and incubation. Media contained in culture plates are not protected from contact with the environment. Airborne microorganisms or microorganisms from laboratory worker hands can lodge on agar media and form colonies. Steps that can be taken to minimize contamination include inoculating cultures within a laminar airflow hood and examining cultures without removing the lids of culture plates. Identification of colonies as contaminants is aided by noting growth on uninoculated areas of agar media.

Blood culture isolates should be saved by the laboratory for at least 1 month. Such practice permits further testing of isolates during epidemiologic investigation of outbreaks.

BODY FLUIDS

Recognition of infections in closed-cavity body fluids (e.g., cerebrospinal, synovial, pleural, pericardial, and peritoneal fluids) is just as important as detecting microorganisms in the bloodstream. The task can be easier with body fluids, in that microscopic examination of smears is a productive option. If the quantity of specimen submitted for testing is more than 1 mL, and not viscous or clotted, it should be concentrated by centrifugation before analysis. Smears and cultures should be prepared from resuspended sediments. Antigen detection can be performed on specimen supernatants.

MICROSCOPY

Gram-stained or **acridine orange–stained smears** should be part of the workup of all patients with suspected body fluid infections. Examination of smears prepared by cytocentrifugation yield more accurate results than smears prepared from conventional centrifugation sediments. Results should be ready in less than 30 minutes. When microorganisms are seen, selection of initial antimicrobial therapy can be guided by the Gram reaction of the organisms detected. Not every culture-positive body fluid is positive by Gram stain or acridine orange stain. Negative reports must be interpreted in the context of clinical findings and other laboratory results (e.g., cell count and differential, glucose and protein concentrations).

Body fluid smears for fungi and acid-fast bacteria are notoriously insensitive. Negative results are virtually meaningless. Positive results should be viewed with some skepticism unless several microorganisms are seen.

ANTIGEN DETECTION

Following their introduction to the laboratory, there was a tendency to order bacterial antigen detection tests on every cerebrospinal fluid sample submitted to the laboratory. The reasoning was that results could be available much sooner than from culture and a diagnosis could be made before the patient was admitted to the hospital. The reality is that antigen testing is expensive and time consuming.

Because positive results cannot predict the antimicrobial susceptibility of microorganisms detected, they have little bearing on modifying empirical antimicrobial therapy. The transition from expensive, potentially toxic, broad-spectrum therapy to cheaper, safer, narrow-spectrum therapy usually awaits growth of microorganisms in culture and determination of antimicrobial susceptibility results. The other difficulty with wholesale testing of body fluids, to reiterate a point made earlier, is a reduction in the positive predictive value of results. When a large majority of specimens tested are negative, the majority of positive results may be falsely positive.

There are specific situations in which body fluid antigen detection can be clinically useful (Table 14–2). If an infected patient has received a partial course of antimicrobial therapy, the culture may be falsely negative. Antigen detection may be the only way to determine the etiology of infection. If clinical evaluation suggests the possibility of meningococcal infection, positive results may trigger prompt antimicrobial prophylaxis for at-risk contacts of the patient.

Decisions regarding antigen testing should not be made until the body fluid cell count, differential, glucose, protein, and Gram stain results are known. If the hematology and chemistry results are incompatible with bacterial infection, antigen detection is unnecessary. Also, if the Gram stain results are positive, antigen detection is usually not necessary.

CULTURE

Body fluid specimens should be inoculated to 5% sheep blood agar and chocolate agar for growth of *Haemophilus influenzae* (Color Plate 79) and *Neisseria gonorrhoeae*. Cultures should be examined, if possible, after 12 hours of incubation. Positive results should be reported to clinicians immediately. Isolates from synovial fluid should be saved for at least

---

TABLE 14–2. INDICATIONS FOR BODY FLUID ANTIGEN DETECTION

Partial treatment with antimicrobial agent

Selection of appropriate empirical antimicrobial therapy for a child at the age threshold between neonatism and infancy

Prompt administration of prophylactic antimicrobial therapy to close contacts of a patient with meningococcal infection

---

1 month in case special antimicrobial susceptibility testing becomes necessary.

URINE

The microbiology laboratory is often asked to diagnose urinary tract infection. Success is contingent on the care with which specimens are collected and delivered to the laboratory. Specimens must not be contaminated with periurethral flora during collection, and microbial growth during transport to the laboratory must be prevented. Failure to comply with either practice can ruin the diagnostic value of specimens. See the discussion in Chapter 13 on collection and transport of urine specimens for specific recommendations.

MICROSCOPY

Microscopic examination of unstained urine sediments or of gram-stained smears is often the first laboratory evidence of infection. Seeing at least one organism per oil immersion field of uncentrifuged urine suggests the presence of greater than 100,000 cfu/mL. The Gram stain cannot be relied upon to estimate colony counts less than 100,000 cfu/mL.

Smears should be examined for the presence of leukocytes as well as microorganisms. The finding of many microorganisms in the absence of leukocytes in an immunologically normal host suggests specimen contamination. On the other hand, the presence of leukocytes without any microorganisms may still reflect infection, and such specimens should definitely be cultured.

SCREENING TESTS FOR EVIDENCE OF INFECTION

Several rapid screening tests are available to aid the diagnosis of urinary tract infection. They furnish useful information to clinicians, especially those practicing in locations without immediate laboratory support. They are potentially beneficial to the laboratory in helping decide which specimens warrant the time, effort, and expense of culture. The principal shortcoming of the rapid screening tests described below is their inability to detect specimens with colony counts less than 100,000 cfu/mL in a consistent manner. (See also Chapter 19.)

Leukocyte Esterase

The **leukocyte esterase (LE) test** is a 2-minute screen for the presence of neutrophil granulocytes. The test thus screens for pyuria instead of bacteriuria. A positive result, evidenced by pinkish-purple color development (Color Plate 80), correlates with >10 leukocytes per mm^3. A false-positive result can occur in patients infected with *Trichomonas vaginalis*. The test does not detect lymphocytes. Obviously, the test is ineffective for screening specimens collected from neutropenic patients.

Urinary Nitrite

The **nitrite test (NO$_2$)** is also part of the standard urine dipstick and is a 1-minute screen for microbial reduction of urinary nitrate to nitrite. Best results are obtained from tests of first morning specimens when microbial colony counts are at their highest and plenty of time for conversion of dietary nitrate to nitrite has elapsed. The test is falsely negative with specimens harboring microorganisms that (1) lack the nitrate reductase system or (2) further reduce nitrite to ammonia or nitrogen gas. A positive result is signified by pinkish-red color development (see Color Plate 80).

Colorimetric Filtration

Either bacteriuria or pyuria may be detected in less than 2 minutes by **colorimetric filtration.** Specimens are passed through a filter that traps both microorganisms and leukocytes. Safranin dye is then used to stain trapped material. Any degree of pinkness against the white background of the filter indicates a positive result. Specimens that contain precipitates or urinary pigments interfere with test performance and interpretation.

CULTURE

Culture continues to be the mainstay for laboratory diagnosis of urinary tract infection. Clean catch, catheterized, and suprapubic aspirate specimens are acceptable for culture. Bagged specimens from young infants are acceptable for culture only when refrigerated or inoculated to media less than 30 minutes after collection. Under no circumstances are Foley catheter tips suitable for culture. Specimens may be inoculated immediately after collection using a commercial dipslide device, or they may be delivered to the laboratory for conventional culture.

Colony counts are determined by inoculating measured amounts of urine to culture media. With dipslides, this is accomplished by immersing agar-coated slides in urine, with adherence of quantitative amounts of specimen to the agar surface. Conventional culture calls for use of a calibrated loop or micropipette to transfer 0.001 mL or 0.01 mL of urine to agar media. The urine is streaked over the entire agar surface, using the colony count technique.

Media selection is dictated by the microorganisms most likely to cause infection: enteric gram-negative bacilli, enterococci, and staphylococci. Urine specimens routinely are inoculated to a medium selective for gram-negative bacilli (e.g., MacConkey or EMB agars) and a medium that supports the growth of gram-positive cocci (e.g., nonselective 5% sheep blood agar, selective CNA or CLED + polymyxin B agar). When unusual urinary tract etiologies are under consideration (e.g., *Neisseria gonorrhoeae*, *Haemophilus* spp), the laboratory must be informed so that appropriate media are inoculated.

Cultures are incubated overnight at 35°C under aerobic conditions. Because the most commonly encountered pathogens grow rapidly, cultures need not be incubated for longer periods. However, if slow-growing organisms are being sought or specimens with positive Gram stains are culture negative after 1 day, lengthier incubation is indicated.

General guidelines for interpreting culture results on clean-catch or catheterized specimens are as follows:

- Colony counts of a single organism at greater than 100,000 cfu/mL are indicative of infection.
- Colony counts between 10,000 and 100,000 cfu/mL may be indicative of infection.
- Colony counts less than 10,000 cfu/mL are usually not indicative of infection.
- Specimens yielding growth of more than one organism generally suggest that contamination with periurethral or fecal flora has occurred.

It must be remembered, however, that the above guidelines were developed following study of a specific patient population—namely, the first morning void from asymptomatic adult females. Specimens collected later in the day from symptomatic infected patients or infected patients partially treated with antimicrobial therapy may exhibit colony counts as low as 100 cfu/mL. Clinically significant colony counts from adult males and children also may be less than 100,000 cfu/mL. Detection of any microorganisms in suprapubic aspirates is direct evidence of infection.

RESPIRATORY TRACT SPECIMENS

The respiratory tract comprises the upper (mouth, nose, nasopharynx, pharynx, trachea) and lower (bronchus, bronchiole, lung) respiratory tracts. Diagnosis of infection is complicated by the wide variety of microorganisms colonizing the upper respiratory tract. When infection occurs in the upper respiratory tract, the etiologic agent(s) must be recognized among numerous saprophytic, but potentially pathogenic, microorganisms. Collection of specimens from the lower respiratory tract without contamination by upper respiratory tract flora is virtually impossible unless an invasive procedure bypassing the mouth, pharynx, and trachea is used. Interpretation of culture/smear results from the respiratory tract is difficult at best.

MICROSCOPY

Microscopy is not very useful in diagnosing infections of the upper respiratory tract. Save for noting the presence of inflammatory cells or finding a heavy predominance of a single morphotype, smear results are usually noncontributory. Gram-stained aspirates from walled-off abscesses or from patients with sinusitis may be useful, if specimens can be collected without extraneous flora contamination.

On the other hand, microscopic examination of lower respiratory tract specimens can be helpful. Sputa from patients with pneumonia may be evaluated by Gram stain to assess the quality of specimens before further processing. Specimens exhibiting more than 25 squamous epithelial cells per low power field are heavily contaminated with saliva and probably not worth the time, effort, and expense of culturing. Sputa from patients with tuberculosis may be acid-fast stained to obtain a rapid, presumptive diagnosis. Microscopic examination of bronchoalveolar lavage, lung aspirate, and lung biopsy specimens generally produces a high yield. Specimens may be Gram stained to diagnose bacterial infections, acid-fast stained to diagnose mycobacterial infections, calcofluor-white stained for fungal infections, or toluidine-blue stained for *Pneumocystis* infections. (See also Chapter 19.)

ANTIGEN DETECTION

Microbial antigen detection for diagnosis of respiratory tract infections is practiced widely, following an increase in the number of commercially available products. Currently, there are literally dozens of FDA-licensed assays available for detection of Group A streptococcal antigen in pharyngeal swabs alone. Other organisms for which antigen detection reagents are available include *Bordetella pertussis*, *Legionella pneumophila*, *Chlamydia trachomatis*, *Pneumocystis carinii*, influenza virus, parainfluenza virus, adenovirus, and respiratory syncytial virus (RSV).

Latex particle agglutination assays, rapid enzyme immunoassays (EIA), rapid immunochromatographic assays, and an optical immunoassay are currently on the market for detection of Group A streptococcal antigen. Results are available in less than 10 minutes with most of these tests. The main deficiency of these products is a lack of sensitivity compared to carefully performed cultures. Most assays have difficulty detecting fewer than 10,000 cfu of Group A streptococci on a consistent basis. Positive results reported by trained, experienced testers are generally reliable, but negative results should be confirmed by culture.

Detection of *B. pertussis, L. pneumophila, C. trachomatis, P. carinii*, respiratory syncytial virus, influenza virus A and B, and parainfluenza virus 1–3 antigens is achieved primarily by direct or indirect fluorescent antibody. The specimens of choice are nasopharyngeal swabs *(B. pertussis)*, nasopharyngeal secretions (*C. trachomatis*, influenza A and B virus, parainfluenza virus 1–3, and respiratory syncytial virus), and tissue impression smears or lung aspirates (*L. pneumophila* and *P. carinii*). *B. pertussis* and *L. pneumophila* antigen assays are significantly less sensitive than culture, and negative results should be confirmed by culture. *P. carinii* cannot be grown in culture. Antigen detection results are available in 2 hours or less.

NUCLEIC ACID PROBES

A DNA probe assay for rapid detection of Group A streptococcal ribosomal RNA is commercially available. Experience suggests that the DNA probe assay is more sensitive than the antigen detection assays. The probe is labeled with a chemiluminescent signal-generating molecule known as **acridinium ester.** A luminometer is necessary for reading assay results. Assay time is approximately 70 minutes.

Two commercially available nucleic acid target amplification–based DNA probe assays are licensed by the FDA for testing acid-fast smear positive specimens for the presence of *Mycobacterium tuberculosis*. One uses the principle of transcription-mediated amplification (TMA), and the other is based on the polymerase chain reaction (PCR). The manufacturers of these assays are improving the performance of their products so that they can be used for testing AFB smear-negative specimens in the future. Until then, the clinical usefulness of these assays is limited.

Experimental nucleic acid probe assays for detecting *B. pertussis* DNA in nasopharyngeal specimens have been described. These assays, which entail target amplification by PCR, appear significantly more sensitive than antigen detection or culture.

CULTURE

The methods used for culture of respiratory tract specimens vary with the pathogens being pursued. Cultures for aerobic bacteria, anaerobic bacteria, mycobacteria, fungi, and/or viruses may need to be inoculated.

Aerobic Bacteria

Most aerobic bacteria that cause respiratory tract infection are cultivable using standard media and incubation conditions. The following paragraphs address several essential pathogens for which special media or incubation conditions are necessary.

Group A *Streptococcus* (GAS) is the primary cause of bacterial pharyngitis and is a microorganism that most microbiology laboratories and many physician offices routinely culture. These bacteria are mildly fastidious and carry out an aerotolerant, anaerobic mode of metabolism. They require media richly supplemented with nutrients. Their growth rate is maximal under anaerobic conditions. Anaerobic incubation also enhances beta hemolysis (Color Plate 81) produced by the oxygen-labile GAS exoenzyme streptolysin O and suppresses the growth of competing, obligately aerobic respiratory flora. Published data indicate that selective media yield higher numbers of positive cultures than nonselective media. Selective media, however, do reduce the growth rate of GAS, and cultures on these media should be incubated at least 36 hours before they are reported as negative. In summary, maximal detection of GAS in throat cultures requires inoculation of selective media and anaerobic incubation for at least 36 hours. Other culture conditions risk false-negative results from specimens harboring small numbers of GAS.

Neisseria gonorrhoeae is a cause of pharyngitis in individuals who engage in oral-genital contact. *N. gonorrhoeae* is readily cultured from these patients if selective media (e.g., modified Thayer-Martin agar) and an incubation atmosphere containing 5 to 10% CO_2 is used (Color Plate 82). See the section on genital tract specimens that follows.

Arcanobacterium haemolyticum is a cause of pharyngitis mostly in adolescents and young adults. The microorganism grows poorly on 5% sheep blood agar and, as such, is not readily detected in cultures for Group A streptococci. *A. haemolyticum* grows much better on media containing human or rabbit blood, forming wide zones of beta hemolysis around the colonies. Cultures may be incubated aerobically or anaerobically, and the addition of 25 µg/mL of trimethoprim/sulfamethoxazole to culture media inhibits the growth of nonpathogenic flora.

Corynebacterium diphtheriae is primarily of historical interest in the United States but remains an important cause of disease in areas of the world where immunization rates are low. This microorganism causes a pseudomembranous pharyngitis that can lead to complications like myocarditis, neural demyelination, and renal tubular necrosis. Pharyngeal specimens should be inoculated to Loeffler media slants in preparation for microscopic examination and to a cystine-tellurite agar plate for culture. After overnight incubation, growth from the Loeffler medium is smeared, stained with methylene blue, and examined for coryneform bacteria containing metachromatic granules. Cystine-tellurite agar plates are examined after 24 to 48 hours for growth of black or gunmetal-gray colonies. Isolates biochemically confirmed as *C. diphtheriae* should be tested for production of diphtheria toxin.

Bordetella pertussis, the cause of whooping cough, is a microorganism that is exquisitely sensitive to the toxic effects of materials found in collection swabs and growth media. The microorganism fails to grow on standard blood or chocolate agar plates for this reason. Specimens for culture should be collected from the nasopharynx and placed immediately in protective transport medium, such as 1% casamino acids broth or semisolid Regan-Lowe agar. Most laboratories today inoculate specimens to standard Regan-Lowe agar, which contains activated charcoal to neutralize growth inhibitory substances and 10% horse blood as a source of nutrients. Cultures should be incubated in a humid aerobic environment for at least 5 days. Supplementation of the atmosphere with 5 to 10% CO_2 is unnecessary. Most isolates form visible colonies in 3 to 5 days. Bordet-Gengou agar is an alternative to Regan-Lowe agar but is less desirable because of its 1-day recommended shelf life. Classically described "cough plates" fail to detect many positive patients and should not be used.

Streptococcus pneumoniae is the major cause of bacterial pneumonia in adults. The organism is not especially difficult to grow or identify. Inoculation to 5% sheep blood agar is very helpful; zones of alpha hemolysis (greening of the medium) form around the colonies. The colonies exhibit a characteristic centrally dimpled appearance due to autolysis of the oldest cells in the population (Color Plate 83).

Specimens from children and adults with cystic fibrosis should be inoculated to media that enable detection of *Pseudomonas aeruginosa, Staphylococcus aureus, Haemophilus influenzae,* and *Burkholderia cepacia.* The combination of 5% sheep blood, chocolate, MacConkey or EMB, and OFPBL or PC agars is minimally sufficient for this purpose. Optional use of selective media for *S. aureus* (e.g., mannitol salt agar) and *H. influenzae* (bacitracin-chocolate agar) help avoid overgrowth of these organisms by mucoid strains of *P. aeruginosa.* Mannitol salt agar, in addition, aids detection of thymidine-dependent strains of *S. aureus* that may escape notice on 5% sheep blood and chocolate agars. The recommended selective media for growth of *B. cepacia* (PC and OFPBL agars) are commercially available from major media manufacturers.

Legionella species are causes of opportunistic pneumonia in patients with underlying immunosuppressive or chronic pulmonary diseases. Like *B. pertussis,* legionellae grow best on media containing activated charcoal to neutralize toxic materials. Buffered charcoal yeast extract agar supplemented with alpha-ketoglutaric acid is the medium of choice. The medium may be made selective for *Legionella* spp by including antimicrobial agents (e.g., cefamandole, polymyxin B, and anisomycin) during preparation. Cultures should be incubated for at least 5 days at 35°C in a humid, aerobic environment.

Mycoplasma pneumoniae is the main cause of atypical pneumonia in adolescents, young adults, and adults. Members of the genus are bacteria that lack cell walls. The absence of cell walls renders them osmotically fragile. Accordingly, special provision must be made to provide these microorganisms with an isotonic transport and culture environment (e.g., by adjusting the NaCl or glucose concentration to achieve isotonicity). *M. pneumoniae* also has growth requirements for sterols and nucleic acid precursors. These are usually met by including animal serum and yeast extract in culture media. Growth of other bacteria can be minimized by adding antimicrobial agents that kill by inhibiting cell wall synthesis (e.g., penicillins or cephalosporins). Media (e.g., PPLO broth supplemented with 10% yeast extract, 20% horse serum, and 1000 units/mL penicillin) should be incubated aerobically for 4 weeks at 37°C. Broth media should be examined for any color changes indicating acidification (a sign of *M. pneumoniae* growth). Presumptively positive broth cultures should be subcultured to suitable agar media for confirmation of mycoplasmal growth. Agar subcultures should be incubated in an aerobic atmosphere supplemented with 5 to 7% CO_2. Agar subcultures should be examined under a dissecting microscope for the presence of colonies exhibiting a "fried egg morphology." *M. pneumoniae* colonies are hemadsorption-positive. Gram-stained smears of colony microorganisms should yield no reaction.

Chlamydia trachomatis is a cause of lower respiratory tract infections in newborn infants. Culture techniques for this microorganism are described in the section dealing with the genital tract.

Chlamydia pneumoniae (TWAR agent) was recently established as a pathogen of the lower respiratory tract. The microorganism causes infections similar in clinical presentation to *Mycoplasma pneumoniae*. It is more difficult to culture from clinical samples than is *C. trachomatis*. Specimens should be inoculated to appropriate cell lines such as HL and HEp-2. The McCoy and HeLa-229 cell lines that support the growth of *C. trachomatis* do not support the growth of *C. pneumoniae*. Specimens should be centrifuged onto cycloheximide-treated cell monolayers and incubated at 37°C in a 5 to 7% CO_2-enriched atmosphere for up to 7 days. Positive cultures are recognized by staining cell monolayers with fluorescently labeled monoclonal antibodies directed against *C. pneumoniae* antigens.

Anaerobic Bacteria

Anaerobic bacteria constitute the majority of the nonpathogenic upper respiratory tract flora. These microorganisms can become involved in infectious processes as opportunists (e.g., the stuporous alcoholic who aspirates saliva or respiratory secretions and develops pneumonia). Proof that anaerobes are causing infection in the respiratory tract demands that specimens for culture be collected in a careful manner. The cardinal requirement is to *avoid contamination with microorganisms from the upper respiratory tract.* Only under these circumstances can one assume that anaerobes grown in culture are contributing to infection.

Specimens should be transported to the laboratory and cultures inoculated and incubated according to the guidelines discussed earlier. Respiratory tract cultures from patients with anaerobic infections frequently yield growth of obligate anaerobes mixed with facultative anaerobes and aerotolerant anaerobes. As a result, a great deal of care must be taken by laboratory technologists to isolate each organism in pure culture and then determine its oxygen requirement. Because most anaerobes grow at slower rates than aerobes, a significant amount of time may pass before final culture results are available. Clinicians must be patient with the laboratory during this process.

Identification of anaerobes is based on Gram-stain reaction and morphology, biochemical test results, and, when necessary, gas-liquid chromatographic analysis of glucose fermentation endproducts or cell membrane fatty acids. Once isolated in pure culture, most anaerobes can be identified in less than 24 hours.

Anaerobes frequently implicated in respiratory tract infections include *Prevotella/Porphyromonas* spp, *Fusobacterium* spp, *Peptostreptococcus* spp, *Actinomyces* spp, and *Veillonella* spp. These microorganisms are susceptible to standard antimicrobial agents and, except under unusual circumstances, do not require antimicrobial susceptibility testing. However, bacteria within the *Prevotella/Porphyromonas* spp can exhibit beta-lactamase-mediated penicillin resistance. To be on the safe side, anaerobic gram-negative rods should be tested for penicillinase production upon initial isolation, so that penicillin resistance, if present, can be reported promptly to clinicians.

Mycobacteria

The lower respiratory tract is the site of most human mycobacterial infections. Culture of sputum or specimens obtained directly from the lungs is required to confirm infection and to obtain organisms for antimicrobial susceptibility testing. The specimen digestion and decontamination steps necessary to maximize culture yield from sputa were discussed earlier. Respiratory tract specimens not contaminated with upper respiratory tract flora do not benefit from decontamination.

The species of mycobacteria that most often cause pulmonary infection are *M. tuberculosis, M. avium, M. intracellulare, M. kansasii, M. szulgai, M. malmoense, M. fortuitum,* and *M. chelonei.* Many laboratories today rapidly identify *M. tuberculosis* isolates with a DNA probe directed against the microorganism's ribosomal RNA. Other laboratories use the more traditional approach of demonstrating positive niacin production and nitrate reduction results, and negative heat-stable catalase results. Identification of *M. avium, M. intracellulare,* and *M. kansasii* isolates can also be made rapidly by DNA probe. Definitive identification of the other species requires biochemical testing. Antimicrobial susceptibility testing of mycobacteria is frequently referred to another laboratory.

Fungi

Fungal infections of the respiratory tract often are diagnosed initially by microscopic examination. The identification of specific etiologic agents, however, is not possible until positive cultures are available. Infections may be benign (e.g., *Candida albicans* infection of a neonatal palate) or life-threatening (e.g., *Aspergillus fumigatus* pulmonary infection in an immunosuppressed patient). Quite a number of fungi can colonize the upper respiratory tract on a temporary or permanent basis. Thus, interpretation of culture results from specimens contaminated with upper respiratory flora can be just as difficult with fungal cultures as it is for aerobic or anaerobic bacterial cultures.

Yeast infections of the upper respiratory tract occur in immunologically incompetent hosts (e.g., patients with underlying immunosuppressive conditions) and in individuals receiving broad-spectrum antibacterial therapy. In the latter situation, growth of resident yeasts is not suppressed by growth of bacteria. Infections usually start in the mouth; in rare instances they advance to the throat, esophagus, and the gastrointestinal tract. *Candida albicans* is the leading cause of these infections and is easily detected by routine bacterial and fungal cultures.

Yeast infections of the lower respiratory tract may be acquired by inhalation (e.g., *Cryptococcus neoformans*), aspiration (*C. albicans* pneumonia in the neonate), or hematogenous spread (*Candida* pneumonia in the immunosuppressed patient). Obtaining definitive evidence of *Candida* lung infection is complicated by the microorganism's normal presence in the upper respiratory tract; specimens collected directly from the lung are often necessary. *C. neoformans* lung infection often is undiagnosed, and the microorganism remains undetected until disseminated infection occurs. When suspected, pulmonary cryptococcal infection can be confirmed by culture or examination of lower respiratory secretions with India ink preparations.

Histoplasma capsulatum, Blastomyces dermatitidis, Coccidioides immitis, and *Paracoccidioides brasiliensis* are dimorphic fungi that grow either as yeasts (37°C) or molds (≤30°C) (Color Plate 84). Because most laboratories routinely incubate fungal cultures at less than or equal to 30°C, these microorganisms generally are first detected growing as molds. Colonies are visible after as few as 3 days of incubation (*C. immitis*) to as long as 3 weeks (*P. brasiliensis*). Once conidia formation occurs, these fungi pose dangers to laboratory workers because careless handling of cultures may lead to inhalation of conidia. Definitive identification of any of the dimorphic fungi requires laboratory demonstration of both the yeast and mold phases of growth.

Aspergillus fumigatus, A. flavus, and *A. niger* are three species of *Aspergillus* that can cause fatal disseminated infections in immunocompromised patients. These fungi grow readily on bacteriologic and fungal media. They form visible colonies within 3 days of incubation. Identification is contingent on recognizing characteristic conidial structures and colony morphologies.

The zygomycetes (*Mucor* spp, *Rhizopus* spp, *Rhizomucor* spp, and *Absidia* spp) may cause opportunistic infection in the lungs. They are also noteworthy for their propensity in diabetic patients to colonize nasal and facial sinus cavities and then invade the brain (rhinocerebral mucormycosis). These fungi grow extremely rapidly on routine media, quickly filling the culture vessel with woolly aerial mycelia. The zygomycetes form sporangia and sporangiospores rather than conidia. They are differentiated from one another microscopically. Characteristic features include the presence and location of rhizoids and the structural attributes of their sporangia.

Viruses

A number of DNA and RNA viruses are pathogenic to the respiratory tract and cause a variety of infections. Infectious processes localized to the upper respiratory tract include pharyngitis, laryngitis, laryngotracheobronchitis (croup), and rhinitis (the common cold). Among the infections of the lower respiratory tract are bronchitis, bronchiolitis, and pneumonia. Antigens of respiratory syncytial virus (RSV), the most common cause of viral bronchitis, bronchiolitis, and pneumonia in young children, are readily detected by immunofluorescence and enzyme immunoassay. Antigens of influenza A and B viruses, parainfluenza viruses 1–3, and adenovirus can also be detected by immunofluorescence. Viral culture, using the techniques described earlier, is the most common approach toward detecting agents not recognized by antigen assays.

To facilitate determining the etiology of respiratory viral infections in antigen-negative specimens, the laboratory should be able to culture influenza and parainfluenza viruses, RSV, and adenoviruses in immunocompetent hosts, and cytomegalovirus, herpes simplex virus, and varicella zoster virus in immunologically compromised hosts. Proper specimen collection and transport are essential to the success of these activities. Conventional culture or shell vial culture techniques can be used.

GENITAL TRACT SPECIMENS

Genital specimens from patients at risk of sexually transmitted diseases represent a significant workload for many microbiology laboratories these days. Advances in technology over the last 25 years have made it possible for the laboratory to diagnose *Chlamydia trachomatis,* herpes simplex virus, human papilloma virus, *Haemophilus ducreyi,* and *Mobiluncus curtisii*-associated infections, as well as those caused by *Neisseria gonorrhoeae, Treponema pallidum,* and *Trichomonas vaginalis.* Infection due to each of these agents is detected by separate techniques. It is the clinician's responsibility to inform the laboratory as to which organism(s) are suspected in a particular patient.

MICROSCOPY

Gram stain is the laboratory method of choice for diagnosis of gonococcal urethritis in males. A thin smear prepared from urethral discharge is heat- or methanol-fixed, stained, and examined under oil immersion magnification for intracellular and extracellular gram-negative diplococci. A positive result is definitive evidence of gonorrhea. Results can be available in less than 20 minutes and, when read by an experienced microscopist, are as sensitive and specific as culture. Gram stain of cervical and vaginal discharge in females yields only presumptive evidence of gonorrhea if intracellular gram-negative diplococci are found. That is because nonpathogenic species of *Neisseria* may be normally present in the female genital tract. Many laboratories deem Gram stains of cervical or vaginal discharge inappropriate test requests for this reason.

The saline wet preparation is the most commonly performed test for diagnosis of vaginal and urethral trichomoniasis (Color Plate 85). A small drop of discharge is suspended in sterile normal saline and examined under low power for the presence of motile trophozoites. Results are available within 5 minutes but fail to detect trichomonads in more than 25% of culture-proven cases.

Cervical and urethral scrapings of epithelial cells from patients with possible *C. trachomatis* infection may be stained with Giemsa or iodine reagents to demonstrate intracytoplasmic inclusion bodies (Color Plate 86). Giemsa stain may be used to detect chlamydial elementary bodies as well. However, the sensitivity of these staining methods is not great and most laboratories today perform more sensitive antigen detection, DNA probe, and/or culture tests.

Microscopic diagnosis of herpes simplex virus genital infections can be achieved with use of the **Tzanck prep.** Scrapings from genital lesions are Giemsa-stained and examined for the presence of multinucleated giant cells (Color Plate 87). Confusion of herpes simplex lesions with those produced by varicella zoster virus must be avoided, as the latter lesions also yield positive Tzanck preps. The sensitivity of the Tzanck prep is low—negative results do not rule out herpesvirus infection—but the specificity, or the believability of positive results, is high.

Diagnosis of syphilis can be made by dark-field examination of freshly collected transudates from the chancres of primary infection or the condyloma lata of secondary infection. The lesions should be gently abraded with dry gauze to elicit production of transudate, and a drop of it placed on a microscope slide. If necessary, a drop of saline may be mixed with the specimen. The prep should be coverslipped and examined promptly under a microscope equipped with a dark-field condenser. Positive specimens display motile, tightly coiled spirochetes that flex and rotate around their longitudinal axes (Fig. 14–1).

Gram stains or wet mounts of vaginal discharge may be examined for the "clue cells" (epithelial cells coated with large numbers of bacilli) of bacterial vaginosis (Color Plate 88). Occasionally, Gram stains reveal the

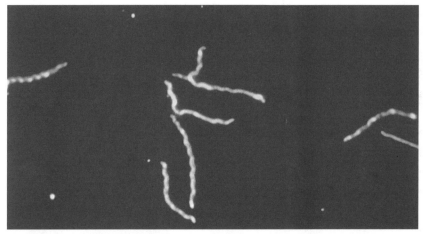

FIGURE 14–1. Dark-field microscopy of *Treponema pallidum*. (Reprinted with permission from Gower Medical Publishing, Ltd., London.)

faintly stained curved rods of a different microorganism, *Mobiluncus* spp. This gram-positive anaerobe is thought to be the etiologic agent of the infection. Smear results are ready in less than 20 minutes and are more sensitive and specific than cultures for *Gardnerella vaginalis,* a bacterium that was previously thought to be the cause of this infection.

Gram stains of vaginal discharge may also reveal fungal elements: budding yeasts, pseudohyphae, and/or true hyphae (Fig. 14–2). When fungal elements predominate, the patient, in most instances, is infected with *Candida albicans.* It is not necessary to see true hyphae in the specimen before a presumptive diagnosis of candidiasis is made. Observation of large numbers of any of the stages of yeast growth is suggestive.

Chancroid is caused by *Haemophilus ducreyi,* a facultatively anaerobic gram-negative rod. Lesions begin as erythematous papules, which progress to pustules that ulcerate within a few days. Approximately 50% of patients develop painful inguinal lymphadenopathy (buboes), which may drain noninfectious pus spontaneously. Examination of Gram-stained pus may reveal the bacilli of *H. ducreyi,* displaying the characteristic "school of fish" morphology.

The **Papanicolaou (Pap) smear** of cervical cells collected from the squamocolumnar cell junction is a popular means of recognizing signs of human papilloma virus (HPV) infection of the cervix. However, the Pap smear is merely a screening test. Diagnosis and treatment of HPV infection based on a suspicious smear (one displaying koilocytosis) is discouraged. Suspicious smears should prompt further colposcopic examinations, DNA probe testing, or biopsy-dependent evaluation.

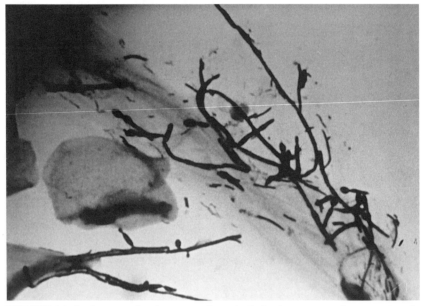

FIGURE 14–2. Gram-stained smear of vaginal discharge revealing yeast cells, pseudohyphae, and hyphae of *Candida albicans.*

ANTIGEN DETECTION

Detection of gonococcal antigens in genital tract specimens can be accomplished by particle agglutination and enzyme immunoassay methods. The assays have worked well with male urethral specimens, but no better than much less expensive Gram stains of the same specimens. Immunofluorescence assays have also been developed but have been unable to differentiate *N. gonorrhoeae* from related *Neisseria* species in a reliable manner. All of the assays lack sensitivity in detecting gonococcal antigens in female specimens. Negative results require confirmation with a more sensitive test method. Another drawback of these assays is their inability to identify penicillin-resistant strains. Only when penicillin resistance is so prevalent that initial therapy covers resistant strains is antigen detection likely to prove useful.

Detection of *C. trachomatis* antigens in genital tract specimens is commonly performed in laboratories these days. Several assay methods are in use, including immunofluorescence, enzyme immunoassay, immunochromatography, and optical immunoassay. Testing by immunofluorescence requires less than 30 minutes, whereas the other assays require between several minutes and 2 hours. The accuracy of antigen detection results from any of the methods is highly dependent on the quality of specimens. *C. trachomatis* is an intracellular pathogen of columnar epithelial cells, and unless these cells are present in specimens, the yield of positive results will be low. The attraction of antigen detection assays is the rapidity of results compared to culture, but culture is more sensitive, especially when specimens from asymptomatically infected individuals are tested. Antigen detection is most accurate for symptomatic individuals from populations with a high incidence of infection. Negative antigen results from asymptomatic individuals should be confirmed by a more sensitive method.

Scrapings from genital lesions can be stained with immunofluorescent or immunoperoxidase reagents or tested by enzyme immunoassay for herpes simplex virus antigens. The sensitivity of these assays is contingent on the quality of the specimens tested. One advantage of the immunoperoxidase method is that an ordinary light microscope can be used to examine stained smears, whereas a microscope equipped with ultraviolet illumination is necessary for the immunofluorescent method. The enzyme immunoassays are lengthier than the microscopic assays, taking as long as 4 hours to perform.

Commercial antigen detection methods for diagnosis of *Trichomonas vaginalis* infection are based on immunofluorescence and require use of a microscope equipped to provide ultraviolet illumination. The assays are more sensitive than saline wet preparations but more time consuming to perform (approximately 30 minutes). Accordingly, a batch mode of testing is all that is feasible for most laboratories, negating the advantage of providing results while patients are waiting.

NUCLEIC ACID PROBES

Assays to detect *Neisseria gonorrhoeae* or *Chlamydia trachomatis* ribosomal RNA in urogenital swabs involve the use of nucleic acid probes. A strong attraction of these assays is that both pathogens can be looked for simultaneously. The probes are labeled with a chemiluminescent signal-generating ligand, necessitating the use of a luminometer to obtain results. Assay time is less than 2 hours.

DNA probe assays for *N. gonorrhoeae* and *C. trachomatis* that call for amplification of target nucleic acid sequences before testing have become available. Amplification methods in use include the polymerase chain reaction, the ligase chain reaction, and transcription-mediated amplification. An appealing feature of these assays is their ability to diagnose infections from testing urine. The sensitivity of urine testing is almost as high as genital specimen testing and is superior to the sensitivity of the nonamplification assays just described. Admittedly, the cost per test is also higher, but testing can be completed within one work shift.

A diagnostic approach for identifying HPV infections entails probing for DNA of types 6, 11, 16, 18, 31, 33, and 35 in cells obtained from the squamocolumnar junction. If screening tests are positive, specific typing tests can be performed to elucidate whether HPV types 6/11, 16/18, or 31/33/35 are present. The DNA probe assay is considerably more sensitive than the Pap smear or colposcopy.

CULTURE

Culture is the primary method for laboratory diagnosis of many sexually transmitted infections. *N. gonorrhoeae, C. trachomatis,* and herpes simplex virus cultures are performed routinely by large numbers of laboratories. Cultivation of *Trichomonas vaginalis, Haemophilus ducreyi, Ureaplasma urealyticum,* and *Mycoplasma hominis* is practiced in a few laboratories and is available from most reference laboratories.

N. gonorrhoeae propagate more slowly than other genital tract microorganisms, so cultures on nonselective media predictably become overgrown by nonpathogenic resident flora. Fortunately, several selective media are available (e.g., modified Thayer-Martin, Martin-Lewis, GC-Lect, and NYC agars) that facilitate detection of this microorganism. Occasional strains of *N. gonorrhoeae* fail to grow on selective media because of the borderline sensitivity to vancomycin (especially on Martin-Lewis agar, which has the highest vancomycin concentration of the aforementioned media). Some laboratories inoculate nonselective chocolate agar with selective media to enable detection of vancomycin-sensitive strains. Cultures must be incubated in an aerobic atmosphere enriched with 5 to 10% CO_2 for 72 hours to achieve maximal isolation rates. The use of "candle jars," in which CO_2 levels are raised to higher levels by candles burning to extinction, is satisfactory but less than optimal. Suspicious colonies of oxidase-positive, gram-negative diplococci must be confirmed as *N. gonorrhoeae* by additional tests. The laboratory must be careful to differentiate *N. gonorrhoeae* from *N. meningitidis, N. lactamica,* and *Kingella denitrificans,* all of which grow well on *N. gonorrhoeae*–selective media. Another *Neisseria* species, *N. cinerea,* sometimes grows on selective media and is very similar to *N. gonorrhoeae* in its biochemical test profile. The essential difference is the ability of *N. cinerea* to grow on nutrient agar, whereas *N. gonorrhoeae* is unable to do so. Numerous commercial metabolic, immunologic, and DNA probe–based assays specific for *N. gonorrhoeae* are also available as confirmatory tests.

C. trachomatis is an obligately intracellular parasite that requires host cell adenosine triphosphate (ATP) as an energy source. Specimens should be placed in chlamydial transport medium (e.g., sucrose phosphate medium), brought to the laboratory, and inoculated to cycloheximide-treated McCoy cells. Inoculation consists of centrifuging specimens onto cells growing on coverslips or on the bottoms of microtiter tray wells. Cultures should be incubated at 37°C in an aerobic atmosphere containing 5% CO_2. Cultures are examined for chlamydial growth after 48 to 72 hours by staining for elementary and reticulate bodies with fluorescent antibody conjugates or staining for glycogen inclusion bodies with iodine or Giemsa reagents. Some laboratories blindly passage cultures negative after 72 hours of incubation by homogenizing the cell monolayers and using the suspensions to inoculate fresh McCoy cells.

Cell culture is the most sensitive method for diagnosis of herpes simplex virus (HSV) genital infection. Fluid specimens collected from young vesicular lesions yield the highest rate of positive cultures. The positivity rate falls rapidly as the lesions age and reach the crusted stage. As is the case with most viruses, specimens in transport medium should be stored at 4°C before culture, rather than at −20°C because the freeze-thaw process reduces the viability of HSV populations. HSV grows well in most human or primate established cell lines, displaying visible cytopathic effect in as little as 24 hours. The majority of positive cultures are detected in less than 3 days, and blind passage of negative cultures is rarely fruitful. Because of the expense and lack of clinical importance in most situations, most laboratories do not routinely perform serotyping of HSV isolates. When the situation warrants, serotyping should be referred to a laboratory experienced with interpreting test results because there is a high degree of antigen overlap between serotypes I and II.

The clinical significance of detecting *U. urealyticum* and *M. hominis* in the genital tract is still uncertain. These organisms are recoverable in low numbers from a high percentage of asymptomatic women, which makes interpretation of positive cultures difficult. Relationships between the presence of *U. urealyticum* in pregnant women and infertility and low birth weight, and between *M. hominis* and pelvic inflammatory disease have been described, but definitive evidence of causality does not exist. Cultures for genital mycoplasma must be inoculated to osmotically protected media to avoid lysis. Media for recovery of *Ureaplasma* contain antimicrobial agents (e.g., penicillin and lincomycin) to inhibit growth of *M. hominis* and other bacteria. Media must be maintained at a pH less than 7.0. *M. hominis* culture media contain penicillin and are maintained at a pH greater than 7.0 to prevent growth of *U. urealyticum*. Cultures may be performed in broth or on agar. Broth cultures contain a pH indicator to signal occurrence of growth. Agar cultures may be inoculated from positive broth cultures or directly from specimens. They may be incubated aerobically or anaerobically in an atmosphere containing 5% CO_2. Growth is monitored by scanning the agar surface through a dissecting microscope. Both organisms grow rapidly in broth and on agar, with positive cultures evident in less than 5 days.

The value of *Gardnerella vaginalis* cultures is dubious. The organism is part of the normal vaginal flora and can be the predominant isolate from cultures of vaginal discharge specimens that are negative for routine pathogens. Current evidence points toward fastidious anaerobic gram-positive rods (i.e., *Mobiluncus* spp.) as the true cause of *nonspecific vaginosis*. Physiologic and chemical changes in the vaginal environment that encourage rampant growth of *G. vaginalis* may be the after effect of *Mobiluncus* infection. The clinical diagnosis of nonspecific vaginosis correlates better with microscopic findings of curved rods and "clue cells" than with positive cultures for *G. vaginalis* (see Color Plate 88).

Yeast vaginal infections are almost always caused by *Candida albicans*, a normal inhabitant of the gastrointestinal tract. Cultures for *C. albicans* are not difficult to perform. This yeast grows extremely well on routine bacterial as well as fungal media. Heavy growth of *C. albicans* from vaginal specimens is strong evidence of infection. Interpretation of culture results is difficult when only small numbers of yeast colonies are found. Such findings usually suggest colonization rather than infection of the vagina. Yeast isolates can be confirmed as *C. albicans* by demonstrating their ability to form "germ tubes" after 2½ hours incubation in rabbit plasma at 37°C.

Culture is the most sensitive laboratory assay for detection of *Trichomonas vaginalis* but requires several days to obtain final results. Specimens should be inoculated to one of several *Trichomonas*-selective media that inhibit the growth of genital bacteria (e.g., Trichosel broth or Diamond's medium). Cultures should be incubated at 35°C under anaerobic conditions for 7 days, although most positive cultures will be apparent within 48 to 72 hours. Aerobic incubation of semisolid tubed media may be used instead of anaerobic incubation, provided that specimens are inoculated below the surface of the medium. Positive cultures are recognized by a color change in some media and by appearance of turbidity in other media. Cultures also may be examined microscopically for motile trophozoites.

Haemophilus ducreyi is the causative agent of *chancroid*, a sexually transmitted infection resulting in formation of genital ulcers. *H. ducreyi* are nonmotile, pleomorphic gram-negative bacilli that have a nutritional requirement for hemin ("X factor"). Lymph node aspirates from patients with suspected chancroid should be inoculated to selective, nutritionally enriched media. Media that can suffice include the following: Hammond gonococcal medium (gonococcal agar base containing 5% fetal calf serum, 1% bovine hemoglobin, 1% CVA enrichment, and 3 µg/mL vancomycin), Fildes-enriched gonococcal medium (gonococcal agar base containing 5% Fildes reagent, 5% horse blood, and vancomycin), and enriched Mueller-Hinton agar (Mueller-Hinton agar base containing 5% chocolatized horse blood, 1% CVA enrichment, and vancomycin). Vancomycin is added to these media to prevent the growth of gram-positive cutaneous flora. Cultures should be incubated at 33 to 35°C for 72 hours in an aerobic atmosphere containing 5 to 10% CO_2. Recovery rates are higher when cultures are incubated at 33°C instead of 35°C.

GASTROINTESTINAL TRACT SPECIMENS

The majority of gastrointestinal tract specimens submitted to the microbiology laboratory for testing are for diagnosing the etiology

TABLE 14–3. MECHANISMS OF BACTERIAL DIARRHEA

Preformed Toxin Ingested; Organisms Absent from Feces:

Staphylococcal food poisoning
Clostridium botulinum

Intraluminal Multiplication Causes Accumulation of Toxin, Which Causes Diarrhea:

Cholera (*Vibrio cholerae*)
Traveler's diarrhea (*Escherichia coli*)
Pseudomembranous colitis (*Clostridium difficile*)
Some shigellas
Other *Vibrio* species
Clostridium perfringens

Organisms Damage Tissue Directly:

Typhoid (*Salmonella typhi*)
Other salmonellas
Some shigellas
Staphylococcal pseudomembranous colitis
E. coli infants ("enteropathogenic" species)
Yersinia species
Campylobacter jejuni

of diarrhea. Table 14–3 outlines mechanisms responsible for bacterial diarrhea. The discussion in this section will center on laboratory procedures useful in identifying agents that cause diarrhea. (See also Chapter 19, Stool Analysis.)

MICROSCOPY

Microscopic analysis of stool specimens is a frequent request. Detection of inflammatory cells with Gram or methylene blue stains steers the clinician toward the mucosally invasive pathogens (e.g., *Salmonella, Shigella, Campylobacter*), rather than the noninvasive agents (e.g., rotavirus, Norwalk agent, *Yersinia, Vibrio*). A modified Gram-stain procedure, in which dilute carbol fuchsin is substituted for safranin, has been used successfully to identify the curved gram-negative rods of *Campylobacter* spp. in stool smears.

Detection of most gastrointestinal tract parasites is accomplished by microscopy. Specimens may be examined directly in wet mount, or chemically extracted and concentrated by centrifugation before examination. In the latter case, ethyl acetate (or other similar solvent) is added to preserved specimens to extract soluble fatty material from the stool, leaving parasites present in the aqueous phase. The parasites are then sedimented by centrifugation and identified in wet mount preparations (see Color Plates 67, 68, and 89).

Protozoan parasites are more difficult to detect and identify in direct or concentrated wet mounts than are helminths. To increase the yield of positive findings, smears from preserved stools can be stained with trichrome or iron hematoxylin reagents that differentially stain the nucleus and cytoplasm of protozoan cysts and trophozoites. Not only is the contrast between protozoa and background debris heightened, making them easier to find, but nuclear structure is delineated, facilitating accurate identification.

The protozoan *Cryptosporidium parvum* is a veterinary pathogen that also infects humans, especially immunocompromised patients and children in daycare centers. The stage of the microorganism found in stool, the **oocyst,** is approximately the size of a yeast cell. It is readily distinguished from yeast cells by its lack of budding forms and the presence of four internal sporozoites (best visualized in wet mount by phase contrast microscopy). The oocysts are acid-fast when stained by the modified procedure commonly used for recognizing *Nocardia* spp. Smears prepared directly from preserved or concentrated stools yield satisfactory results. Yeast cells either are not acid-fast or stain in a homogeneous fashion. Cryptosporidial oocysts, on the other hand, stain unevenly, with the sporozoites having greater color intensity than the rest of the oocyst.

Another enteric agent closely related to *C. parvum* is *Cyclospora cayetanensis*. This protozoan was at first thought to be a colorless variant of blue-green algae. It was first referred to as a cyanobacterium-like body (CLB). The oocysts of *C. cayetanensis* are approximately twice the size (8 to 10 µ diameter) of those of *C. parvum* (4 to 5 µ diameter) and stain less dependably with modified acid-fast reagents. The presence of unstained oocysts in heavy infections can be recognized by seeing oocyst "ghosts," unstained bodies the size of *Cyclospora* oocysts. Another oocyst property aiding in their recognition is their autofluorescence. Microscopic examination of *C. cayetanensis* oocysts with ultraviolet illumination reveals bluish-white fluorescent structures.

In some centers with large virology laboratories, electron microscopy may be the method of choice for detection of enteric viruses. Stool suspensions are spotted on copper grids, negatively stained with solutions of phosphotungstic acid or uranyl acetate, and examined under an electron microscope for virus particles (Fig. 14–3). The size, shape, and structural characteristics of the particles contribute to the identification of the agent.

ANTIGEN DETECTION

Enzyme immunoassays (EIA) and **particle agglutination assays (PAA)** are widely used for diagnosis of rotaviral gastroenteritis. The EIAs provide results in 2 to 4 hours that are nearly as sensitive as those from

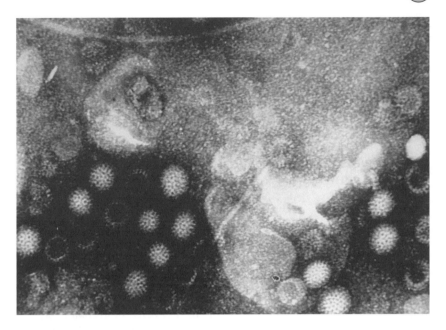

FIGURE 14–3. Electron micrograph of negatively stained rotavirus particles. (Reprinted with permission from Gower Medical Publishing, Ltd., London.)

electron microscopy. Specificity of results from neonates has been problematic for EIAs that do not include a negative control. The PAAs furnish results in less than 10 minutes, but they are not as sensitive as the EIAs or electron microscopy.

An EIA has also been developed for identifying adenovirus type 40/41 antigens in stool. Although the assay performs well, most laboratories have found the incidence of adenovirus gastroenteritis to be too low to justify purchasing the reagents, which have a limited shelf life.

PAAs for detection of *Salmonella* and *Shigella* antigens are available. The assays are currently intended for screening overnight enrichment broth cultures for these antigens. Antigen-positive broths are then subcultured to agar media for further workup. Studies evaluating direct LPA testing of stools and rectal swabs for *Salmonella* and *Shigella* antigens have yielded disappointing results.

An **indirect immunofluorescence assay (IFA)** for visualizing both *Giardia lamblia* cysts and *Cryptosporidium parvum* oocysts using monoclonal antibodies is commercially available. The test has demonstrated sensitivity superior to and specificity equal to that of conventional ova and parasite examination. Results are ready in less than 1 hour, but require a microscope equipped to provide ultraviolet illumination. EIAs that detect *Giardia lamblia* antigen in 60 minutes are available. These assays, like IFA, are more sensitive than standard microscopic examination.

Ready to be licensed for diagnostic use in the near future is an EIA for identification of *Helicobacter pylori* antigens in stool. The limited information available suggests that the assay is very effective, but costly.

TOXIN DETECTION

Quite a number of gastrointestinal pathogens produce toxins that are the microorganism's primary virulence factors. Diagnostic assays have been developed for some of these toxins, including those produced by *Clostridium difficile, C. botulinum, Vibrio cholerae, Staphylococcus aureus,* and *Escherichia coli,* which may produce an enterotoxin and a Shiga-like toxin. Only the assays for *C. difficile* enterotoxin (toxin A) and cytotoxin (toxin B), and for *E. coli* Shiga-like toxin are commercially available in the United States. Requests for other toxin assays need to be processed by reference or research laboratories.

C. difficile toxin A, the enterotoxin thought to be the actual agent of disease, can be identified using several 1- to 2-hour EIAs. Assay results may be read manually or with the aid of a spectrophotometer. Studies indicate that the toxin A EIAs are comparable to or somewhat less sensitive than the more cumbersome toxin B assay.

The *C. difficile* toxin B assay determines the cytotoxigenic properties of stool filtrates on cell cultures. Cytotoxic activity that is neutralizable with specific *C. difficile* antitoxin indicates a positive result. Testing calls for filtering of stools and may require as long as 48 hours before results are ready.

A popular particle agglutination assay for *C. difficile* actually detects neither *C. difficile* toxin A nor toxin B, but an antigen unrelated to its pathogenicity (glutamate dehydrogenase) instead. The test is rapid, requiring less than 20 minutes. However, the credibility of positive results is questionable in that some harmless species of *Clostridium* also produce the antigen detected. Similar membrane EIAs offer 15-minute identification of *C. difficile* common antigens in stool. The accuracy of these membrane EIAs is on a par with the LPA assay previously described.

Escherichia coli producing Shiga-like toxin (SLT) have the ability to kill host cells by interfering with protein synthesis. Because the genes conferring SLT production are bacteriophage-mediated, they are widely distributed among the various serotypes of *E. coli* that comprise the bacteriophage host range. The enterohemorrhagic *E. coli* (EHEC) are a subgroup of the Shiga-like toxin–producing strains and harbor a virulence plasmid containing genetic elements specific for the EHEC hemolysin. EIAs for detection of *E. coli* Shiga-like toxins were recently introduced. These assays are able to diagnose infection caused by serotype O157:H7 of *E. coli* (an agent incriminated in *hemolytic-uremic syndrome*), as well as any of the other serotypes capable of producing

Shiga-like toxins. The available data on the performance of these assays are very encouraging.

CULTURE

In most regions of the United States, routine stool cultures are intended to recover *Salmonella* spp, *Shigella* spp, *Yersinia enterocolitica*, and *Campylobacter jejuni*. Identification of *Vibrio* spp, *Aeromonas* spp, *Clostridium difficile*, or enteropathogenic, enterotoxigenic, enterohemorrhagic, enteroinvasive, or enteroadherent *Escherichia coli* usually requires a special request.

Salmonella spp and *Shigella* spp grow on MacConkey (MAC), *Salmonella-Shigella* (SS), Hektoen Enteric (HE), and xylose-lysine-desoxycholate (XLD) agars as non–lactose fermenting colonies (Color Plate 91). Lactose fermenting colonies (e.g., *Escherichia coli, Klebsiella* spp, and *Enterobacter* spp) are differentiated from non–lactose fermenters by their color because the acidic waste products of lactose fermentation cause pH indicators in these media to change color. *Salmonella* also reduces $Na_2S_2O_3$ to H_2S gas, which reacts with Fe^{+++} in SS, HE, and XLD agars to form insoluble FeS_3. The black precipitate of FeS_3 gives these colonies a black color (Color Plate 92). Because other microorganisms can form colonies that resemble *Salmonella* and *Shigella*, suspicious colonies must be definitively identified and serologically confirmed before final reports are issued. Enrichment broth media such as Selenite C, Selenite F, GN, and Tetrathionate broths promote growth of *Salmonella* spp and, in some cases, *Shigella* spp, while inhibiting growth of other flora. These media are incubated for 8 to 24 hours after inoculation and subcultured to one of the selective agar media above. The utility of enrichment broths is greatest when searching for low numbers of *Salmonella* and *Shigella* in specimens (e.g., when searching for asymptomatic carriers of *S. typhi*).

Y. enterocolitica is also a non–lactose fermenter but, because of its psychrophilic (cold-loving) characteristic, grows at a slower rate than most enteric gram-negative rods at 35 to 37°C. Because some strains are inhibited by enteric media or are easily overgrown by other flora, selective media have been developed for isolation of *Y. enterocolitica*. Cefsulodin-Irgasin-Novobiocin (CIN) agar is perhaps the most widely used. If culture results are not needed quickly, 30-day cold enrichment of stool in refrigerated saline increases the yield of positive cultures. In some instances cold enrichment is so effective that nonpathogenic serotypes of *Y. enterocolitica* are recovered, leading to errant diagnoses.

C. jejuni cannot grow on the media used for isolation of *Salmonella, Shigella*, or *Yersinia*, and require a microaerophilic atmosphere: 5% O_2, 10% CO_2, 85% N_2 is optimum. Several agar (e.g., Skirrow's medium and CVA) and broth (e.g., Campy thioglycollate) media for recovery of *Campylobacter* are commercially available. Alternatively, specimens can be inoculated to agar media overlaid with sterile 0.45-micron cellulose acetate filter membranes. The thin, corkscrew-shaped, motile campylobacters are able to pass through the pores in the membranes and form colonies on the underlying agar surface. Because *C. jejuni* is thermophilic (heat-loving), primary culture media can be incubated at temperatures greater than 37°C. The recommended incubation temperature of 42°C prevents growth of most enteric flora, yet allows *C. jejuni* to grow. Whether a selective medium or selective filtration is used, little if any growth of other microorganisms should occur. This is essential since campylobacters grow at slower rates than most other microorganisms in stool. They could be missed very easily if other organisms overgrow the culture.

When cultures for *Vibrio* spp. are indicated, a highly selective medium such as thiosulfate-citrate-bile salts (TCBS) agar should be inoculated. Very few stool microorganisms other than *Vibrio* spp and *Enterococcus* spp grow on TCBS agar. Alkaline peptone water serves as a suitable enrichment medium for low numbers of vibrios in stool.

Members of the *Aeromonas hydrophila* group (*A. hydrophila, A. caviae,* and *A. veronii* biotype sobria) are acknowledged as causes of enterotoxin-mediated gastroenteritis. They grow well on MacConkey agar; lactose fermenting strains are morphologically indistinguishable from *E. coli.* They are oxidase positive, however, which sets them apart from the *Enterobacteriaceae.* Enterotoxigenic strains tend to be beta-hemolytic on 5% sheep blood agar. A selective medium, 5% sheep blood agar with 10 µg/mL ampicillin, may be used to improve detection rates.

C. difficile, the major cause of *enterocolitis* associated with antimicrobial agents, is an obligate anaerobe that is not difficult to grow in culture. A selective medium, cycloserine-cefoxitin-fructose agar (CCFA), is available to augment isolation rates. The clinical significance of culture results, however, remains controversial. Toxigenic strains of *C. difficile* can be recovered from asymptomatic individuals, especially young children. On the other hand, cytotoxin-positive, culture-negative specimens from symptomatic individuals may be encountered. At this point, the EIA for toxin A and the cytotoxin assay for toxin B are the preferred methods for laboratory diagnosis of disease. Culture has been relegated to an adjunctive role.

Etiologic diagnosis of diarrhea caused by disease-producing *E. coli* is a difficult challenge for most laboratories. The antisera needed for serotyping enteropathogenic strains are either unavailable or too expensive. Assays for enterotoxigenic, enteroinvasive, or enteroadherent *E. coli* are difficult to establish and not available from commercial sources. Stool cultures for the most prevalent serotype of enterohemorrhagic *E. coli* (O157:H7) can be aided by inoculating MacConkey-sorbitol agar. O157:H7 strains are unable to ferment sorbitol, but nearly all other *E. coli* serotypes do. Sorbitol-negative *E. coli* can be screened for production of O157 somatic antigen and H7 flagellar antigen with commercially available antisera. The limitation of this strategy is that serotype O157:H7 is just one of more than a dozen serotypes known to produce Shiga-like toxins. Thus, the preferred method for laboratory diagnosis of entero-hemorrhagic colitis is an assay for Shiga-like toxins.

CUTANEOUS SPECIMENS

Cutaneous infections generally result from invasion by microorganisms colonizing the superficial layers of the skin or from microorganisms originating from the external environment. At times, cutaneous manifestations are the first symptoms of disseminated infections. Many skin and soft-tissue infections can be diagnosed clinically and treated empirically with antimicrobial agents. Nevertheless, the laboratory must be prepared to assist clinicians with these infections when situations call for laboratory support.

Bacterial infections of the skin can be minor and self-limited (e.g., folliculitis, pyoderma, furuncles), cause major discomfort to patients (e.g., animal or human bite infections, cellulitis, erysipelas, carbuncles, decubitus ulcers), or serve as the source of generalized sepsis (e.g., burn infections). In some situations, cutaneous findings are signals of disseminated infection (e.g., the petechial rash of gonococcal or menin-gococcal sepsis). Gram stain, culture, and antimicrobial susceptibility test results may be necessary for optimal patient management.

Superficial fungal infections of the skin, hair, or nails are known as *dermatophyte infections* (i.e., ringworm). Laboratory confirmation is some-times necessary when dermatophytic lesions cannot be distinguished from those produced by bacterial, mycobacterial, or parasitic agents.

Viral skin infections can be acquired exogenously (e.g., primary herpes simplex virus infection) or endogenously (e.g., reactivation of herpes simplex or varicella virus infections). The laboratory may be requested to confirm diagnosis of these infections when therapeutic or infection control decisions must be made. The rashes of systemic viral infections (e.g., rubella, rubeola, exanthema subitum, erythema infectiosum) occur frequently, but rarely require laboratory investigation of their etiology.

Mycobacterial cutaneous infections (e.g., swimmer's granuloma) usu-ally are caused by species unable to grow at internal body temperature. *M. marinum*, *M. ulcerans*, and *M. haemophilum* all fall into this category.

MICROSCOPY

Microscopic examination of cutaneous specimens provides information that can result in a presumptive diagnosis and initial antimicrobial therapy. Specimen Gram stains can confirm their purulent nature and limit the spectrum of possible bacterial etiologies. KOH preparation of skin scrapings or hair/nail clippings are frequently all that is needed to identify fungal dermatophyte infections. Examination of Tzanck preparations of vesicular lesions detect the multinucleated giant cells characteristic of infections caused by herpes simplex and varicella zoster viruses.

ANTIGEN DETECTION

Antigen detection methods, for the most part, are not applicable to rapid diagnosis of bacterial and fungal cutaneous infections. Use of particle agglutination assays for detection of Group A streptococcal antigen in cellulitis specimens has been described, but any advantage such testing would have over Gram stain is questionable.

Immunofluorescence or enzyme immunoassay detection of viral antigens in skin, on the other hand, has proved useful in early determination of the cause of infection. Identification of maternal herpes simplex virus genital infection late in pregnancy, recognizing herpes simplex virus lesions in newborn infants, and diagnosing varicella zoster infection in health care settings are situations in which these rapid diagnostic tools are valuable.

CULTURE

Culture of cutaneous lesion aspirates is the method of choice for definitive laboratory diagnosis of bacterial infections. Specimens should be inoculated to 5% sheep blood and chocolate agars for growth of streptococcal, staphylococcal, and *Haemophilus* organisms. Anaerobic cultures should be considered in patients with puncture wounds (e.g., animal bites) or when crepitus is evident. Such specimens must be transported under conditions compatible with survival of obligate anaerobes.

Dermatophyte fungi (*Trichophyton* spp, *Microsporum* spp, and *Epidermophyton floccosum*) can be cultivated on routine fungal media, including those containing cycloheximide. Cultures need to be incubated at 25 to 30°C to permit growth of fungi inhibited at body temperature. Cultures should be incubated for at least 3 weeks to detect slowly growing species. Specialty media intended for detection of dermatophytes—that is, dermatophyte test media (DTMs) are commercially available. DTM is selective for dermatophytes and contains a pH indicator that changes color from yellow to red when these fungi grow.

Material from cutaneous lesions suspected to be of mycobacterial origin should be inoculated to solid (e.g., Lowenstein-Jensen medium, 7H10 agar, 7H11 agar) and/or liquid (7H9 or Dubos broth) media. At least one set of media should be incubated at 30 to 33°C to allow thermotolerant species to grow.

Cultures for herpes simplex virus should be inoculated to cell cultures that support rapid lytic growth of the virus (e.g., primary human embryonic, primary human diploid, primary rabbit kidney, or primary mink lung cell lines). Inoculated cells should be incubated at 37°C for 7 days, although most positive cultures will be evident in less than 5 days. In vitro culture of varicella zoster virus is possible, but the yield of positive results is lower than that from immunofluorescent antigen detection assays.

WOUND, TISSUE/BIOPSY SPECIMENS

Wound infections usually follow a breach of the host's skin due to trauma. Pathogens originate from the environment or are derived from endogenous colonized sites. Laboratory identification of etiologic agents is conditional on examining specimens from the actual site of infection. Too often, material sent for laboratory analysis is inadequate. An example of an inadequate specimen is a wound swab obtained by simply rubbing the superficial surface of a wound. Such a specimen will contain large numbers of colonizing microorganisms that are inconsequential to the patient's infection. Gram stain and culture reports may mislead clinicians into prescribing inappropriate antimicrobial therapy.

A recurring problem with tissue/organ infections is collection of insufficient material for the laboratory examinations requested. When this occurs, the laboratory must allocate specimens into portions so tiny that the validity of negative test results is questionable. When specimen quantity is less than desired, clinicians should be asked to prioritize test requests to allow the laboratory to perform as many tests well as possible.

MICROSCOPY

Microscopic examination of wound and organ specimens can provide extremely useful data. Results can be available within minutes to guide initial patient management. Microscopic findings that do not correlate with culture results can suggest additional laboratory studies that would not have been considered otherwise. Most bacteria causing wound/tissue/organ infections can be seen during examination of Gram-stained material. Acid-fast and fungal stains are indicated when the patient history suggests mycobacterial or mycologic infections, although the number of organisms present may be below the sensitivity of microscopy.

CULTURE

Cultures of wound, tissue, and organ specimens provide definitive diagnostic information and the information required to monitor the success of selected therapies. Cultures for routine bacterial pathogens should include inoculation of 5% sheep blood agar, MacConkey or EMB agar, and chocolate agar.

The fungi most likely to cause wound and organ infections grow quite well on standard fungal media. In fact, many are detectable in routine bacterial cultures. To re-emphasize a point made earlier, fungal cultures should always include media incubated at 25 to 30°C to permit growth of fungi that are inhibited at internal body temperature. Culture plates and tubes may be incubated at 35 to 37°C also to hasten detection of fungi capable of growth at body temperature.

Wound infections are sometimes caused by rapidly growing mycobacteria (Runyon Group 4) of the **fortuitum-chelonei** complex. These organisms form visible colonies on routine bacterial media, if cultures are held for 5 to 7 days. Since only enrichment broth cultures of wounds are typically incubated that long, these mycobacteria often are detected initially by Gram stains of turbid broths. Morphologically, they resemble diphtheroids (*Corynebacterium* spp). The laboratory must be alert and not automatically consider such results as indicative of skin contamination. An acid-fast stain of the broth is the logical next step in the workup of such cultures.

Some slowly growing mycobacteria also may cause wound infections. The advice given earlier for fungal wound cultures also holds for mycobacterial wound cultures. These cultures must include media incubated at 25 to 30°C, because *M. marinum* and *M. ulcerans* do not grow at 35 to 37°C.

Organ cultures from patients with suspected miliary tuberculosis or disseminated *M. avium* or *M. intracellulare* infection should be handled as routine mycobacterial cultures, with one exception. Digestion and decontamination procedures are not needed if the specimen was collected from a body site not colonized with normal flora.

EYE/EAR SPECIMENS

Diagnosis of eye and ear infections are a challenge to laboratories in that the quantity of specimen submitted for testing often is small and the list of possible pathogens is large. Clinicians can help by informing the laboratory of the list of suspected pathogens.

Ocular infections encountered with greatest frequency include orbital cellulitis, conjunctivitis, blepharitis, keratitis, and endophthalmitis. Specimens commonly submitted for testing include conjunctival swabs, corneal scrapings, and needle aspirates of intraocular fluid and pus.

Ear infections occur in the outer, middle or inner ear. Outer ear infections are similar to wound and skin infections and are caused by the same spectrum of microorganisms. The presence of cerumen in the ear canal may predispose patients to colonization with bacteria and fungi, whose presence can result in minor irritation. The middle and inner ears ordinarily are sterile sites and become infected following entry of organisms from the nasopharynx or occasionally via hematogenous spread.

MICROSCOPY

The Gram stain contributes toward diagnosis of eye and ear infections by supplying information about etiologic agents. The microscopist should keep in mind that smears from sites with exposure to the surroundings (e.g., conjunctival and corneal scrapings, outer ear swabs) may exhibit small numbers of cutaneous flora. Thus, pathogens may be found in the midst of several microorganism morphologies.

Mycobacterial infections of the eyes and ears may be diagnosed by performing one of the acid-fast stains discussed earlier. Negative smears, however, do not rule out infection because the number of organisms present may be less than the sensitivity of the staining method.

The Giemsa stain, although not often performed by the microbiology laboratory, can be used for diagnosis of chlamydial conjunctivitis and trachoma. Most laboratories presently rely on detection of *Chlamydia trachomatis* antigen by direct immunofluorescence for rapid diagnosis of ocular infections (see below).

Diagnosis of fungal infections of the eye and ear can be facilitated by staining specimens with calcofluor white or related dyes. However, negative smears should be confirmed by culture before fungal infection is eliminated as a diagnostic possibility.

ANTIGEN DETECTION

Direct immunofluorescence using fluorescein-labeled monoclonal antibodies is currently the antigen detection test of choice for identifying ocular chlamydial infections. Frank pus should not be examined with this assay. Instead, the ideal specimen is obtained by gentle abrasion of the conjunctival membranes. Published experience with these assays has been favorable. Positive specimens generally exhibit abundant numbers of elementary bodies that are easily recognized.

CULTURE

Culture continues as the "gold standard" for determining the etiology of eye and ear infections. Routine bacterial culture methods are satisfactory for growing and identifying the common pathogens (e.g., nontypable *Haemophilus influenzae*, *Streptococcus pneumoniae*, *Staphylococcus aureus*,

Group A *Streptococcus, Branhamella catarrhalis, Neisseria gonorrhoeae, Pseudomonas aeruginosa,* and members of the Enterobacteriaceae family). Concern over less common pathogens may require communication with the laboratory. The laboratory should be prepared to handle such situations. Inoculation of special media, incubation of cultures under nonstandard conditions, or forwarding specimens to reference laboratories are options for consideration.

Routine culture methods for *Chlamydia trachomatis* (described earlier) enable recovery of this organism from ocular specimens. Viral infections of the conjunctiva and cornea call for inoculation of cell cultures that support growth of at least the herpes viruses and the adenoviruses. Of interest is the increasing concern over corneal infections caused by free-living amoebae (e.g., *Acanthamoeba* spp) in users of extended-wear soft contact lenses. Culture for these organisms can be set up using a homemade nonnutritive agar to which has been added a dense suspension of heat-killed *Escherichia coli.*

SUGGESTED READING

Bartlett, JG: Community-acquired pneumonia: Current status. Infect Dis Clin Pract 4(4 Suppl):S223–S231, 1995.

Black, CM: Current methods of laboratory diagnosis of *Chlamydia trachomatis* infections. Clin Microbiol Rev 10:160–184, 1997.

Burns, JW, and Greenberg, HB: Viral gastroenteritis. Infect Dis Clin Pract 3:411–417, 1994.

Falagas, ME, and Gorbach, SL: IDCP guidelines: Sexually transmitted diseases, part I. Infect Dis Clin Pract 4:407–418, 1995.

Falagas, ME, and Gorbach, SL: IDCP guidelines: Sexually transmitted diseases, part II. Infect Dis Clin Pract 5:6–11, 1996.

Falagas, ME, and Gorbach, SL: IDCP guidelines: Sexually transmitted diseases, part III. Infect Dis Clin Pract 5:85–93, 1996.

Falagas, ME, and Gorbach, SL: Practice guidelines: Urinary tract infections. Infect Dis Clin Pract 4:241–257, 1995.

Feigin, RD, McCracken, GH, and Klein, JO: Diagnosis and management of meningitis. Pediatr Infect Dis J 11:785–814, 1992.

Garcia, LS, and Shimizu, RY: Medical parasitology: Update on diagnostic techniques and laboratory safety. Lab Med 24:81–88, 1993.

Harrison, HR, and Alexander, ER: Chlamydial infections in infants and children. In Holmes, KK, et al (eds): Sexually Transmitted Diseases, ed 2. McGraw-Hill, New York, 1990, pp 811–820.

Hines, J, and Nachamkin, I: Effective use of the clinical microbiology laboratory for diagnosing diarrheal diseases. Clin Infect Dis 23:1292–1301, 1996.

Hooton, TM, and Stamm, WE: Diagnosis and treatment of uncomplicated urinary tract infection. Infect Dis Clin N Amer 11:551–582, 1997.

Larsen, SA, Steiner, BM, and Rudolph, AH: Laboratory diagnosis and interpretation of tests for syphilis. Clin Microbiol Rev 8:1–21, 1995.

Pfaller, MA: Application of new technology to the detection, identification, and antimicrobial susceptibility testing of mycobacteria. Amer J Clin Pathol 101:329–337, 1994.

Reimer, LG, Wilson, ML, and Weinstein, MP: Update on detection of bacteremia and fungemia. Clin Microbiol Rev 10:444–465, 1997.

Shulman, ST: Streptococcal pharyngitis: Diagnostic considerations. Pediatr Infect Dis J 13:567–571, 1994.

Storch, GA: The diagnosis of viral infections. Infect Dis Clin Pract 2:1–20, 1993.

Townsend, GC, and Scheld, WM: Clinically important trends in bacterial meningitis. Infect Dis Clin Pract 4:423–430, 1995.

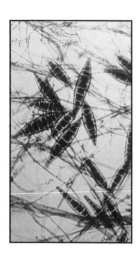

15

Serologic Diagnosis of Infectious Diseases

DETECTION OF MICROBIAL ANTIGENS

Detection of microbial antigens by immunoassay was discussed in detail in Chapters 13 and 14. Antigen detection provides direct evidence as to the etiology of infection and, in almost every instance, is preferred for diagnosis of infection over antibody detection, which furnishes only indirect evidence of infection.

DETECTION OF MICROBIAL ANTIBODIES

Depending on the situation and the infectious agent, antigen detection assays or culture techniques are either not available or have such poor yields that detection of specific antibodies is diagnostically more useful. In still other circumstances, it is desirable to obtain evidence of past infection or immunization against an infectious agent. The immunocompetent host responds to most infections or immunizations by producing antibodies that are detectable in the bloodstream. Occasionally the detection of antibodies in other body fluids (e.g., cerebrospinal fluid) can be of diagnostic importance.

The assays discussed in this chapter are those performed most frequently in the average serology laboratory. Many other assays are available, and the reader is referred to other texts for a more comprehensive treatment of the subject.

CLASSES OF ANTIBODIES

As was discussed in Chapters 4 and 7, immunoelectrophoretic separation of human serum proteins identifies the five classes of immunoglobulins: **IgG, IgM, IgA, IgD,** and **IgE.** Only IgG, IgM, and IgA are formed in response to infection and are the subject of the remainder of this section.

IgM antibodies generally appear in serum 1 to 2 weeks after onset of infection and usually persist for 2 to 3 months (Fig. 15–1). Detection of infectious agent-specific IgM antibody in serum is consistent with current or very recent infection in the host. Diagnosis of **congenital infection** in the newborn may be accomplished by demonstrating organism-specific IgM in the cord blood or in the newborn infant's bloodstream. Such IgM

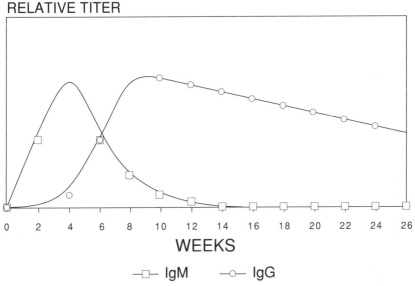

APPEARANCE OF HUMAN IgG AND IgM IN SERUM
FOLLOWING ONSET OF INFECTION

RELATIVE TITER

WEEKS

—□— IgM   —○— IgG

FIGURE 15–1. Appearance of human immunoglobulins in serum following onset of infection.

must have been produced by the infant because the IgM molecule is pentameric and too large to cross the fetal placenta. The presence of organism-specific monomeric IgG in the cord blood or infant's blood-stream may indicate passively acquired maternal antibody.

Serum IgG antibody titers typically begin rising 2 to 3 weeks after infection and may persist at detectable levels for life. Because of these variable periods of elevation, detection of organism-specific IgG in a single serum may not be useful for diagnosis of current or recent infection. Much more useful are simultaneous assays of paired sera collected at least 2 and preferably 4 weeks apart. Demonstration of at least a fourfold rise (or fall) in titer of specific IgG to an organism during the interval between each specimen collection is serologic verification of a recent infection. A twofold rise (or fall) in titer is not a significant change and could be attributable to minor variations in test performance. It is mandatory that both specimens be tested in the same run with the same lots of reagents if titer comparisons are to be meaningful.

IgA antibodies are formed in response to infections of cells with secretory activity (e.g., the cells lining the respiratory, gastrointestinal, and genitourinary tracts). Secretory IgA is released at the sites of infection, and serum IgA is found in the bloodstream. The standard serology laboratory infrequently measures secretory or serum IgA specifically, so further discussion in this chapter will be limited to IgG and IgM assays.

SEPARATION OF IgM FROM IgG

IgM-specific antibody assays are subject to difficulties that the serology laboratory must take measures to avoid:

- **False-negative IgM** results may occur if the patient's serum contains both IgG- and IgM-specific antibodies directed against the antigen(s) of interest. Such a situation could happen if an infant has mounted an IgM response while still carrying maternal IgG. Because IgG usually has a greater avidity for antigens than IgM or may be present at much higher titers than IgM, competition between the two antibody classes for a limited number of antibody-binding sites on the assay antigens could result in an apparent negative IgM result.
- **Rheumatoid factor** (IgM antibodies directed against the heavy chain of IgG immunoglobulin) may also interfere with assays for IgM specific antibodies, particularly in sera from infants who have serologically responded to maternal IgG. Organism-specific maternal IgG in the sera of noninfected infants may react with assay antigens. Rheumatoid factor in the same specimens can bind to the newly formed immune complexes, leading to the inference that organism-specific IgM is present in the specimens (**false-positive IgM** result).

The false-negative and false-positive IgM results described above can be prevented by separation of IgM and IgG immunoglobulins from each other prior to performing the immunoassay. Specimen pretreatment steps may include **ion exchange chromatography** using inexpensive, disposable minicolumns (e.g., Quik-Sep, Isolab, Inc., Akron, OH), sucrose gradient ultracentrifugation, affinity chromatography using protein A–coated Sepharose beads, or reaction of sera with precipitating goat anti–human IgG antisera (e.g., Serum Pretreatment Reagent, M. A. Bioproducts, Walkersville, MD). Perhaps the most successful approach is the use of **antibody capture assays,** in which the solid phase component of an enzyme immunoassay or radioimmunoassay is coated with antibody directed against the mu chain of the IgM molecule. After absorption of IgM from the specimen by the capture antibody, non-IgM antibodies are removed from the assay vessel by washing. The major disadvantage of the antibody capture assay is that it is not amenable to assay methodologies other than enzyme immunoassay or radioimmunoassay.

METHODS FOR DETECTION OF ANTIBODIES

The serology laboratory has at its disposal a large variety of assay methodologies for detection of antibodies. The first assays developed were tedious, labor-intensive, and often required more than 24 hours to obtain results. In the last few decades, most of these assays have been replaced by simpler, more rapid methods. Nevertheless, a few of the older assays are still practiced and, in some cases, remain the serologic test of choice.

Immunoprecipitation

The first **immunoprecipitation** assays detected antibodies in solution and yielded a qualitative indication of the presence of antibodies. Assays were performed in test tubes or capillary tubes and generally required incubation for several hours to overnight. The standard assay endpoint was visual flocculation of the antigen suspension.

Performance of immunoprecipitation assays in a gel matrix represented a major step forward in assay technology. **Immunodiffusion assays** enabled identification of specific precipitin bands that increased the diagnostic value of test results. Important information could be gleaned from a single test using the **Ouchterlony double immunodiffusion assay,** a method in which precipitin lines of identity, partial identity, or nonidentity facilitated comparison of patient's sera to reference sera (Fig. 15–2).

The development of **immunoelectrophoresis** and **counterimmunoelectrophoresis** methods for detection of infectious agent antigens and antibodies has been the crowning achievement, thus far, in immunopre-

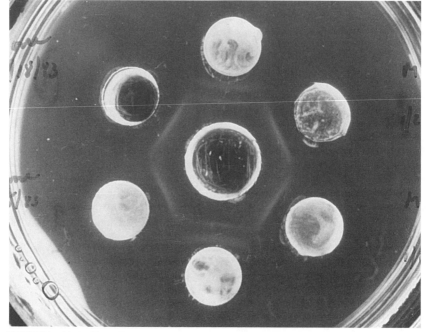

FIGURE 15–2. The Ouchterlony double immunodiffusion assay. Note white precipitin lines of identity compared with reference sera.

cipitation technology. Directed flow of antigens and antibodies toward each other through a gel matrix under the influence of an electric field dramatically increases the sensitivity of precipitation assays and drastically shortens the time to assay results. See Chapter 13 for more discussion of counterimmunoelectrophoresis.

Complement Fixation

One of the first of a new generation of more sensitive antibody assays developed more than 30 years ago, the **complement fixation test** is based on the inactivation (fixation) of complement following binding of complement factors to antigen-antibody immune complexes. Once bound, the complement is not available to induce lysis (hemolysis) of antibody (hemolysin)-coated sheep erythrocytes, which are added to the assay tubes to detect immune complex formation (Fig. 15–3).

The complement fixation test is tedious and time consuming. Titrations of antigen, hemolysin, and complement must be performed prior to actual specimen testing. The test procedure itself is a 2-day undertaking. Despite development of simpler, more rapid, more sensitive assay

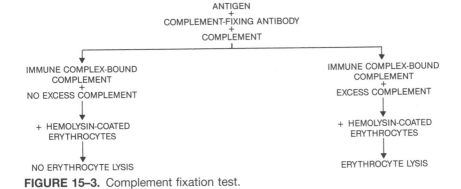

FIGURE 15–3. Complement fixation test.

methods, complement fixation is still the test of choice for serologic confirmation of certain infectious diseases. For the most part, only large-scale reference laboratories set up complement fixation tests today, because of the complexities of the procedure.

Neutralization

Neutralization assays, in which the infectivity of a microorganism or the activity of a toxin is neutralized by specific antibody (Fig. 15–4), are rarely performed for diagnostic purposes. Rather, because these assays often require several days to complete, testing is restricted to screening populations of patients for immunity or past exposure to infectious agents. Almost all neutralization assays performed today are designed to detect antibodies to viruses, subsequent to infection or immunization with the agent.

Neutralizing antibodies commonly prevent viral infection of the host or nullify toxin activity by blocking adherence of the virus or toxin to its target. Consequently, these antibodies generally are considered protec-

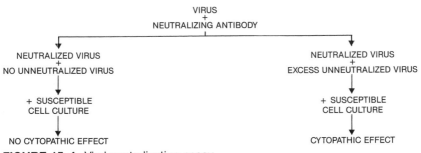

FIGURE 15–4. Viral neutralization assay.

tive; in the case of new vaccine preparations, efficacy frequently is predicted by measuring neutralizing antibodies generated.

Particle Agglutination/Agglutination Inhibition

Particle agglutination/agglutination inhibition (PA/PAI) assays for detection of infectious agent antibodies have become popular because of the simplicity and speed of the test procedure. In addition, most PA/PAI procedures can detect lower antibody titers than the methods described previously in this chapter.

Commercially available PA assays usually utilize antigen-coated latex particles, charcoal particles, bentonite particles, or erythrocytes. In general, patient serum dilutions are mixed with antigen-coated particles on a glass slide, placed on a mechanical rotator for 2 to 10 minutes, and examined for macroscopic particle agglutination. The PA assays for antibodies are very similar in principle to the latex particle agglutination assays for microbial antigens described in Chapter 13, with the obvious exception that the particles are coated with antigens instead of antibodies.

A handful of assays are still in use in which the agglutinating particles are cells of the infectious agent itself. The sensitivity of such assays is usually low because of the extremely small size of the cells: very large numbers of particles must aggregate before agglutination is macroscopically visible. The specificity of these assays is often poor as well because of the large diversity of antigens present on the cell surface, some of which are shared or cross-react with antigens of related organisms.

Most PAI assays are based on competition between antibody-coated particles and serum antibodies for a limited number of soluble antigen–binding sites. Antigens that have reacted with serum antibodies are unable to bind to antibody-coated particles, so particle agglutination is inhibited. In the case of some PAI assays, the competition for antigen is between serum antibodies and nonantibody sites on particles that have a high affinity for the antigen (e.g., hemagglutination inhibition assays for antibodies directed against the hemagglutinin of hemagglutinating viruses).

Immunofluorescence

Immunofluorescence assays for infectious agent antibodies require the use of either a microscope equipped to provide ultraviolet illumination or an instrument capable of detecting the fluorescence of a reaction mixture with an ultraviolet light–equipped fluorometer (e.g., FIAX System, International Diagnostic Technology, Inc., Santa Clara, CA). Assays for antibodies are of **indirect fluorescent antibody (IFA)** assay type, in contrast to the **direct fluorescent antibody (DFA)** assays for antigens described in Chapter 13. IFAs typically require less than 4 hours to perform, with most of the time occupied by hands-off incubation periods.

An IFA differs from a DFA procedure in that the antibody component of the antibody-fluorescent dye conjugate is an anti–human IgG or IgM instead of an anti–infectious agent antibody. The presence of the anti–human antibody conjugate in the assay method necessitates an extra procedural step, and thus a longer time period before test results are ready. The IFA procedure is performed by applying a dilution of the patient's serum to a smear containing the infectious agent or infected cells expressing antigens of the infectious agent. After suitable incubation and careful rinsing, the smear is flooded with the anti–human IgG or IgM antibody conjugate. A second incubation-rinse cycle follows, and then the smear is examined microscopically or with instrumentation for ultraviolet light–induced fluorescence.

The sensitivity of an IFA is superior to that of a DFA because of the signal amplification resulting from reaction of the antibody conjugate with the first antigen-antibody complex. Only one antibody conjugate molecule is present per DFA antigen-antibody complex. However, each IFA antigen-antibody complex may bind several antibody conjugate molecules, giving rise to a much stronger fluorescent signal.

The increased sensitivity of IFAs does not come without a price. IFAs are less specific than comparable DFAs, primarily due to nonspecific retention of antibody conjugate. Other disadvantages of the IFA procedure are the same as for the DFA: a requirement for specialized equipment to perform the assay and a need for an experienced microscopist, if immunofluorescence is detected manually.

Enzyme Immunoassay

The use of the **enzyme immunoassay (EIA)** for detection of infectious-agent antibodies has grown rapidly during recent years. The major reasons are that EIAs lend themselves well to automation and instrumentation and, together with radioimmunoassays, are the most sensitive of the antibody detection assays discussed in this chapter. EIAs for antibodies are usually indirect assays that depend on use of an anti–human IgG or IgM antibody-enzyme conjugate. The relationship between direct and indirect EIAs is analogous to the relationship between direct and indirect fluorescent antibody assays described in the previous section of this chapter.

Indirect EIA procedures require 2 to 24 hours to complete. A popular EIA procedure involves incubating a dilution of the patient's specimen with antigens of the infectious agent attached to a solid phase (e.g., a plastic bead or paddle, or the walls of a microtiter tray or tube). The solid phase is then carefully rinsed and bathed in a solution of the anti–human antibody-enzyme conjugate. The incubation-rinse cycle is repeated, followed by addition of the enzyme substrate. Enzyme-antibody conjugate bound to the solid phase via interaction with immune complexes catalyzes conversion of the substrate to a colored endproduct, which is detected with the unaided eye or with the help of a spectrophotometer. The degree of color development directly correlates with the amount of antibody present in the specimen.

In certain situations, a **competitive EIA** is more appropriate for antibody detection. In this case, a dilution of the patient's specimen is mixed with a precisely measured quantity of enzyme-antibody conjugate directed against the same antigen as the patient's antibody. The antibody conjugate and the patient's antibody compete for a limited number of antibody-binding sites found on antigens attached to the solid phase. The solid phase is carefully rinsed and bathed in enzyme substrate. The amount of color development inversely correlates with the amount of antibody present in the specimen.

The advantages and disadvantages of EIAs for antibody detection are the same as those for antigen detection described in Chapter 13.

Radioimmunoassay

Development during the 1960s and 1970s of commercially available **radioimmunoassay (RIA)** techniques for antigen and antibody detection was a major advance in the serologic diagnosis of infectious diseases. The strongest appeal of the RIAs was the tremendous increase in sensitivity compared to the other assay methods that were then in vogue. RIAs continue to be used today but at declining rates, owing to the inconvenience and expense of radioactive waste disposal and the increasing availability of comparably sensitive EIA methods.

Direct and indirect RIA procedures are identical in principle to the direct and indirect enzyme immunoassay procedures discussed in the previous section, with two important exceptions: (1) the endpoint reading of an RIA requires a gamma or beta scintillation counter, and (2) proper handling of radiolabeled reagents and disposal of radioactive waste requires extra precautions to protect the laboratory workers and the environment.

SEROLOGIC DIAGNOSIS OF SPECIFIC INFECTIONS

The rest of the chapter will address detection of antibodies that facilitates diagnosis of specific infections. Most of the assays described are routinely available in serology laboratories; some are performed only in central reference laboratories.

BACTERIAL INFECTIONS

Most bacterial infections are readily diagnosed by culture. Serologic tests for bacterial antibodies are primarily used for seroprevalence surveys of large populations for documentation of past infection, or for diagnosis of current or recent infection in patients whose cultures are negative (e.g., patients who have been partially treated with broad-spectrum antimicrobial agents, or patients with fever of unknown origin for longer than 2 to 3 weeks). Other serologic tests have unique applications, which will be discussed on an individual basis. Table 15–1 lists the commonly performed serologic assays for bacterial infection and the results that suggest recent or current infection.

TABLE 15–1. COMMONLY PERFORMED SEROLOGIC TESTS FOR DIAGNOSIS OF RECENT BACTERIAL INFECTIONS

Organism	Test	Clinically Significant Result*
Streptococcus pyogenes	Antistreptolysin O	≥1:240
	AntiDNAase B	≥1:240
	Antihyaluronidase	≥1:512
Salmonella typhi	Widal test (S. typhi)	≥1:160
Legionella pneumophila	Indirect immunofluorescence	≥1:256
Treponema pallidum	Rapid plasma reagin	Positive
	VDRL	Positive
	FTA-ABS (IgG or IgM)	Positive
Borrelia burgdorferi	Indirect immunofluorescence (IgG)	≥1:64
	Enzyme immunoassay	Positive
	Western blot (IgG)	≥4 of 9 bands
	Western blot (IgM)	≥2 of 9 bands
Helicobacter pylori	Enzyme immunoassay	Positive
Mycoplasma pneumoniae	Cold agglutinins	≥1:128
	Complement fixation	≥1:32
	Enzyme immunoassay	Positive
Rickettsia rickettsii	Weil-Felix (OX-19)	≥1:320
	Indirect immunofluorescence (IgG)	≥1:64
Ehrlichia chaffeensis	Indirect immunofluorescence (IgG)	≥1:64
Bartonella henselae	Indirect immunofluorescence (IgG)	≥1:128

*Titers greater than or equal to those displayed in this table or four-fold or greater rises in titer between acute and convalescent sera are only suggestive of recent infection by all of the agents listed. Titers less than those displayed in the table do not rule out infection.

Streptococcal Infections

Streptococcus pyogenes (Group A streptococci) infections are the only streptococcal infections for which antibody detection is clinically useful. In particular, a confirmed diagnosis of poststreptococcal acute rheumatic fever or acute glomerulonephritis requires serologic documentation of a recent *S. pyogenes* infection.

Screening tests are available that simultaneously detect antibodies to five different streptococcal enzymes: streptolysin O, DNAase B, hyaluronidase, NADase, and streptokinase. Demonstration of a fourfold or greater rise in antibody titer is considered evidence of recent infection.

The **antistreptolysin O (ASO) test** is an enzyme neutralization procedure performed when it is desirable to know whether the ASO titer specifically is elevated or rising. The test setup involves mixing patient serum dilutions with a specific quantity of streptolysin O. After appropriate incubation, washed human Type O erythrocytes are added, and the tubes are reincubated and examined for hemolysis. The ASO titer is the highest dilution of serum that completely prevents lysis of the erythrocytes. A clinically significant ASO titer is greater than or equal to 1:240 (greater than or equal to 240 Todd Units) in a single specimen, or a rise in titer of at least two dilutions between acute and convalescent specimens. Because of the complicated dilution scheme used in performing the ASO test, a two-dilution rise in titer is not equivalent to a fourfold rise. The greatest value of the ASO test is serologic confirmation of acute rheumatic fever following *S. pyogenes* pharyngeal infection. The test is unreliable for diagnosis of acute glomerulonephritis following *S. pyogenes* skin infection.

The **anti-DNAase B (ADB) test** is also an enzyme neutralization assay. Dilutions of the patient's serum are mixed with a standard amount of streptococcal DNAase B and incubated. Substrate DNA is then added, and after a second period of incubation, the DNA is checked for depolymerization. Depolymerized DNA can be identified by loss of alcohol precipitability or by a loss or change in color of a DNA-dye complex (e.g., DNA-methyl green). The assay endpoint is the highest dilution of the patient's serum that retains sufficient ADB activity to prevent DNA hydrolysis.

The ADB test detects antibodies produced after both pharyngeal and skin *S. pyogenes* infections and thus is superior to the ASO test for serologic confirmation of poststreptococcal acute glomerulonephritis. In addition, ADB antibodies persist longer than ASO antibodies and can serve as proof of recent *S. pyogenes* infection when the ASO titer has fallen to normal levels. A single specimen ADB titer of greater than or equal to 1:240 is considered elevated, but more convincing evidence of antecedent infection is demonstration of a two-dilution increment or greater rise in titer between acute and convalescent sera.

One final enzyme neutralization assay for streptococcal antibodies is the **antihyaluronidase test (AHT).** The AHT is performed by incubating dilutions of the patient's serum with streptococcal hyaluronidase, followed by addition of potassium hyaluronate. After further incubation, hydrolysis of hyaluronate is recognized by failure of a clot to form upon addition of 2N acetic acid. The AHT endpoint is the highest dilution of the patient's serum in which a definite clot forms.

The AHT, like the ADB test, is positive subsequent to either pharyngeal or skin *S. pyogenes* infection. A fourfold or greater rise in titer between acute and convalescent sera is regarded as documentation of recent *S. pyogenes* infection. Most serologists find ADB test results easier to interpret than AHT results and reserve the AHT for circumstances when a third-line test is called for.

Salmonellosis

The **Widal test,** an assay for *Salmonella typhi* antibodies in which salmonella organisms are agglutinated by patient sera, was first used in 1896. The test is performed by mixing serum dilutions with killed salmonella suspensions harboring known O (somatic) and H (flagellar) antigens. The assay endpoint is the highest dilution of patient serum that causes visible agglutination of the salmonella suspension.

In parts of the world where the incidence of typhoid fever is low, and competent facilities for recovery of *S. typhi* in cultures are available, there is little justification for performing the Widal test. The reason is that the serologic response to *S. typhi* O and H antigens may not be very impressive in immunologically naive populations and may not reach titers suggestive of infection. Furthermore, blood, bone marrow, stool, and bile cultures, when performed with up-to-date methods, are more reliable than the Widal test for diagnosis of typhoid fever or the *S. typhi* carrier state. In locales where typhoid fever is endemic or epidemic, or where facilities for culture of *S. typhi* are not available, the Widal test remains a valuable diagnostic tool. Patients with histories of salmonella infection are immunologically primed to respond with antibodies directed against *S. typhi* antigens, and O and H antibody titers rise quickly to clinically meaningful levels. Serodiagnosis of typhoid fever is based on a fourfold or greater rise between acute and convalescent antibody titers, or a single titer that is significantly higher than the mean baseline titer for the population.

The Widal test is not recommended for diagnosis of infection caused by other species or bioserotypes of *Salmonella* because of interpretive difficulties caused by serologic cross-reactions.

Legionellosis

The **indirect fluorescent antibody (IFA) test** for identifying circulating antibodies to *Legionella pneumophila* was at one time the method of choice for diagnosis of legionellosis (Legionnaire's disease). Now, however, the IFA test has been relegated to secondary status by the development of a direct fluorescent antibody test for *Legionella* antigens in lower respiratory specimens (see Chapter 13) and by the availability of selective media for recovery of *Legionella* organisms from specimens harboring mixed respiratory flora.

The IFA test for *L. pneumophila* antibodies is performed by flooding smears of heat-killed serogroup 1 (Philadelphia 1 strain) organisms with serial dilutions of the patient's serum. The smears are incubated, carefully washed, and exposed to polyvalent anti–human IgG, IgM, or IgA antibodies conjugated with fluorescein isothiocyanate (FITC). After another round of incubation and careful washing, the slides are coverslipped and examined microscopically using ultraviolet illumination. The assay endpoint is the highest dilution of the patient's serum that results in organisms exhibiting at least 1+ fluorescence.

A positive *L. pneumophila* IFA test in patients with a compatible history of pneumonia is demonstration of at least a four-fold rise in titer between acute and convalescent sera, with the latter specimen showing a titer of greater than or equal to 1:128. Alternatively, if paired specimens are not available, a single titer greater than or equal to 1:256 is presumptive evidence of recent infection.

Syphilis

Because *Treponema pallidum* cannot be grown on artificial culture media, the only ways in which the laboratory can help diagnose syphilis is to visualize the organisms by dark-field microscopy or direct fluorescent antibody staining and to detect antibodies in serum and cerebrospinal fluid. Two categories of antibodies may be sought: (1) **nontreponemal antibodies** (reagin), which are directed against lipid-containing antigens from damaged host cells (or perhaps the treponemes themselves), and (2) **treponemal antibodies,** which are directed against surface antigens of *T. pallidum.*

The nontreponemal antibody assay used most often today is the **rapid plasma reagin (RPR)** test. The qualitative RPR test is a screening assay in which the patient's undiluted serum is mixed with cardiolipin-coated charcoal particles on a cardboard slide. After mechanical rotation for a specified length of time, the test is examined for macroscopic agglutination of the charcoal particles. When a quantitative RPR test is performed, serial dilutions of the patient's serum are prepared, and the endpoint is the highest dilution of the patient's serum that results in charcoal particle agglutination.

The **Venereal Disease Research Laboratory (VDRL)** test is still performed by a few laboratories when testing serum and is the only assay recommended for testing cerebrospinal fluid (CSF). The VDRL test differs from the RPR test in that the cardiolipin antigen is complexed with lecithin and coated onto cholesterol-containing particles. In addition, complement must be heat-inactivated at 56°C for 30 minutes prior to serum testing, and flocculation of the cholesterol particles must be read microscopically. The VDRL is not as sensitive as the RPR or the treponemal antibody tests. This characteristic is the reason that the VDRL test is recommended for testing CSF because of the high likelihood of contaminating CSF with minute quantities of reagin or trepenomal antibody–positive blood during lumbar puncture. The VDRL test is less likely to yield falsely positive results with CSF.

The treponemal antibody tests in widespread use today are the **fluorescent treponemal antibody–absorbed double stain (FTA-ABS DS) test,** the **microhemagglutination–*T. pallidum* test (MHA-TP),** and the **hemagglutination treponemal test for syphilis (HATTS).** Use of these tests is usually limited to confirmation of positive nontreponemal antibody test results (VDRL or RPR).

The FTA-ABS DS test is an IFA assay. Prior to testing, patient serum is heat-inactivated and absorbed with "sorbent," which removes antibodies to commensal treponemes that could cause false-positive results. The treated serum is applied to a smear of *T. pallidum* on a microscope slide, incubated, and carefully rinsed. A tetramethyl-rhodamine isothiocyanate (TMRITC)–tagged anti–human immunoglobulin antibody conjugate is added, and the slide is reincubated and rerinsed. Finally, a fluorescein isothiocyanate (FITC)–labeled antitreponemal antibody is added as a counterstain, and the slide is reincubated, rerinsed, and coverslipped. The smear is examined under a microscope using ultraviolet illumination. Treponemes first are located on the slide using the FITC filter system, and then reaction of the treponemes with serum antibodies is ascertained by converting the microscope to the TMRITC filter system. A positive result is indicated by observing TMRITC-fluorescing treponemes on the smear.

The MHA-TP and HATTS assays are both hemagglutination tests performed in the wells of microdilution trays. Sheep (MHA-TP) or turkey (HATTS) erythrocytes that have been sensitized with *T. pallidum* antigens are mixed with "sorbent"-treated patient serum. As a negative control, nonsensitized erythrocytes are mixed with treated patient serum in a separate well. After suitable incubation, the erythrocytes in the wells are examined for agglutination. A positive result is indicated by hemagglutination of the sensitized erythrocytes and no hemagglutination of the nonsensitized erythrocytes.

The nontreponemal antibody tests are used primarily for screening patients for syphilis and for monitoring the therapeutic response during antimicrobial treatment for syphilis. A positive RPR or VDRL test in a patient not being treated for syphilis should be confirmed by a test for treponemal antibodies because many patient conditions can result in "biologically false-positive" nontreponemal antibody test results (Table 15–2). Nontreponemal antibodies appear 1 to 4 weeks after infection and remain elevated until antimicrobial therapy begins or, in some cases,

TABLE 15–2. CAUSES OF FALSE-POSITIVE SEROLOGIC TESTS FOR SYPHILIS

Infectious Diseases

Leprosy
Tuberculosis
Pneumococcal pneumonia
Subacute bacterial endocarditis
Chancroid
Scarlet fever
Leptospirosis
Relapsing fever
Rat-bite fever (*Spirillum minor*)
Rickettsial disease
Malaria
Trypanosomiasis
Vaccinia (vaccination)
Mycoplasma pneumonia
Measles
Chickenpox
Lymphogranuloma venereum
Hepatitis
Infectious mononucleosis
Lyme disease
Early HIV infection

Noninfectious Diseases

Drug addiction
Any connective disease disorder
Rheumatoid heart disease
Blood transfusions (multiple)
Pregnancy
"Old age"
Chronic liver disease

Reprinted from Mandell, GL, Douglas, RG, Jr., and Bennett, JE (eds): Principles and Practice of Infectious Diseases, ed 3. John Wiley, New York, 1990, p 1804, with permission.

when the patient enters the late phase of the infection (Fig. 15–5). Once effective antimicrobial therapy has begun, the nontreponemal antibody titer starts to decline, often reaching undetectable levels before the completion of treatment.

The treponemal antibodies are the first to appear following infection, and they remain elevated in most patients for life. FTA-ABS DS antibodies appear slightly before MHA-TP and HATTS antibodies. The principal use of the treponemal antibody tests is to confirm positive nontreponemal antibody test results. Since treponemal antibody test results are reported qualitatively only, and since titers, even if they were determined, are affected very little by antimicrobial therapy, these tests are of no value for monitoring the patient's response to antimicrobial therapy.

Diagnosis of congenital *T. pallidum* infection can be troublesome because infants born of infected mothers passively acquire nontreponemal and treponemal maternal IgG antibodies. Theoretically, assays for IgM-specific *T. pallidum* antibodies could identify congenitally infected infants, but a reliable IgM-specific assay has not yet been recognized by the Sexually Transmitted Diseases Branch of the Centers for Disease Control and Prevention (Atlanta, GA). The best available laboratory option is to perform serial nontreponemal antibody tests on infant sera for 3 to 6 months and observe for increasing or disappearing antibody levels.

Lyme Disease

Lyme disease is a zoonotic infection spread to humans via the bite of a deer tick. The causative agent, *Borrelia burgdorferi*, is very difficult to grow in culture, and diagnosis of infection is commonly the result of serologic confirmation of the physician's clinical impression, often supplemented by a history of a tick bite or the appearance of the characteristic **erythema chronicum migrans** rash. Commercially available IFA and EIA procedures have been developed to detect *B. burgdorferi* antibodies, but they have a tendency toward cross-reaction with other spirochetal antibodies

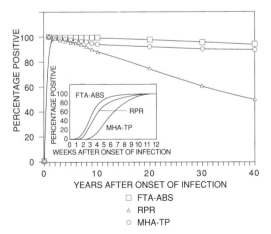

FIGURE 15–5. Appearance of nontreponemal and treponemal antibodies in patients with untreated syphilis.

(e.g., *B. recurrentis, T. pallidum,* and *Leptospira* spp), and their results have a less than desirable predictive value for infection. More reliable are the Western blot IgG- and IgM-specific antibody assays performed by a limited number of regional or national reference laboratories.

Current recommendations call for a two-step protocol for serodiagnosis of Lyme disease. The first step is a screening test employing a sensitive EIA or IFA for *B. burgdorferi* IgG or IgM antibodies. Screening test–negative specimens require no further testing. New specimens collected 2 to 4 weeks later should be screened if patients with initially negative results continue to display symptoms consistent with Lyme disease. Specimens that are positive or equivocal on the screening test should be retested with the confirmatory **Western blot (WB)** procedure. If specimens are collected within the first 4 weeks of disease, Western blot assays for both IgG and IgM antibodies should be performed. Specimens collected after 4 weeks of disease should be tested for IgG antibodies only.

Helicobacter pylori Infections

Persuasive evidence has accumulated implicating *Helicobacter pylori* as the primary cause of antral gastritis and peptic ulcer disease. Furthermore, an epidemiologic link between *H. pylori* infection and gastric carcinoma has been established.

Tests developed for diagnosis of infection include the rapid urease test, the ^{13}C urea breath test, culture, and serology. The main disadvantage of the urease and culture tests is the requirement for biopsy material obtained during endoscopy. The breath test is noninvasive but very expensive to perform. Serologic assays can be performed on plasma or serum, furnish results rapidly, and are relatively inexpensive. A promising but expensive *H. pylori* antigen test performed on stool has also been developed and should be available in the near future.

EIAs for *H. pylori* IgG, IgM, and in some cases even IgA antibodies have been developed by a large number of manufacturers. The difficulty is in determining which patients have clinically significant infection because as many as 60% of elderly adults in underdeveloped countries exhibit serologic evidence of infection.

The correlation between clinical gastritis, the presence of *H. pylori* in the stomach, and elevated serum levels of *H. pylori* antibodies is strong. Thus, clinicians and laboratorians should be selective about which patients are tested serologically, to maximize the predictive value of test results. Positive results in a compatible clinical setting should justify an empirical course of antimicrobial therapy. Antibody levels should fall significantly following suitable treatment. Infected patients not treated with antimicrobial agents retain elevated antibody titers, presumably for life.

Mycoplasmal Infections

Infections caused by *Mycoplasma pneumoniae* and *Ureaplasma urealyticum* are best diagnosed by culture. Availability of new media formulations from commercial media manufacturers have made it possible for microbiology laboratories to successfully cultivate these organisms.

Serologic tests for diagnosis of *M. pneumoniae* infections range from the nonspecific **"cold agglutinins" (CA)** test to **complement fixation (CF)** and **enzyme immunoassays (EIAs)** for specific antibodies. The insensitive and nonspecific CA test is relied on less often than in the past; the more accurate CF or EIA tests are performed by larger hospital and major reference laboratories.

The CA test requires that test specimens be maintained at room temperature during separation of serum from clotted blood cells. Storage at refrigerator temperatures result in absorption of agglutinins to erythrocytes. The test is set up by adding washed human group O erythrocytes to dilutions of patient sera, followed by incubation at 4°C. The assay endpoint is the highest dilution of serum that results in reversible hemagglutination, which disappears during incubation at 37°C. Approximately one-half of patients with culture-proven *M. pneumoniae* pneumonia have CA titers greater than or equal to 1:32.

The CF test is performed by mixing serum dilutions with *M. pneumoniae* lipid antigen, followed by addition of complement. Binding of complement to immune complexes is detected by adding hemolysin-coated erythrocytes. After suitable incubation, the tubes or wells are examined for hemolysis. The assay endpoint is the highest dilution of patient serum that results in less than or equal to 30% hemolysis of erythrocytes. A four-fold or greater rise in CF titer between acute and convalescent sera is evidence of recent *M. pneumoniae* infection; a single specimen CF titer greater than or equal to 1:32 in a patient with pneumonia suggests *M. pneumoniae* infection.

The EIA test is an indirect EIA in which *M. pneumoniae* antigen bound to some sort of solid phase (e.g., a plastic paddle) is exposed to patient serum, washed, reacted with anti–human immunoglobulin antibody–enzyme conjugate, washed again, and then exposed to enzyme substrate. A positive assay is indicated by conversion of the colorless substrate to a colored endproduct. Color development may be observed with the unaided eye or with a spectrophotometer.

Rickettsial Infections

Infections caused by *Rickettsia* and *Coxiella* species include the spotted fevers, typhus fevers, scrub typhus, and Q fever. Diagnosis of any of these infections is rarely achieved by culture because the organism is an obligate intracellular parasite that does not grow in cell culture.

Immunofluorescence detection of *R. rickettsii* antigen in the rash of patients with Rocky Mountain Spotted Fever (RMSF) is possible, but not widely practiced. In most instances, rickettsial infections are identified with clinical judgment, taking into account epidemiologic factors, the patient's symptoms, and general laboratory findings. Warthin-Starry stains of lymph node biopsies can be used to gain presumptive diagnosis of cat scratch disease. Specific serologic tests have been developed but are not widely available. Results of these tests, although very accurate, usually are available only after a diagnosis has been made and serve to confirm the physician's clinical impression.

During the past 10 years, two new infectious diseases caused by *Ehrlichia* spp have emerged. **Human monocytic ehrlichiosis** is caused by *E. chaffeensis* (closely related to *E. canis*) and **human granulocytic ehrlichiosis** is caused by an *E. equi*-like organism. The diagnosis of most cases of ehrlichiosis is confirmed serologically by detecting antibodies reactive by immunofluorescence (IF) assay with *E. chaffeensis* (or the surrogate *E. canis*) antigens. Most testing is performed by reference laboratories.

Another new infectious disease, **bacillary angiomatosis,** is caused by the rickettsia-like organism *Bartonella henselae*. This agent has also been implicated as the primary cause of cat scratch disease. Both IF assays and EIAs have been devised to reliably detect antibodies to this agent. A related organism for which diagnostic serologic assays are available from reference laboratories is *B. quintana,* the etiologic agent of trench fever.

One assay that is performed in a large number of laboratories is the **Weil-Felix (WF) test.** The WF test is dependent on cross-reactions that exist between the antigens of certain rickettsiae and those of selected strains of *Proteus vulgaris* and *P. mirabilis*. Suspensions of three *Proteus* strains, OX-19, OX-2, and OX-K, are added to dilutions of patient serum. After appropriate incubation, the tubes are examined for agglutination of the *Proteus* suspension. The endpoint is the highest dilution of the patient's serum that results in bacterial agglutination. Either a four-fold or greater rise in titer between acute and convalescent sera or a single specimen titer of greater than or equal to 1:320 is considered evidence of certain rickettsial infections (Table 15–3).

Other serologic assays for rickettsial antibodies that have been developed include indirect fluorescent antibody, indirect hemagglutination, latex particle agglutination, enzyme immunoassay, and complement fixation. Since these assays are rarely performed in routine laboratories, they will not be discussed in this chapter.

FUNGAL INFECTIONS

Assays for fungal antibodies are of little or no use for diagnosis of superficial fungal infections or infections in immunocompromised patients unable to mount a significant humoral immune response.

TABLE 15–3. INTERPRETATION OF WEIL-FELIX TEST RESULTS

Infection	*Proteus* Suspension		
	OX-19	OX-2	OX-K
Epidemic typhus	++++	+	0
Murine typhus	++++	+	0
Spotted fever group	++++	+	0
	+	+++	0
Brill-Zinsser disease	±	±	0
Scrub typhus	0	0	+++
Q Fever	0	0	0
Rickettsialpox	0	0	0

Detection of fungal antibodies can play a key role, however, in immunocompetent patients with longstanding invasive infections. Serology may be the only diagnostic option in patients who cannot tolerate the invasive procedures necessary for collection of suitable specimens. The assay methods used, for the most part, were described at the outset of this chapter. Table 15–4 lists the commonly performed serologic assays for fungal infection and the results that suggest recent or current infection. Following is a discussion of selected tests presently used to detect antibody responses to frequently encountered invasive fungal infections.

Aspergillosis

Immunodiffusion furnishes valuable information for diagnosis of *Aspergillus* infection in hosts capable of mounting an antibody response. The majority of patients with allergic bronchopulmonary aspergillosis or pulmonary aspergilloma have *Aspergillus* precipitins in their blood. Diagnosis of invasive aspergillosis resulting from pre-existing infection in the recently immunosuppressed host can also be aided by detection of serum antibodies. Antibody testing in patients with longstanding iatrogenically induced or disease-related immunosuppression is of little value.

Sera may be screened initially for genus-specific (and then, if positive, for species-specific) *Aspergillus* precipitins. *A. fumigatus, A. flavus,* and *A. niger* cause more than 95% of *Aspergillus* infections and should be included if species-specific testing is conducted. Immunodiffusion gels should be incubated for 48 hours at room temperature in a humid chamber. Positive specimens should exhibit precipitin lines of identity

TABLE 15–4. COMMONLY PERFORMED SEROLOGIC TESTS FOR DIAGNOSIS OF RECENT FUNGAL INFECTIONS

Organism	Test	Clinically Significant Result*
Aspergillus spp	Immunodiffusion	Positive
	Complement fixation	≥1:32
Blastomyces dermatitidis	Enzyme immunoassay	≥1:32
	Immunodiffusion	Positive
	Complement fixation	≥1:32
Candida spp	Immunodiffusion	Positive
	Latex particle agglutination	≥1:8
Coccidioides immitis	Immunodiffusion	Positive
	Complement fixation	≥1:32*
Histoplasma capsulatum	Immunodiffusion	Positive
	Complement fixation	≥1:32
	Latex particle agglutination	≥1:32

*Disseminated infection.

with positive control specimens placed on the same gel. Negative specimens should exhibit no precipitin lines and no lines of identity with controls.

The complement fixation test for *Aspergillus* antibodies, though providing very specific results in new or recent infections, is not as sensitive as immunodiffusion and is regarded as a second-line test. Positive results are best demonstrated by a four-fold or greater rise in titer between acute and convalescent specimens.

Blastomycosis

Serologic diagnosis of blastomycosis in culture negative patients or in patients whose cultures are still incubating is best accomplished by EIA. EIA results are positive in more than 75% of infected patients. The former tests of choice for serodiagnosis of blastomycosis were immunodiffusion, which is positive in fewer than 30% of infected patients, and complement fixation, which is positive in fewer than 10%. All three tests demonstrate excellent specificity.

An EIA titer of greater than or equal to 1:32 in a single specimen or with at least a four-fold rise in titer between acute and convalescent specimens is indicative of recent or current *Blastomyces dermatitidis* infection. Titers of 1:8 or 1:16 are suggestive of infection.

Candidiasis

Most infections caused by *Candida* spp are easily diagnosed by culture. The organism grows readily on routine culture media and, even when causing disseminated infection, can be recovered from the bloodstream efficiently and rapidly. Detection of *Candida* antibodies can help determine the clinical significance of *Candida* isolated from culture in patients at risk of invasive infection. However, patients at risk of invasive infection frequently are immunodeficient and may not be able to mount a detectable antibody response. Thus, negative *Candida* serologies may not rule out systemic candidiasis.

Immunodiffusion, immunoelectrophoresis (IEP), and latex particle agglutination (LPA) assays for antibodies directed against mannan (cell wall polysaccharide) or cytoplasmic protein antigens are relied on most often. The immunodiffusion method yields qualitative results and requires as long as 3 days of incubation at room temperature in a humid chamber. Serum precipitins in positive specimens must show lines of identity with positive control specimens. The IEP assay, while technically demanding to perform, provides results that better differentiate between mucocutaneous and invasive infection. The LPA assay yields quantitative results and requires only a few minutes to perform. An LPA titer of greater than or equal to 1:8 is suggestive of invasive infection; lower titers indicate early invasive infection, mucocutaneous infection, or colonization.

Coccidioidomycosis

Serologic tests for *Coccidioides immitis* antibodies are helpful for diagnosis and for monitoring the efficacy of antifungal therapy. Assay methods used include tube precipitation (TP), LPA, CF, and immunodiffusion (ID). The CF test has been the most widely used and serves as the reference method for comparative studies.

The quantitative CF and qualitative ID assays use heat-labile factors present in coccidioidin (a skin test antigen) as their antigens. Any CF antibody titer is presumptive evidence of infection, with titers greater than or equal to 1:32 suggesting disseminated infection. Positive CF titers less than or equal to 1:8 that are corroborated by positive ID results indicate recent infection. CF titers rise with advancing infection and decline with successful therapy; they can be used to monitor the status of the patient.

The quantitative TP and LPA assays use heat-treated coccidioidin as their antigens. The TP and LPA assays become positive earlier in the course of infection than the CF and ID assays. The TP assay, however, can require as long as 5 days before results are completed. The LPA assay is much more rapid than the TP assay, requiring less than 10 minutes to perform. The LPA assay is more sensitive than the TP assay, but less specific. TP and LPA antibodies usually disappear within 6 months, regardless of the patient's status.

Histoplasmosis

CF, ID, and LPA assays for antibodies to *Histoplasma capsulatum* are presently available. One of the antigens used for these tests is histoplasmin, which, unfortunately, cross-reacts to varying degrees with antibodies directed against *Blastomyces, Coccidioides,* and *Paracoccidioides.* Positive results must be interpreted in the context of the patient's epidemiologic history and clinical findings. Moreover, since histoplasmin skin testing causes transiently elevated antibody titers, patients with positive results must be questioned about past exposure to skin test antigens.

The CF test alternatively may be performed using an intact yeast cell antigen suspension. Antibody titers in infected patients rise sooner and are generally higher with the yeast cell antigen than with histoplasmin. A titer of greater than or equal to 1:32 is strong presumptive evidence of infection; a titer of 1:8 or 1:16 is presumptive evidence of infection. A four-fold or greater rise in titer between acute and convalescent sera is convincing evidence of infection.

The ID test is read after 24 hours or more incubation at room temperature in a humid chamber. When positive, the ID test provides a qualitative indication of infection if precipitin bands in patient sera form lines of identity with positive control specimens. The M band is usually the first to appear and provides inferential evidence of a recent skin test or current or past infection. The H band, if it appears, correlates with active infection.

The quantitative LPA test is also a 24-hour test and is conducted in tubes. The antibodies detected by LPA rise very quickly after onset of infection, so the LPA test usually is positive before the CF and ID tests. A titer greater than or equal to 1:32 is indicative of recent infection, but false-positive results attributable to cross-reactive antibodies or a recent skin test are possible.

PARASITIC INFECTIONS

None of the parasitic agents discussed in this section can be cultured readily by microbiology laboratories. Infections are diagnosed either by direct visualization of the agent itself or by detection of antibodies in patient specimens (Table 15–5). Thus, serologic testing plays a critical role in diagnosis of parasitic infections.

TABLE 15–5. COMMONLY PERFORMED SEROLOGIC TESTS FOR DIAGNOSIS OF RECENT PARASITIC INFECTIONS

Organism	Test	Clinically Significant Result
Entamoeba histolytica	Indirect hemagglutination	≥1:256
	Counterimmunoelectrophoresis	Positive
	Enzyme immunoassay	Positive
Toxoplasma gondii	Indirect immunofluorescence	≥1:64
	Enzyme immunoassay	Positive
Cysticercosis	Indirect hemagglutination	≥1:128
	Enzyme immunoassay	≥1:160
Toxocara spp	Enzyme immunoassay	≥1:32
Trichinella spiralis	Bentonite flocculation	≥1:5
	Enzyme immunoassay	Positive

Amebiasis

Diagnosis of dysentery and extraintestinal infection due to *Entamoeba histolytica* is greatly facilitated by serologic testing. More than 85% of infected patients possess detectable serum antibodies. Asymptomatic intestinal carriers of *E. histolytica* exhibit much lower rates of seropositivity. Microscopic examination of stained stool smears or concentrated stool suspensions is much more reliable for documenting asymptomatic carriage.

Indirect hemagglutination (IHA), counterimmunoelectrophoresis (CIE), indirect immunofluorescence (IIF), and EIA are the methods used most often to detect *E. histolytica* antibodies. The IHA procedure is performed by mixing dilutions of patient serum with erythrocytes coated with *E. histolytica* antigens. A titer greater than or equal to 1:256 is strongly suggestive of extraintestinal amebiasis. CIE, IIF, and EIA offer qualitative serologic evidence of amoebic infection and require specialized equipment for test performance.

Toxoplasmosis

Past or present *Toxoplasma gondii* infections are almost always diagnosed serologically. Baseline prenatal laboratory testing of pregnant women in high risk areas should include a screen for *T. gondii* antibodies. Infants showing signs of congenital infection, whose mothers are of unknown serologic status, should be tested for *T. gondii* IgM antibodies. The assay methods widely used in serology laboratories today include IIF and EIA.

The **Sabin-Feldman dye exclusion assay,** once the reference method for detection of *T. gondii* antibodies, is now performed rarely.

An advantage of the IIF and EIA tests is that IgG- or IgM-specific antibodies can be assayed. The laboratory must be careful, as pointed out earlier in the chapter, to pretreat specimens to separate IgM- from IgG-specific antibodies, if an IgM-specific assay is to be run. The IIF test is performed by flooding smears of *T. gondii* trophozoites with patient serum dilutions, followed by careful rinsing and staining with an anti–human immunoglobulin conjugated with a fluorescent dye. The smears are examined microscopically using ultraviolet illumination. Observation of fluorescent trophozoites indicates a positive result (Color Plate 90). An IgG titer of greater than or equal to 1:1024 in an adult suggests recent infection. Any detectable IgM in a neonate (as long as placental rupture did not occur before birth) or an IgM titer of greater than or equal to 1:64 in an adult is proof of recent infection.

The EIA is performed by adding a dilution of patient serum to a solid phase (plastic bead, walls of a tube or microtiter tray well) precoated with *T. gondii* antigen. After suitable incubation, the solid phase is carefully rinsed and reincubated with anti–human immunoglobulin conjugated with an enzyme. After a second rinse step, the enzyme substrate is added to the solid phase. A positive result is recognized by qualitatively detected or quantitatively measured color development. Modified EIAs performed by automated instruments are also available and are used by laboratories with large test volumes.

Cysticercosis

Ordinarily, humans serve as the definitive host for the pork tapeworm, *Taenia solium,* and the only stage of the life cycle present in humans is the adult worm in the gastrointestinal tract. Cysticercosis is a complication of *T. solium* infection, in which humans instead serve as an intermediate host and larval cysts form in tissues or organs.

Because symptomatic cysticercosis often results from cyst formation in difficult-to-biopsy vital organs (e.g., the brain), diagnosis frequently is accomplished radiologically or by demonstrating *T. solium* antibodies in serum. The most reliable serologic assay in current use is **indirect hemagglutination (IHA),** available from a small number of reference laboratories only. Serial dilutions of patient sera are mixed with tanned erythrocytes sensitized with *T. solium* antigens and examined for hemagglutination. A titer greater than 1:128 is clinically significant. False-positive reactions occur commonly in patients with echinococcosis.

Echinococcosis

Echinococcus granulosus is a tapeworm of dogs in which the usual intermediate host is an herbivore (e.g., sheep). Occasionally, humans, upon ingesting *E. granulosus* ova, serve as accidental intermediate hosts and echinococcal cysts may form in vital organs (e.g., liver and lungs). Symptomatic infections are customarily diagnosed by radiologic or diagnostic imaging methods, with echinococcal serology providing important adjunctive evidence.

As for cysticercosis, the test of choice for serodiagnosis of echinococcosis is IHA. A clinically significant IHA titer is greater than or equal to 1:128. Cross-reactions are commonplace in patients with a history of cysticercosis.

Toxocariasis

Toxocara spp roundworms of domestic animals (e.g., dogs and cats) can accidentally infect humans who ingest ova from fecally contaminated environments. Migrating larvae traverse the tissues and organs of the body, causing a disease known as visceral larva migrans. Many years after infection, a minority of patients experience ocular manifestations of infection, leading to visual impairment.

Detection of *Toxocara* antibodies enables the most precise diagnosis of infection. Attempting to demonstrate migratory larvae in tissue or organ biopsies has a low yield. The serologic test of choice is an EIA utilizing larval antigens obtained from embryonated *Toxocara* ova. Diagnostic titers in patients with visceral organ involvement and ocular involvement are greater than or equal to 1:32 and greater than or equal to 1:8, respectively.

Trichinellosis

Trichinellosis (trichinosis) is pursuant to human ingestion of meat containing encysted larvae of *Trichinella spiralis*. The larvae excyst, mature to the adult stage, and then produce new larvae, which migrate to striated muscle tissue of humans. There, cyst formation ensues, and when the number of cysts is sufficiently large, the symptoms of trichinellosis become evident. Diagnosis of trichinellosis is based on patient history, clinical findings, radiologic observation of calcified cysts, and, if necessary, a positive *T. spiralis* serology.

The **bentonite flocculation test** is the standard assay for serodiagnosis of trichinellosis. Serial dilutions of patient sera are mixed with a suspension of bentonite (clay) particles sensitized with *T. spiralis* larval antigens and examined for flocculation of the particles. A four-fold or greater rise in titer between acute and convalescent specimens or a single titer greater than 1:5 in a symptomatic individual is clinically significant.

VIRAL INFECTIONS

The preferred methods for diagnosis of viral infections are culture and direct detection of viral antigens or nucleic acid in clinical specimens. Serologic tests for viral antibodies (Table 15–6) are favored mainly in the following situations:

- Congenitally infected neonates, in whom IgM-specific antibody assays can lead to a speedy diagnosis
- Patients infected with viruses that are very difficult or impossible to culture
- Patients or patient populations in whom past evidence of infection is sought
- Screening of blood or organ donors

Many of the antibody assays to be discussed are similar for multiple agents: only the specificity of the antibody-binding antigens changes from test to test. To avoid repetition, only the assay characteristics that affect interpretation of test results will be discussed.

Herpes Simplex Virus Infections

Two serotypes of herpes simplex virus, types I and II, cause human infections. Virtually all adult sera contain detectable antibodies to one or both serotypes. Even so, individuals possessing these antibodies are still susceptible to repeated bouts of infection. Antibody studies are not useful for predicting immunity to infection but can be helpful in identifying congenitally infected neonates or patients scheduled for iatrogenic immunosuppression (chemotherapy or radiation therapy) who are at risk of life-threatening recurrence of infection.

Assay methods used include enzyme immunoassay (EIA) and indirect immunofluorescence (IIF). Both methods enable testing for IgM-specific antibodies, provided measures to prevent interference from organism-specific IgG or rheumatoid factor are implemented (see the specimen pretreatment regimens described earlier in the chapter). Detection of any amount of herpes simplex virus IgM antibody in cord blood (without early placental rupture) or in serum of the nontransfused neonate is evidence of congenital infection.

Characterization of herpes simplex virus serotype antibody specificity is also possible. Obtaining such information is practical during epidemiologic studies and may be necessary if type-specific antiviral therapy becomes reality. The recommended method is **indirect hemagglutination inhibition (IHAI)** testing of the patient's serum versus tanned erythrocytes sensitized with type I and type II herpes simplex virus antigens.

TABLE 15–6. COMMONLY PERFORMED SEROLOGIC TESTS FOR DIAGNOSIS OF RECENT VIRAL INFECTIONS

Organism	Test	Clinically Significant Result
Herpes simplex virus types 1 and 2	Indirect immunofluorescence	≥1:80
	Enzyme immunoassay	Positive
Human herpesvirus type 6	Indirect immunofluorescence	≥1:40
	Enzyme immunoassay	Positive
Varicella zoster virus	Complement fixation	≥1:256
	Enzyme immunoassay	Positive
	Anticomplement immunofluorescence	≥1:4
Cytomegalovirus	Indirect immunofluorescence	≥1:80
	Enzyme immunoassay	Positive
Epstein-Barr virus	Heterophile antibody	≥1:80
	Indirect immunofluorescence (VCA)	≥1:20
	Indirect immunofluorescence (EA)	≥1:20
	Anticomplement immunofluorescence (EBNA)	≥1:20
Rubella virus	Hemagglutination inhibition	≥1:8
	Latex particle agglutination	≥1:10
	Enzyme immunoassay	Positive
Parvovirus	Indirect immunofluorescence	≥1:256
	Enzyme immunoassay	Positive
	Radioimmunoassay	Positive
Hepatitis A virus (IgG/IgM)	Enzyme immunoassay	Positive
Hepatitis B virus		
Surface antigen	Enzyme immunoassay	Positive
Surface antibody	Enzyme immunoassay	Positive
Core antibody (IgG/IgM)	Enzyme immunoassay	Positive
e antigen	Enzyme immunoassay	Positive
e antibody	Enzyme immunoassay	Positive
Hepatitis C virus	Enzyme immunoassay	Positive
Hepatitis D virus	Enzyme immunoassay	Positive
Human immunodeficiency virus types 1 and 2	Enzyme immunoassay	Positive
	Western blot	Positive
Human T-lymphotropic virus type 1	Enzyme immunoassay	Positive
	Immunoblot	Positive
	Radioimmunoprecipitation	Positive

Human Herpesvirus Types 6, 7 and 8

Three new human herpesviruses identified in recent years have been named **HHV-6, HHV-7,** and **HHV-8.** HHV-6 is genetically related to cytomegalovirus (CMV) and is now recognized as the cause of the childhood illness **roseola,** also referred to as "exanthem subitum" or "sixth disease." HHV-6 has also been associated with other febrile illnesses in children, pneumonitis in organ transplant recipients, and progression of human immunodeficiency virus (HIV) infection. HHV-7 is serologically related to HHV-6 and appears to cause a roseola-like infection in children. HHV-8 has been associated with Kaposi's sarcoma and lymphoma in AIDS patients.

Serologic testing for HHV-6 antibodies can be done by EIA and IIF. Because HHV-6 is related to both CMV and HHV-7, cross-reaction with antibodies to those agents is a possibility. Development of assays with greater specificity for HHV-6 is necessary before serologic testing becomes routine. Serologic assays for HHV-7 and HHV-8 antibodies are not available commercially.

Varicella Virus Infections

Diagnosis of varicella virus infection usually is based on a history of exposure to an infected individual and clinical recognition of the characteristic rash. Diagnosis of recent infection is possible by demonstration of a four-fold or greater rise in complement fixation antibody titers in acute and convalescent sera, provided that a simultaneous rise in cross-reacting antibodies to herpes simplex virus did not occur, or by detection of IgM-specific antibodies directed against the virus.

The most frequent rationale for seeking varicella virus antibodies is to determine the immune status of individuals with negative or uncertain histories of infection in the past. Enzyme immunoassay (EIA) is more sensitive than complement fixation for determining immune status and is the most commonly used method today. A positive EIA IgG result in a patient not recently transfused nor administered varicella-zoster immune globulin is evidence of past infection and is predictive of immunity. A positive EIA IgM result is evidence of current or recent infection. Occasional patients with low antibody titers experience reinfection. Production of serum antibodies does not prevent the occurrence or recurrence of herpes zoster (shingles).

Other useful assay methods for documenting past infection are the **fluorescent antibody to membrane antigen (FAMA)** and the **anticomplement immunofluorescence (ACIF)** tests. These assays are technically more demanding to perform and read, and they generally are available in reference laboratories only.

Cytomegalovirus Infections

Cytomegalovirus (CMV) can cause serious or life-threatening infection in neonates and immunocompromised hosts. Congenital infection may be acquired *in utero* or through exposure to virus during the birthing process. The source of infection in iatrogenically immunocompromised individuals (e.g., organ transplant recipients) is often the organ itself, when harvested from a CMV-seropositive donor. CMV-infected patients with underlying immunocompromising diseases (e.g., AIDS) are usually victims of reactivated latent infection or transfused blood products from CMV-seropositive donors.

Culture is the method of choice for diagnosis of CMV infection. Testing for CMV antibodies (in hosts capable of manufacturing antibodies), however, yields results much sooner than culture, and detection of IgM-specific antibodies is diagnostic of current or recent infection. Furthermore, serologic studies are necessary to elucidate the CMV-immune status of organ or tissue donors and recipients.

EIA and IIF are the most commonly performed serologic tests for CMV antibodies. Both methods enable detection of IgM-specific antibodies for diagnosis of congenital infection and provide accurate indication of past infection. More complex, equally helpful assays for CMV antibodies (e.g., complement fixation, anticomplement immunofluorescence, indirect hemagglutination) are also available, usually from reference laboratories.

Detection of IgM-specific CMV antibodies or demonstration of rising IgG titers in serial specimens from neonates are diagnostic of congenital infection. Confirmation of distant CMV infection in donors and recipients of blood, tissue, or organs is sought by screening single serum specimens for IgG antibody.

Epstein-Barr Virus Infections

Epstein-Barr virus (EBV) causes most cases of infectious mononucleosis and has been implicated as a cause of Burkitt's lymphoma and nasopharyngeal carcinoma. EBV is difficult to culture and even when successfully grown does not prove patients are currently infected. EBV, like the other members of the herpesvirus family, becomes latent after primary infection, and recovery of virus from asymptomatic individuals is possible at any time thereafter. The preferred methods for laboratory diagnosis of EBV infections are assays for heterophile and EBV-specific antibodies.

Heterophile antibodies agglutinate erythrocytes obtained from a variety of animals. The commonly performed slide tests for infectious mononucleosis are rapid assays for sheep or horse erythrocyte-agglutinating heterophile antibodies in sera preabsorbed with guinea pig kidney to remove serum sickness antibodies and antibodies to Forssman antigen. A heterophile antibody titer greater than 1:40 in a symptomatic patient is diagnostic of infectious mononucleosis.

The heterophile antibody response in children is less dependable than in adolescents and adults, probably because of the milder course of disease seen in the young. When evaluating symptomatic children or heterophile antibody–negative adults, assays for EBV-specific antibodies may be very helpful (Fig. 15–6). Antibodies to **EBV viral capsid antigen (EBV-VCA)** rise early in illness (IgM class) and persist for life (IgG class). Antibodies to **EBV early antigen (EBV-EA)** are the first to appear; they disappear 3 to 6 months after onset of infection. IgG antibodies to **EBV nuclear antigen (EBNA)** rise late in infection (after 6 months) and persist for life.

Indirect immunofluorescence is the assay method most frequently used for detection of EBV-specific antibodies. A positive EBV-VCA IgM antibody titer is diagnostic of current or recent EBV infection. A positive EBV-EA antibody result in a patient with existing EBV-EBNA antibodies indicates a relapse of previous infection. Positive EBV-VCA IgG and EBV-EBNA antibody titers suggest a history of EBV infection in the indefinite past.

Rubella Virus Infections

Serologic evidence of **rubella virus (RV)** infection assumes tremendous importance when congenital infection in neonates is being considered.

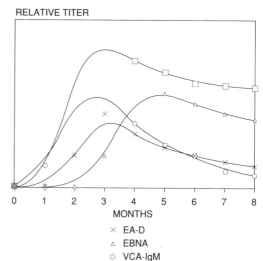

APPEARANCE OF SERUM EBV ANTIBODIES
FOLLOWING ONSET OF INFECTION

FIGURE 15–6. Appearance of Epstein-Barr virus antibodies in serum after onset of infection.

× EA-D
△ EBNA
○ VCA-IgM
□ VCA-IgG

Culture diagnosis of infection is time consuming and difficult. Because serologic testing can be accomplished rapidly and accurately, results from the serology laboratory play a key role in the physician's decision-making process.

Hemagglutination inhibition (HI), although seldom performed by laboratories today, remains the standard by which modern RV antibody tests are judged. HI is labor intensive, requires specimen pretreatment to remove inhibitors of hemagglutination, and is not as sensitive as the newer tests. The most popular test methods today include **passive hemagglutination (PHA),** in which tanned erythrocytes are sensitized with RV antigens; LPA; and EIA. Detection of HI titers greater than or equal to 1:8 is considered evidence of immunity. Lower-titered positive results from the newer, more sensitive assays may or may not indicate immunity.

The EIA for RV antibodies can be modified to detect only IgM-specific antibodies, an assay vital to the diagnosis of congenital rubella syndrome in neonates. Specimens must be pretreated to physically separate IgM from IgG to avoid interference from rheumatoid factor (false-positive results) or competition for assay antigens from IgG-specific RV antibodies (false-negative results). Alternatively, IgM capture EIAs can be used to avert these same problems. Please refer to the section earlier in this chapter on separation of IgM from IgG for a more complete discussion of the subject. Detection of any level of IgM-specific RV antibodies in the neonate constitutes proof of congenital infection.

Parvovirus

Only one of the **human parvoviruses, B19,** has been shown to be a human pathogen. Serology has been the mainstay for diagnosis of infection, with EIA or RIA methods enjoying the greatest use. Both methods lend themselves well to detection of IgM-specific antibody (diagnosis of acute or recent infection) and IgG-specific antibody (diagnosis of past infection). Test kits can be obtained from commercial sources, and reference testing service is available from a number of regional laboratories.

Hepatitis

Diagnosis of hepatitis A, B, C, or D in the laboratory is dependent on immunologic detection of specific antibodies or antigens. Both EIA and RIA procedures are used.

Hepatitis A Virus

Assays for total and IgM-specific **hepatitis A virus (HAV)** antibodies are routinely available. IgM-specific antibodies rise early in infection and disappear within 2 to 3 months. IgG-specific antibodies rise more slowly and persist for life. The assay for total HAV antibody is best used as a screen for past infection and documentation of immunity in persons visiting high-risk areas or engaging in high-risk occupations. The IgM-specific antibody assay is useful for diagnosis of current infection. As explained earlier, measures should be taken to avoid false-positive and false-negative results due to rheumatoid factor and competing IgG-specific antibody.

Hepatitis B Virus

A variety of serologic tests are available for diagnosis of **hepatitis B virus (HBV)** infection and for elucidation of the infectivity and prognosis of patients (Fig. 15–7). Commercially available tests include EIA and RIA assays for hepatitis B surface antigen (HB_sAg), hepatitis B surface antibody (HB_sAb), hepatitis B core antibody (HB_cAb), IgM-specific hepatitis B core antibody (HB_cAb-IgM), hepatitis B e antigen (HB_eAg), and hepatitis B e antibody (HB_eAb).

In the natural history of HBV infection, the HB_sAg test is the first to become positive, and it remains positive until the patient mounts an HB_sAb response. HB_sAb titers, if present, persist for life. Shortly after the appearance of HB_sAg in the serum, HB_eAg becomes detectable and remains present until HB_eAb is produced. HB_cAb-IgM is manufactured shortly after HB_sAg and HB_eAg are detectable in the serum and is the first

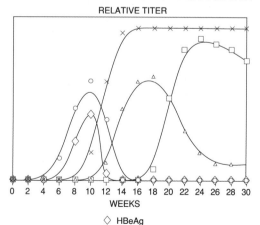

FIGURE 15–7. Appearance of hepatitis B virus antigens and antibodies in serum following infection.

of the HBV antibodies to rise in titer. Shortly thereafter, lifetime production of HB$_c$Ab-IgG commences.

The presence of HB$_s$Ab and HB$_e$Ab in serum indicates immunity to HBV infection because of previous infection or, when HB$_s$Ab alone is present, immunization against HBV. Persons whose sera remain positive for HB$_s$Ag and HB$_e$Ag for extended periods are infectious to others and are at risk of the serious complications of HBV infection. The assays for HB$_c$Ab and HB$_c$Ab-IgM are extremely useful for diagnosis of HBV infection during the "window" period between the disappearance of HB$_s$Ag and the appearance of HB$_s$Ab. When HB$_c$Ab-IgM is being assayed, potential interferences from rheumatoid factor and competing HB$_c$Ab-IgG must be avoided (see the section on Separation of IgM from IgG).

Hepatitis C Virus

The parenterally acquired infection formerly known as non-A, non-B hepatitis has now been established to be caused primarily by **hepatitis C virus (HCV).** Very soon after its discovery, a first-generation EIA for IgG antibody to an HCV cloned peptide (c110-c) was developed. Since then, second- and third-generation assays incorporating mixtures of recombinant antigens to detect a broader range of antibodies have become available. Positive results can be confirmed by use of the **recombinant immunoblot assay (RIBA),** which is available from selected reference laboratories. False-positive results, while uncommon, still are encountered even with use of third-generation assays. False-negative results were more common with first-generation assays than they are with second- and third-generation assays, but they still occur. The window period of several weeks between infection and the appearance of detectable antibodies is the main reason for false-negative results.

Hepatitis D Virus

Hepatitis D virus (HDV) (delta hepatitis virus) is a defective virus that can only coinfect patients already experiencing active HBV infections. Diagnosis of HDV infection is best accomplished by detection of HDV antibodies via EIA in serum.

Human Immunodeficiency Virus Infections

Human immunodeficiency virus type 1 (HIV-1) is the causative agent of AIDS. During the natural course of infection, HIV-1 antigens are detectable in serum shortly after onset of infection (Fig. 15–8). Several weeks to months later, HIV-1 antigens become undetectable and HIV-1 antibodies appear. Prior to the patient's death, during the final phase of infection, HIV-1 antibodies may no longer be found in serum, and HIV-1 antigens once again appear.

Serologic testing for HIV-1 infection is achieved by detecting IgG

APPEARANCE OF ANTIGEN AND ANTIBODIES
DURING HIV–1 INFECTION

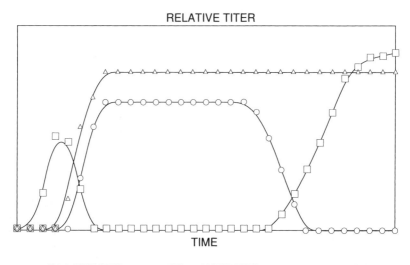

FIGURE 15–8. Appearance of human immunodeficiency virus 1 (HIV-1) antigens and antibodies in serum during infection.

antibodies using EIA as a screening test and Western blot (WB) or IF as confirmatory tests (Fig. 15–9). Available EIAs were developed initially for testing donated blood products and for that reason are exquisitely sensitive, even at the expense of some specificity. For that reason, confirmatory testing of EIA-positive specimens is absolutely essential prior to informing patients of their seropositivity. Among low-seroprevalence populations, most EIA-positive specimens are found to be falsely positive by followup testing.

Serologic diagnosis of HIV-1 infection in infants born of infected mothers is complicated by the presence of maternally derived HIV-1 IgG antibodies in the infants' bloodstream. Conventional EIA, WB, or IF assays are unable to distinguish infant antibodies from maternal antibodies. Nevertheless, it is important to determine which infants are infected for therapeutic reasons because only 15 to 25% of infants born to infected mothers turn out to be infected. One solution, which has been successful in infants 6 months of age or older, is to screen for HIV-1 IgA antibodies in serum. IgA antibodies do not cross the placenta, and those in infant sera displaying HIV-1 reactivity presumably were manufactured by the infant in response to HIV-1 infection. Unfortunately the IgA assay is much less sensitive in infants younger than 6 months and cannot be relied on to rule out infection.

Assays for HIV-1 antigens (p24 especially) are commercially available in test kit format, and in some cases results facilitate early diagnosis of HIV-1 infection. In infants born of infected mothers, detection of HIV-1 antigens would seem to be a logical means of identifying infected infants. The difficulty is that test results can be falsely negative when HIV-1 antibody is present. Since maternal antibody is inevitably present at high titer, the sensitivity of the antigen test is low in high-risk infants. Techniques like **acid dissociation of HIV-1 antigen-antibody complexes** have improved the sensitivity of the antigen test, but this still fails to identify most infected infants immediately after birth. See Chapter 8 for further discussion.

Serologic diagnosis of **HIV-2 infection** can also be performed by EIA and confirmed by Western Blot assays. The greatest use of these assays has involved testing of donated blood products.

Human T-Lymphotropic Virus Type 1

The causes of **adult T-cell leukemia/lymphoma** and **tropical spastic paraparesis** have been strongly associated with **human T-lymphotropic virus type 1 (HTLV-1).** Because HTLV-1 infection can be transmitted via donated blood products, the FDA in the United States has mandated for several years that HTLV-1 antibody screening take place on all products, using a licensed EIA. Positive antibody screening tests should be confirmed by immunoblot (IB) or radioimmunoprecipitation assays (RIPA).

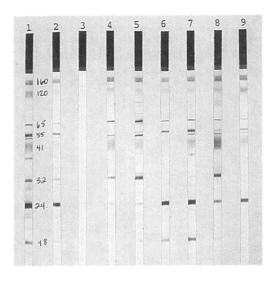

FIGURE 15–9. Western blot used in confirming human immunodeficiency virus infection. Lanes 7, 8, 9 show bands in the p24, GP41, GP120, or GP160 region (i.e., positive test results). Lanes 3, 4, without bands in these locations, are negative. Lane 1 identifies the molecular weight numerical markers.

SUGGESTED READING

Ayoub, EM: Immune response to group A streptococcal infections. Pediatr Infect Dis J 10:S15–S19, 1991.

Braden, CR, and Klempner, MS: Serologic tests for the diagnosis of Lyme disease. Infect Dis Clin Pract 2:317–324, 1993.

Cederna, JB, and Stapleton, JT: Hepatitis A virus. In Murray, PR, et al (eds): Manual of Clinical Microbiology, ed 6. American Society for Microbiology, Washington, DC, 1995, pp 1025–1032.

Herrmann, JE: Immunoassays for the diagnosis of infectious diseases. In Murray, PR, et al (eds): Manual of Clinical Microbiology, ed 6. American Society for Microbiology, Washington, DC, 1995, pp 110–122.

Hollinger, FB, and Dienstag, JL: Hepatitis B and D viruses. In Murray, PR, et al (eds): Manual of Clinical Microbiology, ed 6. American Society for Microbiology, Washington, DC, 1995, pp 1033–1049.

Larsen, SA, Steiner, BM, and Rudolph, AH: Laboratory diagnosis and interpretation of tests for syphilis. Clin Microbiol Rev 8:1–21, 1995.

Proffitt, MR, and Yen-Lieberman, B: Laboratory diagnosis of human immunodeficiency virus infection. Infect Dis Clin N Amer 7:203–220, 1993.

Sim, JG, Kim, EC, and Seo, JK: The role of serology in the diagnosis of *Helicobacter pylori* infection in children. Clin Pediatr 458–462, 1995.

Storch, GA: The diagnosis of viral infections. Infect Dis Clin Pract 2:1–20, 1993.

Wilber, JC: Hepatitis C virus. In Murray, PR, et al (eds): Manual of Clinical Microbiology, ed 6. American Society for Microbiology, Washington, DC, 1995, pp 1050–1055.

Wilkinson, HW: Serodiagnosis of *Legionella pneumophila* disease. In Rose, NR, et al (eds): Manual of Clinical Immunology, ed 3. American Society for Microbiology, Washington, DC, 1986, pp 395–398.

Wilson, M, and Arrowood, MJ: Diagnostic parasitology: Direct detection methods and serodiagnosis. Lab Med 24:145–149, 1993.

Winn, W, Jr: Legionella. In Murray, PR, et al (eds): Manual of Clinical Microbiology, ed 6. American Society for Microbiology, Washington, DC, 1995, pp 533–534.

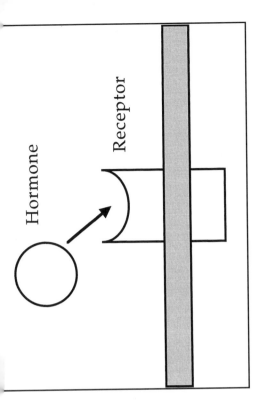

Hormone

Receptor

The Endocrine
System

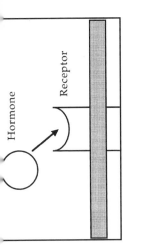

16

Laboratory Interpretation of Endocrine Tests

GENERAL PRINCIPLES

The endocrine system consists of different glands that secrete various hormones directly into the blood. Some of these hormones are regulatory in that they stimulate the secretion of metabolically active hormones from other glands. The secretion, and thus the concentration, of each hormone is under continuous feedback control in normal physiologic conditions. Consequently, the concentration of each hormone in the circulation should fall within a predictable range in the healthy state. Diagnosis of endocrine disorders is made possible largely through the direct measurement of individual hormones in serum.

MECHANISMS OF ACTION

Peptide or protein hormones and catecholamines cannot pass through the lipid membrane of a cell on their own because of either large molecular size or polarity with molecular charge that makes them insoluble in lipid. Consequently, to have an influence, they must

739

interact with receptors on cell surfaces. Whether a hormone in the circulation will be effective at a particular tissue site depends on the presence of receptor molecules specific for that hormone on cell surfaces. The receptor molecule for a given hormone will recognize no other hormone. As the hormone binds to the correct receptor in the cell membrane, the cell is stimulated through a series of activation steps resulting in the synthesis of a "second messenger" that transmits the stimulation signal intracellularly. Examples of these second messengers are adenosine 3',5'-monophosphate (cyclic AMP, cAMP), inositol phosphate, and calcium ions.

Some hormone receptors extend from the extracellular side through the cell membrane to interact with a guanine nucleotide-binding protein **(G protein)** on the cytoplasmic side of the membrane. Binding of hormone to receptor promotes an association with the G protein, which then gives up a molecule of guanine diphosphate (GDP) and picks up another molecule of guanine triphosphate (GTP). This complex interacts with adenylate cyclase in the cytoplasm to convert adenosine triphosphate (ATP) to cAMP (Fig. 16–1). This second messenger cAMP diffuses throughout the cytoplasm, where it activates enzymes called **cAMP-dependent protein kinases;** these are able to phosphorylate other proteins that control cell processes such as cell respiration, ion transport, transcription, protein synthesis, DNA synthesis, and cell growth, thereby effecting action of the hormone in that cell. The intracellular concentration of cAMP is regulated by the enzyme **phosphodiesterase,** which converts it to AMP, which no longer is able to stimulate protein kinase activity. The pituitary hormones ACTH, FSH, LH, and TSH, as well as human chorionic gonadotropin, parathyroid hormone, catecholamines, and glucagon generate cAMP by this mechanism.

An analogous series of reactions occurs for some other hormones (releasing factors, ADH) in which binding to the receptor and interaction with a G protein results in activation of the enzyme phospholipase C, which generates inositol phosphate. This molecule causes release of intracellular calcium ions, which activate protein kinase C. Through this type of reaction and also by binding to calmodulin, calcium ions act as a second messenger. Still another mechanism for hormone action involves binding to a receptor that stimulates tyrosine kinase activity directly without a second messenger. Insulin and some growth factors act through this mechanism.

A completely different mechanism of hormone action is employed by steroid and thyroid hormones that are able to move directly across the cell membrane. Steroid hormones bind to receptor molecules in the cytoplasm and are transported to the cell nucleus, where the activated complex of hormone and receptor stimulates mRNA transcription of specific genes. Thyroid hormone similarly stimulates transcription by interacting with receptors in chromatin of the nucleus.

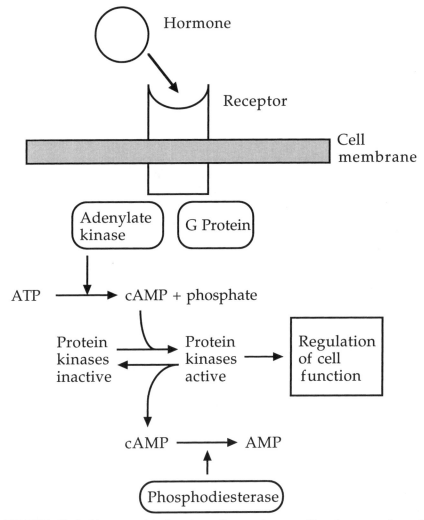

FIGURE 16–1. Hormone binding to cell receptor, resulting in generation of second messenger cAMP. Phosphodiesterase further degrades cAMP to down-regulate hormone stimulation.

CONTROL OF HORMONE SECRETION

The majority of endocrine functions are regulated through the pituitary gland, which in turn is controlled by secretions from the hypothalamus. The posterior part of the pituitary secretes some hormones that have direct effects on end organs (vasopressin and oxytocin). From its anterior part it secretes a group of stimulating hormones that circulate to other endocrine glands and cause those glands to secrete hormones that then directly affect end organs.

Because of the tight feedback control among all these secretions, it should theoretically be possible to measure concentrations of only one hormone in each feedback loop in order to detect an endocrine disorder. However, in clinical practice it is frequently desirable to measure multiple hormone levels in order to rule out even minor abnormalities that might be the only chemical sign early in the course of endocrine disease. In addition, the measurement of hormones from both the pituitary and those organs it stimulates can assist in determining whether an endocrine disorder is primary to the final secreting gland (e.g., thyroid, adrenal cortex, gonad), to the pituitary, or even to the hypothalamus. It is also possible to interrupt the feedback loop for diagnostic purposes by administering a drug in a stimulation test to determine more precisely at which level apparent endocrine failure has occurred.

PITUITARY-HYPOTHALAMIC AXIS

The normal pituitary gland is a 1-gram sphere of tissue located inferior to the midbrain, and connected to it by a short stalk. The main body of the pituitary is contained in a small bony structure called the sella turcica and is adjacent to the chiasm of the optic nerve. Because of these anatomic relationships, enlargement of the pituitary due to tumor may present initially with loss of vision in some quadrants of the visual field; skull x-rays can show erosion of the sella turcica due to tumor extension.

The pituitary secretes numerous hormones and is sometimes called the "master gland" of the body. The anterior lobe, or **adenohypophysis,** consists of specialized secretory epithelial cells. The tropic hormones that it secretes in turn stimulate endocrine secretion by the adrenal gland **(adrenocorticotropic hormone, ACTH),** thyroid gland **(thyroid-stimulating hormone, TSH),** and gonads **(follicle-stimulating hormone, FSH; luteinizing hormone, LH)** (Fig. 16–2). The anterior pituitary also secretes human **growth hormone (GH),** which directly affects skeletal growth and overall metabolism. It also secretes **prolactin,** which stimulates breast growth and milk production. The posterior lobe (through which the pituitary is attached to the brain) is of neuroectodermal origin and is referred to as the **neurohypophysis.** It secretes **antidiuretic hormone (ADH,** also called **vasopressin),** a polypeptide hormone that increases blood pressure and also regulates water excretion by decreasing urine flow at the level of renal tubules (see Chapter 10). In addition, the posterior pituitary secretes **oxytocin,** an octapeptide that stimulates uterine contractions during labor and release of milk from the lactating breast.

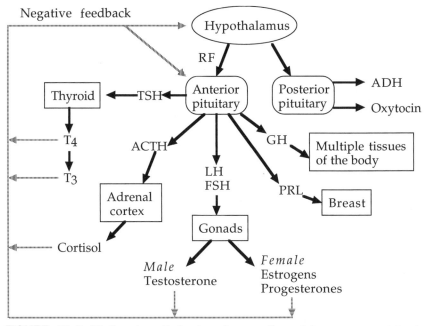

FIGURE 16–2. Pituitary-hypothalamic axis secretion of hormones and feedback control. RF = releasing factors; TSH = thyroid-stimulating hormone; ACTH = adrenocorticotropic hormone; LH = luteinizing hormone; FSH = follicle-stimulating hormone; PRL = prolactin; GH = growth hormone. Solid lines indicate stimulation; dashed lines indicate inhibition.

The pituitary does not function as an autonomous master: adenohypophyseal hormones are released only after stimulation by hypothalamic hormones, and the two major secretory products of the posterior hypophysis are actually synthesized by the hypothalamus. The neurohypophysis acts only for storage and ultimate release of vasopressin and of oxytocin.

HYPOTHALAMIC HORMONES

The hypothalamus regulates pituitary function in response to physical cues provided by circulating hormone levels and other messages carried in the blood. In addition, hypothalamic secretions can be influenced by drugs or psychiatric disorders that affect higher neurologic levels. Not all the hypothalamic regulators or releasing factors are fully understood. Some of the well-characterized hypothalamic hormones are shown in Table 16–1. These releasing factors are secreted by the hypothalamus into

TABLE 16–1. HORMONES PRODUCED BY THE HYPOTHALAMUS

Hypothalamic Product	Target Effect
Gonadotropin-releasing hormone (GnRH, LHRH)	Stimulates pituitary to release FSH and LH
Thyrotropin-releasing hormone (TRH)	Stimulates pituitary release of TSH
Corticotropin-releasing hormone (CRH)	Stimulates pituitary release of ACTH
Growth hormone releasing-inhibiting hormone (somatostatin)	Inhibits pituitary release of hGH
	Inhibits secretion of insulin, glucagon, gastrin
	Diminishes gastric acid production
	May diminish parathyroid hormone, calcitonin, renin production
Vasopressin (antidiuretic hormone, ADH)	Allows water resorption in distal convoluted tubules, collecting ducts in kidney
	Raises blood pressure by vasoconstriction
Oxytocin	Stimulates myometrial contractions
	Releases milk from lactating breast

FSH = follicle stimulating hormone; LH = luteinizing hormone; TSH = thyroid-stimulating hormone; ACTH = adrenocorticotropic hormone; hGH = human growth hormone; RH = releasing hormone.

a venous blood supply that then passes directly to the adenohypophysis through a portal circulation. Consequently, the lag time from hypothalamic secretion to pituitary stimulation is very short. In addition, the local concentration of the releasing hormones at the adenohypophysis is much higher than systemic levels of those hormones once they have been thoroughly mixed into the circulation. For that reason, it is not generally feasible to assay for the releasing factors in samples of blood in the evaluation of endocrine disease. However, several of these short-chain peptides have been synthesized in the laboratory and are available commercially for use in provocative diagnostic stimulation tests.

ANTERIOR PITUITARY HORMONES

The secretory cells of the anterior pituitary are described by their staining characteristics and secretory products as **acidophil, basophil,** and **chromophobe cells.** Pituitary hormones are classified by chemical configuration into three groups:

- **Polypeptides** with intramolecular disulfide bonds, such as growth hormone and prolactin. They share a partial amino acid sequence that also occurs in placental prolactin, a hormone present only during pregnancy.

- **Glycoproteins** such as TSH, FSH, and LH. All three share a common subunit (alpha chain), and each has another distinctive peptide chain with a carbohydrate portion (beta subunit). The placental hormone chorionic gonadotropin has the same alpha subunit and its own distinct beta chain.
- **Single-chain peptides** without disulfide bonds. ACTH is the major example, but products of the intermediate portion of the pituitary fall into this group.

In fact, several different active molecules are derived from cleavage of a single large prohormone molecule called **pro-opiocortin**. This natural precursor is split into two smaller molecules, **corticotropin (ACTH)** and **beta-lipotropin**. The first of these products, corticotropin, is the active form of ACTH. It can also be split further to yield a melanocyte-stimulating hormone, the one designated **alpha-MSH**. The intermediate beta-lipotropin is also further degraded into **gamma-lipotropin, beta-endorphin** (a natural neural modulator that induces analgesia through its chemical similarity to morphine), and another melanocyte-stimulating hormone, **beta-MSH**. It is possible that other undiscovered hormone activities may reside in proteolytic cleavage products of pro-opiocortin.

Radioimmunoassays have been used for many years to measure the pituitary hormones in blood. Advances in monoclonal antibody technology and enzyme labeling have made modern assays possible for many of these hormones using automated instrumentation without radioisotopes. Thus most laboratories should have available rapid measurements for at least TSH and human chorionic gonadotropin (hCG) and perhaps also for FSH and LH. Corticotropin (ACTH) is a more labile material and few laboratories attempt to measure it but prefer to send samples for occasional ACTH measurements to reference laboratories. ACTH measurements tend to be requested far less frequently than the other pituitary hormones, partly because of the widespread availability of more easily performed cortisol assays. The tropic hormones are discussed below in the sections that consider the activities of their target glands. The rest are described in the following sections.

GROWTH HORMONE

Growth hormone (GH), a polypeptide with a molecular size of 21,500 daltons, is the only hormone present in substantial amounts in the pituitary gland itself. It shares structural similarities with prolactin and chorionic somatomammotropin. It is secreted in episodic bursts, most prominently during early sleep and also a few hours after eating or after exercise. Basal (fasting) levels in the serum of adults are less than approximately 7 ng/mL; after stimulation, GH levels are expected to rise by 5 to 7 ng/mL to a peak of greater than 10 ng/mL. Although GH exerts its most conspicuous physiologic effects during the growth phases of infancy and childhood, serum levels are the same for adults and for children, except for elevated levels at birth and in the first few months of life. In adulthood, GH has continued actions to promote soft tissue and bone growth through stimulation of protein synthesis.

Excessive GH production causes signs and symptoms in both children and adults, but the deficiency state is more apparent in children. Stimuli that induce the release of GH include exercise, hypoglycemia, and protein in the diet. It also is released by acute starvation and by oral contraceptives because of estrogen content. Decreases of GH are typically found in obesity and in corticosteroid therapy. Pharmaceutical preparations of recombinant GH synthesized from the cloned human gene are now available for replacement therapy in cases of deficiency. Previously GH could only be obtained by extracting it from the pituitaries of hundreds to thousands of cadavers. The human product is no longer deemed safe because some recipients developed Creutzfeld-Jakob disease (CJD), an untreatable spongiform encephalopathy presumably transmitted from a small number of the donors through pooled preparations of cadaveric GH. The present availability of synthetic GH will help those patients with genuine deficiency states, but it appears that it also has a large illicit market among athletes and others who want to increase body and muscle mass surreptitiously for competition.

Metabolic Effects

Growth hormone stimulates synthesis of RNA and in so doing effects an increase in protein synthesis and anabolic metabolism. Growth hormone stimulates the liver to produce proteins called **somatomedins.** Previously, one of these was called "sulfation factor" because it stimulated the incorporation of sulfate into cartilage, but it also promotes DNA, RNA, and collagen synthesis. Subsequent studies have shown that the somatomedins are structurally similar to insulin; accordingly they are currently referred to as **insulin-like growth factors (IGFs).** The concentrations of IGFs are more constant in the circulation over the course of the day than are the peaks and valleys of GH. IGF levels are influenced by the nutritional status of an individual, with low levels occurring in malnutrition. IGFs mediate the effect of GH on skeletal growth. The net effect is increased synthesis of RNA, DNA, and protein with increased sulfation of cartilage constituents locally at sites of bone growth. **IGF-1** (previously called "somatomedin C") has additional insulin-like activity in that it inhibits lipolysis and stimulates adipose tissue to metabolize glucose.

Growth hormone also affects energy metabolism by mobilizing fatty acids from fat stores that travel by the circulation to muscle cells where they can be used during exercise. Under chronic GH influence, hepatic glucose output rises (i.e., antagonist of insulin action) and transport of amino acids into peripheral cells is enhanced. Growth hormone also increases renal cortical blood flow and glomerular filtration rate, with the kidneys excreting more calcium and less phosphate than usual. Net nitrogen balance becomes positive under excess GH action because of increased protein synthesis that retains nitrogen in the body.

Deficiency States

Children with GH deficiency have very small stature but normal body proportions. Children with growth retardation should be screened for GH deficiency, which may be congenital or acquired. If other pituitary hormones besides GH are reduced, deficient thyroid, adrenal, and gonadal development will also be noted (panhypopituitarism). Pituitary dwarfism is uncommon, an estimated 150 to 200 new cases being diagnosed annually in the United States. Pituitary tumors and craniopharyngiomas account for a third of these; another third result from other kinds of pituitary damage. Isolated deficiency of GH with apparently normal levels of other hormones causes only one-third of pituitary dwarfism. Measurement of IGF-1 is useful in the diagnosis of growth disorders in children because it is low whenever GH is deficient. A normal value of IGF-1 indicates normal stimulation by GH, even when direct measurement of GH is undetectable or otherwise equivocal. Low levels of IGF-1 should be followed up by other testing such as stimulation tests (see below) to evaluate GH secretion more directly.

Isolated GH deficiency causes no recognizable syndrome in adults. If other tropic hormones are also deficient, hypogonadism tends to occur first, followed by declining thyroid function. Hypoadrenalism is usually the last to develop. Tumors cause 50% of adult hypopituitarism; gradually evolving vascular or idiopathic changes account for most of the rest.

Excessive Production

Excessive GH stimulation of the actively growing skeleton causes long bones to continue enlarging, producing tall stature with eunuchoid proportions **(pituitary gigantism).** Hypersecretion of GH occurs more often in adults than in children; eosinophilic or chromophobe cell tumors are the usual cause. The pathognomonic physical appearance of acromegaly results from thickening of the bones of the skull (especially frontal bossing and enlargement of the jaw) and of the hands and feet. Internal organs, skeleton, and heart muscle also hypertrophy; nerves and cartilage often enlarge to produce nerve compression and joint disorders. Because of its anatomic location near the optic chiasm, enlargement of the pituitary with a tumor can cause selective visual impairment. In addition, excess secretion of GH can lead to diabetes mellitus due to its antagonism with insulin. Diagnosis of pituitary adenoma is often aided by computed tomography (CT) or magnetic resonance imaging (MRI) of the skull to detect destruction of the sella turcica and extension of the gland beyond normal dimensions.

Laboratory Evaluation

Growth hormone is quantitated in serum by methods such as radioimmunoassay and more recently with immunoassays using chemiluminescence. Single determinations are typically done on fasting morning samples. Many events stimulate GH secretion: low serum glucose levels, dopamine and other neurotransmitters, exercise or stress, and many other physiological and pharmacologic agents. Measurement of baseline serum GH level alone can be misleading. Normal individuals may have low to undetectable levels, and hypersecreting individuals may have values that fall within the normal range. More useful than baseline measurement is information gained by observing the effects of stimulation in cases of suspected deficiency or suppression in situations of excessive production.

Provocative Tests to Encourage Growth Hormone Secretion

Hypoglycemia to levels below 50 mg/dL causes GH levels to rise tenfold or more in most normal individuals. Giving insulin to provoke hypoglycemia must be done under careful medical supervision, with provision for treatment if the patient becomes symptomatic. Intravenous administration of L-dopa or the amino acid arginine also induces predictable secretory surges. GH-releasing hormone is also available for stimulation studies. A typical stimulation test for GH would include samples at baseline (time 0) and at intervals of 15, 30, 45, 60, 90, and 120 minutes, although individual protocols vary in precise timing.

A successful stimulation test in a person with normal pituitary function results in an incremental rise in GH of at least 5 to 7 ng/mL above baseline. A smaller rise suggests partial hormone deficiency; no rise coupled with undetectable baseline level indicates inability to secrete GH. Patients respond idiosyncratically to the different stimuli, so it is desirable to attempt two or three different stimulation tests before concluding that the pituitary is unresponsive.

Hyperglycemia suppresses GH secretion in normal persons but not in those with autonomous or elevated hormone levels. The diagnosis of acromegaly can be made if serum GH levels are repeatedly above 10 ng/mL, even if some decline occurs after glucose infusion. Whereas normal persons increase GH secretion after receiving L-dopa, persons with acromegaly may reduce their GH output.

PROLACTIN

Prolactin is a single-chain polypeptide with three disulfide bonds and molecular weight of about 22,000. It is unique among known hormones in that prolactin secretion is not driven by positive stimulation, but rather is continuous unless suppressed by a specific inhibitory control mechanism. Pituitary lactotropic acidophil cells secrete prolactin; their number increases under the influence of estrogen during pregnancy. **Prolactin-inhibiting factor (PIF)** is released from the hypothalamus; PIF is either dopamine or under the control of dopaminergic neurons. Consequently administration of L-dopa can suppress secretion of prolactin. Circulating prolactin levels rise in patients with reduced dopamine levels, with damaged hypothalamic function, or with anatomic separation of the pituitary from the hypothalamus. In men and nonpregnant women, secretion occurs in bursts that result from sleep, stress, and hypoglycemia. Physiologic functions of prolactin include the stimulation of breast growth and milk production as well as steroidogenesis in the adrenals and gonads, metabolism of carbohydrates and fat, vitamin D metabolism, and aspects of fetal development.

Concentrations of prolactin in blood rise in response to exercise, sleep, stress, anxiety, hypoglycemia, sexual intercourse, pregnancy, and nipple stimulation (suckling). Thyrotropin-releasing hormone (TRH) also stimulates prolactin release, which can be used as a clinical, provocative test to evaluate stores and secretion capacity. Measurement of prolactin is applied to the evaluation of galactorrhea and amenorrhea and to the diagnosis of prolactinomas (acidophil adenomas), which are the most common disorder involving excess pituitary secretion. The major diagnostic distinction to be made in cases of hyperprolactinemia is between a hypothalamic dysfunction and an autonomous prolactinoma, in which case the levels of prolactin tend to be much higher. In addition to the physiologic influences on prolactin secretion, a number of drugs, including psychotropics, antihypertensives, and estrogen, can elevate prolactin. The drug bromocriptine causes a decrease of prolactin and is used to treat disorders with abnormally elevated prolactin.

PANHYPOPITUITARISM

Global pituitary deficiency, when it occurs, usually develops very gradually. Hormone deficiency may be the presenting sign, or evidence of intracranial disease may prompt evaluation that uncovers hormonal dysfunction. The most common cause is pituitary destruction by tumors, frequently eosinophil or chromophobe adenoma of the pituitary or tumors of nearby structures. Vascular damage, notably postpartum pituitary necrosis **(Sheehan's syndrome)**, may occur without acute clinical changes, and months or years may elapse before functional deficiencies develop. Many cases that manifest as hypopituitarism are probably due to hypothalamic problems. If purified releasing-factor preparations are available, hypothalamic failure can be distinguished from pituitary failure by administering pituitary stimulants.

DIAGNOSTIC APPROACHES

A useful test for evaluating the hypothalamic-pituitary axis is administering insulin to provoke hypoglycemia. Besides inducing GH release, hypoglycemia below 50 mg/dL also stimulates ACTH release; with normal pituitary and adrenal function, plasma cortisol should rise to 20 µg/dL or more. Patients with poorly controlled diabetes, ischemic heart disease, epilepsy, or severely inadequate adrenal function should not be exposed to the risk of profound hypoglycemia.

An acquired form of apparent hypopituitarism is **anorexia nervosa,** or self-induced starvation. However, several striking differences exist between true panhypopituitarism and this form of acquired metabolic imbalance (Table 16–2).

PATIENT CARE CONSIDERATIONS

Pituitary hypofunction is suspected when target gland functions are defective. The first line of investigation consists of history, physical examination, and preliminary tests to evaluate gonadal, thyroid, and adrenal activities. Clinical findings that should arouse suspicion include abnormalities of skeletal growth, retarded or accelerated sexual matura-

TABLE 16–2. DISTINCTION BETWEEN HYPOPITUITARISM AND ANOREXIA NERVOSA

Characteristic	Panhypopituitarism	Anorexia Nervosa
Age	Any age	Adolescence or early adulthood
Sex distribution	Slight preponderance of females	F:M = 9:1 or more
Cachexia	Rare	Frequent
Body hair	Diminished or absent	Present
Circulating GH	Low	Normal or high
TSH and thyroid function	Low	Normal

GH = growth hormone; TSH = thyroid-stimulating hormone.

tion, disappearance of previously established sexual function, thyroid or adrenal insufficiency, disorders of fluid regulation, galactorrhea, and neurologic signs suggesting intracranial disease.

Once target gland hormones are found to be deficient, both pituitary and end-organ activity should be evaluated. Of the pituitary hormones, TSH, FSH, and LH are the easiest to measure. Measurement of ACTH may not be available on site and so may not be used as much. More detailed investigation may include measuring prolactin, specific gonadal hormones, and GH. Stimulation tests can provide definitive differential information, but they are often inconvenient, expensive, or uncomfortable, and should be performed only to obtain clearly defined and necessary information.

POSTERIOR PITUITARY HORMONES

The hypothalamus synthesizes ADH (arginine vasopressin) and oxytocin, which are then transported in secretory granules via neuronal axons to the posterior pituitary (neurohypophysis), where they are stored until stimulation for release. Both of these hormones are nonapeptides (containing nine amino acids) that have very similar chemical structures (Fig. 16–3). ADH has two major actions: altering the permeability of renal collecting tubules to water and causing vasoconstriction. This latter property can be used therapeutically in von Willebrand's disease as arginine vasopressin will also release von Willebrand factor from storage granules in vascular endothelium. Oxytocin stimulates contraction of the uterus and also the lactating breast. Oxytocin can be used therapeutically to induce labor. Its function in males is unknown.

ANTIDIURETIC HORMONE AND REGULATION OF BODY WATER

Despite wide variations in metabolic conditions, serum osmolality normally remains within a very narrow range, 285 to 310 mOsm/liter. Urinary excretion of solutes and water contributes most importantly to this equilibrium. Many uncontrolled variables affect the quantity of solutes to be excreted, so the amount of water excreted with the solutes is the major point of osmotic regulation. Urine volume in healthy individuals can range from 500 to 2000 mL/day.

The amount of water the kidneys excrete is determined by ADH acting on the distal convoluted tubule and collecting ducts. Cells are normally rather impermeable to water; without ADH, the large volume of water in hypo-osmolar tubular fluid passes unaltered to be excreted as highly dilute urine. ADH acts on renal tubular epithelial cells to allow water

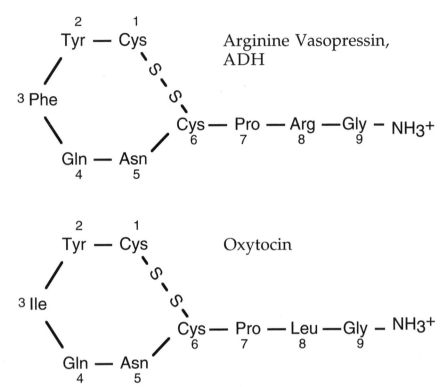

FIGURE 16–3. Amino acid sequences of the cyclic peptide hormones antidiuretic hormone (ADH, arginine vasopressin) and oxytocin, which are secreted by the posterior pituitary.

from the tubules to be drawn toward the hypertonic interstitial fluid of the medulla, which exerts a countercurrent concentrating effect (see Chapters 10 and 19). Without ADH, urine has an osmolality of about 50 mOsm/liter. With maximum ADH secretion, osmolality reaches 1100 mOsm/liter; additional concentration to 1400 mOsm/liter can be achieved during severe water deprivation when slow tubular flow allows maximum countercurrent concentrating effect.

Control of Osmolality

Stimulus of ADH release arises from osmoreceptors in the hypothalamus; an increase in extracellular osmolality causes these receptors to send nerve impulses to cells of the posterior pituitary, which then release ADH. Baroreceptors that sense blood volume also stimulate ADH release. Usually ADH is secreted when plasma/serum osmolality rises above 285 mOsm/liter. Psychogenic stimuli also affect ADH levels, but the mechanism is unclear. During periods of water deprivation the thirst reflex (to drink upon dehydration) and ADH secretion (to decrease water loss) act in concert to stabilize water status. Osmoregulatory centers in the hypothalamus respond to changes as modest as 2% of serum osmolality. Diminished blood volume provokes ADH secretion without change in osmolality, but the threshold for ADH stimulation is 10% volume loss. Cholinergic drugs, barbiturates, morphine, nicotine, and histamine stimulate ADH release, whereas alcohol and the phenytoin drugs inhibit ADH secretion. Incidentally, secretion of the other posterior pituitary hormone, oxytocin, is also inhibited by alcohol, which has been used intravenously for stopping premature labor.

Renal Function

Antidiuretic hormone is not the only regulator of urine volume and concentration. Destruction of renal tissue, especially the juxtamedullary nephrons where ADH plays its most significant role, impairs renal concentrating ability, as does diminished glomerular filtration rate. If there is a large solute load to be excreted, urine volume and concentration will both be high, relatively independent of ADH status. This occurs with the osmotic diuresis caused by hyperglycemia, mannitol, or radiographic contrast media. Alterations of renal tubular mineralocorticoid activity also cause high-concentration diuresis. Abnormal intake of fluids (**psychogenic polydipsia,** or compulsive water drinking) causes very low-concentration diuresis; as massive volumes of fluid pass through the tubules, tubular epithelium temporarily loses its responsiveness to ADH.

DIABETES INSIPIDUS

Diabetes insipidus occurs when ADH secretion or response is inadequate. Other causes for excessive urine output are referred to as **polyuria.** Pituitary-hypothalamic regulation of ADH may be impaired because of trauma, neoplastic or inflammatory destruction of tissue, or surgical ablation of the pituitary. However, most diabetes insipidus is described as idiopathic because no clearly defined lesion can be found. Characteristic of the condition is daily excretion of 3 liters or more of urine with osmolality consistently below 300 mOsm/kg or specific gravity below 1.010. The body responds to fluid loss by increasing fluid intake, so the patient consumes a correspondingly large amount of water. The average ADH concentration in healthy adults is 2.3 to 3.1 pg/mL of serum; in diabetes insipidus, ADH may be unmeasurable. However, direct measurement is rarely available, so the diagnosis of ADH deficiency is usually made by observing urine responses to alterations of body fluid.

Concentration Testing

Overnight water deprivation is the first step. After 8 to 12 hours without fluid intake, normal individuals preserve normal serum osmolality and excrete urine with 800 mOsm/kg or more; in ADH deficiency, urine osmolality does not rise above 300 mOsm/kg. As body water diminishes, urine concentration increases until a plateau is reached and no further concentration occurs. In normal persons, this usually occurs after 16 to 18 hours without water intake. With massive urinary water loss, water deprivation for 4 to 8 hours may produce the concentration plateau, but if ADH is deficient, urine osmolality continues to be low while serum osmolality increases. Patients must be observed carefully throughout the test, partly to prevent the patient with severe ADH deficiency from collapsing with dehydration and partly to prevent the patient with psychogenic polydipsia from surreptitiously consuming fluid.

Once the concentration plateau has been reached, administering exogenous ADH (aqueous vasopressin) provides additional diagnostic information. If there is primary ADH deficiency, administration of vasopressin causes urine osmolality to increase substantially. If the problem is renal insensitivity to ADH (nephrogenic diabetes insipidus), exogenous vasopressin has little effect. If the problem is psychogenic polydipsia, serum osmolality remains normal with water deprivation, peak urine osmolality is well above serum osmolality, and exogenous vasopressin causes little further concentration. Differential observations are shown in Table 16–3.

These tests should be done only after other causes for polyuria have been excluded, especially hyperglycemia, uremia, and such electrolyte disturbances as hypercalcemia, hypokalemia, excessive electrolyte or diuretic therapy, and renal disorders of bicarbonate and sodium excretion.

INAPPROPRIATE SECRETION OF ANTIDIURETIC HORMONE

Excessive urine concentration relative to serum osmolality can occur with impaired hypothalamic-pituitary regulation or, more often, when there are excessive levels of ADH-active material of nonpituitary origin. This is called the **syndrome of inappropriate ADH secretion (SIADH).** Characteristic findings are low serum osmolality and low serum sodium at a time when urine is hypertonic and contains excreted sodium. Hyponatremia may be masked by dehydration, and with severe sodium depletion, urine sodium levels may diminish, but the hallmark finding is urine osmolality inappropriately high for serum levels of sodium and osmolality (see Chapter 19).

Measuring ADH levels is rarely necessary for diagnosis. Because kidney or adrenal disease can produce hyponatremia and abnormal urine

TABLE 16-3. DIFFERENTIAL DIAGNOSIS OF POLYURIA

	Urine Osmolality (mOsm/kg)		Serum Osmolality (mOsm/kg)		Effects of Exogenous ADH After Plateau
	Average	Plateau	Average	Plateau	
Normal individuals	300–800	~1600	280–295	<300	Very little
Osmotic diuresis	High	High	High	High	Very little
Diabetes insipidus	<300	<300	Normal or ↑	>300	Urine osmolality increases
Nephrogenic diabetes insipidus	<300	<300	Normal or ↓	>300	Very little
Primary polydipsia	<300	Variable but above serum levels	Normal	Normal	Very little

findings, it is important to document that BUN and electrolytes other than sodium are all normal. Sodium depletion from chronic gastrointestinal tract or kidney disease must be ruled out, as well as the low-sodium, high-blood-volume conditions of cirrhosis and cardiac failure. When other causes of hyponatremia have been eliminated and serum sodium has been raised to 125 mEq/liter or more to protect the patient against symptomatic hyponatremia, a water loading test can confirm the diagnosis of SIADH.

Water Loading

Water loading involves giving 1000 mL of water orally and then collecting hourly urine and serum samples for 5 hours. Normal results are urinary excretion of 600 mL or more in 4 hours, with urine osmolality falling below that of serum, nearly always to levels below 180 mOsm/kg. In SIADH, serum osmolality falls, but urine does not become appropriately dilute; urine osmolality remains higher than serum values, usually higher than 230 mOsm/kg.

Inappropriate ADH secretion syndrome was initially demonstrated in cases of ectopic hormone production by bronchogenic carcinoma; this is still the most common tumor-associated cause. Many other tumors have also been found to cause the syndrome. The causes of SIADH are listed in Table 16–4.

LABORATORY MEASUREMENT OF ADH

The laboratory measurement of ADH (frequently listed as vasopressin) in serum entails an initial extraction either with an organic solvent or by column chromatography to remove interfering substances and to concentrate ADH for quantitation by radioimmunoassay. ADH measurements are not commonly requested and are generally performed only in reference laboratories because of the complexity of the procedure. Any request for ADH measurement should be accompanied by measurement of serum osmolality for proper interpretation; the reference range for ADH is 0 to 2 pg/mL when osmolality is less than 285 mOsm/L, and 2 to 12 pg/mL when osmolality is greater than 290 mOsm/L.

Although most clinical conditions with ADH abnormalities may be diagnosed by measuring electrolytes and osmolality in serum and urine, quantitation of ADH has some utility in distinguishing between central (hypothalamic) diabetes insipidus (low or absent ADH), in which ADH production or release is deficient, and nephrogenic diabetes insipidus (normal or elevated ADH), in which the kidneys fail to respond.

TABLE 16–4. CAUSES OF THE SYNDROME OF INAPPROPRIATE ANTIDIURETIC HORMONE SECRETION (SIADH)

Tumors
Bronchogenic carcinoma
Thymoma
Lymphoma
Pancreatic carcinoma
Gastrointestinal carcinoma

Pulmonary disease
Tuberculosis
Pneumonia

Central nervous system disorder
Brain tumor (secondary stimulation)
Abscess
Meningitis
Inflammatory disorder

Endocrine abnormality
Thyroid
Adrenal

Drugs
Chlorpropamide
Thiazide diuretics
Vincristine
Clofibrate

ADRENAL GLAND

The adrenal, like the pituitary, has two functionally and embryologically distinct portions. The outer portion or cortex is of mesodermal origin and secretes several essential steroid hormones that assist in maintaining homeostatic processes of life. The inner region or medulla derives from ectoderm, and its secretions are involved in the regulation of acute responses of the entire body to stimuli from the environment.

STEROID HORMONES

Adrenal cortical hormones are steroids, compounds whose basic structure is the cyclopentanoperhydrophenanthrene ring, a 17-carbon skeleton derived from cholesterol (Fig. 16–4). The cortex secretes three types of

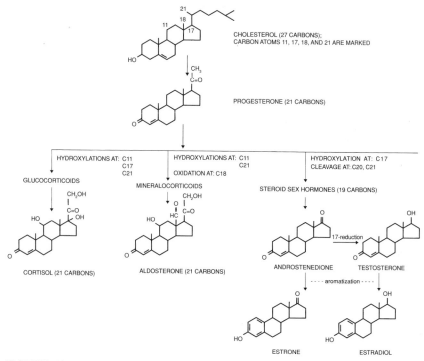

FIGURE 16–4. Key intermediates of steroid biosynthesis from cholesterol.

steroids: (1) the **glucosteroids,** or **glucocorticoids,** 21-carbon steroids that affect intermediary carbohydrate metabolism; (2) the **mineralocorticoids,** 21-carbon steroids that promote renal K^+ excretion and increase water retention by enhancing renal Na^+ retention; and (3) the **adrenal androgens,** 19-carbon steroids that the liver converts into the potent male hormone testosterone; although unmodified, they also have a modest effect on secondary male sex characteristics.

Glucocorticoids

The pituitary **adrenocorticotropic hormone (ACTH)** stimulates glucocorticoid production. The pituitary secretes ACTH episodically when it is stimulated by falling levels of the circulating active glucocorticoid, by stress, or by cycles of sleeping and waking. **Cortisol** is the predominant glucocorticoid. Of circulating cortisol, 90% is in an inactive fraction bound to proteins, primarily **cortisol-binding globulin (CBG),** and also a small amount to albumin. Physiologic activity arises only from the unbound or free fraction of cortisol, which is capable of leaving the blood stream to affect target cells and also to be excreted in the urine.

Urinary Metabolites

The liver degrades all the glucocorticoids to metabolites excreted in urine, where they are measured as a collective group called **17-hydroxycorticosteroids (17-OHCS).** These compounds, which have hydroxyl groups at C-17 and C-21 and a ketone group at C-20, react with phenylhydrazine to form a yellow compound. This reactivity is called the **Porter-Silber reaction,** and 17-OHCSs are referred to as Porter-Silber chromogens. This method allows simple urinary quantitation and is an indirect measure of excessive plasma glucocorticoids.

ALDOSTERONE AND THE RENIN-ANGIOTENSIN SYSTEM

Secretion of aldosterone, the predominant mineralocorticoid, occurs when cells in the region of the adrenal gland called the **zona glomerulosa** are stimulated by angiotensin. Diminution of blood volume causes specialized kidney cells to produce renin, which initiates a sequence of steps that eventuate in angiotensin production. Aldosterone influences the transport of ions across cell membranes of the renal tubules to retain sodium and chloride and to excrete potassium and hydrogen ions. By increasing sodium retention, aldosterone causes retention of water that expands blood volume (and, as a side effect, also increases blood pressure). Restoration of blood volume suppresses the renin-angiotensin axis with reduction in production of aldosterone in a complete feedback loop mechanism.

ACTH can also stimulate aldosterone production, but this pathway does not significantly contribute to overall concentrations of aldosterone. Increased body potassium or decreased body sodium enhances the reactivity of the renin-angiotensin system, and high serum potassium seems to stimulate aldosterone production directly. Aldosterone is extracted from serum or urine and then measured by radioimmunoassay. **Primary aldosteronism** (aldosterone elevation or **Conn's syndrome**) is usually due to benign adrenal adenoma or to hyperplasia of the adrenal cortex. With aldosteronism, the exchange of ions normally facilitated by aldosterone results in hypertension (excess intravascular fluid volume secondary to retained sodium) and in potassium depletion.

ADRENAL ANDROGENS

Both men and women secrete adrenal androgens, although their normal physiologic role is not clear, considering the much larger amounts of similar hormones secreted by the gonads. Secretion from the adrenal is controlled by ACTH, not by gonadotropins. Production of ACTH is regulated only by glucocorticoid concentrations; circulating androgens do not affect ACTH release. Androgens of both adrenal and testicular origin are metabolized to 19-carbon compounds called **17-ketosteroids (17-KS).** In women and children, urine 17-KS levels directly reflect adrenal androgen production. In men, about one third of urinary 17-KS derive from testicular steroids.

The C-21 steroids (cortisol and its many metabolites and associated compounds) can be converted by chemical oxidation to form 17-ketosteroids. These urinary metabolites, referred to as **17-ketogenic steroids (17-KGS),** are sometimes used as a measure of overall glucocorticoid metabolism. Elevation of urinary 17-KGS indicates tumor or hyperplasia of the zona fasciculata and reticularis of the adrenal cortex.

The following outline summarizes the derivation of urinary steroid hormone metabolic products:

Glucocorticoids → 17-hydroxycorticosteroids
Glucocorticoids → 17-ketogenic steroids
Mineralocorticoids → not detected by colorimetric methods
Androgens → 17-ketosteroids
(women and children: adrenals)
(men: adrenals and testes)

MEASURING HORMONES IN THE CIRCULATION AND URINE

Circulating plasma hormone levels are affected by their rates of secretion and degradation; the level of binding protein also influences their concentration in blood. The adrenal gland secretes cortisol in short bursts; binding to CBG allows an equilibrium of free and bound hormone so that a fairly uniform concentration of the unbound, physiologically active form is presented to the tissues of the body. Urinary free cortisol is a convenient means by which to estimate the free fraction of cortisol in the circulation because only that portion of cortisol passes through glomerular filtration. A single measurement of ACTH or of cortisol concentration in plasma may be quite misleading because values change significantly with episodes of secretion or inactivity during a 24-hour period. Bursts of cortisol secretion occur most frequently at night; consequently, plasma cortisol levels are consistently higher on awakening in the morning than later in the day.

All the adrenal hormones and the hormones that regulate their secretion are conveniently measured by RIA or other immunoassays. These direct and specific measurements for cortisol and aldosterone in plasma or serum are very useful for screening and in establishing diagnoses, but frequently urine testing is especially useful when androgen-producing conditions such as adrenal tumors or defects of steroid synthesis are suspected. Urine tests have the advantage of being more complete and therefore capturing all the adrenal products secreted into the blood and then excreted into the urine in a 24-hour period. This timed collection assures the physician of not missing a peak period of hormone concentration, as might occur from the mistiming of a single plasma collection. In addition, it is more reliable to follow serial 24-hour samples of urine to determine response to pharmacologic manipulations than it is to obtain the blood samples. In order to ensure complete 24-hour urine collection or to validate results on partial collections, it is necessary to measure the level of creatinine in the urine collection. Normal values for blood and urine hormone concentrations and for urinary metabolites are shown in Table 16–5.

TESTS OF PITUITARY-ADRENAL AXIS

Concentrations of glucocorticoids are controlled by ACTH secretion, which, in turn, depends on the amount of adrenal hormones in the circulation (see Fig. 16–2). Two provocative tests are available to measure the integrity of this feedback control mechanism. In the **dexamethasone suppression test,** the pituitary senses high levels of circulating hormones and should respond by curtailing ACTH production, which leads to diminished excretion of steroid metabolites (Fig. 16–5). In the **metyrapone test,** hormone synthesis is blocked (Fig. 16–6). The pituitary responds to this induced hormone deficiency by producing more and more ACTH, which in turn stimulates the adrenal to synthesize more and more of the inactive steroid intermediates.

DEXAMETHASONE SUPPRESSION TEST

This test may be performed whenever there is evidence of unexplained excessive glucocorticoid secretion. Both dexamethasone and 9-alpha-

TABLE 16–5. ADRENAL HORMONES AND METABOLITES

Hormone or Metabolite	Reference Range
Plasma cortisol	
8:00 A.M.	9–24 µg/dL
4:00 P.M.	3–12 µg/dL
Urine-free cortisol	20–100 µg excreted in 24 hr
Plasma aldosterone	1–5 ng/dL (patient supine, normal Na$^+$ and K$^+$ intake)
Urine aldosterone	2–10 µg excreted in 24 hr (normal Na$^+$ and K$^+$ intake)
Urine 17-hydroxycorticoids	2–10 mg excreted in 24 hr
Urine 17-ketosteroids	
Men	7–25 mg excreted in 24 hr
Women	4–15 mg excreted in 24 hr

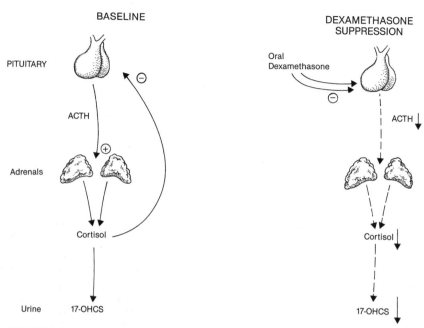

FIGURE 16–5. Dexamethasone suppression of the pituitary-adrenal axis. The normal response is suppression of ACTH, cortisol, and 17-hydroxycorticosteroids (17-OHCS, measured in urine by the laboratory).

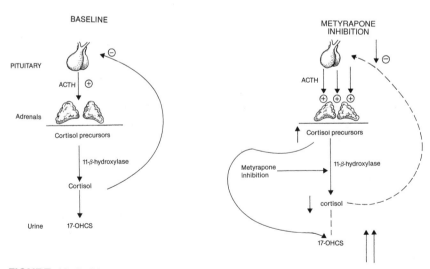

FIGURE 16–6. Metyrapone inhibition test for pituitary ACTH reserve secreting capacity.

fluorohydrocortisone are potent glucocorticoids that influence adrenal and pituitary function without causing significant quantitative change in urinary steroid (17-OHCS) excretion. Either drug could be used for this test, but 9-alpha-fluorohydrocortisone produces sodium retention, which is an undesirable side effect. Following baseline determination of 17-OHCS excretion over a 24-hour period, 0.5 mg of dexamethasone is given orally every 6 hours for 2 days. The theory is that dexamethasone is a potent analog of cortisol and so can be effective in suppressing the pituitary secretion of ACTH when given in small doses that do not contribute significantly to the measurement of urinary steroids. In patients with a normally responsive pituitary-adrenal axis, steroid production should drop in response to decreased ACTH stimulation, usually to 2.5 mg or less per 24 hours, on the second day of medication (see Fig. 16–5). When the urinary excretion of 17-OHCS does not fall in response to dexamethasone administration, there may be excessive ACTH stimulation or autonomous activity of the adrenals. Phenytoin anticonvulsants and phenobarbital, which induce hepatic mixed-function oxidases, may cause excessively rapid degradation of dexamethasone, thereby reducing its physiologic effect and causing apparent failure of hormone suppression.

Patients with **melancholia**—a psychiatric affective disorder of endogenous depression—may have excess stimulation through the hypothalamic-pituitary-adrenal axis with high excretion of 17-OHCS similar to Cushing's syndrome. This excretion is not suppressible by dexamethasone in depression and has been used in the past as an ancillary diagnostic test.

High-Dose Dexamethasone Test

Patients with Cushing's syndrome from any cause fail to reduce steroid excretion after the total dosage of 4 mg over 2 days. In cases of adrenal hyperfunction, it is often possible to distinguish bilateral hyperplasia from adrenal tumor by repeating the dexamethasone test with a higher dosage. In patients with bilateral hyperplasia, administration of 2 mg of dexamethasone every 6 hours for 2 days usually produces a fall in 17-OHCS excretion to 50% or less of the basal value; whereas excretion in patients with adenomas is unaffected by the total dosage of 16 mg. Patients with Cushing's syndrome associated with pituitary gland tumors may have suppressed steroid excretion after the larger dose of dexamethasone, but not after the smaller one.

Rapid Dexamethasone Test

To avoid the disadvantages of prolonged medication and the pitfalls of repeated 24-hour urine collections, a rapid screening test of dexamethasone suppression has been employed. In this simplified version, 1.0 mg of oral dexamethasone is given at midnight, and in the morning plasma cortisol is measured, and a 5-hour urine specimen is tested for 17-OHCS and creatinine. Normal subjects should have no more than 5 µg/dL of cortisol in this suppressed 8:00 A.M. plasma sample, and excrete no more than 4 mg of 17-OHCS per gram of creatinine in the period from 7:00 A.M. to noon.

METYRAPONE TEST

This test measures the ability of the pituitary gland to respond to declining levels of circulating cortisol. An 11-beta-hydroxylation enzymatic reaction in the adrenal cortex is required to convert precursor steroids into cortisol (see Fig. 16–4). Metyrapone (SU 4885) inhibits this. When this drug is given, cortisol levels decline, while the precursor products (which are not able to suppress ACTH) accumulate (see Fig. 16–6). If plasma cortisol levels remain high, at 20 µg/dL or more, the test results are invalid because cortisol has not been adequately suppressed, and expected stimulation of ACTH cannot occur. If cortisol declines and the pituitary is normally responsive, increasing ACTH levels cause acceleration of efforts at synthesis and further accumulation of the precursor substances, which react chemically in the test for urine 17-OHCS. Conversion of these precursors to cortisol is blocked by the drug. Therefore, when the pituitary adrenal axis is normal, excess stimulation of ACTH occurs, leading to excess excretion of urinary 17-OHCS.

Urine is collected in 24-hour aliquots during and for one day after oral administration of 500 or 750 mg of metyrapone every 4 hours for 24 hours. The 24-hour excretion of 17-OHCS on the last day of collection should be at least double the baseline excretion in normal individuals. The primary use of this test is in adrenocortical deficiency to assess the capacity of the pituitary to secrete ACTH. Because the result will be abnormal if the adrenals cannot respond to stimulation, this test should be done only if the ACTH stimulation test gives normal results (see section discussion of Addison's disease). Chlorpromazine interferes with normal response to metyrapone and should not be given during the testing period. Drugs that induce hepatic mixed-function oxidases (such as phenobarbital and phenytoin) increase the degradation of administered metyrapone and prevent it from achieving the desired effect.

ADRENAL CORTICAL MALFUNCTION

Adrenal cortical diseases fall into four major categories: too much corticosteroid **(Cushing's syndrome),** too little corticosteroid **(Addison's disease),** too much mineralocorticoid **(hyperaldosteronism, Conn's**

syndrome), and too much adrenal androgenic activity. None is very common, but their symptoms and ancillary laboratory findings can occur frequently—sometimes as part of an adrenal syndrome or in association with other conditions. Disease of the adrenal-pituitary axis must be distinguished from more common and sometimes less specific conditions because effective therapy is available for most adrenal malfunctions.

Cushing's Syndrome

Excessive production of adrenal steroids occurs for one of two reasons: excessive ACTH stimulation (resulting in adrenal hyperplasia) or autonomously active adrenal tumors. About 70% of cases of Cushing's syndrome result from pituitary oversecretion of ACTH due to pituitary adenomas or hyperfunctioning groups of cells called **microadenomas.** With continuous high-level ACTH stimulation, the adrenal glands undergo bilateral hyperplasia, producing glucocorticoids and mineralo-corticoids at levels that would suppress ACTH production if pituitary function were normal.

In up to 5% of cases of Cushing's syndrome, excess ACTH has a nonpituitary origin, coming from nonendocrine malignant tumors, most often small-cell carcinomas of the lung or carcinoid tumors. Approxi-mately one fourth of cases of Cushing's syndrome result from adrenal neoplasms, either benign adenomas or carcinomas.

Clinical Observations

In Cushing's syndrome, the metabolic and endocrine abnormalities reflect both glucocorticoid and mineralocorticoid excess. Interrelated abnormalities of glucose and protein metabolism lead to elevated blood glucose, reduced glucose tolerance, and muscle wasting. Redistribution of adipose tissue results in truncal obesity and thin extremities. Abnormal lipid metabolism leads to hypercholesterolemia and accelerated arterio-sclerosis. Since ACTH stimulates aldosterone production, many patients with Cushing's syndrome have hypertension, excessive urinary loss of potassium, and hypokalemic alkalosis. Androgen excess may cause virilism in women. Extreme emotional lability also frequently accompa-nies glucocorticoid excess.

Differential Diagnosis

Cushing's syndrome must be distinguished from simple obesity, in which diabetes mellitus, hypertension, and lipid abnormalities are often present as well; these can include ovarian causes of virilism in women or hypothyroidism and can range from normal reaction mechanisms to severe physiologic stress. The critical diagnostic finding is continuous high-level cortisol secretion unresponsive to stimuli that normally suppress cortisol production. Table 16–6 outlines common findings and differential laboratory observations in Cushing's syndrome.

TABLE 16–6. CUSHING'S SYNDROME

FEATURES THAT CHARACTERIZE CUSHING'S SYNDROME

Clinical Observations	Laboratory Findings
Truncal obesity with thin extremities	Elevated urine 17-OHCS and 17-KS
Abnormal glucose tolerance	Urine free cortisol ≥80 µg/24 hr
Hypertension	Loss of diurnal change in cortisol production (evening level >50% of morning
Hirsutism and menstrual disorders in women	level)
Easy bruisability	
Osteoporosis	

FEATURES THAT DISTINGUISH ETIOLOGIC CATEGORIES OF CUSHING'S SYNDROME

	17-OHCS Excretion	17-KS Excretion	Response to High-Dose Dexamethasone	Response to Metyrapone	Remarks
Pituitary disorders	High	High	17-OHCS excretion drops 50%	17-OHCS excretion rises excessively	Skin pigmentation prominent
Ectopic ACTH secretion	Very high (4 × normal)	High	None	Unpredictable	Hypokalemia often severe Skin pigmentation prominent Malignancy may cause generalized wasting
Adrenal adenoma	High	Normal	None	None	Opposite gland becomes atrophic
Adrenal carcinoma	High	Very high (4 × normal)	None	None	

Excessive excretion of urinary-free cortisol is the best single indicator of hyperadrenocorticism. Loss of normal late-afternoon drop in serum cortisol is also highly suggestive. Excess urinary levels of 17-OHCS and 17-KS are not unique to Cushing's syndrome and may be seen in all the conditions just mentioned. A high serum cortisol level is not, by itself, diagnostic because high levels of estrogens may elevate concentrations of the cortisol-binding globulin in serum, thereby producing high absolute levels of cortisol; however, with increased binding protein, free hormone (the form that enters the urine) does not increase.

Establishing the Etiology

The adrenal-pituitary axis must be tested to establish the cause of adrenal hyperfunction. Reliable measurement of ACTH greatly simplifies this process; however, ACTH assays suffer from technical difficulties and lability of the hormone. For those reasons, indirect tests are usually employed. Persistently high ACTH levels with high cortisol levels point to pituitary overactivity or ectopic ACTH production; low ACTH levels indicate autonomous adrenal activity. It is often possible to suppress pituitary hypersecretion by raising levels of circulating glucocorticoids to extremely high concentrations. High-dose dexamethasone testing usually reduces urinary 17-OHCS excretion by 50% or more when pituitary hyperactivity exists. The expected rise in urinary 17-OHCS after metyrapone administration occurs in pituitary Cushing's syndrome, often to an exaggerated degree. If ACTH is secreted by nonpituitary neoplasms, dexamethasone has no effect at any dose; metyrapone sometimes and unpredictably induces additional ACTH production. Both types of hormonal tests give negative results when hypersecretion results from adrenal adenomas or carcinomas.

The relative concentrations of urinary 17-OHCS and 17-KS may offer clues to the etiology of Cushing's syndrome. Both 17-OHCS and 17-KS are increased when ACTH stimulation is excessive; with adrenal gland adenomas, androgen levels are often normal, so urinary 17-KS concentrations remain normal. Conversely, adrenal carcinomas tend to cause 17-KS levels significantly higher than 17-OHCS levels, a reflection of malignant differentiation. Nonpituitary ACTH produces especially high levels of 17-OHCS, with less pronounced effect on 17-KS.

Addison's Disease

Adrenal corticosteroids are necessary to maintain life. As a deficiency **(Addison's disease)** develops, there is increasing but rather nonspecific debility, with loss of weight and muscle strength; hyperkalemia, sodium depletion, and hypotension; gastrointestinal disturbances; and inability to maintain normal glucose levels. There is often overall dirty-gray pigmentation of the skin, most marked on pressure points and recent scars. This pigmentation occurs if the pituitary responds normally to declining glucocorticoid levels because secretion of **melanocyte-stimulating hormone (MSH)** and ACTH are closely linked.

Adequate adrenal hormone production is essential to withstand acute physiologic stress, such as trauma, severe infection, burns, surgical procedures, and overwhelming emotional response. In patients with unsuspected or borderline adrenal hypofunction, acute physiologic or emotional stress may unmask the deficiency and precipitate acute hypotension, hypoglycemia, hyponatremia, muscle cramps, and severe gastrointestinal disturbances. Table 16–7 outlines clinical and laboratory findings in Addison's disease.

Diagnostic Observations

Urine levels of 17-OHCS and 17-KS are only moderately effective in screening for adrenal hypofunction, although normal values rule out the diagnosis of adrenal insufficiency. Urinary excretion of steroid metabolites may be low in patients with cachexia, hypothyroidism, liver disease, or severe psychic depression, although free cortisol levels are usually normal. High serum potassium and low serum levels of sodium, bicarbonate, and glucose are contributory but nonspecific findings.

If a patient has low blood cortisol levels, low urinary free cortisol, and low urinary metabolites, pituitary function and adrenal response to ACTH must be evaluated. If ACTH is high while adrenal hormones are low, there is primary adrenal malfunction; low ACTH values point to the much less common problem of pituitary deficiency. In lieu of the direct measurement of ACTH, exogenous purified or synthetic ACTH can be given to assess the capacity of the adrenals to respond to ACTH. By this

TABLE 16–7. ADDISON'S DISEASE: DEFICIENT ADRENAL CORTICOSTEROID PRODUCTION

Clinical Observations:	Cause:
Weight loss, muscle wasting	Disordered glucose metabolism
Salt craving, muscle cramps	Sodium loss, hyperkalemia
Hypotension, especially postural	Small, hypoactive heart
	Disordered fluid metabolism
Pigmentation of skin	Excess pituitary tropic hormone
Laboratory Findings:	**Cause:**
Low plasma cortisol	Diminished secretion
Low urine 17-OHCS	Diminished cortisol secretion
Low urine 17-KS (in female)	Diminished secretion of adrenal androgens
High serum K^+, low Na^+	Diminished aldosterone secretion
Low blood glucose	Diminished cortisol secretion
Adrenal, thyroid, or gastric autoantibodies	Autoimmune derangement

means, it may be possible to distinguish between primary hypoadrenalism and hypopituitarism. The dose of ACTH and the timing of sample collections for measuring response must be carefully monitored.

Hormones and Hormonal Response

The first test uses a single intravenous dose of ACTH. If plasma cortisol rises 10 µg/dL or more in one hour, the diagnosis of adrenal deficiency has been excluded. If there is no response to a single dose of ACTH, repeated daily doses are given for 3 to 5 days to prime the adrenals in case they have become hypoplastic from lack of ACTH stimulation but are otherwise normal. Adrenal insufficiency is established if this maneuver does not provoke a twofold or greater increase in urine 17-OHCS excretion.

Pituitary function is difficult to evaluate without direct measurements of tropic hormones. Gonadal and thyroidal hormones are easier to measure than ACTH; hypoadrenalism of pituitary origin can sometimes be established by demonstrating low levels of these other stimulatory hormones. Patients with hypopituitarism lack the hyperpigmentation characteristic of excess ACTH secretion (i.e., accompanying MSH secretion). Mineralocorticoid deficiency is usually less striking with hypopituitarism than with adrenal gland dysfunction because the major stimulus to aldosterone production is the renin-angiotensin system, which remains intact.

Etiology

The single most common cause of adrenal hypofunction is administration of exogenous steroids. Production of ACTH is suppressed by steroidal therapy used in treating autoimmune diseases, in many anticancer regimens, and in immunosuppressive therapy. The adrenal gland, deprived of physiologic stimulation, undergoes atrophic changes, which may be quite severe and can persist for many months after therapy is discontinued. A patient with prolonged reduction of adrenal function may develop acute adrenocorticoid deficiency if severe physiologic stress occurs during the recovery phase.

In years past, Addison's disease frequently arose from tuberculous destruction of the adrenal gland. Today most adrenal hypofunction is idiopathic. In some patients, autoantibodies to adrenal tissue antigens suggest an autoimmune etiology. Patients with idiopathic adrenal dysfunction often have antibodies to thyroid and gastric antigens also, pointing to polyendocrine immune disorders. Infectious diseases such as tuberculosis can cause adrenal destruction. Other conditions that destroy the gland or damage its function include hemorrhagic damage in meningococcal or other bacteremic conditions (Waterhouse-Friderichsen syndrome); replacement of glandular tissue by metastatic neoplasms, especially lung cancer; primary or secondary amyloidosis with deposition of the amyloid protein; and hemochromatosis with deposition of iron.

Diagnostic Challenge Test

If the differential diagnosis is borderline adrenal activity versus borderline pituitary activity, it may be useful to stress the pituitary-adrenal axis to gather definitive diagnostic information. First it is necessary to establish that the adrenal gland is capable of producing glucocorticoids. The metyrapone test stimulates ACTH release by blocking cortisol synthesis; if the pituitary responds normally, urinary excretion of 17-OHCS metabolites increases. Absence of this 17-OHCS surge indicates pituitary unresponsiveness, provided that adrenal capability has already been established.

A more direct challenge to the pituitary is the insulin administration test. Physiologic stress is an extremely potent stimulus to ACTH production. Failure of insulin-induced hypoglycemia (serum glucose of 50 mg/dL or less) to induce ACTH release establishes the diagnosis of pituitary dysfunction. If ACTH is not measured directly, pituitary response to stimulation must be inferred by measuring cortisol production; a normal response consists of an increment of 6 µg/dL or more, to total levels of 20 µg/dL or more. The insulin test constitutes a genuine metabolic stress. Many clinicians believe that it imposes an unacceptably great risk on the patient, while others believe that the test, done under careful medical supervision, is the most sensitive way available to evaluate pituitary function.

Hyperaldosteronism

Excessive aldosterone production may be the inappropriate result of primary adrenal hyperfunction, or it may be an appropriate response to pathologic changes in blood volume and electrolyte regulation, in which case it is considered **secondary hyperaldosteronism.** Diagnosis of primary hyperaldosteronism (Conn's syndrome) requires demonstration that aldosterone is excessive and that the renin-angiotensin system is unresponsive. Conn's syndrome is usually due to a solitary benign adenoma. Less frequently it may result from generalized bilateral hyperplasia of the aldosterone-secreting glomerulosa cells or of the adrenal cortex.

Laboratory Findings

Presenting features of primary or secondary hyperaldosteronism are low serum K^+ (below 3 mEq/liter), high urinary K^+ excretion (above 50 mEq/day), and hypertension. There is excessive excretion of urine with alkaline pH, low specific gravity (about 1.010), and often proteinuria. Serum Na^+ and bicarbonate are high-normal or slightly elevated.

Excessive aldosterone production can be demonstrated by measuring the effects of the aldosterone antagonist spironolactone, which allows serum potassium levels to rise and urine potassium to drop to less than

20 mEq/24 hours. This spironolactone response rules out renal dysfunction, diuretic excess, and systemic electrolyte disturbances as causes of deranged potassium metabolism but does not explain why aldosteronism exists. It simply confirms aldosterone excess. Table 16–8 summarizes clinical and laboratory findings.

Increased levels of circulating Na^+ and expanded extracellular fluid volume suppress aldosterone production and reduce potassium excretion in normal persons. If hypokalemia and alkalosis persist after 4 days of sodium-augmented diet, it indicates persistent aldosterone secretion independent of renin-angiotensin control. In primary hyperaldosteronism, plasma renin levels are low and unresponsive to increased sodium levels.

Autonomous aldosterone overproduction can be documented by measuring baseline and challenge levels of plasma aldosterone. After infusion of 2 liters of normal saline solution, plasma aldosterone levels should drop to 5 ng/dL. Another way to demonstrate integrity of the negative feedback loop is to administer a synthetic mineralocorticoid (fludrocortisone acetate [Florinef]) for 3 days. Except in autonomous hyperaldosteronism, plasma aldosterone levels should fall to 4 ng/dL or below. Aldosterone levels are normally only about one-thousandth those of cortisol in serum.

Renin-Angiotensin System

Interrelationships of the renin-angiotensin system are outlined in Figure 16–7. Renin acts on renin substrate (an alpha-2-globulin normally present in plasma) to release the fragment angiotensin I (10 amino acids long). Angiotensin I is further modified to the octapeptide

---

TABLE 16–8. HYPERALDOSTERONISM: EXCESSIVE STIMULUS TO K^+ EXCRETION AND Na^+ RETENTION

Clinical Observations:

Hypertension
Increased urine volume
Muscle dysfunction, from K^+ loss

Laboratory Findings:

Serum K^+: <3 mEq/liter
Urine K^+: >50 mEq/24 hr
Alkalosis, usually moderate
Urine pH elevated, specific gravity no higher than 1.010

Test Results:

Sodium loading (200 mEq/day) causes accentuated hypokalemia and alkalosis
Spironolactone antagonizes aldosterone, reduces urine K^+ to <20 mEq/24 hr

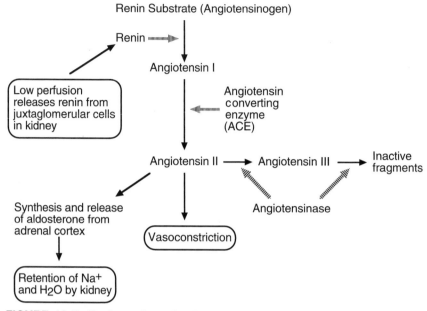

FIGURE 16–7. Renin-angiotensin-aldosterone system. Broken arrows indicate proteolytic actions.

angiotensin II by **angiotensin-converting enzyme (ACE)** derived primarily from the lungs. This enzyme is the site of action for the ACE inhibitor class of antihypertensive medications. Angiotensin II is the vasoactive substance directly responsible for elevating blood pressure; blocking its synthesis ameliorates hypertension due to renin excess. Angiotensin II is further degraded to angiotensin III and still smaller inactive fragments by angiotensinase. Angiotensin III apparently also affects release of aldosterone.

Assessment of the renin-angiotensin system is often part of a hypertension work-up. There are several other factors that contribute to the development of hypertension through the separate mechanisms of vasoconstriction or blood volume expansion. Primary hyperaldosteronism causes hypertension and low renin levels. Many hypertensive patients have high serum aldosterone levels that are secondary to high renin levels. Treatment with propranolol or other beta-adrenergic blocking agents often reduces renin levels, corrects the electrolyte and fluid disturbances, and permits normalization of arterial blood pressure. Renin measurement is technically demanding, and several different procedures are available. Correct interpretation requires detailed knowledge of the patient's electrolyte status, diet over the preceding several days, exposure to diuretic agents, and posture for the 4 hours preceding the test.

High-renin aldosterone excess (secondary hyperaldosteronism) can be distinguished from renin-system unresponsiveness (primary hyperaldosteronism) by observing the effects of electrolyte and volume manipulation on aldosterone levels and serum and urine electrolytes. Administering vasopressin expands blood volume. In high-renin states or in normally responsive individuals, volume expansion reduces renin-angiotensin activity, suppresses aldosterone secretion, and promotes sodium excretion. Volume expansion thus causes increased urine sodium and decreased serum sodium; with low-renin states, slight hypernatremia may follow volume expansion. Synthetic mineralocorticoid (fludrocortisone acetate) is also useful in distinguishing primary from secondary hyperaldosteronism. Fludrocortisone acetate reduces aldosterone stimulation, allowing 50% or more reduction in aldosterone secretion after 4 days if the adrenal is normally responsive. Table 16–9 summarizes the distinction between primary and secondary hyperaldosteronism.

Renin measurements are often performed on specimens collected during catheterization studies from several different locations such as inferior vena cava, left renal vein, right renal vein, and peripheral blood to help localize a site of abnormally high renin production. With expansion of ambulatory medicine, patients with hypertension are likely to be screened for excess renin production using a single measurement on peripheral blood. Laboratory measurement of renin activity is based on production of angiotensin I in a serum sample during an incubation

TABLE 16–9. PRIMARY VERSUS SECONDARY HYPERALDOSTERONISM

Diagnostic Manipulation	Renin-Independent (Primary)	High-Renin (Secondary)
Volume depletion:	Aldosterone secretion remains high	Aldosterone secretion falls
80 mg furosemide or assuming upright posture in patients with: Normal Na$^+$ intake No diuretics for 3 weeks No antihypertensives for 1 week		
Mineralocorticoid administration:	Aldosterone secretion remains high	Aldosterone secretion falls
10 mg deoxycorticosterone every 12 h × 6 *or* 400 µg fludrocortisone acetate 3 times/day		

period. It is a complex and demanding assay generally done in reference laboratories.

Essential hypertension has been classified as low, normal, and high renin, which guides drug therapy. Roughly 15% of patients with essential hypertension have high renin generally due to kidney disease, such as atherosclerosis, affecting the renal arteries. Even when their hypertension is controlled medically, patients with high renin tend to do worse; high renin is also a risk factor for myocardial infarction.

Adrenal Virilism

Adrenal virilism occurs either because of enzyme defects that distort normal patterns of synthesis or because of hormone-secreting tumors. The clinical signs of adrenal virilism vary with age and sex. Among these are the inappropriate appearance of masculine traits in prepubertal children of either sex; virilization in mature women; and, less easily recognized, accentuation of the male secondary sex characteristics in mature men.

Defective Synthesis

Congenital adrenal virilism results from any of several inborn enzymatic defects in cortisol synthesis. As glucocorticoids are normally synthesized, many preliminary products are 19-carbon steroids with androgenic properties. If normal cortisol production is blocked by enzyme deficiencies, ACTH secretion continues at a high level, producing glandular hyperplasia that results in continuing high levels of the precursor substances. A number of different genetically determined defects have been implicated.

Despite the inborn nature of the disease, symptoms may become manifest at any time, although most cases are recognized at birth or in early childhood. The effect of massive doses of androgenically active steroids in utero is masculinization of the female infant, who may appear to be a pseudohermaphrodite. In the male infant there is macrogenitosomia. If aldosterone production is impaired along with cortisol synthesis, there may be sodium loss and potassium retention in the so-called salt-losing type of adrenal virilism.

Laboratory Findings

Principal laboratory findings in adrenal virilism include increased levels of plasma and urine 17-KS and high levels of circulating ACTH. The most common defect, that of inadequate 21-hydroxylation, produces high levels of pregnanetriol, a 21-carbon steroid. Because this compound is measured in the 17-KGS, in these cases there will be high levels of 17-KGS but low 17-OHCS.

In most patients with congenital adrenal hyperplasia, the gland remains sensitive to ACTH stimulation. Exogenous ACTH further elevates the already high levels of 17-ketosteroids, but 17-OHCS levels do not rise. A rare form of the syndrome arises from a defect in 11-beta-hydroxylation, which causes 17-OH precursors of cortisol to accumulate, analogous to the situation in which normal individuals receive metyrapone. In this form, 17-OHCS levels are elevated, and increased mineralocorticoid activity and hypertension are present.

Tumors
Occasional cases of adrenal virilism in adults are due to late manifestation of congenital enzyme defects; however, more often they are due to hyperplasia or tumor. Benign androgenic hyperplasia, in which 17-ketosteroids are elevated but 17-OHCS are normal, is rarely seen. Adrenal virilization usually is due to carcinoma, and generally there are increased 17-OHCS levels in addition to the high levels of 17-ketosteroids.

Patient-Care Considerations

Full-blown Cushing's syndrome and Addison's disease are virtually unmistakable, but mild adrenal hyperfunction or hypofunction is difficult to distinguish from other common system complexes that affect metabolism of the body. Thyroid disease is particularly misleading; screening tests for adrenal function are less readily available than those for thyroid malfunction. True adrenal disorders occur significantly less often than thyroid aberration, but this should not blunt the edge of suspicion.

Artifactual Laboratory Findings
Many artifacts affect screening tests. The Porter-Silber reaction for 17-OHCS may be depressed by urine glucose levels. Patients taking estrogens, meperidine, morphine, pentazocine, or phenytoins may have falsely low 17-OHCS results. Estrogens alter routes of steroid degradation, so pregnant women or those taking estrogens have low 17-OHCS excretion despite the increased total serum cortisol values that accompany increased cortisol-binding globulin. Spironolactone, quinidine, chloramphenicol, and such psychoactive drugs as chlorpromazine, meprobamate, and the monoamine-oxidase inhibitors cause artifactually high 17-OHCS levels. Estrogens, pregnancy, barbiturates, phenytoins, and liver disease also affect the metabolic pathways that lead to 17-KS excretion. Urine 17-KS levels are artifactually low in the presence of these drugs; the penicillins and erythromycins cause falsely high 17-KS excretion values, as do the drugs mentioned that elevate 17-OHCS results.

Levels of 17-OHCS are truly elevated in obesity, hyperthyroidism, and acromegaly, reflecting increased secretion and turnover rather than true hyperfunction. Urinary free cortisol is usually normal in these conditions. Patients taking diuretics or those with high salt intake may increase free cortisol excretion without having functional hyperadrenalism.

Severe renal disease affects all the urine tests. If creatinine clearance is less than 50 mL/minute, all urinary screening tests may confuse rather than illuminate the assessment of adrenal function.

Challenge Testing

Many problems can occur with dynamic functional tests, especially those that take several days. With oral dosages, the patient must take every dose at the appropriate time; vomiting or malabsorption must be ruled out. Intramuscular injections may give misleading results if absorption is irregular or circulation poor. Altered renal function—excretory failure, increased diuresis, or inappropriate volume expansion—can alter the expected drug effects. Altered liver function—especially induction of mixed-function oxidases by drugs like alcohol, barbiturates, and phenytoins—may increase drug degradation and divert metabolites from their expected pathways.

Interfering Drugs

Before adrenal function is vigorously examined, interfering drugs must be eliminated. Diuretics, anticonvulsants, psychoactive drugs, and oral contraceptives are especially likely to interfere. For optimal baseline conditions, these drugs should be stopped two weeks before definitive tests are undertaken. Other pharmacologic hazards include chronic laxative use, prolonged diarrhea, and large-scale licorice intake, all of which cause hypokalemia on a nonadrenal basis. Before testing the renin-angiotensin-aldosterone axis, the patient should be given potassium to correct systemic hypokalemia if it is present.

Previous steroid medications severely depress adrenal function. Daily doses of 15 mg of prednisone or its equivalent can leave the adrenal gland hyporesponsive for months; several weeks to a month are needed to recover from doses of 5 to 10 mg. Detailed medication history is important in any patient needing endocrine evaluation, but especially when adrenal function is in question.

Psychophysiologic Problems

Physiologic stress powerfully stimulates the adrenal-pituitary axis, appropriately provoking adrenal hypersecretion. Endocrine evaluation should be postponed in patients who have recently undergone trauma, surgical procedures, severe infection, or burns. Emotional trauma rarely causes confusingly high hormone levels, but could produce a problem in distinguishing borderline normal from modestly increased function. Because stress should consistently increase adrenal output, cortisol levels below 15 µg/dL in a severely ill patient should arouse the suspicion of underlying adrenal hypofunction.

The myriad physiologic abnormalities created by adrenal dysfunction complicate clinical care of the patient. Muscle weakness, fatigue, and emotional instability complicate both hyperfunction and hypofunction, requiring empathetic support. Infections are poorly tolerated in both conditions. In Cushing's syndrome, glucocorticoid excess suppresses inflammatory and immune defenses; in hypoadrenalism, a minor infectious stimulus can precipitate dangerous addisonian crisis. Because patients with adrenal gland damage remain vulnerable to stress throughout life, they should be carefully instructed about increasing steroid dosage during times of physical or emotional stress. Changing urine output is diagnostically significant. Increasing volume can indicate incipient diabetes mellitus in hyperadrenalism or point to increased sodium excretion and depressed concentrating ability in hyperaldosteronism. Decreased output may reflect impaired renal perfusion and declining blood pressure in adrenal hypofunction.

ADRENAL MEDULLA

The **adrenal-medulla,** comprising one tenth of the gland volume and totally surrounded by cortical epithelium, belongs to the sympathetic nervous system. The adrenal medulla secretes epinephrine (adrenaline), the "fight-or-flight" hormone, after generalized sympathetic stimulation or in response to hypoglycemia or arterial hypotension. The adrenal medulla also produces norepinephrine (noradrenaline), whose physiologic effects differ somewhat from those of epinephrine (Table 16–10).

TABLE 16–10. FEATURES OF SYMPATHETIC CATECHOLAMINES

	Epinephrine	Norepinephrine
Production site	Adrenal gland	Adrenal gland
		Peripheral nerve endings
Storage and metabolism	Little tissue storage	Stored in tissue; tyramine
	Rapid degradation	provokes release
		Major source of urine
		metabolites
Urine excretion	<20 µg/24 hr	<100 µg/24 hr
Representative actions		
Heart rate	Increases	Decreases
Arterial blood pressure	Increases	Increases
Peripheral vascular	Decreases	Increases
resistance		
Skin and renal blood flow	Decreases	Decreases
Splanchnic blood flow	Increases	Decreases
Blood glucose level	Increases	Increases slightly
Association with chromaffin-cell tumors	Rarely predominant catecholamine	Often predominant or only hormone
	Not found with paragangliomas	Secreted by paragangliomas

Most systemic norepinephrine is manufactured by sympathetic nerve endings, but some is secreted by the adrenal medulla.

Catecholamine Metabolism

The catecholamines are chemically very similar; epinephrine has one more methyl group than does norepinephrine (Fig. 16–8). Synthetic

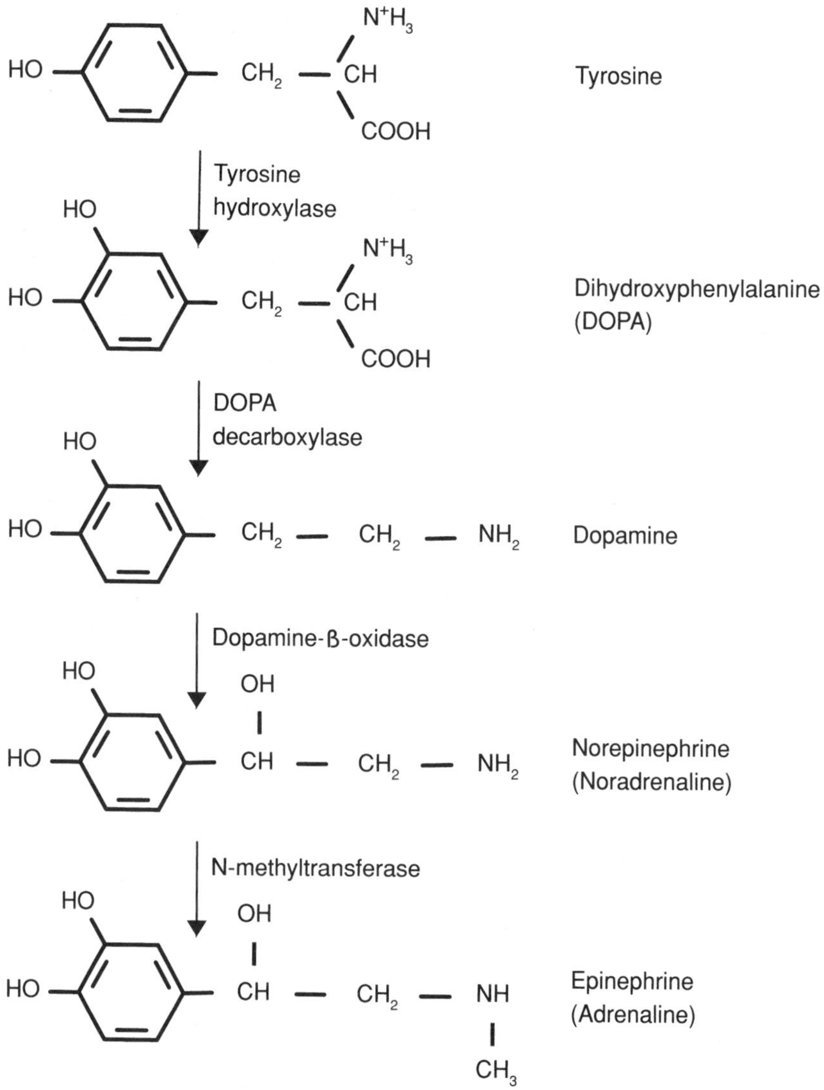

FIGURE 16–8. Biosynthesis of catecholamines.

pathways begin with tyrosine and progress through the intermediate compounds dihydroxyphenylalanine (DOPA) and dopamine. Degradative pathways involve the enzyme monoamine oxidase that affects dopamine, norepinephrine, and epinephrine. Circulating catecholamines are metabolized to eventual excretion of metanephrine and normetanephrine in the urine. The predominant catecholamine metabolite in urine is **vanillylmandelic acid (VMA),** which derives largely from norepinephrine secreted and metabolized at nerve endings.

Catecholamines can be measured by fluorimetric methods, but more sensitive and specific analysis is done with catecholamine fractionation by high pressure liquid chromatography. Plasma concentrations of epinephrine and norepinephrine are affected by body positioning (lower values when supine compared to standing); accordingly samples should be collected after 30 minutes in a stable position. Urinary excretion of these hormones and their metabolites can also be useful for clinical evaluation. Measurements should be done as 24-hour urine excretions rather than on isolated random specimens: such random samples may be misleading if they are obtained during peaks or valleys of excretion. Reference values for plasma and urinary levels are given in Table 16–11.

TABLE 16–11. REFERENCE RANGES FOR CATECHOLAMINES AND METABOLITES

Plasma

Dopamine	<30 pg/mL
Epinephrine	
Supine	<110 pg/mL
Standing	<140 pg/mL
Norepinephrine	
Supine	70–750 pg/mL
Standing	200–1700 pg/mL

Urinary Excretion/24 Hours

Epinephrine	<120 µg
Norepinephrine	15–80 µg
Dopamine	65–400 µg
Homovanillic acid	<15 mg
Vanillylmandelic acid	1.0–6.5 mg
Metanephrine	<0.4 mg
Normetanephrine	<0.9 mg

Pheochromocytoma

The only clinically significant disease of the adrenal medulla is the catecholamine-secreting tumor **pheochromocytoma.** Hormonally active tumors also develop in nonadrenal sites. About 10% of catecholamine-producing tumors originate from neuroectodermal cells in sympathetic paraganglia. Pheochromocytomas may release hormones continuously or intermittently; symptoms occur paroxysmally in about one half of cases, whereas sustained abnormalities characterize the other half. Arterial hypertension is the most conspicuous event; approximately 0.5% of newly diagnosed cases of hypertension are due to pheochromocytomas. Since this tumor is treatable by surgery, it is very important to diagnose it accurately at an early stage in order to prevent some of the consequences of severe hypertension.

Diagnostic Findings

Pheochromocytoma classically presents with paroxysmal episodes of hypertension, headache, tachycardia, vascular instability, and feelings of apprehension. Other presentations include sustained hypertension of varying degree; episodic or postural hypotension in a hypertensive patient; weight loss, fever, and hypermetabolism; or episodes of hypotension, tachycardia, and dizziness that mimic hypoglycemic attacks.

Diagnosis depends on demonstrating excessive catecholamine secretion. When hormone secretion occurs continuously, urinary excretion of catecholamines and their metabolites is unambiguously elevated above reference values. If the hormone is released episodically, it is important to collect urine during and after symptomatic attacks, because urinary findings may be normal between attacks. If urinary findings unequivocally demonstrate elevated hormone activity, it is inappropriate to perform further provocative testing, which may be uncomfortable or even dangerous.

Clonidine Suppression Test

Clonidine is a compound that decreases the release of catecholamines from sympathetic postganglionic neurons. When a small oral dose (0.3 mg) is administered, base-line levels of catecholamines are decreased by 25% in normal persons and those in whom there is an elevated endogenous excess of catecholamines from stress. In contrast, in those persons with a pheochromocytoma in whom there is autonomous production of catecholamines, no suppression occurs.

The present method for determination of each specific catecholamine fraction in plasma is high-performance liquid chromatography (HPLC) with electrochemical detector. Measurement in plasma avoids the artifacts and uncertainties of measuring urine metabolites and, in several series, has been shown to give the best distinction between presence and absence of a tumor. The patient must be at rest, in a supine position, and free of any external stress or stimulation when blood is drawn.

Patient-Care Considerations

Although less than 1% of newly diagnosed hypertension is due to pheochromocytoma, routine screening for catecholamine secretion is probably worthwhile because this form of hypertension can be effectively treated. Episodic elevation or depression of blood pressure should direct clinical suspicion toward pheochromocytoma, as should episodes of tachycardia or reflex bradycardia. The symptoms of pheochromocytoma may resemble those of other conditions, as partially listed in Table 16–12; because catecholamine-producing tumors are relatively uncommon, they may not figure prominently in the list of differential diagnoses.

Drug Effects

Many drugs affect urinary catecholamine measurements, as summarized in Table 16–13. Dopamine given therapeutically is metabolized and excreted like endogenous dopamine and causes elevated levels of urine metabolites. Alpha-methyldopa *(Aldomet)*, a common antihypertensive drug, increases urine levels of free catecholamines but does not affect the metabolites VMA and metanephrine. Monoamine-oxidase inhibitors increase urine metanephrine but decrease VMA excretion. Patients taking monoamine-oxidase inhibitors may have increased tissue catecholamine levels even in the absence of pheochromocytoma; methamphetamines may also influence tests used for pheochromocytoma.

Sympathetic catecholamines elevate blood lipid levels; clofibrate, a lipid-lowering drug, may be given to patients who subsequently undergo evaluation for pheochromocytoma. Since clofibrate depresses urinary VMA excretion, this drug should be discontinued before testing.

TABLE 16–12. CONDITIONS WITH WHICH PHEOCHROMOCYTOMA MAY BE CONFUSED

Condition	Findings in Pheochromocytoma
Hypoglycemic attacks	Blood glucose normal or high
Diabetes mellitus	Weight loss disproportional to degree of glycosuria
Malignant carcinoid syndrome	5-HIAA (a serotonin metabolite) normal
Hyperthyroidism	T_4, ^{131}I-uptake normal
Anxiety attacks, psychosis	No specific laboratory discriminants

TABLE 16–13. ARTIFACTS THAT ALTER CATECHOLAMINE FINDINGS

	Plasma		Urine	
	Catecholamines	E and NE	Metanephrine and Normetanephrine	VMA
Caffeine, bananas, nuts, etc.				↑
MAO inhibitors			↑	↓
Alpha-methyldopa		↑	nl	nl
Dopamine	↑	↑	↑	↑
Severe stress	↑	↑	↑	↑
Chlorpromazine			↑	
Clofibrate				↓
Quinidine		↑		
Isoproterenol		↑		

E = epinephrine; NE = norepinephrine; VMA = vanillylmandelic acid; MAO = monoamine oxidase; nl = normal.

The traditional artifact said to influence VMA levels is diet; bananas, nuts, cereal grains, tea, and coffee are said to raise urine VMA levels, causing false-positive rates as high as 10 to 15%.

Pharmacologic agents used to treat hypertension affect autonomic nervous system activity. Ganglionic blockers like hexamethonium and adrenergic blockers and vasodilators of the hydralazine type increase norepinephrine. Beta blockers like propranolol may have unpredictable or variable effects.

The 24-hour urine specimen for catecholamine evaluation should be acidified to between pH 2 and pH 3 by adding 12 to 15 mL of concentrated hydrochloric acid to the empty specimen container before collection.

Psychophysiologic Problems

Patients with pheochromocytoma are susceptible to acute hypertensive episodes that are always unpleasant and sometimes life-threatening. In especially labile patients, attacks can result from minor postural changes or palpation of flanks or abdomen during physical examination. Other reported precipitating events include exercise, straining at stool, intraperitoneal distension from a full bladder or a full stomach, and sexual activity. Many procedures that occur in hospitals can readily trigger an attack, so it is important to have potent antihypertensive blocking agents available whenever there is manipulation of a patient with known or suspected pheochromocytoma.

Physiologic stress elevates catecholamine levels; the patient's baseline condition must be considered when evaluating urine or plasma findings. Myocardial infarct or cerebrovascular accident can be the presenting symptom of hitherto unsuspected pheochromocytoma; on the other hand, these events can independently elicit catecholamine secretion at levels suggestive of pheochromocytoma. Strenuous exercise induces significant increase in hormone levels, but this should rarely complicate diagnosis.

THYROID GLAND

The thyroid gland synthesizes its hormones from iodine and the essential amino acid tyrosine. Most of the body's iodine enters through the alimentary tract as iodide (I^-), but it may also enter through the lungs or skin. Of the iodine that enters the body, approximately one third enters the thyroid gland, and the remaining two thirds of it leaves the body in urine.

METABOLISM OF THYROID HORMONES

In the thyroid gland, enzymes oxidize iodide to organic iodine, which is incorporated into monoiodotyrosine and diiodotyrosine. These one- and two-iodine-containing compounds are building blocks for the active thyroid hormones thyroxine (T_4), which has four iodine molecules, and triiodothyronine (T_3), which has three (Fig. 16–9).

TRIIODOTHYRONINE AND THYROXINE

There is more T_4 than T_3 in serum, but T_3 is far more significant physiologically. Normal serum contains 5.5 to 12.5 µg/dL of thyroxine. It is converted by peripheral nonthyroidal tissues to T_3 by removal of one iodine residue (see Fig. 16–9). Triiodothyronine has a normal range in the circulation of only 100 to 200 ng/dL; however, T_3 exerts the majority of thyroidal hormone effects, and T_4 may serve no direct endocrine activity until converted to T_3.

Thyroxine has a half-life of one week in the circulation, whereas T_3 has a half-life of only about 1 day. Approximately one-third of thyroxine produced is converted to T_3. Removing an iodine atom from the other ring results in reverse T_3 (rT_3), which has its three iodines at the 3, 3', and

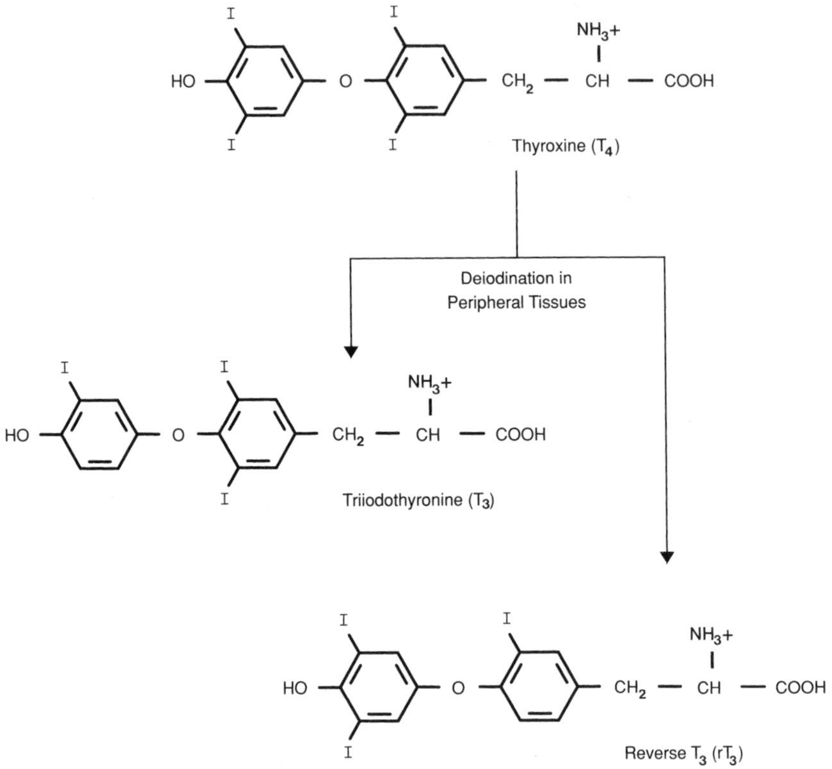

FIGURE 16–9. Chemical structures of the thyroid hormones.

5′ positions, instead of the 3, 5, and 3′ positions of active T_3. Reverse T_3 has no recognized physiologic function.

Both T_3 and T_4 are extensively bound to serum proteins, mostly to thyroxine-binding globulin (TBG) but also to albumin and prealbumin (see Proteins in Chapter 9). Although 99.97% of T_4 and 99.7% of T_3 circulate in bound form, physiologic activity results only from the unbound or free molecules of the hormones. Thyroxine is more tightly bound to TBG than is T_3, thus accounting for the respective half-lives of these two similar molecules.

PITUITARY-HYPOTHALAMIC RELATIONSHIP

The thyroid gland responds with the production of thyroxine on stimulation by the anterior pituitary hormone TSH, also called thyrotropin. Pituitary production of TSH follows stimulation of that gland by the hypothalamic peptide called TRH, which responds to active levels of free

T_3 and T_4 in blood perfusing the hypothalamus. When hormone levels are low, TRH provokes TSH secretion, which then accelerates all aspects of thyroidal iodine metabolism and hormone production.

EFFECTS OF THYROID HORMONES

Control of oxygen consumption is the most conspicuous biologic effect of the thyroid hormones, a physiologic variable measured in simplest fashion by the basal metabolic rate. Thyroid hormones also influence carbohydrate and protein metabolism, the mobilization of electrolytes, and the conversion of carotene to vitamin A. Although the mechanism is not known, thyroid hormones are essential for development of the central nervous system, and the thyroid-deficient infant suffers irreversible mental damage called **cretinism.** The thyroid-deficient adult may have slowed deep-tendon reflexes and diffuse psychomotor retardation, but these changes are reversible with hormone replacement therapy.

FACTORS THAT DECREASE THYROID ACTIVITY

Genetically determined enzyme deficiencies may interfere with iodine metabolism at any step, causing congenital goiter (enlargement of the thyroid gland). Much more frequently depressed thyroid function results from external causes. Exogenous thyroid hormone suppresses hormone production by depressing TSH levels. Drugs of the thiocyanate and perchlorate groups interfere with iodide concentration, whereas thiourea and thiouracil prevent incorporation of thyroidal iodine into organic compounds. The antithyroid effects of iodine are not fully understood but probably include inhibition both of iodine binding and of hormonal release. Radioactive iodine has the additional effect of selectively irradiating hormonally active tissue, owing to its uptake by the actively functioning gland.

Blood Chemistry Values

Thyroid hormones affect the synthesis, degradation, and intermediate metabolism of adipose tissue and circulating lipids, and abnormalities of endocrine function are reflected in altered lipid levels. In hyperthyroidism, degradation and excretion increase more than synthesis, resulting in low circulating levels of cholesterol, phospholipids, and triglycerides; hypothyroidism slows catabolism more than it affects synthesis, and hypercholesterolemia and hypertriglyceridemia reliably accompany myxedema. Increased serum cholesterol levels may be an early indicator of impending hypothyroidism; however, hypothyroidism secondary to pituitary failure does not cause lipids to rise. In an obviously hypothyroid patient, a normal serum cholesterol level should direct attention to the pituitary. Cholesterol levels drop to normal within 2 or 3 weeks after successful therapy for hypothyroidism has been initiated.

In severe hypothyroidism, serum levels of muscle-associated enzymes tend to rise. Total creatine kinase (CK) and lactate dehydrogenase (LDH) values rise moderately, and isoenzyme partition reveals skeletal muscle to be the source. Spinal fluid proteins (predominantly albumin) rise to 50 to 200 mg/dL in hypothyroidism.

Table 16–14 lists laboratory findings affected by thyroid hyperfunction and hypofunction.

MEASURING THYROID ACTIVITY

Thyroxine and Triiodothyronine

Automated immunoassays are widely used for the separate measurements of T_4 and T_3. The antibodies in these assays are highly specific, so there is no significant cross-reactivity between T_4 and T_3 in their quantitation. Measurement of T_4 has long been a first-round test in screening for thyroid disease by detection of a level either abnormally high or abnormally low. Triiodothyronine measurements are useful in confirming suspected thyroid abnormality, but they can also be diagnostic in rare situations of hyperthyroidism with low or normal T_4 and high

TABLE 16–14. EFFECTS OF THYROID DYSFUNCTION ON NONTHYROID TESTS

Hypothyroidism

Increased serum cholesterol, triglycerides
Increased serum carotene (yellow skin discoloration)
Increased serum levels of muscle enzymes: CPK, AST, LDH
Increased serum prolactin
Normochromic anemia, hemoglobin around 10 g/dL
Increased capillary fragility
Increased spinal fluid protein
Decreased urinary excretion of 17-KS, 17-OHCS

Hyperthyroidism

Increased skin temperature, pulse rate, pulse pressure
Decreased serum cholesterol, triglycerides
Increased serum levels of aminotransferases and alkaline phosphatase
Altered glucose insulin relationship
Increased proportion of lymphocytes in differential white count
Increased urinary calcium excretion

T_3 as an isolated finding. Triiodothyronine levels may also be used for monitoring thyroid replacement therapy consisting of T_3.

Thyroxine-Binding Globulin and Free Hormone

The concentration of binding protein affects serum levels of T_3 and T_4, but the physiologic thyroid status is reflected only by the amount of free active hormone present. When total T_3 or T_4 levels are abnormal, it is important to evaluate the major thyroid-binding protein, TBG. It is possible to measure TBG levels directly by RIA, but the usual test for TBG activity is the T_3 uptake test. The T_3 uptake test reflects the quantity of TBG present and the quantity of hormone attached to it (i.e., its degree of saturation with thyroid hormone).

Hormone Uptake

In the T_3 uptake procedure, a known amount of radiolabeled T_3 is added to the test serum. (A different nonisotopic reagent is now also used in place of T_3 for a chemically equivalent automated immunoassay that is termed "T uptake.") Endogenous thyroid hormone does not ordinarily fully saturate TBG, so binding sites are available to combine with the reagent T_3. Labeled T_3 binds to TBG to a degree inversely proportional to the amount of endogenous hormone already bound. If endogenous T_4 levels are low, many TBG sites will be free to react with the labeled T_3; if much T_4 is present, few TBG sites will be available to bind labeled T_3.

Results are determined by measuring labeled T_3 remaining after all available sites on the TBG have been filled. High residual radioactivity means that endogenous hormone levels were high and few TBG sites were available to combine with the radiolabeled T_3; low residual activity means that numerous binding sites were unoccupied by endogenous hormone and thus were available to combine with the radiolabeled T_3. Resin or some other solid-phase indicator is used to detect residual activity. The results are expressed as percent of radioactivity left unbound; normal values depend on the individual method used (e.g., 25 to 35% by some methods and 35 to 45% by others). In hyperthyroidism, both T_4 and T_3 uptake have large numerical values; in hypothyroidism, both have low values.

Factors Affecting Thyroxine-Binding Globulin

Estrogens increase the amount of TBG in serum, whereas androgens and glucocorticoids depress TBG synthesis. In pregnant women and in patients taking exogenous estrogens or with endocrine-secreting tumors, T_3 uptake values are low (in response to elevated concentrations of TBG), simulating hypothyroidism. Conversely, seemingly hyperthyroid high uptake occurs in patients taking androgens or adrenocorticosteroids, owing to depressed levels of TBG.

Low TBG concentration and consequent high uptake results are seen if overall protein levels are low, as for example, in severe liver disease or in protein-losing conditions like nephrotic syndrome or protein-losing enteropathy. Salicylates and the phenytoin anticonvulsants bind to TBG in competition with thyroxine. Patients taking these drugs have high residual T_3 uptake because binding sites are occupied by these nonhormonal agents.

Administration of heparin causes an elevation of free fatty acids in the circulation from breakdown of triglycerides by post-heparin lipoprotein lipase activation. These free fatty acids then bind to TBG and displace thyroid hormone. The T_3 uptake is very sensitive to heparin administration, with falsely high values.

Free Hormone Level

Physiologic thyroid status is little affected by altered TBG levels despite abnormal measured values for total hormone. It is now standard that some measurement of free hormone level must be part of a detailed thyroid investigation. It is difficult to measure free T_4 or T_3 directly because the quantities are so small and the interference from the preponderant bound fraction is so large. The ultimate reference method for free T_4 is by equilibrium dialysis, but this method requires special equipment and expertise available in only a few laboratories. Another method is putative RIA for free T_4, although this method suffers extensively from interference due to T_4 loosely bound to albumin. The most commonly used method for free T_4 is the **free thyroxine index (FTI,** a unitless number) that is calculated as the product of (the measured T_4) × (the value of T_3 uptake). This calculation takes into account both absolute hormone level and the binding capacity of TBG. For example, if a patient has $T_4 = 9.5$ µg/dL (reference interval 4.0 to 12.0 µg/dL), and T_3 uptake 30% (reference interval 25 to 35%), the FTI = $9.5 \times 0.30 = 2.85$ (reference interval 1.0 to 4.2); these values are all euthyroid (i.e., normal thyroid status). The FTI is sometimes referred to as the "T_7."

Clinical Application

The FTI is low in hypothyroidism and high in hyperthyroidism (Fig. 16–10). The index is normal in pregnancy, when measured hormone and TBG are both high (low T_3 uptake), and in patients taking salicylates or phenytoin drugs who have low measured hormone levels and low TBG (high T_3 uptake). Exogenous L-thyroxine, taken at doses to produce a euthyroid state, causes a high FTI because total circulating T_4 and degree of TBG saturation are both high, although in this instance the level of total T_3 is normal.

Stimulation of Thyroid-Stimulating Hormone

Thyroid activity is regulated by the body's perceived need for hormone. If inadequate thyroid hormone circulates in the free fraction, the hypothalamus produces TRH, which provokes rising TSH levels to

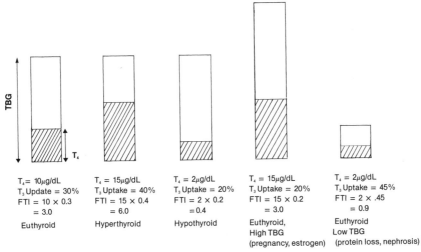

FIGURE 16–10. Examples of T_4 and TBG (thyroid-binding globulin) in different states affecting the FTI (free thyroxine index). The vertical bars represent concentrations of the TBG and T_4.

stimulate thyroid output. Measuring TSH provides useful information about both thyroid and pituitary function.

Immunoassays for TSH have become extraordinarily specific for TSH through the application of monoclonal antibodies. However, in some highly unusual circumstances, it is possible for extremely high levels of FSH, LH, or hCG to show some cross-reactivity in the assay for TSH. For the most part, TSH assays have become highly standardized and available on automated immunoanalyzers with assay times well under 1 hour (compared with at least 48 hours assay time only a decade ago).

Values of TSH are given in international activity units, the normal range being roughly 0.5 to 5.0 µU/mL. Current trends in TSH assay development have emphasized the lower end of this range in order to distinguish small amounts of TSH from true 0 levels for detection of the depression of TSH, which occurs in hyperthyroidism and secondary hypothyroidism. The level of TSH is consistently elevated in primary hypothyroidism; the TSH assay has its greatest value in distinguishing primary thyroid deficiency from hypothyroidism secondary to pituitary dysfunction. Levels of TSH also help distinguish true hypothyroidism from a functionally euthyroid condition with low thyroid hormone levels.

Immunoassays for TSH have been divided into generations according to their sensitivity of measurement at low levels. First-generation assays could quantitate TSH at elevated concentrations and were used for diagnosis of hypothyroidism; at best, their sensitivity was roughly 1.0 µU/L. Second-generation assays can measure TSH down to 0.1 or 0.2 µU/L. Third-generation assays aim for sensitivity of 0.01 to 0.02

μU/mL; fourth-generation assays should detect in the range of 0.001 to 0.002 μU/L. Most TSH assays now in use have sensitivities somewhere intermediate between second- and third-generation. Theoretically, the ability to distinguish between a very low amount of TSH and absolutely none at all should be useful for diagnosing hyperthyroidism (complete suppression of TSH). However, after several years of clinical use, it now appears that the sensitivity of third-generation assays may be too great for general clinical practice as there is overlap between ranges of thyroidal and nonthyroidal diseases. This aspect of thyroid testing will certainly change even more as clinical needs are balanced against analytic improvements.

Hypothalamic Stimulation

Purified preparations of TRH are available, making it possible to evaluate the entire thyroid-pituitary-hypothalamus feedback loop. Within 15 to 30 minutes after administration of TRH, TSH levels should rise by a factor of 2.5 to 4 and return to baseline within 2 to 4 hours. In euthyroid controls, TRH-induced TSH secretion elevates T_3 and T_4 by 50 to 75% within 1 to 4 hours.

Levels of TSH fail to rise in response to TRH stimulation in primary hypopituitarism and in states of altered thyroid homeostasis. When TRH administration elicits no TSH response in a hyperthyroid patient, it indicates that thyroid hormone production is behaving autonomously. In a hypothyroid patient with low baseline TSH levels, a subnormal response to TRH indicates pituitary dysfunction but does not distinguish between primary hypopituitarism and changes secondary to severe psychiatric depression or malnutrition.

Radioiodine Uptake

The rate at which the thyroid absorbs and metabolizes iodine reflects the level of glandular activity. Measuring thyroidal uptake of radioiodine (^{131}I) has been a popular screening test for thyroid function. Radioactivity is determined by external counting at varying intervals after an oral dose of ^{131}I. In addition, a scan is made to determine the distribution of ^{131}I within the thyroid (e.g., homogeneous, hot nodules, cold nodules). With hyperthyroidism, high uptake is seen at 1 to 6 hours, and usually at 24 hours. Some hyperthyroid patients have normal or low values at 24 hours because excessively rapid uptake and turnover eliminate the test material. Hypothyroid individuals have diminished uptake at all intervals. In normal persons, 5 to 30% of the oral dose remains detectable over the gland after 24 hours.

Artifacts

Radioiodine uptake testing suffers from many artifacts. If the body contains unusually large amounts of iodine, the administered iodine is diluted in a large pool of unlabeled element, and measured uptake is spuriously low. The rates of absorption from the gastrointestinal tract and excretion through the kidneys also affect uptake measurements. A further drawback is that the patient is exposed to a radionuclide, ^{131}I, having a half-life of 8 days.

Limited Usefulness

With the widespread availability of accurate hormone measurements, ^{131}I uptake is not a necessary screening procedure. However, the test has continuing use in evaluating already demonstrated hyperthyroidism and also in the evaluation of thyroid nodules as potentially neoplastic versus simply hyperfunctioning. If administration of exogenous T_3 or T_4 fails to suppress elevated ^{131}I uptake, it indicates autonomous thyroid function of the sort seen in functioning adenomas and Graves' disease. If radioiodine is to be used for treating hyperthyroidism, it is easier to calculate the appropriate dose if it is known what level of isotope uptake exists.

Thyroid Antibodies

Antibodies to various thyroid-related antigens usually accompany thyroiditis and diffuse **hyperthyroidism,** or **Graves' disease,** and may occur in hypothyroidism or thyroid carcinoma. The thyroid autoantibodies most often measured are those directed against thyroglobulin and against the microsomal antigen of thyroid epithelial cells. Agglutination tests, using tanned red cells coated with the specific antigen, or thyroid tissue slices for indirect immunofluorescent staining are readily available.

Clinical Correlations

Microsomal antibodies correlate extremely well with histologic changes of thyroiditis; thyroglobulin antibodies are moderately reliable in thyroiditis. Titers above $1:32$ for microsomal antibodies or above $1:100$ for thyroglobulin antibodies point so strongly to autoimmune thyroiditis that biopsy is virtually unnecessary unless there is reason to suspect carcinoma. Patients with Graves' disease who have microsomal antibodies have an increased likelihood of becoming hypothyroid after therapy. Many patients with primary hypothyroidism have low to moderate antibody titers, suggesting that immune-mediated tissue destruction may cause atrophic gland changes.

Long-Acting Thyroid Stimulator

The immunoglobulin formerly known as "long-acting thyroid stimulator (LATS)" is one of the biologically unique autoantibodies whose effect is to stimulate the target cell. Now called **thyroid-stimulating immunoglobulins (TSIg or TSI),** these antibodies react with the cell-surface receptor that usually combines with TSH. The thyroid-stimulating immunoglobulin reacts with the receptors, activates intracellular enzymes, and promotes epithelial cell activity that operates outside of the feedback regulation for TSH.

Table 16–15 summarizes information about widely available tests used to evaluate thyroid activity.

THYROID DISORDERS

Hypothyroidism

With thyroid deficiency, there is generalized hypometabolism, a syndrome often called **myxedema.** Lethargy, constipation, dry skin and hair, and, in premenopausal women, excessive menstrual bleeding commonly occur. These symptoms are so nonspecific that they do not pinpoint thyroid disorder. More specifically associated with hypothyroidism are slowed tendon reflexes, coarse skin texture, facial puffiness, cold intolerance, decreased sweating, impaired memory, and slowing of speech and motor activity. Many of these symptoms also characterize depressive states, but in hypothyroidism weight remains stable or increases, whereas in depression weight loss commonly occurs. Systolic and diastolic blood pressures are often high, but heart rate is slow, often below 60 beats per minute.

The diagnostic laboratory finding is decreased serum T_4 associated with low T_3 uptake. Serum T_3 is normal in 20 to 30% of hypothyroid patients and low in many nonthyroid conditions (see "Euthyroid Sick" Syndrome), so this measurement adds little to the diagnostic evaluation. Epithyroid ^{131}I uptake is low, but the test is rarely needed for diagnosis. Levels of TSH are three or more times greater than normal, except in those rare cases when hypothyroidism results from pituitary dysfunction. Administering thyrotropin-releasing hormone allows evaluation of pituitary responsiveness. Antibodies to thyroglobulin or microsomal antigen occur in up to 20% of hypothyroid patients, but seldom at high titers.

Congenital hypothyroidism results in irreversible, severe mental retardation and characteristic body changes termed **cretinism.** This disorder is wholly preventable with the lifelong administration of thyroid hormone beginning soon after birth. For that reason under state laws, all newborns are now screened by heel-stick blood samples for low levels of T_4 with confirmation by TSH assay. In addition to this program being an outstanding humanitarian effort, the cost to society for mass screening is much less than the cost for lifelong institutionalized care for untreated cases (roughly 1 in 7000 births).

TABLE 16-15. TESTS OF THYROID FUNCTION

Test	Frequently Used Abbreviation	Variable Measured	Normal Range	Notes
Protein-bound iodine	PBI	Serum iodine content	3.5–8 µg/dL	Useful if nonhormonal iodine is to be measured
Thyroxine measured by immunoassay	T_4RIA	Serum thyroxine content	4–12 µg/dL	Usual screening measurement
Triiodothyronine by immunoassay	T_3	Serum triiodothyronine content	70–190 ng/dL	
Free thyroxine index	FTI	Calculation, based on serum T_4 and binding capacity of TBG	(method dependent)	Product of T_4 concentration and T_3 uptake
T_3 resin uptake	RT_3U	% of labeled T_3 left unbound by TBG in test serum	25–35%	
T_3 uptake ratio	RT_3UR	Comparison of T_3 between test serum and pooled normal serum	0.8–1.35	
Thyroid-binding globulin	TBG	Serum TBG concentration		
Thyroid-stimulating hormone	TSH	Serum levels of pituitary hormone	1–10 µIU/mL	Used in assessment of free T_4. Normal range varies in different laboratories
Epithyroid ^{131}I uptake	RAIU	% of tracer dose present in thyroid gland	5–30% at 24 hours	Scan pattern important: diffuse vs. nodular; hot vs. cold nodule
Reverse triiodothyronine	rT_3	Serum content of $3,3'5'$-T_3	38–44 ng/dL	Not metabolically active; frequently elevated in nonthyroidal illness
Thyroid antibodies		Autoantibodies to thyroglobulin, thyroid microsomes	None detected	Used to assess autoimmune thyroiditis
Thyroid-stimulating immunoglobulin or	TSIg	Antibody to TSH receptor; may stimulate thyroid	None detected	For assessing Graves' disease
Long-acting thyroid stimulator	LATS			

Hyperthyroidism

The thyroid may produce excessive hormone from local nodular areas of hyperfunctioning tissue (adenomas and toxic nodular goiter) or from overall hyperactivity (diffuse toxic goiter, Graves' disease). Graves' disease usually occurs at younger ages than toxic nodular goiter; both are more common in women than in men. Nervousness, fatigue, weight loss despite normal or increased appetite, heat intolerance, and increased sweating are nonspecific symptoms reflecting generalized metabolic hyperactivity. Atrial fibrillation is commonly encountered in hyperthyroidism, especially above the age of 60 years, because of cardiac excitation from elevated thyroid hormone. In Graves' disease, but not in toxic nodular goiter, there is often excessive prominence of the eyes (exophthalmos) and widening of the palpebral fissures. Some patients develop eye changes before metabolic changes occur, a condition called **euthyroid Graves' disease.**

Laboratory Findings

Both T_3 and T_4 are high in most types of hyperthyroidism, with high T_3 uptake and very high free T_4 or free thyroxine index. Epithyroid ^{131}I uptake is high, sometimes so rapid that normal or low activity remains at 24 hours, the entire dose having been turned over in the first 6 to 12 hours. Levels of TSH are suppressed to nonmeasurable values. Characteristically absent is the drop in endogenous thyroid activity that should follow administration of exogenous thyroid hormone. Many patients with Graves' disease have in their serum TSIg, but there is poor correlation between measured TSIg level and functional hormonal status.

A subclass of hyperthyroidism, reflecting perhaps 5% of thyrotoxic patients, is so-called T_3 thyrotoxicosis. These patients have normal T_4 and FTI, but increased levels of T_3. In patients with high T_4 levels, T_3 is also expected to be high. Testing of T_3 levels can be very helpful in a patient who is clinically hyperthyroid but has normal total T_4 and FTI.

Stimulation by Chorionic Gonadotropin

The chemical structure of TSH resembles that of **human chorionic gonadotropin (hCG).** Patients with high hCG levels from hydatidiform mole, choriocarcinoma, or embryonal carcinoma of the testis sometimes manifest hyperthyroidism. Extended diagnostic work-up is not indicated, unless the thyroid manifestations persist after removal of these reproductive tract neoplasms.

Thyroiditis

The thyroid is rarely attacked by acute inflammation, but lymphocytic infiltration and fibrosis occur fairly often. The histologic appearance is that of immune-mediated chronic inflammation; this condition, called

lymphocytic thyroiditis or **Hashimoto's disease,** is often associated with glandular enlargement. High titers of antibodies to thyroglobulin and microsomal antigen are pathognomonic of lymphocytic thyroiditis. Hormonal levels may be normal when the goiter is first noted, but as tissue destruction progresses, the patient often becomes hypothyroid. Measurements of T_4 are usually normal when the disease first develops, but even at this point there is usually follicular damage that allows nonhormonal iodine to enter the circulation. Measurement of PBI may be useful if this is suspected; a high PBI value associated with normal or low-normal T_4 values is suggestive of follicular disruption.

Subacute Thyroiditis

Subacute thyroiditis can occur in localized epidemics, indicating that a viral agent may be responsible. The disorder begins as a sore throat with fever and progresses to involve one or both lobes of the thyroid, which become enlarged and tender to palpation or on swallowing. Thyroid biopsy reveals inflammatory cell infiltrates with subsequent resolution as focal scarring. In a small number of cases, the thyroid can atrophy, leading to irreversible hypothyroidism.

The PBI is generally elevated and the ^{131}I uptake is decreased because the inflamed thyroid does not take up iodine but releases organic iodine compounds into the circulation. With sufficient thyroid destruction, the T_4 can also be elevated with a brief period of functional hyperthyroidism. Patients having this disorder should be expected to recover and require little more than rest or anti-inflammatory medication (aspirin; steroids in severe cases).

"Euthyroid Sick" Syndrome

Severe illness may induce laboratory and clinical findings strongly indicative of hypothyroidism. Patients with neoplastic disease, diabetes mellitus, burns, trauma, cardiovascular conditions, liver disease, renal failure, or prolonged infections often have low serum levels of T_3 and T_4 and systemic changes consistent with profound hypometabolism. However, treatment for myxedema could be catastrophic in these debilitated patients.

Two changes seem to underlie the abnormal hormonal measurements. Serum prealbumin drops rapidly in severe illness, and the fall in prealbumin diminishes hormone-binding capacity. In addition, the amount of T_4 deiodinated to T_3 falls significantly, while there is an increase in the metabolic pathways leading to the inactive product, reverse T_3. Active hormone diminishes, but so does binding capacity, resulting in a normal FTI. Some severely ill patients do have a low FTI but are metabolically euthyroid. In such cases, demonstration of normal TSH levels documents the euthyroid state. If determination of reverse T_3 level is available, the diagnosis of "euthyroid sick" can be confirmed by showing that reverse T_3 is elevated.

Patient-Care Considerations

Iodine Artifacts

Assays specific for serum hormones are not affected by iodine intake; this simplifies testing for thyroid abnormalities because it is no longer crucial to ascertain to what medications or diagnostic procedures the patient has recently been exposed.

Epithyroid radioiodine uptake or **radioactive iodine uptake (RAIU)**— measurement is affected by whole-body iodine stores. The patient should be questioned as to use of suntan preparation, cough syrups, vaginal suppositories, and other proprietary medications, many of which contain iodine and may cause factitiously low RAIU results for 1 to 4 weeks. Radiographic contrast media have more prolonged effects, which persist for periods that range from several weeks to several months, or even years. Products used for intravenous pyelography tend to have shorter-lasting effects than those used for cholecystography or bronchography. If the patient's history includes these procedures, the request for RAIU should include very specific information about the time, place, and nature of the tests performed.

Factors Affecting Thyroxine

Circulating T_4 level is directly affected by quantity and activity of thyroid-binding proteins; the quantity of proteins present, their affinity for hormone, and the presence of exogenous hormone or other drugs that bind to proteins will all affect the measured total. Table 16–16 lists drugs

TABLE 16–16 CONDITIONS THAT AFFECT HORMONAL BINDING

Increased TBG, Low RT$_3$U

Pregnancy, estrogen therapy, oral contraceptives, acute intermittent porphyria, heroin, methadone, acute liver damage, genetic abnormalities of TBG

Decreased TBG, High RT$_3$U

Androgens, glucocorticoids, nephrosis, cirrhosis, malnutrition, protein-losing enteropathy, genetic abnormalities of TBG

Reduced Binding In Vivo, High RT$_3$U

Phenytoins in high doses, salicylates in high doses, renal failure, severe illness or stress that depresses prealbumin levels

TBG = thyroid-binding globulin; RT_3U = resin uptake of T_3.

and conditions that should be evaluated when T_4 results are abnormal. Use of the FTI helps compensate for artifacts introduced by these factors, but it is useful to know that potential interfering conditions exist.

Ingesting thyroxine causes high serum T_4 values and depresses RAIU. "Factitious hyperthyroidism" occurs in patients (often working in a medical environment) who take thyroid preparations without prescription or in excessive doses. The combination of high T_4 levels and low RAIU should provoke suspicion of self-medication.

Index of Diagnostic Suspicion

Both hyperthyroidism and hypothyroidism cause nonspecific changes in many organ systems, often of insidious onset. Both conditions occur more often in women than men, by a factor of at least 4 to 1. Although persons of any age can be affected, peak occurrence of thyroid diseases is between the ages of 30 and 60. Emotional disturbances are often incorrectly invoked to explain the fatigue, constipation, emotional blunting, and cold intolerance of hypothyroidism, and conversely, the nervousness, tremor, sleep disturbances, and weight changes of hyperthyroidism. A family history of hyperthyroidism or other thyroid disorders is often present; it may be diagnostically revealing to inquire whether other family members have had similar problems.

It is by no means clear how commonly hypothyroidism occurs. Many women are given thyroid medication on rather flimsy documentation. Conversely, attributing symptoms to emotional disturbance or encroaching old age has probably deprived many older women of potentially curative medical intervention. Patients who undergo therapy for hyperthyroidism have a lifelong increased risk for developing thyroid hypofunction. Organ-specific autoimmune diseases tend to run in families. Many cases of hypothyroidism and glandular shrinkage seem to represent the end stage of autoimmune thyroid change. A family history of thyroid hypofunction or hyperfunction, or pernicious anemia, of adrenal or parathyroid gland dysfunction, or of nonviral and nontoxic liver diseases should arouse suspicion of immune-mediated thyroid destruction.

SCREENING FOR THYROID DISEASE

Current recommendations are based on the case-finding strategy in which patients who are seeing a physician for any reason are also tested for other possible abnormalities. This strategy is intended to be more efficient than screening all individuals whether they have any symptoms or not. The case-finding approach to detecting thyroid disease consists of testing the following individuals:

- all females 50 years of age or older seeking medical care
- all geriatric inpatients on admissions, and then every 5 years

- any patient 50 years of age or older visiting a medical facility for other than minor illness; repeat every 5 years
- all adults with newly diagnosed dyslipidemia, which may in fact be secondary to hypothyroidism

Screening for thyroid disease in asymptomatic adults or children is considered not to be cost-effective; thus screening is best applied to the special groups listed here. Care should be taken in the interpretation of thyroid tests in critically ill patients and those receiving medications that might in themselves alter thyroid results.

The specific test now recommended to screen for thyroid disease is a third- or fourth-generation-sensitive TSH immunoassay. Measuring TSH allows detection of primary hypothyroidism (in which TSH is high), secondary or tertiary hyperthyroidism (in which TSH is below reference range or below detection limit), and hyperthyroidism (in which TSH is low because it is suppressed). Recent advances in the sensitivity of TSH measurements at low levels have made TSH a better test than T_4 for distinguishing thyroidal illness from some nonthyroidal illnesses that can cause alterations in circulating T_4. Abnormally low TSH values (e.g., less than 0.1 U/mL) should be confirmed by searching for an elevation of total thyroid hormone or preferably of free hormone such as free thyroxine index, or measurement by equilibrium dialysis.

PARATHYROID GLANDS

CALCIUM AND PHOSPHORUS METABOLISM

Calcium and phosphorus constitute the mineral portion of bone. **Calcium** in its ionized form critically affects neuromuscular excitability, blood coagulation, transmembrane transport of sodium and potassium, and secretory activity of exocrine glands. **Phosphates** are essential elements of energy storage compounds, nucleic acids, nucleotides, phospholipids, and other complex molecules vital to the structure, function, and replication of cells. Many interacting systems involving primarily the small intestine, the kidneys, and bone contribute to calcium and phosphorus homeostasis.

PARATHYROID HORMONE

Both minerals enter the body by absorption in the small intestine. Unabsorbed calcium and phosphorus are excreted in the feces, but changing levels of dietary absorption and of urinary excretion control the quantities present in the body. **Parathyroid hormone (PTH,** also called

parathormone), the secretory product of the parathyroid glands, exerts the most significant modulating influence. Vitamin D metabolites are also important; calcitonin, a hormone secreted by C (chief)-cells in the thyroid, has both direct and indirect effects on bone and kidneys to reduce circulating levels of calcium.

The net result of PTH action is maintenance of adequately high serum calcium levels. The action of PTH on bone is to release calcium into the bloodstream (Fig. 16–11); phosphates and protein-matrix constituents are also mobilized. In the kidney, PTH promotes tubular reabsorption of Ca^{2+} and depresses phosphate reabsorption, leading to reduced calcium excretion and increased phosphate loss. In addition, PTH causes the kidney to secrete less H^+ and excrete more HCO_3^-, with retention of both H^+ and Cl^-. Parathyroid hormone enhances renal production of active vitamin D metabolites, causing increased calcium absorption in the small intestine. The physiologic effects of PTH are summarized in Table 16–17.

Secretion of PTH occurs when serum calcium levels are low; high serum calcium suppresses parathyroid secretion. Normal serum calcium levels remain within a rather narrow range of 9 to 11 mg/dL (4.5 to 5.5 mEq/L or 2.3 to 2.8 mmol/L).

VITAMIN D

Vitamin D is a general term embracing several fat-soluble sterols that enter the body in inactive form and are sequentially transformed into

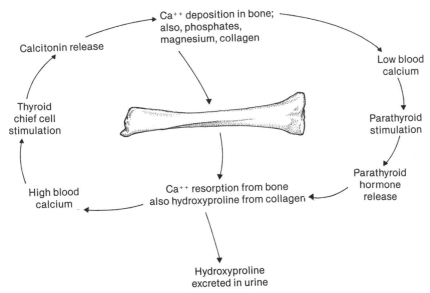

FIGURE 16–11. Hormonal regulation of mineral turnover in bone.

TABLE 16–17. EFFECTS OF PARATHYROID HORMONE*

Mobilizes Ca^{2+} and phosphate from bone
Increases phosphate excretion by decreasing renal phosphate reabsorption
Decreases calcium excretion by increasing renal calcium reabsorption
Decreases renal H^+ secretion, causing increased bicarbonate excretion and chloride retention
Enhances renal hydroxylation of vitamin D_3
Increases calcium absorption from gut, through effect on $1,25\text{-}(OH)_2D_3$

*Overall result is elevation of serum Ca^{2+} and increased urinary phosphate excretion.

biologically active material. Biologically, the most important compound is **1,25-dihydroxycholecalciferol [1,25-$(OH)_2D_3$]**. All the precursors derive from diet and are absorbed in the intestine. Some of these must be activated by ultraviolet rays absorbed through the skin, but others are in metabolizable form when ingested.

Vitamin D precursors undergo a first hydroxylation in the liver and are then converted by the kidney to the dihydroxy form. The renal product travels through the bloodstream to its target organs, small intestine and bone. Absorption of dietary calcium and phosphate is increased by $1,25\text{-}(OH)_2D_3$, which also enhances the effect of PTH in mobilizing skeletal calcium and phosphorus. Low serum phosphate levels promote renal production of $1,25\text{-}(OH)_2D_3$; hypocalcemia stimulates production of PTH, which then enhances renal synthesis of $1,25\text{-}(OH)_2D_3$.

CALCITONIN

High serum calcium levels induce calcitonin production by the thyroid. Calcitonin inhibits the osteoclasts that reabsorb bone so that calcium continues to be laid down but is not reabsorbed to enter the blood. The physiologic role of calcitonin is somewhat enigmatic. Patients with medullary carcinoma of the thyroid and very high calcitonin levels do not have abnormal calcium metabolism, nor do patients whose thyroid gland has been removed.

LABORATORY TESTING

Evaluation of parathyroid function and calcium and phosphorus metabolism starts with measurement of serum calcium, phosphorus, and PTH, but often expands to include investigation of alimentary, renal, and acid-base function.

Calcium and Phosphorus

Calcium is measured in several ways, previously mostly by atomic absorption spectrophotometry, but now usually by dye binding. In the bloodstream, calcium binds to circulating proteins, predominantly albumin. Serum calcium levels include both protein-bound and free ionized calcium; only the ionized portion has biologic significance. Roughly one half of the total serum calcium is in the ionized form. Patients with low serum proteins have low total calcium levels but are not physiologically hypocalcemic because their ionized fractions can remain normal. A simple approximation to correct calcium values for decreases in serum albumin is to expect that calcium should fall roughly 1.0 mg/dL for each 1.0 g/dL drop in albumin. Calcium also forms complexes with various anions in the circulation, notably citrate, phosphates, and oxalate; most anticoagulants prevent blood from clotting by chelating calcium, so plasma cannot be used for calcium determinations unless it is heparinized.

Ionized Calcium

Ionized calcium can be measured with an ion-selective electrode, giving a result expressed in milliequivalents or millimoles. Blood pH affects the proportions of bound and ionized calcium. As pH falls, the ionized fraction increases, whereas specimens with high pH because of carbon dioxide loss have reduced ionized calcium. Measured results will be affected by the patient's pH status, by venous stasis during phlebotomy (low pH, increased ionized fraction), by nervous hyperventilation (loss of carbon dioxide, decreased ionized fraction), and by careless handling of the specimen.

Phosphates

Phosphorus is measured in terms of phosphate; the result cannot be expressed in milliequivalents because different phosphate groups normally present at physiologic pH have different valences. Phosphate levels are somewhat higher in children than in adults and tend to be significantly higher at night than in the morning.

Urine Levels

Urinary excretion of calcium and phosphorus reflects a balance of physiologic variables, including dietary intake, body mass, and intrinsic renal function. It is rarely necessary to measure urine calcium or phosphorus except to evaluate suspected renal tubular disorders.

Diet has an enormous effect on urinary calcium excretion. High intake of carbohydrate and protein increases calcium excretion; dairy products cause high urine levels of both calcium and phosphate. Urinary calcium excretion varies also with time of day, relation to meals, and level of physical activity. A 24-hour excretion study is necessary to provide useful quantitative information.

Bone Metabolism

Mineral turnover in bone is evaluated indirectly. Bone resorption involves both minerals and protein matrix, allowing the amino acids normally confined to the osteoid to enter the circulation (see Fig. 16–11). **Hydroxyproline** is an amino acid found only in collagen; 57% of body collagen exists in the skeleton. Circulating hydroxyproline levels and urinary hydroxyproline excretion rise with increased bone resorption. For this reason, urinary hydroxyproline excretion is measured as an index of bone turnover. When skeletal growth is rapid, hydroxyproline excretion is high; children have much higher normal values than adults. Very high dietary intake of meat or of gelatin prepared from collagen can elevate urine hydroxyproline in the absence of bone pathology.

Alkaline phosphatase (ALP) is an enzyme associated with osteocyte activity, primarily bone deposition. When there is evidence of mineral turnover, it can be useful to measure ALP as an index of bone deposition and hydroxyproline as an index of dissolution. Growing children normally have high ALP levels. Men generally have more skeletal mass than women and, on average, have slightly higher normal ALP levels.

Parathyroid Hormone

The secreted parathyroid hormone consists of 84 amino acids (so-called intact form) that are cleaved before secretion by the chief cells from a 115-amino-acid peptide prohormone. The hormonal activity of PTH derives from its amino (N)-terminus of residues 1 to 34 of the intact molecule. The carboxy (C)-terminal portion of PTH is biologically nonfunctional. The intact PTH molecule is normally cleaved in the circulation, resulting in different PTH molecular species. The intact PTH molecule has a half-life in the circulation of five to ten minutes, whereas the C-terminal fragment has a half-life of one to two hours. Because the C-terminal fragment is not functionally active, it is more appropriate to measure the intact or N-terminal PTH in a patient to elucidate parathyroid activity. In addition, the C-terminal fragment is normally cleared by the kidney, but in renal failure it can rise to very high levels that have no physiologic or diagnostic significance. For these reasons, to properly interpret the measurements, it is essential to know what PTH assay is being performed.

Cyclic Adenosine Monophosphate

Parathyroid hormone affects kidney and bone cells by stimulating intracellular adenylate cyclase activity through cell-surface receptors. Increased adenylate cyclase activity releases cyclic adenosine monophosphate (cAMP) into the circulation and thence into the urine. Although plasma levels of cAMP are somewhat variable and difficult to measure accurately, urine levels expressed as micromoles of cAMP/gram of creatinine vary little with exercise, diet, and posture; this can be useful in investigating altered hormonal physiology. In addition to PTH, glucagon and the catecholamines increase cAMP excretion; but ADH, insulin, and growth hormone do not.

Vitamin D Metabolites

Recently developed analytic techniques permit far more accurate and discriminating measurement of vitamin D metabolites than the old, time-consuming bioassay that showed only overall biologic effects. The metabolite most easily measured is 25-hydroxycholecalciferol [25-$(OH)D_3$], the monohydroxylated form that leaves the liver for subsequent dihydroxylation by the kidney. Laboratory measurement of vitamin D is commonly done with extraction from serum followed by quantitation using competitive binding assays. Pronounced exposure to sunlight increases levels of 25-$(OH)D_3$ but not of the dihydroxylated compound.

Table 16–18 summarizes variables measured to evaluate PTH activity and calcium metabolism.

Calcitonin

Measurements of calcitonin (also called thyrocalcitonin) in serum are generally reserved for evaluation of medullary carcinoma of the thyroid, which secretes calcitonin at concentrations roughly proportional to tumor

TABLE 16–18. REFERENCE RANGES FOR TESTS INVOLVED IN CALCIUM METABOLISM

Measurement	Reference Range
Serum	
Parathyroid hormone	
C-terminal/midregion PTH	(see individual laboratory reference range)
N-terminal/intact PTH	
Calcium	9–11 mg/dL or 4.5–5.5 mEq/liter; 2.3–2.8 mmol/liter
Inorganic phosphorus	2.4–4.4 mg/dL
Alkaline phosphatase	25–80 IU/liter (adults)
25-$(OH)D_3$	20–30 ng/mL
1,25-$(OH)_2D_3$	2–5 ng/mL
Urine	
Calcium	50–250 mg/24 hr
Hydroxyproline	10–50 mg/24 hr (adults)
cAMP	2–6 μmol/g creatinine/24 hr

mass. After surgical excision of that tumor, serum calcitonin levels are used to monitor for recurrence. Calcitonin can also be used as a screening test for affected members of families with multiple endocrine neoplasia (MEN) type 2, which involves medullary carcinoma of the thyroid as well as hyperparathyroidism and pheochromocytoma. Elevations of calcitonin may also occur in some patients with carcinoma of the lung or breast, islet cell tumors, or carcinoid tumors. Patients with the preneoplastic state of parafollicular cell (thyroid C-cell) hyperplasia also demonstrate elevations of calcitonin. Standardized conditions with infusion of calcium or pentagastrin may be very useful as provocative tests for eliciting elevations of calcitonin in medullary carcinoma of the thyroid that are more readily interpreted than random collections. Calcitonin is generally measured by radioimmunoassay.

DISORDERS CAUSING INCREASED SERUM CALCIUM

Clinical Events

Hypercalcemia (serum calcium consistently above 12.5 mg/dL) causes changes in the nervous system, the alimentary tract, and the kidneys. Nonspecific neurologic symptoms like irritability and memory loss are combined with muscle weakness that results from altered neuromuscular transmission and calcium-induced hypokalemia. Peptic ulcer occurs fairly commonly, possibly because high calcium levels promote secretion of gastrin, which promotes gastric acid secretion. Nonspecific symptoms like anorexia and constipation are even more frequent and, along with the neurologic symptoms mentioned above, often lead to a diagnosis of depression or neurosis. High urine solute load produces high urine volume. With hypercalcemia, hypercalciuria, and phosphaturia, kidney stones frequently develop. Bone lesions are common as bone minerals are mobilized and the protein matrix dissolves.

Parathyroid Hormone Levels

Excessive PTH production may occur in primary hyperparathyroidism, usually due to a solitary adenoma; or as a secondary parathyroid response to depressed serum calcium levels. Classically, hypercalcemia and high PTH occur in both conditions; but actually, either calcium or PTH or both may fall within or near the normal range. Relative values are, in these cases, more important than absolute figures. In normal individuals, PTH will be low if serum calcium is high; a normal or high-normal PTH level in the presence of elevated or high-normal calcium level strongly suggests primary hyperparathyroidism (Fig. 16–12).

The most common cause of secondary hyperparathyroidism is renal disease. Calcium phosphate has limited solubility and precipitates

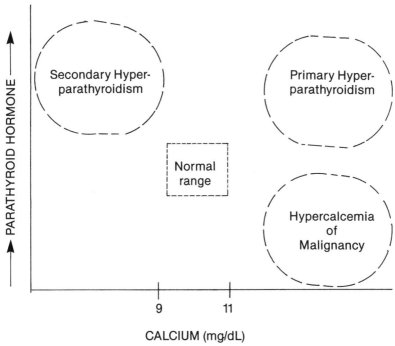

FIGURE 16–12. Graphic display of simultaneous calcium and PTH levels in various disorders. In primary hyperparathyroidism, the elevation of PTH drives calcium levels up. In secondary hyperparathyroidism, the pathologically low calcium stimulates secretion of PTH. In malignancy, lytic lesions of bone or other hormonal actions can elevate calcium independently of PTH, which remains suppressed.

(formation of dystrophic calcification) if the mathematical product between calcium ion and phosphate ion concentrations exceeds a fixed constant (i.e., $[Ca^{2+}] \times [phosphate] = K$). This ionic relationship dictates that serum calcium must decline if serum phosphate increases. With declining renal function, phosphate retention occurs, depressing serum calcium levels and provoking PTH secretion. Another cause for low serum calcium in renal failure is impaired conversion of vitamin D into the physiologically active 1,25-dihydroxy form that promotes absorption of dietary calcium. Parathyroid hormone is a potent stimulus to increased vitamin D conversion. In renal failure, the low serum calcium stimulates PTH secretion, but the kidneys cannot respond by activating vitamin D; the resulting PTH pulls calcium into the blood from bone stores. Patients with renal failure whose serum phosphates are high and whose serum calcium is within the normal range should be evaluated for the possibility of secondary hyperparathyroidism.

Nonparathyroid Conditions

Hyperparathyroidism is not the only cause of hypercalcemia. Malignant tumors—especially multiple myeloma, lymphoma, and cancer of the breast, lung, and kidney—may affect serum calcium in several ways. Some tumors secrete a PTH-like substance (ectopic PTH production); others seem to secrete prostaglandin or vitamin D–like material. Bone metastases can liberate substantial calcium into the circulation. In severe hyperthyroidism, increased bone turnover may elevate serum calcium, serum alkaline phosphatase, urine levels of calcium phosphate, and hydroxyproline—a picture very similar to hyperparathyroidism. Hormone assays readily distinguish these conditions; correcting the hyperthyroidism usually restores calcium metabolism to normal.

With skeletal immobilization or disease, more bone is reabsorbed than deposited, sometimes causing a sharp rise in serum calcium. Intrinsic diseases of bone alter calcium metabolism, and conversely, impaired calcium metabolism adversely affects bone. Distinguishing among primary and secondary causes can become rather difficult.

DISORDERS CAUSING DECREASED SERUM CALCIUM

Clinical Events

When ionized calcium is low, neuromuscular excitability increases; early symptoms are paresthesias or tingling, but muscular twitching or cramping (tetany) and altered myocardial function occur with prolonged or severe calcium depression. Patients with low serum protein levels can have low total calcium levels without symptomatic hypocalcemia. Conversely, total calcium can be normal when systemic alkalosis or hyperventilation depresses ionized calcium sufficiently to cause hypocalcemic symptoms. Hypokalemia produces a somewhat similar clinical picture. Symptomatic hypocalcemia may also occur during therapeutic hemapheresis (see Chapter 8) or in association with massive blood transfusion because of the use of the anticoagulant **citrate** (a calcium chelator, or binder).

Hormone or Vitamin D Deficiency

Most hypocalcemia results from PTH or vitamin D deficiencies due either to low absolute level or to decreased responsiveness. Severe malabsorption syndromes cause hypocalcemia by reducing intestinal calcium absorption; in steatorrhea, calcium malabsorption is further aggravated by decreased absorption of fat-soluble vitamin D and loss of calcium complexed with fatty acids. Widespread fat necrosis may, in acute pancreatitis, trap calcium as deposited calcium soaps and cause relative PTH deficiency.

Most primary hypoparathyroidism results from surgical removal of the glands, either deliberately in treating hyperparathyroidism or inadvertently during other operations on the neck, notably thyroidectomy. **Pseudohypoparathyroidism** is a rare condition characterized by decreased tissue responsiveness to PTH. It frequently results in short stature, rounded face, short and thick neck, mental retardation, and characteristic shortening of the metacarpals and metatarsals. If this syndrome occurs *without* the abnormalities of calcium and phosphorus, it is termed **pseudopseudohypoparathyroidism.**

Although vitamin D is not normally present in most foods, enrichment of it in dairy products has made dietary deficiency of vitamin D rare in the United States; however, impaired absorption is by no means uncommon. Altered metabolism or reduced tissue responsiveness to vitamin D occurs as several rare congenital disorders or as a result of drugs, renal disease, or ectopic tumor products. Phenytoin anticonvulsants and barbiturates affect hepatic hydroxylation of vitamin D and also impair response to $1,25\text{-}(OD)_2D_3$; in severe uremia, calcium absorption is depressed.

So-called vitamin D–resistant rickets is the result of an X-chromosome-linked dominant hereditary disorder in which there is a severe phosphate-losing nephropathy. Short stature and rachitic deformities occur. This condition is treatable with large doses of vitamin D plus a high intake of dietary phosphate.

Table 16–19 lists clinical conditions associated with abnormal serum calcium levels, and Table 16–20 outlines laboratory findings.

Effect of Magnesium

This divalent cation is very important to many physiologic functions, particularly those relating to neurologic and muscular actions. Despite its importance, magnesium homeostasis is not as tightly regulated as that of calcium, and there is no rapid mechanism for the body to restore depleted levels. Magnesium ions interact with PTH to affect calcium metabolism in a manner not clearly understood. Severe hypomagnesemia seems to affect both PTH production and tissue response to PTH. Apparent hypoparathyroidism may resolve if magnesium stores are repleted; hypomagnesemia, by itself or through its effect on PTH responsiveness, can be a cause of tetany. Serum magnesium should be measured whenever hypocalcemia or hypoparathyroidism is evaluated in order to detect concurrent disorder that requires separate correction (see Chapter 9).

TABLE 16–19. CONDITIONS THAT AFFECT SERUM CALCIUM

Causes of Hypercalcemia

Hyperparathyroidism, primary
Hyperparathyroidism, secondary to renal disease
Ectopic production of PTH-like material
Malignant tumors, mechanisms various or unknown
Multiple myeloma
Sarcoidosis, mechanism unknown
Skeletal immobilization
Vitamin D intoxication
Hyperthyroidism
Excessive calcium intake (milk-alkali syndrome)

Causes of Hypocalcemia

Hypoparathyroidism, usually due to operation
Unresponsiveness to PTH (pseudohypoparathyroidism)
Vitamin D deficiency
Unresponsiveness to vitamin D (vitamin D–resistant rickets)
Malabsorption syndromes: calcium, phosphate, vitamin D, or combination
Acute pancreatitis
Therapeutic hemapheresis
Massive blood transfusion

DISORDERS OF PHOSPHATE METABOLISM

The kidneys control phosphate excretion. Severe kidney disease causes phosphate retention and high serum phosphate levels. Elevated serum phosphate levels cause serum calcium to diminish; this effect on calcium stimulates PTH secretion. Chronic renal disease regularly leads to secondary hyperparathyroidism.

Insulin causes phosphate ions to shift from extracellular to intracellular fluid, so serum phosphate levels characteristically drop after meals or after a carbohydrate challenge. Acidity of intestinal contents increases phosphate absorption, and alkalinity causes less phosphate to enter the circulation. Patients taking antacids have low phosphate absorption because antacid medications complex with phosphate to render it unabsorbable.

Increased phosphate excretion occurs with systemic acidosis. Patients receiving insulin for diabetic ketoacidosis may become severely phosphate-depleted because of increased renal loss and insulin-induced shift of phosphate ions to intracellular fluid. Alcohol abuse also depletes body phosphate partly by reducing intestinal absorption, partly by the chronic dietary protein deficiency that frequently occurs, and partly by the systemic acidosis that accompanies alcohol metabolism.

TABLE 16–20. LABORATORY FINDINGS IN DISEASES THAT AFFECT CALCIUM METABOLISM

Disease	Serum				Urine			
	Ca²⁺	Phosphate	ALP	PTH	Ca²⁺	Phosphate	Hydroxyproline	cAMP
Primary hyperparathyroidism	↑↑	→	↑	↑↑	↑	↑	↑↑	↑↑
Renal disease	nl or ↓	↑	nl or ↑	↑	↓	↓	↓	↓
Hypercalcemia of malignant tumors	↑	nl or ↓	nl or ↑	↑ if ectopic; otherwise nl or ↓	↑	nl or ↓	↑	nl
Sarcoidosis	↑	nl or ↓	nl	↓	↑	nl or →	nl	nl
Paget's disease	nl	nl	↑↑	nl	nl or ↑	nl or ↑	↑↑	nl
Vitamin D intoxication	↑	↑	nl	↓	↑	↓	nl	nl
Senile osteoporosis	nl	nl	nl	nl	nl or ↑	nl	nl or ↑	nl
Skeletal immobilization	↑	↑	nl	nl	↑	↓	↑	nl
Primary hypoparathyroidism	↓	↑	nl	↓	↓	↓	nl	↓
Pseudohypoparathyroidism	↓	↑	nl	↑↑	→ or ↓	→ ↓	nl	nl or ↓
Vitamin D deficiency	nl or ↓	↑↓	nl ↑	↑↑	nl or ↓	→ ↑	nl ↑	nl or ↑

ALP = alkaline phosphatase; PTH = parathyroid hormone; cAMP = cyclic adenosine monophosphate; nl = normal.

Patient-Care Considerations

Mild to moderate hypercalcemia is one of the most common abnormalities found on blood chemistry screening batteries. Many events (see Table 16–19) can cause hypercalcemia, and the decision whether to undertake exhaustive investigation can be difficult. As serum calcium rises, there is increasing likelihood that the patient will be symptomatic. At very high levels (16 mg/dL or more), hypercalcemia becomes a potentially life-threatening emergency. Hyperparathyroidism only rarely causes severe hypercalcemia; disseminated malignant disease is the usual cause. Severe hypercalcemia of any cause should be promptly treated by correcting dehydration and increasing calcium excretion.

Although hypocalcemia can cause unpleasant physical and behavioral symptoms, life-threatening hypocalcemia is rare except after removal of the parathyroid glands. Serum calcium should be carefully monitored after operations on the neck, especially on parathyroids or thyroid. The diagnosis of hypoparathyroidism is usually obvious from the clinical history, combined with laboratory information and the signs and symptoms of actual or impending tetany. Careful intravenous infusion of calcium gluconate reverses the immediate problem. Rapidly rising serum levels may precipitate digitalis toxicity in patients receiving digitalis. In symptomatic acute or chronic hypocalcemia, coexisting hypomagnesemia may impair therapeutic response to administered calcium, so the magnesium levels should also be monitored.

Calcium-containing solutions must not be allowed to extravasate because they cause severe tissue damage, nor must they come in contact with blood or plasma because the transfusion product will clot. If calcium ions come in contact with solutions containing phosphates or carbonate, solid precipitaes may rapidly develop.

EVALUATION OF OSTEOPOROSIS

Very recently the Food and Drug Administration has cleared new assays that have promise for evaluating bone turnover. These assays are intended to have greatest application in monitoring the response to therapy in patients who have osteoporosis and in predicting which individuals are at greatest risk for bone fracture. Formerly osteoporosis was assessed clinically by **bone mineral density (BMD)** measurement using dual energy x-ray absorptimetry, which indicates how much calcium is present in the bone. That method is expensive and is sensitive only to bone mass changes that occur over long time periods such as 6 months to a year. In contrast, the new laboratory assays should be capable of reflecting response to therapy after only 2 to 3 months.

Markers of bone formation (primarily osteoblastic action) in serum include bone-specific **alkaline phosphatase (ALP)** and **osteocalcin.** Bone-specific ALP is measured by immunoassay; it has greater specificity than total ALP enzymatic activity, which can come from several other organ sources. Fractionation of ALP isoenzymes typically yields qualitative results; thus, it cannot be used to monitor bone source of ALP quantitatively. Unfortunately the bone-specific ALP immunoassay also has cross-reactivity with some other isoenzymes of ALP. Osteocalcin is a bone matrix protein that binds calcium through negative charges deriving from gamma carboxylic glutamic acid residues that are regulated by vitamin K; thus osteocalcin is a vitamin K–dependent protein.

Markers of bone resorption are based on the breakdown of bone by osteoclasts, giving rise to bone-specific degradation products that are excreted into the urine as small–molecular-weight species. The bone resorption markers include **N-telopeptides (NTx),** which arise from the N-terminal ends of crosslinked type I collagen fibers, and **deoxypyridi-noline cross links (Dpd),** also formed between collagen fibers. Another assay detects cross links from the C-terminal ends of collagen. These markers are all quantitated by immunoassays done on urine samples; it is appropriate to measure creatinine in the same samples to normalize values for variations in urine production and dilution of the marker. Although these assays are new and not yet proven over many years of clinical use, they have been tied into treatment studies with various drugs that are now being investigated in large groups of patients for slowing osteoporosis, especially in postmenopausal women and in patients on long-term corticosteroid treatment. Therapies under evaluation include hormone replacement (estrogen), calcitonin, calcium and vitamin D supplements, and the biphosphonates alendronate *(Fosamax),* etidronate, and pamidronate. These and other treatments of osteoporosis will undoubtedly set the standard of practice to (1) establish the starting levels of BMD (by x-ray) and (2) determine the rate of bone loss by immunoassay of breakdown products. Repeat measurements of the immunoassays every few months may prove very effective in encouraging patients to remain on their therapy because long-term discontinuation could have no other recognizable effect short of bone fracture.

The most serious criticism of assays for bone turnover is that they become abnormal only after major change has already occurred in the bone. Furthermore, measurements on the same patient can vary considerably even without therapy, probably due to alterations in exercise and other normal life factors. Consequently, it is appropriate to remain skeptical about these new assays while waiting for definition of their utility in large clinical trials.

PANCREAS

HORMONES

The endocrine pancreas is scattered as the islets of Langerhans amidst the glands of the exocrine pancreas. Islet cells are known to produce at least three glucose-related hormones. Insulin, produced by beta cells, dominates the metabolic picture. It promotes glucose utilization in many ways: it enhances glucose and potassium entry into most somatic cells; stimulates glycogen synthesis in liver and muscle; promotes conversion of glucose to fatty acids and triglycerides; and enhances protein synthesis, in part from residues of glucose metabolism. Overall, its effects are to promote energy storage and encourage glucose utilization. It exerts its effects by interacting with cell-surface receptors.

Alpha cells produce glucagon, which promotes synthesis and release of glucose, causing blood glucose to rise and reversing the effects of insulin. Delta cells produce somatostatin, a peptide that inhibits secretion of both glucagon and insulin; it also inhibits growth hormone and the pituitary hormones that promote thyroid and adrenal secretion.

Insulin Production

Insulin levels rise when blood glucose rises. Certain amino acids, ketones, and fatty acids also promote insulin secretion, as do rising levels of growth hormone, ACTH, glucagon, gastrin, and secretin. High blood levels of insulin, somatostatin, epinephrine, and norepinephrine inhibit insulin release. Beta cells normally cleave proinsulin to yield insulin and **C-peptide,** both of which are released in equimolar amounts into the circulation. C-peptide is metabolically inactive (and is cleared more rapidly from the circulation than is insulin), but its presence provides an index of beta-cell activity apart from measuring serum insulin, which is affected by administered exogenous hormone. Normal fasting serum insulin levels are 8 to 15 U/mL (0.3 to 0.6 ng/mL). Glucose and insulin concentrations normally vary in parallel. At very low serum glucose levels, insulin may decline to levels below the sensitivity of the test. Serum insulin is measured by radioimmunoassay, but the antibody used also reacts with the inactive precursor form, proinsulin. This becomes significant only when abnormal insulin activity is suspected, or in certain pancreatic tumors that secrete more proinsulin than active hormone.

DIABETES MELLITUS

Diabetes mellitus is a constitutional disorder of carbohydrate metabolism characterized by high blood glucose levels, glycosuria, and after some years of disease, varying clinical complications (atherosclerotic vascular disease, renal disease, neuropathy, retinopathy, etc.). Diabetes mellitus is caused by a defect in insulin secretion, in insulin action, or a combination of the two. The mechanism by which chronic hyperglycemia produces these effects is thought to be nonenzymatic glycation of proteins resulting in tissue damage. Other conditions, diseases, and medications that can affect blood glucose concentration are listed in Table 16–21).

TABLE 16–21. FACTORS AFFECTING GLUCOSE CONTROL

Stress ↑
  Anxiety
  Illness
  Infections
  Trauma
Food consumption ↑
Exercise
Hormonal influences
  Insulin ↑
  Glucagon ↑
  Corticosteroids ↑
  Catecholamines ↑
  Growth hormone ↑
  Estrogen ↑
  Thyroxine ↑
  Aldosterone ↑
Self-monitoring (stabilizes)
Drugs
  Thiazide diuretics ↑
  Oral contraceptives ↑
Alcoholism ↑
Liver disease ↑
Kidney disease ↑

Classification

The classification of diabetes mellitus was redefined in 1997 by an expert committee of the American Diabetes Association. The new classification scheme was established to reflect etiology and pathogenesis, whereas previous classification was based more on type of pharmacological treatment for management of diabetes. The etiologic classification of diabetes mellitus consists of the following:

I. **Type 1 diabetes,** in which beta cells are destroyed, leading to absolute insulin deficiency; most cases are immune mediated although a small percent are idiopathic. This type was formerly called "insulin-dependent diabetes mellitus (IDDM)."

II. **Type 2 diabetes,** which has components of insulin resistance at the tissue level and relative insulin deficiency. It was formerly called "non-insulin-dependent diabetes mellitus (NIDDM)."

III. Specific types including genetic defects of beta-cell function, genetic defects in insulin action, diseases affecting the exocrine pancreas, endocrinopathies (involving other hormones such as GH, cortisol, etc.), drug- or chemical-induced defects, infections, autoimmune disorders, and other genetic syndromes.

IV. **Gestational diabetes mellitus (GDM).**

The terms "IDDM" and "NIDDM" are no longer used. Characteristics of the two major types (1 and 2) of diabetes mellitus are listed in Table 16–22.

Diagnosis

In the document reworking the classification system, the American Diabetes Association also presented new diagnostic criteria and screening recommendations for diabetes mellitus. The new criteria for diagnosis of diabetes mellitus are as follows:

- Symptoms of diabetes (e.g., polyuria, polydipsia, weight loss, blurred vision) plus casual (any time of day, without regard to last meal) plasma glucose concentration ≥200 mg/dL.
- **Fasting plasma glucose (FPG)** (no caloric intake for at least 8 hours) ≥126 mg/dL
- **Two-hour postload glucose (2hPG)** ≥200 mg/dL, using an oral loading dose of 75 g anhydrous glucose dissolved in water.

Diagnosis is made based on satisfying any one of these three criteria followed by confirmation with another criterion on a subsequent day.

TABLE 16–22. THE TWO MAJOR TYPES OF DIABETES MELLITUS

Type 1	Type 2
Accounts for 10–15% of diabetes	Commonest form; about 85% of diabetes
Usually presents in childhood or teens	Usually presents over age 40
Patients usually normal weight or thin	Patients often overweight
Symptoms develop precipitously	Symptoms gradual, or patient is asymptomatic
Ketoacidosis frequent consequence of poor control	Ketoacidosis rare except with severe intercurrent illness
Nonketotic hyperosmolar syndrome does not occur	Nonketotic hyperosmolar syndrome precipitated by renal or cardiovascular insults
No measurable circulating insulin (usually)	Insulin present at low, normal, or even high levels
Insulin receptors unimpaired	Insulin receptors reduced or ineffective
Islet cell antibodies often detectable	No islet cell antibodies
Beta cell mass markedly reduced	Beta cell mass reduced only modestly
No response to oral hypoglycemic agents	Oral hypoglycemic agents often effective
Association with HLA phenotypes: antigens DR3 and DR4 (also B8, B15); heterozygotes DR3/DR4 at especial risk	No association with HLA phenotypes

An intermediate group has also been recognized in which glucose levels do not meet the criteria for diabetes but are too high to be considered normal. This intermediate group is characterized as having:

- FPG ≥110 and <126 mg/dL (normal FPG is <110 mg/dL)
- 2hPG ≥140 and <200 mg/dL (normal 2hPG is <140 mg/dL)

The previous World Health Organization criteria for diagnosis of diabetes mellitus were FPG ≥140 mg/dL and 2hPG ≥200 mg/dL. The new criteria better identify FPG above which microvascular diabetic complications begin to arise and comparability between the abnormal thresholds of FPG and 2hPG. The change in FPG threshold from 140 to 126 mg/dL is definitely substantiated by clinical and epidemiologic findings; it is likely to create some confusion in patients who previously had test results between 126 and 140 mg/dL. FPG is convenient and accurate and so should probably be the most commonly used screening test for diabetes mellitus. It is also now recommended that the following asymptomatic individuals be screened:

- All individuals at age 45 years and older; if normal, repeat every 3 years
- Younger individuals who have the following risk factors:
  1. Obesity
  2. First-degree relative with diabetes
  3. High-risk ethnic group (African-American, Hispanic, Native American)
  4. Had a baby weighing >9 pounds or had gestational diabetes
  5. Hypertension
  6. HDL cholesterol ≤35 mg/dL and/or triglycerides ≥250 mg/dL
  7. Had intermediate glucose measurements previously

Gestational Diabetes Mellitus

In the U.S., gestational diabetes mellitus (GDM) occurs in approximately 4% of all pregnancies. Detection of GDM allows for appropriate diet, therapy, fetal surveillance, and special procedures for delivery. Glucose tolerance normally fluctuates during pregnancy, and so criteria for GDM have been set to identify those women at greatest risk for diabetic complications during pregnancy. Most women with GDM will show return to normal glucose control after delivery, but many remain at risk for developing diabetes later in life.

Screening for GDM consists of plasma glucose measurement 1 hour after a 50 g oral glucose load (usually given as a specially formulated cola-type solution that is commercially bottled for this type of testing). This testing should be done between weeks 24 and 28 of gestation. If the 1-hour plasma glucose is greater than or equal to 140 mg/dL, a full 3-hour oral glucose tolerance test (GTT) should be administered with a dose of 100 g of glucose. The plasma glucose should be less than 105 mg/dL fasting, less than 190 mg/dL at 1 hour, less than 165 mg/dL at 2 hours, and less than 145 mg/dL at 3 hours. Diagnosis of GDM is based on meeting or exceeding any two of these four plasma glucose levels. If the patient cannot retain the oral glucose load and vomits, the GTT is invalid, and sample collection should be stopped; repeat GTT should be scheduled at a later date.

Although this combination of 50 g screening and 100 g confirmatory testing had previously been recommended for all pregnant women, it is now considered unnecessary to do for women under 25 years of age who have normal body weight, no family history of diabetes, and are not members of an ethnic group with high prevalence of diabetes. All other pregnant women should be tested. The American College of Obstetricians and Gynecologists also recommends proceeding directly to confirmatory testing without screening in some populations with very high risk.

Glucose Tolerance Test

Although not a standard part of the new recommendations to screen for and diagnose diabetes except for GDM, **glucose tolerance testing (GTT)** may be used by some physicians for evaluating equivocal cases of hyperglycemia and even hypoglycemia. The oral GTT is affected by many physiologic variables and is subject to many different diagnostic interpretations. Intravenous glucose tolerance testing, which is even more difficult to interpret, is rarely indicated for diagnostic purposes. The patient undergoing a GTT should be in a normal nutritional state; should not be taking salicylates, diuretics, anticonvulsants, steroids, or oral contraceptives; and should not smoke, eat, or drink anything other than water for 12 hours before the test. Carbohydrate depletion and inactivity or bed rest impair glucose tolerance, so a GTT should not be done on bedridden or immobilized patients or on persons taking inadequate diets. The patient should have consumed at least 150 g of carbohydrate daily for 3 days before testing and have had no alcohol intake.

Some workers use a standard dose of glucose (variously 50 g, 75 g, or 100 g), whereas others tailor glucose load to body size, using either 1.75 g/kg body weight or 50 g/m^2 of body surface. Protocols for sampling vary; most workers evaluate at fasting and at 1 and 2 hours; some obtain a third hourly specimen, whereas others include a half-hour and a 1.5-hour specimen as well.

Interpretation

Two hours after a glucose load, blood glucose should return to the fasting level. Persistent elevation at 2 hours is abnormal; a modest 2-hour increment and normal 3-hour level suggest impaired glucose metabolism without overt diabetes. A very sharp rise followed by decline to subnormal levels may occur in hyperthyroidism and alcoholic liver disease. With advancing age, the speed of glucose clearance declines; 2-hour levels in persons who do not have diabetes and those with negative family histories increase an average of 6 mg/dL for each decade over age 30.

Concurrent collection of urine is not essential but is often done. If the glucose is given with large volumes of fluid, collecting urine at 1½ to 2 hours is not difficult, and the results may show how much glucose the patient spills at a given level of hyperglycemia. If glycosuria occurs without hyperglycemia, the patient must be evaluated for abnormal renal tubular function.

Monitoring Diabetic Control

Urine Testing

Observing and quantifying urine glucose levels is the time-honored approach to monitoring blood glucose control. With enzyme-impregnated strips, the patient can easily detect sugar spillage after meals, a significant but rather insensitive index of hyperglycemia. For stable diabetic patients, urine testing allows very satisfactory surveillance of therapy, be it diet, oral hypoglycemic agents, or insulin; however, it must be recognized that urine concentrations of glucose reflect what blood levels were at an earlier time and may not accurately indicate acute changes in glucose regulation.

Blood Glucose Testing

The American Diabetes Association now recommends that diabetic individuals monitor their own blood glucose in fingerstick samples with portable electronic meters that use reagent strips similar to those for urine glucose testing. The immediacy of these test results is extremely important in establishing correct insulin amount for next dose, thereby improving blood glucose control through patient feedback. Self-monitoring of blood glucose has been highly effective in reducing the rate of development of diabetic complications.

Glycosylated Hemoglobin

When exposed to high glucose levels, the hemoglobin molecule irreversibly acquires a glucose moiety on the beta chain. In normal individuals, 3 to 6% of hemoglobin is glycosylated in the form designated A1c. With prolonged hyperglycemia, levels of hemoglobin A1c may rise as high as 18 to 20%. Glycosylation does not impair oxygen-exchanging capacity, but high hemoglobin A1c levels reflect inadequate diabetic control in the preceding 3 to 5 weeks. After normoglycemic levels are stabilized, hemoglobin A1c levels return to normal in about 3 weeks. Periodic measurement of hemoglobin A1c provides information that spot urine checks might miss; insulin-sensitive type-1 patients may have undetected periods of hyperglycemia alternating with postinsulin periods of normoglycemia or even hypoglycemia.

Older red cells, having been in the circulation longer than young cells, have higher hemoglobin A1c levels. In a patient with episodic or chronic hemolysis, circulating blood contains a disproportionately large number of young red blood cells, thus diluting the hemoglobin A1c to spuriously low levels.

Fructosamine

This relatively new procedure is based on measurement of glycosylated serum proteins, primarily albumin, which become linked to glucose analogously to the nonenzymatic formation of glycosylated hemoglobin. This measurement is also referred to as **fructosamine.** Because albumin has a half-life in the circulation of 20 days, the amount of fructosamine reflects hyperglycemic periods within the previous few weeks. Thus blood glucose gives information about immediate control of diabetes, fructosamine about short-term control, and glycosylated hemoglobin about long-term control.

Fructosamine measurements can be particularly useful for monitoring diabetics who also have chronic hemolytic anemias and other conditions of shortened red-cell life span, in which glycosylated hemoglobin is not fully reliable for assessing diabetic control.

Tissue Glycosylation

Increasing evidence correlates ocular, vascular, and neurologic complications of diabetes mellitus with the existence of prolonged or repeated hyperglycemia. Proteins in the retina, peripheral nerves, and the capillary basement membranes appear to undergo the same kind of glycosylation as hemoglobin, thereby suffering irreversible changes in structure and function. Studies in different populations have shown a very sharp and linear rise in the prevalence of diabetic retinopathy above fasting plasma glucose of 126 mg/dL, 2-hour postload glucose of 200 mg/dL, and hemoglobin A1c of 7%. These three laboratory thresholds thus appear to have biological equivalence. Because diabetic individuals may go on to develop substantial complications due to elevations of these parameters years before diagnosis, the American Diabetes Association in 1997 made the changes listed above in the criteria for screening and diagnosing diabetes mellitus.

Efforts to avoid peaks and valleys in blood glucose levels include combination treatment with short-, medium-, and long-acting insulins; institution of more frequent dosage; and the use of devices that permit continuous or automatically pulsed insulin injection. The factors that influence glucose control are shown in Table 16–21.

Abnormalities of Diabetic Control

Diabetic ketoacidosis and hyperglycemia are the two most dangerous complications in patients with type 1. Ketoacidosis occurs much less often in patients with type 2, probably because there is sufficient residual insulin to suppress lipolytic release of the fatty acids that provoke ketosis and its attendant complications. In older patients with type 1, ketoacidosis usually indicates intercurrent illness, especially infections or hormonal imbalance; in younger patients, serious irregularities of glucose homeostasis more often promote ketoacidosis.

Ketoacidosis

The pathophysiology of **diabetic ketoacidosis** begins with pronounced hyperglycemia and insulin deficiency. Hyperglycemia causes excessive serum osmolality, which leads to osmotic diuresis that carries water, glucose, and electrolytes out of the body. Defective glucose utilization and absence of insulin activate metabolic and stress receptors that increase glucagon, epinephrine, and adrenal steroid levels. These have the combined effect of mobilizing amino acids and fatty acids for gluconeogenesis (a process whereby glucose is produced from proteins and fats) and for combustion in anaerobic metabolism, and of mobilizing glucose from glycogen stores (glycogenolysis). The end products of fatty acid metabolism are highly acidic ketone bodies that are excreted in the urine along with water and the cations K^+ and Na^+.

As the blood becomes more acid, respiratory stimulation causes arterial PCO_2 to drop, but since H^+ production continues, total body acidity continues to rise. Serum K^+ levels often rise because potassium cannot enter cells without insulin. Elevated circulating K^+ is used to meet the need for urinary cations as more anions such as ketoacids are excreted, causing severe whole-body potassium loss. As intracellular potassium declines, cells become progressively dehydrated because water leaves the cells to equilibrate with the hyperosmolar serum. Arterial hypotension occurs if dehydration is severe, reducing tissue oxygenation and promoting lactic acid generation in the poorly perfused tissue. Dehydration, acidosis, and potassium deficiency are major threats to life; even with present-day therapeutic regimens, ketoacidosis causes mortality as high as 5 to 10%. During the correction of diabetic ketoacidosis with intravenous administration of fluid, insulin, and potassium, it is common practice to monitor blood levels of glucose, ketones, osmolality, blood gases, electrolytes, anion gap, BUN, and white count (to detect possible infection).

The differential diagnosis of diabetic ketoacidosis includes hypoglycemic coma, lactic acidosis, nonketotic hyperosmolar coma, and drug-induced comas. Differentiating features are shown in Table 16–23 (see also Anion Gap, Chapter 10).

Nonketotic Hyperosmolar Syndrome

Older people with type 2 diabetes sometimes experience pronounced hyperglycemia without the lipolytic and electrolyte derangements resulting from absolute insulin deficiency. This clinical presentation differs from ketoacidosis. Blood glucose may achieve astronomic levels, as high as 1500 to 2000 mg/dL; with serum osmolality so high, the kidneys respond with osmotic diuresis. Unless there is abundant fluid intake, water loss outstrips solute excretion, and serum osmolality

TABLE 16–23. DIFFERENTIAL DIAGNOSIS OF COMA IN PERSONS WITH DIABETES

	Diabetic Ketoacidosis	Hypoglycemia	Lactic Acidosis	Nonketotic Hyperosmolar Syndrome	Salicylate or Other Poisoning
Blood Levels of					
Glucose	↑↑	↓↓	Normal	↑↑↑	Normal
Ketones	↑↑	Absent	Absent	Absent	Absent to ↑↑
Osmolality	↑↑	Normal	Normal or ↑	↑↑↑	Normal
pH	↓↓	Normal	↓↓	Normal	↓
HCO$_3^-$	↓↓	Normal	↓↓	Normal	↓
Na$^+$	↓	Normal	Normal	Normal or ↑*	↓
K$^+$	Variable	Normal	Normal	Normal	Normal
Anion gap	↑↑	Normal	↑↑↑	Normal	↑ or ↑↑
Urea nitrogen	↑*	Normal	Normal or ↑*	↑*	Normal or ↑*
WBC	↑	Variable	Variable	↑	Variable
Urine Levels of					
Glucose	↑↑	Absent	Absent	↑↑↑	Absent
Other reducing substances	Absent	Absent	Absent	Absent	↑↑
Ketones	↑↑	Absent	Absent or ↑	Absent	↑
Respiration	Air hunger	Normal	Air hunger	Normal	Variable
Dehydration	↑↑	Absent	Absent or ↑	↑↑↑	Variable

*Largely due to dehydration.

further increases. Intracellular dehydration and reduced plasma volume cause widespread and functional abnormalities, leading to severe hypotension and deep stupor or coma. The drop in glucose utilization is often precipitated by infection, cerebrovascular accidents, acute endocrine imbalance, or the effects of drugs like diuretics, phenytoins, or propranolol. Therapy is directed toward maintaining intravascular volume and sodium concentration to prevent hypovolemic shock. Special care must be given to the electrolytes (especially potassium) to prevent cardiac arrhythmias. Administration of insulin and correction of the glucose elevation is secondary to establishing blood pressure and circulatory support. Laboratory monitoring should include frequent measurements in blood of glucose, osmolality, sodium, potassium, hematocrit, and other electrolytes.

HYPOGLYCEMIA

The symptoms of acute hypoglycemia result from increased epinephrine secretion induced by rapidly falling glucose levels. Sweating, trembling, weakness, and anxiety are prominent, with subsequent alterations of consciousness. Gradually developing hypoglycemia provokes headache, irritability, and lethargy. A common cause of hypoglycemia is insulin overdosage in patients with unstable type 1 diabetes mellitus. It is important that these patients learn to recognize early symptoms of hypoglycemia and keep available some source of sugar they can take to abort impending hypoglycemia. Table 16–24 lists causes of hypoglycemia.

TABLE 16–24. CAUSES OF HYPOGLYCEMIA

Insulin or oral hypoglycemic overdose
Reactive hypoglycemia
   Inappropriate insulin release after a meal (early diabetes)
   Rapid intestinal transit time and altered course of glucose absorption
Fasting hypoglycemia
   Tumor: insulinoma of pancreatic beta cells or extrapancreatic
   Liver failure: defective gluconeogenesis
   Low glycogen stores
   Alcohol ingestion, chronic
   Endocrine insufficiencies
     Pituitary: growth hormone
     Adrenal

Diagnosis and Distinctive Forms

The nonmedical press has popularized the idea that unrecognized hypoglycemia causes much nervousness, weakness, anxiety, headache, and irritability; many patients believe themselves to suffer from a constitutional tendency to hypoglycemia. True symptomatic hypoglycemia should be diagnosed only when blood glucose levels are demonstrated to be below 50 mg/dL at the time that symptoms occur; it should also be shown that correcting the blood sugar level abolishes the symptoms.

Two patterns of hypoglycemia are recognized. **Postprandial hypoglycemia,** occurring several hours after eating, appears to result from delayed or exaggerated response to the insulin secreted in response to dietary blood sugar rise. **Fasting hypoglycemia,** in contrast, occurs after 10 or more hours without food; it reflects either failure to mobilize glucose appropriately or persistence of excessive insulin secretion despite declining physiologic stimulation.

Postprandial Hypoglycemia

Postprandial hypoglycemia may occur as an early event in developing type 2 diabetes mellitus, representing disproportion between pancreatic function and cellular insulin receptors. A few patients with gastrointestinal malfunction have rapid, exaggerated blood sugar rise just after eating, leading to exaggerated insulin secretion, which causes blood glucose to plummet. Most postprandial hypoglycemia, however, has no demonstrable physiologic cause and is considered functional. Symptomatic episodes tend to last no more than 30 minutes and to resolve even without carbohydrate intake.

Postprandial hypoglycemia can be diagnosed by a 5-hour glucose tolerance test with samples taken every 30 minutes. It is important for the patient to report subjective symptoms so that a specimen can be drawn to coincide with the symptoms. If symptoms become severe, glucose should be given and the test terminated, but blood glucose level should be documented at the time of maximum symptoms.

Additional information can be gained by measuring insulin and cortisol secretion relative to blood glucose levels. If reactive hypoglycemia is part of developing diabetes mellitus, excessive insulin production can be shown; whereas in functional hypoglycemia, the amount of circulating insulin is appropriate for the changing blood sugar levels. Physiologically significant hypoglycemia stimulates adrenal secretion of cortisol; within 90 minutes after a hypoglycemic trough, cortisol levels can be shown to increase at least twofold in patients with true hypoglycemia.

Fasting Hypoglycemia

Fasting hypoglycemia nearly always has pathologic significance. Tumors are one source of excessive or autonomous insulin production. The tumor may arise in pancreatic beta cells (insulinoma), or there may be some other epithelial neoplasm with ectopic hormone synthesis. Liver disease is a major cause of fasting hypoglycemia; occasionally, the enzymes involved in gluconeogenesis are defective, but more often the problem is widespread hepatocellular necrosis due to tumor or to surgical or traumatic tissue destruction. Chronic alcoholics who stop ingesting carbohydrates frequently become hypoglycemic because their glycogen stores are low and accumulating ethanol metabolites interfere with gluconeogenesis. Diabetic patients taking either insulin or oral hypoglycemics are especially liable to alcohol-induced hypoglycemia.

Fasting hypoglycemia is detected by measuring blood glucose after 12 or 24 hours without food. Normal women seem to withstand lower fasting levels than men. In men, fasting hypoglycemia is diagnosed if blood sugar declines to 50 mg/dL or below after prolonged fasting, but in women the diagnostic threshold may be as low as 35 mg/dL. Since fasting hypoglycemia may result from overproduction of insulin or undermobilization of glucose, measuring serum insulin levels allows diagnostic distinction. Insulin secretion should decline as blood glucose levels fall; failure to do so indicates insulin-producing tumor.

Factitious Hypoglycemia

A significant issue in evaluating hypoglycemia is self-administered insulin. This **factitious hypoglycemia** occurs without consistent relationship to eating; it tends to occur in women with neurosis who have access to insulin and syringes, from either a diabetic family member or employment in a medical setting. In such patients, normal results are found in glucose tests performed under observation that prevents self-medication. Also diagnostic is demonstration of high serum insulin levels and low C-peptide levels. Injectable insulin preparations are purified to remove C-peptide. Injected insulin elevates immunoreactive insulin levels and suppresses endogenous pancreatic secretion, thereby eliminating the physiologic source of normally present C-peptide.

SUGGESTED READING

Adachi, JD, et al: Intermittent etidronate therapy to prevent corticosteroid-induced osteoporosis. N Engl J Med 337:382, 1997.

Bauer, DC, and Brown, AN: Sensitive thyrotropin and free thyroxine testing in outpatients. Arch Intern Med 156:2333, 1996.

Danese, MD, et al: Screening for mild thyroid failure at the periodic health examination: A decision and cost-effectiveness analysis. JAMA 276:285, 1996.

Franklyn, JA, et al: Comparison of second and third generation methods for measurement of serum thyrotropin in patients with overt hyperthyroidism, patients receiving thyroxine therapy, and those with nonthyroidal illness. J Clin Endocrinol Metab 78:1368, 1994.

Garnero, P, et al: Comparison of new biochemical markers of bone turnover in late postmenopausal osteoporotic women in response to alendronate treatment. J Clin Endocrinol Metab 79:1693, 1994.

Gerlo, EAM, and Sevens, C: Urinary and plasma catecholamines and urinary catecholamine metabolites in pheochromocytoma: Diagnostic value in 19 cases. Clin Chem 40:250, 1994.

Gertz, BJ, et al: Monitoring bone resorption in early postmenopausal women by an immunoassay for cross-linked collagen peptides in urine. J Bone Miner Res 9:135, 1994.

Glenn, GC, and the Laboratory Testing Strategy Task Force of the College of American Pathologists: Practice parameter on laboratory panel testing for screening and case finding in asymptomatic adults. Arch Pathol Lab Med 120:929, 1996.

Inzucchi, SE: Growth hormone in adults: Indications and implications. Hosp Pract 32:79, 90, 95, 1997.

Laragh, JH: Renin profiling for diagnosis, risk assessment, and the treatment of hypertension. Kidney Int 44:1163, 1993.

Magiakou, MA, and Chrousos, GP: Corticosteroid therapy, nonendocrine disease, and corticosteroid withdrawal. Curr Ther Endocrinol Metab 6:138, 1997.

Malchoff, CD, and Carey, RM: Adrenal insufficiency. Curr Ther Endocrinol Metab 6:142, 1997.

Nelson, JC, Weiss, RM, and Wilcox, RB: Underestimates of serum free thyroxine (T_4) concentrations by free T_4 immunoassays. J Clin Endocrinol Metab 79:76, 1994.

Niccoli, P, et al: Interest of routine measurement of serum calcitonin: Study in a large series of thyroidectomized patients. The French Medullary Study Group. J Clin Endocrinol Metab 82:338, 1997.

O'Brien, T, et al: Hyperlipidemia in patients with primary and secondary hypothyroidism. Mayo Clin Proc 68:860, 1993.

Oelkers, WK: Hypopituitarism. Curr Ther Endocrinol Metab 6:27, 1997.

Peplinski, GR, and Norton, JA: The predictive value of diagnostic tests for pheochromocytoma. Surgery 116:1101, 1994.

Pittman, JG: Evaluation of patients with mildly abnormal thyroid function tests. Am Fam Physician 54:961, 1996.

Report of the expert committee on the diagnosis and classification of diabetes mellitus. Diabetes Care 20:1183, 1997.

Sawin, CT, et al: Low serum thyrotropin concentrations as a risk factor for atrial fibrillation in older persons. N Engl J Med 331:1249, 1994.

Surks, MI, et al: American Thyroid Association guidelines for use of laboratory tests in thyroid disorders. J Am Med Assoc 263:1529, 1990.

Urban, MD, and Kogut, MD: Adrenocortical insufficiency in the child. Curr Ther Endocrinol Metab 6:147, 1997.

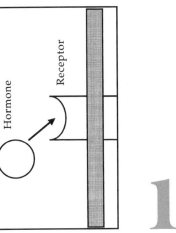

17

Reproductive Endocrinology

GENERAL PHYSIOLOGY

In both men and women, the gonads serve both endocrine and reproductive functions. Sperm and ova derive from germinal epithelium; embryologically distinct secretory epithelium produces testosterone in men, and estrogens and progesterone in women.

The pituitary hormones that regulate endocrine secretion and thereby affect reproductive function are the same in men and women. These tropic hormones are called, in both men and women, **follicle-stimulating hormone (FSH)** and **luteinizing hormone (LH),** although the **follicle** and the **corpus luteum** are unique to the ovary in women. Pituitary function, in turn, is controlled by a hypothalamic hormone called **gonadotropin-releasing hormone (GnRH)** or **luteinizing hormone-releasing hormone (LHRH);** hypothalamic secretion occurs when levels of the gonadal hormones decline. These complex physiologic interactions are collectively designated the **hypothalamic-pituitary-gonadal axis** (see Chapter 16). Evaluation of individual parts of this axis is made possible by the availability of immunoassays for measurements and the availability of purified hormones, hormone stimulators, and hormone antagonists for diagnosis and treatment.

The gonads differentiate early in fetal life; external genitalia and secondary sex characteristics are influenced by hormones secreted by the fetal gonads. Ambiguous or failed sexual differentiation may occur if chromosomally determined enzyme abnormalities alter the synthetic pathways necessary for normal steroid formation (see Fig. 16–4). Aberrations of these synthetic pathways may accentuate or depress anatomic and sexual development in fetal life or in the prepubertal child. Discriminating the syndromes caused by congenital disorders of sexual differentiation is a complex process that requires quantitation of several steroid hormone intermediates and end products in order to diagnose specific enzyme deficiencies.

GONADAL FUNCTION IN MEN

In males, testosterone is produced by the **Leydig cells,** epithelial cells located in the testes among the seminiferous tubules. The seminiferous tubules contribute 75% of total testicular volume and produce the sperm. **Testosterone** production is stimulated by pituitary LH; spermatogenesis is partially controlled by FSH stimulation, but the presence of testosterone is also necessary. Circulating testosterone levels influence the secretion of the single hypothalamic hormone (GnRH) that affects both FSH and LH secretion. Isolated elevation of FSH can occur if testosterone production is normal but the germinal epithelium fails to produce spermatozoa; isolated overproduction of LH rarely occurs.

GONADAL FUNCTION IN WOMEN

In females, FSH promotes maturation of the germinal follicle, causing estrogen secretion and allowing the ovum to mature (follicular phase). At the midpoint of the cycle, there is a surge of LH secretion that induces ovulation and release of the ovum from the ovary into the peritoneal cavity from whence it migrates into the fallopian tube and to the uterus. In addition, there are morphologic changes and secretory activation (called **luteinization,** or **luteal phase**) in the epithelial cells that secrete progesterone. Rising estrogen levels at this time inhibit FSH production and seem to stimulate LH production. As progesterone levels rise, LH drops off sharply. Estrogen secretion peaks just before midcycle, drops rather sharply with ovulation, and then rises to a plateau that falls off just before menstruation begins. Progesterone levels are low in the first half of the cycle and rise sharply at ovulation to a high plateau that persists until shortly before menstruation (Fig. 17–1).

The surge of LH levels in serum and then into urine by clearance through the kidney has been employed for detection of the time of ovulation in women who have difficulty becoming pregnant. New over-the-counter ovulation tests are based on colorimetric enzyme immunoassays for LH incorporated into dipsticks to be used on morning

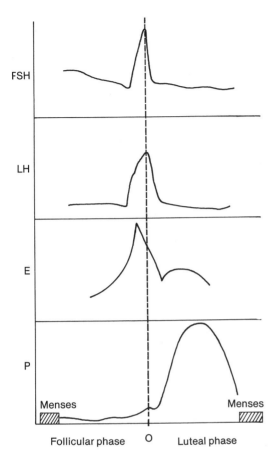

FSH

LH

E

P

Menses   Menses

Follicular phase   O   Luteal phase

FIGURE 17–1. Hormone cycle levels during the menstrual cycle.

urine samples. After repeated days of negative testing during the first half of a menstrual cycle, a woman can use this assay's detection of LH to time intercourse to maximize the possibility of fertilizing a recently ovulated ovum.

GONADAL HORMONES AND THEIR METABOLISM

All the sex hormones are steroids, converted from precursor molecules through cholesterol to their final forms (see Fig. 16–4). **Progesterone** is an active steroid and also serves as a precursor for later steps. **Testosterone** is derived from progesterone; **estrogen** arises through structural alteration of the testosterone molecule. Both men and women have substantial amounts of circulating androgens. The adrenals secrete hormones capable of transformation into androgens, and the ovary, under LH stimulation, elaborates steroids that peripheral tissues convert to androgenically active compounds. Of the estrogens, **estradiol (E_2)** is physiologically the most important; **estrone (E_3)** and **estriol (E_1)** have less potent hormonal effects.

PUBERTAL AND SENESCENT CHANGES

Before puberty, there are low levels of both gonadotropins and sex hormones. During childhood, FSH is somewhat more conspicuous than LH, and FSH levels rise first as puberty approaches. Surges of FSH and later of LH occur first during sleep; as puberty advances, daytime levels of gonadotropin rise. After the reproductive years, secretion of sex hormones declines and gonadotropin levels rise due to less feedback inhibition from diminished concentrations of those steroid hormones. In older women, FSH levels rise more markedly than LH levels; in men, both tropic hormones increase gradually. Table 17–1 gives expected ranges for the different hormones at different ages.

URINARY METABOLITES

Measurement of urinary metabolites has long been used to indicate overall hormonal function; it is still useful despite current availability of specific assays for serum hormone levels. Urinary excretion accounts for 70 to 95% of total estrogen produced; reports are given either as total estrogens or as the proportions of E_1, E_2, and E_3 present. Progesterone activity is reflected by urine **pregnanediol** (the excretory product of progesterone). Testosterone does not contribute a specific metabolite to urine; urinary 17-ketosteroids (17-KS) reflect both testosterone and adrenal hormones, and 17-KS is most often measured to evaluate adrenal function. Excreted testosterone can be measured directly by radioimmunoassay. Table 17–2 gives expected ranges of commonly measured urine metabolites.

AMENORRHEA

The failure of a woman to have menstruation is designated **amenorrhea.** In **primary amenorrhea,** a woman has never had menstrual periods, owing to disease or delayed maturation of the hypothalamus, pituitary, or

TABLE 17-1. REFERENCE RANGES FOR SERUM HORMONE LEVELS

	Prolactin (ng/mL)	FSH (mIU/mL)	LH (mIU/mL)	Testosterone (ng/mL)	Estradiol (ng/dL)	Progesterone (ng/dL)
Children	1–20	5–10	5–10	0.12–0.16	<2	
Adult men	1–20	10–15	5–20	3.9–7.9	1.6–2	<100
Adult women	1–25			0.25–0.67		
Early in cycle		5–25	5–25		1.8–2.4	37–57
Midcycle		20–30	40–80		16.6–23.2	Rising
Luteal phase		5–25	5–25		6.3–7.3	332–1198
Menopausal women	1–20	40–250	>75	0.21–0.37		10–22

TABLE 17-2. REFERENCE RANGES FOR URINARY HORMONE EXCRETION

	Estrone (µg/day)	Estradiol (µg/day)	Estriol (µg/day)	Pregnanediol (mg/day)	17-KS (mg/day)
Children	0.2–1	0–0.2	0.3–2.4	<1	<2*
Adult men	3.4–8.2	0–0.4	0.8–7.5	<1.4	9–22
Adult women					
Early in cycle	4–7	0–3	0–15	1–1.5	6–15
Luteal phase	11–31	4–14	13–54	3–6	6–15
Menopausal women	0.8–7.1	0–2.3	0.6–6.8	<1.4	6–15

*Increases, in both sexes, as puberty approaches.

ovaries. In this situation, there is also generally absence of secondary sexual characteristics. **Secondary amenorrhea** arises after a woman has had normal cycling but then develops disease of the hypothalamic-pituitary-gonadal axis that results in disruption of the normal hormonal cycles. In addition, the differential diagnosis of primary amenorrhea includes congenital anomalies such as imperforate hymen or absence of the uterus and also the syndrome of testicular feminization. Causes of secondary amenorrhea also include pregnancy, excessive athletic activity, menopause, and systemic diseases (e.g., leukemia, other organ disease of a severe nature, malnutrition).

STIMULATION TESTS

The hypothalamic-pituitary-gonadal axis can be studied by administering stimuli known to affect specific interactions. The progesterone-withdrawal test, used to evaluate amenorrhea, is an example. Bleeding occurs when the estrogen-stimulated endometrium experiences a drop in hormonal stimulation. In the normal cycle, the progesterone surge that follows ovulation inhibits gonadotropin secretion, and hormone levels decline. This is called **withdrawal bleeding.** The physiologic condition can be simulated in the test of progesterone-stimulated withdrawal bleeding.

If hypothalamic-pituitary feedback is intact, administering intramuscular progesterone or giving a course of oral progesterone induces bleeding in a uterus already exposed to adequate estrogen levels. If a woman is amenorrheic but responds with bleeding to progesterone administration, the problem is usually failure of ovulation. Several different problems can cause failure of the bleeding response to progesterone. Estrogen production may be inadequate, either from primary ovarian failure or from inadequate pituitary secretion of gonadotropin; hypothalamic dysfunction can cause defective gonadotropin secretion and reactivity; or the uterus could be abnormal. These possibilities can be distinguished by repeating the progesterone dose after stimulating the endometrium with externally available estrogen. At this point, failure to bleed indicates unresponsive endometrium; the woman who does bleed after this regimen probably has either ovarian failure or inadequately responsive hypothalamic-pituitary activity. Specific measurement of estrogens and gonadotropins resolves the diagnostic choice.

CLOMIPHENE EFFECT ON GONADOTROPINS

Clomiphene is a potent synthetic antiestrogen that blocks the uptake of steroid hormones into the hypothalamus. In patients with normal hypothalamic-pituitary function, clomiphene increases gonadotropin secretion by preventing the hypothalamus from recognizing normally inhibitory levels of estrogen or testosterone. After 5 days of clomiphene, both LH and FSH should rise substantially, usually to 50 to 100% over baseline. In anovulatory women whose ovaries are normal, clomiphene often enhances gonadotropin production sufficiently that ovulation is induced. Accordingly, clomiphene is employed for treatment of ovulatory failure to enable women whose husbands are fertile to become pregnant.

Inadequate gonadotropin response to clomiphene indicates either hypothalamic or pituitary dysfunction. It is sometimes possible to discriminate these states if purified GnRH is available. If gonadotropins rise after GnRH administration, the pituitary is normal, but hypothalamic function is impaired; absent gonadotropin response points to a pituitary abnormality. In patients with deficient pituitary gonadotropin secretion, it is important to evaluate levels of other pituitary hormones to diagnose impending or established pituitary disease.

CHORIONIC GONADOTROPIN

Human chorionic gonadotropin (hCG) is a placental glycoprotein hormone with physiologic effects very similar to those of LH. Administration of hCG is used to evaluate testicular reactivity. In a man with low testosterone levels, a rise in testosterone after hCG administration indicates normal testes but depressed hypothalamic-pituitary function; failure to respond to hCG suggests primary testicular dysfunction. Administration of hCG is not useful for female patients because there is no single measurable endpoint after LH stimulation.

LABORATORY TESTS OF GONADAL FUNCTION

Assessment of gonadal function can be useful for different conditions occurring at various ages. The infant or child with ambiguous sexual differentiation requires a complex evaluation to delineate specific enzyme deficiencies. In adults, the indications for endocrine evaluation are failure to experience sexual maturation at puberty or older; failure of fertility, either lifelong or developing after initial establishment of fertility; and change in sexual characteristics. These changes may be perceived as alteration of reproductive functions or of secondary sex characteristics, notably feminization in a man or masculinization in a woman, but also include accentuation of isosexual characteristics.

Most endocrine evaluations are undertaken for gonadal hypofunction. Primary hypofunction means failure of initial maturation. Secondary sex characteristics develop only slowly; men fail to achieve erectile and/or ejaculatory capacity, and women fail to experience menstruation. Secondary hypofunction means regression of sexual functions that have already developed normally. Tables 17–3 and 17–4 outline expected findings in different categories of sexual dysfunction with an organic basis.

GONADAL HYPERFUNCTION

Congenital enzyme deficiencies are rare; these cause hormonal imbalances that may induce striking structural and functional abnormalities. Most congenital problems are detected and evaluated early in life, but a few enzyme defects are subtle enough to escape detection until the age at which puberty should occur. In adults, hormonal overactivity is nearly always due to tumor of either the gonads or the gonadotropin-producing organs.

SEMEN ANALYSIS

Evaluation of involuntary infertility is not the only indication for semen analysis. Demonstrating normal seminal fluid is virtually diagnostic of normal hypothalamic-pituitary-testicular activity; normal results on this relatively simple, inexpensive examination can forestall the need for more complex and expensive procedures. Sperm counts are also essential in establishing the success of vasectomy.

It is essential to analyze a fresh specimen (no more than 1 hour old) to obtain meaningful results for liquefaction and sperm motility. The other measurements are less sensitive to delay in analysis (Table 17–5). Specimens may be obtained by masturbation at the physician's office or at home, but in the latter case care must be taken to transport it to the laboratory quickly and at a temperature between 25 and 32°C. Semen samples may also be obtained from sexual intercourse by use of a condom: spermicidal agents may have an immediate harmful effect on sperm motility. Before collecting the specimen, the patient should have refrained from ejaculation for at least 2 days in order to demonstrate optimal sperm production, but preferably no more than 5 days so as to avoid including aged sperm.

Findings and their significance are presented in Table 17–5. The most important findings relate to sperm number, sperm motility, sperm morphology, and also whether there is evidence of infection (white blood cells). Male infertility can result from inadequate numbers of sperm, from impaired sperm motility, and also from a large proportion of aberrant sperm forms (e.g., abnormal sperm heads or tails). In addition, a coagulum of fibrin that forms in the ejaculate must liquefy to release the sperm so that it can migrate and fertilize the ovum.

Text continued on page 838

TABLE 17–3. DIAGNOSTIC LABORATORY FINDINGS IN FEMALES

Condition	Secondary Sex Characteristics	Urine 17-KS	Serum LH	Serum FSH	Serum Estradiol	Serum Progesterone	Other
Precocious puberty	Advanced for age	Normal for stage	↑	↑	↑	↑	Bone age advanced
Feminizing tumors	Normal or enhanced	Normal	→	→	↑	→	Leiomyomas, uterine bleeding frequent
Masculinizing tumors	Diminished or virilized	↑	→	→	→	→	
Primary amenorrhea syndromes							
Turner's syndrome	Infantile	→	↑	↑	→	→	(–) sex chromatin, or karyotypic mosaic
Hypopituitarism	Infantile	→	→	→	→	→	→ growth hormone level; (–) response to GnRH

(Continued)

833

TABLE 17–3. DIAGNOSTIC LABORATORY FINDINGS IN FEMALES *(Continued)*

Condition	Secondary Sex Characteristics	Urine 17-KS	Serum LH	Serum FSH	Serum Estradiol	Serum Progesterone	Other
Hypogonado-tropism	Infantile	Normal	↓	↓	↓	↓	Normal growth hormone level: (+) response to GnRH
Adrenogenital syndrome	Masculinized or advanced or ambiguous	↑	↑	↓	↓	↓	Glucocorticoid and mineral-ocorticoid abnormalities
Secondary amenorrhea*							
Polycystic ovary (Stein-Leventhal)	Diminished or slight virilization	↑	↑	Normal or ↓	↓	↓	Plasma and urine testosterone increased Urine estrone increased GnRH → ↑↑LH (+) response to clomiphene
Hyperprolactinemia	Normal or galactorrhea	Normal	Normal or ↓	Normal	↓	↓	Serum prolactin ↑ Bromocriptine suppresses prolactin secretion

Pituitary hypofunction	Normal or diminished	Normal	→	→	→	→	Progesterone withdrawal (+) only with added estrogen (−) response to GnRH
Hypothalamic dysfunction	Normal or diminished	Normal	→	→	→	→	Progesterone withdrawal (+) only with added estrogen (+) response to GnRH
Ovarian failure	Normal or diminished	Normal	←	←	→	→	Progesterone withdrawal (+) only with added estrogen
Dysfunctional bleeding with anovulation	Normal	Normal	→	Normal or →	←	→	(+) progesterone withdrawal No luteal surge of progesterone

*Pregnancy is the most common cause of secondary amenorrhea. Test for human chorionic gonadotropin before pursuing further investigations.

TABLE 17–4. DIAGNOSTIC LABORATORY FINDINGS IN MALES

Condition	Testicular Size	Urine 17-KS	LH	FSH	Testosterone	Other
Precocious puberty	Advanced for age	↑ for age	↑	↑	↑	Advanced bone age
Adrenogenital syndromes	Small	↑	Normal	Normal	Normal	Glucocorticoid or mineralocorticoid abnormalities
CNS dysfunction	Advanced for age	↑ for age	↑	↑	↑	Skull roentgenograms may be abnormal
Testicular tumors	Asymmetric	Normal or ↑	→	→	↑	
Delayed puberty syndromes						
Hypogonadotropism (Kallman's syndrome)	Small or cryptorchid	Normal or →	→	→	→	(+) response to GnRH (−) response to clomiphene Disorders of smell common Eunuchoid skeletal proportions
Hypopituitarism	Small	Normal or →	→	→	→	(−) response to GnRH ↓ growth hormone levels Skeletal proportions not eunuchoid

Infertility syndromes

	Testes					Comments
Klinefelter's syndrome	Small	→	Normal or ↑	↑	Normal or →	(+) sex chromatin Azoospermia
Postviral orchitis	Normal or small	Normal	Normal or ↑	Normal or ↑	Normal	Azoospermia Testicular biopsy diagnostic
Varicocele	↑ or asymmetric	Normal	Normal	Normal	Normal	Semen examination normal or only slightly abnormal
Failure of germinal epithelium	Normal or small ("Fertile eunuch")	Normal	Normal	↑	Normal	Azoospermia Testicular biopsy diagnostic
Testicular failure	Normal or small	→	→	Normal	→	(+) response to GnRH (+) response to hCG
Hypothalamic-pituitary dysfunction	Normal	Slight ↓	→	→	→	GnRH response distinguishes pituitary from hypothalamic problem (+) response to hCG Sperm number declines more than volume of seminal fluid
Testicular dysfunction	Normal or small	Slight ↓	↑	↑	→	(−) response to hCG Sperm number and semen volume both low

TABLE 17–5. EXAMINATION OF SEMINAL FLUID*

Observation	Normal Findings	Interpretation
Volume	2–5 mL	Increased volume is often associated with reduced fertility.
Color	White, grayish, pale yellow	Specimen should not contain blood, pus, or mucus.
Consistency	Viscid, coagulates promptly	Excessive fluidity suggests specimen is not fresh or has abnormal composition.
Liquefaction	Liquefies in 20–60 min	Persistent coagulum may impair motility.
Sperm number*	60–150 million/mL	Below 20 million/mL, fertility is much reduced.
Sperm motility†	60% or more show good movement	Low percent of motile sperm or rapid fall-off in motility is often associated with reduced fertility.
Sperm morphology‡	<30% abnormal forms	RBCs, WBCs are also abnormal findings.
Fructose	Present	Seminal vesicles produce fructose; if sperm are absent, presence of fructose documents patency of ejaculatory ducts.
pH	7–7.7	Increased acidity suggests excessive admixture with prostatic fluid.

Adapted from Davajan, V, and Israel, R: Infertility: Causes, evaluation, and treatment. In DeGroot, LJ, et al (eds): Endocrinology. Grune & Stratton, New York, 1979, pp 1459–1472.

*Well-mixed, liquefied specimen is diluted and immobilized sperm counted in hemocytometer. Several counts on each specimen should be averaged. A single individual may have great variation over time; in doubtful cases, at least 3 different specimens should be examined.

†Estimated by examining a drop of well-mixed, undiluted, liquefied specimen.

‡Estimated by examining fixed, stained preparation.

PATIENT-CARE CONSIDERATIONS

Specimen Artifacts

Immunoassays for gonadotropins and for the steroid sex hormones do not have many artifactual interferences because of the high degree of specificity from the reagent antibodies (frequently monoclonal). Steroid hormone levels are stable, so the blood or urine samples require no special precautions. Spectrophotometric analysis of urine metabolites is more subject to artifact, as discussed in the section on 17-ketosteroids (Chapter 16) because various chromogens can interfere with a detection step based simply on absorption of light at a particular wavelength. For example, the laxative agents senna and phenolphthalein may color the urine and interfere with urine estrogen measurement.

Psychological Issues

Evaluating endocrine and sexual function is enormously stressful for most people, both men and women. Sexual function is markedly affected by exogenous stress, anxiety, depression, and most other psychic disturbances; the events that may be causing or triggering the problem are then made worse by the process of evaluation. A supportive, nonjudgmental, sympathetic attitude is essential in helping the patient through this experience.

Pathophysiological Relationships

Many physiological and pharmacological events affect hormones of the hypothalamic-pituitary-gonadal axis. Hypoglycemia can induce increased prolactin secretion; hypothyroidism, by stimulating thyrotropin-releasing hormone, is a potent stimulus to hyperprolactinemia (see below). Alcoholism and severe liver disease of any type raise functional estrogen levels in men; these conditions also cause low testosterone levels. In anorexia nervosa, low gonadotropin levels depress sexual appearance and function; these are among the first abnormalities noted, but other pituitary hormones often decline as the condition progresses. Depressed steroidogenesis is one of the many physiologic derangements caused by uremia. Some of the conditions that affect sexual functioning are shown in Table 17–6.

EVALUATION OF INFERTILITY

Infertility occurs in approximately one out of every five couples who attempt to conceive a child. The clinical evaluation of this disorder attempts to determine whether both the man and woman are capable of gametogenesis, transporting the gametes (sperm in men, ovum in women) to sites of fertilization, and implantation of the fertilized egg into the endometrium. Evaluation of the man consists primarily of semen analysis for sperm count, motility, and morphology, along with ejaculate volume and liquefaction. Qualitative aspects of sperm function can be

TABLE 17–6. ARTIFACTS AFFECTING SEXUAL FUNCTION

Effect	Drugs	Other
Increased prolactin secretion	Reserpine	Exercise
	α-Methyldopa	Stress
	Phenothiazines	Sleep
	Haloperidol	Pregnancy
	Metoclopramide	Thyroid-stimulating hormone
	Estrogens	Hypoglycemia
		Liver disease
Decreased gonadotropins		Anorexia nervosa
		Depression
		Renal disease
Gynecomastia	Spironolactone	Liver disease
	Cimetidine	
Male impotence	Ganglionic blockers	Stress
	Narcotics	Depression
	Tricyclic antidepressants	
	Clonidine	

assessed by egg penetration tests using oocytes from mammalian sources such as hamsters. This test examines the ability of a male's sperm to penetrate the egg as an indicator of how efficient that sperm would be in fertilizing a human egg.

Sperm can be immobilized and made nonfunctional by antibodies directed against sperm head, body, or tail. Their presence in a woman may cause infertility. Sperm antibodies may be detected in the serum or the cervical mucus of the woman. Although abnormalities of semen analysis may explain infertility, they do not necessarily exclude the possibility of fertility unless no sperm are present.

Laboratory evaluation of the woman is directed toward determining both the existence and timing of ovulation. This occurrence is identified by the surge in LH that occurs in serum and in urine at the time of or just prior to ovulation (see Fig. 17–1). Rapid test kits are now available over-the-counter for self-testing of urine by women in their own homes to pinpoint the day of ovulation. This knowledge then allows for synchronization of sexual intercourse to optimize the chance for fertilization to occur. If no ovulation occurs, it can sometimes be induced by biochemical manipulation of the pituitary to release larger than normal amounts of FSH and LH. This effect can be achieved by administration of synthetic estrogens (e.g., clomiphene) that interfere with the normal feedback inhibition to the pituitary, or by administration of synthetic gonadotropin-releasing hormone that directly stimulates the pituitary.

Much infertility in women who are ovulating is due to scarring of the fallopian tubes (as from previous pelvic infection) and cannot be detected by laboratory means. These tubes are not capable of transporting the fertilized ovum to a site for implantation. This condition can be better evaluated by laparoscopy and sometimes can be reversed surgically.

Anovulatory females may be further examined for chromosomal abnormalities as well as general medical and endocrine disorders that can preclude normal functioning of the pituitary and ovaries. In particular, galactorrhea may indicate a prolactin-producing adenoma of the pituitary that interferes with normal feedback mechanisms.

Some infertility does remain unexplained even after complete physical and laboratory examination of both partners in a couple. If gametogenesis does occur in those individuals, they may achieve childbirth by in vitro fertilization using their own gametes followed by embryo transfer into the woman's uterus for implantation and completion of pregnancy. If only one member of the couple is capable of gametogenesis, they may resort to use of banked sperm or oocytes from other donors.

PREGNANCY AND LACTATION

PHYSIOLOGY

Fertilization occurs within several days of ovulation at the midpoint of the menstrual cycle. The fertilized ovum floats down the fallopian tube into the uterus, where it implants on the prepared secretory endometrium. Shortly after implantation, on the 21st to 23rd day of the cycle, chorionic gonadotropin production begins. Because hCG is a glycoprotein hormone that is unique to the developing placenta (and some tumors), pregnancy tests are based on the detection of hCG in serum or urine. Its small size permits it to pass directly into the urine from the circulation.

DIAGNOSIS OF PREGNANCY

General Principles

Before immunoassays became available in the 1960s, tests for pregnancy employed bioassays using animals (rabbits, rats, and frogs). Immunoassays for hCG are still standardized in terms of equivalent bioactivity as IU/L or mIU/mL. The hCG molecule is dimeric, consisting of one alpha subunit that cross-reacts with the alpha subunits of the pituitary protein hormones (e.g., TSH, LH, FSH, ACTH) and also of one beta subunit that is unique to hCG and confers antigenic individuality. The beta subunit of hCG does have considerable homology with the beta subunit structures of TSH, LH, and FSH, which leads to the requirement for exacting antibody reactivities for assay purposes. However, hCG does have a unique region of 30 amino acids at its carboxyl terminus that confers immunologic identity.

In the first two decades of immunoassays, only polyclonal antisera were available for standard use. This practice made it necessary to immunize animals with highly purified beta subunits in order to avoid contaminating antibodies directed against alpha subunits. For that reason, the assay became associated with assessment of beta-hCG, although in fact the molecule being measured was assumed to have both alpha and beta subunits. Pregnancy screens were available as the rapid slide test and the more lengthy tube test, both of which employed polyclonal antibodies. There was substantial interference from LH in particular. For more sensitive and specific results, there has also been available a radioimmunoassay for beta-hCG with detection limits down to around 5 mIU/mL.

In the last decade, the development of monoclonal antibodies as diagnostic reagents (particularly for hCG) has been rapid. Many of these monoclonal-based assays use two different antibodies, one against the alpha subunit and one against the beta subunit, in a sandwich that captures the whole hCG molecule on a solid phase. Detection or quantitation of hCG is then generally accomplished by a color indicator reaction mediated by an enzyme (e.g., alkaline phosphatase) linked to the second antibody. Quick automated analyzers using these reagents are now capable of accurate and reliable quantitation of hCG down to the range of 2 to 5 mIU/mL within an assay time of several minutes.

Manufacturers may use differing international standards to calibrate the secondary standards supplied in kits for performance of these hCG assays. Most assays for hCG are now calibrated against the Third International Standard but the Second International Standard, which was widely used in the past, may be the calibrator for some assays still in use. Unfortunately because these two sets of international standards differ, measured values of hCG should not be interchanged between laboratories using assays calibrated against different international standards. The Third International Standard is roughly twice the Second. The laboratory performing the test will provide the reference range appropriate for that assay.

Interpretation

Early in pregnancy, concentrations of hCG in maternal serum rise quickly, with a doubling time of roughly 2 days during the first few weeks as the trophoblastic tissues increase in size. Values of 25 to 50 mIU/mL are encountered 1 week after conception. Within 10 to 12 weeks, hCG values will peak at 150,000 to 200,000 mIU/mL and then gradually fall to normal plateau values of 10,000 to 50,000 mIU/mL in the second and third trimesters (Fig. 17–2). A later-term pregnancy in which there is a sudden drop in hCG from the plateau may indicate threatened abortion.

If the measured value in urine is negative, but clinical examination indicates possible pregnancy, the test should be repeated in 2 days. Urine pregnancy tests may be negative even though serum tested at the same time is positive because the serum assay is more sensitive, being optimized for the protein matrix found in serum. Furthermore, the hCG in urine of a newly pregnant woman may be diluted to nondetectable levels by high urine flow; a negative hCG result in urine should be followed by measurement of specific gravity to determine whether the urine was sufficiently concentrated.

There is very little or no need to quantitate hCG for diagnosing most pregnancies, and consequently qualitative screening tests for hCG are now widely available over the counter for home use. These tests should be reserved for screening purpose because any woman obtaining a positive result ought to seek prenatal care; in addition, a woman with a negative self-test but continuing symptoms of pregnancy also ought to

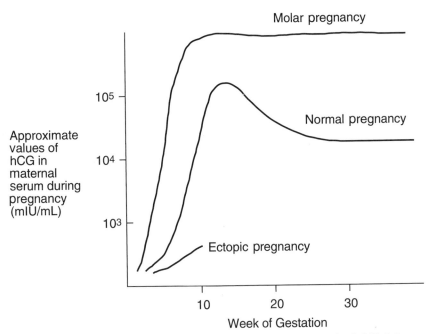

FIGURE 17–2. Serum values of human chorionic gonadotropin (hCG) follow a predictable early rise in normal pregnancy, peaking at 10 to 12 weeks, followed by a lower plateau. Ectopic pregnancies have much lower hCG values and do not go to term. Molar pregnancies and other trophoblastic malignancies can have very high values of hCG, considerably beyond those encountered in normal pregnancy.

seek medical advice. Former assays based on polyclonal antibodies or those that otherwise have high cross-reactivity with LH and FSH may yield false-positive results for hCG in women past the menopause.

Concentrations of hCG are typically lower in ectopic pregnancy than in intrauterine pregnancy of the same gestational age (see Fig. 17–2). In one series of suspected ectopic pregnancies, hCG levels were less than 4000 mIU/mL in 85% of true ectopic cases but in only 13% of viable intrauterine pregnancies. Frequently the hCG will be quite low in ectopic pregnancy, in the range of 10 to 100 mIU/mL; hCG may also be nondetectable in ectopic pregnancies that experience necrosis of chorionic tissue. Further clinical evaluation for ectopic pregnancy entails abdominal or transvaginal ultrasound examination to locate and size the embryo. This information is also useful to establish the volume of the secreting tissue and expected level of hCG for that gestational age versus the amount actually measured. Once an ectopic pregnancy is terminated by medical or surgical means, the half-life of the remaining hCG is 3 to 7 days. Recently it has been found that additional assessment for ectopic pregnancy is available through quantitation of serum progesterone: high values indicate viability, lower values suggest risk.

Human chorionic gonadotropin is produced by tumors of trophoblastic origin (choriocarcinoma) as well as by some seminomas, embryonal carcinomas, and nonendocrine carcinomas such as hepatoblastomas and bronchogenic carcinomas. Because a number of molecular alterations can occur, assays for hCG exhibit variations in reactivity for patients with these tumors. In addition to the complete hCG molecule with alpha and beta subunits, the beta subunit may be elaborated without the alpha subunit. This beta subunit may escape detection by immunoassays that employ a sandwich technique with separate antialpha and antibeta antibodies. More recent immunoassays utilize antibodies that recognize separate antigenic sites on the beta subunit; these assays can detect both intact hCG and the beta subunit alone. Other molecular variants include two nicked forms that may lack a portion of the C-terminal segment of the beta subunit; additional variants arise because of alterations in the amount of glycosylation at six sites on the beta subunit and at two sites on the alpha subunit. Every assay for hCG shows somewhat different reactivities for the different molecular species of hCG, each of which may vary among different patients. Accordingly, serial measurements of hCG for monitoring malignancy should be done with the same assay method.

PLACENTAL HORMONES

Besides chorionic gonadotropin, the placenta secretes estrogens, progesterone, and human placental lactogen (hPL). All of these can be measured in the maternal blood stream or urine. Pregnancy-related hormones are measured as a means to assess fetal well-being and to evaluate the effects of therapy intended to improve fetal development.

Relationships to Pregnancy

Each of these hormones follows its own quantitative curve at various stages of pregnancy. Total estrogen excretion increases progressively throughout pregnancy, rising most sharply after the 30th week. Pregnanediol, the excretory product of progesterone, rises steadily until 30 to 34 weeks, and then remains level or falls slightly. Human placental lactogen rises steadily throughout much of pregnancy, maintaining a high plateau during the last trimester. The range of normal values is wide for all the hormones, and, even for a single individual, pronounced variation occurs from day to day.

Because we do not have an accurate description of how these hormones or their metabolites influence fetal development, or which aspects of fetoplacental function they represent, it is difficult to know which tests are useful for prenatal medical care. It is still more difficult to interpret a single result obtained by testing an apparently normal pregnant woman who suddenly develops bleeding, fever, toxemia, or other worrisome signs. Given the range of normal variation, it is almost essential that each woman serve as her own control. In following a high-risk pregnancy, sequential values should be obtained to construct a curve for that individual pregnancy; marked departure from that established norm indicates a change in fetal or placental development. When a previously normal woman unexpectedly has clinical problems, it may be necessary to extrapolate from only a few results as the best guide to interpretation.

Estriol

Maternal **estriol** derives partly from the placenta and partly from the fetal adrenal glands. Estriol levels in maternal urine are also influenced by the woman's excretory function and urine volume. Urinary estriol correlates fairly well with fetal growth rate; pregnancies with an anencephalic fetus have consistently low levels because pituitary aplasia causes fetal adrenal gland hypofunction. When serial estriol levels are available, a sharp downward trend on a day-to-day basis indicates probable fetal difficulty. This can be defined as a drop of 30 to 40% below previous levels, observed on 2 consecutive days, or a fall of 35% or more, on a single day, from the average of the preceding 3 days' values. Frequent sampling is especially useful in women with hypertension or impending toxemia. Diabetic women often show such wide swings in value that a valid downward trend is hard to document until it is too late to help the fetus; nevertheless, these women should be followed to provide as early an indication of fetal distress as possible. A sharp rise in free (unconjugated) estriol occurs normally when delivery is imminent.

Progesterone

Pregnanediol is the most easily measured metabolite of progesterone, but there is only modest correlation between pregnanediol levels in urine and circulating plasma progesterone. In pregnancy, progesterone derives entirely from the placenta, with no fetal contribution. Urinary pregnanediol levels drop with severe placental dysfunction, but this occurs too late to allow detection or correction of impending problems. Although urinary pregnanediol levels may remain unchanged despite severe fetal distress, serum progesterone levels can be used to evaluate placental integrity.

Human Placental Lactogen

Although produced by the placenta, **human placental lactogen** exerts its entire known effects on the mother. Like growth hormone, it causes relative insulin resistance and an increased level of circulating free fatty acids. Plasma and urine hPL levels reflect placental size and tend to be high in diabetic mothers. Despite good statistical correlation between hPL levels and placental weight, urinary hPL levels have little predictive values for any individual pregnancy. Plasma hPL levels below 4 μg/mL frequently indicate retarded growth, especially if total estrogen also is low. Levels of hPL fall in toxemia, and declining values sometimes can help in distinguishing incomplete abortion from threatened abortion.

PROLACTIN

Prolactin is a peptide hormone secreted by the anterior pituitary (see Chapter 16). Its role in disorders of sexual function is becoming increasingly apparent. The only known physiologic role of prolactin is to induce milk production in a female breast already stimulated by high estrogen levels; once milk production is established, lactation can continue without supranormal prolactin levels. Prolactin levels rise late in pregnancy, peak with the initiation of lactation, and surge each time a lactating woman suckles. In nonpregnant women, hyperprolactinemia often, but not inevitably, causes inappropriate milk secretion **(galactorrhea)**.

Pathophysiological Relationships

The unstimulated pituitary secretes prolactin at a high, continuous rate. Circulating levels are controlled by inhibition of output, produced by a hypothalamic mediator. The hypothalamic inhibitor is thought to be the CNS transmitter **dopamine;** any agent that antagonizes or depletes dopamine causes prolactin levels to rise. Thyroid-stimulating hormone enhances prolactin release; primary hypothyroidism often causes hyperprolactinemia by provoking TSH hypersecretion. Pituitary adenomas cause enormously elevated prolactin values, and ectopic prolactin may be produced by lung or kidney tumors.

Significant Alterations

Normal men and prepubertal children have prolactin levels that are measurable but lower than those of women. Stress, exercise, and sleep increase prolactin circulation in both men and women, suggesting some still-undefined physiologic role exclusive of lactation. Excessive circulating prolactin disturbs gonadal function in both men and women; women experience amenorrhea and anovulation, whereas in men there is impotence sometimes accompanied by gynecomastia. Although testosterone production may sometimes be suppressed, hyperprolactinemia causes male impotence even at normal testosterone levels.

A wide range of drugs affect dopamine activity and CNS neurotransmission. The first part of Table 17–6 lists prominent ones. High or changing estrogen levels stimulate prolactinemia, an interaction that may explain some of the reproductive dysfunctions observed with oral contraceptives, liver disease, and chronic alcoholism.

NORMAL PHYSIOLOGICAL CHANGES IN PREGNANCY

Pregnancy causes plasma volume in the circulation to increase substantially, plateauing at about 34 weeks. Complex changes in hormonal relationships and sodium regulation produce this volume expansion, which in turn demands increased cardiac and renal workload and leads to dilution of many blood constituents. Measurements made on whole blood, plasma, or serum must be interpreted with this volume increase in mind.

Hematologic System

Red Blood Cells

Red cell production increases during pregnancy but not as much as does plasma volume. If iron stores are adequate, red cell mass increases by 400 to 500 mL, but hemoglobin concentration and hematocrit decline. Hemoglobin concentration below 11 g/dL should be considered abnormally low, even when hemodilution is greatest. Reticulocyte counts rise, especially in the middle trimester; reticulocyte counts of 2 to 5% may result from pregnancy alone without indicating additional hematopoietic stress.

Anemia occurs very commonly during pregnancy, with iron deficiency the most common cause. Red cells are small, hypochromic, and irregularly shaped; serum iron levels are low, with low transferrin saturation; and bone marrow iron is absent.

Megaloblastic anemia also is common. The fetus drains off substantial amounts of folic acid and modest amounts of vitamin B_{12}. In addition, the mother's tissues absorb more folate and vitamin B_{12} than usual, and there is increased excretion of the dialyzable or free fraction of folic acid. Serum folate levels decline in all pregnancies, but red cell folate levels remain unchanged unless deficiency exists. Both serum and red cell levels of vitamin B_{12} decline in normal pregnancies, a phenomenon also seen in women taking oral contraceptives.

White Blood Cells

In the last half of pregnancy, granulocyte levels rise, but lymphocyte levels remain unchanged, resulting in increases in total white count to as much as 15,000/μL with a relative granulocytosis. Up to 25% of pregnant women have occasional metamyelocytes or myelocytes in the peripheral blood. The hematologic picture often resembles that seen in infection or other tissue stress. There is an increase in the number of neutrophils, giving a positive nitroblue tetrazolium test result; leukocyte alkaline phosphatase values rise, and Dohle bodies are seen not infrequently. These findings must be interpreted with caution. Although it is undesirable to initiate an intensive, expensive search for infection too quickly, it is even worse to overlook acute infection on the grounds that the laboratory findings represent physiologic variation. History, physical findings, and the results of sputum and urine examination should clarify doubtful cases.

The Coagulation System

Fibrinogen levels rise throughout pregnancy, reaching levels of 400 to 600 mg/dL in the third trimester. Plasminogen levels also increase, but total fibrinolytic activity declines. Venous thrombosis occurs more often in pregnant than in nonpregnant women of comparable age and health. This increase in fibrinogen and decrease in relative fibrinolytic activity are laboratory findings that may have no relation to actual incidence of thrombosis during pregnancy. Assayed activities of all the coagulation factors except factors XI and XIII increase somewhat; prothrombin time and partial thromboplastin time may shorten slightly. Mild von Willebrand's disease may show clinical improvement during pregnancy due to increased levels of that factor, which returns to lower prepregnancy levels after delivery.

Serum Proteins

Many proteins increase during pregnancy. The increase is especially striking for thyroxine- and cortisol-binding proteins, so total circulating hormone levels increase significantly during pregnancy. These changes, of course, reflect only bound, inactive hormone levels; the free hormone concentrations are expected to remain normal.

Serum concentrations also rise during pregnancy for beta-lipoproteins, transferrin, ceruloplasmin, alpha-1-antitrypsin, several complement components, and a pregnancy-associated protein that migrates as an alpha-2-macroglobulin. The elevation of **ceruloplasmin** (a copper transport protein) frequently confers a green tint to plasma or serum (the combination of normal yellow chromogens in serum plus blue from copper). A twofold rise in fibrinogen levels causes the erythrocyte sedimentation rate to increase. Levels of IgG and IgA decline, but IgM concentrations remain unchanged. Serum albumin concentration falls by as much as 0.5 to 0.8 g/dL. Hemodilution causes part of this drop, as does a slight reduction in synthesis despite acceleration of albumin degradation.

The Endocrine System

Thyroid Gland

Plasma concentration of thyroxine-binding globulin (TBG) increases markedly with pregnancy. The rise begins shortly after fertilization and continues until it reaches an elevated plateau at 12 weeks. Failure to initiate this rise after fertilization suggests hypothyroidism or estrogen deficiency, conditions that severely reduce the likelihood of successful pregnancy. Plasma thyroxine levels rise along with the TBG, but TBG increases more than the hormone does. This means that the level of TBG saturation declines. In vitro tests of T_3 uptake and free thyroxine index fall into the nonpregnant hypothyroid range during normal pregnancy (see Fig. 16–10). The increase in circulating thyroxine affects only the bound fraction; the active, free fraction does not increase. Values for total thyroxine fall into the hyperthyroid range during normal pregnancy; levels of TSH remain normal in euthyroid pregnant women.

Many pregnancy-associated changes in thyroid tests parallel those seen when nonpregnant women take estrogens (e.g., oral contraceptives). Both conditions simulate, in some respects, the laboratory findings of hyperthyroidism, but significant differences exist (Table 17–7). Pregnant women can become hyperthyroid, and hyperthyroid women can become pregnant. If a pregnant woman has thyroxine levels above 12 µg/dL or T_3 uptake in the euthyroid range, the free thyroxine index is likely to be elevated because of true hyperthyroidism. To avoid diagnostic confusion in thyroid testing during pregnancy, screening for thyroid disease should

TABLE 17–7. THYROID FUNCTION TESTS IN PREGNANCY AND ESTROGEN ADMINISTRATION COMPARED WITH HYPERTHYROIDISM

Test	Pregnancy/Estrogen Administration	Hyperthyroidism
Total T_4	Increased	Increased
Thyroxine-binding globulin	Increased	Normal
T uptake	Increased (due to elevated TBG)	Increased (due to increased T_4)
Free T_4	Normal	Increased
Total T_3	Increased	Increased
Free T_3	Normal	Increased
TSH	Normal	Suppressed in primary; increased in secondary or tertiary hyperthyroidism

be done with a highly sensitive TSH assay that remains unaffected by pregnancy (see Chapter 16).

Adrenal Glands

Both cortisol and cortisol-binding protein increase with pregnancy, but the relation between bound and free hormone is less clear-cut than with bound and free thyroid hormone. Cortisol values remain elevated throughout the day, and there is flattening of the usual diurnal curve. Women taking oral contraceptives have an elevated morning peak for free cortisol but do not have elevated round-the-clock levels. The rate of cortisol production actually declines slightly, but the plasma half-life is increased during pregnancy, and there is exaggerated response to ACTH stimulation. It may be difficult to diagnose adrenal hyperfunction during pregnancy, but suppression of steroid secretion following dexamethasone administration persists in normal pregnancy. Cortisol levels in the "normal" range and failure of ACTH response indicate diminished adrenal function during pregnancy.

Aldosterone, the sodium-conserving, potassium-depleting hormone of the outermost part of the adrenal cortex, is increased throughout pregnancy. Pregnancy produces a cumulative total sodium retention of about 500 to 900 mEq, but plasma volume increases beyond this level, and there is a decline in effective osmolality because of sodium retention. Because the increases in plasma volume, cardiac output, and glomerular filtration rate combine to impose a huge sodium load on the pregnant woman's kidney, it is essential to rely on the aldosterone mechanism to retain sufficient sodium. During pregnancy, the flexibility of aldosterone production declines. Urinary sodium loss rises if excessive sodium is present, but when sodium deprivation occurs, inappropriate sodium loss occurs before sodium retention readjusts. The increased aldosterone activity does not generally cause potassium wastage.

Hormones Affecting Carbohydrate Metabolism

During pregnancy, insulin production increases, but the need for insulin increases simultaneously. The combined effects of increased cortisol, increased estrogen, increased progesterone, and circulating placental lactogen reduce the entry of glucose into cells and increase the circulation of free fatty acids. In normal pregnancies, compensatory insulin production counteracts these tendencies, and fasting blood glucose levels remain in the normal range or even drop slightly. Glucose absorption diminishes somewhat; oral glucose tolerance curves are essentially normal, but there is slight progressive increase in the time required for serum glucose levels to peak.

The metabolic stress of pregnancy may push the pancreas beyond its ability to respond, unmasking a latent diabetic state. This disorder of gestational diabetes is due to insufficient insulin secretion that occurs only during pregnancy and reverts to normal when pregnancy terminates. Many women with gestational diabetes have abnormal glucose tolerance curves between pregnancies but do not have glycosuria or fasting hyperglycemia unless some other stress supervenes. Such women can eventually become overtly diabetic after many years (see Chapter 16).

Glycosuria during pregnancy does not necessarily indicate gestational diabetes. Pregnancy imposes such a glucose load on the tubular reabsorptive capacity that glycosuria is a common event and need not, on a single random specimen, set off a major search for diabetes. More significant is consistent glycosuria or glycosuria in older women, in obese women, in women with a family history of diabetes, or in those with a history of bearing deformed babies or babies weighing over 9.5 pounds.

Monitoring of glucose during pregnancy traditionally has been done with dipsticks on timed urine specimens at home and with blood glucose measurements at the physician's office. Modern methods include the use of personal glucose meters for self-monitoring of blood glucose on fingerstick blood samples and glycosylated hemoglobin (which is less useful for pregnancy in which metabolic state is changing on a week-by-week basis).

Renal Function

Both absolute blood volume and the relative renal blood flow increase in pregnancy. The glomerular filtration rate increases by as much as 50%, and response to altered posture or to sodium load becomes exaggerated. Because of increased filtration, increased amounts of electrolytes, proteins, vitamins, and nitrogenous products pass through the tubules.

Urinary loss of sodium, calcium, protein, and urea increases, causing a small but consistent drop in serum levels of these constituents. In a woman in the last half of pregnancy, serum calcium or urea in the "high-normal" range should be considered abnormal.

Throughout pregnancy, the calyces, renal pelves, and ureters are widened and slack. Urine flow slows, and complete emptying becomes more difficult. These factors contribute to the increased susceptibility to urinary tract infections during pregnancy.

Liver Function

The most conspicuous pregnancy-associated change in standard "liver function tests" is a twofold to fourfold rise in serum alkaline phosphatase. The placenta manufactures a specific alkaline phosphatase isoenzyme that is not expressed in other normal tissues of the body (see Chapter 11). The hepatobiliary forms of alkaline phosphatase do not increase, and circulating aminotransferase levels do not change in normal pregnancy.

The liver is largely responsible for the increased production of proteins during pregnancy. The binding proteins are most conspicuous in this regard. Cortisol- and thyroxine-binding proteins increase significantly; testosterone-binding protein, ceruloplasmin, and transferrin also increase. Fibrinogen rises to double the prepregnancy levels. However, albumin manufacture does not seem to increase. Because albumin degradation increases and plasma volume expands, failure to increase synthesis causes circulatory levels to drop by as much as 0.5 to 0.8 g/dL or more.

Creatine Kinase

Following contractions of the uterus during normal vaginal delivery of the fetus, there is release of **creatine kinase (CK)** from the myometrium into the maternal circulation. Because CK from the myometrium is almost entirely comprised of the BB isoenzyme form, the maternal serum will show normal CK-MM plus a band of CK-BB in varying amounts in the first several hours after delivery. This finding is expected and should not be confused with other organ damage such as acute brain injury without clinical evidence of such disorder. It is also important to recognize that some methods for CK-MB give falsely positive results with CK-BB, so that in the situation of suspected postpartum myocardial infarction, interpretation of CK isoenzyme testing should be done with appropriate consultation from laboratory staff.

Summary of Pregnancy-Associated Changes

Table 17–8 lists the alterations in laboratory values that most commonly occur in normal pregnancies.

TABLE 17–8. ALTERED LABORATORY RESULTS IN NORMAL PREGNANCY

Test	Alteration	Demonstrated or Possible Reason
Hematology		
Hemoglobin	Falls but not lower than 11 g/dL	Plasma volume expands more than RBC mass
WBC	Mild neutrophilia; no lymphocytosis	Similar response seen with stress, strenuous exercise
Platelets	Slight decrease or no change	Plasma volume expansion
Reticulocytes	Rise to 2–5%	RBC mass increases
Blood volume	Rises by 40–50%	Increase in plasma and red cells
Serum iron	Falls modestly, even if stores are adequate	Loss to fetal blood supply Increased plasma volume Supplementation is desirable
Iron-binding capacity	Increases	Estrogen-induced increase in protein synthesis
Folate levels	Serum concentration falls; RBC concentration should be constant	Fetal use; estrogen-associated folate block Supplementation is desirable
Erythrocyte sedimentation rate	Increases markedly	Elevated fibrinogen levels
Coagulation		
Fibrinogen	Rises about 50%	? Acute phase reaction
PT and PTT	Normal or slightly shortened	Increased factor levels affect tests relatively little
Plasminogen	Increases	?
Antithrombin III	Decreases moderately	Comparable effect seen with estrogen therapy
Fibrin split products	Increased slightly	? Effect of increased plasminogen and decreased antithrombin III ? Effect of fibrin deposition in placenta
Chemistry		
Serum albumin	Decreases by as much as 1 g/dL	Increased degradation; hemodilution
Immunoglobulins	IgG, IgA drop	? Increased degradation ? Altered immunologic responsiveness
Serum alkaline phosphatase	Increases by 200–300%	Placental alkaline phosphatase in serum
Serum cholesterol	Increases 30–40%	? Effects of placental hormones
Serum free fatty acids	Increases 50–60%	? Effects of placental hormones, altered insulin reactivity

(Continued)

TABLE 17–8. ALTERED LABORATORY RESULTS IN NORMAL PREGNANCY *(Continued)*

Test	Alteration	Demonstrated or Possible Reason
Serum creatinine	Decreases	Hemodilution; increased glomerular filtration
Plasma bicarbonate	Decreases by 10–15%	Compensation for chronic hyperventilation
Urine glucose	Mild glycosuria with normal blood sugar levels	Lowered renal threshold
Renal function	GFR increases; concentrating capacity decreases	Mobilization of retained fluid
Endocrine		
Thyroid tests	T_4 increased	Estrogen-associated rise in binding protein
ACTH	Markedly decreased in early months	Unknown
Serum total cortisol	Increased	Estrogen-associated rise in binding protein
Serum testosterone	Increased	? Increased ovarian synthesis
Parathormone	Increased	Unknown; ionized calcium levels normal
Aldosterone	Progressive increase	Altered plasma volume, renal sodium load
Renin-angiotensin	Increased in latter half	With ↑ Na or ↑ blood pressure, level decreases

PRENATAL ASSESSMENT OF THE FETUS

Amniocentesis and Percutaneous Umbilical Blood Sampling

Amniocentesis permits specific laboratory analysis of many critical variables for pregnancy and delivery by direct examination of the amniotic fluid surrounding the fetus. With aseptic technique and ultrasonic scanning to locate the placenta and to guide the insertion of the needle, the risk to mother and fetus is minimal. Hemorrhage that threatens fetal well-being occurs rarely, but there is significant risk that fetal cells will enter the mother's circulation and possibly immunize her to fetal red cell antigens. Women with Rh-negative blood who undergo amniocentesis should receive Rh immune globulin after each procedure (see Chapter 8).

In early and mid pregnancy, amniocentesis is done to detect congenital disorders that would impose excessive suffering on the infant and family. These procedures must be done early enough that, if the findings are positive and the family wishes to terminate the pregnancy, abortion can safely be undertaken. Alternatively, foreknowledge of the congenital abnormality can be useful in guiding family counseling and even appropriate early medical or surgical care if abortion is not elected. Later in pregnancy, amniocentesis is done to monitor fetal health, so that intrauterine intervention can be undertaken (if possible and indicated) or a rational decision can be made about premature delivery. Some of the common indications for amniocentesis are shown in Table 17–9.

In addition to amniocentesis, which provides information on fetal status by diffusion out of the circulation, direct sampling of fetal blood is now done in many modern centers by **percutaneous umbilical blood sampling (PUBS)** (see Appendix C). However, the procedure can only be performed after 20 weeks of gestation. Using continuous sonographic monitoring, the needle is inserted into the umbilicus near its junction with the placenta. This procedure is applicable to collecting samples for direct measurement of such determinants as bilirubin (for hemolytic disease) and specific antibody titers to infectious agents (e.g., to establish intrauterine infection). (See also Appendix C and Table C–1.)

Chorionic Villus Sampling

Chorionic villus sampling (CVS) is a method employed in the first trimester of gestation for the diagnosis of genetic defects in the fetus. It

---

TABLE 17–9. INDICATIONS FOR AMNIOCENTESIS

Early (14–16 weeks)
Culture fetal cells for chromosome anomalies

Early and mid pregnancy
Bile pigment level in amniotic fluid, for hemolytic disease
Alpha-fetoprotein level in amniotic fluid, for neural tube defects
Examine fetal cells for genetically determined abnormalities:
Tay-Sachs disease
Other biochemical defects
Hemoglobinopathy
Thalassemia

Late 2nd, 3rd trimester
Lecithin/sphingomyelin ratio, for pulmonary maturity
Creatinine level in amniotic fluid, for renal maturity
Bile pigment level in amniotic fluid, for hemolytic disease

consists of intrauterine biopsy of placental tissue (fetal origin) by suctioning through thin plastic tubing. Results from CVS may be erroneous due to contamination with maternal cells. When it was first introduced as a clinical procedure, there was substantial concern about the risk of inducing spontaneous abortions of normal fetuses from application of CVS. After several years of practice, it now appears that CVS carries about a 1 to 2% increased risk of abortion compared to a 0.5% risk from amniocentesis; CVS may also be associated with fetal limb abnormalities. On the other hand, the advantage of CVS over amniocentesis for diagnosis of fetal genetic abnormality is that CVS can be performed much earlier in the pregnancy. Accordingly, decisions to terminate pregnancy in cases of abnormalities can be made much earlier in the pregnancy when that procedure is safer for the mother. The primary indication for diagnostic amniocentesis or CVS is advanced maternal age.

Karyotyping for Chromosomal Abnormalities

The fetal cells from a successful amniocentesis or CVS specimen can be cultured for chromosomal analysis. **Karyotyping** involves separation and analysis of individual chromosomes photographed during the metaphase of mitosis. Fine resolution of chromosomal abnormalities is done with digitized image analysis on computers. Each of the 22 pairs of autosomes, the X chromosome, and the Y chromosome can be identified and examined. Karyotyping, augmented by staining or banding techniques, allows not only enumeration of chromosome number but also detection of morphologic changes like translocation from one chromosome to another, deletion, inversion, and rings.

Culturing the cells and preparing the karyotype takes 4 to 6 weeks. Potential problems include culturing contaminant cells of maternal origin, failure to culture the cells successfully due to improper or inadequate specimen collection and processing, artifacts or in vitro problems causing ambiguous results, and interpretational difficulties arising from genetic mosaicism. It is customary to perform replicate analyses to increase the likelihood of achieving diagnostic results. Because this procedure is highly specialized and requires a great deal of expertise to perform and interpret, most hospital laboratories will send specimen requests to a regional reference laboratory that routinely handles many karyotyping analyses.

The method itself consists of growing cells (e.g., amniotic fibroblasts or peripheral blood cells) on coverslips in tissue medium and then exposing them to colchicine to hold cell divisions in metaphase when the chromosomes are condensed into recognizable forms. Approximately 10 to 20 metaphases are photographed, and the actual diagnostic karyotype is read from at least three representative metaphases. High-resolution banding is now frequently employed to map particular abnormalities more precisely. Usual reagents for this technique include **giemsa** (for **G-banding**) and **quinicrine** (for **Q-banding**). Centromeric banding is also employed.

Modern methods of karyotyping also include fluorescent-labeled DNA probes that are specific for regions of individual chromosomes; this technique is termed **fluorescent in situ hybridization (FISH).** The resulting microscopic image shows dots of fluorescence where the DNA probe binds. In FISH using probes for the centromere of a specific chromosome, it is possible to determine how many copies of that chromosome are present in a cell, in interphase cells as well as metaphase cells. Using probes for regions of different chromosomes labeled with different colored dyes, it is possible to demonstrate translocation between chromosomes when the different colors lie adjacent to one another instead of being dispersed through the nucleus.

Disorders of Number or Form

Chromosomal aberrations occur frequently. Of fetuses spontaneously aborted in the first trimester, 50 to 60% have abnormal chromosomal complement. In stillborn infants, the incidence is 5%, and 1 in 200 liveborn infants has some chromosomal abnormality. Trisomy of chromosome 21 and abnormal numbers of X chromosomes are by far the most common events (Table 17–10).

TABLE 17–10. CHROMOSOMAL ABNORMALITIES

	Karyotype*	Clinical Findings
Klinefelter's syndrome	XXY (47)	Female appearance, mental retardation
Turner's syndrome	XO (45)	Short stature, webbed neck, amenorrhea
Double Y male	XYY (47)	Tall, aggressive behavior
Triple X female	XXX (47)	Mental retardation
Fragile X	XY, XX (46)	Mild to severe mental retardation
Down's syndrome	Trisomy 21 (47)	Mental retardation, flat facies, dysplastic phalanges
Edward's syndrome	Trisomy 18 (47)	Mental retardation, skull abnormalities, multiple organ defects
Patau's syndrome	Trisomy 13 (47)	Skull and brain defects, cardiac and other organ defects
Cri du Chat syndrome	XX, 5p– (46, deletion on chromosome 5) XY, 5p–	Mental retardation, small skull and brain, cry like a cat's mewing

*Total number of chromosomes in parentheses.

Autosomal aneuploidy consists of a change in the number of autosomal chromosomes, usually the presence of three chromosomes **(trisomy)** instead of the single pair of a particular chromosome (most often chromosome 18 or 21). Sex chromosome alterations include Turner's syndrome, which is XO (i.e., single X chromosome without Y or other X) and Klinefelter's syndrome (more than one X chromosome per cell in conjunction with a Y, such as XXY or XXXY).

Translocations arise as parts of one chromosome exchange with parts of other chromosomes. As long as there is no net loss or gain of genetic material (i.e., a balanced translocation), this abnormality is essentially normal. However, if such an abnormal chromosome is passed on to offspring along with two copies of the normal chromosome, there is a net increase of genetic material that functionally acts as aneuploidy with possible phenotypic expression of mental retardation or other congenital malformation.

Mosaicism arises when an individual has at least two different cell types, each with a different chromosomal complement. For example, Turner's syndrome patients can have some cells that are normal XX or XY plus a critical mass of cells that are XO.

The risk of chromosomal aberration increases with advancing maternal age, which is the primary indication for fetal karyotyping. Although Down's syndrome **(trisomy 21)** is the most familiar problem affecting offspring of older mothers, incidence of all the other chromosomal abnormalities also increases with age. For an unselected woman aged 20, there is a 1 in 200 or less risk of any abnormality, and a 1 in 2000 risk of Down's syndrome. These figures increase to 1 in 100 for any defect and 1 in 300 for Down's syndrome for a 35-year-old mother, and to 1 in 20 and 1 in 40, respectively, for a mother aged 45 years. Most obstetricians perform chromosomal analysis on the fetus of any pregnant woman aged 35 or older.

Couples of any age who have already had one chromosomally abnormal child should have CVS, amniocentesis, or PUBS in subsequent pregnancies, as should couples in which either partner is a carrier of a balanced translocation defect. Aborted fetuses can also be karyotyped to determine whether the parents are likely to have a chromosomal aberration that will manifest itself in subsequent pregnancies.

The diagnosis of genetic disorders is becoming much more precise; genes responsible for known hereditary disorders have been identified and cloned. Molecular genetic techniques will greatly enhance diagnostic sensitivity and ultimately counseling and management. Table 17–11 is a partial list of cloned genes responsible for known hereditary disorders.

Sex-Linked Diseases

Many disorders transmitted by abnormal genes on the X chromosome cause severe, lifelong suffering. Common examples are hemophilia and Duchenne's muscular dystrophy, but there are many others, including chronic granulomatous disease and Lesch-Nyhan syndrome. Families

TABLE 17–11. PARTIAL LIST OF MAPPED GENES RESPONSIBLE FOR KNOWN HEREDITARY DISORDERS

Genes	Chromosome	Disorder
Antithrombin II	1q	Antithrombin II deficiency
Fucosidase	1p	Fucosidosis
Protein 4.1	1p	Elliptocytosis-I
Glycocerebrosidase	1q	Gaucher's disease
Uroporphyrinogen decarboxylase	1p	Porphyria cutanea tarda
Medium-chain acyl-CoA dehydrogenase	1p	Medium-chain acyl-CoA dehydrogenase deficiency
α-Spectrin	1q	Elliptocytosis-2, spherocytosis
Carbamylphosphate synthetase deficiency	2p	Carbamylphosphate synthetase deficiency
Apolipoprotein B	2p	Hypobetalipoproteinemia, premature atherosclerosis?
α_1(III)-Procollagen	2p	Ehlers–Danlos syndrome type IV
Protein C	2	Thrombophilia due to protein C deficiency
β-Propionyl-CoA carboxylase	3q	Propionic acidemia type II
Transferrin	3q	Atransferrinemia
Fibrinogen α, β, and γ	4q	Dysfibrinogenemias
β-Hexosaminidase	5q	Sandhoff's disease
Factor XIII	6p	Factor XIII deficiency
Steroid 21-hydroxylase	6p	Congenital adrenal hyperplasia
Complement factor 2	6p	C2 deficiency
Complement factor 4	6p	C4 deficiency
Plasminogen	6q	Thrombophilia due to plasminogen variant
Argininosuccinate lyase	7q	Argininosuccinic aciduria
β-Glucuronidase	7q	Mucopolysaccharidosis VII
α_2(I)-Procollagen	7q	Osteogenesis imperfecta, Ehlers–Danlos syndrome type VII A2
Plasminogen activator	8p	Thrombophilia due to plasminogen activator deficiency
Carbonic anhydrase	8q	Renal tubular acidosis with osteopetrosis
Thyroglobulin	8q	Hereditary congenital hypothyroidism
Argininosuccinate synthetase	9q	Citrullinemia
Fructose-1-phosphate aldolase	9q	Fructose intolerance
Ornithine aminotransferase	10q	Gyrate atrophy
Steroid 17-hydroxylase/ 17,20-lyase	10	Congenital adrenal hyperplasia

(Continued)

TABLE 17–11. PARTIAL LIST OF MAPPED GENES RESPONSIBLE FOR KNOWN HEREDITARY DISORDERS *(Continued)*

Genes	Chromosome	Disorder
Insulin	11p	Diabetes mellitus due to abnormal insulins
β-Globin	11p	Sickle cell anemia, β-thalassemia
γ-Globin	11p	Hereditary persistence of fetal hemoglobin
Parathyroid hormone	11p	Familial hypoparathyroidism (one form)
Catalase	11p	Acatalasemia
Apolipoprotein A1, C3, and A4	11q	Premature coronary artery disease
Muscle glycogen phosphorylase	11q	McArdle's disease
Porphobilinogen deaminase	11q	Acute intermittent porphyria
Pyruvate carboxylase	11q	Pyruvate carboxylase deficiency
von Willebrand factor	12p	von Willebrand's disease
Triosephosphate isomerase	12p	Triosephosphate isomerase deficiency
Phenylalanine hydroxylase	12q	Phenylketonuria
Retinoblastoma gene	13q	Retinoblastoma
Factor VII	13q	Factor VII deficiency
Factor X	13q	Factor X deficiency
α-Propionyl-CoA carboxylase	13	Propionic acidemia type I
α_1-Antitrypsin	14	α_1-Antitrypsin deficiency
Liver phosphorylase	14	Hers' disease (glycogen storage disease VI)
α_1-Hexosaminidase	15q	Tay–Sachs disease
P-450 side-chain cleavage enzyme/20,22-desmolase	15	Lipid adrenal hyperplasia
α-Globin	16p	α-Thalassemia
Tyrosine aminotransferase	16q	Tyrosinemia type II
Lecithin–cholesterol acyltransferase	16q	Lecithin–cholesterol acyltransferase deficiency
Growth hormone	17q	Isolated familial growth hormone deficiency
α_1(I)-Procollagen	17q	Osteogenesis imperfecta, Ehlers–Danlos syndrome type VII A1
Complement factor 3	19p	C3 deficiency
Apolipoprotein E, C2, and C1	19q	Dyslipoproteinemia
Low-density-lipoprotein receptor	19q	Familial hypercholesterolemia

(Continued)

TABLE 17–11. PARTIAL LIST OF MAPPED GENES RESPONSIBLE FOR KNOWN HEREDITARY DISORDERS (Continued)

Genes	Chromosome	Disorder
Adenosine deaminase	20q	Severe combined immunodeficiency due to adenosine deaminase deficiency
Cystathionine β-synthase	21q	Homocystinuria
Steroid sulfatase	Xp	X-linked ichthyosis
Ornithine transcarbamylase	Xp	Ornithine transcarbamylase deficiency
Chronic granulomatous disease gene	Xp	Chronic granulomatous disease
Gene for Duchenne's muscular dystrophy	Xp	Duchenne's muscular dystrophy
α-Galactosidase	Xq	Fabry's disease
Phosphoglycerate kinase	Xq	Phosphoglycerate kinase deficiency
Hypoxanthine guanine phosphoribosyltransferase	Xq	Lesch–Nyhan syndrome
Factor IX	Xq	Hemophilia B
Factor VIII	Xq	Hemophilia A
Green/red cone pigment	Xq	Color blindness
Glucose-6-phosphate dehydrogenase	Xq	Glucose-6-phosphase dehydrogenase deficiency

Adapted from Antonarakis, A: Diagnosis of genetic disorders. N Engl J Med 320:155, 1989.

who know the woman to be a carrier of an abnormal gene may prefer to avoid having affected children by restricting themselves to female offspring. Selectively aborting all male fetuses inevitably means sacrificing some who would have been normal, but with early prenatal sex determination, the family at least has information on which to base their decision.

The disorder termed **fragile X syndrome** is characterized by the tendency of the X chromosome to break in cells cultured in special medium depleted of folate. The phenotype of fragile X is mental retardation in affected males and perhaps also in females with a single normal X in addition to the abnormal fragile X. The incidence of mental retardation due to fragile X is 1 in 1500 males and 1 in 2500 females, making it the most common form of inherited mental retardation. The molecular basis of the fragile X chromosome is gene expansion from one generation to the next of a repetitive DNA sequence (the trinucleotide repeat CGG). Carriers may have a gene with 50 or more repeats that expand in an affected individual to over 200 repeats. This knowledge of the actual molecular disorder has made DNA analysis using Southern blot or polymerase reaction the preferred method for detecting fragile X.

Other acquired chromosomal abnormalities are discussed in considering diagnoses of leukemias (see Chapter 4).

Inborn Errors of Metabolism

There are many hundreds of genetically determined disorders (Table 17–11). Many arise from defects or deficiencies of enzymes, receptor molecules, or other essential proteins. If the abnormal activity can be identified in fetal cells obtained through amniocentesis, CVS, or PUBS, the congenital metabolic deficiency can, at least in theory, be diagnosed while the fetus is still in utero. Many errors of lipid, carbohydrate, and amino acid metabolism can be identified in the fetus early enough to permit decision about abortion. Modern diagnostic techniques include detection of abnormal genes in fetal cells by specific DNA analysis for point mutations, deletions, or change in DNA sequence before it is even expressed as a protein. DNA analysis is extremely specific and, for that reason, it must be performed with a highly purified nucleic acid probe that will react with no other gene. In some disease states for which the abnormal gene is not yet precisely identified, investigators take advantage of genetic linkages between the disease of interest and some other known gene on the same chromosome. In this type of analysis, it is necessary to study a complete kindred in order to establish whether a fetus will be affected with the disease based on the genetic linkage present in that family. This analysis is termed **restriction fragment length polymorphism (RFLP).** However, progress in mapping genes through the Human Genome Project has made feasible specific DNA probes for a wide range of genetic abnormalities. Probably within a decade, essentially all genetic diseases will be understood at the DNA level; testing should then be possible directly through probe or sequence analysis, making indirect studies of genetic linkage with RFLP unnecessary.

In most cases, the indication for specific prenatal analysis is birth of an affected infant from an earlier pregnancy. Most of these conditions are autosomal-recessive traits, becoming manifest only when the child of two heterozygous carriers receives a double dose of the abnormal gene. Most of these deleterious genes occur only rarely in an unselected population, and ordinarily parents do not know they are carriers until an affected child is born.

A few genes occur rather commonly in specific populations. Notable examples are the gene for Tay-Sachs disease in Jews of central European origin, the genes for hemoglobinopathies in blacks, and the gene for beta-thalassemia in persons of Mediterranean or Eastern origin.

Tay-Sachs Disease

Tay-Sachs disease (deficiency of hexosaminidase A) can be identified in utero by assay of the specific enzyme activity, and the carrier state can also be reliably detected. In Jews from central Europe (Ashkenazic Jews), the gene has a frequency of 1 in 30, making the risk of an affected infant $1/30 \times 1/30 \times 1/4 = 1/3600$ for any child of this descent. High yields can be expected from screening young people for asymptomatic possession of the gene, followed by prenatal examination of any pregnancy involving two carriers.

Sickle Cell Disease

The situation with sickle cell disease, the condition caused by an abnormal amino acid substitution in the beta globin chain giving rise to hemoglobin S, is more difficult. The abnormal gene is very common, present in 1 out of every 10 American blacks. The carrier state is easy to diagnose reliably, but prenatal diagnosis of the 1 affected pregnancy in 400 $(1/10 \times 1/10 \times 1/4)$ is difficult because fetal red cells contain predominantly hemoglobin F $(\alpha_2\gamma_2)$ with only traces, if any, of adult hemoglobin $(\alpha_2\beta_2)$. Fetal red cells must be examined, not amniotic fluid or readily accessible superficial cells. In some centers that specialize in high-risk pregnancies, PUBS or fetoscopy can be used to obtain fetal cells during the second trimester. Neither of these techniques is available on a widespread basis.

Recent advances in DNA sequence analysis and gene probing have made it possible to detect the gene for hemoglobin S distinct from that for hemoglobin A in DNA isolated from the fetus. This technique is not limited by failure to synthesize adult hemoglobin at early fetal age because the same genes are present at all fetal ages. Although still largely an investigational procedure, gene detection of hemoglobinopathies has potential for prenatal diagnosis in the near future.

Thalassemia

Accurate prenatal diagnosis of alpha- or beta-thalassemia is yet more specialized. Although the gene is fairly common, specific tests for heterozygous beta-thalassemia are not in general use; carriers are detected only when mild anemia is observed and detailed investigation pursued. Even if both parents are known to carry a beta-thalassemia gene, the tests that must be done on the fetal red cells for protein analysis are highly demanding. Accurate prenatal diagnosis has been achieved in a few instances, but this will not soon become a routine procedure. More likely to become standard, if only in reference laboratories, is the gene probe analysis for detection of the thalassemias. The difficulty with any specific gene test is that there are multiple different thalassemias, and a negative test for one by gene probe analysis does not exclude any of the others.

Cystic Fibrosis

Cystic fibrosis, an autosomal recessive disorder, causes severe pulmonary disease because of abnormally thick mucus that causes plugging of bronchi with persistent secondary bacterial infections in affected individuals. It has other manifestations with secretion of thick mucus that obstructs pancreatic and bile ducts and also excess loss of electrolytes through sweat. Cystic fibrosis occurs in about 1 in 2000 births (about 1 in 17,000 in blacks and very rarely in Asians). Thus the carrier rate of an abnormal cystic fibrosis gene in whites is about 1 in 20. In one of the most sophisticated pieces of joint clinical and molecular research, the gene for cystic fibrosis has been mapped on chromosome 7 and its DNA sequence completely determined. A single mutation resulting in the deletion of a phenylalanine from position 508 (ΔF_{508}) of the protein encoded by this gene has been found to account for about three-quarters of cases; multiple other different mutations account for the remainder. Cystic fibrosis carrier detection has not been possible until now because the actual defective protein/enzyme had been unknown. It is now feasible to test for the majority of carriers by DNA analysis, but unless the particular mutation affecting a kindred is known, it is necessary to test for many different mutations throughout the gene.

Neural Tube Defects

Defects of neural tube development and closure account for 10% or more of serious fetal malformations. **Meningomyelocele** and **spina bifida** are the most common examples. **Anencephaly** is the most extreme occurrence. Although these conditions cannot clearly be shown to have a genetic basis, recurrence risk after an initial affected pregnancy is 3 to 5%, and the offspring of affected parents also run a 3 to 5% risk. After two affected pregnancies, likelihood of subsequent fetal abnormality is many times higher. Dietary supplementation of folic acid for pregnant women can reduce the incidence of neural tube defects. **Alpha-fetoprotein (AFP)** measurement and ultrasonic techniques make accurate prenatal diagnosis possible in most cases.

Alpha-Fetoprotein

The fetal liver synthesizes **alpha-fetoprotein (AFP),** a glycoprotein that is the major serum protein through much of fetal development. Peak production occurs at 13 weeks and declines progressively thereafter. After the immediate postnatal period, elevated serum AFP levels occur only with conditions of abnormal cell multiplication (e.g., malignancies such as hepatocellular carcinoma). During normal pregnancy, maternal serum contains minute amounts of AFP that pass from the fetus to the mother. Amniotic fluid contains modest amounts, thought to derive largely from fetal urine. Normal values for maternal serum and amniotic fluid levels rise with gestational age and are also elevated in pregnancies with multiple fetuses; therefore, it is important to know the gestational age to avoid inaccurate false-positive or false-negative interpretations of AFP data.

Screening in Pregnancy

If the fetal neural tube fails to close properly (usually it closes at about 4 weeks), large quantities of AFP enter the amniotic fluid, presumably because permeable tissues like choroid plexus have direct access to the exterior. This is the equivalent of cerebrospinal fluid (an ultrafiltrate of plasma that contains substantial amounts of AFP) leaking into the amniotic fluid. Elevated amniotic fluid levels usually produce excessive AFP in maternal serum. The best time to screen maternal serum for AFP is 13 to 16 weeks because fetal production peaks during this period, and subsequent confirmatory tests can readily be done if screening results are suggestive. If a second serum test result is also abnormal, ultrasound and/or amniocentesis is indicated. With open neural tube defects, amniotic fluid AFP is dramatically elevated. AFP is measured by immunoassay, and results are reported as **multiples of the median (MoM)** for a population of pregnant women at the same week of gestation. The MoM may be adjusted according to maternal weight, race (blacks have slightly higher values), number of fetuses (the value doubles with twins), and diabetes mellitus (lower than normal). The risk of having a neural tube defect is generally based on a cutoff of 2.0 for the AFP MoM, resulting in 3 to 4% of abnormally high values on the screening test that should be further evaluated.

An additional confirmatory test performed on the amniotic fluid is determination of **acetylcholinesterase (AChE)** enzyme activity. Acetylcholinesterase is secreted into CSF in an age-dependent manner. Because none is present normally, the presence of this neural AChE in amniotic fluid is evidence for neural tube defect. Acetylcholinesterase must be distinguished from pseudocholinesterase (PChE) (see Chapter 11), which is also expected to be present. The method for detecting these two enzyme activities involves electrophoresis in polyacrylamide gels followed by staining for enzyme activity with a colorimetric substrate. The reference value is negative (no AChE activity in amniotic fluid).

Abnormal Results

Because fetal serum has AFP levels 100 times those of amniotic fluid, it is critical to avoid contaminating the specimen with fetal blood. Analyzing the specimen for fetal hemoglobin helps clarify possible contamination. Values will be abnormally high in multiple gestations, in cases of fetal death, or if estimated gestational age is incorrect. With ultrasound, these conditions can be resolved. True elevations occur in pregnancies complicated by congenital nephrosis, obstructive anomalies of the digestive tract, and closure problems of the abdominal wall.

Serum screening, active surveillance of high-risk pregnancies, and accurate AFP measurements have combined to produce excellent case-finding results. The modest AFP elevation caused by closed spina bifida is the usual cause of false-negative results. False-positive results are usually due to contamination with fetal blood or to hemorrhage into the amniotic sac occurring before the examination.

Triple Test for Down's Syndrome

The combination of three separate markers has proven useful in assessing risk of a pregnancy for Down's syndrome in the "triple test." These measurements are AFP, hCG, and estriol in the serum of a pregnant woman. In cases of fetal Down's syndrome, maternal AFP tends to be about 30% low, hCG tends to be about twice expected, and estriol tends to be decreased. The results of these individual measurements are combined with other factors such as maternal age, family history, diabetes mellitus, and gestational age to establish a composite risk for Down's syndrome and other fetal defects as well.

Multifactorial Defects

Normal results on amniocentesis and chromosomal analysis do not guarantee birth of a healthy infant. Most of the common congenital defects cannot be attributed to a single enzyme deficiency or chromosomal aberration. Ultrasonic techniques and fetoscopy have greatly expanded the possibilities for accurate prenatal diagnosis, along with newer techniques such as chorionic villus sampling and biopsy, from which multiple studies of proteins, enzymes, and genes are feasible. Many more diagnostic procedures for prenatal application will likely emerge in the near future as molecular probe reagents become available for the prevention or amelioration of birth defects.

ESTIMATION OF FETAL WELL-BEING

An important indication for amniocentesis is to estimate fetal maturity and detect deteriorating intrauterine condition. The goal is to balance the risks of premature delivery against the risks of continuing exposure to progressive intrauterine problems. Prompt delivery may be desirable in hemolytic disease of the newborn, in pregnancies complicated by maternal diabetes or pre-eclampsia, or when clinical and technical monitoring indicate fetal distress of unknown causes.

Hemolytic Disease

Rapid antibody-mediated destruction of fetal red blood cells imposes tremendous hematopoietic burden on the fetus. If erythropoiesis cannot keep place, the fetus may become dangerously anemic. The bilirubin generated as cells are destroyed does not endanger the fetus because it is cleared into the maternal circulation, but amniotic fluid bile pigment levels provide an index to the severity of the process (see Chapter 8).

Pregnancy in any woman known to have an IgG antibody against red cell antigens should be examined by amniocentesis at 24 to 48 weeks. Large quantities of pigments absorbing at wavelength 450 nm indicate the presence of bilirubin from significant red cell destruction. The degree of fetal danger can be correlated with bile pigment levels at different gestational ages by using Liley graphs (see Chapter 8). If the fetus is severely affected, intrauterine transfusion may be considered, or early delivery, if the infant proves mature enough by further testing. The application of PUBS has enabled direct analysis of fetal hemoglobin concentration or hematocrit and, consequently, accurate determination of the extent of fetal hemolytic disease. (See Appendix C.)

Lecithin/Sphingomyelin Ratio

The leading killer of premature infants is respiratory distress syndrome, also called "hyaline membrane disease." Immature lungs commonly collapse shortly after birth because respiratory movements cannot overcome the forces of surface tension that make alveolar membranes adhere to one another. This collapse of small alveolar air spaces is a consequence of the physical property that small bubbles of air in liquid naturally tend to coalesce into larger ones. **Surfactant** is a substance that reduces surface tension of liquid, thereby stabilizing small bubbles. If sufficient surfactant material lubricates the alveolar surfaces, the alveoli do not collapse and respiration with exchange of gases occurs normally. Neonates at risk of developing respiratory distress are now treated with intratracheal doses of synthetic surfactant soon after birth.

Surfactant activity depends on physical interactions between complex lipid molecules. The lipid concentration in amniotic fluid reflects the lipids present in intrapulmonary secretion, making it possible to estimate pulmonary surfactant levels from analysis of the amniotic fluid. The lipids that give the most information are **lecithin (L), sphingomyelin (S), and phosphatidylglycerol (PG).**

Sphingomyelin in the amniotic fluid remains fairly constant throughout pregnancy, in the range of 4 to 6 mg/dL. Lecithin rises slowly during the first two trimesters and sharply at about 35 weeks. At 30 to 34 weeks, lecithin concentration is usually about 6 to 9 mg/dL. The absolute values for lecithin and sphingomyelin are less important than the ratio between them. Mature lung function correlates strongly with L/S ratios of 2 or above. Infants born with amniotic fluid L/S ratios below 1.5 have a 70% risk of respiratory distress syndrome. With an L/S ratio between 1.5 and 2, the risk is 40%; at a ratio of 2 or above, the risk of respiratory distress syndrome is 1% to 2%. At a ratio of 3 or greater, respiratory distress is highly unlikely. Mature values of the L/S ratio can reach as high as 8 at term. Fetal blood, maternal blood, and meconium (fetal feces released into the amniotic fluid by fetal distress) can cause technical interference because of the lipid content of those body fluids.

Thin-layer Chromatography

Quantitation of the L/S ratio by **thin-layer chromatography (TLC)** entails rapid processing of the amniotic fluid with centrifugation to remove cells and other particulate matter, extraction with organic solvent, concentration, and sample application to a thin-layer plate. TLC is based on separation of lecithin and sphingomyelin by migration of an organic solvent along the thin-layer plate; relative amounts of these two substances is then calculated from measurements of spot areas or intensities using densitometry. TLC is very laborious, requires special expertise, and takes several hours to perform. Nevertheless, TLC methods were used in the earliest clinical assays for L/S ratio and are still used in many laboratories.

Foam Stability Index

Instead of measuring the concentrations of chemical analytes, the **foam stability index (FSI)** is based on the functional ability of pulmonary surfactant in amniotic fluid to stabilize bubbles in foam. It is performed by mixing amniotic fluid with different concentrations of ethanol to eliminate other potential surface-active substances such as protein or bile salts. The mixtures are shaken, and the tubes are examined visually for the presence of bubbles; the highest concentration of ethanol demonstrating bubbles is reported. Values of FSI at or above 0.47 are considered mature.

Fetal Lung Maturity by Fluorescence Polarization Assay

Fluorescence polarization has been applied to a commercial assay, the TDx fetal lung maturity (FLM) test (Abbott Laboratories). The method is based on changes in the angle of polarization of fluorescence emitted from a dye following rotational diffusion. The polarization is influenced by the binding of the dye to surfactant and to albumin in an amniotic fluid sample. This analysis is automated and so has excellent precision. The TDx FLM has attained great popularity owing to its ease of performance and widespread use of the TDx for other assays.

OTHER TESTS OF FETAL GROWTH AND MATURATION

In recent years, it has become feasible to detect **phosphatidylinositol (PI)** and **phosphatidylglycerol (PG)** routinely by two-dimensional thin-layer chromatography and also by specific immunoassay (for PG). Phosphatidylglycerol is detectable in amniotic fluid 2 to 6 weeks before full term, and PI appears a few weeks before PG. The presence of PG in amniotic fluid indicates fetal pulmonary maturity; in combination with a mature ratio of L/S, it virtually rules out the possibility of respiratory distress syndrome (RDS). Conversely, the absence of PG is a strong indicator for high risk of RDS over the next week or more. Consequently, absence of PG would lead an obstetrician to defer delivery if possible until the fetal lungs have had further opportunity to mature. Absence of both PG and PI indicates risk of RDS continuing for 3 or 4 weeks.

Creatinine concentration in amniotic fluid rises steadily in the last half of pregnancy, as the fetal kidneys mature. Levels of 2 mg/dL or above generally correlate with adequately mature renal function. If the L/S testing and creatinine measurement give divergent results, the index of pulmonary maturity carries far greater clinical weight.

Epithelial cells shed into the amniotic fluid reflect the maturation of skin and skin appendages. Increasing numbers of shed cells contain stainable fat as sebaceous glands mature. Some workers have attempted to correlate the number of lipid-stainable cells with fetal maturity, but this task has proven difficult to perform and of questionable significance.

Surfactant forms particles that are lamellar bodies with volumes between 2 and 20 femtoliters; this size range corresponds to platelets in blood. A lamellar body count can be done on amniotic fluid with standard hematology analyzers; larger numbers of lamellar bodies in amniotic fluid predict greater fetal lung maturity. This assay is rapid but not yet standardized.

SUGGESTED READING

Ashwood, ER: Evaluating health and maturation of the unborn: The role of the clinical laboratory. Clin Chem 38:1523, 1992.

Baird, DT: Amenorrhoea. Lancet 350:275, 1997.

Batrinos, ML, and Panitsa-Faflia, C: Clinical syndromes of primary amenorrhea. Ann N Y Acad Sci 816:235, 1997.

Brown, WT: Perspectives and molecular diagnosis of the fragile X syndrome. Clin Lab Med 15:859, 1995.

Carson, SA, and Buster, JE: Ectopic pregnancy. N Engl J Med 329:1174, 1993.

Cartwright, PS: Diagnosis of ectopic pregnancy. Obstet Gynecol Clin North Am 18:19, 1991.

Comhaire, F, and Vermeulen, L: Human semen analysis. Hum Reprod Update 1:343, 1995.

Czeizel, A, and Dudás, I: Prevention of the first occurrence of neural-tube defects by periconceptional vitamin supplementation. N Engl J Med 327:1832, 1992.

Del Valle, GO, et al: Interpretation of the TDx-FLM fluorescence polarization assay in pregnancies complicated by diabetes mellitus. Am J Perinatol 14:241, 1997.

Emancipator, K, Bock, JL, and Burke, MD: Diagnosis of ectopic pregnancy by the rate of increase of choriogonadotropin in serum: Diagnostic criteria compared. Clin Chem 36:2097, 1990.

Field, NT, and Gilbert, WM: Current status of amniotic fluid tests of fetal maturity. Clin Obstet Gynecol 40:366, 1997.

Haddow, JE, et al: Prenatal screening for Down's syndrome with use of maternal serum markers. N Engl J Med 327:588, 1992.

Jackson-Cook, C, and Pandya, A: Strategies and logistical requirements for efficient testing in genetic disease. Clin Lab Med 15:839, 1995.

Kant, JA, et al: Molecular diagnosis of cystic fibrosis. Clin Lab Med 15:877, 1995.

Katznelson, L, and Klibanski, A: Prolactinomas. Cancer Treat Res 89:41, 1997.

Mavroudis, K: Clinical syndromes of secondary amenorrhea. Ann N Y Acad Sci 816:241, 1997.

Moore, TR: Clinical assessment of amniotic fluid. Clin Obstet Gynecol 40:303, 1997.

Ombelet, W, et al: Sperm morphology assessment: Historical review in relation to fertility. Hum Reprod Update 1:543, 1995.

Palomaki, GE, Knight, GJ, and Haddow, JE: Human chorionic gonadotropin and unconjugated oestriol measurements in insulin-dependent diabetic pregnant women being screened for fetal Down syndrome. Prenat Diagn 14:65, 1994.

Reece, EA: Early and midtrimester genetic amniocenteses: Safety and outcomes. Obstet Gynecol Clin North Am 24:71, 1997.

Ross, HL, and Elias, S: Maternal serum screening for fetal genetic disorders. Obstet Gynecol Clin North Am 24:33, 1997.

Santolaya-Forgas, J, et al: Pregnancy outcome in women with low midtrimester maternal serum unconjugated estriol. J Reprod Med 41:87, 1996.

Sasi, K, et al: Prenatal diagnosis for inborn errors of metabolism and haemoglobinopathies: The Montreal Children's Hospital experience. Prenat Diagn 17:681, 1997.

Stern, JJ, Voss, F, and Coulam, CB: Early diagnosis of ectopic pregnancy using receiver-operator characteristic curves of serum progesterone concentrations. Hum Reprod 8:775, 1993.

Stranc, LC, Evans, JA, and Hamerton, JL: Chorionic villus sampling and amniocentesis for prenatal diagnosis. Lancet 349:711, 1997.

Wapner, RJ: Chorionic villus sampling. Obstet Gynecol Clin North Am 24:83, 1997.

Wolf, AS, Marx, K, and Ulrich, U: Athletic amenorrhea. Ann N Y Acad Sci 816:295, 1997.

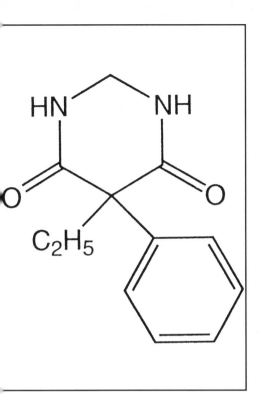

Section Seven

Miscellaneous

18

Therapeutic Drug Monitoring and Toxicology

![chemical structure]

PRINCIPLES OF DRUG KINETICS

Measurement of drug concentrations in blood enables clinicians to adjust dosages of medications to achieve desired therapeutic benefits while avoiding potentially toxic side effects. The route of drug administration to a patient is either **enteral** via the gastrointestinal tract (orally or by rectum) or **parenteral** through intravenous or intramuscular injections. The extent to which a drug can be successfully absorbed from the gastrointestinal tract and be therapeutically active is termed its **bioavailability.** The factors that go into determining the bioavailability include the chemical form of the drug itself (e.g., as a salt with another chemical), other agents used in compounding the tablets or liquid medication, its physical form and how easily it can be disrupted and dissolved by the normal processes of digestion, and the absorptive capacity of the patient's intestines. The most immediate route for drug delivery is intravenous because there is essentially no delay for bolus administration of a drug before it reaches its highest or *peak level* in the circulation (Fig. 18–1). From there, its concentration gradually falls as it is metabolized (generally by the liver), taken up by tissues (where it can react with receptors on cells

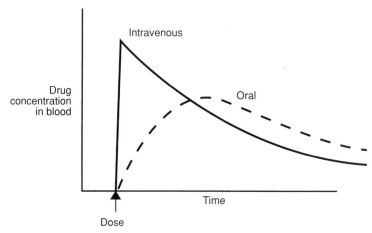

FIGURE 18–1. Idealized kinetics of drug clearance after a single dose.

and achieve its therapeutic effect), and cleared from the body (by biliary or urinary excretion).

The locations where the drugs are effective are in the body tissues, not generally in the blood. However, it is much more convenient to measure drug concentrations in blood than in tissues, and standard values for therapy are based predominantly on levels in serum because of convention and the convenience of utilizing serum for analysis. Nevertheless, it must be kept in mind that drugs diffuse widely through the body, frequently reaching higher concentrations in tissues than in blood, depending on a drug's chemical nature, particularly its relative solubilities in aqueous versus lipid solvents. This relationship between tissue and blood levels is termed the **distribution space.** A large distribution space indicates that much more of the drug moves into the tissues than stays in the circulation.

The rate at which a particular drug is cleared from the circulation is dependent not only on the type of drug itself, but also on a patient's capacity to metabolize and excrete it. The time needed for the body to reduce the drug concentration by one half from the peak level is commonly referred to as that drug's **half-life** (Fig. 18–2). The half-life is important because it establishes guidelines for how frequently medication should be administered. For example, a drug with a half-life of 1 to 2 hours would drop below therapeutically effective levels between successive doses if it were given only once a day. Conversely, if a drug has a half-life of a day, there would be little point in administering it several times per day when once a day would probably suffice to maintain stable levels over time.

If the route of administration is oral, the time required for absorption from the gastrointestinal tract delays the peak level until approximately 1 to 2 hours after the oral dose. **Intramuscular (IM)** administration also

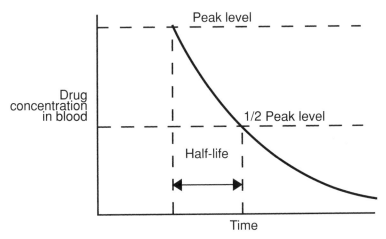

FIGURE 18–2. Half-life of a drug in the circulation.

has an absorption phase, but the IM route is more typically used for one-time (single) dosages such as immunizations, whose kinetics of absorption are not usually of concern medically. When medication is given periodically at regular intervals, the drug concentration in blood goes through a regular series of peaks and troughs (Fig. 18–3). From the time a drug is first given, the values of the peaks and troughs increase with each dose until they reach a plateau or steady state, after which subsequent peaks remain roughly the same and subsequent troughs are also similar.

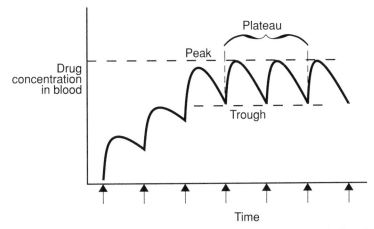

FIGURE 18–3. Kinetics of drug concentration in blood with regularly administered doses (arrows).

To be meaningful, collection of specimens for therapeutic monitoring of drug levels must be coordinated with the timing of doses. It is conventional to measure **peak levels** (at a time after administration to allow for absorption) or **trough levels** (immediately prior to next dose) and not at intermediate points between peaks and troughs. Knowledge of drug levels at these points permits the physician to assess degree of therapeutic effectiveness or potential toxicities. If measurements are made at other times, it is not always possible to relate those values to the correct plan of therapy.

REASONS FOR THERAPEUTIC DRUG MONITORING

The primary reasons for monitoring drug levels are to establish (1) whether a patient is receiving a sufficient dosage of medication to produce a desired therapeutic effect, and (2) whether the dosage is too great and is likely to produce undesired toxic effects. Within the context of clinical management, several unknown factors about a patient may prompt a physician to request the measurement of drug levels. Included among these are the bioavailability of the drug in that particular patient, who may have idiosyncrasies of absorption from alterations of gastric and pancreatic secretions, diminished absorptive surface in the intestine, and prolonged or greatly accelerated transit time of intestinal contents during which absorption must occur. In addition, there may be greatly altered metabolism or clearance of many drugs, usually due to disorders of the liver or kidneys, although simple congestive heart failure can also affect drug clearance by not delivering normal blood flow to those organs. Distribution spaces can also be quite different from those expected due to substantial volumes of body fluid accumulated as ascites or even large amounts of body fat.

At times, other drugs (e.g., aspirin, erythromycin, phenobarbital) or substances (e.g., alcohol, tobacco) taken by patients will affect the metabolism of a drug of interest. This can happen because of displacement of that drug from binding proteins in the blood and acceleration of its clearance or enhancement of its activity in the free, non-protein-bound fraction. In addition, the other substance can directly affect metabolism by tying up hepatic enzymes, thereby blocking the drug metabolism, or conversely by inducing synthesis of more of those enzymes and so speeding up the metabolism.

Finally, there is the issue of patient **compliance** or **noncompliance.** There is always an element of uncertainty as to whether a patient has fully understood and accepted the instructions for taking medication at home and has successfully complied with the physician's orders to take prescribed doses at specific times. In this situation, therapeutic monitoring can lead to an understanding of why a patient may not be responding as expected to standard dosages.

Not all drugs are regularly measured as part of medical care. If an easily observed physical or physiologic response (e.g., blood pressure) can be measured as an indicator of drug action, there is very little purpose in quantitating its level in serum. Furthermore, there may be no need to monitor drug levels if that medication has little or no toxicity even at high concentrations. This latter concept is expressed as the **therapeutic index,** which relates the blood levels at which drug toxicities occur compared with the levels needed to achieve desired therapeutic effects.

To understand the therapeutic index, consider the following contrasting examples demonstrated in Figure 18–4. Drug A has a high therapeutic index (the ratio of the threshold of toxicity to minimal therapeutic level) with a relatively wide **therapeutic range** (the difference between highest and lowest effective dosages), whereas drug B has a low therapeutic index and narrow therapeutic range, owing to toxicities at levels close to the minimal therapeutic level. Drugs with therapeutic indices similar to that of drug A can generally be administered without concern for toxicities because the desired therapeutic effects can be achieved at dosages and concentrations in the blood well below those levels that cause side effects. An example of this type is penicillin, which interferes with a specific step of bacterial cell wall synthesis but has no effect on human metabolism. Some individuals, of course, are allergic to penicillin, but that side effect is of a different kind and is not considered a standard drug toxicity. Conversely, drugs similar to drug B can be expected to produce the same symptoms of toxicity in virtually all individuals when the drug concentration in blood exceeds a toxic level that is not too far above levels at which the therapeutic effects are achieved. For such drugs, it is desirable to monitor the drug's physiologic effects on a patient whenever possible (such as the control of cardiac arrhythmias or of heart rate with antiarrhythmics; prolongation of plasma clotting times with

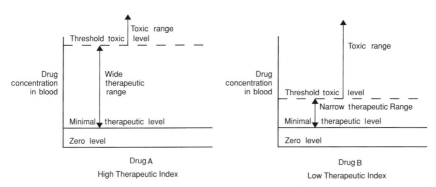

FIGURE 18–4. Depiction of therapeutic versus toxic levels of drugs and therapeutic index.

anticoagulant therapy: prothrombin time for coumadin, partial thrombo-plastin time for heparin). In addition, it is frequently advantageous to measure drug concentrations in unstable or otherwise unpredictable patients to prevent the development of excessively high levels that would almost certainly lead to toxicities.

METHODS OF DRUG ANALYSIS

Traditional methods for the detection and quantitation of drugs in patient samples have been relatively laborious, have required a great deal of highly specialized equipment, and have been relatively slow even in those institutions that had the luxury of on-site analysis. Fortunately, immunoassays have emerged that are applicable to the measurement of many drugs with low therapeutic indices and for which quantitation is important in planning therapy. Nevertheless, many drugs remain for which no commercial assays are available; these must be quantitated by other methods.

Spectrophotometry is one of the traditional methods still in use for many drugs that have unique absorption spectra. Many new, complex drugs with unusual chemical bonds and properties can frequently be measured by spectrophotometry after extraction from serum or other biologic fluid. The drug is then placed into a solvent or derivatized in such a way as to maximize the absorption peaks. An older method for barbiturate determination depended on the shift in its absorption spectrum from its ionized form at pH 10 to that at pH 14. This differential measurement is performed on a scanning spectrophotometer. Assuming a compatible chemical structure that manifests absorption of ultraviolet or visible wavelengths of light, spectrophotometry remains an important method for quantitating drugs for which specific immunoassays are not commercially available. Spectrophotometry is employed in the measurement of acetaminophen, and the differential method is applied to quantitation of toxically altered hemoglobin species (methemoglobin from oxidation induced by nitrites, sulfonamides, phenacetin; sulfhemoglobin from phenacetin; carbon monoxide intoxication). Nitroprusside administration (for management of acute and severe hypertension) can be monitored indirectly by spectrophotometric measurement of its metabolite, thiocyanate.

One of the limitations of direct or differential spectrophotometry is the possibility that a drug has no significant absorption properties or that therapeutic concentrations are far below the threshold of detection by standard optical means. To amplify the optical signal or to create one indicating the presence of a drug, specific reagents are mixed with the sample to be tested and then read at characteristic wavelengths. Using this technique, salicylates form a purple color with maximum absorption at 540 nm when mixed with ferric ions.

Various chromatographic methods are useful for detection of many drugs and other small compounds such as normal metabolic products of the body. Chromatographic methods have the special advantage of identifying the metabolites of drugs that are characteristic of drug ingestion. **Thin-layer chromatography (TLC)** is used extensively for toxicologic screening of blood and urine. In this method, small molecules are carried along a solid support layer by a solvent that moves by capillary attraction uniformly across a whole plate. When the advancing edge of the solvent reaches a certain point, the TLC plate is examined by exposing it to several standard stains and to ultraviolet light. Drugs are identified according to how far they have migrated and to how they appear with each of the stains. To positively identify an unknown substance by TLC, it is necessary to run a standard or a series of standard drugs in parallel with the unknown sample. As a method, TLC has tremendous power in demonstrating the presence of a multitude of drugs of abuse. It is a lengthy procedure, however, and requires an authentic standard (which may be unavailable for new street drugs) of the drug in question to establish an absolute identification of that agent. Thin-layer chromatography is applicable for the detection of drugs, but it is not used for quantitation of substances.

Gas chromatography (GC) is used for the quantitation of many drugs that are volatile or that can be chemically derivatized into volatile form. The alcohols are resolved separately by GC, as are their metabolites. Barbiturates can also be separately resolved according to their solubility properties.

High-performance liquid chromatography (HPLC) can be applied to a wide variety of drugs depending on the type of column used, the solvent system, and the detector (which can be based on chemical properties of the analytes in addition to simple optical absorbance). HPLC can be highly quantitative, but the procedure takes a relatively long time for analysis and requires expensive equipment that involves a great deal of maintenance. It does have tremendous advantages in quantitation of a vast array of drugs for which immunoassay or other assays are simply impractical or even impossible. Reagent costs of HPLC assays are typically quite low (for solvents only).

A device called a **mass spectrometer (MS)** can be added onto the effluent end of GC, enhancing its capability. By this means, unknown peaks (drugs) initially detected by the GC can be fragmented into characteristic pieces by the MS for absolute identification of the unknown substance. The mass spectra exhibited by even simple compounds can be highly complex. These "fingerprint patterns" are then compared with other known patterns in a collection or library derived from previous analyses. These comparison studies are best accomplished by an automated computer system. GC-MS is considered to be the ultimate for confirmation of drug identity, albeit an expensive option that is usually available only through specialized reference laboratories.

Some other methods with specific applications are flame photometry or ion selective electrodes for measurement of lithium, co-oximetry for detection of carbon monoxide, and assays that use reagent enzymes to quantitate materials such as ethanol.

IMMUNOASSAYS

The introduction of automated immunoassays has made it feasible for virtually every clinical laboratory to perform drug measurements that previously might have been possible only through far more complex HPLC methods. The basic element common to all these assays is an antibody specifically reactive with a particular drug. In many instances the antibody will also react with metabolites of the parent drug. Although such cross-reactivity makes the assay less specific, it could also be useful clinically to detect all the metabolites that are biologically active. Both polyclonal and monoclonal antibodies have been adapted to drug immunoassays. The earliest examples of these methods were **radioimmunoassays (RIA),** which depend on having a radiolabeled drug as a reagent. The concentration of a drug in a sample is determined by the extent to which that drug binds to the antibody, thereby displacing the radiolabeled drug reagent. An RIA requires the physical separation (e.g., by centrifugation) of radiolabeled drug bound to the antibody from radiolabeled drug still unbound at the end of an incubation period (usually 1 to several hours). Radioimmunoassay procedures also require scintillation or gamma counters to determine the amount of radioactivity in each assayed sample. Most of the pipetting steps are done manually, which introduces a source of potential error. Thus, use of RIAs for measurement of drug concentrations has many of the same disadvantages that HPLC has: relatively long assay times, expensive dedicated equipment, and almost continuous involvement of highly skilled labor.

Within the last several years, many different technologies have emerged for immunoassays that have been adapted to automated instrumentation (cutting down on some of the labor need) and that use principles of the reactions for detecting free and bound drug without a distinct separation phase (termed **homogeneous assays).**

One such methodology uses an enzyme (e.g., glucose-6-phosphate dehydrogenase) to which a molecule of the drug is linked in a location near the active site of the enzyme. If there is drug in the test sample, the reagent antibody binds to it, and the marker enzyme activity remains high since less reagent antibody is available to bind to the marker drug-enzyme complex. An automated instrument is then used to measure the amount of enzyme activity, which is directly proportional to the amount of drug present in the sample being assayed. This procedure is the EMIT method patented by the Syva Corporation (Palo Alto, California).

Another method makes use of the properties of fluorescent materials to emit light in the same polarization coordinates as the exciting light source. Small molecules such as free drug can rotate before light emission, thereby giving rise to a different angle of polarization. Larger molecules such as antibodies are restricted in their rotation. Consequently, the binding of the marker drug to antibody can be quantitated by the angle at which the emissions occur. This method of fluorescence polarization immunoassay is used extensively by Abbott Laboratories (Illinois) on the TDX analyzer.

Another method uses small particles or beads coated with the drug of interest. Addition of antibody to the drug causes the particles to agglutinate, as can be determined optically. If a sample premixed with the antibody contains some of that drug, the antibody will bind to it, and less agglutination of the particles occurs in the second stage of the assay.

The use of these methods and variations on their principles permit rapid quantitation without the time-consuming step of phase separation. Recently the use of chemiluminescent labels has been applied to automated immunoassays, improving analytic sensitivity and precision.

INDIVIDUAL DRUGS

The following sections discuss some of the most commonly administered and monitored drugs and also many that are commonly abused. These drugs have been chosen for presentation because of their frequent use in clinical medicine today. Other drugs that are frequently prescribed have been specifically excluded if therapeutic monitoring is not available or is not necessary. This list of drugs that are monitored routinely in practice is small indeed when compared with the total number of drugs usually available from a pharmacy (2000 to 3000 drugs in most hospitals).

The fundamental source book for information about prescription drugs sold in the United States is the *Physicians' Desk Reference (PDR)*, which is updated annually. It indexes drugs by manufacturer, by brand and generic name, and by product category. It also includes a pictorial product identification guide that allows comparison of unknown medications according to tablet (or package) size, shape, color, and markings. The bulk of the *PDR* consists of reprinted product inserts that detail each drug's content, its pharmacology, indications, contraindications, dosage information, recognized adverse effects, and appropriate precautions. In other countries, similar pharmaceutical indices are also available.

ANTIASTHMATIC DRUGS

Theophylline

Drugs of the **methylated xanthine class** (theophylline, caffeine, and theobromine) (Fig. 18–5) have several physiological actions: to relax smooth muscle, to stimulate cardiac muscle, to stimulate the nervous

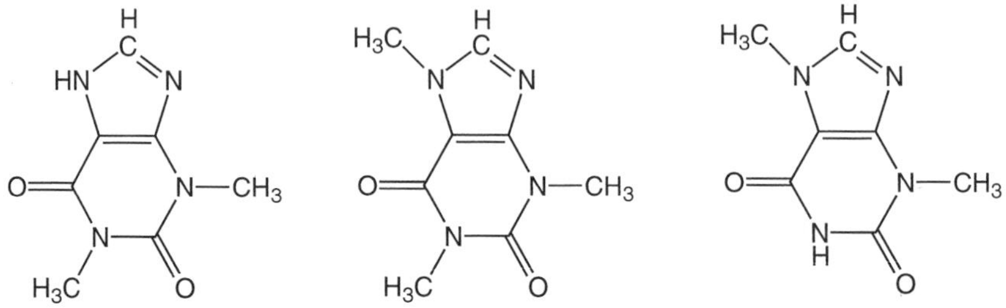

Theophylline   Caffeine   Theobromine

FIGURE 18–5. Chemical structures of the methylated xanthines theophylline, caffeine, and theobromine.

system, and to induce urine formation by the kidney (diuresis). These naturally occurring drugs vary in their specific actions on each of the target organs. The drug **theophylline** has an action more specific to the relaxation of bronchial smooth muscle, which is a desirable effect for the treatment of symptoms of bronchospasm in asthma. Theophylline is found naturally along with caffeine in tea leaves. **Caffeine** is abundant in coffee beans and is frequently added to soft drinks. **Theobromine** is found with caffeine in the seeds of cocoa. Although there is some bronchial-relaxing action from caffeine and theobromine, these two compounds do not have as potent an action as does theophylline in bronchodilatation. They also have undesired side effects (particularly in stimulating the nervous system and the heart) that limit their effective medical use in treatment of asthma.

Theophylline can be administered intravenously for correction of acute exacerbations of asthma or orally for the prevention of acute asthmatic episodes. Oral preparations are available as liquid for quick absorption or as tablets with longer periods for peak absorption. In addition to widespread use for asthma, theophylline also has applications for the treatment of patients with chronic obstructive lung disease, in which there are components of bronchoconstriction. In newborns, the disorder of neonatal apnea (episodes of failure to have spontaneous respirations) can be treated with theophylline due to its ability to stimulate respiration, probably directly through the central nervous system. The levels of theophylline in the blood necessary to treat neonatal apnea are significantly lower (under 10 μg/mL) than those necessary to treat asthmatic symptoms.

Theophylline is widely distributed in extracellular fluid and tissues without entry into red blood cells. Desired therapeutic range for theophylline in serum is 10 to 20 μg/mL. Over that range there is continuously increasing improvement of pulmonary function (frequently quantitated as the 1-second forced expiratory volume—FEV_1) with increasing concentration of theophylline. Unfortunately, toxic symptoms such as nausea, vomiting, and abdominal irritation can occur at levels of theophylline above 20 µg/mL, and above 30µg/mL seizures, cardiac arrhythmias, respiratory arrest, or cardiac arrest may occur. Because of these toxicities, theophylline cannot simply be given indiscriminately. The best predictor of theophylline toxicity is the blood level of the drug and not early signs or symptoms of toxicity.

The mechanism of action of theophylline is to induce smooth muscle relaxation by inhibition of the intracellular enzyme phosphodiesterase, which degrades 3',5'-cyclic AMP (cAMP), the second messenger or mediator of many peptide hormone actions (see Chapter 16). High levels of cAMP cause the smooth muscle around bronchioles to relax, and theophylline allows concentrations of cAMP to build up by inhibiting phosphodiesterase.

Another drug class frequently used alone or in conjunction with theophylline is that of the **beta-adrenergic agents** such as **epinephrine** (usually given by subcutaneous injection to break an acute bronchospasm), **metaproterenol** *(Alupent),* or **albuterol** *(Salbutamol, Ventolin, Proventil).* These latter two drugs can be administered orally in liquid solution or as inhalants. Albuterol has a greater specificity for the beta-2-adrenergic receptors located in the bronchiolar smooth muscle and less affinity for the adrenergic receptors (beta-1) that are found in myocardium. These adrenergic agents also work by increasing intracellular levels of cAMP, as does theophylline, but the adrenergic agents result in an increase in the rate of cAMP production rather than a decrease in its rate of degradation. For that reason, the adrenergic agents and theophylline are synergistic in their effects and can be used in combination to produce a greater therapeutic result, while avoiding the toxicities associated with too great a dose of either drug alone.

Asthmatic symptoms of bronchoconstriction and excess mucus production with wheezing and coughing can be induced by several stimuli: allergens, exercise, cold, emotion, or infection. A common chemical mediator of asthma is histamine, which is found in mast cells in the lungs and is released by one or more of those stimuli. Both theophylline and the adrenergic agents have pharmacologic action that is effective after the physiological step of histamine release. Modern therapeutic approaches to management of asthma have the goal of preventing the release of histamine by administration of glucocorticoid steroids or other medications that modulate the immune response. In severe acute asthmatic attacks, oral prednisone is administered for several days to stabilize the inflammatory response in the patient's lungs. Daily maintenance therapy has shifted in recent years from oral theophylline or aerosol bronchodilators to aerosol inhalers with potent steroids. Although theophylline dosing requires therapeutic monitoring of concentrations in blood, the use of steroids does not.

The half-life of theophylline in the circulation differs according to the preparation and route of administration. Intravenous infusion of theophylline allows the full dose to be available immediately to the liver for metabolism and fastest clearance. Oral administration delays the peak level by 1 to 2 hours. Liquid solutions of theophylline taken by mouth are absorbed much faster than special slow-absorbing solid formulations of theophylline that dissolve over a period of hours in the intestine (*Slo-Phyllin, Theo-Dur*). These latter slow-absorbing preparations are particularly useful in achieving relatively constant blood levels of theophylline between doses spaced up to 12 hours apart.

The age and medical status of the patient can also play a major role in serum half-life. For a given dose of theophylline (usually calculated initially on the basis of body weight), children before puberty have a shorter half-life of the drug (2 to 10 hours, mean of roughly 4 hours) than do older children and adults (4 to 16 hours, mean of roughly 9 hours). Neonates and premature infants can have half-lives for theophylline of 24 to 30 hours. These differences in clearance rates are due primarily to variation in the metabolism of theophylline by the liver. Theophylline is metabolized by oxidation and methylation in the liver to inert products that are then excreted into the urine. An immature liver cannot enzymatically convert theophylline as efficiently as a mature one. Conversely, individuals who smoke cigarettes typically induce more enzyme formation and are able to metabolize theophylline more rapidly than nonsmokers. Patients with liver dysfunction or cardiac abnormalities that compromise the delivery of blood to the liver have a prolonged theophylline half-life. The macrolide antibiotics (e.g., erythromycin) compete with theophylline for the hepatic enzymes. Consequently, administration of these antibiotics along with theophylline can prolong its half-life. Fever by itself apparently can also reduce hepatic metabolism of theophylline. Gastrointestinal disturbances such as vomiting or diarrhea may also lend a factor of uncertainty as to how much theophylline has actually been absorbed from a given oral dose, even though the patient has been successfully managed on a maintenance dose for months or years. Increases of dosage of theophylline may be amplified out of proportion in the blood level due to saturation of the metabolic clearance pathways. For example, to achieve a doubling of the blood level, it may only be necessary to increase the dose by 25 to 50%. This process obviously should be monitored, so as to avoid slipping into a toxic range.

CARDIAC DRUGS

Digoxin

Cardiac glycosides have been used for many years in the form of dried leaves from the foxglove plant to treat the disease termed **dropsy (pedal edema).** The cardiac glycosides contain a steroid nucleus to which are attached sugars plus an unsaturated lactone ring. **Digoxin** differs from digitoxin by a hydroxyl group at position 12 (Fig. 18–6). Because of that

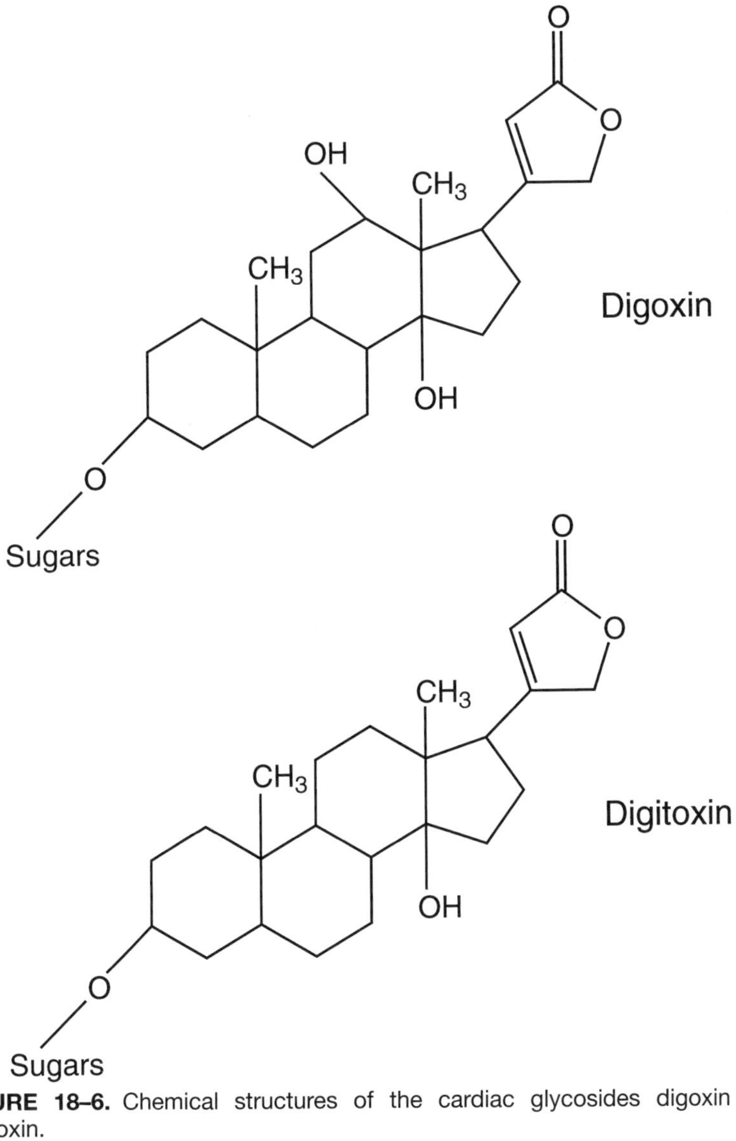

FIGURE 18–6. Chemical structures of the cardiac glycosides digoxin and digitoxin.

chemical difference, only about one-fifth of digoxin in serum is bound to proteins, whereas about 97% of digitoxin is bound to proteins. Coupling that phenomenon with tissue distributions of the two drugs and their interactions with receptors, it is necessary to achieve about tenfold the concentration of digitoxin to achieve the same pharmacologic effect as from a particular concentration of digoxin.

The action of cardiac glycosides such as digoxin is twofold. First, these agents increase the force and velocity of myocardial contraction, thereby reversing the pathologic effect of congestive heart failure. In this clinical setting, a diuretic is also commonly administered in order to reduce body water and electrolyte load. In that instance, the possible induction of hypokalemia (low serum potassium) and hypomagnesemia (low serum magnesium) may heighten the sensitivity of myocardial muscle to irritation from digoxin with development of cardiac arrhythmias. Interestingly, the second major clinical use of digoxin is for the control of cardiac arrhythmias by limiting conduction of pulses through the atrioventricular (AV) node during atrial fibrillation or flutter. Because of the possibility that a cardiac arrhythmia may be due either to underdosing of digoxin (digitalization) or to overdigitalization, the actual diagnosis and plan of action may rest entirely on chemical measurements of digoxin concentration and electrolytes. The toxicities resulting from digoxin overdose include premature ventricular contractions, atrial-ventricular dissociation with complete heart block, paroxysmal atrial tachycardia, ventricular fibrillation, congestive heart failure, gastrointestinal effects (nausea and vomiting), and neurologic effects (headache, fatigue, disorientation, visual disturbances, and convulsions). In addition to electrolyte abnormalities, hypothyroidism, severe ischemic heart disease, and diminished renal function also predispose to toxicities from the cardiac glycosides. The diagnosis of intoxication with digoxin should also include electrocardiogram as well as laboratory examinations.

Digoxin is generally given orally, although intravenous bolus administration is also available to achieve rapid digitalization of patients to control critical cardiac dysfunction. Absorption from the gastrointestinal tract is usually satisfactory to achieve therapeutic levels, although the efficiency of absorbing different compounds (e.g., digoxin versus digitoxin) can vary considerably. Initial digitalization of a patient not previously taking a cardiac glycoside may be achieved by administering a loading dose followed by regularly spaced maintenance doses intended to keep blood levels within a prescribed range. There are many ways to accomplish this initial digitalization, including a combination of sufficient intravenous and oral doses to arrive at therapeutic concentrations quickly while taking care to avoid toxicities to a diseased (and thus sensitized) heart.

To perform correct therapeutic monitoring of cardiac glycosides, it is necessary to know which form the patient is receiving because the therapeutic range for each drug can be markedly different. For example, the range for digoxin is 0.5 to 2.0 ng/mL; for digitoxin, the range is 10 to 25 ng/mL. Thus, a reading of 5.0 ng/mL would be toxic for digoxin but subtherapeutic for digitoxin. In addition, the timing of blood collection after last dose can be critical to interpretation of digoxin levels. The half-life of digoxin is roughly one and a half days in persons with normal renal and hepatic function. Most of the digoxin is excreted unmetabolized in the urine. Digitoxin has a much longer half-life of up to 5 days with a substantial portion metabolized in the liver and excreted in bile. These clearance times mean that single oral daily doses are probably adequate to maintain blood levels within therapeutic range at all times. With oral doses, the blood level climbs slowly to ultimate steady-state values. However, intravenous administration of digoxin results in an immediate and very high circulating level before the drug equilibrates in the tissues of the heart, where it has pharmacologic effect. Contrary to the case of theophylline, a sudden rise in digoxin level in the blood does not have an immediate therapeutic effect. In fact, there is a distribution phase in which intravenously administered digoxin moves quickly out of the blood and into the tissues. Digoxin then is eliminated much more slowly from the body. Thus, it is erroneous to collect a blood specimen for digoxin measurement soon after intravenous digoxin infusion because the value obtained will be high, but it cannot be interpreted as toxic. The proper protocol to use in monitoring intravenous digoxin therapy is to wait *at least 6 hours* after bolus injection and then collect the blood. This precaution need not be so stringently applied with oral dosing of digoxin. (In our experience, mistimed collection of blood samples for digoxin measurement too soon after intravenous bolus administration is the single most frequently encountered error in therapeutic drug monitoring. Not only does it produce results that are impossible to interpret, but it puts unnecessary financial burdens on patients and medical institutions.)

Antiarrhythmic Agents

The use of digoxin to control cardiac arrhythmias is limited to atrial (supraventricular) arrhythmias: digoxin blocks the conduction of atrial-generated impulses through the AV node to the ventricles. However, it is the ventricular arrhythmias that are potentially more serious than the atrial ones because they may lead to sustained rhythmic disorders such as ventricular tachycardia, fibrillation, or asystole, which can be fatal. For these, several different antiarrhythmic agents are therapeutically monitored frequently. These drugs include **disopyramide** *(Norpace),* **lidocaine, procainamide, quinidine,** and **amiodarone.** They generally are effective in the control of both atrial and ventricular arrhythmias, although not all are approved for both kinds. The ventricular arrhythmias of concern are unifocal and multifocal premature ventricular contractions, paired ventricular contractions, and episodic ventricular tachycardia.

Although there are variations in the precise mechanisms of each one, the antiarrhythmic drugs decrease membrane excitability and increase conduction times, thereby decreasing cardiac automaticity (inappropriate and disordered excitation of the heart in local regions, out of the normal sequence of transmission from atrium to ventricle). By prolonging the time for cardiac membrane excitability, the force of contraction is improved.

Disopyramide

Generally **disopyramide** is reserved for use in ventricular arrhythmias. It also exhibits some anticholinergic effects that may add to its antiarrhythmic action by blocking vagal stimulation of the sinus node. Its side effects are due largely to its anticholinergic properties, including dryness of mouth, nose, throat, and eyes; urinary retention; blurred vision; abdominal bloating and pain; constipation; hypotension; syncope; and mental depression. Rarely, a cardiac arrhythmia may also be induced. Therapeutic concentrations are in the range of 3 to 5 µg/mL, with toxicity possible above 7 µg/mL. Clearance is primarily via the liver and kidneys, with a half-life of 4 to 10 hours in individuals who have normal hepatic and renal function.

Lidocaine

In addition to being a cardiac antiarrhythmic drug, **lidocaine** also has been used clinically as a local anesthetic *(Xylocaine)* for many years. It now is widely used for treatment of ventricular arrhythmias that arise after acute myocardial infarction or from other myocardial damage or irritation. It is useful for counteracting the arrhythmias induced by digoxin toxicity. Lidocaine toxicity is manifested by cardiovascular findings of hypotension, bradyarrhythmias, or asystole and by a wide array of central nervous system changes, including paresthesias, confusion, dysarthria, agitation, convulsions, and coma.

Therapeutic concentrations of lidocaine are 1.5 to 5 µg/mL, with potential toxicity above that range. Lidocaine may be 70% or more bound to albumin and alpha-1-acid glycoprotein (AAG) in serum. Patients who do not show expected clinical response to normally therapeutic concentrations of lidocaine and are not toxic may have elevated circulating levels of AAG that bind and keep lidocaine inactive. These patients may require higher than usual therapeutic levels to show a response. Plasma half-life is 1 to 2 hours, with metabolism and clearance by the liver. Patients with hepatic failure may have markedly prolonged half-life of lidocaine.

Quinidine

A plant alkaloid that derives from the cinchona bark, **quinidine** has been recognized for over 200 years for its action as an antiarrhythmic. It has cardiac depressant properties that limit cardiac excitability, conduction, automaticity, and (although not always desirable) contractility. Quinidine is now employed for both supraventricular and ventricular arrhythmias. It has the undesired effect of increasing the ventricular response (i.e., enhancing the conduction of impulses through the AV junction). Therefore, quinidine administration may be deferred until digoxin can be given to block this undesired AV conduction enhancement in cases of atrial flutter or fibrillation. Quinidine has many clinical applications, both for treatment and prevention (e.g., prior to elective electric shock cardioversion or after acute myocardial infarction) of arrhythmias.

Side effects of quinidine may occur in one-fifth to one-third of patients. Primary symptoms of toxicity affect the gastrointestinal tract with anorexia, nausea, vomiting, abdominal irritability, and diarrhea. These toxic effects can arise from either oral or intravenous administration of quinidine. The syndrome **cinchonism** consists of blurred vision, disturbed hearing with tinnitus, vertigo, and nervous tremor from excess combination therapy with quinidine and digitalis. Because of its long-term use, quinidine has many other recognized (albeit somewhat rare) adverse effects, including hypersensitivities with fever, rash, thrombocytopenia, and even anaphylactic shock. Cardiac side effects include arrhythmias.

Therapeutic levels of quinidine are 2.3 to 5 µg/mL with potentially toxic levels above 5 µg/mL. Half-life is 2 to 16 hours (average, 6 hours) with metabolism and clearance by the liver.

Procainamide (Pronestyl)

This drug has very potent actions in controlling both supraventricular and ventricular arrhythmias. **Procainamide** is typically used for patients with life-threatening arrhythmias who have not achieved satisfactory results from lidocaine. It can be administered either orally or intravenously, but has a short half-life that necessitates frequent dosing to maintain therapeutic levels. Procainamide is converted by acetylation in the liver to N-acetylprocainamide (NAPA), which is also fully active and recirculates into the blood. Procainamide and NAPA are cleared by the kidneys with different half-lives: 3 to 5 hours for procainamide and 6 to 10 hours for NAPA. Thus, as a patient receives successive doses of procainamide, NAPA levels continue to build up. Immunoassays for procainamide do not detect NAPA; consequently, separate quantitation of NAPA is necessary. The total effective concentration should be calculated as the sum of procainamide plus NAPA and should be in the range of 10 to 30 µg/mL.

Not all patients acetylate procainamide at the same rate, which has unfortunate implications for predicting patient drug response. Some individuals with large amounts of hepatic N-acetyltransferase are termed "fast acetylators," and produce substantially more NAPA for a given level of procainamide than do individuals with smaller amounts of the transferase ("slow acetylators"). The situation is made more complex in renal failure, in which levels of procainamide may be greatly exceeded by those of NAPA due to failure of clearance. It can be very useful for the clinician planning dosage schedules to determine the specific kinetics of procainamide clearance for each patient by measuring drug levels two or three times during a single dose cycle.

Adverse effects of procainamide include bradycardia, hypotension, arrhythmias, nausea, vomiting, and mild neurologic symptoms of malaise and confusion. Long-term use of procainamide may result in systemic lupus erythematosus, which is usually reversible within months of discontinuing the drug.

Amiodarone

Amiodarone *(Cordarone)* is an antiarrhythmic drug used to treat life-threatening ventricular tachyarrhythmias that have been unresponsive to other, less toxic agents. It is typically administered only to hospitalized patients. Serum half-life is extremely variable, ranging from 13 to over 100 days, so monitoring is important when the administration period is lengthy. Amiodarone is eliminated through hepatic excretion. Side effects include pulmonary fibrosis, deterioration of congestive heart failure, neuromuscular weakness or tremor, and thyroid abnormality. Therapeutic range is 1.0 to 2.5 µg/mL.

ANTIBIOTICS

Most antibiotics act specifically against bacterial metabolic processes that are unique to bacteria and that do not have exact counterparts in the human host. Because they tend to be metabolically inert in humans, large amounts of many antibiotics can be administered to patients without adverse effects. **Penicillins, cephalosporins,** and **erythromycin** fall into this category, although idiosyncratic drug reactions are possible (often on an allergic basis), in which adverse effects are not related to antibiotic concentration. However, some antibiotics have been found to have toxic effects with predictable regularity if their concentrations remain high in the blood for an extended time. These toxic effects are not directly related to the drug's antibacterial action. Because it is necessary to achieve prolonged minimal inhibitory concentrations of antibiotics in blood and infected tissues in order to treat infections effectively, close therapeutic monitoring for toxicity is required.

One class of antibiotics for which therapeutic monitoring is essential is the **aminoglycosides.** These antibiotics have a broad spectrum of antibacterial activity but have special utility for many gram-negative infections. **Gentamicin** and **tobramycin** are chemically similar aminoglycosides and have parallel antibacterial actions. The aminoglycosides act by attaching to bacterial ribosomes, thereby interfering with bacterial protein synthesis. Bacterial resistance may be acquired by transfer of an R factor that encodes an enzyme capable of inactivating the antibiotic. Because of the variety of enzymes, each with slightly different inactivating properties, such resistance to one aminoglycoside may not inhibit other aminoglycosides. **Kanamycin** and the chemically similar **amikacin** are sometimes effective even when there is resistance to gentamicin or tobramycin. These sensitivities must be individually determined on each bacterial isolate in separate culture. The normal route of excretion of aminoglycosides is through the urine (see also Chapter 13).

Experts disagree about the appropriate parameter to monitor in aminoglycoside therapy: peak levels, trough levels, both levels, or the integrated area under the concentration-time curve. For moderate infections, lower levels of amikacin and kanamycin may be sufficient (peak, 20 to 25 µg/mL; trough, 1 to 4 µg/mL), but life-threatening infections may require higher levels (peak, 25 to 30 µg/mL; trough, 5 to 8 µg/mL). Above peaks of 30 µg/mL and troughs of 8 µg/mL, toxicity may occur. For gentamicin and tobramycin, these levels are scaled down slightly, with therapeutic peaks of 6 to 10 µg/mL and troughs of 0.5 to 1.5 µg/mL; toxicity can occur at peaks above 12 to 15 µg/mL and troughs >2 µg/mL.

Aminoglycosides cause two primary toxicities: **ototoxicity** (nerve deafness) in which the eighth cranial nerve may be irreversibly damaged, and **nephrotoxicity** due to proximal renal tubular damage. Nephrotoxicity can be looked for as a rise in blood urea nitrogen (BUN) and creatinine in serum. If caught early, nephrotoxicity may be reversible by discontinuing the antibiotic. A better means of predicting toxicity before onset is to monitor drug levels directly and to lower dosage accordingly if necessary. Special consideration should be given to patients with renal failure, whose ability to clear aminoglycosides is severely impaired. These antibiotics may be very useful for treating infections acquired from peritoneal dialysis or other procedures, and these patients should certainly have aminoglycoside levels measured.

Recently a new approach for administering large doses of aminoglycosides on an infrequent basis has gained acceptance. This administration technique (termed "once-daily" aminoglycosides) is designed to optimize concentration-dependent bactericidal action and also to take advantage of the postantibiotic effect of aminoglycosides absorbed by bacteria. In addition, nephrotoxicity is apparently reduced with this dosing because uptake of aminoglycosides into kidney tissue is saturable, so less frequent dosing leads to less accumulation in renal tubules. Less frequent dosing of aminoglycosides does not require therapeutic monitoring; if it is performed, peak values will ostensibly appear toxic, and trough levels may be undetectable.

Normal serum half-life of gentamicin for adults is 0.5 to 3 hours, with older individuals showing even longer half-lives (up to 15 hours). Amikacin's half-life normally ranges from 1 to 7 hours.

Vancomycin is a tricyclic glycopeptide antibiotic with a broad spectrum of antibacterial activity. It works by inhibiting bacterial cell wall synthesis and also affects membrane permeability and RNA synthesis. Its therapeutic range is 18 to 26 µg/mL for peak and 5 to 10 µg/mL for trough levels. Vancomycin may have potential for ototoxicity and nephrotoxicity, especially when administered with aminoglycosides.

Vancomycin should be reserved for use intravenously in patients with serious infections due to sensitive staphylococci or other gram-positive bacteria. It is poorly absorbed from the gastrointestinal tract, and so oral vancomycin can be used to treat pseudomembranous colitis caused by *Clostridium difficile*. Vancomycin has been used extensively for treating many infections in high-risk patients such as those receiving chemotherapy or having indwelling catheters. It is also used for prophylaxis in many arenas such as cardiac and orthopedic surgery. Unfortunately, vancomycin-resistant enterococci now appear regularly in response to such widespread use.

ANTIEPILEPTIC DRUGS

Antiepileptic drugs are used to treat seizure disorders. In the unmedicated state, seizures may occur with great frequency or only occasionally. If they are frequent, the dosage of an anticonvulsant drug can be clinically titrated based on its success in reducing the frequency of seizures or in eliminating them altogether. However, if a patient has only a few seizures per year without medication, reduction in seizure frequency is not feasible as an endpoint by which to adjust dosage. In this instance, it is particularly desirable to have information regarding blood levels of an anticonvulsant drug in order to document adequate medical control.

The choice of which anticonvulsant drug to administer is guided by the clinical situation: for example, petit mal seizures, grand mal seizures, or seizures due to acute injury or alcohol withdrawal. The major anticonvulsant drugs in clinical application today are **phenytoin** *(Dilantin)*, **barbiturates (phenobarbital** and **primidone** *[Mysoline]*), **diazepam** *(Valium)*, **carbamazepine** *(Tegretol)*, **ethosuximide** *(Zarontin)*, and **valproic acid** *(Depakene)*.

Phenytoin

Phenytoin is the anticonvulsant drug most frequently prescribed for control of seizure disorders (Fig. 18–7). Variations in the metabolism of phenytoin between different individuals can lead to widely different serum levels after oral doses. For that reason, therapeutic monitoring of

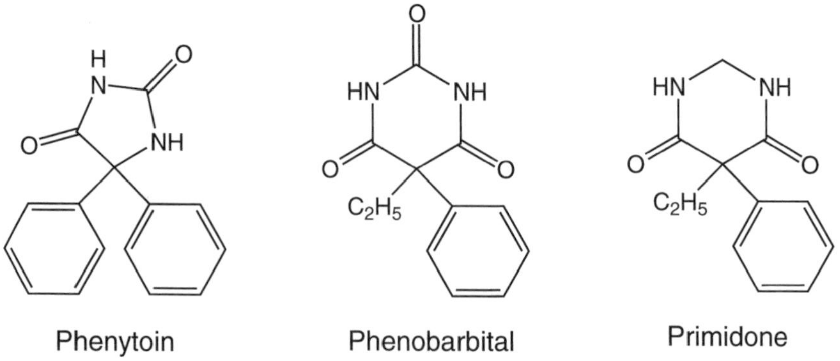

Phenytoin   Phenobarbital   Primidone

FIGURE 18–7. Chemical structures of the antiepileptic drugs phenytoin, phenobarbital, and primidone.

phenytoin is widely applied. This drug has been used for over 50 years as an anticonvulsant in tonic-clonic epilepsy, as well as in focal seizures and the more complex seizures such as psychomotor. It is frequently used in treatment of status epilepticus (i.e., the acute state of an uncontrolled seizure) to achieve rapid control. It is apparently not effective for relieving petit mal seizure activity. Although the cellular and biochemical mechanisms of its action are not known, phenytoin is recognized to depress seizure activity, especially in motor cortex of the brain.

Phenytoin can generally be used as the sole agent for treating patients with epilepsy. Those who remain refractory to phenytoin alone may be treated with an additional anticonvulsant drug. Therapeutic levels of phenytoin in serum are in the range of 10 to 20 μg/mL, with toxicity potentially occurring at concentrations above 20 μg/mL. The half-life of phenytoin in adults is 20 to 40 hours, whereas in children it is 4 to 11 hours, owing to differences in metabolic clearance by the liver. Premature neonates can have a much longer half-life for phenytoin (e.g., 75 to 140 hours).

The metabolism of phenytoin consists of hydroxylation and conjugation with glucuronic acid (parahydroxyphenylhydantoin or HPPH) in the liver, followed by excretion into the urine. Because the capacity of the liver to metabolize phenytoin is limited, increments in dosage can saturate the hepatic pathways, leading to unexpectedly high blood levels of the drug. Thus adjustment of dosage should be done with therapeutic drug monitoring for guidance.

After a half-century of clinical use, phenytoin has many well-recognized clinical side effects. The immediate toxicities of overdose are primarily related to the central nervous system and include blurring of vision, nystagmus, dysarthria, ataxia, and drowsiness progressing to coma or to cardiac conduction disturbance. Long-term adverse effects include skin changes (acne and hirsutism), gingival hyperplasia (leading to dental problems), lymphoid hyperplasia (which may be confused with lymphoma), interference with hepatic metabolism of vitamin D (resulting in impaired calcification of bone and osteomalacia), and hypersensitivity reactions. There is some thought that phenytoin may have adverse effects on peripheral nerves and on cells of the cerebellum. It almost certainly has some teratogenic action, resulting largely in cleft lip and cleft palate when used in pregnancy.

Absorption of phenytoin can be affected by the formulation of the drug preparation and by its route of administration. Phenytoin is available as a sodium salt in liquid suspension or as tablets (including chewable ones for children). It is generally well absorbed in the small intestine. Acid in the stomach keeps phenytoin relatively insoluble, and it is not absorbed until it reaches the more alkaline conditions of the small intestine. Peak levels occur about 3 to 9 hours after oral administration. Parenteral administration is also complicated by phenytoin's solubility properties. Intravenous administration of phenytoin is recommended to control acute seizure activity, taking care that the rate of administration is slow enough to avoid disturbance of respiration and cardiac conduction.

Within the blood, about 90% of phenytoin is protein bound. The remaining amount is free and representative of the active drug fraction. Bilirubin or various drugs (e.g., salicylates, valproic acid, sulfonylureas, dicumerol, and phenylbutazone) can interfere with the binding of phenytoin to the major plasma protein, albumin. Thus a seemingly therapeutic level of total (free plus protein-bound) phenytoin in serum may actually be toxic if the concentration of albumin is reduced (e.g., liver or renal failure) or if the patient is receiving other drugs. To determine the active drug level, it is possible to prepare a protein-free filtrate of serum and measure the free phenytoin level (therapeutic range 1 to 2 μg/mL) directly in it by immunoassay.

Diazepam

Diazepam is a sedative drug and a member of the benzodiazepine class of tranquilizers (Fig. 18–8). It is used extensively as a hypnotic agent, as an antianxiety agent, or as a muscle relaxant (for skeletal muscle spasms). It is also frequently used for the immediate control of seizure activity by intravenous injection in the emergency situation or in acute alcohol withdrawal. Diazepam has dramatic short-term effects on the central nervous system, but it is not useful for long-term management of seizure disorders. Furthermore, it has strong potential for abuse and the development of drug dependence. Clinically diazepam is used largely for rapid control of acute seizure activity, followed by a change to another anticonvulsant such as phenytoin.

Diazepam is metabolized to the active compound **nordiazepam.** Drug levels are calculated as the sum of diazepam plus nordiazepam concentrations (determined by HPLC). Therapeutic range is up to about 2 μg/mL, with toxicities (central nervous system depression; cardiac and respiratory arrest) potentially occurring at levels above 5 μg/mL.

Alprazolam *(Xanax)* (see Fig. 18–8) is a related triazolobenzodiazepine that has short-acting antidepressant and anxiolytic actions. It is used to treat disorders such as agoraphobia and panic attacks. Peak blood levels occur roughly 1 hour after oral administration. Therapeutic levels are 10 to 50 μg/L in serum. Toxicities appear at levels above 75 μg/L. Both diazepam and alprazolam have high potential for abuse.

Phenobarbital and Primidone

These two barbiturates are frequently used for the treatment of generalized tonic-clonic seizure activity, psychomotor seizures, and focal epileptic seizures, but not in petit mal seizures. **Primidone** is converted in the body to **phenobarbital,** and thus the action and monitoring of these

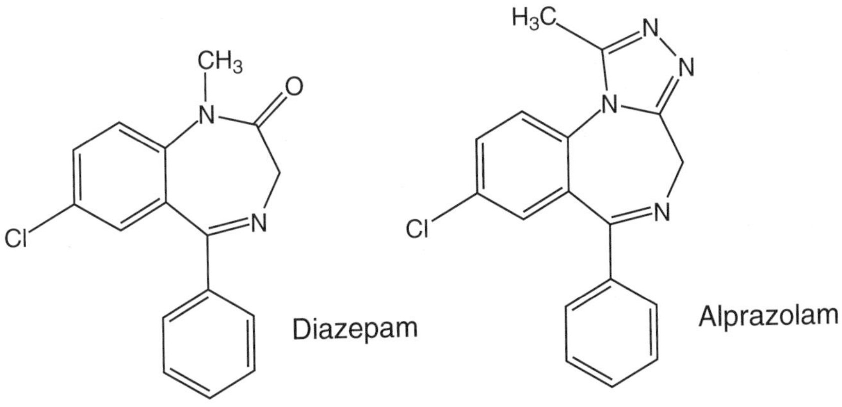

FIGURE 18–8. Chemical structures of the benzodiazepine diazepam and the triazolobenzodiazepine alprazolam.

two drugs are considered to be very much the same (see Fig. 18–7). The drug action of both primidone and phenobarbital is a decrease in the threshold of nerve cell stimulation in the motor cortex, thereby inhibiting spread of electrical activity (discharge) from a focus of epileptic activity in the brain.

These drugs have a sedative side effect, although they may induce the paradoxical effect of hyperactivity in children. Additional adverse effects from excess dosing include nausea, vomiting, vertigo, ataxia, lethargy, and coma. Tolerance to these side effects increases with chronic therapy. There is potential for drug abuse and dependency with barbiturates.

Metabolism of primidone and phenobarbital occurs in the liver with hydroxylation and conjugation to sulfate or glucuronic acid, followed by renal excretion. The half-life of phenobarbital is from 50 to over 100 hours. The half-life of primidone ranges from 3 to 20 hours. Therefore, in primidone therapy, monitoring can be accomplished either by measuring levels of both drugs, or by relying on phenobarbital levels alone.

After oral administration, there is good absorption from both the stomach and small intestine, with peak levels occurring 2 to 20 hours later. Therapeutic levels for adults are roughly 20 to 40 µg/mL (phenobarbital) and 5 to 12 µg/mL (primidone), with slightly lower levels being effective in children.

The many potential interactions between phenobarbital and other drugs can occur as the result of inducing hepatic enzymes that enhance drug metabolism or in response to competing with hepatic enzymes, thereby slowing drug metabolism. Excretion is facilitated by alkalinization of the urine. Acidification of urine by co-administration of valproic acid can delay phenobarbital clearance. For these reasons, it is essential to establish correct dosage of primidone and phenobarbital by monitoring serum concentrations when other drugs are co-administered.

Other barbiturates commonly used in clinical practice include intermediate-acting amobarbital and butabarbital and short-acting pentobarbital and secobarbital. The onset and duration of action of the different barbiturates is related to how each distributes throughout the body, largely according to its relative membrane solubility.

Carbamazepine

Carbamazepine is chemically similar to the tricyclic antidepressants. It is effective for controlling grand mal and psychomotor seizures, but its particular advantage is in relieving the pain associated with trigeminal neuralgia. Its mechanism of action is probably related to a reduction in synaptic transmission in the spinal cord. For that reason it is also used in treating seizures in which there are components of pain.

The side effects of carbamazepine include neurologic alterations related to drug levels (visual and vestibular changes; ataxia; nausea and vomiting), and chronic adverse reactions such as rash, hematologic failure (agranulocytosis), and hepatic failure.

Metabolism of the drug is by way of the liver, and its half-life is 5 to 25 hours. Carbamazepine can induce its own metabolism in the liver, thereby reducing effective bioavailable levels, while a patient remains on what was a previously therapeutic regimen. As with other anticonvulsants whose clearance is dependent on protein-binding, hepatic function, and co-administration of other drugs, therapeutic monitoring of carbamazepine is a requisite to establishing correct dosages.

Therapeutic levels of carbamazepine range from 8 to 12 µg/mL but are slightly lower if the patient is also receiving another anticonvulsant.

Ethosuximide

Ethosuximide (a succinimide) has primary clinical use for the control of petit mal (or absence) seizures. These absence disorders consist of incidents in which the patient has brief loss of awareness without convulsion. They may be associated with minor motor actions such as body motion, shift in position, blinking of the eyes, or a habitual action. These petit mal seizures occur without warning and last a few seconds each. There is a strong correlation with a unique high voltage spiking pattern on the electroencephalogram for confirmation of diagnosis. Patients who have petit mal seizure activity may also suffer from grand mal seizures and thus require ethosuximide and other anticonvulsant therapy concurrently.

Adverse effects include gastrointestinal disturbances that improve with chronicity of therapy (as do mild mental changes), although psychotic episodes have been associated with ethosuximide. Other chronic adverse effects include rash and, rarely, leukopenia.

The liver probably metabolizes ethosuximide into multiple inactive compounds that are then excreted into the urine. Clearance is slower in children than in adults, so that children can achieve therapeutic concentrations with lower dosages. The drug's half-life is about 60 hours for adults and 30 hours for children. The therapeutic range for ethosuximide is 40 to 100 µg/mL, with potential toxicity above 100 µg/mL.

Valproic Acid

Valproic acid is chemically unusual as an anticonvulsant in that it consists of a simple branched fatty acid (an eight-carbon carboxylic acid) without a nitrogen atom or aromatic group. It is thought to act by increasing concentrations of the inhibitory neurotransmitter gamma-aminobutyric acid (GABA) in the brain. Valproic acid is used clinically to control a broad spectrum of seizures including grand mal, petit mal, and complex partial.

Valproic acid is absorbed well after dosing with capsules or syrup, and it can also be administered rectally. Its side effects are primarily related to gastrointestinal disturbances, and it may cause pancreatitis. Valproic acid is extensively metabolized by the liver and excreted into the urine. Parent drug half-life is 5 to 20 hours. It interacts with a variety of other drugs. For instance, used in conjunction with phenobarbital, valproic acid inhibits hepatic metabolism; concomitant use with phenytoin displaces the latter from plasma proteins.

Therapeutic monitoring of valproic acid is complicated by its volatility: it may evaporate from a serum sample kept in the open. It is conveniently measured either by gas liquid chromatography or by immunoassay. Therapeutic levels of valproic acid are 50 to 100 µg/mL.

Gabapentin

Gabapentin *(Neurontin)* is 1-(aminomethyl)cyclohexaneacetic acid, an anticonvulsant that has recently come into clinical use. It is chemically similar to the neurotransmitter GABA, but it does not interact with the GABA receptor nor does it interfere with other GABA functions; its mechanism of action is unknown.

Gabapentin is administered orally. Its bioavailability decreases with increasing dose, but with the usual doses of 300 to 600 mg three times a day, bioavailability is roughly 60% with no effect from food. It circulates mostly unbound to plasma proteins. Gabapentin is not metabolized in humans, but rather is excreted unchanged in the urine. Its half-life can range from 6.5 hours in patients with normal creatinine clearance to over 50 hours in patients with renal impairment. Hepatic disease apparently causes no change in gabapentin clearance.

Gabapentin is used to treat partial seizures in patients over 12 years of age for adjunctive therapy with other antiepileptic drugs. It is generally administered without monitoring serum concentrations, but monitoring can be useful in renal failure or in other clinical situations in which absorption and clearance are atypical. Quantitation is done using gas chromatography. The therapeutic range of gabapentin is 2 to 15 mg/L in serum. Adverse effects most commonly include somnolence, dizziness, ataxia, fatigue, and nystagmus.

Lamotrigine

Lamotrigine *(Lamictal)*, a phenyltriazine, is chemically unrelated to other currently used antiepileptic drugs. It has also recently come into clinical use. Its mechanism of action as an anticonvulsant is unknown but may involve an effect on sodium channels, thereby stabilizing nerve membranes and reducing presynaptic release of the amino acids glutamate and aspartate. Lamotrigine is recommended as adjunctive therapy with other drugs for treatment of partial seizures in adult patients.

Oral doses are readily absorbed, with peak plasma levels occurring between 1.4 and 4.8 hours after administration, unaffected by food. Lamotrigine is metabolized in the liver through conjugation with glucuronic acid and excreted in the urine along with a smaller amount of the parent drug. Metabolism of lamotrigine is hastened by enzyme-inducing antiepileptic drugs such as carbamazepine, phenobarbital, primidone, and phenytoin; valproic acid apparently does not induce those enzymes. Consequently, therapeutic monitoring may be necessary to achieve desired levels when used in combination with other drugs. Lamotrigine is quantitated in serum samples using HPLC. The therapeutic range of lamotrigine is 0.5 to 9.0 mg/L.

Dose-related adverse reactions to lamotrigine include dizziness, ataxia, diplopia, blurred vision, nausea, and vomiting; serious skin rash has also been observed with lamotrigine use.

AGENTS OF CHEMOTHERAPY AND IMMUNOSUPPRESSION

Methotrexate

Many chemotherapeutic agents are presently used for the treatment of neoplasia. For almost all of these drugs, no direct monitoring of blood levels is available except through research protocols in which highly specialized techniques and equipment are used to establish the kinetics of drug concentrations. It is generally assumed that at least minimally therapeutic concentrations are achieved based on dosages that are adjusted according to body weight or body surface area. Toxicities are typically evaluated by regular screening with the CBC (for depression of leukocytes and platelets due to bone marrow toxicity) and with multiphase serum chemistry panels to gauge specific organ damage (e.g., liver and renal function tests). The electrolytes potassium and magnesium may also be depleted after successive doses of cisplatinum. Because toxicity is an expected feature of cancer chemotherapy, comparability of actual levels from patient to patient is not necessarily sought. Instead, possibly lethal side effects are avoided by titrating dosage according to the actual toxicities experienced.

Methotrexate is unusual in that a specific compound (leucovorin, folinic acid) bypasses the effect of methotrexate and thus can be used to minimize toxicities after a period of treatment of malignant cells in the body (Fig. 18–9). Methotrexate inhibits the enzyme dihydrofolate

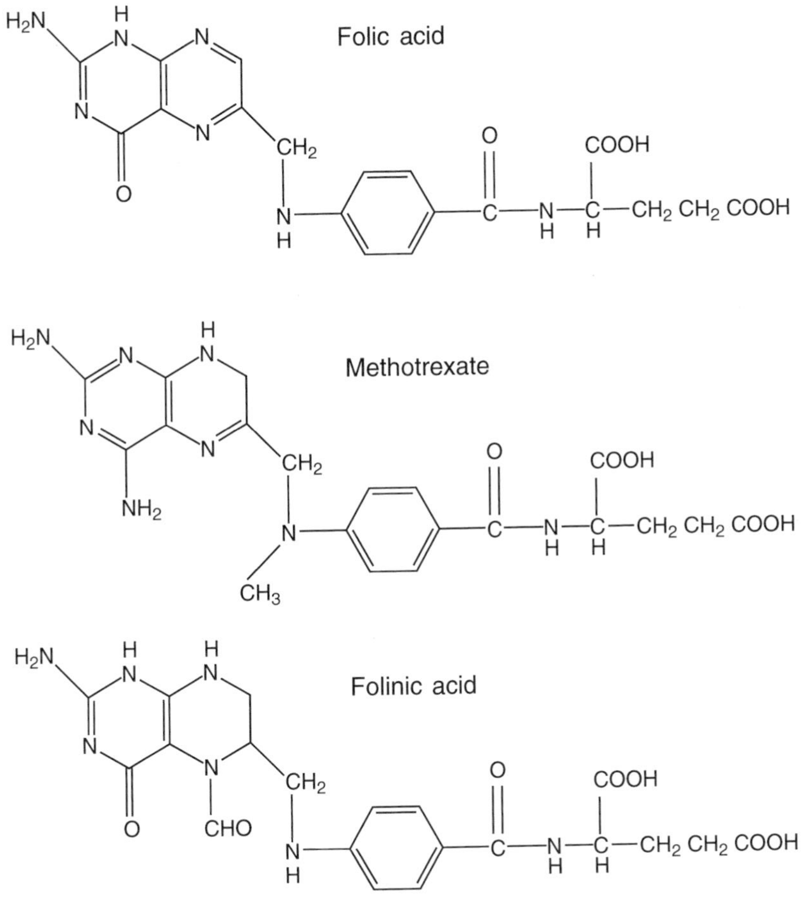

FIGURE 18–9. Chemical structures of the vitamin folic acid, the antimetabolite methotrexate, and the rescue agent folinic acid (leucovorin).

reductase, thereby blocking the metabolism of folic acid to tetrahydrofolate, which in turn is involved in the synthesis of DNA precursors (thymidylate) (see also Chapter 2, Folic Acid Metabolism). In methotrexate therapy, the drug level is assessed at approximately 24 or 48 hours after administration. During that period, both malignant and normal tissues are exposed to methotrexate, but the malignant cells have greater sensitivity to the drug's effect owing to their more frequent nuclear divisions. After this treatment time, leucovorin may be administered to prevent continuing damage to normal cells **(leucovorin rescue)** as long as the serum concentration of methotrexate exceeds a toxic threshold of 0.01 µmol/L. The duration of therapy and other variables are adjusted according to protocols for different solid tumors as well as hematologic malignancies. Methotrexate may also be administered intrathecally to treat leukemic infiltration of the brain, especially in children. Lower doses of methotrexate have been used recently to treat psoriasis and rheumatoid arthritis.

Particular concerns with methotrexate therapy include individual drug clearance rates (predominantly renal), abrupt changes in a patient's clearance rate due to acute renal toxicity, and third-space accumulation of methotrexate that delays its clearance from the body (e.g., in ascites fluid).

Although the minimum cytotoxic concentration in serum is roughly 0.01 µmol/L, adjustment of dose and "rescue therapy" with leucovorin are determined according to the individual cancer chemotherapy protocol. Measurement is done in serum by immunoassay.

Cyclosporine

Cyclosporine *(Sandimmune)* is the major immunosuppressive drug used for prevention of rejection of allogeneic organ transplants. It is a cyclic peptide molecule containing 11 amino acids that are heavily covered with aliphatic side groups, making the drug highly lipophilic. The family of different cyclosporins (e.g., A, C, G, etc.) arises from substitution of different amino acids into the ringed molecule. A single unique amino acid with a side group of seven carbon atoms and one double bond is apparently absolutely necessary in order for a cyclosporin to be immunosuppressive. **Cyclosporin A** is referred to as "cyclosporine" by standard nomenclature.

Cyclosporine selectively inhibits the cellular immune response by blocking production of **interleukin-2 (IL-2),** a growth factor or stimulator of T lymphocytes. These T cells are responsible for the infiltration and rejection of transplanted solid organs (such as kidney, liver, heart, lung, and pancreas) from donors who have different histocompatibility antigens on their cell surfaces than the recipients have on theirs (see Chapter 8, HLA Antigens and Antibodies). Cyclosporine is also administered to bone marrow transplant patients to prevent graft-versus-host disease (GVHD), in which transplanted lymphocytes attack tissues of the recipient.

Cyclosporine exerts its immunosuppressive action by binding to the intracellular protein cyclophilin, one of a group of similar proteins designated **immunophilins** (Fig. 18–10). Another immunosuppressive agent, the macrolide **tacrolimus** *(Prograf)* has an action similar to that of cyclosporine, inhibiting T-cell immunity. Tacrolimus (formerly "FK506") binds to a different immunophilin termed **FK506 binding protein.** These immunophilin-drug complexes interact with the proteins calcineurin and calmodulin to prevent the transcription of interleukin-2 in T cells, thereby leading to suppression of T cells. The precise biochemical action of immunophilins in this process is not proven, although they do exhibit peptide isomerase (or rotamase) activities that are inhibited by both cyclosporine and tacrolimus. Tacrolimus is currently used in a restricted number of transplant centers; it is monitored with immunoassay in whole blood samples.

T lymphocytes normally act in the body to destroy foreign organisms such as fungi, viruses, and some bacteria (e.g., mycobacteria). However, down-regulating the T-lymphocyte response with cyclosporine to prevent rejection of foreign tissues (allogeneic organs) also reduces the ability of the body to counteract infection by these organisms. This acute toxicity of cyclosporine leaves a patient particularly susceptible to infection with *Candida*, cytomegalovirus, or other herpesviruses that are present in latent form in most individuals. Another acute toxicity from cyclosporine is

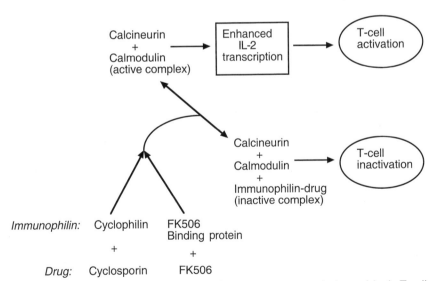

FIGURE 18–10. Mechanism by which immunosuppressant drugs block T-cell activation through inhibition of interleukin-2 (IL-2) transcription.

impairment of renal function, which can be irreversible after months or years of therapy.

A typical clinical problem in cyclosporine administration is to determine whether a rise in serum creatinine is due to acute rejection of a transplanted kidney (because of insufficient immunosuppression) or to toxicity from excess levels of cyclosporine. Within this clinical context, the possibility of infection frequently arises when an immunosuppressed patient develops fever, cough, and other symptoms that could be caused by bacteria (potentially treatable with antibiotics) or by fungi or viruses (for which immunosuppression should be lowered). Thus, physicians caring for transplant patients are constantly monitoring for signs of rejection, toxicity, and infection in order to adjust dosages of different medicines.

Measurement of cyclosporine in the blood is particularly useful in distinguishing between toxicity and rejection and also in guiding strategy for combating infections. The techniques for routine monitoring of cyclosporine have evolved rapidly since widespread use of cyclosporine began in 1983. Two types of assay are available. The first is HPLC, which allows quantitation of cyclosporine parent drug and its individual metabolites separately. The second is immunoassay, which generally is sensitive to cyclosporine as well as those metabolites that are antigenically similar and so does not distinguish between parent drug and metabolites. Controversy has existed regarding which of these approaches is better for monitoring cyclosporine administration and determining the likelihood of therapeutic effect versus toxicity. Some metabolites have both therapeutic and toxic effects, and thus it would seem prudent to have a measurement that reflects both. Some transplant programs have attempted to concentrate on parent drug measurements by HPLC, but most centers now use a fluorescence polarization immunoassay for cyclosporine because of its ease and standardization between institutions. This assay measures parent drug and metabolites in a single reported value.

One other unique characteristic of cyclosporine that has an impact on sample type, collection, and processing is the drug's marked affinity for a binding protein present in most cells, including erythrocytes. Although most other drugs are distributed throughout blood plasma and are excluded from the cellular elements of blood, a substantial amount of cyclosporine in blood is contained within the erythrocytes. This cell-bound fraction varies with the patient's hematocrit. In addition, the ratio of cyclosporine in cells to that in plasma varies with the temperature at which a blood sample is stored, with lower temperature favoring even greater cellular uptake. The net result of this effect is to lend considerable variation to levels of serum cyclosporine concentration, depending on the ambient temperature at which a blood sample is clotted, stored, and centrifuged. To overcome this problem, most laboratories measure cyclosporine in whole blood with lysis of the erythrocytes to yield whole blood cyclosporine content.

Cyclosporine is administered in an oil base, usually orally, but it can also be given intravenously. It is extensively metabolized and then excreted predominantly in bile. Its half-life in blood is roughly 20 hours. Therapeutic trough levels of cyclosporine are in the range of 250 to 800 ng/mL for whole blood, or 50 to 300 ng/mL in plasma. Above these ranges, toxicities may occur, with development of renal impairment, neurologic damage and tremor, hirsutism, hypertension, or gingival hyperplasia. To prevent these toxicities, and especially the long-term deterioration of renal or hepatic function, immunosuppressive regimens have been developed to use reduced dosages of cyclosporine in combination with prednisone and azathioprine ("triple therapy"), minimizing the potential side effects from each drug.

ANALGESICS

The drugs included in this category (Fig. 18–11) are **acetaminophen** (*Tylenol*), **acetylsalicylic acid (aspirin)**, **ibuprofen** (*Advil, Motrin, Nuprin*),

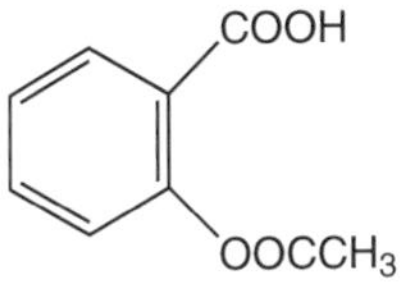

Acetylsalicylic acid

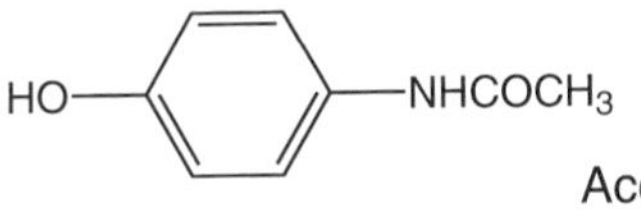

Acetaminophen

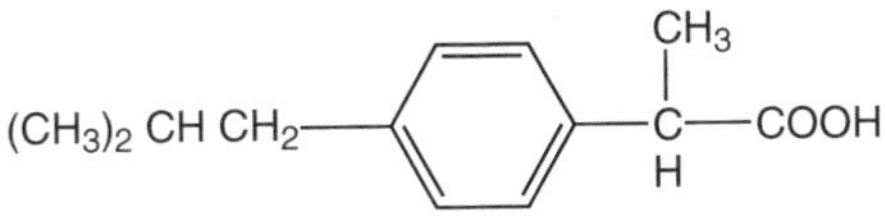

Ibuprofen

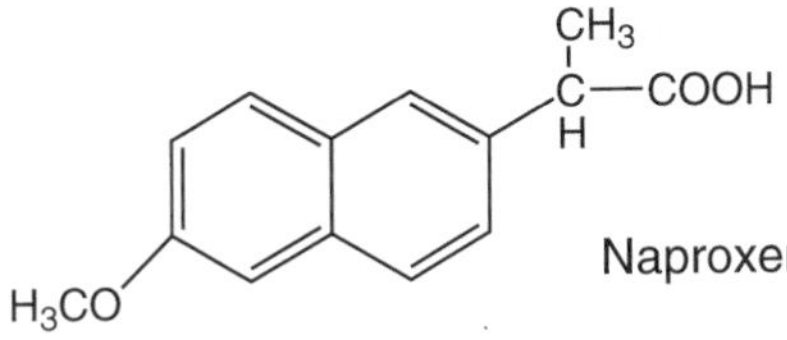

Naproxen

FIGURE 18–11. Chemical structure of common analgesic drugs.

naproxen *(Naprosyn, Aleve, Anaprox)*, **phenylbutazone** *(Butazolidin)*, **propoxyphene** *(Darvon)*, and other salicylate preparations. These analgesic agents are used for relief of pain not severe enough to require narcotic treatment. In the clinical use of analgesics, there is generally no need to measure these drug levels, but in cases of unknown drug overdose, all of these medications can be detected in a drug screen performed on serum, urine, or gastric fluid. Quantitation is frequently applied in cases of excess acetaminophen or salicylate ingestion.

Caution should be taken when interpreting levels of salicylate, acetaminophen, and ibuprofen to make certain that the units of measurement are properly understood. For many years the units were expressed as mg/dL; today many laboratories report values as mg/L (or µg/mL). Numerically these units differ by a factor of 10. Nontoxic values reported as mg/L may be confused with toxic values in units of mg/dL from older nomograms (e.g., Fig. 18–12), which are commonly referred to in medical and pediatric textbooks.

Salicylate

The various preparations of **salicylate** (salicylic acid, sodium salicylate, and acetylsalicylic acid) have the same effect of relieving pain (analgesic),

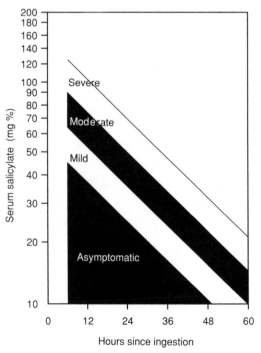

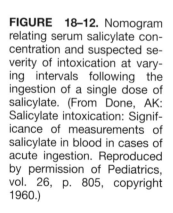

FIGURE 18–12. Nomogram relating serum salicylate concentration and suspected severity of intoxication at varying intervals following the ingestion of a single dose of salicylate. (From Done, AK: Salicylate intoxication: Significance of measurements of salicylate in blood in cases of acute ingestion. Reproduced by permission of Pediatrics, vol. 26, p. 805, copyright 1960.)

reducing fever (antipyretic), and diminishing inflammation (anti-inflammatory). Normal use of salicylate provides 325 mg/tablet as the over-the-counter medication aspirin (ASA). Children who take aspirin for upper respiratory infection of viral etiology are at increased risk of developing Reye's syndrome (acute hepatic fatty degeneration and encephalopathy) even at doses that would not normally be measured. High-dose aspirin is frequently prescribed to treat the pain and inflammation of rheumatoid arthritis. Therapeutic concentrations of salicylate in serum at high dosages are 2 to 20 mg/dL, and the measurement is performed as a colorimetric reaction with ferric ions read spectrophotometrically. The therapeutic level for treatment of headache is 5 mg/dL. Even at low doses, salicylates may lead to hemorrhagic tendencies in patients taking coumadin-type anticoagulants because the anticoagulant is displaced from serum albumin by the salicylate molecules. Aspirin also inhibits platelet aggregation and has been recommended to reduce the risk of myocardial infarction, although chronic use increases the risk of hemorrhagic stroke and of other bleeding complications.

Salicylate overdose can be a very serious medical situation and one in which monitoring of serum concentrations plays a major role in predicting the extent of toxicity. A large proportion of childhood poisoning is due to salicylate ingestion, probably because of the availability of aspirin in virtually every home and the casual attitude toward aspirin use, so that small children may ingest a whole bottle of tablets. The initial physiologic effect of overdose is heightened respiration with resultant respiratory alkalosis. This early phase is followed by metabolic acidosis. Other symptoms are gastrointestinal irritation, hemorrhage, tinnitus, mental changes, coma, and death. Levels over 30 mg/dL may be toxic, with severe toxicity and death at levels of 50 to 100 mg/dL. In following salicylate overdose, the actual level is important as well as the rate of fall in salicylate concentration determined by serial measurements (see Fig. 18–12). Prolonged serum half-life (>20 hours) indicates greater chance of serious toxicity.

Acetaminophen

Acetaminophen is an inhibitor of prostaglandin metabolism that is used clinically to relieve pain and to reduce fever. It is different from aspirin in that it lacks anti-inflammatory action. Its metabolism consists largely of conjugation to sulfates or glucuronates in the liver with excretion into urine. Overdose can result in fatal hepatic failure. Acetaminophen binds to hepatic proteins, leading to hepatocellular necrosis. Initial symptoms of overdose are nausea, vomiting, and abdominal discomfort. If there is hepatic necrosis, liver enzymes become elevated in serum after a few days. Hepatic coma and necrosis ensue with prolonged drug half-life (>12 hours) (Fig. 18–13). Thus serial measurements of acetaminophen are routinely employed to

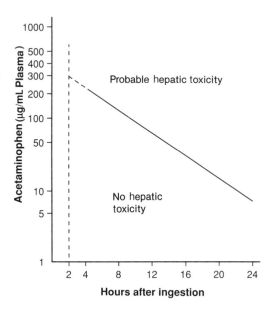

FIGURE 18–13. Semilogarithmic plot of plasma acetaminophen levels versus time. (From Rumack, BH, and Matthews, H: Acetaminophen poisoning and toxicity. Reproduced by permission of Pediatrics, vol. 55, p. 871, copyright 1975.)

establish prognosis. Specific treatment is with acetylcysteine, which appears to reverse or prevent further hepatic injury.

The therapeutic range of acetaminophen in serum is up to 25 μg/mL, with toxicity possible above 50 μg/mL. Between 100 and 300 μg/mL, hepatic necrosis may occur in up to one-half of cases; above 300 μg/mL, virtually all patients will have hepatic necrosis. Acetaminophen at lower levels may also cause hepatic necrosis if ingested with alcohol.

Ibuprofen

Ibuprofen (see Fig. 18–11) has analgesic and anti-inflammatory actions. Toxicities include nausea, vomiting, abdominal pain, diarrhea, dizziness, blurred vision, and even edema. Overall, ibuprofen has a much lower risk of toxicities than salicylates or acetaminophen. The therapeutic range is 10 to 50 μg/mL, with toxicities occurring above 100 μg/mL.

Naproxen

Naproxen has recently been made available without prescription as an analgesic, antipyretic, and anti-inflammatory agent. Toxicities include nausea, abdominal pain, constipation, headache, dizziness, drowsiness, and tinnitus. Skin rash may occur. Acute ingestion of even very large amounts of naproxen appears to cause only minor episodes of these symptoms. Therapeutic range is 30 to 90 mg/L. Because of its relatively low potential for toxicity, naproxen is not often quantitated.

PSYCHIATRIC DRUGS

Lithium

Lithium (Li) is an element that forms monovalent cations that are effective in the control of manic-depressive disorders. It is administered orally and distributes with sodium in body fluids. It is eliminated in the urine. Peak levels occur 1 to 4 hours after ingestion, with a half-life of 1 to 2 days. Toxicities include acute mental changes, nephrogenic diabetes insipidus, hypothyroidism, cardiac arrhythmias, and cardiovascular impairment. Therapeutic levels of lithium in serum are roughly 0.8 to 1.4 mEq/L. Toxicity can occur at levels as low as 1.5 mEq/L, with severe effects or death at 3 to 5 mEq/L. Measurement is by flame photometry or more recently by ion-selective electrodes.

Sedatives and Minor Tranquilizers

The sedatives include **ethchlorvynol** *(Placidyl)*, **glutethimide** *(Doriden)*, **meprobamate** *(Miltown)*, **methaqualone** *(Quaalude)*, and **methyprylon** *(Noludar)*. They are used for sedation or hypnotic effects. These agents are not often quantitated to monitor therapy but are frequently encountered in drug screens for overdose or abuse.

The minor tranquilizers (primarily benzodiazepines) include **chlordiazepoxide** *(Librium)*, **diazepam** *(Valium)*, **flurazepam** *(Dalmane)*, **oxazepam** *(Serax)*, and **nordiazepam** *(Tranxene)*. These agents are used to treat anxiety, as hypnotics, to relieve muscle spasms, to control seizure activity acutely, and as premedication for anesthesia. Monitoring can be performed but is not usual. Toxic drug screens pick up these drugs, which can be abused.

Major Tranquilizers

These agents (phenothiazines) include **chlorpromazine** *(Thorazine)* and **thioridazine** *(Mellaril)*, which are used to treat psychotic disorders, nausea and vomiting, anxiety, muscular tetany, manic symptoms, and aggressive behavioral disorders. They also may be of use in the symptomatic management of acute intermittent porphyria. A major side effect is tardive dyskinesia, which may be irreversible. Hematologic disorders, hypotensive effects, cholestatic jaundice, pseudo-parkinsonism, and other motor or behavioral changes are also possible. Therapeutic monitoring is sometimes done to verify the effectiveness of dosage regimens, but it is not usually a part of phenothiazine therapy.

Tricyclic Antidepressants

These agents are **amitriptyline** *(Elavil),* **nortriptyline** *(Pamelor),* **imipramine** *(Tofranil),* **desipramine** *(Norpramine),* **doxepin** *(Sinequan),* **trimipramine** *(Surmontil),* and **maprotiline** *(Ludiomil)* (a tetracyclic molecule). These drugs are variations on a basic tricyclic structure (Fig. 18–14). They are employed clinically for the long-term treatment of depressive illness that is severe, pathologic, and characterized by depressed mood, insomnia, irritability, lack of concentration, energy loss, and feelings of guilt leading to catatonia or suicide. The range of therapeutic concentrations is limited, with excessively high doses not being psychiatrically effective. The therapeutic concentration for each drug is probably slightly different, but roughly in the range of 100 to 300 ng/mL. Drug monitoring should be used if a patient fails to respond to standard doses and

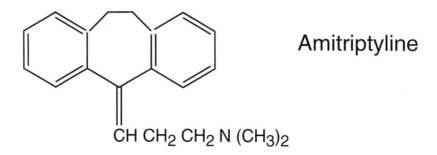

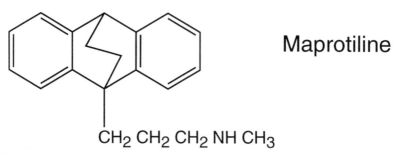

FIGURE 18–14. Chemic al structures of a tricyclic antidepressant (amitriptyline) and a tetracyclic one (maprotiline).

treatment. Monitoring of tricyclic antidepressants has been somewhat limited in the past, but its use is increasing as monitoring techniques are becoming available and gain acceptance, especially on psychiatric services.

Measurement is by HPLC. Considering that therapy will probably be lifelong for severe psychiatric disorders, measurement of tricyclic antidepressant levels on occasion is a prudent part of management for virtually all such patients.

Fluoxetine

Fluoxetine *(Prozac)* (Fig. 18–15) is an antidepressant whose action is to block the uptake of serotonin at nerve endings, thereby increasing serotonin levels in the brain. It is effective in treating depression and has gained considerable public recognition. Other clinical applications include obsessive-compulsive disorders and recent trials in obesity and bulimia. The drug is administered once daily. Because its half-life is long, missing a daily dose is usually without consequence. Therapeutic monitoring is not typically necessary; the dosage may be titrated by the observed psychiatric effect. The therapeutic range of fluoxetine is 90 to 300 ng/mL.

Another antidepressant of the serotonin uptake inhibitor class is **sertraline** *(Zoloft)* (see Fig. 18–15). The therapeutic range of sertraline is 30 to 200 ng/mL.

DRUGS OF ABUSE AND TOXICOLOGIC ANALYSIS

Patient Evaluation and Specimen Collection

The evaluation of patients for the presence of drugs of abuse in serum, urine, or other body fluids (e.g., gastric aspirate) frequently carries with it legal implications. This type of analysis is commonly requested on patients who are comatose or intoxicated and who present as acute medical emergencies to hospitals. In these cases, a history from family members, friends, or witnesses, or the finding of medicine bottles containing remainders of the ingested material is information that may assist in determining the substance involved in an overdose. Physical examination should be complete, specifically looking for vital signs, indication of trauma (e.g., head injury, abdominal tenderness), cardiovascular and pulmonary status, and neurologic examination (e.g., alertness and attention, coma, hallucinations, seizures, hyperactivity). Specific physical signs of toxicologic influence include size of pupils, odor of breath, skin color, and ventilatory status. In cases of suspected drug overdose, immediate laboratory examination should include CBC (to assess red cell content for oxygen-carrying capacity and white cells for

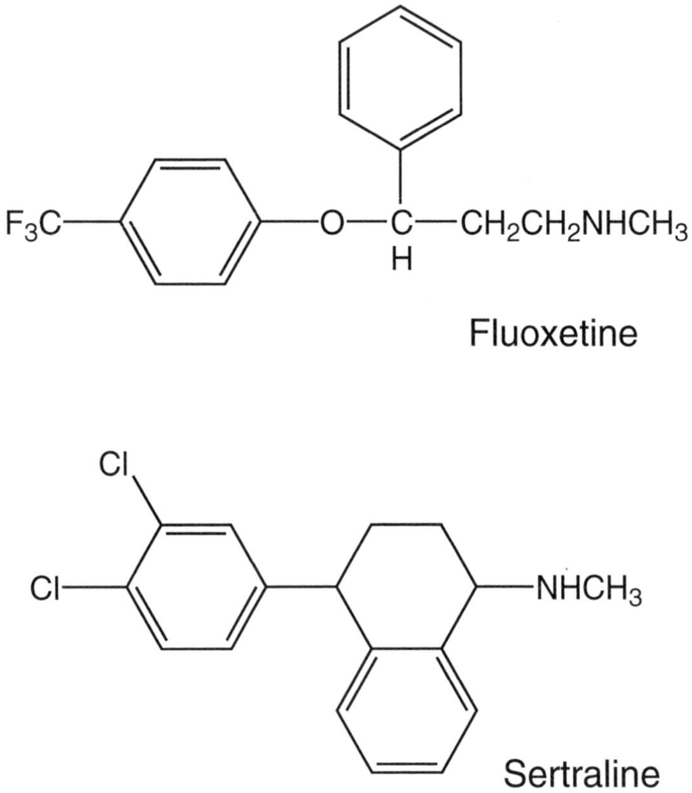

FIGURE 18–15. Chemical structures of the serotonin uptake inhibitors fluoxetine and sertraline, which are antidepressants.

infection); serum electrolytes, glucose, and BUN (for metabolic and fluid balance assessment); urinalysis (for ketones and glucose); and blood gas measurement if respirations are depressed.

Early in the evaluation and treatment of a comatose patient, it is common practice to administer a test dose of the narcotic antagonist **naloxone** *(Narcan)*. If the patient responds with an improvement of symptoms (e.g., increased level of consciousness, improved respirations, dilatation of constricted pupils), it is then presumed that the patient has taken an overdose of a narcotic substance and will require further doses of naloxone to maintain satisfactory clinical status after the test dose wears off.

Laboratory toxicologic evaluation is best done on both blood and urine. Examination of blood has the advantage of identifying currently circulating drugs and of potentially quantitating them when appropriate for prognosis, design of treatment plan (e.g., intravenous fluids and diuresis versus hemodialysis or hemoperfusion; administering specific drug antagonists), and monitoring the success of treatment and drug removal by serial blood levels. In contrast, one advantage of using urine for toxicologic analysis is that it reflects more completely the composite of drugs that have been ingested over a longer period than is detectable with blood specimens. In addition, most drugs are cleared from the body into the urine and thus become more concentrated and easier to detect in urine than in blood. Aspiration of gastric contents or examination of vomitus may reveal tablets or capsules from which the ingested drug can be identified by shape, color, and markings. Other ingested materials obtained from gastric fluid will be in high concentration (before absorption) and therefore even easier to identify by chemical analysis than they would be in blood or urine.

In addition to identification of the agent responsible for acute intoxication in emergency room patients, toxicologic analysis is increasingly being applied to screen for drug use as a condition of employment in sensitive positions of responsibility. Aside from the issues of civil rights, human rights, invasion of privacy, and so on, which may be used to legally invalidate the actual laboratory test results, it is essential to preserve and guarantee the legal integrity of appropriately collected specimens. For use as medicolegal evidence, a chain of custody must be established for a specimen, with written documentation and the signatures of persons responsible for its collection and handling continuously through the stage of analysis and reporting of result. This process must guarantee that there is no opportunity for surreptitious substitution of a specimen from a different person and no introduction of contaminating substances. Each stage of the chain of custody may be called into question in court during a trial. In this light, it is relatively simple to guarantee the validity and authenticity of blood samples obtained by venipuncture. Collection of urine may be observed, but it is traditionally done by the patient alone in a rest room, thus allowing for substitution of a "clean sample" from another individual or for introduction of a small amount of soap that causes some tests to yield false-negative results by elevating the pH. Current regulations for these collections often stipulate that urine temperature be measured to confirm that it was warm enough to have been freshly voided (96.5 to 100.5°F) and not a cold sample brought from the outside. Another stipulation that is sometimes enforced is that the urine sample be collected in the presence of a witness. Tamper-free containers have also been designed to prevent opening after a urine sample has been sealed.

Alcohols

Ethyl alcohol (ethanol, grain alcohol) is the most commonly abused substance in the United States, and probably the entire world. It exhibits a range of actions on the central nervous system extending from sedative to anesthetic; ingestion impairs judgment and thinking and alters behavior. Legal definitions have been established through "presumption laws" for drunk driving. With a blood alcohol concentration of <50 mg/dL (0.05%), the individual is presumed not to be under the influence of alcohol. For levels between 50 and 100 mg/dL (0.05 to 0.1%), no presumption is established, but other evidence such as behavior is taken into account. When blood alcohol concentration is >100 mg/dL (0.1%), the person is presumed legally to be under the influence of alcohol; some states have set this limit at 80 mg/dL (0.08%). Ethanol distributes in the water phase of both plasma and erythrocytes. Because the water content of erythrocytes is lower than that of plasma, plasma or serum concentrations of ethanol are approximately 12% higher than in whole blood drawn at the same time. For uniformity, alcohol is generally measured in whole blood samples, although it can also be done in serum or plasma.

At low alcohol levels there may be CNS excitation or euphoria, but at higher levels there is progression to coma (at 250 to 400 mg/dL) and possible fatality. The effect of alcohol is greater for a given level when it is increasing. Particularly dangerous is the combination of alcohol and sedatives (benzodiazepines, barbiturates), with extreme risk of accidental death from respiratory depression. Chronic alcohol abuse leads to cirrhosis of the liver and degeneration of the brain and of skeletal muscles. Alcoholics frequently have vitamin and other nutritional deficiencies. Acute treatment of alcohol withdrawal includes injection of thiamine (vitamin B_1). In addition, such patients may require treatment with diazepam to ameliorate seizure activity in delirium tremens. Women alcoholics in the childbearing years run the risk of having low–birth weight infants with mental retardation and other birth defects (fetal alcohol syndrome, an irreversible congenital disorder). Nutritional and metabolic studies have clearly demonstrated that ethanol also causes hypertension.

Ethanol causes diuresis by inhibiting secretion of antidiuretic hormone from the posterior pituitary (neurohypophysis). It also inhibits secretion of oxytocin by the posterior pituitary and for this reason has been used for stopping uterine contractions (initiated by oxytocin) in premature labor (tocolysis).

Ethanol diffuses freely into body fluids and is partially cleared into the urine and other body excretions. Clearance of alcohol is by zero-order kinetics (i.e., at a constant rate independent of concentration). Its major metabolic pathway is conversion to acetaldehyde by alcohol dehydrogenase in the liver (Fig. 18–16). Acetaldehyde is then converted to acetate by acetaldehyde dehydrogenase. The headache, flushing, and other symptoms of a "hangover" are largely due to the effects of acetaldehyde before it is metabolized, as well as to alterations in water and electrolyte concentrations. The drug **disulfiram** (*Antabuse*) specifically inhibits the enzyme acetaldehyde dehydrogenase, leading to accumulation of acetaldehyde and toxic symptoms that discourage a patient from ingesting alcohol while on that preventive medication. Persons congenitally deficient in acetaldehyde dehydrogenase similarly have intolerance to alcohol because of the effects of acetaldehyde.

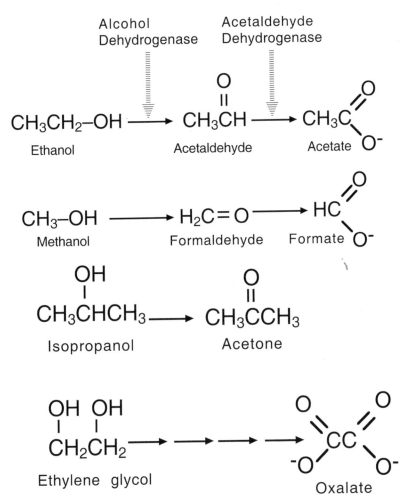

FIGURE 18–16. Enzyme-catalyzed metabolism of alcohols by the liver.

Chronic alcohol abusers may intentionally or accidentally ingest other alcohols when ethanol is not available or when it is contaminated with these other substances. These alcohols include methanol (wood alcohol), isopropanol (rubbing alcohol), and ethylene glycol (antifreeze), which all have associated toxicities. Their metabolism in the body parallels that of ethanol, using the same enzymes (see Fig. 18–16).

Assays for blood alcohol are generally of two types: *gas liquid chromatography (GLC)*, which provides quantitation plus qualitative identification of the alcohol and some metabolites and *enzymatic assay,* which uses alcohol dehydrogenase as a reagent and usually quantitates the sum of all alcohols present in a sample without distinguishing them or identifying metabolites. In cases of unknown acute alcohol intoxication, it is essential to identify the alcohol present in order to plan therapy. For example, treatment of methanol intoxication consists of administering ethanol to block further formation of formaldehyde while waiting for unmetabolized methanol to clear from the body by renal excretion. Obviously, in ethanol intoxication, one would not administer more ethanol, but merely give supportive therapy while the ethanol metabolizes and clears.

Specimens for alcohol analysis include blood, urine, and exhaled breath (for immediate analysis by breath meter). Alcohol in blood samples may be analyzed even after considerable delay if the specimen tube remains sealed, because blood lacks the enzymes that metabolize it.

DRUG SCREENING

Unlike the ingestion of alcohol (which is frequently evident from symptoms, history, breath odor, etc.), ingestion and overdose of other substances of abuse may not be readily apparent without toxicologic analysis to identify the ingested drug. The agents routinely screened for are conveniently grouped according to their overall pharmacologic actions (Table 18–1). Benzodiazepines, methaqualone, and barbiturates were discussed earlier in this chapter. All three can be detected by enzyme immunoassay or fluorescence polarization immunoassay.

Opiates

These narcotic drugs derive from a natural product of the opium poppy pod. They are used clinically for relief of pain. Chemical modification of the natural products yields **heroin** and **hydrocodone.** Fully synthetic opioids are **meperidine** *(Demerol)* and **methadone,** which may not be as readily detected by immunoassays as are the other opioids. These agents

TABLE 18–1. DRUGS OF ABUSE COMMONLY DETECTED IN SCREENING TESTS

Ethanol
Sedative-hypnotic: benzodiazepines, methaqualone
Depressant: barbiturates, opiates
Stimulant: amphetamines, cocaine
Hallucinogen: cannabinoids, phencyclidine, lysergic acid
  diethylamide

are highly addictive, and continued use is expected to produce physical addiction. Absorption is efficient from the gastrointestinal tract or mucosal surfaces; they can also be administered parenterally. Opiate metabolism includes conjugation and renal excretion of parent drug and metabolite. Positive results on qualitative analysis can be confirmed by thin-layer chromatography or GC-MS to identify the specific opiate ingested or injected. Cross-reactivity in the immunoassay can occur with high concentrations of **meperidine** *(Demerol)*. **Propoxyphene** *(Darvon)* is a nonnarcotic congener of methadone that is commonly used for relief of mild to moderate pain.

Many medications (particularly those from foreign formularies) contain opiates that can show up as true-positive results on opiate screening of urine. In that instance, an individual may test positive (e.g., on a pre-employment screen) without specific knowledge of having ingested opiates compounded with other drugs. It is also now well recognized that eating poppy seeds (as on rolls) may result in a positive urine screening test for opiates.

Amphetamines

This class of drugs is sympathomimetic and has direct stimulant activity on the central nervous system as well as on myocardium. Their valid medical applications are limited: narcolepsy, minimal brain dysfunction, and as diet pills in obesity. They are extensively abused by individuals who are trying to stay awake for long periods (e.g., students, long-distance truck drivers). Addiction leads to need for greater doses in order to achieve similar effects. Enzyme immunoassay is used for detecting amphetamines (generally taken orally) and methamphetamines (taken intravenously). There can be cross-reacting interference from ephedrine or phenylpropanolamine, which are present in over-the-counter medications. Confirmation testing is performed with GC-MS.

Cocaine

This potent stimulant derives from the leaf of the coca plant (genus *Erythroxylon*) indigenous to South America. **Cocaine** has a powerful stimulating effect on the central nervous system that includes stimulation of the cerebral cortex, as well as lower brain centers, and nervous activity. Administration systemically results in increased motor activity, mental excitation, and a sense of increased ability to perform physical work (probably due to the lessening of fatigue rather than direct skeletal muscle action).

With brain stem stimulation, respiration rate increases and vomiting may be induced. The phase of stimulation is followed by depression of both mental state and respirations that can lead to death. Cardiac excitation occurs with actions of cocaine on overall sympathetic tone. However, cocaine can cause sudden death due to direct toxicity on myocardium. Treatment of acute cocaine overdose is supportive, with administration of a short-acting barbiturate intravenously.

The only valid medical use of cocaine is as a topical anesthetic, with primary application in ophthalmology for anesthetization of the cornea. Cocaine causes local vasoconstriction as well as blockage of nerve conduction at the site of administration.

The illicit use of cocaine is a major public health problem because of addiction. It has an instantaneous onset of action and brief clearance requiring repeat dosing. The method of abuse may be by nasal mucosa (snorting, sniffing) or by intravenous injection. The free-base form of cocaine called **crack** is also taken by smoking. Immunoassays and thin-layer chromatography are configured to detect cocaine's primary metabolite, **benzoyl ecgonine,** present in urine.

Cannabinoids

The naturally occurring **cannabinoids** (cannabis) are **marijuana** (from the flowers of the hemp plant) and **hashish** (from the resin of hemp). Marijuana, which is extensively used in the United States, consists of multiple psychoactive substances, with the predominant drug being Δ^9-**tetrahydrocannabinol (THC).** Marijuana is rapidly absorbed by the oral mucosa on smoking and slightly less well from oral ingestion. The THC is metabolized in part to Δ^9-tetrahydrocannabinol carboxylic acid (THC-CA), which is excreted into the urine.

THC produces altered states of consciousness, a decrease in aggression, hallucinations, and moods of well-being and of being "high." Clinical applications have included control of emesis during chemotherapy and reduction of ocular pressure in glaucoma. Marijuana has widespread popularity as a recreational drug; physical or psychological addiction is probably not a significant problem. Long-term smoking of marijuana can lead to severe destructive pulmonary disease from inhalation of the burned ash and toxic products similar to that encountered in cigarette use. THC is lipophilic and distributes into body fat deposits, from which it is gradually liberated over a period of days after the last dose.

Enzyme immunoassays detect THC-CA in urine. There is cross-reactivity with some anti-inflammatory agents of nonsteroidal nature; other false-positives may occur in up to 5% of samples for unknown reasons. To define the actual presence of THC, it is necessary to follow the screening immunoassay with confirmatory analysis by GC-MS. One interesting twist of the analysis is that passive inhalation (of the smoke from an active user nearby) can also yield detectable levels of THC. Another consideration is whether an individual is actually under the influence of marijuana at the time of testing positive, or if the positive test is a result of use sometime in the last several days. The medicolegal issues of drug screening are clearly important with marijuana, which is so widely used, is so easily detected (sometimes with false-positive results), and has such controversy regarding its actual deleterious effects.

Phencyclidine and Lysergic Acid Diethylamide

Phencyclidine, also known as "PCP" and "angel dust," was developed and used as an anesthetic until recognition of its adverse mental effects. It produces strong hallucinatory effects with a stimulatory component and may lead to violent, uncontrolled, and irresponsible behavior. Phencyclidine is now available from illegal synthesis in small drug laboratories, and in part, from its use as a veterinary anesthetic.

Phencyclidine is lipophilic and accumulates in body fat stores with frequent use. It is excreted in acid urine, but much less so in alkaline urine. Excretion in detectable quantities can continue for a week or more after the last dose. Detection is by immunoassay as part of a drug screen on urine samples.

The hallucinogen **lysergic acid diethylamide (LSD)** can be identified by HPLC or immunoassay of serum or urine.

POISONING

Accidental or intentional (suicidal, homicidal) ingestion of poisonous substances or the breathing of toxic gases requires rapid diagnosis to administer a proper antidote and to follow with correct therapy. Ingested material such as acid or alkali can usually be defined by the verbal account of the patient, family, or a witness and can be substantiated by a quick check on the substance's pH if some of it is available. Hydrocarbon (gasoline, kerosene) ingestion may also be obvious from its odor. The following agents have more specific laboratory procedures associated with their identification.

Gases

Carbon Monoxide

Carbon monoxide (CO) arises as a result of incomplete combustion of carbon-containing (organic) material in fires, gasoline engines, and cigarette smoke. It has a higher affinity for hemoglobin than does oxygen, and by binding to hemoglobin (as carboxyhemoglobin), it impairs the capacity of hemoglobin to deliver oxygen to tissues of the body. This toxicity is exacerbated by anemia and by diminished cardiac output in patients with heart disease. Symptoms of CO toxicity are headache, fatigue, mental confusion, nausea, and severe neurologic impairment due to hypoxia leading to coma and death.

Analysis for carbon monoxide is performed on whole blood that is anticoagulated (generally with EDTA). Samples are secure from deterioration if sealed to prevent exposure to air. Methods are spectrophotometry and co-oximetry. Results are expressed as the percent of hemoglobin present as carboxyhemoglobin (percent saturation with CO). Because of the ubiquitous nature of CO in our fossil fuel-burning and tobacco-smoking society, healthy urban nonsmokers may have levels up to 2% and smokers up to 7%. Many laboratories report low levels (up to 3%) as nondetectable. Heavy smokers may have levels to 15% or greater depending on how deeply they inhale the smoke.

Toxic symptoms of CO poisoning arise at 20% with progression of symptoms to convulsions, coma, and death at 60%. Treatment consists of removing the patient from the CO source rapidly and maintaining respirations with adequate ventilation and oxygen support to allow the CO to dissociate from hemoglobin and diffuse away.

Cyanide

Cyanide in the form of ions (CN$^-$) is used in chemicals in industrial applications. In the form **hydrocyanic acid (HCN, prussic acid),** it is used as a rodenticide and an insecticide. Cyanide has the odor of bitter almonds. It also occurs naturally bound to the substance amygdalin, which is present in seeds of stone fruits (apricots, peaches).

Cyanide binds avidly to the heme-containing molecules of oxygen transport and utilization in cells: hemoglobin and cytochrome oxidase. The result is poisoning of respiration at the cellular level. Cyanide is rapidly metabolized to **thiocyanate (SCN$^-$)** in the liver. Thiocyanate has some toxicity but less than does cyanide. Thiocyanate's half-life is about 1 week, with clearance by the kidneys. Acute ingestion of cyanide can be fatal in a matter of minutes when it is taken in large amounts (e.g., a cyanide capsule). Lower-level exposures cause headache, nausea, tachypnea, tachycardia, unconsciousness, convulsions, and death. Cyanide poisoning can be treated with sodium nitrite or sodium thiosulfate to tie up the cyanide groups.

Securely sealed whole blood samples are used to detect cyanide by spectrophotometry. Cyanide is present at nontoxic low levels (0.2 μg/mL) in healthy individuals exposed to industrial pollution, cigarette smoke, and some vegetables (e.g., brussel sprouts). Symptoms may appear with levels above 2 μg/mL, and death can occur at levels above 5 μg/mL. There is not always a strict relationship between blood levels of cyanide and toxicity (especially with acute ingestion) because it is the amount of cyanide bound to cytochrome oxidase within cells of the body that is important physiologically. Thiocyanate levels in blood are more useful for documenting chronic exposures.

The drug **nitroprusside** *(Nipride)* is used intravenously to treat severe hypertension in acute care situations. Each molecule of nitroprusside contains five cyanide groups, and the drug yields cyanide in the body with comparable toxicities. For that reason, nitroprusside must be administered cautiously, with frequent monitoring of blood pressure to titrate dose. Nitroprusside use is also sometimes checked for toxicity by measuring cyanide and thiocyanate concentrations.

Heavy Metals

All metals can be toxic if ingested in large quantities and absorbed in their ionized forms. Analysis of trace metals in biologic samples may require ashing of the sample by burning, followed by specific chemical procedure for detection of the metallic ions. A qualitative screening procedure, the **Reinsch test,** has been used widely in the past for detecting the presence in a sample of any one of several heavy metals: **antimony, arsenic, bismuth, mercury,** and **selenium.** It consists of interacting the sample with metallic copper wire, which demonstrates a color change when it is oxidized by those metallic ions. Today most metals can be quantitated by atomic absorption spectrophotometry, anodic stripping voltametry, or inductively coupled plasma mass spectrometry, which can quantitate several different metals simultaneously.

Iron

Iron-containing tablets and solutions are commonly present in the home for iron (Fe) supplementation in the diet. In that environment, children are particularly prone to accidental ingestion of large amounts of iron, resulting in toxicity. Doses of 150 mg/kg can cause serious toxicity; 200 mg/kg or more can cause death. Within an hour after ingestion, there is gastrointestinal toxicity with pain and bloody diarrhea. After absorption, there is wider toxicity to the liver and nervous system. Treatment consists of removing unabsorbed tablets from the stomach and removing absorbed iron from the body by chelation with deferoxamine.

Laboratory evaluation should include serum electrolytes, glucose, and BUN. Iron concentration in the serum is an excellent measure to use for documenting the absorption of iron. When the iron-binding capacity (transferrin) becomes saturated, the excess free iron is toxic. Iron concentrations in serum above 700 µg/dL lead to serious symptoms, and above 1000 µg/dL, they may be lethal. Free iron is removed from the circulation by the liver, where it is toxic and can lead to cirrhosis in the long term (see also Chapter 2).

Lead

Lead (Pb) has no physiologic role in the body, but it is frequently absorbed because of the presence of lead in paints; gasoline (formerly); storage batteries, from which it is released on burning; some eating utensils, plates, and ceramics; and drinking water from lead pipes or from lead in the solder used to join copper plumbing. In the body, lead deposits in bone and also accumulates in erythrocytes and other tissues. Toxicities of lead include damage to the kidneys and brain (encephalopathy) and interference with the biosynthesis of heme, which is required for production of hemoglobin (see Chapter 2, Sideroblastic Anemias).

Several laboratory findings can indicate lead poisoning: basophilic stippling in red cells on a peripheral blood smear, mild anemia, increased erythrocyte protoporphyrin, increased excretion of gamma-aminolevulinic acid, and increased excretion of coproporphyrin. Blood for direct measurement of lead must be collected into specially treated tubes to avoid contamination from lead in the glass. Lead is measured in whole blood (lead is contained largely in erythrocytes) by flameless (graphite furnace) atomic absorption spectrophotometry or by anodic stripping voltametry. Normal individuals have levels less than 20 µg/dL; levels greater than 30 µg/dL are probably abnormally high and potentially toxic; above 70 µg/dL is considered definite evidence of lead poisoning. Current practice is to keep lead exposure very low in children; for children under 16 years of age, blood lead should be less than 10 µg/dL. Intermediate levels are interpreted in conjunction with erythrocyte protoporphyrin measurements.

Arsenic

Arsenic (As) is used in commercial preparations of insecticides, pesticides, and herbicides. These arsenical compounds sometimes contaminate food supplies, leading to accidental poisoning. Shellfish from the ocean also contain significant amounts of arsenic. Industrial exposures occur in metal-working plants. Arsenic has also been used as a poison with homicidal intent. Arsenic is the most frequent agent of heavy metal poisoning (both intentional and accidental), and rapid diagnosis by laboratory tests is essential for therapy.

The toxicity of arsenic occurs as the result of inhibiting sulfhydryl enzymes throughout the body. Acute ingestion causes gastrointestinal irritation with vomiting and diarrhea. Ingestion of greater amounts can cause neurologic impairment with seizures, coma, and death. Chronic ingestion results in accumulation of arsenic in tissues and damage to brain, nerves, kidneys, and gastrointestinal tract. Arsenic has a high affinity of binding for keratin, leading to high concentrations in hair and nails with characteristic white striae across the fingernails **(Mees lines).**

Diagnosis of arsenic poisoning is usually made or confirmed by direct measurement (by flameless atomic absorption spectrophotometry) of arsenic in blood (for acute or recent exposure) and in urine, hair, or nail clippings (for chronic exposures). For reference values, consult the laboratory actually performing the test.

Cadmium

Cadmium (Cd) poisoning can result from ingestion of acidic foods stored or prepared in metal containers composed of or lined with cadmium. Industrial exposures (e.g., in battery manufacture) are generally by inhalation of cadmium fumes. There may be destruction of type I epithelial cells in the lung with pneumonitis and decreased resistance to bacterial infections in the lung. Cadmium accumulates in renal tubule cells causing tubular damage. There is also development of hypertension.

Diagnosis is established with a careful history relating development of symptoms to exposures. Measurements of cadmium in blood and urine are available, but these may not be useful if the cadmium level has fallen after recent acute exposure. Renal toxicity may be demonstrated by measuring the enzyme **gamma-glutamyltransferase** (released from damaged tubule cells) in urine.

Mercury

Many compounds that contain mercury (Hg) are used in industry and farming. Biologic interactions of mercury occur with covalent bond formation to sulfur in proteins, thereby inactivating many enzymes. Inhalation of metallic mercury vapors causes pulmonary damage. Ingestion of mercury salts leads to gastrointestinal damage. Later toxicities affect the kidneys, brain, nerves, bone marrow, and gastrointestinal tract. Diagnosis depends on recognizing characteristic physical signs (e.g., neurologic findings, dementia) and on measuring mercury in blood or urine.

Organic mercury comes from such sources as seafood in the diet. Toxicity from organic mercury generally affects the central nervous system. Organic mercury is found in erythrocytes, and so whole blood samples are used to document exposure. Inorganic mercury exposure usually derives from industrial uses. Inorganic mercury effects are more peripheral, especially on the gastrointestinal tract and the kidney. Urine is used to demonstrate inorganic mercury exposure.

Aluminum

Aluminum (Al) is abundant in the Earth's crust and is widely present in the environment. It has no recognized biologic role. Aluminum toxicity has been noted in patients who receive long-term hemodialysis for treatment of chronic renal failure. Dialysis solutions contribute the aluminum, which crosses dialysis membranes to the patient's circulation. Aluminum is also a constituent in many antacid preparations. Aluminum deposits occur in the brain, causing an encephalopathy, and in bone, leading to osteodystrophy. The major route for excretion of aluminum is through the biliary tract. Chelation therapy with deferoxamine enhances aluminum clearance in urine. Suspicion of aluminum toxicity can be confirmed by measurement in serum, urine, and tissue by flameless atomic absorption spectrophotometry.

Bromide

The halide bromide was once used widely as an analgesic, but it has been removed from such formulations in the United States because of toxicities. Occasionally patients may ingest medications containing bromide from other countries and develop toxicities (*bromism*) including fever, rash, and neurologic abnormalities. Bromide can be measured in serum by spectrophotometric methods. Patients receiving iodine therapy may have falsely elevated bromide results. Unless it is specifically considered in the differential diagnosis, bromide intoxication may be missed, as it is not suggested by other laboratory findings.

SUGGESTED READING

Alak, AM: Measurement of tacrolimus (FK506) and its metabolites: A review of assay development and application in therapeutic drug monitoring and pharmacokinetic studies. Ther Drug Monit 19:338, 1997.

Baumann, P: Pharmacokinetic-pharmacodynamic relationship of the selective serotonin reuptake inhibitors. Clin Pharmacokinet 31:444, 1996.

Belfer, RA, et al: Emergency department evaluation of a rapid assay for detection of cocaine metabolites in urine specimens. Pediatr Emerg Care 12:113, 1996.

Brodie, MJ, and Dichter, MA: Established antiepileptic drugs. Seizure 6:159, 1997.

Brubacher, JR, and Hoffman, RS: Salicylism from topical salicylates: Review of the literature. J Toxicol Clin Toxicol 34:431, 1996.

Burkhart, KK, and Kulig, KW: The other alcohols—methanol, ethylene glycol, and isopropanol. Emerg Med Clinics N Am 8:913, 1990.

Clarkson, TW: The toxicology of mercury. Crit Rev Clin Lab Sci 34:369, 1997.

Done, AK: Salicylate intoxication: Significance of measurements of salicylate in blood in cases of acute ingestion. Pediatrics 26:800, 1960.

Eilers, R: Therapeutic drug monitoring for the treatment of psychiatric disorders. Clinical use and cost effectiveness. Clin Pharmacokinet 29:442, 1995.

Fabbri, LM, et al: Oral vs. inhaled asthma therapy: Pros, cons and combinations. Drugs 52 (suppl 6):20, 1996.

Fraser, AD: New drugs for the treatment of epilepsy. Clin Biochem 29:97, 1996.

Fruman, DA, Burakoff, SJ, and Bierer, BE: Immunophilins in protein folding and immunosuppression. Fed Am Soc Exp Biol J 8:391, 1994.

Harvey, B: New lead screening guidelines from the Centers for Disease Control and Prevention: How will they affect pediatricians? Pediatrics 100:384, 1997.

Hickman, PE, Potter, JM, and Pesce, AJ: Clinical chemistry and post-liver-transplant monitoring. Clin Chem 43:1546, 1997.

Hsiung, CS, et al: Minimizing interferences in the quantitative multielement analysis of trace elements in biological fluids by inductively coupled plasma mass spectrometry. Clin Chem 43:12, 1997.

Jeffes, EW, and Weinstein, GD: Methotrexate and other chemotherapeutic agents used to treat psoriasis. Dermatol Clin 13:875, 2995.

Jortani, SA, and Valdes, R: Digoxin and its related endogenous factors. Crit Rev Clin Lab Sci 34:225, 1997.

Kershner, RP, and Fitzsimmons, WE: Relationship of FK506 whole blood concentrations and efficacy and toxicity after liver and kidney transplantation. Transplantation 62:920, 1996.

Khoschsorur, G, et al: Rapid, sensitive high-performance liquid chromatographic method for the determination of cyclosporin A and its metabolites M1, M17 and M21. J Chromatogr B Biomed Appl 690:367, 1997.

Kunsman, GW, et al: Phencyclidine blood concentrations in DRE cases. J Anal Toxicol 21:498, 1997.

Mason, JW: A comparison of seven antiarrhythmic drugs in patients with ventricular tachyarrhythmias. N Engl J Med 329:452, 1993.

Miles, MV, et al: Special considerations for monitoring vancomycin concentrations in pediatric patients. Ther Drug Monitor 19:265, 1997.

Minton, NA, and Henry, JA: Acute and chronic human toxicity of theophylline. Hum Exp Toxicol 15:471, 1996.

Rumack, BH, and Matthews, H: Acetaminophen poisoning and toxicity. Pediatrics 55:871, 1975.

Saitz, R, Friedman, LS, and Mayo-Smith, MF: Alcohol withdrawal: A nationwide survey of inpatient treatment practices. J Gen Intern Med 10:479, 1995.

Salach, RH, and Cash, JM: Methotrexate: The emerging drug of choice for serious rheumatoid arthritis. Clin Ther 16:912, 1994.

Shih, ML, Korte, WD, and Clark, CR: Multicomponent spectroscopic assay for hemoglobin and ferrihemoglobin species in methemoglobin treatment of cyanide poisoning. J Anal Toxicol 21:543, 1997.

Singh, BN: Amiodarone: The expanding antiarrhythmic role and how to follow a patient on chronic therapy. Clin Cardiol 20:608, 1997.

Spina, E, Pisani, F, and Perucca, E: Clinically significant pharmacokinetic drug interactions with carbamazepine. An update. Clin Pharmacokinet 31:198, 1996.

Sugarman, JM, Rodgers, GC, and Paul, RI: Utility of toxicology screening in a pediatric emergency department. Pediatr Emerg Care 13:194, 1997.

Treon, SP, and Chabner, BA: Concepts in use of high-dose methotrexate therapy. Clin Chem 42:1322, 1996.

Tulkens, PM: Pharmacokinetic and toxicological evaluation of a once-daily regimen versus conventional schedules of netilmicin and amikacin. J Antimicrob Chemother 27 (Suppl C):49, 1991.

Weiss, B: Long ago and far away: A retrospective on the implications of Minamata. Neurotoxicology 17:257, 1996.

Williams, RH, and Erickson, T: Evaluating toxic alcohol poisoning in the emergency setting. Laboratory Medicine 29:102, 1998.

Yukawa, E: Optimisation of antiepileptic drug therapy. The importance of serum drug concentration monitoring. Clin Pharmacokinet 31:120, 1996.

19

Laboratory Assessment of Body Fluids

URINALYSIS

The kidneys perform many metabolic as well as excretory functions and facilitate removal from the body of nitrogenous and other metabolic byproducts. They maintain meticulous homeostasis of fluid, electrolyte, and acid-base status. The kidneys receive approximately 20% of the cardiac output, equal to almost a liter of blood every minute. Through filtration, reabsorption, and secretion, the kidneys daily excrete 1.6 to 1.8 liters of urine in the adult; 2 to 5 mL/kg per hour in children. These volumes may vary considerably depending on the state of hydration of the patient. Because different parts of the kidneys perform different functions, the site and nature of many kidney disorders can be inferred from a differential evaluation of selective aspects of urine and metabolic regulation.

THE PHYSIOLOGY OF URINE FORMATION

The individual functioning units of the kidneys are called **nephrons;** each kidney contains 1 to 1.5 million individual nephrons. Each nephron

924

consists of a capillary tuft, the **glomerulus,** and an elongated epithelium-lined conduit called the **tubule.** The tubule has anatomically and functionally distinct segments designated the **proximal convoluted tubule,** the **Loop of Henle,** and the **distal convoluted tubule.** At their ends, the distal tubules widen into receptacles called **collecting ducts,** which empty into the collecting system of the kidney.

Renal Filtration

Renal filtration occurs when the systemic blood flows through the glomeruli. The filtration rate depends on arterial blood flow, systemic arterial blood pressure, and internal flow pressure within the kidney. The same blood that is filtered through the glomeruli also carries oxygen and nutrients to the kidneys and participates in the metabolic exchanges generated by functioning renal cells. Renal blood flow critically affects homeostasis, the maintenance of the "internal environment," and whole-body metabolism.

Water and dissolved minerals of small molecular size, primarily electrolytes, freely pass through the glomerular filter. The filter retards passage of proteins. This process of separating colloid from crystalloid is called **ultrafiltration.** Filtration is critically dependent on the systemic blood pressure, which allows greater perfusion and is resisted by the colloid osmotic pressure and the peripheral resistance of the **glomerular pores** (endothelial cells, basement membrane, and epithelial cells); these discriminate by restricting the passage of cells and large molecules. Blood cells and most circulating proteins are therefore prevented from entering the glomerular filtrate. About 125 mL of filtrate is generated every minute, or about 140 L of water daily. Glucose, urea, sodium, potassium, bicarbonate, chloride, and many enzymes, hormones, and other constituents have virtually the same concentration in plasma and in the unmodified glomerular filtrates. Tubular epithelial cells modify the filtrate to affect homeostasis and excretion.

Secretion and Absorption

The proximal tubule is mainly reabsorptive. Returned to the bloodstream are large quantities of water along with glucose, amino acids, urates, calcium, and whatever protein leaks through the glomerular filter. The proximal tubule also salvages large quantities of electrolytes, notably sodium, chloride, and bicarbonate. The complex of functions performed by the Loop of Henle results in the reabsorption of water and sodium. The distal tubule performs the delicate regulation of sodium, potassium, bicarbonate, phosphate, and hydrogen ions. Final control over water excretion occurs in the collecting ducts.

The outer portion of the kidney, the **cortex,** contains the glomeruli and the convoluted tubules, both proximal and distal. All the collecting ducts and most of the Loops of Henle are in the interior of the kidney, the **medulla.**

The renal medulla is unique among tissues because its extracellular fluid is hypertonic to plasma. The medullary interstitial fluid contains electrolytes in far higher overall concentration than exists in plasma. These electrolytes, which originate in the fluid passing through the Loop of Henle, are actively transported into the interstitial fluid. The hypertonic interstitial environment in the medulla regulates the reabsorption of ions at different levels of the Loop, as well as the passive absorption of water in the collecting ducts.

Urine Formation

When the number and function of all constituent parts of the kidney are normal, renal function can be understood on the basis of the functional components of the nephron. The glomeruli remove the materials that need to be excreted and prevent the loss of proteins and cells into the urine. Tubules reabsorb solutes that must be conserved; regulate sodium, potassium, and bicarbonate concentrations; and excrete or preserve hydrogen ions as needed. The collecting ducts, in the hypertonic medulla, regulate the amount of water conserved or excreted. Each of the activities can be evaluated by appropriately selected laboratory tests. Renal function tests include the examination of the urine (urinalysis); examination of the blood to measure substances affected by renal function; and dynamic measurements of blood flow, urine formation, and substance excretion.

LABORATORY EVALUATION OF THE URINE

Urinalysis is probably the oldest clinical laboratory practice and usually involves gross observation and assessment of general appearance, dipstick analysis, and microscopic assessment. It is still one of the most commonly performed laboratory tests, both in the clinical laboratory and in the physician's office. A urine sample is readily obtainable, and in certain clinical situations can provide extremely useful information. Readily available dipsticks combined with microscopic evaluation and culture can provide important indicators of disease. Urinalysis is also used as a screening test for the general state of health, a practice that is of uncertain utility in young, otherwise healthy, asymptomatic people. It is, however, critically important that, when urinalysis is performed, an appropriate specimen be collected. Modern urinalysis now also includes quantitative testing of analytes in urine using liquid chemistry performed on automated analyzers.

Obtaining the Specimen

Accurate urinalysis must begin with a good-quality specimen. Vaginal, perineal, and urethral secretions in women and urethral contaminants in men may compromise urinalysis findings. Mucus, proteins, epithelial cells, and microorganisms wash into the urinary system from the urethra and adjacent tissues. Patients should be instructed to void the first few milliliters of urine before beginning the collection. In most cases the patient, male or female, should gently cleanse the urethral meatus with a swab and then a rinse. For a "clean catch" specimen, a requisite for urine culture (see Chapter 14), more diligent cleansing is indicated. Women who are menstruating or who have heavy vaginal secretions should insert a clean tampon before collecting the specimen. Occasionally it is necessary to catheterize to obtain an uncontaminated specimen.

Although specimens collected randomly during the day are satisfactory for many purposes, the most informative specimen is the first urine voided in the morning. Overnight urine reflects a prolonged period without fluid intake, so formed elements are concentrated.

Artifacts

Delay between voiding and urinalysis impairs the validity of results; analysis should be performed no later than 4 hours after collection. Formed elements in urine (the sediment) begin deteriorating within 2 hours. Dissolved urates or phosphates may precipitate, obscuring the microscopic examination of other elements. Bilirubin and urobilinogen may be oxidized if there is prolonged exposure to light. Bacteria begin to multiply if the specimen is not refrigerated, causing misleading results not only for microbiologic examination but also for pH. Protein levels change relatively little, but glucose levels may drop and ketones, if present, may dissipate with prolonged standing.

Appearance

Freshly voided normal urine is clear to slightly hazy and colored yellow by the pigments urochrome and urobilin. The intensity of the color parallels the degree of concentration. Very dilute urine is almost colorless. Very concentrated urine is dark yellow or almost amber. Table 19–1 lists the pathologic and nonpathologic conditions that affect urine color. Turbidity usually results from crystallization or precipitation of urates (in acid urine) or phosphates (in alkaline urine) (see later). Urates and phosphates occasionally precipitate as urine collects in the bladder, but precipitation usually occurs as the voided specimen cools to room or refrigerated temperature.

TABLE 19–1. DIFFERENTIAL CAUSES OF URINE COLORATION*

Color Observed	Pathologic Causes	Nonpathologic Causes	Screening Procedures
Red	1. Hemoglobin 2. Myoglobin 3. Porphobilinogen 4. Porphyrins	Many drugs and dyestuffs Beets, rhubarb, senna	Positive test for occult blood with 1 and 2 Ehrlich's reagent (+) for 3 UV Fluorescence for 4
Orange	1. Bile pigments	Drugs for urinary tract infections, especially pyridium Other drugs including phenothiazines Carrots	Yellow foam when bilirubin is present HCl intensifies color if due to pyridium Careful drug and diet history
Yellow	1. Highly concentrated urine 2. Bilirubin 3. Urobilin	Phenacetin, cascara, nitrofurantoin	Specific gravity for 1 Yellow foam for 2
Green	1. Biliverdin 2. Bacteria, especially *Pseudomonas*	Vitamin preparations Psychoactive drugs Proprietary diuretics	Bilirubin usually also present for 1 Positive culture and microscopic examination for 2 Careful drug history
Blue	None	Proprietary diuretics Nitrofurans Levodopa	Careful drug history
Brown	1. Acid hematin 2. Myoglobin 3. Bile pigments	Nitrofurans Some sulfa drugs Levodopa	Occult blood test (+) for 1 and 2 Bilirubin test usually (+) for 3 Careful drug history Color intensifies with standing for 1,2,3,4
Black or brownish-black	1. Melanin 2. Homogentisic acid 3. Indicans 4. Urobilinogen 5. Methemoglobin	Cascara Iron complexes Phenols	Ferric/chloride (+) for 1,2 Ehrlich's reagent (+) for 4 Occult blood test (+) for 5 Copper sulfate reduction (+) for 2

*Cloudiness from urates (acid urine) and phosphates (alkaline urine) may occur normally.

Urinalysis should begin with the visual observation of color and general appearance. On random collections, volume is irrelevant. With timed collections, the accurate measurement of volume is an important consideration. The degree of concentration is measured by determining the specific gravity or osmolality. After dipstick examination for preliminary chemical tests, the specimen is examined microscopically for formed elements such as red blood cells, white blood cells, epithelial cells from the kidney or bladder, casts, and bacteria.

Dipsticks

Reagent strips (dipsticks) are available with single or multiple test sections. In most laboratories and offices, the usual screening tests are those for pH, sugar, protein, hemoglobin, and ketones. Additional tests available using reagent strips are listed in Table 19–2. Reagent strips with these five to ten test selections are widely used.

Use of Dipsticks

Reagent strips have enormously simplified urinalysis, but they do require some care. The strips should be stored tightly covered in a cool place protected from moisture, light, and chemical fumes. Each strip should be observed before use to ensure that unwanted color changes have not occurred. The strip should remain in the specimen long enough for optimal wetting but not so long that reagents are washed away. The strip should be blotted to remove excess moisture and examined in a good light after an appropriate time interval. Color changes are interpreted by comparison with a reference color chart, usually on the container label. Unpredictably, inaccurate results occur if the colors are read too early or

TABLE 19–2. CHEMICAL URINALYSIS TESTS COMMONLY AVAILABLE ON REAGENT STRIPS

Specific gravity
pH
Glucose
Protein
Ketones
Blood
Bilirubin
Urobilinogen
Nitrite
Leukocyte esterase

too late, or if the lighting is poor. Reading of dipsticks by an automated instrument is preferable to doing so visually, to minimize errors in timing and to yield the most accurate and sensitive results.

Interpreting Results

The results of strip testing are usually reported as a battery. For abnormal results, confirmatory quantitative tests may be appropriate. If confirmatory tests do not agree with screening results, the strips and their use should be reviewed. It is important to scrutinize all results for internal consistency to avoid misinterpretation. Urine specimens with an elevated glucose content should have high specific gravity. If ketones are present, there should be an acid pH. Brown, red, or smoky urine specimens should be observed for the presence of bilirubin and hemoglobin. If hemoglobin is present, the presence or absence of red cells in the sediment should be noted specifically. In some instances, a discrepancy in findings indicates unusual clinical events; more often discrepancies suggest poorly controlled dipstick technique. Tables 19–3 through 19–13 outline some of the principles, limitations, and the significance of the screening tests routinely performed on urine samples.

Formed Elements in the Urine

Urine Microscopy

Microscopic examination is needed to observe cells and other particulate material. The most common technique is to centrifuge part of the specimen and examine a drop of the wet sediment. Stains are sometimes used to enhance detail and visibility. A few laboratories use phase microscopy. Results are traditionally reported in semiquantitative terms as subject material seen on low-power (100×) or high-power (440×) fields. This approach is not very accurate or always reproducible, but the results are still adequate and useful in most clinical settings. For more precise quantification, it is possible to use a counting chamber and relate these findings to urine volume and concentration.

Normal Findings

Examination of urine sediment can usually demonstrate the presence of white blood cells (Color Plate 93); red blood cells (Color Plate 94); epithelial cells of upper or lower urinary tract origin; casts; crystals; and infectious organisms such as bacteria, yeasts, trichomonas, and cytologically transformed cells indicative of neoplastic or virus infections. Normal individuals have occasional (0 to 2 per high-power field) white cells in their urine sediment and occasional (1 to 3 per high-power field) red cells. Epithelial cells from the urethra and bladder are not uncommon, particularly if the specimen includes the entire voided volume rather than the preferred midstream portion. Crystals or amorphous precipitates

text continues on page 934

TABLE 19–3. FACTORS INTERFERING WITH URINE DIPSTICK INTERPRETATION*

	False-Negative	False-Positive	Comment
Glucose	Elevated urinary ascorbate concentrations	Oxidizing agents in urine containers	Ketone bodies reduce sensitivity of test Reactivity of test decreases as specific gravity increases Newer preparations minimize false-negative with ascorbate
Bilirubin	Elevated urinary ascorbate concentrations	Phenazopyridine	Sensitivity lowered by ascorbate
		Etodolac	Sensitivity lowered by elevated urine nitrite Indoxyl sulfate interferes with both negative and positive
Ketone		Pigmented urine (trace or less)	No reaction with β-hydroxybutyrate or acetone
		Large amount levodopa metabolites	Red to red-orange colors with phenylketone in urine ophthalein compounds, distinguishable from 2-Mercaptoethane sulfuric acid color (MESNA)
Specific gravity		Significant glycosuria Radiocontrast media	Note some new indicators not affected as previously by nonionic particles or radiocontrast Very alkaline urine may read low Elevated values may occur with significant proteinuria (>100 mg/dL)

*This table incorporates data drawn from several commercially available dipsticks. Individual preparations may differ in terms of test reagents used, and therefore, clinical settings in which false or ambiguous readings occur may vary. The package insert always should be reviewed in each individual instance.

(Continued)

TABLE 19–3. FACTORS INTERFERING WITH URINE DIPSTICK INTERPRETATION

	False-Negative	False-Positive	Comment
Blood	Formalin urine preservation	Oxidizing agents in urine container Microbial peroxidase with UTI	
pH		Highly alkaline urine	False lowering of pH if urine spills from protein region of dipstick
Protein	Bence Jones protein, globulin not detected	Urine contamination with quaternary ammonium compounds (skin cleansers, chlorhexidine) Phenazopyridine Polyvinylpyrrolidone infusion (blood substitute) Gross hematuria	
Urobilinogen	Formalin	p-Aminosalicylic acid, sulfonamides, PABA Phenazopyridine (with non-Ehrlich reagent)	The absence of urobilinogen cannot be determined with this test

Nitrite	Infecting organisms lacking nitrate → nitrite reductase Short bladder transit time limiting nitrate → nitrite reduction Ascorbate concentrations ≥25 mg/dL	Meds discoloring urine red or which make red in acid medium
Leukocytes	High urine tetracycline levels	Decreased activity with high glucose concentration (>3 g/dL), high specific gravity, high oxalic acid concentration Interference from nitrofurantoin, gentamicin, cephalexin, and high albumin concentrations (>500 mg/dL)

Data from Ames, Multistix reagent strips, tests for glucose, bilirubin, ketone, specific gravity, blood pH, protein, urobilinogen, nitrite, and leukocytes in urine. Boehringer Mannheim Diagnostics, Chemstrip, urinalysis tests for leukocytes, nitrite, pH, protein, glucose, ketones, urobilinogen, bilirubin, and blood in urine. Rose, BD: Pathophysiology of Renal Disease, McGraw-Hill, New York, 1986.

From Kokko, JP: Approach to patient with renal disease. In Bennett, JC, and Plum, F (eds), Cecil Textbook of Medicine, ed 20. WB Saunders, Philadelphia, 1996, p 512, with permission.

TABLE 19–4. CAUSES OF ALTERATIONS OF URINARY pH*

Finding and Condition	Causes and Comments
Alkaline:	
Postprandial "alkaline tide"	Normal finding in specimens voided shortly after meals
Vegetarianism	Meats produce fixed acid residue, vegetarian diet does not
Systemic alkalosis	Look for severe vomiting, hyperventilation, excess alkali ingestion
Urinary tract infection	*Proteus* or *pseudomonas* splits urea to CO_2 and ammonia
Alkalinization therapy	Used to prevent crystallization of uric acid, oxalate, cystine, sulfonamides, streptomycin
Stale specimen	Very high pH and ammoniacal odor suggests bacterial overgrowth. If true infection exists, sediment should have white blood cells
Renal tubular acidosis	Impaired tubular acidification causes inappropriately high urine pH with systemic acidosis and low serum HCO_3^-
Acid:	
Ketosis	Diabetes, starvation, febrile illness in children
Systemic acidosis	Except with impaired renal tubular function, respiratory or metabolic acidosis provokes intense urine acidity and increased NH_4^+ excretion
Acidification therapy	Used in treating urinary tract infections, and to prevent precipitation of calcium carbonate or phosphates, or magnesium ammonium phosphate

*Reference interval 4.8–7.8. Standard reagent strip indicators can differentiate pH values to within 0.5 units; usual range is 4.8 to 7.8. Urine pH changes in response to plasma pH; acidosis is associated with excretion of an acid urine due to acid secretion and base conservation, whereas in alkalosis there is an alkaline urine due to base excretion and acid conservation. The normal pH of a fasting individual is 6.0.

usually have little significance unless there is a history of stones or therapy with drugs known to crystallize in the kidneys.

Dysmorphic red cells in the urine sediment are a highly specific indicator of glomerular bleeding. Under phase contrast microscopy, these cells may show cytoplasmic blebs and appear to have "Mickey Mouse" ears, or other shapes. These dysmorphic erythrocytes also have substantially smaller mean cell volumes than erythrocytes in blood.

Casts

Casts are cylindrical masses of protein that form in renal tubules and are washed through into the urine. These are subclassified according to their morphologic appearance and composition. The **protein matrix** is a

text continues on page 939

TABLE 19–5. TESTS FOR SUGARS* IN URINE

	Clinitest ("Benedicts Solution") Tablets†	Glucose Oxidase Strips
Sugars detected (minimum concentration)	Glucose (25 mg/dL) Galactose Lactose Fructose Maltose Pentose	Glucose (50 mg/dL)
False-positive	Ascorbic acid Homogentisic acid Many antibiotics Phenothiazines Salicylates Levodopa X-ray contrast media	Hydrogen peroxide or hypochlorite in container
False-negative	Bacterial infection	Ascorbic acid Homogentisic acid Large amounts of salicylates Bacterial infection Hydroxyindoleacetic acid

*Sucrose is not detected by either test. It is rarely found in urine except for occasional instances when patient has deliberately added table sugar to urine sample.
†Screening test for all reducing sugars.

TABLE 19–6. SIGNIFICANCE OF SUGARS IN URINE

Glycosuria with High Blood Sugar

Diabetes mellitus

Other endocrine disorders: Acromegaly, Cushing's syndrome, hyperthyroidism, pheochromocytoma

Pancreatic disease: Advanced stages of cystic fibrosis, hemochromatosis, severe chronic pancreatitis, carcinoma

Central nervous system dysfunction: Asphyxia; tumors or hemorrhage, especially involving hypothalamus

Massive metabolic derangement: Severe burns, uremia, advanced liver disease, sepsis, cardiogenic shock

Drug induced: Corticosteroids and ACTH; thiazides; oral contraceptives

Glycosuria without Elevated Blood Glucose

Renal tubular dysfunction

Pregnancy (must be carefully distinguished from gestational diabetes)

Nonglucose Sugars in Urine

Galactose: Detecting galactosemia in newborn period may prevent irreversible CNS and liver damage. Galactose spills into urine only if milk is being taken.

Fructose: Essential fructosuria is rare, benign condition. Hereditary fructose intolerance produces severe hypoglycernia with CNS and liver problems occurring only after eating sucrose, fruits, vegetables, or potatoes.

Pentose: Very high fruit intake may cause pentosuria in normal persons. Benign genetic condition, more common in Jews; must be distinguished from diabetes mellitus.

TABLE 19–7. TESTS FOR PROTEIN IN URINE

	Reagent Strip	Heat and Acid	Sulfosalicylic Acid
Proteins detected (concentration)	Albumin (5–10 mg/dL)	Albumin (5–10 mg/dL) Globulins Bence Jones (clears with boiling)	Albumin (0.25 mg/dL) Globulins Bence Jones Glycoproteins
Proteins missed	Globulins Bence Jones		
False-positive	Skin disinfectants (also cause very high pH)	Phosphates and urates may confuse interpretation Drug metabolites: tolbutamide, sulfonamide, high-dose penicillin White blood cells Red blood cells	Same as heat and acid Also cephalothin, chlorpromazine
False-negative	Very dilute urine Very high salt concentration	Highly buffered alkaline urine	Same as heat and acid

TABLE 19–8. SIGNIFICANCE OF PROTEINS* IN URINE

Minimal Proteinuria (<0.5 g/day):
Following exercise or in highly concentrated urine, in healthy persons
Fever, severe emotional or thermal stress, in otherwise healthy persons
Postural proteinuria: Young adults may spill protein while ambulatory but not when recumbent
Hypertension
Renal tubular dysfunction, including genetic and drug-induced
Polycystic kidneys
Lower urinary tract infections
Hemoglobinuria with severe hemolytic transfusion reaction, paroxysmal cold hemoglobinuria, paroxysmal nocturnal hemoglobinuria

Moderate Proteinuria (0.5–3 g/day):
Chronic glomerulonephritis, moderate
Congestive heart failure
Diabetic nephropathy, mild
Pyelonephritis
Multiple myeloma (Bence Jones protein and other proteins)
Pre-eclampsia

Marked Proteinuria (>3 g/day):
Acute glomerulonephritis
Chronic glomerulonephritis, severe
Lipoid nephrosis
Diabetic nephropathy, severe
Amyloid disease
Lupus nephritis

*Usually predominantly albumin. Bence Jones protein, hemoglobin, and myoglobin are significant nonalbumin proteins sometimes present.

TABLE 19–9. TESTS FOR HEMOGLOBIN* IN URINE

	Orthotolidine (Reagent Strip or Wet Test)	Benzidine
Substance detected	Intact RBCs Hemoglobin Myoglobin	Carcinogenic: not used for routine testing
False-positive	Oxidizing agents (peroxide, hypochlorite in container)	
False-negative	Ascorbic acid Formaldehyde Reduced sensitivity: very high specific gravity; high concentration nitrite	

*Based on peroxidase activity of heme, which catalyzes oxidation of indicator chromogen.
RBC = red blood cells.

TABLE 19–10. SIGNIFICANCE OF HEMOGLOBINURIA

Nature of Hemoglobin	Other Findings
Intact Red Cells Present in Sediment*; No Casts	
Contamination with menstrual blood	Clots, mucus in urine
Vigorous exercise, in normal individuals	History of exercise
Trauma at any part of urinary tract	History of trauma
Cystitis	WBCs, often bacteria, in urine
Renal calculi	Characteristic pain pattern
	X-ray or ultrasound demonstration of stone
Kidney or bladder tumors	Urine cytology may be helpful
Anticoagulant excess	Bleeding diathesis, drug history
Malignant hypertension	Elevated blood pressure
Sickle-cell trait or disease	Often proteinuria
	No urinary abnormalities
	Hemoglobin S in circulating blood
Hemorrhagic cystitis	Cyclophosphamide chemotherapy

*Dysmorphic RBCs suggest glomerular bleeding. *(Continued)*

TABLE 19–10. SIGNIFICANCE OF HEMOGLOBINURIA *(Continued)*

Nature of Hemoglobin	Other Findings
Intact Red Cells Present; Red Cell or Granular Casts; Proteinuria	
Acute glomerulonephritis	Elevated blood pressure, oliguria
	History of infection or allergen exposure
Chronic glomerulonephritis	May have low serum complement
	Renal biopsy important
Lupus nephritis	Positive history and diagnostic signs for lupus
	Serum anti-DNA level high, C3 and C4 low
	Fever, joint pain often accompany
Goodpasture's syndrome	Hemoptysis usually precedes kidney involvement
	Serum antibodies to glomerular basement membrane
Polyarteritis	Multiple cells and casts in sediment
	Multiorgan involvement
	Hypertension may develop
	Immune complexes in circulation
Allergic nephropathy (Henoch-Schönlein purpura)	Purpuric skin rash
	Nephrotic syndrome may develop
No Intact Red Cells in Sediment	
Red cell lysis because of delay in examination	Occurs most rapidly in dilute urine
Traumatic rupture of circulating red cells	History of pounding exercise (marching, karate chops, etc.)
Hemolytic transfusion reaction	History of transfusion within preceding 2 weeks (usually several hours, or 2–3 days)
	Red cell antibodies present
	Acute drop in blood pressure
Transfusion of hemolyzed blood	Improper freezing and thawing of transfused product
Paroxysmal cold hemoglobinuria	Positive test for biphasic cold antibody
Paroxysmal nocturnal hemoglobinuria	Positive Ham's acid hemolysis test
	Hemosiderinuria often present
Nonimmune hemolysis	Prosthetic heart valves
	Thrombotic thrombocytopenic purpura (TTP) or hemolytic-uremic syndrome
Myoglobin present; not hemoglobin	History of crushing injury or other severe trauma to muscle
	Alcoholic or congenital myopathy
	Serum CPK levels very high

TABLE 19–11. TESTS FOR URINE BILIRUBIN*

	Diazo Reaction (Tablet or Dipstick)	Fouchet's Test (Acidified Ferric Chloride)
False-positive	Chlorpromazine	Aspirin metabolites Urobilin or indican Urobilinogen
False-negative	Ascorbic acid High levels of nitrites Oxidation of bilirubin, if examination is delayed more than 4 hours	Oxidation of bilirubin, if examination is delayed
Remarks	Tablet test more sensitive than dipstick (0.2–0.4 mg/dL, compared with 0.05–0.1 mg/dL)	Many compounds give assorted colors in FeCl$_2$ test (see Table 16–18)

*Only the direct-reacting, posthepatic form of bilirubin enters the urine. There must be a 25-fold increase in bilirubin before a positive test is noted on urinalysis strip.

glycoprotein produced by renal epithelial cells called the **Tamm-Horsfall mucoproteins.** Slow tubular flow, acidic pH, and low volume with high protein content predisposes to protein aggregation, but even normal urine specimens contain a modest number of clear protein (hyaline) casts (Color Plate 95). Any particulate or cellular matter present in abnormal tubular conditions readily adheres to the sticky proteinaceous matrix.

TABLE 19–12. SCREENING TESTS FOR URINE UROBILINOGEN*

	Ehrlich's Aldehyde Reaction (Multistix, Urobilistix)	Azo Dye Reaction (BMC Chemstrip)
False-positive	Porphobilinogen 5-Hydroxyindoleacetic acid Phenothiazines Sulfonamides Para-aminosalicylic acid	Red urine from any cause
Remarks	Unreliable if urine bilirubin level is high Sensitivity level 1.3 mg/dL	Sensitivity level 0.4 mg/dL

*Urobilinogen rapidly oxidizes to nonreactive urobilin. Negative urine screening test is normal. Elevated level indicates increased intestinal content of bilirubin, usually from hemolysis or liver disease.

TABLE 19–13. SCREENING TEST FOR URINE NITRITES*

False-Positive

Red urine from any cause.
In vitro bacterial metabolism, if examination is delayed.

False-Negative

Vegetarian diet provides insufficient nitrate.
Antibiotic therapy alters bacterial metabolism.
Infecting organism may not metabolize nitrate.
Urine not in bladder requisite 4–6 hours.
Level of ascorbic acid is high.

---

*Based on observation that most urinary tract pathogens convert urine nitrate to nitrite; positive result interpreted as indicating urinary tract infection. Organisms such as gonococcus, *Mycobacterium tuberculosis*, and *Streptococcus faecalis* are non–nitrate reducers.

The cellular constituents of casts most often include red cells, white cells, and tubular epithelial cells, either intact or in various stages of disintegration. Sometimes there may be entrapped crystals or masses of hemoglobin, myoglobin, hemosiderin, or other substances. When casts contain recognizable cells or other materials, they are described by the constituent: for example, as red cell casts (Color Plate 96) or white cell casts (Color Plate 97). Recognition becomes more difficult as cells disintegrate into granular particles or debris, and many casts are described simply as granular (Color Plate 98).

Interpretation The presence of casts signifies abnormal conditions within the renal parenchyma and may be described as an "active sediment." Cells in the urine sediment cannot readily be assigned to kidney, bladder, or urethral origin, but finding cells trapped in tubular protein provides proof of renal origin. Lower urinary tract abnormalities may, of course, be present at the same time. **White cell casts** always indicate inflammation (usually infection) involving the tubules, the peritubular tissue, or the glomeruli. **Red cell casts** usually derive from damaged glomeruli. **Mixed or granular casts** may represent combinations of inflammation or hemorrhage, or may indicate that damaged tubular lining cells have disintegrated and sloughed into the lumen. Clinical correlates of different types of casts are given in Tables 19–14 and 19–15.

TABLE 19–14. CASTS IN URINE SEDIMENT (REFERENCE RANGE <1/LPF)

Type of Cast	Appearance	Etiologic Conditions
Hyaline	Clear, colorless, structureless ↓ R.I.	Normal people after strenuous exercise Congestive heart failure Diabetic nephropathy Chronic renal failure (glomerulonephritis and pyelonephritis, but not predominant form)
Red cell	Cell outlines visible, may be pigmented ↑ R.I.	Acute glomerulonephritis Lupus nephritis Goodpasture's syndrome Subacute bacterial endocarditis Renal infarct
White cell	Nucleated cells present ↑ R.I.	Acute pyelonephritis Interstitial nephritis Lupus nephritis
Epithelial cell	May be hard to distinguish from WBC cast ↑ R.I.	Tubular necrosis Cytomegalovirus infection Toxicity from heavy metals, salicylates Transplant rejection
Granular	Coarse or fine granules, with or without cell fragments ↑ R.I.	Rarely in normal subjects Nephrotic syndrome Pyelonephritis Glomerulonephritis Transplant rejection Lead toxicity
Waxy casts	Broad, structureless, refractile, sharply outlined Ends may appear "broken off"	Severe tubular atrophy Renal failure Transplant rejection
Bacterial casts	May be misdiagnosed as granular casts May co-exist with white cell casts	Pyelonephritis
Fatty casts	Contain spherical highly refractile fat droplets that may demonstrate "Maltese cross appearance under polarized light"	Proteinuria Nephrotic syndrome

R.I. = refractive index; LPF = low-power field.

TABLE 19–15. MISCELLANEOUS CELLS IN URINE

Cells	Appearance	Etiologic Conditions
Neutrophils	• May appear smaller or larger than RBCs depending on urine tonicity • May contain ingested particles	Infections (particularly acute) Inflammatory disorders
Eosinophils	Not normally present	Interstitial nephritis
Lymphocytes	A few lymphocytes ± Increased lymphocytes ++	May be normal Renal transplant rejection
Mononuclear cells	± ------------- ++ in number	Chronic inflammation
Histiocytes	May contain ingested material (oval fat bodies)	Radiation therapy Nephrosis Lipidemia Infections
Epithelial cells	Squamous, transitional, cuboidal, columnar • Renal tubular cells Polyhedral or elongated Twice as large as PMN May have microvilli • Ingested lipids may appear as a Maltese cross under polarized microscopy • Hemosiderin granules	Renal tubular or lower urinary tract disorders Acute tubular recurrent viral infection Renal transplant rejection
Spermatozoa	4–6 μ Head may be separated from tail	Postprostatectomy Postejaculation
Squamous epithelium	Large 30–50 μ +++ in number	Vaginal, perineal, urethral infection
Mesothelial (transitional)	Renal pelvis → bladder 6× size of RBC Spherical, ovoid, or polyhedral, ± in number or clusters	Normal Can indicate urinary tract pathology or occur postcatheterization

LABORATORY ASSESSMENT OF RENAL FUNCTION

Urinalysis obviously provides information about the kidneys. The term "renal function tests" implies evaluation of the dynamics of excretion, secretion, and osmolar regulation (see also Chapter 10). Since excretory and secretory functions control the osmolar content of urine, these activities are closely interrelated. The renal activity most studied is **clearance,** the relationship between renal excretory mechanisms and the circulating blood levels of the excreted material. Clearance studies generally reflect the overall level of glomerular functioning and reflect the ability of the kidneys to "clear" the plasma of a specific substance.

Clearance Principle

After solutes pass through the glomerulus into the tubule, they may pass unaltered through the entire nephron. Some or all of the material may be reabsorbed for return to the blood, or the tubular epithelium may modify or add to the solute load already present. If a substance passes unaltered through the nephron, the quantity excreted reflects exactly the amount that entered the glomerulus. One can use this principle to determine the amount of fluid flowing through all glomeruli into the tubules in a given time, thus measuring the **glomerular filtration rate (GFR).**

If the concentration of the solute in the *blood* is known, the volume of urine in a predetermined time is measured, and if the concentration of the solute in the *urine* is known, the clearance rate of this solute by the kidney can be calculated as the removal of that substance from plasma into urine over a fixed time. Clearance calculations represent the volume of plasma that would contribute all the solute excreted, assuming all material entering the glomerulus is cleared from the plasma and is excreted in an unmodified way into the urine.

Calculation
The formula for calculating clearance is:

$$C = \frac{[U]V}{[P]}$$

where:

C = Plasma clearance in mL/min
V = The milliliter volume of urine excreted during the measured period (mL/min)
$[U]$ = Solute concentration in the urine
$[P]$ = The solute concentration in the plasma at the midpoint of the collection

For example, if the urine concentration of creatinine is 196 mg/dL when the plasma creatinine is 1.4 mg/dL and urine volume is 1500 mL in 24 hours (1440 min), then the volume of plasma cleared of that concentration of creatinine in 1 minute (C) is

$$\frac{196 \text{ mg/dL} \times 1500 \text{ mL/1440 min}}{1.4 \text{ mg/dL}} = 146 \text{ mL/min}$$

Clearance is expressed in milliliters per minute, representing the volume of plasma that would be totally cleared of the solute in 1 minute.

Plasma concentration and clearance are inversely proportional; as clearance of a substance declines, its concentration in the circulating plasma increases. Variables that affect clearance include the number of nephrons functioning, the efficiency with which they function, and the amount of blood entering the nephrons.

Clearance can be calculated for almost any substance, but only a few such measurements are clinically useful (Table 19–16). Substances like sodium, potassium, hydrogen ions, and water are affected by so many different physiologic reactions that many unknown variables distort attempts to correlate urinary excretion with plasma concentration.

Creatinine Clearance

Creatinine is the metabolite best suited for calculating reliable clearance figures and has replaced other methods such as urea clearance. Creatinine is a product of the breakdown of creatine, a nitrogen-containing compound found largely in muscle. Creatine is phosphorylated by the enzyme **creatine phosphokinase (CPK),** also called creatine kinase (CK), into a high-energy phosphate compound that participates in energy-requiring metabolic reactions. In any one individual, the amount of creatinine generated from creatine turnover tends to remain constant. The quantity generated and excreted is proportional to muscle mass and is usually higher in men than in women. The quantity of creatinine excreted by a single individual remains fairly constant from day to day. Because the quantity of creatinine excreted does not vary much within the urine volume, it is customary to estimate whether successive 24-hour urine collections are complete by comparing the creatinine excretion in each specimen.

Artifacts Creatinine clearance is an excellent measurement of renal function because a uniform quantity is generated and excretion depends only on urinary filtration. One drawback is that tubular cells secrete small amounts of creatinine into the filtrate, producing clearance values about 10% higher than those for inulin (the **reference research method**) (Table 19–17). This is relatively insignificant at normal flow rates, but when filtration levels decline because of declining renal function, the tubular contribution becomes proportionately much larger. With severely damaged kidneys, a single figure for creatinine clearance may give an incorrect impression that clearance rates are fairly good. If serial determinations are done, however, the sequence of clearance figures provides an excellent indication of changing renal function.

Procedure The creatinine clearance test is easy to perform. Urine is collected for a specific period, often 24 hours, but shorter periods are acceptable if there is good hydration and adequate urine output. The total amount of creatinine excreted is measured, and plasma creatinine is determined at some point during the collection period. The calculated clearance is reported as milliliters per minute per $1.73 m^2$ of body surface

TABLE 19-16. RELATIVE CONCENTRATIONS OF SUBSTANCES IN THE GLOMERULAR FILTRATE AND IN THE URINE

	Glomerular Filtrate (125 mL/min)		Urine (1 mL/min)		Concentration of Urine/Concentration of Plasma (Plasma Clearance per min)
	Quantity/min	Concentration	Quantity/min	Concentration	
Na^+	17.7 mEq	142 mEq/L	0.128 mEq	128 mEq	0.9
K^+	0.63	5	0.06	60	12
Ca^{2+}	0.5	4	0.0048	4.8	1.2
Mg^{2+}	0.38	3	0.015	15	5.0
Cl^-	12.9	103	0.134	134	1.3
HCO_3^-	3.5	28	0.014	14	0.5
$H_2PO_4^-$ } HPO_4^{2-} }	0.25	2	0.05	50	25
SO_4^{2-}	0.09	0.7	0.033	33	47
Glucose	125 mg	100 mg/dL	0 mg	0 mg/dL	0.0
Urea	33	26	18.2	1820	70
Uric acid	3.8	3	0.42	42	14
Creatinine	1.4	1.1	1.96	196	140
Inulin	—	—	—	—	125
Diodrast	—	—	—	—	560
PAH	—	—	—	—	585

From Guyton, AC: Textbook of Medical Physiology, ed 7. WB Saunders, Philadelphia, 1986, p 407, with permission.

TABLE 19–17. CREATININE CLEARANCE TEST

Normal Range

85–125 mL/min (men)

75–112 mL/min (women)

Effect of Age on Normal Function

Ages 50–75, subtract 5 mL for each 5–year interval

Over age 75, subtract 8 mL for each 5–year interval

Causes for Overestimation of Calculated Figure

Reduced creatinine production (malnutrition, starvation, cirrhosis, muscle wasting, prolonged bed rest)

Artifacts that Lower Calculated Figure

Incomplete urine collection

Bacterial multiplication in collecting vessel

Ketones, barbiturates, PSP, BSP in urine at higher levels than in plasma .

Causes for Reduced Creatinine Clearance

Acute: Shock, hypovolemia, nephrotoxic chemicals, acute glomerulonephritis, malignant hypertension, eclampsia

Chronic: Glomerulonephritis, pyelonephritis, hypertensive nephrosclerosis, polycystic kidneys

area. Clearance values decline with age in a seemingly normal population, and normal women have somewhat lower values than normal men (see Tables 19–17, 19–18).

When a quick estimate of renal capacity is needed and there is no opportunity to collect an adequately timed urine specimen, an approximate figure for creatinine clearance can be derived from the serum creatinine level alone, using the formulas shown in Table 19–18. These formulas are empirically derived and are useful over an age range from 20 to 80 years. The bedside calculation gives enough information to determine medication schedules or to interpret other diagnostic tests in the light of impaired but relatively stable renal function.

Pathophysiologic Correlations Normal kidneys have a large safety margin. Many nephrons can be lost without losing excretory capacity for nitrogenous wastes. As creatinine clearance declines, plasma creatinine levels rise very little until about half the functioning nephrons are gone. If the loss occurs slowly, the remaining nephrons hypertrophy to counterbalance the loss, and as many as two-thirds of the original number may be lost before plasma creatinine begins to rise sharply (see also Chapter 9). Values rise more rapidly with acute damage to renal blood flow or glomerular activity.

Blood urea concentration is less stable than creatinine concentration and gives a rough index of renal functions. Prerenal causes for uremia

TABLE 19–18. ALTERNATIVE FORMULAS USED TO ESTIMATE CREATININE CLEARANCE (mL/min) BASED ON SERUM CREATININE MEASUREMENT*

1.
$$\frac{[U_c]V}{[P_c]}$$

2.
$$\frac{(140 - age\ [yrs])\ (weight\ [kg])}{72\ (serum\ creatinine)}$$

(Values for women are 0.85 of above formula)

*These equations are reliable only in patients with stable renal function who are not obese or edematous.

U_c = concentration (mg/mL) of creatinine in urine; P_c = concentration (mg/mL) of creatinine in plasma (or serum); V = volume of urine in mL/min.

such as excessive protein or hemoglobin breakdown or fever with dehydration either have no effect on plasma creatinine or cause creatinine levels to rise quite slowly. If creatinine concentration is normal in a patient with elevated blood urea, a nonrenal (prerenal) cause for the uremia should be sought.

With initially normal or near-normal glomerular function, a true rise in plasma creatinine of 0.5 mg/dL represents as much as a 40% change in the glomerular filtration rate. Normal plasma creatinine levels are low; the figure varies with laboratory and method, but is never higher than 1.5 mg/dL. With severely impaired kidneys, plasma creatinine varies much more with small changes in clearance, and the confidence limits of the test have less relative effect on the absolute values observed. Table 19–17 outlines significant and artifactual events that affect creatinine clearance.

Blood Urea Nitrogen: Creatinine Ratio

The ratio of blood urea nitrogen (BUN) to serum creatinine is normally about 10:1. This value is increased in prerenal causes (e.g., dehydration, hypotension) to more than 15:1 because of augmented tubular reabsorption of urea in the presence of a decreased glomerular filtration rate. Postrenal causes of an elevated BUN are associated with a BUN/creatinine ratio of less than 15 because increased tubular reabsorption of urea occurs with stasis, but BUN rise is proportionately greater than that of creatinine. A high BUN/creatinine ratio may also be seen in patients with reduced muscle mass, compromised renal function with a high-protein diet, tissue destruction, and myopathies associated with thyrotoxicosis or Cushing's syndrome. A decreased BUN/creatinine ratio may occur with decreased urea production, as may be seen in liver disease, a low-protein diet, or with hemodialysis because urea dialyses more readily than creatinine.

Other Renal Function Tests

Renal Blood Flow

The **para-aminohippuric acid test (PAHA)** uses a dye that is removed and filtered during a single passage through the kidney (Table 19–19).

Tubular Function

Different tubular segments perform different functions, and there are many ways to evaluate these. Measuring maximum tubular transport (Tm) for different materials also provides valuable physiologic insights but has little applicability to individual clinical situations. More appropriate for diagnostic use are the comparative measurements of serum and urine levels of substances like glucose, phosphates, amino acids, hydrogen ions, bicarbonate, ammonium ions, and standard electrolytes; this allows inferences about how renal tubular function affects metabolism. Collectively, loss of excessive amounts of these substances constitutes Fanconi's syndrome. Glycosuria at normal blood glucose levels, for example, indicates proximal tubular dysfunction. Inappropriate secretion of bicarbonate, sodium, and potassium indicates distal tubular dysfunction, as does failure to appropriately excrete acidic or alkaline urine (see section on Acid-Base Regulation in Chapter 9). A rough indication of functioning tubular mass is derived from testing the excretion of phenolsulfonphthalein (PSP), although this test is not commonly used (see Table 19–19).

Concentrating Ability

Urine concentrating ability and osmolality reflect functioning of the collecting tubules, the Loops of Henle, and the interstitium of the renal medulla. The normal kidney can concentrate urine to an osmolality four times that of plasma (if there is a need to conserve fluid) and can dilute urine to an osmolality one-fourth that of plasma (when excess water must be excreted). Normal plasma osmolality is approximately 285 mOsm/kg. Urine volume bears considerable relationship to urine concentration, but the association is far from absolute. Table 19–20 lists events that affect the quantity of urine excreted.

Physiology (Osmolality and Osmolarity)

The concepts of **osmolarity** (dissolved solutes per liter of solution) and **osmolality** (dissolved solutes per kilogram of body weight) have been discussed in Chapter 10, Fluid and Electrolyte Balance. Osmolality may

TABLE 19–19. ADDITIONAL RENAL FUNCTION TESTS

Test	Measures	Method	Reference Range
PAHA	Renal plasma flow	Clearance of dye	600–700 mL/min
PSP	Renal tubular function	Excretion of dye proportional to renal tubular mass	1200 mL blood flow/min >25% in urine in 15 min 55–75% in urine in 2 hr
Filtration fraction		GFR/RPF	17–21% males 17–23% females
Urine sodium in oliguric renal failure (mEq/L)			<20: pre-renal >40: renal
Fractional Electrolyte Excretion			
F_{Na}, F_{Cl}	Differentiate etiologies of hyponatremia and salt-losing states	Blood and urine electrolyte measurement (spot urine)	<1: pre-renal failure >1 (usually >3): SIADH, acute tubular necrosis, salt-losing nephropathy, adrenal insufficiency
24-Hour Excretion of Potassium (mEq/L)			
F_K	Differentiate etiologies of hypokalemia and hyperkalemia		>40 suggests renal loss, aldosterone excess, diuretics, renal artery stenosis <40 suggests aldosterone deficiency, poor intake, GI loss

PAHA = para-aminohippuric acid; PSP = phenolsulfonphthalein; GFR = glomerular filtration rate; RPF = renal plasma flow; SIADH = syndrome of inappropriate antidiuretic hormone; F_{Na} = fractional sodium excretion; F_{Cl} = fractional chloride excretion; F_K = fractional potassium excretion.

Fractional excretion for an analyte (x) is calculated using the formula:

$$F_x = ([U_x/P_x]/[U_{Cr}/P_{Cr}]) \times 100$$

Where U_x = urine concentration; P_x = plasma concentration; Cr = creatinine.

TABLE 19–20. CONDITIONS THAT AFFECT URINE VOLUME

Acute Oliguria* (↓ Urine Volume)	Acute Polyuria (↑ Urine Volume)	Chronic Polyuria (↑ Urine Volume)
Dehydration	Overhydration	Diabetes insipidus: ADH
Hypovolemic shock	Diabetes mellitus	deficit, psychogenic,
Hypotension	Diuretic phase of recovery	nephrogenic
Massive edema or ascites	from renal failure	Chronic renal failure
Heat stroke	Diuretic therapy	Diabetes mellitus
Nephrotoxic drugs	Osmotic diuresis	Glucocorticoid deficit or
Acute glomerulonephritis		excess
Malignant hypertension		Hyperparathyroidism
Eclampsia		Salt-losing nephritis
Obstruction of pelvis, ureter, bladder outlet		Compulsive water drinking

*Oliguria: <400 mL urine/24 hours—adults
15–20 mL/kg/24 hours—children
Anuria: <100 mL urine/24 hours

be measured in the serum or the urine by freezing point depression. Comparative measurements of serum or plasma and urine osmolality can give an indication of prerenal and renal disorders causing hypertonic and hypotonic states. Osmolality can be calculated with the following formula:

$$\text{Osmolality (mOsm/kg water)} = 2[\text{Na+}] + \text{Glucose}/18 + [\text{BUN}]/2.8$$

where:

Na is measured in milliequivalents per liter; glucose, in milligrams per deciliter; and BUN, in milligrams per deciliter.

Normally the urine-to-serum osmolality ratio is at least 1:1 and after controlled fluid intake, it should reach 3:1. If this value is consistently less than 1:1, it indicates distal tubular disease, whereas if this ratio is consistently greater than 1:1, it indicates that too much solute is in the urinary filtrate and that there is glomerular disease.

Urine osmolality is regulated by the reabsorption of water and electrolytes at two different sites in the nephron, the Loop of Henle and the collecting tubules. In the Loop of Henle, water and electrolytes re-enter the blood in quantities determined only by physical principles of diffusion, concentration, and flow rates. In the collecting tubules, however, water crosses the tubular epithelium into the hypertonic medium of the medulla only if antidiuretic hormone (ADH) renders the epithelium permeable to water. The rate at which urine flows through the tubules also influences reabsorption. Adequate osmolar regulation requires that the medulla remain persistently hypertonic, that the pituitary respond to changes in systemic osmolality, and that the tubular epithelium respond to the effects of ADH. It is also required that filtrate flow through the system slowly enough that water and solutes can respond to the osmotic gradient.

Pathologic Events

Osmotic diuresis occurs when the solute load in the filtrate is high relative to the hypertonic medullary environment. Mannitol or other injected solutes promote water loss because high plasma osmolality pulls water into the blood from the tissues, and then high urine osmolality causes the filtrate to move rapidly through the collecting tubules. Hyperglycemia produces osmotic diuresis by the same mechanism, except that the osmotically active material is endogenous, not infused.

If functioning nephrons are lost, the reduced number of remaining nephrons must handle the entire solute load. Each residual nephron experiences an increased osmotic burden, imposing an internal form of osmotic diuresis. For this reason, the nephrons that remain lose responsiveness to osmotic stimuli. With progressive impairment, there is progressive inability to concentrate, and the urine never achieves osmolality above that of plasma. Dilutional capacity is also lost, and the kidneys have difficulty excreting excessive circulating water.

Concentration Defects

Tests of renal concentrating ability can often detect renal damage that is not yet severe enough to elevate urea or creatinine levels. With severe loss of concentrating ability, urine's specific gravity remains fixed at about 1.010, corresponding to the plasma osmolality of 285 mOsm/kg. In normal metabolic conditions, the body generates a daily solute load of 600 to 800 mOsm, largely representing sodium chloride, urea, and fixed acids that must be excreted. If urine cannot be concentrated, the solute load requires a urine volume of 1.5 to 2.0 L a day for adequate elimination. Normal people increase urine concentration during the night. The patient with failing kidneys continues to excrete a large volume of dilute urine at night and must get up at night to urinate, a condition called **nocturia.** The concentrating ability may diminish when there is selective damage to the medulla or to the tubular epithelium, even if total kidney function is not affected. Inflammation in the medulla can impair concentration, as does altered epithelial response to ADH.

Concentration Tests   The simplest test of renal concentrating ability is the measurement of the specific gravity or osmolality of a first-voided morning urine specimen. If there is no excess protein, glucose, or macromolecule (such as radiographic contrast medium), a specific gravity of 1.025 or osmolality of 850 mOsm/kg indicates that the kidneys have adequate concentrating ability. If spot-checking the morning urine reveals no specimen with adequate osmolality, the patient should be studied under conditions of controlled fluid intake.

Overnight (12 to 14 hours) restriction of all fluid intake provokes increased concentration to about 75% of maximal ability. Maximal concentration should occur after 24 hours without fluids. An alternative method to assess urine-concentrating ability is by injecting 10 units of vasopressin followed by urine collection for 1 to 2 hours. Urine specific gravity should equal or exceed 1.020. The differential diagnosis of impaired concentrating ability is shown in Table 19–21. This includes renal diseases, failure to secrete ADH (diabetes insipidus), failure to respond to ADH, and psychogenic **polydipsia** (compulsive water drinking).

It is important to observe the patient closely during water deprivation, largely to ensure that the patient does not become dehydrated and partly to prevent surreptitious ingestion of fluids. Continuous massive excretion of a dilute urine depresses concentrating ability. If a patient had been overhydrated for days or weeks, several days of normal fluid intake should be imposed before the water deprivation test is done. Tests of

TABLE 19–21. URINE CONCENTRATING ABILITY

	Specific Gravity	Osmolality
Maximal urine dilution	1.010	285 mOs/kg
Normal metabolic activity	1.010–1.025	600–800 mOs/kg
Vasopressin concentration test	≥1.020	≥750 mOs/kg
Maximal urine concentration	1.030	>850 mOs/kg

Conditions that Impair Concentrating Ability

Renal Diseases

Pyelonephritis
Acute or chronic glomerular failure
Nephrogenic diabetes insipidus
Renal tubular acidosis

Metabolic Disturbances

Osmotic diuresis (especially diabetes mellitus)
Hypokalemia
Hypercalcemia (especially hyperparathyroidism)
Lithium use
Ethanol use
Prolonged overhydration
Severe hypoproteinemia

Systemic Diseases Affecting Renal Medulla

Multiple myeloma
Amyloidosis
Sickle cell anemia or sickle trait

dilutional ability are rarely done. They expose the patient to the risk of water intoxication and produce no useful information beyond that obtained with a concentration test and other indices of renal function.

Urine Sodium Excretion The syndrome of inappropriate antidiuretic hormone secretion (SIADH) is discussed in Chapter 16. Table 19–22 links the differential diagnosis of hyponatremia to urine sodium excretion.

Fractional Sodium Excretion Fractional sodium excretion (FNa), also called the **renal failure index,** may provide useful information on whether acute renal insufficiency is prerenal or parenchymal.

$$FNa = \frac{Urine\ Sodium \times Plasma\ Creatinine}{Urine\ Creatinine \times Plasma\ Sodium}$$

A value of less than 1.0 suggests a prerenal (underperfusion) cause, whereas a value greater than 1.5 is more likely due to acute tubular necrosis.

SPECIAL MEASUREMENTS

Innumerable substances found in urine can be measured if circumstances warrant it. This section discusses a few of the more commonly measured urine constituents.

TABLE 19–22. DIFFERENTIAL DIAGNOSIS OF HYPONATREMIA (Na <130 mEq/L): RELATIONSHIP TO URINE SODIUM EXCRETION

Urine Sodium	Differential Diagnosis
>20 mEq/L	Acute renal failure
	Chronic renal failure
	Syndrome of inappropriate antidiuretic hormone (SIADH)
	• Malignant neoplasms: lung, pancreas, prostate
	• Leukemia
	• Lymphoma
	• CNS disorders: tumors, injury, infection
	• Porphyria
	• Pulmonary disorders: tuberculosis, fungi
	Glucocorticoid deficiency
<10 mEq/L	Cirrhosis
	Nephrotic syndrome
	Hyperlipidemia
	Hyperproteinemia

Bilirubin and Urobilinogen

Bilirubin, a breakdown product of hemoglobin, is produced by reticuloendothelial cells scattered throughout the body (see Figs. 2–10 and 2–11, and Chapter 12). As initially produced, bilirubin is not soluble in water; it becomes water soluble after conjugation by the liver. Only the water-soluble posthepatic form can enter the urinary filtrate, so bilirubinuria occurs only when the plasma has high levels of conjugated bilirubin. For an overview of the physiology see Chapter 12 and Figure 12–1.

Urine Findings

Although urine normally contains small amounts of urobilinogen, it is perfectly normal to get negative or trace results on screening (reagent strip) tests, and there is no lower limit to the normal excretion range. Quantitation of urobilinogen in the urine is seldom performed and requires a timed urine specimen (usually 2 hours). If Ehrlich's aldehyde reagent is used, the results are expressed in Ehrlich Units or in mg/dL. Porphobilinogen and 5-hydroxyindoleacetic acid (5-HIAA) are other abnormal urine constituents that react with Ehrlich's reagent. Before an elevated urobilinogen level can be evaluated, these substances must be excluded. Bilirubin is never present in normal conditions. The relationships between serum and urine bilirubin and urine urobilinogen are shown in Table 19–23 (see also Chapter 2).

TABLE 19–23. RELATIONSHIP BETWEEN BILIRUBIN AND UROBILINOGEN LEVELS

Pathologic Conditions	Serum Bilirubin	Urine Bilirubin	Urine Urobilinogen
Hemolysis	↑ indirect Normal direct	Negative	Increased
Early hepatocellular damage	Normal indirect Normal or slightly ↑ direct	Negative	Increased
Moderate-to-severe hepatocellular damage	↑ indirect ↑ direct	Increased	Increased
Obstruction of bile ducts, extrahepatic or intrahepatic	Normal indirect ↑ direct	Increased	Negative

Hemoglobin Precursors

If heme synthesis is deranged, precursor metabolites accumulate because the entire sequence of reactions cannot be completed. It is possible to infer which reaction is blocked by measuring which precursors accumulate. Precursor compounds evolve in the following order, beginning with glycine and succinyl coenzyme A (CoA) as raw materials: delta-aminolevulinic acid (ALA), porphobilinogen, uroporphyrinogen, coproporphyrinogen, and protoporphyrin, which chelates ferrous iron to become heme (see Fig. 2–2A). These substances may variously accumulate in red blood cells, urine, or feces; different disorders have different patterns of excess. Porphobilinogen and ALA react with Ehrlich's reagent and are measured chemically. The later porphyrins are detected by fluorescent techniques and are quantified by spectrophotometry or fluorometry.

Types of Porphyria

The **porphyrias** are a group of disorders characterized by a deficiency or defect in the enzymes involved in porphyrin metabolism and heme synthesis. Depending on the nature of the enzyme deficiency, precursor substances accumulate, and the conditions are classified according to the predominant defect and the major organ system involved. These conditions can be inherited or acquired. The major categories of genetically determined porphyria are **erythropoietic porphyrias,** in which the major diagnostic abnormalities occur in red cell chemistry, and **hepatic porphyrias,** in which the heme precursors are found in urine or feces. In acquired disorders, precursors accumulate more in urine and feces than in red cells. Erythropoietic porphyrias are very rare, as are most of the inherited hepatic porphyrias, except in certain ethnic groups.

Urine Findings

The most significant inherited derangement of heme synthesis is **acute intermittent porphyria (AIP),** an autosomal dominant inherited disorder that affects as many as 1 in 1000 American whites and usually becomes apparent in early or middle adulthood. This condition is characterized by acute intermittent abdominal pain and neurologic manifestations. The diagnostic finding in AIP is elevated urinary porphobilinogen, a compound that is colorless when fresh but turns dark red on standing. Another screening test during the acute attack is the Watson-Schwartz test, which is based on the property that porphobilinogen is insoluble in chloroform and butanol and remains in the aqueous phase of the separation.

Lead poisoning is the most common acquired porphyria. Among other effects, lead inhibits the enzyme necessary to convert ALA to porphobilinogen. As ALA accumulates, increased quantities are excreted in the urine. Severe alcoholic liver disease is sometimes associated with an acquired form of hepatic porphyria. This type is associated with skin manifestations, blister formation, and particular sun sensitivity. Table 19–24 shows classifications of porphyrias based on the responsible organ or clinical manifestations. Table 19–25 shows the diagnostic findings in the different porphyrias.

Collecting the Urine Specimen

Urine for porphyrin measurements should be alkalinized with 7.5 g (0.5 g/100 mL) of sodium carbonate for the 24-hour collection. However, most important to preserving specimens for porphyrin analysis is adequate refrigeration and protection from light. ALA deteriorates rapidly on exposure to light, with as much as 40 to 60% of the compound lost after 24 hours in the light. Uroporphyrin and coproporphyrin exhibit an orange-red fluorescence if exposed to ultraviolet light.

Nitrogenous Compounds

Urea and creatinine are the major nitrogen-containing compounds in the urine. The quantity of urea generated reflects all the many avenues of protein metabolism: dietary intake, urea absorbed from bacterial activity in the gut, protein metabolized as enzymes, and structural proteins

---

TABLE 19–24. CLASSIFICATIONS OF PORPHYRIAS

Classification by Responsible Organ

Erythropoietic:
   Congenital erythropoietic porphyria (Günther's disease)
Erythrohepatic porphyria (erythropoietic protoporphyria)
Hepatic:
   Acute intermittent porphyria
   Variegate porphyria (mixed porphyria)
   Hereditary coproporphyria
   Porphyria cutanea tarda

Classification by Clinical Manifestations

Porphyrias that produce cutaneous manifestations without neurological disease:
   Congenital erythropoietic porphyria
   Erythrohepatic porphyria (erythropoietic protoporphyria)
   Porphyria cutanea tarda
Porphyria that produces neurological disease, but no cutaneous manifestations:
   Acute intermittent porphyria
Porphyrias that can produce cutaneous and neurological disease:
   Variegate porphyria
   Hereditary coproporphyria

From Tschudy, DP: The porphyrias. In Williams, WJ, et al (eds): Hematology, ed 3. McGraw-Hill, New York, 1983, p 693, with permission.

TABLE 19–25. DIAGNOSTIC FINDINGS IN PORPHYRIAS

Condition	Urine	Feces	Other
Hepatic Porphyrias, Congenital			
Acute intermittent porphyria	PBG ↑↑, ALA ↑↑	Normal	Episodic occurrence Estrogens, alcohol, barbiturates may provoke attacks Neurologic symptoms prominent
Porphyria cutanea tarda*	UP ↑, CP ↑ ALA and PBG normal	CP ↑, PP ↑↑	Fluorescence of specimens obtained by liver, skin biopsies Exacerbated by sunlight
Variegate porphyria	ALA ↑, PBG ↑	CP ↑, PP ↑↑	Episodic occurrence Neurologic and skin symptoms
Porphyrias, Acquired			
Lead poisoning	ALA ↑, CP ↑	Normal	ALA-dehydrase levels low
Liver disease	ALA normal or ↑, PBG normal UP ↑, CP ↑	UP ↑, CP ↑	Skin lesions. exacerbated by sunlight Other liver functions abnormal
Erythropoietic Porphyrias, Congenital			
Uroporphyria	UP ↑↑, CP ↑	CP ↑	UP, CP both ↑↑ in red cells Severe skin lesions Hemolysis, tissue defects, early death
Protoporphyria	Normal	CP ↑, PP ↑, UP normal	PP ↑↑ in red cells Moderately severe skin photosensitivity May have liver damage

ALA = delta-aminolevulinic acid; PBG = porphobilinogen; UP = uroporphyrin; CP = coproporphyrin; PP = protoporphyrin.
*Porphyria cutanea tarda usually has familial occurrence, but association with alcohol use or exposure to benzenes or other drugs suggests acquired features as well.

undergoing normal turnover and protein that must be excreted if there is abnormal cellular turnover or destruction. It is rarely necessary to measure the excretion of urea. With impaired renal excretory mechanisms, rising blood urea levels are more sensitive and more easily measured than declining levels of urea excretion.

Creatinine

Creatinine excretion, conversely, constitutes a useful index of renal activity and of uniform urine collection (see earlier discussion on clearance). Each individual excretes a quantity of creatinine each day that depends more on the total muscle mass than on muscular activity or the level of protein metabolism, although these do have a modest effect. Impaired excretory capacity reduces the efficiency of plasma clearance, but daily excretion changes very little from one day to another. Once a careful 24-hour urine collection has established an individual's creatinine excretion level, creatinine measurement can be used to determine whether other 24-hour collections are complete. Women usually excrete 0.8 to 1.7 g and men, 1.0 to 1.9 g. If a 24-hour urine sample contains, for example, only 0.5 g, one can assume that at least half of the day's specimen was lost.

Because urine creatinine levels remain fairly constant, the urine concentration of more variable substances is sometimes expressed in terms relative to creatinine. Thus the excretion of many metabolites is given as grams/gram of creatinine rather than grams/liter of urine or grams/24 hours.

Calcium

Urine calcium excretion varies with serum calcium concentration and with total body calcium load. On a diet containing 0.5 to 1.0 g of calcium daily, normal individuals excrete 200 to 400 mg of calcium (Table 19–26). Increased dietary calcium causes increased excretion, but reducing dietary intake affects urine levels much less. The quantitation of calcium excretion becomes important in evaluating patients with kidney stones and in patients with suspected hyperparathyroidism (see Chapter 16).

Diurnal Variation

Calcium excretion is heaviest just after a meal and lightest at night. If there is concern about progressive hypercalcemia, the test should be done on the first morning specimen, when values are normally low and an increase can most easily be detected. Conversely, the patient concerned about hypocalcemia should test a postprandial specimen, in which there should be abundant calcium.

TABLE 19–26. RENAL FILTRATION AND EXCRETION OF COMMON MINERALS PER DAY

	Filtered and Reabsorbed	Urine Excretion (mg/kg/day)	Range (mEq/L)
Calcium	150	3	5–12
Magnesium	35	1.5	2–18
Phosphate	87	1.3	20–50

Causes of Hypercalciuria

The passage of urine containing excessive amounts of calcium is usually associated with excessive calcium in the plasma (see Chapter 16). The major categories of causes include increased calcium or vitamin D intake, increased calcium mobilization from the bones (e.g., hyperparathyroidism), and decreased calcium reabsorption from the renal tubules.

Calcium homeostasis is discussed in Chapter 16. Under normal circumstances, approximately 10 g calcium are filtered by the kidney daily, and most of this is conserved (see Table 19–26). As will be seen later, a substantial number of patients who present with kidney stones (40%) do have excess urinary calcium.

Amino Acids

Adults normally excrete small amounts of amino acids (less than 200 mg of nitrogen per 24 hours) when dietary intake exceeds absorptive capacity. In general, more than 95% of renal load is reabsorbed in the proximal convoluted tubule. Patients receiving protein hydrolysates or other forms of parenteral alimentation excrete much larger amounts, as do patients with severe liver disease. Excessive quantities of amino acids enter the urine in acquired renal tubular disorders such as those that accompany heavy metal poisoning, Wilson's disease, or the nephrotic syndrome. In all of these circumstances, numerous amino acids are present, with glycine and cystine usually the most prominent. Selective amino acidurias can occur with two types of abnormality: enzyme derangement may cause accumulation of specific amino acids to blood levels that exceed the renal threshold for reabsorption (inborn errors of metabolism), or the specific amino acids may not be reabsorbed from the renal filtrate because of defective absorptive mechanisms at the renal tubular level. An example of an excessive amino acid level in the blood producing aminoaciduria is **phenylketonuria (PKU).** Fanconi's syndrome and cystinuria are renal tubular disorders in which serum amino acid levels are normal, but characteristic combinations of amino acids appear in the urine. In the overflow types of aminoaciduria, excessive serum levels produce excessive excretion.

Ferric Chloride Testing

Many amino acids react with ferric chloride to give distinctive colors. **Ferric chloride testing** is a broad-gauge screening procedure not only for aminoaciduria but also for many abnormal metabolites and drug excretion products in the urine. It is also used as a screening test for patients with PKU to evaluate adherence to dietary control (Table 19–27). The ferric chloride tests can be made somewhat more specific by chemical or physical manipulation, but it remains a screening procedure. The definitive diagnoses require specific identification and measurement of the relevant materials in the blood or urine.

Phenylketonuria

Phenylketonuria (PKU) is the most common of the enzyme abnormalities detected by the presence of excess amino acid in the urine. It occurs

TABLE 19–27. FERRIC CHLORIDE TEST FOR URINE SCREENING

Substance	Color Change
Amino Acids	
α-Ketobutyric acid (oasthouse urine disease)	Purple, fading to red-brown
Homogentisic acid (alkaptonuria)	Rapidly fading blue or green
o-Hydroxyphenylacetic acid	Mauve
o-Hydroxyphenylpyruvic acid	Red-brown, changing to blue or green and then to mauve
p-Hydroxyphenylpyruvic acid (tyrosinosis)	Rapidly fading green
Valine, leucine, and isoleucine (maple syrup urine disease)	Blue
Phenylpyruvic acid (phenylketonuria)	Stable green or blue-green
Imidazole pyruvic acid (histidinemia)	Green
Other Metabolites	
Acetoacetic acid	Red or red-brown
Melanin	Gray, changing to black
Indican (present in Hartnup disease; also intestinal stasis, malabsorption)	Violet or blue
Drugs	
Aspirin, salicylates	Stable red-wine color
Phenothiazine derivatives	Immediate purple-pink
p-Aminosalicylic acid (PAS)	Red-brown
Phenol derivatives	Violet

in about 1 in 20,000 live births and causes irreversible mental deterioration if not detected and treated very early in life. Although definitive diagnosis depends on analyzing serum levels of enzymes and amino acids, the test for phenylpyruvic acid in urine constitutes an effective screening device when performed at a few weeks of age rather than immediately after birth. A reagent strip (Phenistix) is available that detects urine levels of this abnormal metabolite in the range of 15, 40, and 100 mg/dL determined by the reaction color. The **Guthrie technique,** a more sensitive screening procedure that demonstrates elevated phenylalanine levels in the blood, should be used for infants known to be at risk and for those whose urine gives suggestive results. This technique is based on a competitive bacterial culture system that is enhanced by selective amino acids.

Cystinuria

Cystinuria is an autosomal recessive inherited disorder (frequency about 1 in 7000) that is associated with decreased absorption of the amino acid cystine by the proximal renal tubular cells. As a consequence, excessive amounts of cystine accumulate in the urine. This is associated with precipitation in the renal tubules and stone formation. There are distinct disorders of cystine metabolism that have renal complications. Cystinuria is a primary defect in renal tubular transport of the amino acid, whereas **cystinosis** is an inborn error of amino acid metabolism. Cystinuria occurs with approximately the same frequency as PKU. In addition to defects in cystine reabsorption, other amino acids (lysine, arginine, and ornithine) are also excreted in excess in this condition. There are two subcategories of this disorder: one in which all four amino acids are excreted in excess, and a second, in which cystine and lysine are found. The major clinical feature associated with these types is the development of renal calculi (discussed later). Cystine crystals (hexagonal plates) can be easily seen in the first morning specimen. The other amino acids are demonstrated by more sophisticated procedures such as thin-layer chromatography. Cystine crystals may also be demonstrated by the cyanide-nitroprusside test, which detects cystine at a concentration of about 75 to 150 mg/L. A positive result is seen when a red-purple color develops after the addition of sodium cyanide and nitroprusside. False-positive reactions occur with ketonuria and homocystinuria.

Homocystinuria

Homocystinuria results from the deficiency of the enzyme **cystathionine beta-synthase,** which catalyzes the formation of cystathionine from homocysteine and serine. Defects in homocystine metabolism can have profound clinical manifestations that may be associated with mental retardation. This condition may also be detected with a nitroprusside test. In this condition, both homocysteine and methionine accumulate. The cyanide nitroprusside test is a useful screening test and can be monitored to evaluate the effects of dietary restriction.

Cystinosis

This condition is a recessively inherited inborn error of metabolism associated with the accumulation of cystine crystals in many cells. Crystals may be found in the kidneys and eyes and the reticuloendothelial organs such as the bone marrow and the spleen. The clinical manifestation of renal involvement is the development of **Fanconi's syndrome,** which is characteristically an inability to absorb amino acids, phosphorus, potassium, sugar, and water. The frequency of this condition is approximately 1 in 100,000, and the condition may progress to the development of renal failure.

Serotonin Metabolites

Serotonin, a vasoactive substance and neurotransmitter, is produced by the enterochromaffin cells in the gastrointestinal tract, and is normally transported in the platelets. This compound is elaborated by neoplastic cells of carcinoid tumors. The serotonin output of most gastrointestinal tract carcinoid tumors is processed through the liver, where it is degraded. Tumors arising in the bronchial tree or metastatic deposits from gastrointestinal carcinoid tumors secrete serotonin directly into the systemic circulation, where it produces the distressing vascular and bronchospastic symptoms described as the **carcinoid syndrome.**

One of the breakdown products of serotonin is **5-hydroxyindoleacetic acid (5-HIAA).** The traditional diagnostic test for carcinoid syndrome is the demonstration of 5-HIAA in the urine. A nitrosonaphthol reagent is used to measure 5-HIAA in a 24-hour urine specimen stabilized with boric acid or acetic acid. Normal daily excretion is 2 to 9 mg, but in carcinoid syndromes the excretion levels are 50 to 500 mg.

Patients who take reserpine or use guiacolate-containing cough medicine excrete moderate amounts of 5-HIAA; in addition, massive ingestion of bananas, pineapples, avocados, mushrooms, or walnuts causes mild excess urinary excretion.

Serotonin Assay

Blood levels of serotonin can be measured directly in heparinized venous blood using radioimmunoassay or high-performance liquid chromatography. Normal levels of serotonin are 50 to 200 ng/mL in whole blood. High levels of serotonin are present in platelets, so serum assessment is not appropriate. Patients with carcinoid syndrome have values 7 to 15 times higher. If urine testing for 5-HIAA gives diagnostic results, there is no need to perform the serotonin assay; but if urine tests are equivocal or negative in a patient with suggestive clinical findings, a specific assay can be very helpful.

Drug Metabolites

Therapeutic drug monitoring and screening tests are discussed in Chapter 18.

ANALYSIS OF KIDNEY STONES

Renal stones **(calculi)** occur when the concentration of a solute exceeds its ability to stay in solution **(solubility equilibrium).** Calculi precipitate in the urinary tract if excess quantities of the substance are present in the urine or if urine conditions are unfavorable toward maintaining a solution. Successful treatment depends on identifying the precipitated material and then manipulating diet, urine flow, or metabolic conditions so as to keep the material dissolved for excretion.

Chemical Composition

Analyzing the stone is extremely important, especially in the first attack of renal colic, so every effort should be made to retrieve the stone for laboratory examination. Once the composition of the stone is known, the patient should be studied to detect risk factors that can be treated and prevented. Family history and metabolic constitution cannot be altered, but if the underlying problem is clarified, altering intake of foods, fluids, or drugs may prevent the formation of subsequent stones.

In the United States, urine stones usually fall into one of only four major categories. Table 19–28 lists the diagnostic features associated with commonly encountered stones. Most of these stones (up to 75%) are calcium oxalate and/or calcium phosphate. These occur far more often in men than in women, usually in early and middle adulthood. An episodic course is the rule, with clusters of acute episodes alternating with long, unexplained asymptomatic periods. Clinical features may be helpful in predicting which stones are more likely to be found. Patients who have risk factors and clinical signs or symptoms of hypercalcemia are more likely to have calcium oxalate and calcium phosphate stones. These generally form in the usual urinary pH level (6.0 to 6.5). Magnesium ammonium phosphate (struvite) stones account for 15% of all renal stones. These are almost exclusively in patients with recurrent urinary tract infections caused by urea-splitting organisms such as the *Proteus* species. They form in alkaline urine. These large stones distort renal architecture and may alter urine flow patterns.

About 10% of stones are composed of uric acid. Excessive uric acid excretion sometimes occurs in patients with abnormally elevated serum urate levels, but it may also occur in patients with normal blood urate levels. These stones occur in acidic urine.

TABLE 19–28. TYPES OF KIDNEY STONES

Stone Type	Diagnostic Features
Cystine	24-hr cystine excretion markedly increased
	Chromatography shows abnormal amino acid pattern
Magnesium ammonium phosphate	Chronic or recurrent urinary tract infection
	If severe, may have distortion of renal pelvis and calyces
Uric acid	Serum uric acid elevated in 40–50% of patients
	24-hr uric acid excretion increased
	Urine usually persistently acid
Calcium oxalate and calcium phosphate	24-hr calcium excretion increased, especially with high (1000 mg/day) calcium intake
	24-hr oxalate excretion usually high
	24-hr uric acid excretion usually high
	1,25-dihydroxy vitamin D_3 synthesis high
	Parathyroid activity often increased
	Serum calcium and phosphate levels variable

Cystine stones account for 1 to 2% of the stone events and occur only in people with genetic defects of cystine metabolism. The same defect also elevates the urinary excretion of lysine, arginine, and ornithine, but these three amino acids are highly soluble, whereas cystine has very poor solubility. Acid pH and obstructed or altered urine flow further reduce solubility. Cystine stones are especially likely if the urine is consistently acid or highly concentrated, and if infection or surgical intervention has distorted the architecture of the excretory tract. Much rarer constituents of stones are xanthines, glycine, or silicates. Table 19–29 describes how urine should be collected to evaluate stone-forming metabolic abnormalities.

Clinical Manifestations

Renal calculi may be totally asymptomatic or may be associated with the passage of small, particulate material moving from the stone into the ureter and subsequently into the bladder and urethra. Passage through the ureter characteristically produces renal colic, which is excruciating pain radiating from the back to the lower groin. Urethral extrusion of a stone may be associated with hematuria. Large stones may obstruct renal outflow, producing hydronephrosis, or may predispose to recurrent

TABLE 19–29. URINE COLLECTION* TO EVALUATE KIDNEY STONES

Type of Stone	Conditions of Collection	Significant Artifacts
Calcium	Add HCl to maintain low pH	Dietary calcium levels directly affect calcium excretion
		High ascorbic acid intake increases calcium oxalate excretion
		Malabsorption syndromes, jejunoileal bypass increase calcium oxalate excretion
		Thiazide diuretics reduce calcium excretion
Urate	Acidity causes urates to precipitate	Aspirin, glucocorticoids enhance urate excretion
	Add thymol as preservative	High-purine diet (organ meats, shellfish, game birds) produces high urine urates
		Allopurinol reduces urate excretion
Cystine	Acidity causes cystine to precipitate	Dilute urine (high fluid volume) enhances cystine solubility and excretion
	Add thymol as preservative	
Magnesium ammonium phosphate (struvite)	Add HCl to maintain low pH	Urinalysis of fresh specimen should reveal bacteria, WBCs

*A 24-hr urine collection should begin after first voiding in the morning, to eliminate overnight bladder urine. The first morning specimen of the following day is included in the preceding day's specimen. Urine should not be refrigerated because cold temperatures make solutes more likely to precipitate.

urinary tract infections with chronic pyelonephritis and subsequently chronic renal insufficiency. Renal stones are common and occur in about 0.5% of people in the United States. Urinalysis in conjunction with renal calculi is often associated with the presence of hematuria. The absence of red cell casts after a careful search suggests causes other than glomerular or tubular disorder as a cause of bleeding. Clusters of transitional cells may also be seen due to abrasion of the bladder surface by crystals. Crystals are erratically found in the presence of urinary calculi. In some situations, particularly the presence of oxalate crystals, there is said to be a greater likelihood of stone formation. The characteristic morphology of the crystals is shown in Color Plates 99A, B, and C.

Excessive amounts of oxalate in the urine may occur from dietary sources. Oxalate crystals may derive from vitamin C (ascorbic acid) or may occur from dietary vegetables or beverages. Occasionally, in oxalosis, a rare condition, there is an inherited defect in oxalate metabolism.

Uric acid metabolism has already been discussed in Chapter 9. Uric acid crystals may precipitate in acid urine, and large quantities of uric acid crystals are commonly seen in urinary sediment of patients with an acid urine. It is also felt that a urate nidus may serve as a foundation for calcium stones, particularly when the urine output is low.

Treatment

Successful treatment, aimed at eliminating calculus formation, is to promote high fluid intake to produce high urine volume (2500 to 3000 mL/day) and low urine solute concentration. It is often difficult to establish this regimen. The maintenance of high volume is especially difficult at night, when it is particularly important. Alkalinization of the urine with bicarbonate should be attempted in patients with cystinuria and in patients with uric acid stones. All family members of patients with cystine stones should have their urine screened with a sodium nitroprusside test. There is no universal agreement about the value of dietary adjustment. Dairy products contribute calcium to the diet; nuts, tea, and vegetables like rhubarb and spinach contribute oxalates. Organ meats and many shellfish are especially high in purines, the precursors from which uric acid is formed, and moderately high levels exist in all meats, fish, and poultry.

CEREBROSPINAL FLUID

Lumbar puncture and examination of the aspirated spinal fluid is an important diagnostic tool; sometimes this technique is employed to administer drugs (intrathecal therapy) or radiopaque diagnostic agents into the central nervous system (CNS).

ANATOMY AND PHYSIOLOGY

Origin of Cerebrospinal Fluid and Its Contents

The **cerebrospinal fluid (CSF),** originating from the choroid plexus of the intracranial ventricles, occupies these ventricles and the subarachnoid space over the surfaces of the brain and around the spinal cord. The composition of CSF derives from filtration, differential absorption, and active secretion. The CSF provides a fluid medium to enhance the nutrition of the brain, remove metabolic byproducts, and protect against mechanical injury.

The concentration of many CSF electrolytes varies with changes in plasma levels, but some appear to be independent. Most constituents of the CSF are present in equal or lower concentrations than in plasma. Under pathologic conditions, elements ordinarily restrained by the **blood-brain barrier** may enter the spinal fluid and establish higher concentrations. Although not strictly an ultrafiltrate of plasma, the CSF has a paucity of macromolecules such as large proteins (e.g., fibrinogen) and lipoproteins.

Red cells and white cells can only enter the CSF through ruptured blood vessels or by meningeal response to inflammation or irritation. Bilirubin, normally absent from the CSF, may be found in the spinal fluid of nonjaundiced patients after intracranial hemorrhage **(xanthochromia).** The bilirubin is in an unconjugated, prehepatic form, reflecting local hemoglobin catabolism within the central nervous system. If circulating plasma contains large amounts of water-soluble conjugated bilirubin, CSF bilirubin may rise in parallel.

Cerebrospinal Fluid Pressure

The brain, spinal cord, and CSF are enclosed in a rigid container composed of the skull and vertebral column. Normal pressure is maintained by the absorption of CSF in amounts equal to its production through the arachnoid villi and choroid plexus, respectively. Many factors regulate the level of CSF pressure, but central venous pressure is the most important because all reabsorbed fluid drains into the venous system (see later discussion).

Anatomic Relations

Despite continuous production and reabsorption of fluid, and the exchange of substances between the CSF and the blood, considerable stagnation occurs in the lumbar sac. For this reason, the protein concentration and cell count of the lumbar fluid exceed the values found in the ventricular or cisternal fluid. The lumbar sac, however, is the usual site for routine puncture, since in this caudal area only the filum terminale occupies the spinal canal, and damage to the nervous system is unlikely to occur. In children, the spinal cord persists more caudally than in adults, and therefore a low lumbar puncture should be made.

INDICATIONS FOR LUMBAR PUNCTURE

The fluid is usually collected by a needle puncture in the third, fourth, or fifth interlumbar vertebral spaces. Before the test, evaluation needs to be made regarding possible increased intracranial pressure (see below). The patient is generally placed in the left lateral position, and as a rule of thumb, a perpendicular line may be drawn from the posterior superior iliac crest of the pelvis to the midpoint of the spine. This generally represents the third or the fourth interlumbar space, where the needle can be inserted and fluid drained. Careful technique will ensure an atraumatic tap, although occasionally small blood vessels may be injured and may cause bleeding into the fluid, which complicates interpretation (discussed later).

Before undertaking the lumbar puncture, the physician should determine the diagnostic objectives. This will avoid unnecessary manipulation and permit the rational selection of laboratory tests, especially if the volume of fluid obtained is low. Most often, the primary goal of the procedure is to obtain spinal fluid. This goal is paramount in cases of suspected meningitis, in subarachnoid or other intracranial hemorrhage, and to exclude a variety of other diseases. In many patients, spinal fluid pressure is sought to document impairment of CSF flow. With the advent of magnetic resonance imaging (MRI) and computed tomography (CT), increased intracranial pressure can be inferred from noninvasive techniques.

Danger from Increased Intracranial Pressure

Lumbar puncture should be performed with extreme caution, if at all, when intracranial pressure is elevated, especially when papilledema (swelling of the optic disc) is present. Funduscopic examination of the retina (or in some cases, CT scanning) should always be undertaken before performing a lumbar puncture. The reason for caution is that rapid removal of fluid from the sac alters the pressure relationships within the subarachnoid space, and the brain stem can be dislocated from a region of high pressure (within the skull) to a region of low pressure (through the foramen magnum into the spinal canal), a potentially fatal phenomenon known as **herniation** or **coning.**

Other Problems

Serious spinal deformities or extreme age may make lumbar puncture difficult. Infection or severe dermatologic disease in the lumbar area also contraindicate this procedure. Cisternal puncture can be used in such cases, but this procedure requires expertise and should be performed by a neurologist or neurosurgeon.

EXAMINATION OF THE CEREBROSPINAL FLUID

The CSF should initially be examined for general appearance, consistency, and the tendency to clot. Opening pressure should be recorded. A differential cell count should be performed. Protein and sugar concentrations are routine determinations. Other tests performed when the patient's condition dictates include examination of a Gram-stained or acid-fast stained smear of the CSF sediment, culture for pyogenic bacteria, tubercle bacilli, yeasts, or fungi, and serologic tests for syphilis or other organisms. Tests of differential protein composition, and miscellaneous chemical determinations such as bilirubin, urea, lactic acid, and glutamine are also sometimes requested. Characteristics of the normal CSF are given in Table 19–30.

General Appearance

Normal spinal fluid has the clarity and consistency of water. Slight color change may be difficult to note, and it is helpful to compare a sample of CSF with a tube of water. Turbidity signifies the presence of leukocytes in considerable numbers. Haziness begins when 200 to 500 white cells per microliter are present. Yellowish discoloration, called **xanthochromia,** usually signifies previous bleeding, but may occur from high protein levels alone, especially those above 200 mg/dL. The pH of the CSF tends to be slightly lower than that of blood, a pH of 7.34 being normal in CSF, compared with the arterial pH of 7.41.

Blood in Cerebrospinal Fluid

It may be difficult to interpret the significance of fresh blood in the specimen, since damage to an intraspinal vessel may cause a bloody tap, even though the spinal fluid is intrinsically clear. If the blood is due to

TABLE 19–30. CHARACTERISTICS OF NORMAL ADULT CEREBROSPINAL FLUID (CSF)

	CSF Level	Relative to Plasma Level
Pressure	75–200 mm H_2O	
pH	7.32–7.35	Very slightly lower
Total protein	15–45 mg/dL	0.2–0.5%
Immunoglobulins	0.75–3.5 mgm/dL	Less than 0.1%
Albumin/globulin	8:1	3–4 times higher
Glucose	40–80 mg/dL	50–80% of value in blood 30–60 minutes earlier
Lactate	10–20 mg/dL	Approximately equal
Urea (as urea nitrogen)	10–15 mg/dL	Approximately equal
Glutamine	<20 mg/dL	Approximately equal

local trauma, the admixture diminishes as CSF is removed and the fluid in the third tube tends to be appreciably lighter than in the first. If the proportion of blood remains constant, it is probable that the bleeding preceded the puncture.

Subsequent examination of the specimen may clarify the problem of bloody tap versus genuinely bloody fluid. After centrifugation, the supernatant fluid is colorless if the blood came from traumatic lumbar puncture, and is pale to deep yellow if the blood was in the fluid initially. Xanthochromia occurs within 4 to 5 hours after a subarachnoid hemorrhage, and usually clears approximately 3 weeks after the event. Chronic subdural hematoma sometimes stains CSF brown from methemalbumin.

Clotting

When a subarachnoid block has occurred, the fluid may be dark yellow, with a tendency toward rapid and spontaneous clotting, but spontaneous clotting can occur whenever the protein content is high. It is the conversion of fibrinogen to fibrin (see Chapter 5) that produces the clot. Fibrinogen is absent from normal CSF, but protein increases significantly when fibrinogen as well as globulins and increased quantities of albumin cross the blood-brain barrier. The CSF may clot if a traumatic tap allows a large amount of blood and plasma to enter the specimen, whereas bloody CSF from a subarachnoid hemorrhage does not clot.

Cerebrospinal Fluid Pressure

In recumbent adults, the CSF pressure in the lumbar sac varies from 75 to 200 mm of water, with a mean value of 120 mm. If lumbar puncture is performed with the patient seated, the fluid in the manometer normally rises to the level of the patient's neck. Slight elevation of spinal fluid pressure may occur if an anxious patient involuntarily holds his or her breath or tenses his or her muscles. If the knees are flexed too firmly against the abdomen, venous compression may cause spurious elevation, especially in obese patients. Pathologic decrease in CSF pressure is rare, but may occur in conditions of dehydration or following previous aspiration of CSF.

More significant is elevation of CSF pressure, which may be a conspicuous finding in patients with intracranial tumors or purulent or tuberculous meningitis. Less marked elevation, to approximately 250 to 500 mm of water, may accompany low-grade inflammatory processes, encephalitis, or neurosyphilis.

The Queckenstedt Procedure

Because the ventricular spaces, intracranial subarachnoid space, and vertebral subarachnoid space are part of the same closed system, pressure change in one area should be reflected in other areas as well. If local change is not transmitted, the existence of a block can be inferred. In the Queckenstedt test, the jugular veins are compressed while lumbar CSF pressure is monitored. Temporary occlusion of both jugular veins retards venous drainage from the brain; increased intracranial venous pressure is then transmitted throughout the brain causing an acute rise in intracranial CSF pressure. If CSF flow is unobstructed, the pressure elevation is transmitted to the lumbar fluid, which rises in the manometer and then returns to the previous levels when venous occlusion is relieved. A total or partial spinal block is diagnosed if the lumbar pressure fails to rise when both jugular veins are compressed, or if the pressure requires more than 20 seconds to fall after compression is released. This procedure is risky in patients with increased intracranial pressure or with highly reactive carotid baroreceptors. Radiologic examination with contrast material (myelogram) or noninvasive procedures such as CT or MRI give more information and carry less risk.

Opening and Closing Pressure

The removal of cerebrospinal fluid produces a drop in CSF pressure. Although no absolute figure can apply, an expected range of decline is 5 to 10 mm of water for every milliliter of fluid removed from the lumbar sac. If, for example, 10 mL is removed for examination, the closing pressure would be 50 to 100 mm of water less than the opening pressure. A conspicuously small drop in pressure suggests that the total quantity of spinal fluid is increased, as in hydrocephalus. A disproportionately large pressure drop indicates a small CSF pool, which occurs in tumors or blockages in the circulation of the spinal fluid.

Cell Count

Normal spinal fluid is virtually free of cells, although as many as five small lymphocytes per microliter are considered normal. In children, the upper limit of normal may be as high as 20 lymphocytes per microliter. The presence of granulocytes or large mononuclear cells is never normal, nor should red blood cells (RBCs) be present. If RBCs are present in the CSF, it may be due to a hemorrhagic process or to trauma during the puncture. A decrease in the RBCs between the first and the last fluid to be aspirated indicates a traumatic puncture.

Bloody Tap

Sometimes it is necessary to evaluate the leukocyte or protein content of spinal fluid known to be contaminated by traumatic bleeding. A rough rule for correction is that simple contamination adds one or two white cells for every thousand red cells. A bloody spinal fluid that contained, for example, 20,000 RBCs/mL should be expected to contain no more than 30 to 40 white cells derived solely from the recently introduced blood.

Unless the blood has an unusually high white cell count, demonstration of more than 45 cells in such a fluid would indicate preexisting leukocytosis. Bleeding from a traumatic tap introduces approximately 1 mg/dL of protein for every 1000 RBCs/µL.

Differential White Count

When cells are counted, they also should be identified as to type. Spinal fluid submitted for cell counts usually is stained to accentuate the nucleus and permit rapid differentiation between mononuclear cells and granulocytes. For more detailed morphologic study, the centrifuged specimen can be smeared and examined using cytocentrifuge techniques. Table 19–31 lists significant causes for different levels of leukocytosis in the spinal fluid.

Cryptococcus

In occasional cases, an erroneous diagnosis of "moderate number of lymphocytes" may be made if cryptococcal organisms are in the CSF.

TABLE 19–31. CONDITIONS THAT ELEVATE CEREBROSPINAL FLUID CELL COUNT AND PROTEIN

Cell Count

10–200 Cells, Largely Lymphocytes

Most viral meningitis, late neurosyphilis, multiple sclerosis, tumor, cerebral thrombosis

200–500 Cells, Largely Lymphocytes or Mixed

Tuberculous meningitis, choriomeningitis, herpes infection of CNS, meningovascular syphilis

>500 Cells, Largely Granulocytes

Acute bacterial meningitis

Immature Cells

Meningeal leukemia, carcinomatous meningitis

Protein

Mild Elevation, to 300 mg/dL

Viral meningitis, neurosyphilis, subdural hematoma, cerebral thrombosis, brain tumor, multiple sclerosis (rarely >100 mg/dL)

Electrophoretic evidence of ↑ IgG:

Multiple sclerosis, subacute sclerosing panencephalitis, neurosyphilis

Moderate or Pronounced Elevation

Acute bacterial meningitis, tuberculous meningitis, spinal cord tumor, cerebral hemorrhage, intracranial tumor, Guillain-Barré syndrome (ascending polyneuritis)

These yeasts are small and round and may be numerous without provoking a significant cellular response (see also Chapter 14). Cryptococci can sometimes be demonstrated by adding India ink to the spinal fluid, making the cryptococcal capsule stand out as a transparent disk surrounded by the black carbon particles (see Color Plate 65). Immunologic tests for cryptococcal antigens are the most sensitive and accurate means of diagnosing cryptococcal infection (see Chapter 14).

Chemical Tests

Spinal Fluid Proteins

The spinal fluid normally contains very little protein, because serum proteins are large molecules that do not cross the blood-brain barrier. The normal concentration is well below 1% of normal serum levels of 5 to 8 g/dL, and therefore normal values are between 50 and 80 mg/dL. The proportion of albumin to globulin is even higher in spinal fluid than in plasma, because the albumin molecule is significantly smaller and can pass more easily through the endothelial barrier.

Protein concentration may rise for a number of reasons. One source is increased permeability of the blood-brain barrier caused by inflammation. In severe meningitis, all types of serum protein may enter the CSF, including the large molecule fibrinogen. In purulent meningitis, the CSF protein is further increased because bacteria and cells, both intact and disintegrated, contribute protein to the medium (Table 19–32). CSF total protein can be corrected for the presence of blood 1 mg/dL per 1000 red cells/µL if serum protein and red cell count are normal and if assayed on the same CSF specimen. In most disease, cell count and protein concentration tend to change in parallel. In multiple sclerosis, the proportion of IgG rises relative to the other proteins, sometimes with little increase in total protein concentration. This protein may be subjected to electrophoretic techniques and may demonstrate oligoclonal bands (see Chapters 7 and 9). CSF protein electrophoresis always demonstrates a prealbumin band, which is usually not evident in serum.

Elevated Protein Without Cells

When protein concentration rises and relatively few cells are present, degenerative disease of the central nervous system should be suspected. Multiple sclerosis and neurosyphilis may increase the globulin content, adding only a few mononuclear cells. Conditions of subarachnoid blockage, especially when caused by a spinal tumor, permit protein accumulation in the fluid distal to the block, and the fluid may clot on aspiration. Superficially located tumors, notably acoustic neuromas and meningiomas, may cause a moderate increase in CSF protein. Increased capillary permeability breaches the blood-brain barrier allowing plasma proteins increased access to the CSF. This is conspicuous in Guillain-Barré syndrome and may occur in cerebrovascular disease and inflammatory

TABLE 19–32. MAJOR LABORATORY RESULTS FOR THE DIFFERENTIAL DIAGNOSIS OF MENINGITIS

Bacterial	Viral	Tubercular	Fungal
Elevated WBC count	Elevated WBC count	Elevated WBC count	Elevated WBC count
Neutrophils present	Lymphocytes present (neutrophils present very early)	Lymphocytes and monocytes	Lymphocytes and monocytes present
Marked protein elevation	Moderate protein elevation	Moderate to marked protein elevation	Moderate to marked protein elevation
Decreased glucose	Normal glucose	Decreased glucose	Normal to decreased glucose
Elevated lactate	Normal lactate	Elevated lactate	Elevated lactate
Positive bacterial antigen tests (*Haemophilus,* meningococcal)		Pellicle formation	Positive India ink or antigen test with *Cryptococcus neoformans*
Positive Gram stain			

From Strasinger, SK: Urinalysis and Body Fluids. FA Davis, Philadelphia, 1985, p 148, with permission.

processes. Changes in CSF proteins must always be correlated with serum protein levels, which should be concurrently obtained. Table 19–31 summarizes diagnostically significant changes in CSF protein.

Glucose

CSF glucose concentration is normally 50 to 80% of the blood glucose level, but changes in the blood sugar are reflected in the CSF after a 30- to 50-minute lag period. Normal CSF glucose levels are between 45 and 80 mg/dL, but critical evaluation of CSF glucose determination requires comparison against a blood sample (usually 20 mg/dL lower in CSF), if possible, 30 to 60 minutes before the lumbar puncture is done. The most dramatic drop in CSF sugar occurs with purulent meningitis, when the combination of bacterial and leukocytic activity may reduce the CSF glucose to zero (Table 19–33). Glucose metabolism is an active process that continues after the sample has been aspirated, so that sugars should be determined promptly in samples that are suspected to contain granulocytes or microorganisms. Because all types of organisms consume glucose, a decreased sugar content may indicate the presence of bacteria,

TABLE 19–33. CONDITIONS THAT AFFECT CEREBROSPINAL FLUID GLUCOSE

No Significant Change

Viral meningitis, neurosyphilis, brain or cord tumor, cerebral thrombosis, multiple sclerosis, polyneuritis

Moderate Reduction

CNS leukemia, meningeal carcinomatosis, subarachnoid hemorrhage, partially treated bacterial or fungal meningitis (CSF lactate will be high)

Pronounced Reduction

Bacterial meningitis, tuberculous meningitis, fungal meningitis

Artifactual Reduction

Delayed analysis of fluid that contains large numbers of metabolizing cells

fungi, protozoa, or tubercle bacilli. Viral meningitis usually causes only mild reduction, if any, in CSF glucose. Central nervous system leukemia or meningeal carcinomatosis often depresses CSF glucose concentration as well. Table 19–33 summarizes changes in the CSF glucose.

Other Cerebrospinal Fluid Chemistries

Lactic Acid   Because it reflects local glycolytic activity, lactic acid concentration expands the diagnostic information available in the CSF specimens that give ambiguous results. Normal CSF lactate content is 10 to 20 mg/dL. Severe systemic lactic acidosis causes CSF levels to rise in parallel, but an isolated increase of CSF lactate indicates increased glucose metabolism by micro-organisms or leukocytes. In early or partially treated bacterial or fungal meningitis, the CSF cellular population and glucose levels may be difficult to distinguish from those of viral meningitis or diffuse, noninfectious conditions. Lactate levels above 35 mg/dL rarely occur except in bacterial or fungal meningitis. Lactate elevations persist for several days after antibiotic therapy, making this very useful in the differential diagnosis of inadequately treated meningitis. This may augment CSF microbial antigen testing in cases of partially treated meningitis (see also Chapter 14).

Urea   The urea levels in blood and spinal fluid are approximately equal, and CSF urea increases in uremia.

Glutamine   Cerebrospinal glutamine is synthesized in the central nervous system from ammonia and glutamic acid. When blood ammonia levels are high, as they are in conditions of severely altered hepatic blood flow, CSF glutamine levels rise. The complex relationships between hyperammonemia, increased glutamic acid utilization, and alterations of intermediates of oxidative metabolism probably influence the development of hepatic encephalopathy. Glutamine in CSF correlates as well as or better than blood ammonia levels with the degree of hepatic encephalopathy. Glutamine values above 20 mg/dL are considered elevated and values above 35 mg/dL are seen in hepatic encephalopathy.

Enzymes Serum enzymes such as lactate dehydrogenase (LDH), alanine aminotransferase (ALT), and aspartate aminotransferase (AST) have been measured in the spinal fluid and are present in lower concentrations in the CSF than in serum. CSF enzyme levels are not measured under routine conditions and are not generally useful for diagnosing or monitoring patients. The enzyme most often affected is AST, which rises in inflammatory, hemorrhagic, and degenerative diseases of the CNS.

Other Constituents Chloride levels in CSF change passively to compensate for changes in cations and other negatively charged ions. Chloride determination provides no specific diagnostic information. **Calcium** determination in CSF is not particularly useful. The calcium level in CSF is about half of the serum levels, because only the fraction not bound to protein is free to enter the spinal fluid. Calcium in the CSF rises with rising CSF protein levels.

Microorganisms

Significant numbers of bacteria, fungi, or protozoa in the CSF can be identified by examining the stained sediment after centrifugation (see Chapter 14). Whenever there is a question of meningitis or CNS infection, smears of the CSF sediment should be stained with a Gram stain and an acid-fast stain. Failure to isolate organisms on the smear should not be interpreted to mean that organisms are absent, because there must be 10^5/mL in order for them to be demonstrated by this technique. Gram stains are positive in only 80 to 90% of untreated meningitis cases and only 60% of partially treated cases. Unless the cause of CNS disorder is self-evident, steps should be taken to rule out the presence of tubercle bacilli, because tuberculous meningitis can develop insidiously and presents few clear-cut diagnostic signs.

Microbiologic tests performed on the spinal fluid have been considered in Chapter 14, and issues relating to specimen collection and transport were also considered in Chapter 13. As discussed, the spinal fluid should be cultured on several media, to rule out bacteria, fungal, and tuberculous infections and to determine whether more than one organism is present. The meningococcus prefers a high–carbon dioxide atmosphere and special medium to isolate this organism. Sometimes an aliquot of the original sample can be incubated at 37°C for 24 hours, permitting the organisms to multiply in the spinal fluid before incubation on a second set of cultures.

Immunologic techniques are now applied to the detection of microorganisms in the CSF, as was outlined in Chapters 14 and 15. The cryptococcal antigen test uses a strong, specific anticryptococcal antibody to identify antigenic elements that may be in CSF even when organisms are undetectable. Bacterial antigens may also be demonstrated by immunologic methods, as was outlined in Chapter 15. These techniques can give extremely specific documentation of bacterial invasion in little more than 1 hour.

Serologic Tests for Syphilis

Blood tests used in diagnosing syphilis were discussed in Chapter 15. Biologic false-positive results are fairly rare on CSF specimens.

If neurosyphilis is a serious diagnostic consideration, the fluorescent treponemal antigen (FTA) constitutes a more reliable screening test than the flocculation tests such as the VDRL or RPR (see Chapter 15).

PATIENT-CARE CONSIDERATIONS

Explaining the procedure and providing reassurance are more important for lumbar puncture than for almost any other procedure done without general anesthetic. Often the patient has heard tales of catastrophic events during and after spinal taps.

The feeling of pressure and the "pop" when the needle enters the dura may alarm the patient but do not cause persistent discomfort. Occasionally, temporary paresthesias may occur along nerve roots. If the CSF pressure is normal, there is only a very remote chance of complications such as massive hemorrhage or paralysis. Postpuncture headache is the most common adverse effect, occurring in about 25% of patients and lasting anywhere from several hours to several days after the event.

TECHNICAL CONSIDERATIONS AND COLLECTION OF THE SPECIMEN

Positioning the Patient

To expose the interspinal space between the lumbar vertebrae, the spine must be flexed in the most convex possible configuration, but the spine should remain parallel to the surface on which the patient lies, and the greatest pelvic diameter should be perpendicular to this surface.

Posture and intra-abdominal pressure directly influence the CSF, as has already been discussed, so it is important to help the patient relax and partially straighten the legs after the subdural space has been entered. Malpositioned neck flexion may increase jugular venous pressure, causing the CSF pressure to rise, and excessive pressure from the legs against the chest and abdomen causes even greater pressure increases. Apprehensive patients sometimes hold their breath; they should be encouraged to breathe slowly and naturally, but not to the point of hyperventilation. When the needle and manometer are properly positioned, the CSF level should fluctuate several millimeters with respiration.

Postpuncture Headache

The characteristic postpuncture headache is bilateral occipital or frontal and occurs only in an upright position. Lying down promptly relieves this pain and nausea that may occasionally occur. Dizziness and neck and shoulder pain may accompany the headache. The physiology of the postpuncture headache is unclear. Traditionally, it is attributed to extradural leakage of spinal fluid at the puncture site. Using a small-gauge needle and keeping the bevel uppermost so as to separate dural fibers is thought to reduce the incidence and severity of the headache. It is believed that keeping the patient prone after the procedure alters the alignment of tissues along the needle track and seals off routes of leakage. The patient should remain horizontal for 1 to several hours after lumbar puncture, but this varies according to the setting.

Handling the Specimen

Spinal fluid specimens should be transported to the laboratory without delay. It is crucial to maintain sterile technique throughout the procedure and in handling the fluid afterward, especially if the tap was done because infection was suspected. The order in which the specimens were drawn can be important if there is a question of traumatic tap versus hemorrhage. Within 1 hour, red cells within the fluid begin to lyse, imparting spurious coloration to the supernatant, and neutrophils or malignant cells may disintegrate. Bacteria and cells continue to metabolize glucose, and delay in analysis may affect chemical values.

FECAL ANALYSIS

GENERAL CONSIDERATIONS

Fecal examination is often considered a test of default because of the nature of the specimen and esthetic considerations. Unlike urine, blood, and spinal fluid, it cannot be collected on demand, and patients usually dislike collecting and delivering it for examination. Nursing and laboratory personnel tend to share the patient's aversion, and physicians often excuse themselves from contact with the excreta. Yet disease of the gastrointestinal tract is widespread, and examination of the feces helps elucidate many common clinical dilemmas.

Various means of collecting feces are available. The physician performing a rectal examination should sample whatever fecal material is within finger range. This constitutes a random, rather small sample, chiefly important for documenting unsuspected occult bleeding or striking abnormalities of color or consistency. The specimen collected at the time of defecation, constituting a single evacuation, permits a number of tests and inferences. Conditions suggested from single-specimen findings sometimes require further documentation by quantitative tests on timed collections.

THE NORMAL SPECIMEN

The average normal adult excretes 100 to 300 g of fecal material per day. Of this, as much as 70% may be water, and of the remaining material, up to half may be bacteria and cellular debris. Vegetable residues, small amounts of fat, desquamated epithelial cells, and other miscellaneous constituents comprise the rest. The feces are what remain of approximately 10 liters of fluid material entering the gastrointestinal tract each day. Ingested food and fluid, saliva, gastric secretion, pancreatic juice, and bile all contribute to this input; the output depends on a complex series of absorptive, secretory, and fermentative processes.

The small intestine is approximately 23 feet long, whereas the large intestine is between 4 and 5 feet in length. The small intestine degrades ingested fats, proteins, and carbohydrates into absorbable components, and then absorbs them. Pancreatic, biliary, and gastric secretions operate on the lumenal contents to prepare them for active mucosal transport. Other vitally important substances absorbed in the small intestine include fat-soluble vitamins, iron, and calcium. Vitamin B_{12}, after complexing with intrinsic factor, is absorbed in the terminal ileum (see Chapter 2). The small intestine also absorbs as much as 9.5 liters of water and associated electrolytes. The large intestine is shorter and performs less complex functions than the small intestine. The right, or proximal, colon absorbs much of the remaining water. Bacteria within the colonic lumen degrade many of the end products of metabolism, and the distal portion of the colon stores the feces until a convenient time for evacuation.

Normally evacuated feces reflect the shape and caliber of the colonic lumen. The normal consistency is somewhat plastic—neither fluid, mushy, nor hard. The usual brown color results from bacterial degradation of bile pigments into stercobilin, and odor derives from indole and skatole degradation products of proteins. In people with normal gastrointestinal motility who consume a mixed dietary intake, colonic transit time is 24 to 48 hours. Small intestinal contents (chyme) begin to enter the cecum as soon as 2 to 3 hours after a meal, but the process is not complete until 6 to 9 hours after eating.

SPECIMEN COLLECTION

Random specimens are adequate for performing qualitative tests such as the detection of occult blood or microscopic examination for the presence of white cells, yeasts, or parasites. Quantitative determinations require timed specimens varying from 24 to 72 hours.

LABORATORY EXAMINATION

Gross Appearance

Stool examination should evaluate size, shape, consistency, color, odor, and the presence or absence of blood, mucus, pus, tissue fragments, food residues, or parasites. This examination should be done before the patient is exposed to barium or purges.

Alterations in size or shape indicate altered motility or abnormalities of the colonic wall. A very large caliber indicates dilatation of the viscus, whereas excessively small, ribbonlike extrusions suggest decreased elasticity or partial obstruction. Small, round, hard masses accompany habitual, moderate constipation, but severe fecal retention can produce huge, impacted masses with small volumes of pasty material excreted as overflow. Tables 19–34 and 19–35 outline changes that may be observed in the gross appearance of feces.

Diarrhea

Acute, self-limited attacks of mild diarrhea in otherwise healthy adults or older children usually do not warrant further investigation. In infants, the elderly, or anyone in a precarious fluid or nutritional state, diarrhea alone can be dangerous or fatal, and the conditions that provoke the diarrhea can range from trivial to life-threatening. Although today's clinicians possess a broader range of diagnostic tools, many diarrheal illnesses remain undiagnosed. Mucoid or watery diarrhea alternating with constipation is characteristic of an **irritable bowel syndrome** (spastic colon–mucous colitis), a frequently encountered problem that remains difficult to diagnose on physiologic grounds and difficult to treat.

Stool can be cultured for **enteropathogens** and examined microscopically for protozoal parasites. As was mentioned in Chapter 14, the major reason for submitting stool specimens to the microbiology laboratory is for the investigation of diarrhea. Immune electron microscopy has made possible the direct demonstration of viral agents, notably hepatitis, parvo- and rota-like viruses (see Fig. 14–3). **Lactose intolerance** (lactase deficiency) achieving prominence as a common cause of both upper and lower gastrointestinal tract symptoms, is evaluated by the Lactose-H_2 breath test, replacing the older lactose tolerance test. **Pseudomembranous**

TABLE 19–34. DIAGNOSTIC CLUES IN THE APPEARANCE OF FECES

Appearance	Usual Causes	Remarks
Small, hard, dark balls	Constipation	In irritable bowel syndromes, may alternate with watery or mucoid diarrhea
Voluminous, odorous, floating	Malabsorption of fats or protein	Fat excretion of >6 g/day is abnormal. May have primary small-bowel disease, cystic fibrosis, pancreatitis, postgastrectomy syndrome, bile duct obstruction
Loose, contains mucus but no blood	Irritable bowel syndrome. Diffuse superficial inflammation. Villous adenoma	With semiformed stool, often has functional origin
Loose, contains blood and mucus	Inflammatory bowel syndromes. Typhoid, *Shigella, Amoeba* Carcinoma	Blood usually more conspicuous than mucus
Sticky, black, tarry	Upper GI tract hemorrhage	See Table 19–37
Voluminous, watery, little formed material	Noninvasive infections (cholera, toxigenic, *Escherichia coli,* staphylococcal food poisoning). Osmotic catharsis (disaccharidase deficiency, binge-type overeating)	Dehydration, electrolyte derangements may be severe
Loose, contains pus and/or necrotic tissue	Diverticulitis or other abscesses. Necrotic tumor. Parasites	For parasites, examine specimen while still warm
Pasty, grayish-white, little odor	Bile duct obstruction. Barium ingestion	Serum bilirubin usually abnormal

colitis tends to occur in patients with poor intestinal perfusion and in those whose intestinal flora has been disturbed by antibiotics. *Clostridium difficile* is the usual cause; with suitable tests, either the organism or its toxin can be identified in the feces (see also Chapter 14). Table 19–36 summarizes the major clinical considerations in diarrhea.

TABLE 19–35. CONDITIONS THAT INFLUENCE THE COLOR OF FECES

Color	Nonpathologic	Pathologic
Brown, dark brown, yellow-brown	Normal oxidation of bile pigments	
Very dark brown	Prolonged exposure to air Diet high in meat	
Black	Iron, bismuth ingestion	Bleeding from upper GI tract
Gray	Chocolate, cocoa ingestion	Steatorrhea (consistency usually mushy or frothy)
Very light gray	Diet high in milk products Barium	Bile duct obstruction
Green or yellow-green	Diet high in spinach, other greens Laxatives of vegetable origin	Rapid transit time, preventing oxidation of bile pigments
Red	Diet high in beets	Bleeding from lower GI tract

Endoscopic, radiographic, and biopsy procedures, which are beyond the scope of this chapter, are increasingly important in diagnosing intestinal diseases.

Blood in the Stool

Principles of Testing

Tests for blood in biologic specimens exploit the peroxidase activity of heme derivatives in oxidizing organic compounds used as color indicators. Hematin is the hemoglobin metabolite with peroxidase activity, but certain plant enzymes and materials derived from myoglobin are also peroxidase positive. Bleeding into the alimentary tract produces peroxidase-positive hematin in the feces. Large quantities of blood in the upper alimentary tract (25 to 50 mL) produce sufficient acid hematin to darken the feces to a black or tarry appearance, a condition called **melena.** Small amounts of blood that do not affect the appearance of the feces remain undetected **(occult)** unless specific tests are employed.

Tests for occult blood must be sufficiently sensitive to detect small but clinically significant hemorrhage. They should not, however, be so sensitive as to spotlight the 0.5 to 2.0 mL per day that normal people may excrete, or be rendered positive by myoglobin from meat in the diet. As indicators, orthotoluidine has proven too sensitive and benzidine, besides

TABLE 19–36. TYPES OF DIARRHEA

Category	Specific Condition	Other Features
Osmotic	Disaccharidase deficiency (lactose intolerance) Indigestible oligosaccharides in beans, other legumes Saline laxatives	Symptoms follow ingestion of dairy products Abdominal distension, "gas" very common Patient may alternate constipation with laxative abuse History of peptic ulcer symptoms Osmotic effects of antacids
Secretory	Nondigestible sugars in artificial sweeteners Bacterial toxins (cholera, *Escherichia coli,* staphylococcal food poisoning) Enteroactive hormones (gastrin in Zollinger-Ellison syndrome; serotonin, ? others in carcinoid syndrome) Malabsorption syndromes: fat, protein Irritation by bile acids	Dietary history is crucial Epidemiology is more revealing than stool culture Other systemic symptoms are common Foul odor usual sign of calorie or protein malnutrition Follows ileal resection Bacterial overgrowth in small intestine
Altered structure or function	Intestinal resection Enterocolic fistula Irritable bowel syndrome	Apparent from history Complication of diverticular disease or inflammatory bowel disease Pathophysiology remains unclear
Mucosal damage	Inflammatory bowel disease (Crohn's syndrome, ulcerative colitis) Invasive organisms (some *Shigella,* some *Salmonella, Amoeba, Campylobacter*) *Pseudomembranous colitis*	Bleeding, pain, weight loss may accompany Stool cultures useful early in disease Often follows use of broad-spectrum antibiotics May complicate uremia, congestive heart failure; intestinal ischemia

Modified from Gray, GM: Acute diarrhea. In Rubenstein, E, and Federman, DD (eds): Scientific American Medicine. Scientific American, New York, 1981.

being too sensitive, is unacceptable for routine use because it is carcinogenic. Gum guaiac, in various forms, is the most widely used indicator.

Grossly Apparent Bleeding

Guaiac testing is used to detect occult bleeding (see also Chapter 2). Overt bleeding or obvious melena does not require detailed testing, but is important to confirm that red or black pigmentation truly is from blood origin. The general rule is that melena occurs when upper gastrointestinal hemorrhage allows hemoglobin to come in contact with gastric acid, whereas colonic bleeding causes red or maroon stools. However, if transit time is very rapid, blood from the esophagus or stomach may remain red throughout its passage. Conversely, abnormal colonic contents may blacken blood from lower intestinal hemorrhage. Streaks of bright red blood on the stool surface often occur with hemorrhoidal bleeding, but also occur with ulcerative colitis, friable adenomas, or superficially eroded carcinomas. Surface streaking, moreover, may not be the only source of blood. The underlying fecal material may also contain occult blood.

Melena may persist well after active bleeding has stopped. The stool may remain black as long as 5 days without a fresh source of blood, and tests for occult blood may remain positive for several weeks. Table 19–37 lists the common causes of gastrointestinal bleeding and some of the clinical features that distinguish them.

Screening for Occult Blood

The importance of screening feces for occult blood remains controversial. Fecal occult blood testing for the diagnosis of colorectal cancer has a positive predictive value ranging from 2.2 to 50% and sensitivity ranging from 22 to 92%. Large-scale upper or lower gastrointestinal tract hemorrhage is only too obvious clinically. The hope in screening for occult blood is to detect significant lesions when they are asymptomatic or sufficiently mild or localized that treatment can be successful. Peptic ulcer, erosive gastritis, and gastric carcinoma are the usual upper gastrointestinal tract sources of occult blood. Carcinoma or adenomatous polyps of the colon cause most of the lower gastrointestinal tract occult bleeding, although diverticuli are also an important cause.

For screening to be worthwhile, it must be done correctly. Positive results must be investigated even if they prove to be false. False-negative results are more difficult to detect. Guaiac testing on feces obtained during digital examination of the rectum yields relatively little information because diet can cause false-positive results and sampling error can cause false-negative results. The most acceptable procedure for large-scale use has been to give slides or strips to the patient, who then prepares multiple test specimens from the feces passed during several successive days. A meat-free high-bulk diet produces the most suitable specimens. Meat in the diet, bleeding from the gums or nasal passages, and the use of as little

TABLE 19–37. CONDITIONS ASSOCIATED WITH GASTROINTESTINAL BLEEDING

Condition	Usual Age of Occurrence	Severity	Other Features
Upper GI Tract			
Peptic ulcer (gastric or duodenal)	Any, including young children	Variable, from occult to life-threatening	Pain, typical history often absent
Erosive gastritis	Usually adults over age 25	Usually mild; may be very severe	Aspirin, alcohol use often predispose
			Severe uremia, chronic liver disease predispose
Atrophic gastritis	Adults, over age 25	Usually mild	Associated with pernicious anemia, autoantibodies, decreased gastric acidity
Esophageal varices	Adults; children with portal hypertension	Massive, sudden	Common in alcoholic liver disease
			Cirrhosis or portal hypertension always present
Mallory-Weiss tears at gastroesophageal junction	Any, but usually older adults	Variable depending on depth, location of tear	Common in alcohol abusers
Hiatus hernia, esophagitis	Progressively increasing incidence above age 40	Usually mild	Persistent painless bleeding a common cause of iron deficiency anemia in elderly
Small and Large Bowel			
Meckel's diverticulum	Most common in children and young adults	Moderate; stools red or maroon	Caused by peptic ulceration of ectopic gastric mucosa
Polyps	Any age	Usually mild; often intermittent	Diarrhea, mucus in stools sometimes accompany
Infectious diarrheas	Any age	Usually mild or moderate	Amoeba, Shigella, Clostridium difficile

(Continued)

985

TABLE 19-37. CONDITIONS ASSOCIATED WITH GASTROINTESTINAL BLEEDING *(Continued)*

Condition	Usual Age of Occurrence	Severity	Other Features
Inflammatory bowel disease (Crohn's disease, ulcerative colitis)	Adolescents, adults under age 60	Usually mild, but may be massive	Diarrhea, pain, weight loss more common in Crohn's disease than in ulcerative colitis Bleeding more prominent in ulcerative colitis
Diverticular disease	Progressively increasing incidence above age 40	Usually mild, frequently occult	Often asymptomatic, unless inflammation or abscess develops
Vascular malformations	Older adults	Usually mild; may be life-threatening in ~15%	Bleeding often recurrent Often misdiagnosed as peptic ulcer or diverticular disease
Carcinoma	Older adults	Variable, from occult to moderate	Common cause of iron deficiency anemia in older persons Red blood more common with distally located tumors
Rectum and Anus			
Hemorrhoids	Older adults	Usually mild; blood is bright red	May be painless or symptomatic Often associated with constipation
Anorectal fissure	Any age	Usually mild; blood is bright red	Nearly always painful Crohn's disease, anal intercourse may predispose

as 325 mg of aspirin (1 adult tablet/day) may produce positive results without diagnostic significance. Before accepting a positive screening test result, one should repeat the procedure with careful attention to diet.

A false-negative reaction, failure to demonstrate bleeding in a patient with cancer or some other treatable condition, has more significant consequences. Even when six tests are performed, the rate of negative test results in patients later shown to have colon carcinoma or large adenomas is about 20%. The majority of patients with significant lesions have no more than one or two positive results out of six specimens. Besides the fact that bleeding may be intermittent and the sample tested is small, negative results can occur if too much time elapses between applying the sample and performing the test. False-negative results can be due to a low-bulk diet that decreases stool volume and increases intestinal transit time or abnormally large amounts of vitamin C in the diet.

Microscopic Examination

Parasites

General features regarding microbiologic detection in stools have been discussed in the section on Microbiology. The microscopic examination of fecal material may augment observations noted on gross inspection. Parasites and their ova usually require microscopic examination for diagnosis, although adult nematodes or tapeworm segments occasionally may be only too obvious in the gross material (see Color Plates 67, 68, 89). For definitive parasitologic evaluation, the stool specimen must be fresh and the examiner must be experienced. To diagnose and identify amoebae and other motile parasites, the examiner must observe freshly passed material while it is still warm. Bloody or mucus-containing fragments give the best results, and both a saline emulsion and an iodine emulsion should be examined. Concentrating the stool sample also helps in finding helminth ova: their presence in a simple emulsion indicates that large numbers are present (see Chapter 14). A rectal mucosal smear, in preference to whole stool, can better identify chlamydia using an immunofluorescent technique.

Undigested Material

Besides demonstrating parasites, microscopic examination of feces permits rapid screening of digestive efficiency. If visibly striated meat fibers can be seen, proteolysis is inadequate. The significance of fats in a random specimen is less clear. A certain amount of fecal fat is normal, corresponding to 5 to 7% of dietary intake. Recent dietary intake influences the fat content of random or single specimens. A patient with malabsorption problems may restrict fat intake because of anorexia, resulting in normal excretion at the time of examination. Conversely, a metabolically normal patient with abnormally high fat intake may excrete more fat than the expected normal. If there is a reason to suspect abnormal fat metabolism, evaluation of a random specimen should include available information about recent intake.

Cellular Elements

A certain number of epithelial cells may be present in feces, but large numbers of epithelial cells or large amounts of mucus indicate an irritated mucosa. Because white cells are not normal constituents, their presence beyond rare, scattered leukocytes indicates inflammation at some point in the lower alimentary tract or excretory organs. Although large numbers of white cells suggest a fairly serious or extensive inflammatory process, the absence of leukocytes does not mean that inflammation was absent. An inflammatory process deep in the wall or a surface condition that does not attract neutrophils will contribute few leukocytes to the fecal content. Leukemic patients may have inflammatory bowel disease without evidence of leukocyte infiltration due to the marked reduction of absolute numbers of leukocytes.

Unaltered red blood cells, when present, usually come from the anus or the rectum. Intraluminal blood from higher in the gastrointestinal tract experiences damage to the cells even if hemoglobin remains unaltered.

Malabsorption Problems

A variety of disorders may cause excessive fecal fat excretion. Staining a fecal smear to find increased fat globules (normally 0 fat globules are noted per high-power field) is a useful screening device but is nonquantitative. Often the patient's history of bulky, light-colored, floating stools provides the presumptive diagnosis, although in one series of children with celiac disease, 38 out of 40 had excessive fat on a stained smear, while only 21 reported bulky or foul stools. A high index of suspicion is desirable in any child or young adult with persistent irritability, poor growth, and irregular bowel habits. An algorithm for evaluation of malabsorption using a qualitative fecal fat test and serum carotene is presented in Figure 19–1.

Fat Excretion

To quantitate fat excretion, there must be known dietary intake and timed stool collection. The usual technique involves a diet containing 100 g of fat daily with a 3-day stool collection to measure total fat excretion. Excretion of more than 6 g per day is normal, and values may range upwards of 50 g or more. This process is tedious and inaccurate except under controlled metabolic conditions. In pancreatic deficiency, the stool usually contains excessive quantities of undigested protein, because pancreatic proteases also are deficient. Diseases of the liver and biliary tract severe enough to produce steatorrhea usually cause jaundice and abnormalities of blood chemistry before the steatorrhea becomes a diagnostic possibility. **Carotene** is a derivative of fat-soluble vitamin A. It requires an intact lipid absorption process. It is therefore used as a screening test for lipid malabsorption (see Fig. 19–1). Decreased serum concentration of beta-carotene (reference range >0.06 mg/dL) indicates either poor diet or more likely malabsorption.

Carbohydrate Utilization

When celiac disease, nontropical sprue (adult celiac disease), tropical sprue, and infiltrative diseases intrinsic to the small intestine cause steatorrhea, other malabsorptive problems may be present. Carbohydrate absorption is often decreased, exacerbating the patient's nutritional problems. The complete investigation of steatorrhea usually includes one or more studies of carbohydrate metabolism.

D-Xylose Test   A useful screening test for carbohydrate malabsorption is the assessment of the absorption of D-xylose, a pentose monosaccharide. If given orally (25 g in water), the amount excreted in a urine sample collected 5 hours after administration can be measured. Normally, more than 5 g is excreted. Less than this amount is associated with intestinal malabsorption, since xylose does not require pancreatic enzymes for absorption. Appropriate excretion, of course, will require normal renal function. Renal disease, therefore, may cause reduced D-xylose urinary excretion. Blood levels can also be ascertained, to eliminate this possibility when D-xylose excretion is low.

Lactose Intolerance

Most dietary carbohydrates, besides starch, are in the form of **disaccharides** (two simple sugars joined together). For absorption, enzymatic

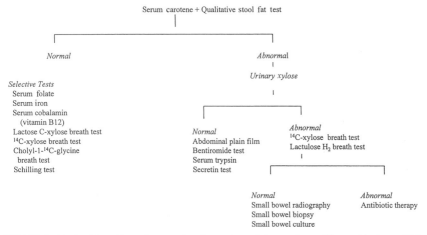

FIGURE 19–1. Algorithm for evaluation of malabsorption. (From Tsokes, PP: Malabsorption. In Bennett, JC, and Plum, F (eds): Cecil Textbook of Medicine, ed 20. WB Saunders, Philadelphia, 1996, p 703, with permission.)

cleavage to simple sugars is necessary. The intestinal mucosa possesses a variety of disaccharidases, several of which can manifest congenital or acquired deficiency. The most common deficiency involves **lactase,** the enzyme that cleaves lactose into its constituent sugars—glucose and galactose. Since intestinal lactase activity declines with age, milk intolerance is far more common in adults than in children (milk is rich in lactose). There is also racial difference in lactase activity. Asians tend to have the lowest levels, Africans only somewhat higher.

Defective lactase activity is associated with diarrhea, abdominal cramping, gas, and general constitutional uneasiness after ingesting milk or milk products. Lactose tolerance is now evaluated by the **lactose-H$_2$ breath test.** The patient drinks 1 g/kg of lactose-H$_2$ (50 g of lactose is the amount present in a quart of milk). An increase in breath H$_2$ (hydrogen) of more than 20 ppm over basal levels indicates lactase deficiency. The older oral lactose tolerance test is no longer recommended. The management of lactose intolerance due to lactase deficiency is either avoidance of dairy products, the use of lactose-free, lactase-pretreated milk, or the provision of some yeasts that contain lactase. These patients do need calcium supplementation.

Protein Loss

There is no satisfactory technique for quantitating fecal proteins. The protein loss with general malabsorption does not require separate documentation. In occasional patients, however, severe fecal protein loss **(protein-losing enteropathy)** may occur.

Proteins within the intestinal lumen are reduced enzymatically to their component amino acids, which are then reabsorbed. If mucosal abnormalities prevent reabsorption, or if protein leakage exceeds the reabsorptive capacity, hypoproteinemia may result. Severe ulcerative colitis, Whipple's disease, disturbances of the lymphatic circulation, and intestinal lymphomas may produce this syndrome, which is suggested by hypoalbuminemia in the absence of hepatic disease or urine protein loss.

Clinical Observations

Patients with severe malabsorption may have low serum albumin levels, partly from general malnutrition and partly from excessive fecal loss. Inadequate absorption of fat-soluble vitamins can produce low vitamin A levels (low serum-carotene levels), coagulation abnormalities caused by vitamin K deficiency, and osteoporosis with elevated heat-labile alkaline phosphatase levels caused by reduced vitamin D activity (see also Appendix A).

Fecal enzyme analysis is not usually performed in suspected pancreatic enzyme deficiencies, except in very young children. The analysis of duodenal aspirates (discussed later) is more informative for the diagnosis of pancreatic disease.

An alternative but also useful test of pancreatic function is the **bentiromide urinary excretion test. Bentiromide** is a synthetic peptide linked to para-aminobenzoic acid (PABA). Chymotrypsin in pancreatic secretions cleaves the bond and PABA is absorbed, conjugated by the liver, and excreted in the urine as arylamines. Normal secretion is more than 57% arylamines per 6-hour urine collection. Pancreatic deficiency is associated with an arylamine excretion of less than 50% of the ingested amount (500 mg of bentiromide). The test is useful in the diagnosis of pancreatic deficiency, assuming creatinine values are <2 mg/dL.

Definitive diagnosis of intestinal mucosal abnormalities can now be made by the histologic examination of biopsy specimens obtained by endoscopy using fiberoptic instrumentation. Biopsy specimens, when available, are especially useful for following the patient's response to therapy because histologic changes in most of the more common problems are reversible.

SPUTUM ANALYSIS

Sputum is the material secreted by the tracheobronchial tree and brought up by coughing. The healthy individual does not normally produce sputum. If sputum is not available, the respiratory tract can be studied by obtaining tracheal secretions or bronchoalveolar lavage specimens, which can be analyzed by a tinctorial or fluorescent stain, antigen tests, or specific nucleic acid probes.

NORMAL PHYSIOLOGY

Mucus secretion is part of the normal bronchopulmonary cleansing. Secretions form a layer perhaps 5 μm thick, immediately overlying the ciliated epithelium. By ciliary action, this semisticky mantle of fluid moves upward toward the oropharynx, carrying with it inhaled particles that have found their way down to the respiratory bronchioles. From the oropharynx the secretions are swallowed, so that the normal person is not aware of their presence. Coughing or expectorating tracheobronchial secretions is abnormal, the quantity of material being roughly parallel to the severity of the malady.

Besides its mechanical cleansing action, mucus attacks inhaled bacteria directly. The antibacterial effect of normal tracheobronchial mucus results largely from its antibody activity, although lysozymes and slightly acid pH conditions also help maintain sterility. The antibodies are predominantly IgA (see Chapter 7) and enter the mucus by direct glandular secretion rather than by transudation from the plasma. Despite the daily inhalation of innumerable organisms, the contents of the lower respiratory tract are sterile in normal individuals (see Chapter 14).

The specifics of response to injury involving the respiratory tract are discussed in this chapter, and issues relating to specimen collection and transport are also discussed in Chapter 13.

It is seldom necessary to collect a pooled sputum specimen. The product of a single coughing episode is more representative of the tracheobronchial tree than is a specimen that partially dries during collection or becomes contaminated with saliva or with organisms from the atmosphere. The specimen should be delivered to the laboratory as promptly as possible. Pooled specimens are, however, sometimes collected when tubercle bacilli are being sought.

GROSS APPEARANCE

Descriptive terms applied to sputum include *mucoid, mucopurulent, frankly purulent, blood-tinged, frankly bloody,* and *dust-flecked.* These characteristics correlate moderately well with the cause of cough. Purulent sputum usually accompanies acute bacterial pneumonias. In a patient with chronic bronchitis, change from mucoid to purulent or mucopurulent sputum indicates bacterial infection overlying a chronic inflammatory process. Gradual progression from scant, sticky sputum to more abundant, loose, purulent material may signal the development of chronic changes such as may occur in bronchiectasis, in which bronchioles are persistently dilated due to inflammatory destruction of the peribronchiolar tissue. Rupture of a pulmonic abscess causes expectoration of abundant purulent, often foul-smelling pus.

BLOOD

Coughing up blood is called **hemoptysis,** and it is always significant. The quantity of blood can range from scant streaks to life-threatening hemorrhage, the latter occurring when a bronchial or bronchopulmonary process erodes through the bronchial wall into a large blood vessel. Table 19–38 lists the diagnostic inferences that can be drawn from bloody sputum.

MICROSCOPIC EXAMINATION

The specimens for optimal diagnosis of pulmonary infections include, but are not limited to, sputum analysis; these are listed in Tables 19–39 and 19–40. The microbiologic findings, culture results, and immunologic techniques that are performed on sputum have been discussed in the earlier chapters (see Chapters 13, 14, and 15) and are summarized in Table 19–40. The formed elements in sputum are best studied by cytologic techniques using the Papanicolaou stain or an appropriate modification. If detailed cytologic examination is not needed, other staining techniques

TABLE 19–38. CAUSES OF BLOOD-STAINED SPUTUM

Appearance	Usual Cause
Uniform "rusty" color, pus present	Pneumococcal pneumonia
Uniform "rusty" color, no pus	Congestive heart failure/mitral valve disease
Bright streaks in viscid sputum	*Klebsiella pneumoniae*
Scant but persistent streaks in mucoid sputum	Bronchogenic carcinoma
Episodic occurrences of small hemorrhages	Tuberculosis
Episodes of large hemorrhages	Cavitary tuberculosis
	Pulmonary infarction
	Fungal pneumonia
Spurious hemoptysis	Bleeding in nose, nasopharynx

are valuable. Leukocytes can be identified on Gram-stained smears, and morphology alone will permit distinction between the polymorphonuclear leukocytes found in infection and eosinophils, characteristic of asthmatic attacks. Wright's stain or other Romanowsky-type stains are helpful in making this distinction. Periodic acid-Schiff (PAS) and silver stains are sometimes applied to sputum in suspected pulmonary alveolar proteinosis. The characteristic compacted protein may be inside mononuclear cells, or free in round or laminated clumps or in aggregates with cleft-like spaces. When round and laminated, these resemble the cysts of *Pneumocystis carinii*. Although both are PAS positive, only *Pneumocystis* takes a silver stain (see Chapter 14). Sudan red staining is useful in detecting lipoid pneumonia. Microbiology laboratories can now also perform same day analysis for *Pneumocystis,* using direct monoclonal fluorescent antibody stains or induced sputum or bronchoalveolar lavage specimens.

Curschmann's spirals can be identified readily on Gram-stained smears. These coiled, mucus filaments, once considered pathognomonic of asthma, are casts of small bronchi and may occur whenever increased mucus production accompanies bronchial obstruction. Since bronchospasm and excessive secretions characterize asthmatic attacks, Curschmann's spirals are particularly to be expected, but they also can occur in other types of acute bronchitis or in bronchopneumonia and may be found in sputum arising from small bronchi adjacent to lung carcinomas. Table 19–41 outlines formed elements that may be seen on microscopic examination.

Bronchoalveolar lavage (BAL), performed during fiberoptic bronchoscopy, is a technique of "flushing" secretions from the lower respiratory tract for the purpose of obtaining material for culture or microscopic study. The test is especially used for the detection of ***Pneumocystis carinii***

TABLE 19–39. SPECIMENS FOR OPTIMAL DIAGNOSIS OF PULMONARY INFECTIONS

Specimen Type	Preferred Specimens for Direct Detection or Culture								
	Bacteria	Legionella species	Chlamydia species*	Mycoplasma species*	Nocardia species	Fungi	Mycobacteria species	Pneumocystis carinii	Viruses
Expectorated sputum	++	+	0–	+	+	+	++	–	+
NaCl-induced sputum	–	–	–	–	+	–	++	++	0–
Nasopharyngeal washes or swabs	–	–	+	+	–	–	–	–	++
Bronchoalveolar lavage, brushings, biopsies	++	++	++	++	++	++	++	++	++
Percutaneous needle aspirate, open lung biopsy	++	++	++	++	++	++	++	++	++

– = not recommended or undocumented; + = acceptable; ++ = preferred.
*Culture not generally available.
From Shelhamer, JH, et al: The laboratory evaluation of opportunistic pulmonary infections. Ann Intern Med 124:585–589, 1996, p 586, with permission.

TABLE 19–40. DIRECT STAINS*, DIRECT TESTS, AND CULTURE AVAILABLE FOR COMMON PULMONARY PATHOGENS†

Organism	Direct Stain	Antigen or Nucleic Acid	Culture	Incubation Duration
Routine bacteria	Gram stain	Not available	Routine methods	3–4 d
Legionella species	Direct fluorescent antibody	PCR‡; urine antigen (RIA)	Special Legionella media (BCYE†)	2–7 d
Fungi	Wet mount or calcofluor white	Serum cryptococcal antigen; Serum/urine histoplasma, antigen PCR§	Mycologic media (e.g., Sabouraud, BHI agar)	6–8 wk
Mycobacteria species	Acid-fast stain	PCR§	Mycobacterial media (Middlebrook 7H 10/11)	≥8 wk
Nocardia species	Modified acid-fast stain	Not available	Blood agar, Sabouraud	4–6 wk
Pneumocystis species	Fluorescent antibody, Giemsa, toluidine blue O	PCR§	Noncultivable organism	
Viruses	Fluorescent antibody for specific viruses**	EIA§ for RSV, Influenza A; FAB for CMV, VZV, HSV	Traditional tissue culture; Shell vial culture††	≥2 wk; 2–5 d
Chlamydia species	None‡‡	PCR§	HL or HEp-2 cells	3–5 d
Mycoplasma species	None	PCR§	Selective media	7–10 d

*Those stains usually done by microbiology laboratories on sputum, bronchoscopic, or biopsy specimens.
†BCYE = buffered charcoal yeast extract; BHI = brain–heart infusion; CMV = cytomegalovirus; EIA = enzyme immunoassay; FAB = fluorescent antibody; HSV = herpes simplex virus; PCR = polymerase chain reaction; RIA = radioimmunoassay; RSV = respiratory syncytial virus; VZV = varicella-zoster virus.
‡The PCR assay is available in a few diagnostic laboratories but is not generally available.
§Research technique.
**Direct fluorescent antibody and EIA are available only for some viruses.
††Influenza A and B; parainfluenza 1, 2, and 3; RSV, CMV, HSV, and VZV are commonly available.
‡‡None for C. pneumoniae.
From Shelhamer, JH, et al: The laboratory evaluation of opportunistic pulmonary infections. Ann Intern Med 124:585–589, 1996, p 586, with permission.

TABLE 19–41. FORMED ELEMENTS SEEN ON SPUTUM MICROSCOPY

Observation	Usual Cause
Numerous squamous epithelial cells	Specimen is mostly saliva, not sputum
Numerous neutrophils, often with intracellular or extracellular organisms	Bacterial or fungal pneumonia
Numerous eosinophils	Asthma or pulmonary hypersensitivity reaction
Numerous neutrophils, abundant mucus, few or no organisms	Chronic bronchitis or bronchiectasis
PAS-positive macrophages	Alveolar proteinosis
PAS-positive rounded bodies that take silver stain	*Pneumocystis carinii*
Lipid droplets in macrophages	Lipoid or aspiration pneumonia
Curschmann's spirals (coiled mucus filaments)	Asthma: obstruction of small bronchi
Charcot-Leyden crystals (pointed eosinophilic masses)	Asthma
Dense, crystalline concretions (may be large enough to be grossly visible)	Broncholithiasis

pneumonitis (PCP), a frequent cause of pulmonary infections in immunosuppressed patients, in particular those with acquired immuno-deficiency syndromes. BAL can be as effective in the diagnosis of PCP as open lung biopsy, but the sensitivity of the test is dependent on the methods used to collect, process, and stain the samples. Testing methods include immunofluorescent-labeled monoclonal antibodies (most sensitive), or stains such as methenamine silver, toludine blue, or Giemsa stains. The diagnostic yield may be improved when BAL is performed with bronchoscopic lung biopsy. (See also Chapters 13 and 14.)

GASTRIC AND DUODENAL CONTENTS

GASTRIC PHYSIOLOGY

The stomach has both mechanical and digestive functions. The mechanical functions are usually evaluated by radiologic, endoscopic, and pressure measurements; they are not subject to direct laboratory investigation. The gastric mucosa has several secretory products—rennin, mucus, and small amounts of nondigestive enzymes—that can be subjected to study but rarely are. The gastric acid is produced by parietal cells of the gastric epithelial lining under the influence of the hormone **gastrin,** secreted by the chief cells of the lower stomach. Gastrin secretion occurs under the influence of parasympathetic stimulation by the vagus nerve and is also induced by the presence of food in the stomach. The quantitation of hydrochloric acid secretion is one of the studies performed in the clinical laboratory.

COLLECTING GASTRIC JUICE

Gastric secretions are collected by aspiration through a tube passed through the mouth or nasopharynx. The tip should be at the most dependent portion of the stomach, without curling or twisting. Most gastric aspiration is performed in the morning after an overnight fast. At this time the stomach should contain no more than 5 mL of clear or opalescent fluid, free of food particles, blood, or bile. The usual bacterial flora has little clinical significance, but tuberculous patients whose sputum contains no organisms sometimes have *Mycobacterium tuberculosis* in overnight gastric contents. Cytologic examination of native gastric juice is usually unsatisfactory, since desquamated cells are poorly preserved. After the gastric contents have been aspirated, gastric washings can be extremely useful in detecting gastric neoplasms.

Hydrochloric acid, along with gastric proteolytic enzymes, is important in initiating protein digestion. In the clinical syndrome of **peptic ulcer disease (PUD),** gastric or duodenal mucosa or both are attacked by these proteolytic activities and by gastric acidity. *Helicobacter pylori* infection, the use of nonsteroidal anti-inflammatory agents, or both factors are responsible for most cases of benign PUD. Standard therapy for PUD consists of proton pump inhibitors and two antimicrobial agents (triple therapy with success rates exceeding 85%). The measurement of gastric acid secretion is valuable in diagnosing the special subgroup of peptic ulcer disease known as **Zollinger-Ellison syndrome.** The hematologic disorder **pernicious anemia** is often characterized by impaired gastric acid production.

Under resting, unstimulated conditions, the stomach secretes a small amount of acid. Increased acidity results physiologically from neural and humoral stimulation. Emotional stimuli and the sight or smell of food can induce gastric acid secretion by stimulating the vagus nerve. Vagal impulses affect the parietal cells directly and induce cells in the antrum of the stomach to produce gastrin, an intense hormonal stimulator of parietal cell activity. Antral gastrin secretion is further enhanced by the distention of the stomach wall or by contact with protein breakdown products. A third but weaker stimulus to gastric acidity occurs when the duodenal mucosa, in contact with intraluminal digestive products, releases humoral activators.

MEASURING GASTRIC ACIDITY

The history of gastric analysis is replete with tubes of various designs and eponyms, different test meals to stimulate acid secretion, and techniques and terms to "express gastric production of HCl." Titration with 0.1 N NaCl and the expression of clinical units have given way to direct determinations of pH and hydrogen ion concentration. The usual procedure is to collect gastric juice for 1 hour in the unstimulated fasting state. The volume and pH are recorded and the total gastric secretion during this period is expressed as **basal acid output (BAO)** in milliequivalents per hour. The BAO is usually 4 to 5 mEq/hour, being somewhat lower in women than in men. The BAO correlates to some degree with body weight.

Stimulation

When the basal output has been established, the parietal cells are exposed to intense stimulation and the resulting acid output is measured. **Histamine** (0.04 mg/kg), **betazole** *(Histalog)* (50 to 100 mg), or **pentagastrin** (6 g/kg) are the stimulants used. Because histamine exerts unpleasant systemic effects on the blood vessels and smooth muscles, any antihistamine should be given 30 minutes before testing. Betazole is a histamine isomer with a preferential effect on gastric secretion and less severe systemic effects. Pentagastrin, a synthetic analog of gastrin, causes the least troublesome and shortest-lived side effects.

The injection of the stimulant is followed by another hour of collection. Sometimes this hour is divided into separate 15-minute collection periods. The total acid secreted in the hour after stimulation is **maximal acid output (MAO).** If the 15-minute periods are reported individually, **peak acid output (PAO)** can be expressed. This is the sum of the two highest consecutive quarterly readings and is therefore somewhat more than half the MAO. Basal and maximal outputs are often compared as the ratio of BAO/MAO. This lies between 0.3 and 0.6, meaning that maximal output is approximately 1.5 to 3.0 times the resting output.

Low Acid Output

If the pH never falls below 6, even after stimulation, the patient has **anacidity.** Strict anacidity would mean no pH below 7.0, but clinically useful correlation with gastric atrophy and pernicious anemia calls for defining anacidity in subcategories. "Achlorhydria" is an older term, originating when titration to pH 3.5 was thought to have physiologic significance. Many workers now use the terms achlorhydria and anacidity interchangeably; attempts to differentiate the two according to rates of pH change are not very useful.

Anacidity indicates defective gastric mucosa. Nearly all adults with pernicious anemia demonstrate anacidity, but half of gastric carcinoma patients will have anacidity, as will very occasional patients with hypoplastic or hypochromic anemia, or with immune-related disorders of the thyroid, stomach, or connective tissue. Anacidity never occurs in peptic ulcer disease. Demonstrating anacidity eliminates peptic ulcer disease as a cause of abdominal pain or bleeding and raises the suspicion of gastric carcinoma. Anacidity alone is insufficient to diagnose pernicious anemia in a patient with megaloblastic anemia, but demonstrating moderate to normal acid secretion is against the diagnosis.

Increased Acid Output

Correlation between acid output and clinical disease is difficult. Normal BAO is 4 to 5 mEq/hour, and the mean figures for MAO range from 16 to 26 mEq/hour. The ratio of BAO to MAO is usually 0.3 or less, and never higher than 0.6 if gastric physiology is normal. The results of acid response testing correlate poorly with the patient's response to medical or surgical treatment.

Zollinger-Ellison syndrome is characterized by a triad of recurrent peptic ulcer disease, non-β-islet cell tumor of the pancreas, and gastric acid hypersecretion. The excessive production of gastrin by these gastrinomas causes high basal acid production: characteristically 10 mEq/hour or more. Because of this continuous gastrin stimulation, pharmacologic stimulation causes little additional increase. Table 19–42 shows a representative normal and abnormal gastric acid analysis.

TABLE 19–42. REPRESENTATIVE NORMAL AND ABNORMAL GASTRIC ACID RESULTS

	Basal Acid Output (BAO) (mEq/hr)	Maximum Acid Output (MAO) (mEq/hr)	BAO/MAO
Normal	2.5	25.0	10%
Pernicious anemia	0	0	0
Gastric carcinoma	1.0	4.0	25%
Duodenal ulcer	5.0	30.0	17%
Zollinger-Ellison syndrome	18.0	25.0	72%

From Strasinger, SK: Urinalysis and Body Fluids. FA Davis, Philadelphia, 1985, p 191, with permission.

Serum Gastrin

After a secretory study shows elevated acid secretion, a serum gastrin is obtained to establish the diagnosis of Zollinger-Ellison syndrome. In addition, a serum gastrin level should always be obtained in a patient with recurrent peptic ulcer disease. Under normal circumstances, acid inhibits gastrin production by the chief cells of the gastric antrum. Patients with the Zollinger-Ellison syndrome, however, have a tumor in the pancreas that increases gastrin production so that serum levels are very high. A high gastrin level can also occur in people with achlorhydria because gastric acid inhibition of the chief cells does not occur (Table 19–43). If a patient has both acid secretion and a serum gastrin of greater than 1000 pg/mL, this is virtually pathognomonic for Zollinger-Ellison syndrome. If serum gastrins are in the midrange (300 to 800 pg/mL), a stimulatory test (using secretin, calcium, or standard meal test) can be performed. Normally, secretin decreases gastrin production; however, in Zollinger-Ellison syndrome there is a paradoxical increase in serum gastrin levels over a 15-minute period.

Most studies of gastric contents are performed to evaluate hypersecretion and in those people with Zollinger-Ellison syndrome.

TABLE 19–43. CAUSES OF ELEVATED SERUM GASTRIN LEVELS (REFERENCE INTERVAL <100 pg/mL)

Level	Causes
>1000 pg/mL	Zollinger-Ellison syndrome*
300–800 pg/mL	History of vagotomy
	Antral G-cell hyperfunction (pseudo Z-E syndrome)
	Gastric outlet obstruction
	Gastroparesis
	Use of acid-lowering medications protein pump inhibitors H_2 blockers
	Atrophic gastritis
	H. pylori infection
	Pernicious anemia
	Renal failure

*<10-fold elevation in serum gastrin with gastric fluid pH <2.5 requires analysis of basal acid output.

DUODENAL FLUID

Collecting duodenal secretions is more difficult and time consuming than gastric aspiration because the tube must be passed beyond the pylorus and located close to the ampulla of Vater. A double-lumen tube is customary, with one portion remaining in the stomach to aspirate gastric acid juice, which, if it passes the pylorus, will contaminate the alkaline duodenal secretions.

When endoscopy is performed with a fiber-optic duodenoscope, it is possible to cannulate the pancreatic duct and collect aliquots of pure pancreatic juice. This technique allows highly specific analysis of enzymes and other proteins.

Physiology

The duodenum normally secretes 1200 to 1500 mL per day of enzyme-rich, clear fluid with a pH of 8.0 to 8.5, containing up to 145 mEq/liter of bicarbonate iron. The pancreatic enzymes split fats, carbohydrates, and proteins—the major constituents being lipase, amylase, trypsin, and chymotrypsin. Secretions of bicarbonate ion and enzymes have different physiologic provocation, although both are mediated hormonally.

When acidic gastric contents enter the duodenum, the falling pH stimulates mucosal cells to produce secretin. Secretin stimulates watery pancreatic secretions with a high bicarbonate content. Enzyme production is provoked by pancreozymin, also elaborated by the small intestinal mucous membrane. The stimulus to pancreozymin secretion, however, is the presence of digestive products in the lumen of the proximal small bowel; distention by volume alone inspires a small amount of pancreozymin secretion, but sustained pancreozymin production is best evoked by polypeptides or micellar fatty acids in the small intestinal contents.

Secretin Testing

Both secretin and pancreozymin are available in pharmacologic forms. Secretin usually is less expensive and gives as good a result as pancreozymin, which is more commonly used in Europe. Prior to intravenous injection, intradermal tests should be given to ensure that there is no sensitivity to these foreign proteins. The procedure involves the passage of an endoscopy tube to the ligament of Treitz at the end of the duodenum. In particular the **secretin test** is the most sensitive test of impaired pancreatic function. Secretin is administered intravenously in a dose of 1 to 2 units per kilogram of bodyweight, after which duodenal fluid bicarbonate is assayed. Normally HCO_3^- concentration greater than 80 mEq/L and a volume greater than 1.8 ml/kg/hr are recovered following secretin stimulation. By assessing bicarbonate production, this test determines the ability of the pancreas to respond to secretin's stimulus. If a patient has a pancreatic carcinoma, there will be a low volume with a normal bicarbonate and a normal amylase. A tumor usually obstructs flow. If the patient has chronic pancreatitis, then there is a low volume and, in addition, a low bicarbonate and a low amylase due to the destruction of the pancreatic parenchyma.

The presence of bile, blood, undigested food particles, and cholesterol crystals in the duodenal fluid is abnormal. Samples are collected at 20-minute intervals. Secretin stimulation normally induces the secretion of 2 to 4 mL of pancreatic juice per kg of body weight, with 90 to 130 mEq/liter of bicarbonate. The secretin test can be useful in documenting progressively declining function if done serially in patients with chronic, progressive pancreatitis.

The use of **endoscopic retrograde cholangiopancreatography (ERCP)** has facilitated the direct study of pancreatic and biliary secretions. This procedure is routinely employed to evaluate the anatomy of the biliary and pancreatic ducts. It requires the passage of an endoscope to the duodenal papilla, and the bile duct or pancreatic ducts are cannulated. Contrast material can be injected, either to outline the anatomy or to assess duct patency.

Biliary drainage with cholesterol crystal analysis is sometimes performed after the administration of the secretagogue **cholecystokinin,** which makes the gallbladder contract. Bile extruded from the duodenal papilla is collected and sent to the clinical laboratory for cholesterol analysis. Approximately 80% of all gallstones seen in the western hemisphere contain cholesterol and may form as a result of the supersaturation of bile by cholesterol. In fact, the presence of any cholesterol crystals in the secretions implies a high concentration of cholesterol and a substantial risk of gallstone formation.

ANALYSIS OF SEROUS FLUIDS

The closed body spaces include the **pleural,** the **pericardial,** and the **peritoneal cavities.** Normally a small amount of serous fluid is present within these spaces to facilitate lubrication between the **body cavity (parietal) membrane** and the **visceral membrane** surrounding the body organs. Fluid may accumulate at one site as a result of many different stimuli. These fluids are studied to distinguish among causes that may be infectious, inflammatory, traumatic, or from primary or secondary malignancies. Symptoms are dependent on the primary cause and the volume and rate of fluid that accumulates. Fluid accumulation may be passive or part of an active inflammatory or neoplastic process. Passive accumulation is simply the leakage of fluid out of blood vessels; it is usually noninflammatory. Distinctions between the passive and active fluid that accumulates in these serous spaces is important in the differential diagnosis of disease. Passive fluid accumulation is termed **transudation,** whereas active mechanisms produce an **exudate.** It is important to differentiate between transudates and exudates, as this distinction may provide clues to the nature of the disease process.

THE MECHANISMS OF PASSIVE FLUID ACCUMULATION

The accumulation of fluid **(effusion)** occurs as a result of a net build-up of **hydrostatic pressure,** forcing fluid through the capillaries out into the tissues (Fig. 19–2). The hydrostatic pressure tends to force fluid out, and this is resisted by the **oncotic pressure** within the circulation. Albumin and proteins in the blood contribute to the oncotic pressure. The hydrostatic pressure at the arterial end usually measures approximately 40 mmHg, and the oncotic pressure measures 25 mmHg; thus the net positive pressure forcing fluid out into the serous spaces is 15 mmHg. If the plasma oncotic pressure is reduced, more fluid is likely to be forced out, and this is a common cause of serous effusion. Normally, at the venous end of the capillary the hydrostatic pressure falls to about 10 mmHg, and the colloid osmotic pressure is maintained at 25 mmHg, counteracting this hydrostatic pressure. Consequently there is a net negative pressure of 15 mmHg at the venous end, tending to draw fluids into the blood vessels. Any process that increases the hydrostatic pressure at the venous end is likely to produce fluid accumulation on a passive basis (see Fig. 19–2). Furthermore, any reduction in plasma oncotic pressure will reduce the amount of fluid drawn into the venous capillary.

Other mechanisms facilitating passive accumulation of fluids, which may be both local and general, are allergic mechanisms increasing capillary permeability or lymphatic obstruction; this, in turn, reduces the amount of extravascular fluid that is cleared by the lymphatic system.

Exudates occur when the membrane or capillary lining is damaged by inflammatory or neoplastic processes. As a result, large proteins and other blood constituents leak out into the spaces and tissues. In active inflammation, there is a higher protein constitution of this fluid. Table 19–44 shows the laboratory differentiation of transudates and exudates.

LABORATORY EVALUATION OF SEROUS FLUIDS

The analysis of serous fluids involves the following.

Gross Appearance

Most normal fluids are clear. Cloudiness implies either high protein content or cellular inflammation. Bloody fluid implies inflammation, damage to blood vessels, or trauma.

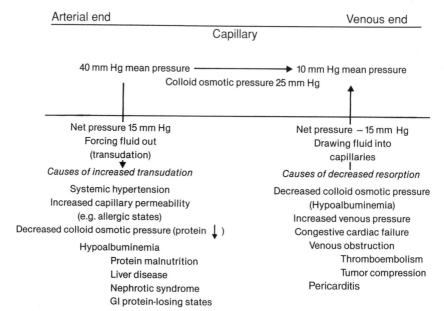

FIGURE 19–2. Etiology and pathogenesis of serous effusions (transudates).

TABLE 19–44. LABORATORY DIFFERENTIATION OF TRANSUDATES AND EXUDATES

	Transudate	Exudate
Appearance	Clear	Cloudy
Specific gravity	<1.015	>1.015
Total protein	<3.0 g/dL*	>3.0 g/dL*
Fluid:serum protein ratio	<0.5	>0.5
Lactic dehydrogenase	<200 IU	>200 IU
Fluid:serum LD ratio	<0.6	>0.6
Cell count	<1000/µL	>1000/µL
Spontaneous clotting	No	Possible

*A lower value of 2.5 g/dL is sometimes used for peritoneal fluid.

Adapted from Strasinger, SK: Urinalysis and Body Fluids, ed 3. FA Davis, Philadelphia, 1994, p 173.

Specific Gravity

This provides an estimation of the protein content. Exudates have a specific gravity greater than 1.015; transudates have a specific gravity less than 1.015.

Cell Counts and Differential Counts

Normally, there may be up to five cells per high-power field. Generally cells, and in particular neutrophils, are not present in normal fluids. A high count or the presence of neutrophils is abnormal. Fluids are also generally sterile, so that the presence of bacteria should be determined and can be easily accomplished with a Gram stain. A positive Gram stain should also be followed by routine culture or special culture, as indicated by the clinical syndrome (see Chapter 14).

Chemical Analysis

Protein levels are higher in exudates than in transudates, and in general the total protein content is less than 3.0 g/dL in a transudate and greater than 3.0 g/dL in an exudate. The presence of the enzyme **lactate dehydrogenase (LDH),** which comes from degenerating cells, is greater than 200 IU/L in an exudate and less than 200 IU/L in a transudate. The ratio with serum LDH should also be determined; this is usually greater than 0.6 in an exudate and less than 0.6 in a transudate. Because exudates contain a substantial amount of protein, including coagulation proteins, exudates may have spontaneous clotting. The reverse, of course, is true for transudates.

A cytologic examination of all serous fluids should be determined, particularly with exudates, where detection of neoplastic cells is of concern.

PLEURAL FLUID

Pleural fluid is obtained by a thoracentesis (pleural tap). The distinction between transudates and exudates is important in analyzing pleural fluid because it may give a substantive clue concerning the cause of the accumulation of fluid (see Table 19–44). Transudates are usually seen in congestive cardiac failure or hypoalbuminemia, whereas exudates are found in lung or pleural malignancies or pneumonia. Again, as is applicable in other serous fluids, the gross appearance of the fluid may be helpful in establishing a diagnosis. If the fluid is turbid, this may suggest an exudate as a result of infection, autoimmune inflammatory process, or malignancy. Blood-stained pleural effusions are seen in cases involving trauma, such as hemothorax, or in pulmonary embolus, malignancy, and tuberculosis. In this situation, it is important to differentiate a traumatic tap from a hemothorax, and again the ratio of red cells to white cells is important, as was discussed in the evaluation of the spinal tap. When the pleural fluid appears cloudy or milky, this may suggest thoracic duct obstruction or damage (e.g., surgical) or lymphatic obstruction, causing a chylous effusion. Cell counts and differential counts may also be helpful in excluding inflammatory, autoimmune, and malignant disease. In general, counts above 1000 cells/µL in pleural fluid are considered abnormal. In bacterial effusions, polymorphonuclear leukocytes are predominant. In tuberculous effusions and those associated with rheumatoid arthritis, there is a predominance of lymphocytes. In malignancy there may be an abundance of all inflammatory cells, with neoplastic cells detected on cytologic examination. Reactive mesothelial cells may be seen in inflammatory and neoplastic disease because these cells, which normally line the pleural cavity, may be desquamated and may show varied morphologic appearance. Malignant mesothelial cells can be seen in mesothelioma of the pleura, particularly in association with asbestos exposure.

Again, chemical analysis will help establish whether the effusion is an exudate or a transudate, determining whether this is a passive accumulation of fluid or part of an active inflammatory or neoplastic disease. Table 19–45 outlines the pleural fluid characteristics in several common pulmonary diseases.

PERICARDIAL FLUID

Under normal circumstances, only a small amount of fluid is present in the pericardial sac (10 to 50 mL). In some inflammatory or neoplastic disease processes affecting the pericardial sac, excessive fluid may accumulate around the heart and impede the cardiac pump (tamponade). Clinical signs such as distended neck veins and distant heart sounds may alert the physician to this occurrence. In this situation, the aspiration of fluid from the pericardial sac can be both therapeutic and diagnostic. Aspiration is often performed under ultrasound guidance. The principles used to evaluate spinal fluid and pleural fluid are also applicable to pericardial fluid. It is important to notice the gross appearance, to get a cell count, differential count, and culture, and to get a chemical analysis to distinguish a transudate from an exudate.

PERITONEAL FLUID

The accumulation of excessive fluid in the peritoneal space is termed **ascites.** Normally the peritoneal sac contains 50 mL of straw-colored clear fluid. Peritoneal fluid may be cloudy in conditions of inflammation or neoplasm, or greenish when bile staining has occurred. Bile staining can

TABLE 19–45. PLEURAL FLUID CHARACTERISTICS IN COMMON DISEASES

Etiology	Appearance	Total WBC (per µL)	Predominant WBC	RBC (per µL)	Protein	Glucose	LDH	Amylase	pH
Transudates									
Congestive heart failure	Clear, straw-colored	<1000	M	0–1000	PF/S <0.5	PF = S	PF/S <0.6 <200 IU/liter	≤S	>7.40
Cirrhosis	Clear, straw-colored	<500	M	<1000	PF/S <0.5	PF = S	PF/S <0.6 <200 IU/liter	≤S	>7.40
Exudates									
Parapneumonic (uncomplicated)	Turbid	5,000–25,000	P	<5000	PF/S >0.5	PF = S	PF/S >0.6	≤S	>7.30
Empyema	Turbid to purulent	25,000–100,000	P	<5000	PF/S >0.5	0–60 mg/dL PF/S <0.5	PF/S >0.6 some >1000 IU/liter	≤S	<7.30
Pulmonary infarction	Straw-colored to bloody	5,000–15,000	P	1,000–100,000	PF/S >0.5	PF = S	PF/S >0.6	≤S	>7.30
Tuberculosis	Straw-colored to sero-sanguinous	5,000–10,000	M	<10,000	PF/S >0.5	PF = S or <60 mg/dL	PF/S >0.6	≤S	< or >7.30
Rheumatoid disease	Turbid, green to yellow	1,000–20,000	M or P	<1000	PF/S >0.5	<30 mg/dL	Often >1000 IU/liter	≤S	<7.30
Carcinoma	Turbid to bloody	<10,000	M	1,000 to several 100,000	PF/S >0.5	PF = S or <60 mg/dL	PF/S >0.6	≤S	< or >7.30
Pancreatitis	Turbid	5,000–20,000	P	1,000–10,000	PF/S >0.5	PF = S	PF/S >0.6	PF/S > 2	>7.30

IU = International units; LDH = lactic dehydrogenase; M = mononuclear; P = polymorphonuclear; PF = pleural fluid; RBC = red blood cells; S = serum; WBC = white blood cells.

From Sahn, SA: Pulmonary disease. In Reller, LB, et al. (eds): Clinical Internal Medicine. Little, Brown, Boston, 1979, pp 106–107, with permission.

(Continued)

be confirmed by the use of a dipstick with a bilirubin test strip. Blood-stained fluid must be distinguished from a traumatic tap, which, as previously mentioned, tends to clear with further fluid collection. Normal red cell counts are less than 100,000 cells/µL, and white cells are usually below 300 cells/µL. Elevations in white cell counts, particularly above 350 neutrophils/µL, are suggestive of bacterial infection.

The differentiation between an exudate and a transudate usually uses a lower cutoff point of 2 to 2.5 g/dL for protein in peritoneal fluid compared with other serous fluids. Other chemical determinations include the evaluation of glucose, amylase, ammonia, and alkaline phosphatase. Glucose levels are reduced in bacterial inflammation, as well as in tuberculous and malignant peritonitis. Amylase levels are elevated in most patients with acute pancreatitis and pancreatic injury. Ammonia levels are increased with perforation of the viscera, including the stomach, bowel, or bladder. Alkaline phosphatase levels are also elevated, often greater than twice the normal serum level in patients with perforation or strangulation of the small bowel. As with other serous fluids, it is important to perform Gram stains for bacterial infection and cytologic examination to check for malignant effusions. Table 19–46 outlines the causes of peritoneal effusion.

The use of the microbiology laboratory in the evaluation of serous effusions has already been discussed in Chapter 14.

Diagnostic peritoneal lavage (DPL) consists of instilling and then aspirating sterile saline solution into the abdominal cavity. The solution is then subjected to chemical analysis and cell counts. DPL is used to evaluate abdominal trauma, establishing whether a patient has intraperitoneal hemorrhage, whether intestines have ruptured, or whether other organ damage may have occurred.

SYNOVIAL (JOINT) FLUID

The mobile synovial joints of the body have a basic structure consisting of a fluid-containing cavity that confers mobility; this is contained within a synovial membrane that synthesizes the lubricant and articulating cartilage. This viscous fluid is a dialysate of blood plasma with added hyaluronic acid; it functions as a lubricant for joints and supplies nutrition to the chondrocytes of the cartilage. The protein content is about 70% albumin, and the total protein is about a third of the plasma value (i.e., 2 g/dL). Inflammatory processes of joints are associated with the leakage of protein, often globulins, into the joint space. Normally only a small amount of fluid is present in a joint cavity, and any accumulation becomes obvious by the swelling, distortion, and pain of the joint. The aspiration of joint fluid **(arthrocentesis)** can be performed from any involved joint, but it is usually performed in the knee joint. Normally only 3.5 mL of fluid is present in the knee. Aspiration of joint fluid is

TABLE 19–46. CAUSES OF PERITONEAL EFFUSIONS

Transudates

Congestive heart failure
Hepatic cirrhosis
Hypoproteinemia (e.g., nephrotic syndrome)

Exudates

Neoplasms
  Hepatoma
  Metastatic carcinoma
  Lymphoma
  Mesothelioma
Infections
  Tuberculosis
  Primary bacterial peritonitis (may be superimposed on
    transudate)
  Secondary bacterial peritonitis (e.g., appendicitis, intestinal
    infarct)
Trauma
Pancreatitis
Bile peritonitis (secondary to ruptured gallbladder or needle
  perforation of bile duct)

Chylous Effusion

Damage or obstruction to thoracic duct (e.g., trauma,
  lymphoma, carcinoma, tuberculosis, parasitic infestation)

Adapted from Kjeldsberg, CR, and Krieg, A: Cerebrospinal fluid and other body fluids. In Henry, JB (ed): Clinical Diagnosis and Management by Laboratory Methods, ed 17. WB Saunders, Philadelphia, 1984, p 484.

usually performed in monarticular effusions or when there is uncertainty as to the cause of a joint disorder. Sterile technique is required to prevent the development of osteomyelitis, and the site of aspiration should be from the area of greatest distention.

Normally, synovial fluid does not form a fibrin clot; however the joint fluid is viscous due to the presence of mucin clots, which can be simply assessed. The *mucin clot test* is unique to joints and is the indirect determination of the hyaluronic acid (mucin) content (discussed below). Inflammation tends to make the fluid less mucoid, and testing for the presence of a mucin clot can assist, particularly in the diagnosis of rheumatoid arthritis.

Under normal circumstances, a heparinized and nonheparinized

TABLE 19–47. SUMMARY OF LABORATORY
FINDINGS IN JOINT DISORDERS

Group Classification	Laboratory Findings
I. Noninflammatory	Clear, yellow fluid Good viscosity WBCs less than 5000 Neutrophils less than 30% Normal glucose
II. Inflammatory	Cloudy, yellow fluid Poor viscosity WBCs 2,000 to 100,000 Neutrophils greater than 50% Decreased glucose Possible auto-antibodies present
III. Septic	Cloudy, yellow-green fluid Poor viscosity WBCs 10,000 to 200,000 Neutrophils greater than 90% Decreased glucose Positive culture
IV. Crystal-induced	Cloudy or milky fluid Poor viscosity WBCs 500 to 200,000 Neutrophils less than 90% Decreased glucose Elevated uric acid Crystals present
V. Hemorrhagic	Cloudy, red fluid Poor viscosity WBCs less than 5000 Neutrophils less than 50% Normal glucose RBCs present

From Strasinger, SK: Urinalysis and Body Fluids, ed 3.
FA Davis, Philadelphia, 1994, p 167, with permission.

specimen should be collected for chemical and immunologic tests. Microbiologic testing and crystal examination are performed from a plain, sterile tube. Table 19–47 is a summary of the laboratory findings from different joint disorders.

Synovial fluid examination also includes appearance, viscosity, cell count, differential count, and crystal identification. The synovial fluid is clear and straw-colored. Principles involved in the analysis of other serous fluids are also applicable to synovial fluids. Cloudy or turbid specimens suggest a bacterial or inflammatory problem. Hemorrhagic fluid may suggest **hemarthrosis** (bleeding into the joint) or a traumatic tap. The **mucin clot,** or **string test,** is an assessment of the hyaluronic acid concentration or the ability of hyaluronic acid to polymerize. It is the assessment of the specimen's ability to form a string of fluid from the tip of the syringe, following withdrawal from the fluid. A string that measures 4 to 6 cm is considered normal. The presence of a mucin clot is determined by the addition of acetic acid. Normally, less than 2000 red cells are present per microliter of synovial fluid, and the white counts are usually below 200 cells/µL. In severe inflammatory conditions, white cell counts can rise to over 100,000 cells/µL. Neutrophils are indicative of an acute bacterial arthritis, whereas an abundance of lymphocytes may indicate a chronic inflammatory process or an autoimmune disease such as rheumatoid arthritis.

Synovial fluid aspiration is especially useful in differentiating septic arthritis from chemical or crystal-induced arthritis. Several types of crystal-induced arthritis occur, the most common of which are those associated with monosodium urate crystals **(gout),** calcium pyrophosphate crystals **(pseudo-gout),** and hydroxyapatite crystals **(apatite arthropathy).** Microscopic examination for crystals is usually performed on a wet slide preparation using both bright-field and polarized light (Table 19–48).

Monosodium urate crystals are birefringent rods or needles. Crystals of calcium pyrophosphate usually occur as birefringent rectangles, rods, or rhomboid structures (Fig. 19–3). Cholesterol crystals may also appear in joint effusions and may complicate the appreciation of both urate and calcium pyrophosphate crystals. They usually have notched edges. Urate crystals are commonly seen in joint effusions during the acute attacks (in up to 95% of patients) and are often seen in joint fluid during the asymptomatic phase (in up to 75% of patients). The diagnosis of acute crystal arthritis is especially suggestive when crystals are found inside leukocytes.

Immunologic studies are occasionally performed on joint fluids and include tests for rheumatoid factor, antinuclear antibody, and complement, and may be useful in elucidating seronegative rheumatoid arthritis (see also Chapter 7). It is also emphasized that both crystal types may be present in the same joint effusion. The interpretation of laboratory data in the differential diagnosis of joint effusion has prompted some clinicians to classify these "typical" patterns in the different diseases into several categories, as shown in Table 19–47.

Because joint effusions are an ultrafiltrate of plasma, they generally contain the same chemical constituents as plasma. In general, glucose levels are not more than 10 mg/dL lower than that of plasma. Lower sugar levels in the joint effusion would tend to suggest a septic arthritis. Synovial fluid lactate levels have been suggested to be a useful test to differentiate between inflammatory and septic arthritis. Synovial fluid lactate levels greater than 7.5 mmol/L are very suggestive of septic

TABLE 19–48. SYNOVIAL FLUID CRYSTALS

Crystal	Shape		Compensated Polarized Light	Location
Monosodium urate	Needles		Negative birefringence	Intracellular and extracellular
Calcium pyrophosphate	Rods Needles Rhombics		Positive birefringence	Intracellular and extracellular
Cholesterol	Notched rhombic plates		Negative birefringence	Extracellular
Apatite	Small needles		May need electron microscope	Intracellular and extracellular
Corticosteroid	Flat, variable shaped plates		Positive and negative birefringence	Primarily intracellular

Adapted from Samuelson, CO, and Ward, JR: Examination of the synovial fluid. J Fam Pract 14:343–349, 1982.

arthritis but may occasionally be seen with rheumatoid arthritis. Microbiologic cultures of synovial fluid should include cultures for *Neisseria, Streptococcus,* and *Staphylococcus.*

SWEAT

The chemical analysis of sweat is infrequently performed, except in the diagnosis of **cystic fibrosis** (a disorder of mucus secretion with occlusion of much of the exocrine glandular functions); this chemical analysis is now augmented by the genetic analysis of the CF mutation. The sweat analysis of electrolytes is a useful test for the presence of cystic fibrosis and is usually performed in children who exhibit recurrent pulmonary infections or those who fail to thrive or have a family history of cystic fibrosis. Cystic fibrosis is one of the most common inherited disorders; it is transmitted as an autosomal recessive trait seen in 1 in approximately 1500 to 2000 white births. Patients with cystic fibrosis characteristically produce sweat with a much higher sodium and chloride content. The usual method is to induce sweat by

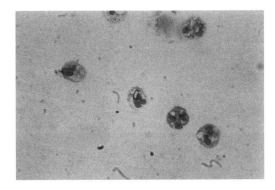

FIGURE 19–3. Polarized calcium pyrophosphate crystals in synovial fluid. Note the intracellular rhombus-shaped crystals (×1000). (From Strasinger, SK: Urinalysis and Body Fluids, ed 3. FA Davis, Philadelphia, 1994, Color Plate 72, with permission.)

iontophoresis, or the introduction of pilocarpine into the skin of the forearm (Gibson and Cook method). The test has many technical difficulties but has a high positive predictive value. The electrolytes are collected with electrolyte-free gauze or filter paper from the stimulated area. More recently, sweat osmolarity has shown a good correlation with sweat electrolytes. Sweat electrolytes may be directly measured by the use of ion-specific electrodes placed on the skin. Normal sweat chloride reference intervals are 5 to 45 mmol/L in children. Values in affected infants are usually greater than 60 mmol/L. Adult values are usually 10 mmol/L higher. The sweat test is an important means of both screening and diagnosing cystic fibrosis. Because of early detection and aggressive management, patients with this disorder have improved survival into the third and even fourth decades.

SUGGESTED READING

Bigner, SH: Cerebrospinal fluid (CSF). Cytology. Current status and diagnostic applications. J Neuropath Exp 51:235–245, 1992.

College of American Pathologists: Introduction to urine sediment. Hematology Manual. CAP, Chicago, 1998, pp 28–36.

Crystal, RG, et al: Bronchoalveolar lavage: the report of an international conference. Chest 90:122–131, 1986.

Dinda, AK, et al: Diagnosis of glomerular hematuria: Role of dysmorphic red cell, GI cell and bright field microscopy. Scand J Clin Lab Invest 57:203–208, 1997.

Fraser, JL, et al: Diagnostic yield of BAL and BLB for detection of *P. carinii*. Mayo Clin Proc 71:1025–1029, 1996.

Gile, VJ: Laboratory evaluation of opportunistic pulmonary infections. Ann Int Med 124:581–591, 1996.

Guyton, AC: Textbook of Medical Physiology, ed 7. WB Saunders, Philadelphia, 1986.

Haber, MH: Pisse prophecy: A brief history of urinalysis. Clin Lab Med 8:415–430, 1988.

Hansel, FK: Cytologic diagnosis in respiratory allergy and infection. Ann Allergy 24:564, 1996.

Horwanitz, PJ, Saladino, MJ, and Dale, JC: Timeliness of urinalysis. Arch Pathol Lab Med 121:667–672, 1997.

Kjeldsberg, CR, and Knight, JA: Body Fluids: Laboratory Examination of Amniotic, Cerebrospinal, Serous and Synovial Fluids: A Textbook Atlas. ASCP, Chicago, 1993.

Kokko, JP: Approach to patients with renal disease. In Bennett, JC, and Plum, F (eds): Cecil Textbook of Medicine, ed 20. WB Saunders, Philadelphia, 1996.

Mandel, N: Urinary tract calculi. Lab Med 17(8):449–458, 1986.

Prayson, RA, and Fischler, DF: Cerebrospinal fluid cytology. Arch Pathol Lab Med 122:47–51, 1998.

Rabinovitch, A, and Cornbleet PJ: Body fluid microscopy in U.S. laboratories. Arch Pathol Lab Med 118:13–17, 1994.

Sahn, SA: The differential diagnosis of pleural effusion. West J Med 137:99, 1982.

Smith, GP, and Kjeldsberg, CR: Cerebrospinal, synovial and serous fluids. In Henry, JB (ed): Clinical Diagnosis and Management by Laboratory Methods, ed 19. WB Saunders, Philadelphia, 1996.

Stagner, SN, and Campbell, GD: Pleural effusions: What you can learn from the result of a "tap." Postgrad Med 91(5):439–454, 1992.

Strasinger, SK: Urinalysis and Body Fluids, ed 3. FA Davis, Philadelphia, 1994.

APPENDIX A

Disorders of Nutrition

CALORIE DEFICIENCY

Persons suffering from starvation in poverty-stricken regions often have combined deficiencies of calories and protein in their diets **(protein-calorie malnutrition)**, but the calorie deficiency is more immediate in its effects. This condition is referred to as **marasmus.** Such individuals appear emaciated with thin and wasted muscles. Physical development of affected children is impaired, and they have the physical manifestations of protuberant abdomens and heads that appear disproportionately large in relation to the thin bodies. Edema is rare in marasmus. Severe calorie deficiency may be fatal in a short time.

PROTEIN DEFICIENCY

A diet with adequate calorie intake but deficient in protein is sometimes encountered in regions of partial famine and in particular when children are weaned from breast milk to a protein-deficient diet. This selective deficiency is termed **kwashiorkor.** It is characterized by generalized edema and hepatomegaly. The children have short stature. Hair changes include loosening of the roots and loss of tensile strength. Pigmentation changes occur in both hair and skin with regions of skin depigmentation and some of hyperpigmentation. Pallor may arise in response to anemia that is usually normocytic and normochromic.

In both marasmus and kwashiorkor, the small intestinal mucosa is atrophic with loss of villi and microvilli, which in turn complicates the ability to absorb nutrients from the diet. The liver shows fatty change that is reversible with restoration of adequate diet. Interestingly, coexisting vitamin deficiencies may be very severe but are not clinically apparent because of generalized reduction in metabolism with calorie or protein deficiency. These deficiencies cause impaired immune responses (e.g., atrophy of thymus in children) which may lead to fatal infections from bacteria, viruses, or parasites. If the deficiency occurs before birth or in the first six months of life, mental development is likely to be adversely affected.

ANOREXIA NERVOSA AND EATING DISORDERS

Eating disorders such as bulimia or anorexia nervosa can lead to abnormalities of nutrition that have serious and fatal consequences. These disorders have a large psychological component in which an individual (usually a woman) essentially starves herself to gratify an urge for control over her own life or to achieve a body image of unusual thinness. Very often these individuals will exercise in addition to dieting in order to maximize weight loss. The resulting starvation can cause tissue damage with release of enzymes from many organs (e.g., liver, muscle, pancreas) in a pattern of tissue injury. Starvation-induced lysis of body fat depots also causes release of stored carotene into the circulation, where it may appear as a very yellow plasma fraction. Other metabolic changes include elevated BUN, but generally normal creatinine (i.e., prerenal azotemia secondary to dehydration), and diminished total body content of phosphorus, potassium, and magnesium. Despite severe starvation, blood glucose tends to remain normal because of the many endocrine factors that act in gluconeogenesis. Death may occur due to the potassium loss, to infection, or to toxic side effects from the drugs sometimes used chronically to induce emesis.

Eating disorders may be exacerbated by the chronic use of laxatives to accelerate weight loss. Until recently, many over-the-counter laxatives sold in the United States contained phenolphthalein as an active ingredient. A simple laboratory procedure for diagnosing laxative abuse is the **phenolphthalein test,** by which the substances are detected in the stool of the patient. The test is performed by mixing 1N NaOH with a stool sample on a piece of white paper. Phenolphthalein (used in the laboratory as pH indicator) turns red at such an alkaline pH. If the stool sample turns red upon alkalinization (positive result), phenolphthalein is presumably present, suggesting laxative abuse. However, a negative result (no color change) does not necessarily rule out laxative abuse because many laxatives do not contain phenolphthalein.

VITAMIN DEFICIENCIES

VITAMIN A

Absorption of fat-soluble vitamins such as **vitamin A** requires intact production of bile to emulsify dietary lipids, lipase from the pancreas to digest the fats and release fat-soluble substances from food, and adequate absorptive surface in the intestine. There are two forms of dietary vitamin A: **retinyl ester** and the **provitamin carotene** (which is split into two molecules of vitamin A) from plants. Vitamin A moves to the liver in chylomicrons and is stored there as retinyl ester. Hydrolysis yields retinol, which is transported through the body attached to retinol-binding protein, which in turn binds to the serum protein prealbumin.

Vitamin A functions as a prosthetic group of photosensitive pigment in rods and cones of the retina. A deficiency affects primarily the rods leading to impaired vision in low intensity light (night blindness). Vitamin A is also involved in the maintenance of epithelial cells in the mucous membranes of the eyes and the cornea, the mucosa of the respiratory, gastrointestinal, and genitourinary tracts, and linings of glandular ducts of the skin. Deficiency of vitamin A can affect all these areas with some dramatic examples being keratomalacia of the cornea and kidney stones arising around the nidus of desquamated epithelium. It is thought that vitamin A may also play a role in protecting against squamous cell carcinomas of the skin, lung, or bladder. Another retinoid, isotretinoin (13-cis-retinoic acid [*Accutane*]) inhibits sebaceous gland action and keratinization and is used clinically in high doses for treatment of acne. It may also be useful in maintaining skin integrity and has been suggested for treatment of wrinkles. Effective doses for treating acne are vastly higher than those normally consumed to prevent vitamin A deficiency; these levels can be teratogenic in the fetus of a woman taking those high doses.

Dietary sources of vitamin A and carotenes are vegetables and fruits; vitamin A is also present at high concentration in cod liver oil. Deficiency of vitamin A can occur due to dietary lack; from malabsorption secondary to biliary, pancreatic, or intestinal disease; or with inadequate stores in the liver or inadequate amounts of prealbumin to transport it to tissues of the body. Very high levels (hypervitaminosis A) may occur in individuals who use excessive amounts of dietary supplement. Toxicities from excess vitamin A include nausea, vomiting, abdominal pain, headaches and other neurologic abnormalities, desquamation of the skin, and (chronically) hepatotoxicity. Excess carotene intake may cause yellowing of the skin but does not result in toxicities.

Vitamin A and carotenes are measured in serum by HPLC; they are light sensitive, so serum samples should be shielded from light either in a special transport tube or covered with aluminum foil.

VITAMIN B COMPLEX

The B complex of vitamins (with the exception of B_{12} and folate) act primarily as cofactors in pathways of energy metabolism. Because of their water solubility, they are cleared from the body too quickly to achieve substantial stores. Deficiencies of B complex vitamins sometimes affect the growth of rapidly dividing cells similarly with overlapping clinical presentations (e.g., rashes, lip and mouth changes). Furthermore the same foods (grains) are usually high in all the B complex vitamins so that a pure deficiency of only one may not often arise. However there are well-described clinical syndromes associated with individual vitamin deficiencies.

Vitamin B_1 (thiamine) is involved in both glycolytic and pentose phosphate pathways of carbohydrate metabolism. The deficiency state is termed **beri-beri.** It can occur with diets in which rice and grains are depleted of thiamine. It can also occur during pregnancy and in alcoholics. There are three forms of beri-beri. The wet form shows primary cardiac failure with peripheral edema (high output failure), in which the myocardium is pale, flabby, and dilated. The dry form is characterized by nerve damage with degeneration of myelin sheaths, peripheral neuritis, paralysis, and atrophy of muscles. This process can extend to the spinal cord and then to the central nervous system. The cerebral form is termed the **Wernicke-Korsakoff syndrome,** in which there are separate components of ataxia and oculomotor nerve derangement secondary to focal hemorrhages and degeneration in nuclei of the thalamus and hypothalamus plus a confabulatory psychosis. Diagnosis is usually made through astute clinical evaluation and confirmed with therapeutic response to thiamine administration.

Vitamin B_2 (riboflavin) participates as part of the cofactor molecule **flavin adenine di (or mono) nucleotide (FAD),** which is involved in the electron transport of oxidative metabolism and the metabolism of short-chain fatty acids. Food sources such as yeast, meats, and legume seeds carry riboflavin in a bound form, whereas milk has free riboflavin that is light sensitive. The body has relatively large stores of riboflavin. Deficiency states are characterized by a greasy and scaling dermatitis, angular stomatitis of the lips, cheilosis (redness, desquamation, and fissuring along the vermillion border of the lips), and a glossitis with a shiny tongue that has lost filiform papillae and may be pebbled.

Niacin (nicotinic acid, sometimes called **vitamin B_3)** is part of the cofactor molecules **nicotinamide adenine dinucleotide (NAD^+)** and **nicotinamide adenine dinucleotide phosphate ($NADP^+$),** which are extensively involved in the electron transport of cellular respiration. Dietary sources are liver, yeast, milk, meats, and whole grains. Deficiency of niacin causes **pellagra,** which is characterized by the three Ds: dermatitis, diarrhea, and dementia.

Vitamin B_6 (pyridoxine) is a cofactor for some very different classes of enzymes: decarboxylases, deaminases, and transaminases; it also is involved in converting tryptophan to nicotinic acid. It is difficult to establish a primary deficiency of vitamin B$_6$ because it is widely available in foods. Processing of foods may destroy the vitamin B$_6$, leading to severe deficiency, especially in infants, if that is their sole dietary source for it. Only the phosphorylated form of vitamin B$_6$ **(pyridoxal-5-phosphate)** is active, and the phosphorylation can be blocked by several drugs including hydralazine, oral contraceptives, penicillamine, and isoniazid (INH); this last drug is given in cases of tuberculosis for periods of months to a year. (Pyridoxal-5-phosphate should be coadministered to prevent a severe deficiency.) Deficiency leads to cheilosis, angular stomatitis, glossitis, dermatitis, polyneuritis, and even anemia in some cases.

Folate (folic acid) and **vitamin B$_{12}$** are thoroughly reviewed in Chapter 2 in the discussion of megaloblastic anemias. Briefly, they are both involved in the synthesis of nucleotide precursors for incorporation into DNA. The rapidly dividing cells of the bone marrow are affected by these deficiencies with the formation of enlarged cells in which the cytoplasm matures out of proportion to the nuclei. In addition to anemia, vitamin B$_{12}$ deficiency causes neurologic deterioration. Dietary sources of folate are largely green vegetables. Conditions of increased bone marrow response to acute anemia or pregnancy may rapidly deplete body stores of folate. Vitamin B$_{12}$ is found in meats. Vegetarians may become deficient only after years of strict meatless diet. Persons with pernicious anemia—in which the stomach does not produce intrinsic factor to bind vitamin B$_{12}$ and thus assist in its absorption—also develop the anemia after body stores are depleted. Inflammatory bowel disease or the intestinal parasite *Diphyllobothrium latum* (tapeworm) may interfere with vitamin B$_{12}$ absorption.

Individuals with low levels of vitamin B$_6$, vitamin B$_{12}$, or folic acid tend to have elevations of **homocysteine** in their blood, owing to the role that those vitamins play in the metabolism of that amino acid. This abnormality is clinically significant because elevated homocysteine is a risk factor for progression of atherosclerosis and occurrence of myocardial infarction. New assays are rapidly emerging for quantitating homocysteine in plasma to help assess risk of coronary artery disease in addition to conventional lipid fractionation. (See also the section on Thrombophilia in Chapter 5.)

VITAMIN C

Vitamin C (ascorbic acid, antiscorbutic factor) was determined to prevent scurvy in sea-going men whose diets lacked vegetable sources of vitamin C for long periods of time. Vitamin C is highly soluble in water and is readily absorbed from the intestines. Body stores can last for months. Vitamin C is particularly rich in the adrenals and in leukocytes. It functions by converting folic acid to folinic acid and also in the maturation and strengthening of collagen, in which lysyl and prolyl residues are hydroxylated. It also serves as a major source of chemical oxidizing and reducing capacity. Deficiency of vitamin C results in vascular fragility, presumably from weak collagen or failure to detoxify some potent vasoactive substances. Scurvy demonstrates excess bleeding around capillaries after minor trauma. There is bleeding into the gastrointestinal tract, kidneys, conjunctivae, and brain, as well as edema and hemorrhage of the gingivae, which then take on a spongy consistency. There may be dental loss and even pathologic fractures plus impaired wound healing and inability to seal off the regions around infections and abscesses. A diagnostic pearl in the differential diagnosis of petechiae is that scurvy results in a perifollicular distribution (around hair follicles), whereas primary platelet defects cause a more random distribution of petechiae. Overdosing of vitamin C has been popular in the lay community for prevention or treatment of the common cold. Although this may be a rather benign therapy in most cases, very high doses may induce the formation of renal calculi by the acidification of urine.

VITAMIN D

Vitamin D is involved in the hormonal regulation of calcium absorption from the intestine and resorption from bone (see Chapter 16). It is a fat-soluble vitamin whose synthesis from cholesterol is catalyzed in part by exposure to the ultraviolet rays of sunlight. Vitamin D is commonly added as a dietary supplement in milk. In order to be biologically active, vitamin D must be successively hydroxylated by the liver (which converts it to 25-hydroxy-vitamin D [25-OH-D]) and by the kidneys (which converts 25-OH-D to 1,25-dihydroxy-vitamin D [1,25-$(OH)_2$-D]). Dietary deficiencies of vitamin D may become more important in winter months with individuals who have minimal sun exposure. A recent study of hospitalized patients in Boston, Massachusetts (a northern latitude with decreased sun exposure in winter months), demonstrated hypovitaminosis D in 57% of hospitalized patients on a general medicine service, suggesting that this deficiency may be more widespread than is commonly assumed. In addition there are complicating factors that also impair hydroxylation, such as malabsorption syndromes (especially of fats), drug interferences with hydroxylation in the liver (e.g., by isoniazid), drug stimulation of hepatic metabolism of vitamin D (e.g., by anticonvulsants), or organ failure (liver or kidney).

The clinical manifestation of vitamin D deficiency is **osteomalacia,** in which there is failure to make or maintain adequate calcification of bone. This condition results in characteristic bony deformities (rickets) in developing children (see Chapter 16); deficiency of vitamin D is also a major risk factor for developing bone loss and fractures in adults. As a fat-soluble substance, vitamin D is carried through the blood complexed with vitamin D-binding protein. Loss of that relatively small protein in severe proteinuria (nephrotic syndrome) contributes to low levels of vitamin D and hypocalcemia due to impaired absorption of calcium. Vitamin D intoxication can occur if excess amounts are taken (usually as medication); the result may include general symptoms of gastrointestinal intolerance as well as hypercalcemia, metastatic calcifications, and formation of renal calculi secondary to the enhanced calcium load cleared through the kidneys.

Vitamin D is also light sensitive; for this reason serum samples should be shielded from light before quantitation by HPLC.

VITAMIN E

Vitamin E (α-tocopherol) is a fat-soluble substance that acts physiologically as an antioxidant, thereby protecting the body from free radicals that could oxidize vitamin A, DNA, and the phospholipid constituents of membranes. Although vitamin E deficiency states have been well characterized experimentally in animals, there is no clear-cut parallel in humans, perhaps because vitamin E is abundant in dietary green vegetables, grains, and oils. Vitamin E deficiency (generally due to malabsorption of fats secondary to biliary abnormality) may be associated with some cases of nerve or muscle deterioration and hemolytic anemia in infants, including defects in membrane maintenance. Other clinical syndromes, such as poor red cell survival in glucose-6-phosphate dehydrogenase deficiency or retrolental fibroplasia in infants treated with high oxygen concentrations, may benefit from vitamin E administration. Because of the general availability of vitamin E in normal diets, true deficiencies are rare. However, this does not mean there is no place for dietary supplementation: recent epidemiologic studies have suggested that diets with extremely high content of vitamin E (typically in response to supplementation with over-the-counter preparations) may help to prevent the progression of atherosclerosis. This protective action is presumably due to its antioxidant effects, specifically its protection of LDL cholesterol from oxidation by free radicals. Although some health food enthusiasts promote large doses of vitamin E daily, no official recommendations now exist for its use in those megadoses.

VITAMIN K

Vitamin K is another fat-soluble vitamin. It was named K because of its role in blood coagulation (*koagulation,* in Danish). It occurs in three different chemical forms: vitamin K_1, phylloquinone; vitamin K_2, menaquinone; and vitamin K_3, menadione (a synthetic form). Vitamins K_1 and K_2 are obtained from green plants and to some small extent from bacteria in the intestine. It is very difficult to produce a vitamin K deficiency by diet alone because there are adequate amounts of vitamin K in most diets. The vitamin K made by intestinal bacteria is probably only a minor source for humans. Vitamin K deficiency may arise in hospitalized patients who have poor appetites and have not eaten well for prolonged periods of time, but generally it occurs only after an additional insult such as intestinal manipulation or antibiotic therapy that would be expected to alter the normal bacterial flora of the gut. Frequently, vitamin K–deficient individuals have biliary tract obstruction that impairs intestinal absorption of fat-soluble substances. Newborns can have vitamin K deficiency, resulting in severe and sometimes fatal hemorrhage in the brain following the trauma of passage through the birth canal. For that reason, it has been standard practice to administer vitamin K to neonates just after birth.

Vitamin K functions in the liver as a cofactor for the post-translational enzymatic conversion of glutamyl residues to γ-carboxyglutamyl residues in the vitamin K–dependent blood clotting factors II (prothrombin), VII, IX, and X plus two other blood proteins (protein C and protein S) that inactivate factors V and VIII in the balance of hemostasis. The bone protein osteocalcin is also vitamin K–dependent. Deficiency of vitamin K is manifested by a hemorrhagic state with seemingly spontaneous bleeding arising from minor trauma. Oral anticoagulant medications such as warfarin are antagonists to vitamin K. Laboratory documentation of their effectiveness is performed with the prothrombin time on plasma (see also Chapters 5 and 6). Direct measurement of vitamin K is rarely needed clinically.

MINERAL DEFICIENCIES

The major mineral for which deficiency states cause concern is *iron*, already considered in Chapter 2 under anemias. Other minerals are utilized by the body in only trace amounts, which are generally well supplied by the abundance of minerals in virtually any diet. However, mineral deficiencies may arise in states such as total parenteral nutrition in which the prepared nutrient solutions perhaps exclude some trace substances such as copper, manganese, selenium, or zinc, which are essential components of many different enzymes. Deficiency of copper and manganese may be inferred because of the crucial nature of the enzymes in which they participate, although syndromes of their lack are not well recognized. (There are well-documented toxicities from their excess.) Selenium deficiency is apparently responsible for a cardiomyopathy common in selenium-deficient regions in China. This disorder, **Keshan disease,** has also occurred rarely in patients maintained for years on intravenous nutrition. Zinc deficiency has occurred in the Middle East because of some restricted diets of cereal grains. It may also be a factor in some syndromes of growth retardation and in slow sexual maturation, impaired wound healing, or anemia.

NUTRITIONAL OVERABUNDANCE

The major nutritional disorders of industrialized society are not those of deficiencies, but rather ones of overabundance and overeating. Major health risks for cardiovascular disease in the United States are related to smoking, high blood pressure, high blood cholesterol, and being overweight. Obesity itself carries a risk of developing hypertension, diabetes mellitus, and atherosclerosis. The evaluation of cholesterol levels and the fractionation of blood lipids as they relate to cardiovascular risk factors are presented in Chapter 9.

Dietary recommendations for the general, healthy public must include the reduction of calories with the goal of losing weight, reducing cholesterol and saturated fats in the diet to lower serum cholesterol, reduction of alcohol intake (which by itself is responsible for elevating blood pressure and for causing damage to the liver, stomach, intestines, and nervous system), and reduction of sodium intake. On this latter point, it is probably true that sodium does not cause high blood pressure, but it can contribute to and exacerbate new or pre-existing hypertension, which may not be recognized by asymptomatic individuals until there is a vascular event. Other recommendations are still evolving; increased intake of potassium, calcium, and some lipids such as linoleic acid, omega fatty acids, and olive oil are examples.

There is now some emphasis on the selective addition of certain dietary constituents such as antioxidant vitamins or fiber with the goal of reducing risk for some cancers. At this time there is not a consensus on these diets, although they probably would not be harmful in the majority of people and may in fact be well worth the effort because they coincide in part with dietary efforts to reduce risk for cardiovascular disease.

HOSPITALIZED PATIENTS

Patients with serious illnesses often develop nutritional problems related to long periods of hospitalization or convalescence during which they have poor appetite or are unable to maintain adequate caloric and protein intake because of malabsorption or other physiologic impairments. For persons suffering from chronic disease, the additional load of inadequate nutrition is likely to lead to other disorders or at least to slow the healing phase of infection or postsurgical recovery. It is clear that such disorders as inflammatory bowel disease, biliary obstruction, pancreatic exocrine failure of cystic fibrosis, and other gastrointestinal disease will have a direct effect on efficiency of absorption. Other organ diseases can also influence general nutritional status; these include the following: cardiac cachexia in persons with heart failure, in which poor blood delivery impairs both absorption and perfusion of tissues; central nervous system disease such as stroke or paralysis, in which a patient cannot feed himself or swallow well; or malignancy that places a major metabolic burden on the body. Furthermore anyone whose nutrition is based on parenteral or intravenous administration of all nutrients (lipid, carbohydrate, protein, vitamins, and minerals) for a prolonged period is at risk for developing both selective deficiencies as well as for having overall lack of protein and calories. Patients on total parenteral nutrition require precise calculations as to daily requirements and close laboratory monitoring to assess optimum metabolic effects.

LABORATORY ASSESSMENT OF NUTRITIONAL STATUS

The ideal marker of general nutritional status should have the characteristic of being sensitive in a roughly quantitative manner to a whole spectrum of nutritional abnormalities from mild to severe. To assist in the early detection of poor nutrition and to monitor the effectiveness of dietary supplementation, such a test should also change quickly in response to dietary defects and corrections. In lieu of such ideal tests, routinely performed procedures should be understood in terms of the insight they provide into nutritional status.

CHEMISTRY PANEL

Formerly, the use of general serum chemistry screening panels was so widespread that it is worth considering the particular biochemical manifestations of poor nutrition.

Glucose

With the exception of disorders such as diabetes mellitus or insulin-secreting tumors, glucose concentrations are generally well maintained within reference ranges despite even severe starvation. Glucose levels are usually monitored very frequently in patients on intravenous fluids as part of assessing overall metabolic balance.

Blood Urea Nitrogen

The source of BUN is the breakdown of protein in the diet. Slight elevations of BUN occur in persons who have a high-protein diet (especially meat) and normal renal function. Dehydration (sometimes seen in starvation or anorexia nervosa) can also lead to elevated BUN with normal serum creatinine (prerenal azotemia) (see Chapter 9). Of course, renal failure causes simultaneous elevations of BUN and creatinine because of the failure to clear those substances from the body.

Creatinine

Normal turnover of creatine in muscle is followed by conversion to creatinine. Thus diet has essentially no effect on serum creatinine concentration. Increased catabolism of muscle can be estimated from the 24-hour urinary excretion of creatinine.

Uric Acid

The dietary source of uric acid is nucleic acids, which are more abundant in meats than in vegetables. Uric acid is excreted by the kidney, but some portion is also reabsorbed there as well. Consequently it is very difficult to alter uric acid levels by diet alone. Elevations are largely due to genetic individuality.

Electrolytes (Na^+, K^+, Cl^-, Bicarbonate)

These substances are normally well controlled by homeostatic processes, and their serum concentrations are largely unaffected by diet. Even excess salt sufficient to complicate hypertension does not typically produce an abnormality detectable by routine analysis. Diuretic therapy can complicate electrolyte metabolism with adverse effects due to loss of total body sodium and potassium that also may not be evident on measurement of serum electrolytes until these substances become severely depleted.

Calcium and Magnesium

These primary divalent cations can be divided into roughly two components each: the free (or ionized, physiologically active) fraction and the protein-bound (inactive) fraction. Any alteration in which there is reduction of serum albumin will also cause a reduction in total calcium and total magnesium because of the smaller amount of the bound fraction, although the physiologically active free fractions remain normal. This condition of itself does not require supplementation. Calcium can be mobilized into the blood from bone to maintain physiologically important concentrations when dietary intake is limited. There is no comparable body store from which to mobilize magnesium, and therefore limited intake of magnesium (e.g., starvation) or excess loss (e.g., prolonged and intense diuretic therapy) may result in profound deficiency of magnesium that impairs neurologic, muscular, and myocardial function. Measurement of serum magnesium may not reflect a deficiency of intracellular stores of magnesium until it becomes quite severe (see Chapter 9).

Phosphorus

This element is used physiologically in the chemical form of phosphate, which is an important constituent of nucleic acids, phospholipids, and intermediates and cofactors of metabolism. Body stores of phosphate are subject to elimination by renal excretion of acid loads. Persons who have inadequate intake of phosphate may therefore encounter problems when they have increased need for it. For example, people who are severely starved (e.g., concentration camp survivors from World War II) may succumb shortly after being started on a high-calorie diet that is low in phosphate. This fatal effect is explained in part by the obligatory need for phosphate whenever glucose molecules enter cells. An analogous effect has been well documented in diabetic individuals being treated for hyperglycemia. Administration of insulin may not be successful in reducing blood glucose in such individuals if they have become acutely depleted of phosphate (and also potassium).

Enzymes

The release of intracellular enzymes into the circulation is usually considered a mark of cellular damage resulting from ischemia, toxicity, or outright necrosis. Starvation may be another means by which cellular membrane integrity is compromised and these intracellular enzymes are released. Although serum enzyme elevations are typically used clinically to identify specific organ damage, elevations of certain of these enzymes can occur simultaneously in cases of severe starvation. Such enzymes include aspartate aminotransferase (AST), alanine aminotransferase (ALT), lactate dehydrogenase, creatine kinase, amylase, alkaline phosphatase, and gamma-glutamyltransferase. These multiple elevations are most likely the result of release from multiple organs, all of whose cellular membranes have become leaky enough to let proteins the size of these enzymes slip out. The major elevations appear to be of AST and ALT, most likely from the liver. Serial measurements of these enzymes should show return to normal after establishing adequate diet if there is no other organ pathology.

Bilirubin

The conjugation of bilirubin requires energy to attach glucuronic acid residues. Consequently starvation may potentially cause a mild hyperbilirubinemia that is reversible after adequate intake is re-established.

Lipids

The measurement of triglycerides, cholesterol, and HDL cholesterol are generally reserved for the evaluation of nutritional overabundance and cardiac risk assessment (see Chapter 9 for lipid fractionation). However, malabsorption or malnutrition can result in marked depression of total cholesterol and all the lipoprotein fractions as well.

Serum Proteins

The concentrations of plasma proteins circulating in blood reflect in part the general state of nutrition of patients. Measurement of total protein is not a reliable index of general nutritional status because concentrations of the individual proteins are influenced by many other factors such as infection, stress, hormones, age, organ dysfunction, and genetic determinants. The most abundant plasma protein is albumin, and its concentration is a good marker of nutritional status; lower levels of albumin are associated with impairment of nutrition. A recent study indicated that patients newly admitted to intensive care units for a variety of different primary illnesses who had serum albumin concentrations below 3.2 g/dL had relatively greater morbidity and mortality. Thus serum albumin measurements can be used to screen for a need for nutritional support among hospitalized patients. Serum albumin measurement is potentially very effective in this format because of the ease and frequency with which it is performed in virtually any laboratory using multichannel analyzers.

HEMATOLOGY PANEL

As in the case of chemistry panel testing, a complete blood count (CBC) is widely available in hospitals, clinics, and physicians' offices. The main information from the CBC to be applied to nutritional assessment has to do with anemia and the particular deficiency based on erythrocyte and leukocyte morphologies. Megaloblastic anemias arise from deficiencies of folate or vitamin B_{12} (presence of hypersegmented polymorphonuclear cells helps to confirm this diagnosis); microcytic hypochromic anemia can arise from iron deficiency; and normocytic normochromic anemias may be a manifestation of general malnutrition involving calorie and protein deprivation.

COAGULATION

The routinely performed plasma coagulation tests are designed to detect deficiencies of all known procoagulant factors. The vitamin K–dependent factors participate in both the prothrombin time (PT) and the activated partial thromboplastin time (PTT) so that deficiency of vitamin K is reflected by prolongation of both the PT and PTT. Because the thrombin time is performed by the addition of exogenous thrombin, it is affected primarily by fibrinogen concentration, but not by endogenous vitamin K–dependent factors. Therefore a normal thrombin time in the presence of long PT and PTT is supportive evidence for vitamin K deficiency.

SPECIAL PROCEDURES

Transferrin

The use of the iron-transport protein transferrin is based on its short half-life (about 1 week) compared with that of albumin (about 3 weeks), which is a reasonably successful marker for poor nutrition. A shorter half-life in the circulation means that transferrin concentrations will respond more quickly to changes in nutritional status than does albumin, a desirable characteristic for a nutritional marker. Transferrin is normally measured directly by immunoassay; it is roughly equivalent to the measurement of iron-binding capacity. One of the potential disadvantages of transferrin levels is that they also can reflect other conditions, in particular being elevated in response to iron deficiency.

Prealbumin

This carrier protein of thyroxine also complexes with retinol-binding protein, which in turn transports vitamin A through the blood. Both of these proteins have half-lives of just under 2 days, which makes them good candidates for nutritional markers, superior to albumin and transferrin. Prealbumin measurements are now becoming more convenient to perform by immunoassays. Falling levels of prealbumin can be used to determine the need for nutritional supplementation in seriously ill patients. After such oral or parenteral support, serial determinations of prealbumin should mark success or failure of the additional feeding.

Vitamin Measurements

The diagnosis of many vitamin deficiencies may rely not on quantitation of vitamin concentrations, but rather on astute clinical evaluation of history and physical examination followed by administration of vitamin supplements that, if successful, help establish the diagnosis. Immunoassays for folic acid and vitamin B_{12} are very useful because they distinguish between these two deficiencies, which have similar manifestations but different treatments. High-pressure liquid chromatography assays are performed for quantitation of vitamins A, B_1 (thiamine), B_2 (riboflavin), B_6 (pyridoxal-5-phosphate), C, D, and E. Vitamin K deficiency is typically documented by prolonged plasma coagulation times that correct with the administration of vitamin K. Because of its cofactor activity for transaminases, B_6 levels can be inferred from the relative correction of serum AST or ALT activity with addition of exogenous B_6.

Tumor Necrosis Factor

Tumor necrosis factor (TNF) is released from monocytes in response to stressful stimuli. TNF acts locally to activate clotting, thereby potentially destroying tumor cells. It also inhibits the enzymatic activity of lipoprotein lipase, which is intimately involved in metabolism at the first step in the breakdown of triglycerides. This inhibition has the effect of starving tumor or other offending cells that need abundant food energy to grow, but it also has the effect of starving the body and may be responsible for the cachexia of cancer and other diseases. TNF measurements are just coming onto the horizon of laboratory medicine. These and other similar tests look promising for future use in quantitating substances that directly control the body's nutritional regulation in addition to present-day procedures that document the end result of nutritional deficiency.

NUTRITIONAL ASSESSMENT FORMULAS

Special formulas have been developed to assess the nutritional status of very sick patients whose dietary intake is limited or impaired by disease (e.g., gastrointestinal disorders, cancer, diabetes, cardiac decompensation, chronic lung disease). These calculations are based on common measurements and include some mathematical weighting factors derived from population studies. One such calculation, the Nutritional Risk Index, is calculated as follows:

$$\text{Nutritional Risk Index} = (1.489 \times \text{serum albumin in g/L}) + 41.7 \times (\text{present weight} \div \text{usual weight})$$

TABLE A–1. INTERPRETATION OF THE NUTRITIONAL RISK INDEX

Nutritional Risk Index	Nutritional Status
>100	Not malnourished
97.5–100	Mild malnourishment
83.5–<97.5	Moderate malnourishment
<83.5	Severe malnourishment

The results of this calculation may be interpreted as shown in Table A–1.

Another calculation is termed the **Maastricht Index.** It is calculated by the following formula:

$$\text{Maastricht Index} = 20.68 - (0.24 \times \text{albumin in g/L})$$
$$- (19.21 \times \text{transthyretin in g/L})$$
$$- (1.86 \times \text{lymphocytes in } 10^6/\text{L})$$
$$- (0.04 \times \text{ideal weight})$$

Values of the Maastricht Index greater than 0
indicate that a patient is malnourished.

Nutritional assessment of critically ill patients has been useful in predicting serious complications during hospital stays and can direct more intense medical support to those patients.

SUGGESTED READING

Bernstein, L, and Pleban, W: Prealbumin in nutrition evaluation. Nutrition 12:255, 1996.

Lonn, EM, and Yusuf, S: Is there a role for antioxidant vitamins in the prevention of cardiovascular diseases? An update on epidemiological and clinical trials data. Can J Cardiol 13:957, 1997.

Miller, RK, et al: Periconceptional vitamin A use: How much is teratogenic? Reprod Toxicol 12:75, 1998.

Naber, THJ, et al: Prevalence of malnutrition in nonsurgical hospitalized patients and its association with disease complications. Am J Clin Nutr 66:1232, 1997.

Stampfer, MJ, et al: Vitamin E consumption and the risk of coronary disease in women. N Engl J Med 328:1444, 1993.

Thomas, MK, et al: Hypovitaminosis D in medical inpatients. N Engl J Med 338:777, 1998.

Verhoef, P, et al: Homocysteine metabolism and risk of myocardial infarction: Relation with vitamins B_6, B_{12}, and folate. Am J Epidemiol 143:845, 1996.

APPENDIX B

Tumor Markers

In contrast to electrolytes, metabolites of many types, and enzymes or other proteins normally released by cells of the body, tumor markers elaborated by neoplastic cells are substances that normally do not appear in the circulation, or if they do, only in small amounts. The spectrum of tumor markers includes a variety of different substances that can be roughly classified as metabolic consequences of a tumor burden, endocrine-associated abnormalities, specific enzyme markers, tumor antigens, and nucleic acid (gene) alterations. To be useful clinically as an efficient predictor or monitor of cancer, a tumor marker should be produced by all tumors of a particular type and be present in the blood of patients in quantities proportional to the mass of the primary tumor and its metastases.

METABOLIC MARKERS OF MALIGNANCY

Standard hematologic and chemistry panels may yield evidence of malignancy even when it is not expected clinically; they are also routinely applied to the monitoring of toxicities from chemotherapy. Invasion and replacement of bone marrow by tumor may cause reduction in numbers of circulating erythrocytes, leukocytes, and platelets. These elements (particularly leukocytes and platelets) are also very sensitive to chemotherapy because of the frequent cell divisions of their precursors in the marrow.

Virtually any of the standard chemistry measurements in serum can show abnormalities related to a malignancy or its metastases. The proliferation of massive numbers of tumor cells carries with it the release of large amounts of uric acid from nucleic acid turnover. The levels of uric acid in serum can be increased substantially in malignancies, particularly when there is lysis of tumor cells resulting from necrosis or chemotherapy. The metabolic state of a cancer patient may also be altered with particularly low levels of serum albumin, prealbumin, cholesterol, and triglycerides. These nutritional abnormalities are the result of general body wasting that may be induced by release from monocytes of the substance designated **tumor necrosis factor (TNF)** (also called **cachectin**). TNF may cause cachexia and block metabolism by inhibition of the enzyme *lipoprotein lipase* in addition to destroying tumor cells locally by initiating clotting. Loss of synthetic capacity in the liver due to extensive hepatic metastases can also cause a drop in albumin and other serum proteins.

Serum enzymes are frequently elevated in malignancy in response to the release of large amounts from a mass of tumor cells (especially lactate dehydrogenase, LD). In addition there may be intrahepatic obstruction of the biliary tract due to metastatic disease, resulting in elevation of serum alkaline phosphatase, gamma-glutamyltranspeptidase, conjugated bilirubin, and total bilirubin (see Chapter 12). In general, these measurements are not tumor specific, but when elevated, they can indicate extensive disease.

ENDOCRINE MARKERS

Before the advent of modern antibody technologies and the definition of many antigens as tumor markers, several different biochemical alterations were recognized to be associated with particular tumor types. Foremost among these were endocrine cancers capable of secreting large amounts of physiologically active hormones in an autonomous manner, unregulated by normal endocrine feedback control (e.g., hypothalamic-pituitary to adrenals, to gonads, and to thyroid). The syndromes of autonomous and excess hormone secretion are discussed under endocrine abnormalities (Chapters 16 and 17).

Some malignancies have been found on occasion to produce hormones inappropriate to the cell type or the organ from which the tumor arose. An example of this inappropriate synthesis is release of ACTH by some carcinomas of the lung, resulting in excess secretion of cortisol by the adrenal cortex, which may present as Cushing's syndrome. Other tumors may disrupt electrolyte balance or water handling in the body by inappropriate secretion of antidiuretic hormone. Cerebellar hemangioblastomas also occasionally secrete excess erythropoietin, which then stimulates overproduction of erythrocytes by the bone marrow (see section on Polycythemias in Chapter 2). This type of hormone secretion by an organ or tissue that deviates from its normal source of production is termed **ectopic.** Unfortunately for diagnostic purposes, these endocrine abnormalities secondary to neoplasia in a nonendocrine organ (ectopic) are not generally efficient tumor markers for detecting all affected patients because they are not uniformly present in all tumors of a given class. In fact, they tend to be the exception rather than the rule. However, their detection has been very instructive in basic and clinical research for the understanding of gene expression. The syndromes they cause in some patients should be recognized so that they may be correctly diagnosed in order to effect proper therapy.

A more successful example of an endocrine tumor marker is the polypeptide hormone **calcitonin,** which is normally secreted by parafollicular cells of the thyroid in response to elevated blood calcium concentrations. Calcitonin is overproduced by *medullary carcinoma of the thyroid* and released into the circulation. Measurement of calcitonin levels in serum (especially following stimulation with intravenous infusion of calcium or pentagastrin) can be used to detect this hereditary carcinoma in previously unaffected relatives of patients who do have it.

ENZYMES

PROSTATIC ACID PHOSPHATASE

The prostate gland normally synthesizes an isoenzyme of acid phosphatase that is unique from the acid phosphatase made in other cells of the body such as platelets. This **prostatic acid phosphatase (PAP)** is never produced in women. Large amounts of PAP appear in the blood with carcinoma of the prostate, particularly when there are metastases. This labile enzyme can be detected through its activity at acidic pH or as an antigen in radioimmunoassay. The enzyme activity measurement is not as sensitive as the antigen measurement for detection of small amounts of PAP in the circulation. Unfortunately, that sensitivity is so great that it detects a positive result in many men who do not have prostate malignancy but may have benign prostatic hypertrophy. For this reason, despite its organ specificity, PAP is not useful as a general cancer screening procedure unless the patient has previously been evaluated for likelihood of malignancy. PAP measurement is very useful, however, for the monitoring of patients for recurrence of tumor after surgery or other ablative treatment for prostatic carcinoma. This enzyme determination is also now complemented with analysis of a completely different substance from the prostate, termed **prostate specific antigen (PSA)** (see below).

CREATINE KINASE

The production of **creatine kinase (CK)** is generally limited to skeletal muscle **(isoenzyme MM),** smooth muscle and brain **(isoenzyme BB),** and myocardium **(isoenzymes MM and MB).** Occasionally there may be ectopic synthesis and release of CK from neoplastic cells (e.g., lung, breast, or ovarian cancers) for unknown biochemical reasons involving cell differentiation. Such atypical CKs are usually detected clinically only if there is another reason to perform CK isoenzyme analysis (e.g., to rule out myocardial infarction when a patient has chest pain). In that instance the ectopic CK is typically detected as the BB isoenzyme (which does not normally circulate in the blood) or perhaps as the MB form. It can be distinguished from release of CK by an acutely injured organ through repeat measurement. An injury pattern consists of changing enzyme concentrations, whereas ectopic CK will remain at approximately the same level for many hours to days or longer, owing to its steady release from the tumor cells. Although CK-BB is a dramatic marker for a patient to have, its presence is not useful for estimation of tumor size or type of tumor because it is found only in exceptional cases. However, in individual cases it may be useful for the clinician to use whatever ectopic enzyme is present as a customized tumor marker for those patients whose tumors happen to release it.

ALKALINE PHOSPHATASE

Enzymes with phosphatase activity at alkaline pH derive from several different tissue sources that may be distinguished by isoenzyme separation or chemical treatment such as heating (see Chapter 11). The major organ sources of alkaline phosphatase in the circulation include liver (biliary tract), bone, and intestine. Metastatic cancer involving the liver typically causes elevation of the liver fraction of alkaline phosphatase in serum. Similarly, primary cancer of bone or tumor metastases to bone can demonstrate elevated bone fraction of alkaline phosphatase. Occasionally a malignancy can make a unique isoenzyme of alkaline phosphatase that is normally synthesized only by the placenta. This placental form is also called the **Regan isoenzyme.** It is very heat stable, allowing it to be readily distinguished from the other isoenzymes.

HUMAN CHORIONIC GONADOTROPIN

A glycoprotein hormone, human chorionic gonadotropin (hCG) is normally secreted during pregnancy by syncytiotrophoblastic tissue of the placenta (see Chapter 17). It is also regularly secreted by certain malignancies of females and males. These include choriocarcinoma and hydatidiform mole in women and testicular carcinomas (germ line) in men. In these instances the amount of hCG in blood is highly representative of the tumor mass. Autonomous production of hCG by these malignant tumors results in markedly elevated levels in serum and urine. Measurement of hCG at low concentrations in serum has particular application in monitoring for recurrence of tumor after surgical removal and chemotherapy. Testicular carcinomas frequently also produce alpha-fetoprotein, which is a convenient companion measurement for monitoring therapy (see below).

Assays for hCG have been performed for many years, initially for the diagnosis of pregnancy and more lately for diagnosis and monitoring of malignancy. The assays available commercially have always done well at quantitating the large amounts of hCG found in pregnancy, but they have not until recently been very good at detecting the small amounts that are present in early malignancy or in early recurrence of treated tumor. In addition there was considerable antigenic cross-reactivity between hCG and the pituitary hormones LH, FSH, and even TSH with many of the assays that utilized polyclonal antibodies. The removal of a testicular malignancy along with a testis (orchidectomy) can upset the normal feedback between pituitary and gonad, leading to elevated concentrations of the pituitary gonadotropins. In this situation it is highly desirable to be confident about the relative lack of cross-reactivity between these molecules in the assays employed.

The technology of antibody production and particularly monoclonal antibodies have worked strongly in favor of both highly specific and highly sensitive immunoassays for the detection of hCG. The nomenclature of these assays has also changed from "beta-hCG," which stands for the subunit of the molecule that has antigenic specificity distinct from LH, FSH, and TSH. Virtually all hCG assays now performed measure the intact molecule that includes both alpha and beta subunits. A small percentage of tumors elaborate only the alpha subunit or only the beta subunit, and accordingly will go undetected by standard hCG assay. These subunits can be separately measured by specific assay, generally through reference laboratories.

Other variations can occur in the hCG molecule due to nicking or truncating. Consequently, different immunoassays for hCG that have been standardized with the same calibrators may yield different results on the same patient due to antigenic variation being measured by monoclonal antibodies with slightly different specificities.

CARCINOEMBRYONIC ANTIGEN

This glycoprotein is an oncofetal antigen, that is, normally abundantly present in fetal life, but absent or greatly diminished in concentration in the adult unless specifically synthesized by an abnormal proliferation of cells. Carcinoembryonic antigen (CEA) has been detected in elevated amounts in patients with malignancies of the gastrointestinal tract (including pancreas), lung, breast, and ovary. Thus it is not tumor specific; its concentration in serum is also dependent on such factors as inflammation and whether the patient is a smoker (higher levels). Because of the inability to distinguish between malignant and benign disease based on CEA levels alone, this procedure cannot be recommended for general cancer screening. However, any very high level does raise some index of suspicion and probably should be followed up with a more rigorous diagnostic evaluation.

For colorectal carcinomas, CEA has become a major monitoring parameter for the early detection of recurrence or relapse after surgical removal of the tumor, radiation, or chemotherapy. Following surgical resection of colon carcinoma, elevated plasma CEA should return to normal after 4 to 6 weeks. Persistent elevation may indicate incomplete resection or the presence of metastases. Some poorly differentiated colorectal malignancies may not show elevated CEA levels, and accordingly a baseline level is necessary to determine whether each patient's tumor is a candidate for this type of monitoring. The other tumor types that variably produce CEA should also be evaluated individually to determine whether CEA monitoring would be appropriate in each case.

One technical note to consider is that immunoassays from different manufacturers have antibodies with somewhat different reactivities for CEA, and therefore some discordance between assay results is sometimes observed. For successful monitoring, therefore, a patient should always have serial serum measurements for CEA performed at the same laboratory where they were begun. Interestingly, the chemical structure of CEA with its sialic acid residues reacts with calcium in such a way as to alter the antigenic reactivity slightly. Thus simultaneously obtained specimens from the same patient collected as serum or into EDTA (which chelates calcium) are expected to give somewhat different CEA values.

Guidelines for the use of tumor markers in breast and colorectal cancer have recently been developed by the American Society of Clinical Oncology (ASCO):

- CEA should not be used as a screening test for colorectal cancer
- CEA may be used preoperatively in patients with colorectal carcinoma if it would assist in staging and planning treatment
- CEA may be used every 2 to 3 months postoperatively if resection of liver metastases would be indicated
- CEA may be used to monitor treatment of metastases

Although these guidelines state that CEA is the marker of choice for monitoring colorectal cancer, they also emphasize the relative nonspecificity of CEA for that malignancy (versus other malignancies, liver disease, kidney disease, effects of therapy, etc.), the lack of effective treatment for many cases with elevated CEA levels (although the elevation correctly predicts poor outcome), and the high cost of extensive testing. Nevertheless, monitoring colorectal cancer patients with CEA has already become standard practice in many regions.

The ASCO guidelines do not recommend CEA for screening, diagnosis, staging, or routine surveillance of patients with breast cancer after initial therapy, nor for monitoring the response of metastatic disease to treatment. However, increasing CEA levels may be used to detect recurrence in the absence of other disease measures.

ALPHA FETOPROTEIN

Alpha fetoprotein (AFP) is the major serum protein in the fetus (analogous to albumin in the adult), with peak values reached at 14 weeks of gestation, thereafter being replaced by albumin. AFP diffuses across the placenta from amniotic fluid and enters the maternal circulation, where it can be used as a marker for neural tube defects in developing fetuses (i.e., increased amounts of AFP in amniotic fluid and elevated levels in maternal serum, adjusted according to week of gestation). AFP is also an oncofetal antigen that is expressed in some germ line tumors (e.g., teratoblastoma and testicular or ovarian carcinomas). AFP is also elevated in the blood of patients with primary hepatocellular carcinoma (hepatoma) and is now used extensively in the diagnosis of liver cancer. Other nonmalignant disease of the liver (e.g., cirrhosis, hepatitis, necrosis) can cause elevations of AFP, as can metastases to the liver from other malignancies.

PROSTATE-SPECIFIC ANTIGEN

Prostate cancer is the most common malignancy of males with over 240,000 new cases diagnosed annually; however, only about 40,000 of those individuals will die from that malignancy. The natural history of prostate cancer in a small proportion of cases is very aggressive with few successful treatment options. The bulk of prostate cancer is much slower to grow, and many cases are discovered incidentally at autopsy of older men who have died from other causes. The promise of early detection is to eradicate the aggressive tumors before they spread; the down side is that most individuals who are detected early stand the risk of complications (including incontinence and impotence as well as infection and even surgical mortality) from surgery that can "cure" the cancer they would not die from anyway. Despite extensive use of screening methods for detection of prostate cancer, there is no evidence that mortality from prostate cancer has been reduced. Consequently, the American College of Physicians recently published a clinical guideline on the early detection of prostate cancer that recommends not to screen men routinely, but only after considering each patient's risks and preferences, and to enroll eligible men in ongoing clinical trials.

Typical screening for prostate cancer includes digital rectal examination of the prostate gland plus serum prostate-specific antigen (PSA) measurement followed by ultrasound examination and needle biopsy for suspicious findings. The use of PSA in screening for prostate cancer has become almost universal in the United States despite the above concerns. In addition, men with benign prostatic hypertrophy may have elevated serum PSA concentrations, leading to a substantial number of false-positive results.

PSA is an enzyme synthesized almost exclusively in the prostate. It is measured as an antigen by immunoassays. Several modifications have been proposed to improve its diagnostic power:

- *Age-adjusted reference ranges* have been proposed, in which the upper limit increases with each decade of life. Concentrations in the serum vary according to prostate volume, which increases with age, thereby leading to further false-positives with only a single reference range (≤ 4.0 ng/mL). Unfortunately, in practice, using multiple reference ranges appears to diminish sensitivity for detection of some cases of prostate cancer.
- *PSA velocity* is derived from annual measurements; an annual increase of 1.0 ng/mL or more can indicate prostate cancer.
- *PSA density* (or *PSA index*) is calculated by dividing serum concentration of PSA by prostate volume (obtained from ultrasound dimensioning). Logically the volume correction should take into account increased release of PSA from benign hypertrophied gland, allowing excess secretion from carcinomas to stand out more clearly. Unfortunately, PSA density has not been very sensitive for detecting cancer in practice.
- *Quantitating free and bound PSA* may be advantageous. PSA is present in serum in three forms: free, complexed with α_1-antichymotrypsin (AACT), and complexed with α_2-macroglobulin (AMG). *Free PSA* and PSA bound to AACT *(bound PSA)* both react with antibodies used in the immunoassay, although to different degrees. PSA bound to AMG does not react with the antibody. Men without prostate cancer tend to have more free PSA than do men with prostate cancer. Consequently, much effort has recently been placed on quantitating free and bound PSA to further enhance diagnostic power. In a recent large clinical series, measurement of the percentage of free PSA did demonstrate some utility in distinguishing benign from malignant prostatic disease, particularly when the total PSA is only moderately elevated in an equivocal range (e.g., 4 to 10 ng/mL).

CANCER ANTIGEN 125

The various substances designated CA are alternatively referred to as **cancer antigens** or **carbohydrate antigens** because their antigenicity derives largely from the carbohydrate portion of their structure. CA 125 is a glycoprotein that is normally found in the adult fallopian tube, endometrium, and endocervix, but not in tissues of other organs including the ovary, breast, and lung. However, it does appear in tumor tissue from a large percentage of ovarian carcinomas and is present in elevated amounts in the serum of these patients as well as those with adenocarcinoma of the cervix or fallopian tube. CA 125 may also be seen in nongynecologic malignancies involving the lung or gastrointestinal tract. Nonmalignant disease such as endometriosis, pelvic inflammatory disease, and even normal ovulation can give rise to elevated CA 125 in as many as 1 to 2% of healthy women. Because of the high prevalence of these conditions, the general use of CA 125 to screen for ovarian cancer would give rise to an overwhelming proportion of false-positive results. Consequently, CA 125 has no role in screening for cancer, but it should be used for monitoring response and possible recurrence in women who have been treated for ovarian cancer. Although some patients show discrepancies between clinical course and serum levels (e.g., some are disease free but have persistently elevated levels of CA 125), the overall relationship is that CA 125 in serum does correlate with tumor (ovarian) size.

CANCER ANTIGEN 15-3

This antigen is measured by application of two distinct monoclonal antibodies (**115D8** and **DF3,** from which the name "15-3" is derived) in a sandwich technique with the antigen serving as linker. The monoclonal antibody 115DB is directed against an antigen of human milkfat globule membranes; DF3 is directed against an antigen from a human breast carcinoma. Thus to react in this assay system, a substance must contain both antigenic sites. This double reactivity ensures some additional degree of specificity. CA 15-3 is often elevated in the serum of patients who have breast cancer and also in some patients with lung cancer or nonmalignant disease. CA 15-3 is not sufficiently specific to be used as a screening test for breast cancer because it may be elevated in 5 to 6% of healthy women and more often in benign diseases such as liver abnormalities. Furthermore, CA 15-3 is not sufficiently sensitive for detecting early-stage breast cancer. In fact, the positive predictive value of

CA 15-3 as a screening test is only 0.7% for stage I and 1.5% for stage II breast cancer. Accordingly, guidelines of the American Society of Clinical Oncology (ASCO) for use of tumor markers in breast cancer recommend CA 15-3 for monitoring the response of metastatic disease only in the absence of other measurement of disease progress. The ASCO guidelines summarize results of patients monitored after treatment for metastatic breast cancer: 66% of patients showed decreases in serum CA 15-3 with responding disease, 73% showed stable levels with stable disease, and 80% showed increasing levels with progressive disease. Thus although CA 15-3 may be useful for monitoring metastatic disease, test results are not infallible and must be considered in concert with other clinical information.

CA 27.29 is another serum test that is used for monitoring metastatic carcinoma of the breast. CA 15-3 and CA 27.29 apparently measure the same antigen, although they react with different epitopes. Accordingly, the limitations in sensitivity and specificity of CA 15-3 also apply to CA 27.29.

CANCER ANTIGEN 19-9

This substance was initially isolated from a cell line derived from a human colorectal carcinoma in an effort to establish a high degree of tumor specificity. Chemically **cancer antigen 19-9 (CA 19-9)** is mucin-glycoprotein-related or identical to the Lewis^A blood group material. It is detectable in normal epithelium of the pancreas, gallbladder, prostate, and stomach. It is shed into the circulation by adenocarcinomas of the pancreas, stomach, gallbladder, colon, ovary, and lung. Its levels in serum are elevated in up to 80% of patients with pancreatic carcinoma, for which it has become an established marker to monitor disease progression; it can be used to differentiate pancreatic cancer from pancreatitis. It is elevated in inflammatory bowel disease, cirrhosis, and rheumatic diseases. CA 19-9 is not recommended for monitoring colorectal carcinomas.

BLADDER TUMOR ANTIGEN

A relatively new assay for detecting bladder cancer by testing urine, **bladder tumor antigen (BTA)** uses two monoclonal antibodies to quantitate human complement factor H-related protein. This protein appears to confer a selective growth advantage to cancer cells that are otherwise susceptible to attack from the immune system. BTA is a quantitative assay that should be used in conjunction with urine cytologic examination. BTA may also be elevated in the urine of patients with genital urinary tract infections, renal calculi, or recent surgery, biopsy, or trauma to the bladder.

FECAL OCCULT BLOOD

Fecal occult blood (FOB) is an examination of feces for the presence of blood as a screening test for colorectal cancer, but it is positive with blood from any source, from bleeding ulcer to hemorrhoids. FOB is often performed by the physician at the time of rectal examination (see Chapter 19). Patients can also collect stool samples (typically from three successive bowel movements) and apply them to test cards, which are then mailed to a testing facility. The test is performed by adding a solution of hydrogen peroxide to the stool sample, which was applied to a piece of filter paper impregnated with guaiac. The hemoglobin exhibits a pseudoperoxidase activity that results in a blue color change that is read visually. Assay sensitivity is improved by rehydrating samples that have dried in transport. Other assays may use a more complicated procedure to detect human hemoglobin in the stool with an immunoassay.

The outcome of yearly screening by FOB is to reduce mortality from colorectal cancer by as much as one-third.

ESTROGEN AND PROGESTERONE RECEPTORS

It has been recognized for almost a century that the growth of some breast cancers is strongly affected by the hormonal status of the patient. Current therapy for breast cancer may involve administration of estrogen or estrogen antagonists, and planning of that therapy includes the determination of the presence of the estrogen receptor in the tumor. The finding of **estrogen receptors (ER)** and **progesterone receptors (PR)** in the tumor cells is predictive of the likelihood that the tumor will respond to manipulative endocrine therapy such as estrogen antagonists (e.g., tamoxifen) or ablation of estrogen secretion sites (ovariectomy). Similar receptors exist in endometrial tissues, and determination of ER and PR status for endometrial carcinoma is also practiced.

ER molecules are probably located in the cell nucleus, where they activate certain genes when combined with molecules of estrogen. The interaction of estrogen with ER stimulates the production of PR. Thus the presence of PR is a strong indicator that the estrogen and ER system is functional. ER positivity is found in about half of breast tumors. Those tumors that are ER-negative appear to grow faster and to have more cell divisions (i.e., greater degree of malignancy). The presence of both ER and PR is associated with a high likelihood that the tumor will respond to endocrine manipulation. However, a small percentage of ER- and PR-positive tumors will not show such a response, perhaps because of a mixture of cell types in the original tumor.

In the past, ER and PR were measured in an extract of tumor tissue that destroyed tissue morphology and did not allow the pathologist to verify that tumor cells were actually included in the segment of tissue biopsy being examined. Today the evaluation of ER and PR is done by immunohistochemical methods using specific monoclonal antibodies to stain cells containing those receptors in thin tissue sections; by this means the pathologist can firmly establish exactly which cells exhibit ER and PR and can be certain that tumor cells are present even in very small biopsy samples taken from the breast.

Other markers have also been proposed as prognostic factors in breast biopsies. These include cathepsin D, DNA ploidy, epidermal growth factor receptor, and HER-2/*neu* oncoprotein. Although these measurements do provide information about tumor aggressiveness, after several years of clinical application it appears that much of that information is redundant and that ER and PR measurements provide adequate information for clinical management of breast cancer.

HUMAN PAPILLOMAVIRUS

This pathogen has been found to be the causative agent of common skin warts, condylomata (venereal warts), and carcinoma of the cervix. The particular manifestation of **human papillomavirus (HPV)** infection depends on the specific virus type; there are more than 50 different types. In the analysis of cervical lesions, HPV types 6 and 11 are generally associated with low-grade malignancy; HPV types 31, 33, and 35 occur in intermediate-grade lesions; and HPV types 16 and 18 are found in the majority of high-grade, rapidly progressing uterine cervical lesions.

HPV from patient samples cannot be cultured in the laboratory. Instead, DNA probes specific for these HPV types are now available for clinical diagnosis performed either on histologic section of cervical biopsy (in situ hybridization) or on dot blot or Southern blot analysis of the DNA extracted from biopsy or cervical smear. The finding of type 16 or 18 may persuade a physician to recommend more definitive and aggressive therapy to a patient at earlier stages in order to prevent cancer progression. Color Plate 100 is an example of adenovirus in lung tissue. The figure demonstrates the technique of in situ hybridization, which preserves normal histologic detail while pinpointing those cells infected by the virus.

GENE REARRANGEMENTS

Proliferations of lymphocytes are generally considered benign if they are polyclonal and malignant if monoclonal in cell origin. A traditional measurement of clonality is the presence of an M-spike of immunoglobulin in the serum of patients with the B-cell (plasma-cell) disorder multiple myeloma (see Chapters 4 and 7). However, such an easily distinguished marker may not always be present, particularly in nonsecretory B-cell disorders such as a lymphoma, and never in T-cell abnormalities. Immunohistochemical staining of lymph node or other tissue biopsies can sometimes detect clonality of B-cell disorders but may only be suggestive in T-cell proliferations. For cases that are difficult to diagnose, it is now possible to perform Southern blot analysis on DNA extracted from the tissue sample or leukemic cells to determine whether there is a clonal population with a single rearrangement of the gene for the T-cell antigen receptor (usually the beta subunit) or of the gene for an immunoglobulin as the B-cell indicator (either the heavy chain constant region or the kappa light chain constant region). In Southern blot analysis, total cellular DNA is extracted from a minimum of approximately 20 million cells. This DNA is then enzymatically digested into fragments of a few thousand base pairs each by **restriction endonucleases,** enzymes that digest DNA and whose cut sites have been mapped onto the genes of interest. These fragments are electrophoresed, and transferred to a membrane (e.g., cellulose nitrate or nylon) that is subsequently hybridized with a labeled DNA probe that will detect only the T-cell or only the B-cell gene. Normal polyclonal DNA will yield a standard set of fragments referred to as the germ line pattern. Maturation and development of a clonal line of lymphocytes will yield a single rearrangement of either the B- or the T-cell gene according to cell lineage. For documentation of recurrence following therapy, the level of sensitivity of this procedure is reported to be down to a content of about 5% clonal cells in an otherwise polyclonal population (Figs. B–1 and B–2). For sensitivity below that level, polymerase chain reaction (PCR) may be used to demonstrate clonal rearrangements in small populations of lymphocytes.

In the leukemic cells of a small percentage of patients with acute lymphoblastic leukemia and a large percentage of patients with chronic myelogenous leukemia, there is a reciprocal translocation between chromosomes 9 and 22, resulting in the abnormality designated "Philadelphia chromosome" (see Chapter 4). This abnormality has diagnostic significance as the translocation brings together a proto-oncogene (c-abl) on chromosome 9 with the breakpoint cluster region (bcr) of chromosome 22. The result is synthesis of a fusion protein derived from these two genetic regions with aberrant enzymatic activity that may be responsible for the development of the leukemia. Although the

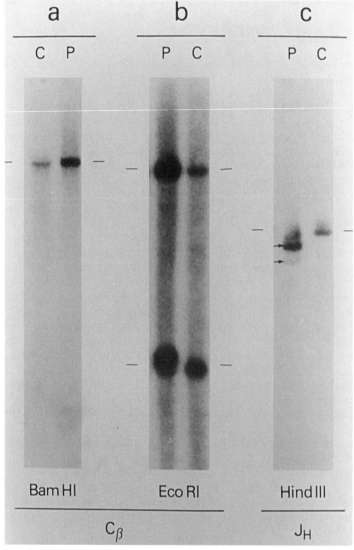

FIGURE B–1. Southern blot analyzing DNA extracted from peripheral blood specimen of a patient (P) with acute lymphocytic leukemia and normal control (C) DNA. Lanes a and b were hybridized with a probe from the constant region of the beta subunit of the T-cell antigen receptor gene (C_β) after digestion with the restriction enzymes BamHI and EcoRI; the T-cell gene was not rearranged. Lane c was hybridized with the immunoglobulin heavy chain joining region gene (J_H) after digestion with HindIII; the extra bands in the patient sample (arrows) indicate gene rearrangements in a clonal B-cell proliferation.

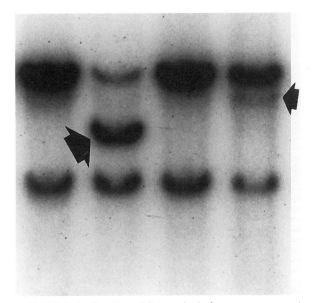

FIGURE B–2. Southern blot analysis for rearrangement of T-cell antigen receptor beta subunit gene using restriction enzyme digestion with EcoRI. Arrows indicate rearranged bands from clonal proliferation of lymphocytes in two different patients. The other bands are normal germ-line unrearranged genes at fragment sizes of 11 kilobases (top) and 4.2 kilobases (bottom).

Philadelphia chromosome can be detected by cytogenetic analysis, it is now possible to detect the rearrangement occurring in the breakpoint cluster region by Southern blot analysis similar to that for B- and T-cell gene rearrangements. It may also be detected by PCR. Bcr-abl analysis has the potential benefits of speed, sensitivity, and accuracy compared with the more traditional examination of chromosomes under a light microscope. Furthermore, DNA analysis may be performed on cells that have lost viability due to storage, whereas cytogenetic testing requires living cells.

Rearrangements resulting from other translocations can also be detected using these techniques, such as the fusion protein resulting from a translocation between the retinoic acid receptor (RARα) on chromosome 15 and the promyelocytic leukemia (PML) oncogene on chromosome 17. This translocation is usually detected by PCR. Table B–1 lists some of the gene rearrangements that can be detected using Southern blotting techniques or PCR and that are useful in oncology.

Fluorescent in situ hybridization (FISH) is a relatively new method that has become quite useful for detecting chromosomal translocations as

TABLE B–1. MOLECULAR DIAGNOSTIC TESTS IN ONCOLOGY

Southern Blotting

Test	Probe	Clinical Implication
Ig heavy chain	J_H SB	Clonality (B-cell lymphomas)
Ig kappa	J_K SB	Clonality (B-cell lymphoma/leukemia)
Ig lambda	C_1	Clonality (B-cell lymphoma/leukemia)
TCR beta	Cb′	Clonality (T-cell leukemias/lymphomas)
TCR gamma	Jg^1	Clonality (T-cell leukemias/lymphomas)
TCR delta	Jd^1	Clonality (T-cell leukemias/lymphomas)
bcl.1	bcl-1,5′, bcl-1.3′	Rearrangement of bcl-1 oncogene
bcl.2	mbr, mcr, 5′3′	Rearrangement of bcl-2 oncogene—follicular lymphoma
bcr/abl	bcr	CML—translocation
c-myc	c-myc5′, 3′	Burkitt's lymphoma

PCR

Test	Probe	Clinical Implication
t(14;18)	bcl_2/IgH	Translocation—follicular lymphoma
t(9;22)	bcr/abl	CML—translocation
p53	SSCP	Tumor suppressor gene mutation
IgH gene	VDJ rearrangement	B-cell leukemias/lymphomas
t(15;17)	rar	APL translocation

APL = acute promyelocytic leukemia; C = constant; CML = chronic myelogenous leukemia; H = heavy chain; Ig = Immunoglobulin; J = joining; PCR = polymerase chain reaction; SB = Southern blotting; TCR = T-cell receptor; t = translocation.

well as other chromosomal alterations such as aneuploidies. FISH is performed using DNA probes labeled with fluorescent dyes that emit visible light of different colors when illuminated with ultraviolet light. The cells of interest are grown in a special medium and are treated with colcemid to arrest cell division in prophase. Cells are then fixed, probed, and examined microscopically. For example, a probe with nucleotide sequences specific to chromosome 9 will bind to chromosome 9 and to any segment of chromosome 9 translocated to another chromosome. Those sites will be identifiable by the color of the fluorescent dye attached to that DNA probe. Similarly a probe specific to chromosome 22 will hybridize to all sites containing chromosome 22 sequences. Consequently, by using FISH, a patient sample with the Philadelphia chromosome should show in individual cells a colored dot for chromosome 9, a different colored dot for chromosome 22, and still another dot with a color mixture of the two dyes, representing the translocated chromosome.

SUGGESTED READING

American College of Physicians: Screening for prostate cancer. Ann Intern Med 126:480, 1997.

American Society of Clinical Oncology Tumor Marker Expert Panel: Clinical practice guidelines for the use of tumor markers in breast and colorectal cancer. J Clin Oncol 14:2843, 1996.

Bezwoda, WR, et al: The value of estrogen and progesterone receptor determinations in advanced breast cancer. Estrogen receptor level but not progesterone receptor level correlates with response to tamoxifen. Cancer 68:867, 1991.

Brawer, MK: How to use prostate-specific antigen in the early detection or screening for prostatic carcinoma. CA—A Cancer Journal for Clinicians 45:148, 1995.

Catalona, WJ, et al: Use of the percentage of free prostate-specific antigen to enhance differentiation of prostate cancer from benign prostatic disease. A prospective multicenter clinical trial. J Am Med Assoc 279:1542, 1998.

Cole, LA, and Kardana, A: Discordant results in human chorionic gonadotropin assays. Clin Chem 38:263, 1992.

Coley, CM, et al: Early detection of prostate cancer. Part I: Prior probability and effectiveness of tests. Ann Intern Med 126:394, 1997.

Coley, CM, et al: Early detection of prostate cancer. Part II: Estimating the risks, benefits, and costs. Ann Intern Med 126:468, 1997.

Ferrante, JM: Colorectal cancer screening. Cancer screening and diagnosis. Med Clin N Am 80:27, 1996.

Lorincz, AT, et al: Human papillomavirus infection of the cervix: relative risk associations of 15 common anogenital types. Obstet Gynecol 79:328, 1992.

Mandel, JS, et al: Reducing mortality from colorectal cancer by screening for fecal occult blood. N Engl J Med 328:1365, 1993.

Montgomery, RC, et al: Prediction of recurrence and survival by post-resection CA 19-9 values in patients with adenocarcinoma of the pancreas. Ann Surg Oncol 4:551, 1997.

Pearson, VAH: Screening for ovarian cancer: A review. Public Health 108:367, 1994.

Ward, BE, et al: Rapid prenatal diagnosis of chromosomal aneuploidies by fluorescence *in situ* hybridization: Clinical experience with 4500 specimens. Am J Hum Gen 52:851, 1993.

Wayne, MS, Cath, A, and Pamies, RJ: Colorectal cancer. A practical review for the primary care physician. Arch Fam Med 4:357, 1995.

APPENDIX C

Perinatal Laboratory Testing

With the advent of percutaneous umbilical cord blood sampling (PUBS), direct access to the fetal circulation is achieved. This affords several management and therapeutic advantages as was mentioned in Chapter 8. Intrauterine transfusions can now be administered directly by the intravascular route. Pure fetal blood samples can be obtained that allow assessment of fetal health.

Fetal blood aspiration is achieved with the insertion of a 20- to 22-gauge spinal needle under ultrasound guidance into the umbilical vessel. The syringe is flushed with sodium citrate or heparin. A standard amniocentesis tray is all that is necessary for the performance of a simple PUBS procedure. For exchange transfusions, more equipment may be needed. Once the umbilical vessel is entered, 0.4 mL of blood is aspirated to clear the anticoagulant solution and then the required blood sample can be obtained in 1–3 mL syringes.

Laboratory confirmation of the purity of the fetal sample can be made by direct electronic determination of the mean erythrocyte cell volume (the MCV is usually 140 fL in the fetus, compared to less than 98 fL in the mother). Other methods include serologic confirmation of Ii status (i is found on cord cells; I on adult cells) and the Kleihauer-Betke acid resistant hemoglobin technique as discussed in Chapter 8. Additional methods to confirm fetal origin of the sample include Doppler analysis, or the APT test. The APT test is used to differentiate adult (maternal) from fetal hemoglobin by applying the alkaline resistance property of hemoglobin F. A small sample of fetal blood when mixed with 1% (0.25N) sodium hydroxide imparts a brownish color to maternal blood (alkaline sensitive) compared to maintenance of the pink color if the sample is of fetal origin (alkaline resistant). Recall that HbF is acid and alkaline resistant, whereas HbA is not. The APT test is a qualitative test only. Table C–1 is a list of indications for performing PUBS.

1048

TABLE C–1. INDICATIONS FOR PERCUTANEOUS UMBILICAL BLOOD SAMPLING

Fetal hemolytic disease
Rapid fetal karyotyping
Congenital infection
Intrauterine growth retardation
Fetal blood gases and acid-base status
Nonimmune hydrops fetalis
Fetal thrombocytopenia
Genetic disorders
Fetal pharmacologic therapy
Evaluation of maternal and fetal therapy
Fetal physiology and pathophysiology

Fetal karyotyping can be performed early in pregnancy by means of applying DNA analytic techniques to samples of chorionic villus or amniotic fluid fibroblasts. However, PUBS allows direct and rapid karyotypic analysis (within 48–72 hours). This is especially useful when the patient is a late prenatal registrant, for legal termination, or when amniocentesis or chorionic villus sampling is ambiguous.

Percutaneous umbilical cord blood sampling in the assessment of fetal anemia caused by alloimmune or autoimmune hemolytic disease can allow an accurate assessment of whether the maternal and fetal blood are antigenetically incompatible and a direct measurement of fetal hematocrit and/or bilirubin level. Formerly amniotic fluid optical density was the only way to characterize the pregnancy risk status (see Fig. 8–7).

PUBS has allowed the calibration of normal fetal hematologic values during gestation. See Tables C–2, C–3.

Fetal platelet counts of less than 50,000/μL are associated with a potential for in utero demise, especially in cases of alloimmune thrombocytopenia. A more logical delivery strategy can also be planned, with cesarean section performed if counts are below 50,000/μL and vaginal delivery being allowed with counts above 50,000/μL, assuming no other contraindications to vaginal delivery exist. A similar strategy can be applied in cases of maternal ITP to determine evidence of fetal thrombocytopenia due to passive transplacental transfer of maternal platelet autoantibody.

Perinatal infections caused by viruses such as cytomegalovirus, toxoplasmosis, rubella, herpes, hepatitis B, or human immunodeficiency virus can be evaluated by prenatal sampling. Prenatal diagnosis of toxoplasmosis is one of the most common indications for the use of PUBS in Europe, particularly France. It can be performed as early as 20 to

TABLE C-2. EVOLUTION OF HEMATOLOGICAL VALUES OF 163 NORMAL FETUSES DURING PREGNANCY (MEAN ± SD) FROM STUDIES PERFORMED WITH A COULTER MODEL S-PLUS II

Wk of Gestation	WBC (×10⁹/liter)	Platelets (×10⁹/liter)	RBC (×10¹²/liter)	Hb (g/100 ml)	Ht (%)	MCV (Fl)	MCH (pg)	MPHC (g/100 mL)	Red Cell Distribution Width
18–20 (n = 25)	4.20 ± 0.83	242.1 ± 34.48	2.66 ± 0.29	11.47 ± 0.78	35.86 ± 3.29	133.92 ± 8.83	43.14 ± 2.71	32 ± 2.38	20.64 ± 2.28
21–22 (n = 55)	4.19 ± 0.84	258.2 ± 53.65	2.96 ± 0.26	12.28 ± 0.89	38.53 ± 3.21	130.06 ± 6.17	41.39 ± 3.32	31.73 ± 2.78	20.15 ± 1.92
23–25 (n = 61)	3.95 ± 0.69	259.43 ± 42.45	3.06 ± 0.26	12.40 ± 0.77	38.59 ± 2.41	126.19 ± 6.23	40.48 ± 2.88	32.14 ± 3.2	19.29 ± 1.62
26–30 (n = 22)	4.44 ± 0.85	253.54 ± 36.6	3.52 ± 0.32	13.35 ± 1.17	41.54 ± 3.31	118.17 ± 5.75	37.94 ± 3.67	32.15 ± 3.55	18.35 ± 1.67

From Forestier, F, et al: Hematological values of 163 normal fetuses between 18 and 30 weeks gestation. Pediatr Res 20:342–346, 1986, with permission.

TABLE C-3. HEMATOLOGICAL DATA OF NORMAL FETUSES*

Wk of Gestation	Lymphocytes (%)	Neutrophils (%)	Eosinophils (%)	Monocytes (%)	Normoblasts (%)
18–20 (n = 25)	80 ± 9	5 ± 2	1.5 ± 2.5	1.5 ± 2	12 ± 8
21–22 (n = 55)	81 ± 7	5.5 ± 3.5	1 ± 1	1.5 ± 1.5	11 ± 7
23–25 (n = 61)	82 ± 6	7.5 ± 4.5	2 ± 2	1.5 ± 1.5	7 ± 4
26–30 (n = 22)	84 ± 6	8.5 ± 2.5	2 ± 1	1.5 ± 1	4 ± 3.5

*Some aspects of fetal differential counts from 18 to 30 wk of gestation of 163 normal fetuses (mean ± SD)
From Forestier, F, et al: Hematological values of 163 normal fetuses between 18 and 30 weeks gestation. Pediatr Res 20:342–346, 1986, with permission.

TABLE C–4. GENETIC DISORDERS IDENTIFIABLE BY PERCUTANEOUS UMBILICAL BLOOD SAMPLING

Disorders of Coagulation and Hemostasis
Von Willebrand's disease
Glanzmann's thrombasthenia
Bernard-Soulier syndrome
Gray platelet syndrome
May-Hegglin syndrome
Radial aplasia thrombocytopenia syndrome
Antithrombin III deficiency
Homozygous C or S deficiency

Red Cell Disorders
Thalassemias
Hemoglobinopathies
Hereditary spherocytosis
Hereditary pyropoikilocytosis
Enzyme deficiencies
Diamond-Blackfan syndrome
Hereditary erythrocyte multinuclearity with
  positive acidified serum (HEMPAS)

Disorders of Metabolism
Duchenne's muscular dystrophy
Familial hypercholesterolemia
Triose phosphate isomerase deficiency
Adrenoleukodystrophy
Alpha$_1$-antitrypsin deficiency
Tay-Sachs disease

White Cell Immunologic Disorders
Chronic granulomatous disease
Chediak-Higashi syndrome
Severe combined immunodeficiency
Wiskott-Aldrich syndrome
Homozygous C3 deficiency

Adapted from Nicolaides, KH: Cordocentesis. Clin Obstet Gynecol 31:123, 1988.

24 weeks. In cases of intrauterine growth retardation, acid-base status, glucose, and lactate levels can be used to determine the metabolic status in the fetuses with intrauterine growth retardation. Future applications of this technology may well be gene transfer, fetal stem cell sampling, and fetal drug therapy. Table C–4 is a list of genetic disorders that can be identified by percutaneous umbilical blood sampling.

SUGGESTED READING

Forestier, F, et al: Hematological values of 163 normal fetuses between 18 and 30 weeks gestation. Pediatr Res 20:342–346, 1986.

Gozzo, ML, et al: Reference intervals for 18 clinical chemistry analytes in fetal plasma samples between 18 and 49 weeks of pregnancy. Clin Chem 44(3):683–685, 1998.

Herson, VC, et al: Placental blood sampling: An aid to the diagnosis of neonatal sepsis. J Perinatol 18(2):135–137, 1998.

King, JC, and Sacher, RA: Percutaneous umbilical blood sampling. In Sacher, RA, and Strauss, RG: Contemporary Issues in Pediatric Transfusion Medicine. American Association of Blood Banks, Arlington, VA, 1989, pp 25–53.

Snijders, R, and Hyett, J: Fetal testing in intra-uterine growth retardation. Curr Opin Obstet Gynecol 9(2):91–95, 1997.

Wilner, JP: Reproductive genetics and today's patient options: Prenatal diagnosis. Mt Sinai J Med 65(3):173–177, 1998.

APPENDIX D

Neonatal Laboratory Testing

Maintenance of life support systems for very premature infants requires continuous laboratory analysis. Because some of these infants have a total blood volume of less than 100 mL, the daily removal of 1 to 2 mL can rapidly deplete the infant's blood volume. Removal of blood for laboratory testing is the most frequent indication for transfusion therapy in the neonatal intensive care unit. The vast majority of these transfusions are given as replacement therapy for numerous laboratory tests necessitated by intensive care management. "Bleeding into the laboratory" can be responsible for losses of over 3 mL/kg/day in the neonatal intensive care nursery.

Laboratory tests that can be performed on microsamples collected using capillary puncture are listed in Table D–1. Several techniques exist for microanalysis and reference ranges vary according to the methods used. One such instrument, popular in neonatology centers, is the Vitros chemistry analyzer (Johnson & Johnson, Rochester, NY). Neonatal and pediatric reference ranges for usual biochemical analytes by this instrument are listed in Tables D–2, D–3, D–4, and D–5. Newborns have lower concentrations of total protein and albumin and higher concentrations of phosphate, bilirubin, and enzymes in serum than older children. Concentrations of urea, glucose, calcium, phosphate, and bilirubin change rapidly after delivery. Another important test performed in the neonatal laboratory is the lecithin-sphingomyelin (L-S) ratio, which was mentioned in Chapter 17.

Because group B streptococcus is an important pathogen in the neonatal period, neonatal laboratories usually perform rapid testing for its presence, as discussed in Chapter 15. Amino acid testing for inborn errors of metabolism (inherited amino-acid defects) was discussed in Chapter 16. It is also becoming apparent, however, that these conditions may be detected at an earlier stage using perinatal sampling (PUBS) as discussed in Appendix C.

TABLE D–1. LABORATORY ANALYTES MEASURED ON MICROSAMPLES

Analyte	Method
Acetone	
Albumin	Bromcresol green
Bilirubin	Dual wavelength reflectance spectrophotometry
Calcium	Arsenazo III dye
Cholesterol	Cholesterol oxidase
Cholesterol, HDL	Dextran sulfate, then cholesterol oxidase
Glucose	Glucose oxidase
Phosphate	Ammonium molybdate
Total protein	Biuret
Triglycerides	Glycerol phosphate oxidase
Urea	Urease
Uric acid	Uricase
ALT	Alanine to pyruvate
ALP	p-Nitrophenyl phosphate
Amylase	Amylopectin
AST	Aspartate to oxaloacetate
Creatine kinase	Creatine phosphate to creatine
GGT	γ-Glutamyl-p-nitroanilide
LDH	Pyruvate to lactate
Lipase	1-Oleoyl-2, 3-diacetylglycerol

Minimum volume 100 μL.

TABLE D-2. REFERENCE INTERVALS (0.025–0.975 FRACTILES) FOR ALBUMIN AND TOTAL PROTEIN

Age	n	Albumin g/L	Total Protein (g/L)
0–5 d, <2.5 kg	30	20–36	38–62
0–5 d, >2.5 kg	93	26–36	54–70
1–3 y	50	34–42	59–70
4–6 y	38	35–52	59–78
7–9 y	74	37–56	62–81
10–19 y	332	37–56	63–86

Reprinted with permission from Clinical Chemistry (1988), Volume 34, No. 8, pages 1622–1625. Copyright American Association for Clinical Chemistry, Inc.

TABLE D-3. REFERENCE INTERVALS (0.025–0.975 FRACTILES) FOR CALCIUM, PHOSPHATE, AND UREA

Age, y	n	Calcium	Phosphate	Urea
		mmol/L		
(0–5 d, >2.5 kg)	50	1.96–2.66	1.50–2.60	
1–3	50	2.17–2.44	1.25–2.10	1.8–6.0
4–6	38	2.19–2.51	1.30–1.75	2.5–6.0
7–9	72	2.19–2.51	1.20–1.80	2.5–6.0
10–11	62	2.22–2.51	1.20–1.80	2.5–6.0
12–13	73	2.19–2.64	1.05–1.75	2.5–6.0
14–15	91	2.29–2.66	0.95–1.75	2.9–7.5
16–19	107	2.22–2.66	0.90–1.50	2.9–7.5

Reprinted with permission from Clinical Chemistry (1988), Volume 34, No. 8, pages 1622–1625. Copyright American Association for Clinical Chemistry, Inc.

TABLE D–4. REFERENCE RANGES FOR SELECTED COMMONLY PERFORMED ENZYME STUDIES IN PEDIATRIC PATIENTS

Age, y	n	ALT	AST	ALP	GGT	CK	LDH
				U/L			
1–3	50	5–45	20–60	145–320	6–19	60–305	500–920
4–6	40	10–25	15–50	150–380	10–22	75–230	470–900
7–9	80	10–35	15–40	175–420	13–25	60–365	420–750
Males							
10–11	27	10–35	10–60	135–530	17–30	55–215	432–700
12–13	31	10–55	15–40	200–495	17–44	60–330	470–750
14–15	26	10–45	15–40	130–525	12–33	60–335	360–730
16–19	40	10–40	10–45	65–260	11–34	55–370	340–670
Females							
10–11	34	10–30	10–40	130–560	17–28	80–230	380–770
12–13	49	10–30	10–30	105–420	14–25	50–295	380–640
14–15	52	5–30	10–30	70–230	14–26	50–240	390–580
16–19	61	5–35	5–30	50–130	11–28	45–230	340–670

Reprinted with permission from Clinical Chemistry (1988), Volume 34, No. 8, pages 1622–1625. Copyright American Association for Clinical Chemistry, Inc.

TABLE D–5. REFERENCE INTERVALS (0.025–0.975 FRACTILES) FOR URIC ACID, TOTAL CHOLESTEROL, AND TRIGLYCERIDES

Age, y	n	Uric acid, µmol/L	Cholesterol*	Triglycerides
			mmol/L	
1–3	49	105–300	1.15–4.70	0.31–1.41
4–6	38	130–280	2.80–4.80	0.36–1.31
7–9	72	120–295	2.90–6.40	0.32–1.46
Males				
10–11	28	135–320	3.25–5.95	0.27–1.55
12–13	32	160–400	3.30–5.95	0.27–1.64
14–15	39	140–465	2.75–5.80	0.38–1.86
16–19	41	235–510	2.85–5.70	0.38–1.58
Females				
10–11	34	180–280	3.30–6.30	0.44–1.58
12–13	40	180–345	3.25–5.55	0.42–1.47
14–15	50	180–345	3.35–5.55	0.43–1.52
16–19	68	180–350	2.75–5.60	0.42–1.58

*Note: To decrease the risk of atherosclerosis, it is recommended for adults that total serum cholesterol should not exceed 5 mmol/L.

Reprinted with permission from Clinical Chemistry (1988), Volume 34, No. 8, pages 1622–1625. Copyright American Association for Clinical Chemistry, Inc.

Recent additions to the armamentarium for neonatal screening include newer assays for evaluation of congenital endocrine problems. For example, congenital hypothyroidism may be predicted by newer immunoassays measuring TSH or thyroxin; congenital adrenal hyperplasia, by similar assays for 17-hydroxyprogesterone; and cystic fibrosis, by trypsin assays. The use of alpha-fetoprotein as a marker of neural tube defects was discussed in Chapter 17.

Despite advances in microtechnology, multiple samples are still associated with the drawing of a substantial amount of blood from these small infants. Several electronic devices have been developed that can facilitate in vivo testing and monitoring. These include catheters (for continuous determinations of Po_2, Pco_2, oxygen saturation, and calcium), transcutaneous electrodes or monitors (for continuous analysis of Po_2, Pco_2, and bilirubin), and breath analysis. The development of both microtechnology and this kind of in situ testing may allow continuous laboratory evaluation of the severely ill neonate with a minimum of blood sampling. Point-of-care testing is also finding its way into neonatal intensive care units and may provide an alternative to traditional blood gas and electrolyte analyzers, with some improvement in turnaround time.

SUGGESTED READING

Blau, N, Duran, M, and Blaskovics, M: Physician's Guide to the Laboratory Diagnosis of Inherited Metabolic Diseases. Chapman & Hall, 1996.

Brown, ER: Metabolic screening. Clin Perinatol 25(2):371–388, 1998.

Lockitch, G, et al: Age and sex specific reference intervals for biochemistry analytes as measured with the Ektachem-700 Analyzer. Clin Chem 38:1622–1625, 1988.

Speidel, B, et al (eds): A Neonatal Vade-Mecum, ed 3. An Arnold Publication, distributed by Oxford University Press, Oxford, 1998.

APPENDIX E

Laboratory Reference Ranges

The reference ranges in this appendix represent reference intervals used at Georgetown University Medical Center in the Department of Laboratory Medicine.* Because reference ranges vary according to the methods used and population demographics, they may vary from institution to institution and should always be reviewed locally. The values given here obviously are not all-encompassing for every analyte.

*From Georgetown University Medical Center, Department of Laboratory Medicine, Washington, DC, March 18, 1999.

TABLE E–1. HEMATOLOGY

Tests	Reference Ranges
CBC (Complete Blood Count)	**(Adults)**
WBC	$4.8–10.8 \times 10^3$ cells/μL
RBC	Male: $4.7–6.1 \times 10^6$ cells/μL
	Female: $4.2–5.4 \times 10^6$ cells/μL
HGB	Male: 14.0–18.0 g/dL
	Female: 12.0–16.0 g/dL
HCT	Male: 42–52%
	Female: 37–47%
MCV	Male: 80–94 fL
	Female: 81–99 fL
MCH	27–31 μg
MCHC	33–37 g/dL
Platelets	130,000–400,000/μL
Differential White Cell Count	
Segs	53–79%
Bands	0–10%
Eosin	0–4%
Lymphs	13–46%
Monos	3–9%
Basos	0–1%
Sedimentation Rate	Below 50 years:
	Male: 0–15 mm/hr
	Female: 0–20 mm/hr
	Above 50 years:
	Male: 0–15 mm/hr
	Female: 0–30 mm/hr

TABLE E–2. COAGULATION

Tests	Reference Ranges
Activated protein C resistance	Ratio of 2–5
Antithrombin III (functional)	87–123%
Antithrombin III (antigen)	22.0–33.0 mg/dL
Bleeding time	Up to 10 min
Cryofibrinogen	Positive test: Cryoprecipitate that dissolves upon heating at 37°C. Negative test: No precipitate visible or cryoprecipitate that does not dissolve at 37°C.
Dilute Russell viper venom	Positive = lupus anticoagulant
Euglobulin clot lysis	Eug. time of >60 min = normal Eug. time of <60 min = abnormal
Factor VIII activity	50–150%
Factor assays: II, V, VII, X, VIII, IX, XI and XII	50–150%
vWF antigen and vWF activity	50–150%
Factor XIII assay	Presumptively normal >15 min Abnormal <15 min
Factor inhibitor assay	Results reported out in Bethesda units (0-0.6). The higher the Bethesda units are, the stronger the inhibitor present.
FSP (fibrin split products)	10 µg/mL or less
Fibrinogen (antigen [RID])	150–548 mg/dL
Fibrinogen (thrombin method)	150–400 mg/dL
Heparin assay (therapeutic)	0.3–0.5 anti-Xa units
Protein C activity	70–130%
Protein S activity	65–140%
Prothrombin time (PT)	11.0–14.5 sec
(INR) International Normalized Ratio	Therapeutic ranges determined by clinical scenario. See Chapter 5.
Reptilase time	Control range should be between 18–22 sec. Patient value should be within ±5 sec of control value.
Thrombin time (TT)	Patient value should be within ±2 seconds of control range (15–20 sec)
Viscosity	Ratio of 1.2–1.8
Partial thromboplastin time (PTT)	24–36 sec

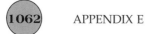

TABLE E–3. CHEMISTRY

Tests	Reference Ranges	
Acetone, serum	Negative	
Albumin	3.5–5.0 g/dL	
Alkaline phosphatase	Children 3–15 years	
	117–390 IU/L	
	Adults	
	31–97 IU/L	
Ammonia serum/plasma	10–65 µmol/L	
Amylase serum/plasma	25–125 U/L	
Amylase urine	0–400 U/L random	
Amylase urine	0–360 U/L 24 hr	
ALT—Alanine aminotransferase (SGPT)	10–40 IU/L	
AST—Aspartate aminotransferase (SGOT)	10–37 IU/L	
Beta-2 microglobulin serum	0.2–2.8 µg/dL	
Beta-2 microglobulin urine	0–370 µg/L	
	Weeks after conception	*U/L*
Beta-HCG serum	1 week	5–50
	2 weeks	40–1,000
	3 weeks	100–4,000
	4 weeks	800–10,000
	5–6 weeks	5,000–100,000
	7–8 weeks	20,000–200,000
	9–12 weeks	10,000–200,000
	2nd Trimester	8,000–50,000
	3rd Trimester	6,000–50,000
	Nonpregnant females	<5
Bilirubin, direct	0.0–0.3 mg/dL	
Bilirubin, total	0.1–1.0 mg/dL	
Blood gases	*Arterial*	*Venous*
pH	7.35–7.45	7.32–7.42
PCO_2 mmHg	35–45	41–51
PO_2 mmHg	80–100	25–40
O_2 SAT	96–97%	40–70%
Blood urea nitrogen (BUN)	6-19 mg/dL	
Calcium ionized whole blood	1.13–1.32 mmol/L (arterial and venous)	
Calcium, total serum	8.4–10.2 mg/dL	
Calcium, total urine	50–150 mg/24 hr	
Carbon dioxide	22.0–30.0 mmol/L	
Carbon monoxide (nonsmoker)	0.5–1.5%	
Carbon monoxide (smoker)	4–9%	
Carbon monoxide, toxic	>20%	
Carbon monoxide, lethal	>50%	
Chloride, serum	101–111 mmol/L	
Cholesterol	140–200 mg/dL	
Cholesterol (HDL)	40–80 mg/dL	

(Continued)

TABLE E–3. CHEMISTRY (Continued)

Tests	Reference Ranges	
Cholesterol (LDL)	Male 20–29 years	79–136 mg/dL
	30–39 years	110–150 mg/dL
	40–49 years	120–162 mg/dL
	50–59 years	125–167 mg/dL
	60–69 years	115–185 mg/dL
	70–150 years	114–172 mg/dL
	Female 20–29 years	82–126 mg/dL
	30–39 years	96–140 mg/dL
	40–49 years	107–148 mg/dL
	50–59 years	115–170 mg/dL
	60–69 years	116–195 mg/dL
	70–150 years	122–176 mg/dL
Creatinine, serum	0.5–1.4 mg/dL	
Creatinine, urine	800–2000 mg/24 hr	
	(15–25 mg/kg/day)	
Creatinine clearance	Male: 90–130 mL/min	
	Female: 80–125 mL/min	
Creatinine kinase (CPK)(CK)	Male: 38–174 IU/L	
	Female: 96–140 IU/L	
Creatinine kinase (MB fraction)	Less than 4.0 ng/mL	
Ferritin	Male: 24–336 ng/mL	
	Female: 11–307 ng/mL	
Follicle-stimulating hormone (FSH)	Midfollicular: 3.85–8.78 mIU/mL	
	Midcycle: 4.54–22.51 mIU/mL	
	Midluteal: 1.79–5.12 mIU/mL	
	Postmenopausal: 16.74–113.59 mIU/mL	
Gamma-glutamyltranspeptidase (GGT)	Male: 8–37 IU/L	
	Female: 5–24 IU/L	
Glucose, fasting	70–105 mg/dL	
Glucose, 2-hour PC or PP	70–110 mg/dL	
Glucose tolerance, fasting	70–105 mg/dL	
Glucose tolerance, ½ hr	120–140 mg/dL	
Glucose tolerance, 1 hr	150–169 mg/dL	
Haptoglobin	37–184 mg/dL	
Iron, total	Male: 42–135 µg/dL	
	Female: 42–135 µg/dL	
Iron, TIBC	260–445 µg/dL	
Lactic acid	0.5–2.2 mmol/L (venous)	
Lactic dehydrogenase (LD)	91–180 IU/L	
Lipase, serum	7–58 U/L	
Luteinizing hormone (LH)	Midfollicular: 2.12–10.89 mIU/mL	
	Midcycle peak: 19.18–103.03 mIU/mL	
	Midluteal: 1.20–12.86 mIU/mL	
	Postmenopausal: 10.87–58.64 mIU/mL	

(Continued)

TABLE E–3. CHEMISTRY *(Continued)*

Tests	Reference Ranges
Magnesium, serum	1.6–2.6 mg/dL
Magnesium, 24-hr urine	12–292 mg/24 hr
Osmolality, serum (freezing point)	0–25D = 270–283 mOsm/kg
	>25D = 289–308 mOsm/kg
Osmolality, urine (freezing point)	0–25D = 50–600
	>25D = 300–900
Phosphorus, urine 24-hr	400–1300 mg/24 hr
Phosphorus, serum	2.7–4.5 mg/dL
Prealbumin	10.0–45.0 mg/dL
Protein, CSF	15–45 mg/dL
Protein, urine	0–165 mg/24 hr
Potassium, serum	3.5–5.0 mmol/L
Potassium, whole blood	3.5–5.0 mmol/L (arterial and venous)
Potassium, urine 24-hr	25–125 mmol/24 hr
Prolactin	Male: 2.64–13.13 ng/mL
	Female (premenopausal): 3.34–26.72 ng/mL
	(postmenopausal): 2.74–19.64 ng/mL
Prostatic specific antigen (PSA)	0–4.0 ng/mL
Rheumatoid factor	0–20 IU/mL
Sodium, serum	135–145 mmol/L
Sodium, urine 24-hr	40–220 mmol/24 hr
Total protein	6.0–8.3 g/dL
Total T_3	87–178 ng/dL
T_3 uptake	32–48.4%
T_4 (thyroxine)	6.1–12.2 µg/dL
T_4 (free) or free T_4	0.71–1.85 ng/dL
Thyroid stimulating hormone	0.34–5.6 µIU/mL
Triglycerides	35–160 mg/dL
Troponin-1	0.0–0.15 ng/mL
Urea nitrogen, urine	12,000–20,000 mg/24 hr
Uric acid, serum	Male: 3.4–7.0 mg/dL
	Female: 2.4–5.7 mg/dL
Uric acid, 24-hr urine	250–750 mg/24 hr
Vitamin B-12	180–914 pg/mL

TABLE E–4. URINALYSIS

Chemical Analysis

Color	Varies
Clarity	Clear
Specific gravity	1.002–1.040
pH	4.5–8.0
Protein	Negative
Blood	Negative
Ketones	Negative
Glucose	Negative
Nitrites	Negative

Microscopic Analysis

Epithelial cells	few/hpf
RBC	0–3/hpf
WBC	0–5 hpf
Bacteria	0–few/hpf

Urine Analytes

Amylase urine	0–400 U/L random
Amylase urine	0–360 U/24 hr
Calcium, total urine	50–150 mg/24 hr
Creatinine, urine	800–2000 mg/24 hr (15–25 mg/kg/day)
Magnesium, 24-hr urine	12–292 mg/24 hr
Osmolality urine (freezing point)	0–25D = 50–600 >25D = 300–900
Phosphorus, 24-hr urine	400–1300 mg/24 hr
Protein, 24-hr urine	0–165 mg/24 hr
Potassium, 24-hr urine	25–125 mmol/24 hr
Sodium, 24-hr urine	40–220 mEq/24 hr
Urea nitrogen, 24-hr urine	12.0–20 g/24 hr

TABLE E–5. TOXICOLOGY (DRUGS)

Drug	Therapeutic	Toxic
Acetaminophen	10–30 µg/mL	>300 µg/mL at 4 hr postingestion >50 µg/mL at 12 hr postingestion
Carbamazepine	4–10 µg/mL	>15 µg/mL
Cyclosporin		>700 ng/mL
Digoxin	0.8–2.0 ng/mL	>2.6 ng/mL
Ethanol	None	>100 mg/dL
Ethosuximide	40–100 µg/mL	>100 µg/mL
Gentamicin	Peak: 5–10 µg/mL Trough: 0–2 µg/mL	>12 µg/mL
Lidocaine	1.5–5 µg/mL	>5.0 µg/mL
Lithium	0.6–1.2 mmol/L	>2.0 mmol/L
Methotrexate	24 hours 5 µMoles/L 48 hours 0.5 µMoles/L 72 hours 0.05 µMoles/L	>0.1 µMoles/L at 48 hr
NAPA	5–30 µg/mL	>40.0 µg/mL
Phenobarbital	15–40 µg/mL	>50.0 µg/mL
Phenytoin	10–20 µg/mL	>25.0 µg/mL
Primidone	5–12 µg/mL	>13 µg/mL
Procainamide	4–10 µg/mL	>12 µg/mL
Quinidine	2–5 µg/mL	>5.0 µg/mL
Salicylate	<20 mg/dL	>30 mg/dL
Theophylline	10–20 µg/mL	>21 µg/mL
Valproic acid	50–100 µg/mL	>100 µg/mL
Vancomycin	Peak: 20–40 µg/mL Trough: 5–10 µg/mL	>80 µg/mL

INDEX

A page number in *italics* indicate a figure. A "*t*" following a page number indicates a table.

A antigen, 367, *368*, 373
Abciximab, 314
Abetalipoproteinemia, hemolysis with, 154
ABO blood group system, 367-371, 370*t*, 373
  antigens and antibodies in, 370*t*, 371
  conditions causing changes in, 373*t*
  HLA typing and, 437
ABO hemolytic disease of the newborn, 421,
  428-429
Absidia, 644
Acanthocytosis, 68*t*
Acetaldehyde, *912, 913*
Acetaminophen toxicity, 903, *903*, 905-906, *906*,
  1066*t*
Acetest tablets, 521
Acetoacetic acid, 521
Acetone, 521, 1062*t*
Acetylcholinesterase, 555-557
Acetylsalicylic acid, 903, *903*, 904-905
Achlorhydria, 998-999, 1000
Acid-base and electrolyte regulation, 499-531
  acid-base disturbance, 517-526, 518-526*t*
  laboratory tests, 505-517
  physiology, 500-505
  renal function and, 505
  water and electrolyte metabolism, 526-531,
  528*t*, 529*t*, 530*t*
Acid dissociation of HIV-1 antigen-antibody
  complexes, 735
Acid-fast stains, 616-617
Acid hemolysis test, 123
Acidosis
  blood gases, 506
  defined, 517
  metabolic, 518*t*, 520-522, 521*t*, 526*t*
  respiratory, 518*t*, 523-525, 526*t*
Acid phosphatase, 84, 545-546, 559*t*, 1033
Acid-resistant hemoglobin test, 150, 423,
  424-425
Acids, 500, 502-505, 998-1000
Acquired bisalbuminemia, 488-489
Acquired immunodeficiency syndrome (AIDS),
  174, 337
  evaluation of, 363
  HHV-8 in, 728
  P. carinii staining, 618-619
Acral cyanosis, 159

Acridine orange stain, 615-616, 667
Acridinium ester, 673
Actin, in RBC membrane, 71, *71*, 127
Activated coagulation time (ACT), 263
Activated partial thromboplastin time
  (aPTT), 281
Acute hemolytic transfusion reactions, 411-413
Acute intermittent porphyria (AIP), 161, 162*t*,
  163, 955
Acute lymphoblastic leukemia (ALL), 191*t*,
  205-206, 208-209
Acute nonhemolytic transfusion reactions,
  413-415
Acute nonlymphocytic leukemia (ANLL), 182
  vs. ALL, 185*t*
  classifications of, 183*t*, 184-186
  etiology and clinical presentation of, 186
  immunophenotyping in, 190*t*
  lab diagnosis and subtype differentiation,
  186-190, 187*t*, 190*t*, 192
Acute phase proteins/reactants, 497-498,
  497*t*, 608
Acute promyelocytic leukemias, 186
Acute respiratory acidosis, 523
Acute transfusion reactions, 408-415
Addison's disease, 764, 767-770, 768*t*, 767-770
Additive effect, 655, *656*, *657*
Adenosine diphosphate (ADP), 248, 535
Adenosine triphosphate (ATP), 447
  chlamydiae, 646
  creatine kinase, 535
Adenylate cyclase, 739, *740*
Adenylate kinase, 538
Adherence factors, 606-607
Administration routes, drug, 873-875
Adrenal androgens, 758, *758*, 759-760
Adrenal gland, 757-783
  adrenal cortical hormones, 757-764, 774-775
  adrenal cortical malfunction, 764-777
  adrenal medulla, 777-783, 777*t*, *778*, 779*t*
  fetal, 845
  pregnancy and, 850-851
  reference ranges, 761*t*
Adrenal virilism, 774-775
Adrenocorticotrophic hormone (ACTH), 742,
  743, 745
  and aldosterone production, 759

Adrenocorticotrophic hormone (ACTH)
(*Continued*)
Cushing's syndrome, 765, 767
exogenous, Addison's disease, 768-769
glucocorticoid regulation, 758, 761
metabolic effect of, 448*t*
metyrapone test, 764
regulation of, 759-760
Aerobic culture, 638, 673-676
Aeromonas spp. culture, 692
Aerotolerant anaerobes, 631, 635*t*
Afibrinogenemia, 288*t*, 296, 495
Agammaglobulinemia, 337
Agar diffusion, 652-653
Agar dilution, 650-651
Agar disk diffusion test, 652-653
Agar disk elution assay, 654
A genes, subgroups of, 370
Agglutination/agglutination methods, 345, *372,*
433, 880
Aggregation, *243,* 244, *245,* 410-411
Agnogenic myeloid metaplasia (myelofibrosis),
120, 184*t*, 193*t*, 198-200
Agranulocytosis, 179-180
Alanine aminotransferase (ALT), 550, 559*t*
in hepatitis C, 419
in liver disorders, 576-578, 576*t*, 577*t*
reference values, 1056*t*, 1062*t*
Albumin, 480, 481-482, *481,* 482*t*
and calcium, 465
liver disease and, 583, 584*t*
liver function tests, 567*t*
nutritional status assessment, 1025-1026
reference values, 1055*t*, 1062*t*
serum analysis, 485-490, 486*t*
Albumin to globulin (A/G) ratio, 480
Albuterol, theophylline with, 883
Alcohol
and acidosis, 522
and folic acid deficiency, 116
and gamma-glutamyltransferase, 557,
574, 579
and hypoglycemia, 823
platelet disorders from, 313, 314
and porphyrias, 163, 955-956, 957*t*
reference ranges, 1066*t*
thrombocytopenia from, 304
toxicity and monitoring, 911-914, *913,* 1066*t*
and triglycerides, 478
Alder-Reilly anomaly, WBCs in, 87
Aldolase, 550, 559*t*
Aldosterone, 759
hyperaldosteronism, 770-774, 771*t*, 772, 773*t*
pregnancy and, 850-851
Alkaline phosphatase (ALP), 545, 546-549, 559*t*,
810-811
bone metabolism, 802
leukocyte, 84, 96
liver, 573-575, 575*t*, 578*t*, 598, *598,* 599
reference values, 1056*t*, 1062*t*
tumor markers, 1034
Alkalosis
blood gases, 506
defined, 517

metabolic, 518*t*, 522-523, 526*t*
and potassium, 513
respiratory, 518*t*, 525, 526*t*
Allergy, 339-340
Allergy testing, 362-363
Alloimmunization, 378, 437-438
Allopurinol, 458, 459*t*
ALP. *See* Alkaline phosphatase
Alpha-1-acid glycoprotein, 497
Alpha-1-antitrypsin (AAT), 588-589
diagnostic significance of, 483*t*
liver disease and, 583
liver function tests, 567*t*
serum analysis, 490-491
Alpha-1-globulins, 481-482, *481,* 482*t*
Alpha-2-globulins, 481-482, *481,* 482*t*
Alpha-2-macroglobulin, 491-492
Alpha chain disease, 234
Alpha-fetoprotein, 587-588, 1037
and hemochromatosis, 165
liver function tests, 567*t*
neural tube defects, 864-866
Alpha granules, of platelets, 242
Alpha lipoprotein, 493
Alpha-methyldopa
and DAT result, 382
and hemolysis, 155, 156*t*
Alpha-thalassemia, 108*t*, 141, 143-145, 150
Alpha-tocopherol, 1021
Alprazolam, 894, *895*
Aluminum toxicity, 921
Amebiasis, serology, 723, 723*t*
Amenorrhea, 828, 830-831, 833*t*
Amino acids, 458
liver regulation, 581
urinalysis, 959-962, 960*t*
Aminoaciduria, in liver disease, 581
Aminoglycosides, 890, 891
Aminolevulinic acid (ALA), 48-49, 111, 160, 163
Aminolevulinic acid synthetase, 49
Aminotransferases/transaminases, 453, 559*t*
biochemistry and tissue sources, 550-551
diagnostic applications, 551-552, *552*
liver-associated, 567*t*, 576-578, 576*t*, 577*t*
Amiodarone, 887, 890
Amitriptyline, 908, *908*
Ammonia, 458, 567*t*, 581-582, 1062*t*
Amniocentesis, 854-855, 855*t*
Amniotic fluid, 866-869
Amniotic fluid analysis, 425-426, *426*
Amphetamines, 915
Amylase, 447, 553-555, 554*t*, 559*t*, 1007*t*, 1062*t*
Amyloidosis, 233-234, 349
Anacidity, gastric, 998-999
Anaerobic culture, 613, 638-639
Anaerobic metabolism, lactic acidosis, 521-522
Anaerobic susceptibility testing, 654
Analbuminemia, 388
Analgesics, 903-907
Anamnestic response, 330, 378, 415
Anaphylactoid reactions, to transfusions, 414
Ancillary testing, 23-25
Androgens, 759-760
adrenal, 758, *758,* 759-760

gonadal function, 826, 832, 836-837*t*, 838, 838*t*
Anemia(s), 46, 47, 102-103, 108*t*, 1015
  aldolase in, 550
  aplastic, 117, 119-120
  Cooley's, 146-147
  corpuscular indices in, 64-65
  fetal, 1049
  hemorrhagic, 123-125
  hypochromic, 103-111, 108*t*
  hypoproliferative, 117, 118*t*, 119-121
  iron deficiency, 72, 103-108, 104*t*, *106*, 107*t*, 108*t*
  Mediterranean, 141, 146-147.
  nutritional status assessment, 1027-1028
  pernicious, 115-116
  during pregnancy, 848
  refractory, 121-122, 202-203
  sickle cell, 136-137, 138*t*
  sideroblastic, 109-110, 109*t*
  spur cell, 154
Anergic response, 352
Angio-immunoblastic lymphadenopathy, 222
Angiopathic hemolytic anemia, 151-152
Angiotensin, renin-angiotensin system, 771-774, *772*
Angiotensin-converting enzyme (ACE), 555, 772
Animal model toxin assay, 630
Anion, defined, 500
Anion gap, 508*t*, 514-515, 515*t*, 520, 521
Anisocytosis, 67, 68*t*
Ankylosing spondylitis, HLA-B27 and, 439
Ankyrin, RBC membrane, 127
Anovulation, 841
Antagonistic effect, 655, *656*, *657*
Anterior pituitary hormones, 744-749
Antiactin, 358-359, 361
Antiarrhythmics, 886-890
Antiasthmatic drugs, 881-884, *882*
Antibiotics, 649, 890-892
Antibodies, 606
  in ABO system, 370*t*, 371
  antiphospholipid, testing of, 359
  to coagulation factors, 320
  cold, 158, 159
  formation without known stimulation, 378-379
  hemophilia, 294
  hepatitis viruses, 596*t*
  maternal, causing HDN, 428-429
  platelet, 398-399
  production of, 88
  response to antigens, 330-331
  Rh, 376-377
  thrombocytopenia from, 305-306
  thyroid, 791-792
Antibody capture assays, IgM-IgG separation, 703
Antibody-dependent cellular cytotoxicity (ADCC), 84
Antibody detection methods, 700-708
Antibody-mediated acute transfusion reactions, 411-413

Antibody screen, for anti-D antibody, 425
Antibody screening test (indirect antiglobulin test), 383-384, 386-387
Anticardiolipin antibody (ACA), 281, 359
Anticoagulants, natural, 260-262, 260*t*
Anti-coagulation factor VIII antibodies, 294
Anticomplement immunofluorescence (ACIF) tests, 728
Anticonvulsants, and folic acid deficiency, 116
Anti-D antibodies, 376-377, 425
Antidiuretic hormone (ADH), 505, 742, 743, *743*, 751-753, *752*
  diabetes insipidus, 753-754
  SIADH, 754, 756, 757*t*
  urine osmolality and osmolarity, 950-951
  water and electrolyte metabolism, 527-529, 528*t*
Anti-DNA antibody testing, 357
Anti-DNAse B (ADB) test, 709*t*, 710
Antiepileptic drugs, 892-898
Anti-GBM, 361
Antigen-antibody equivalence, 332, 341, *342*
Antigen detection, 663
  body fluids, 667-668, 668*t*
  cutaneous specimens, 694
  eye/ear infections, 697
  gastrointestinal tract specimens, 688-690, *689*
  respiratory tract specimen, 672
Antigenic activity (vWF:Ag), 298
Antigens
  hepatitis viruses, 596*t*
  histocompatibility, 336
  principles of, 330-331
  of Rh system, 374
  sputum, 995*t*
Antiglobulin serum (AHG), in antibody screening test, 387
Antiglobulin test (direct Coombs' test), 158, 159-160
Antihemophilic coagulant factor VIII, in platelet adhesion, 243
Antihemophilic factor (AHF), 238-239*t*, 401-402
Antihuman globulin (Coombs') serum test, 158, 159-160, 379-380, *380*
Antihyaluronidase test (AHT), 709*t*, 710-711
Antimicrobial agents, measurement of levels, 658-659
Antimicrobial agent synergy testing, 655, *656*
Antimicrobial susceptibility testing, 647-659
Antimitochondrial (AMA) antibody, 358, 359, 593
Antineuronal nuclear antibodies (ANNA), 362
Antineutrophil cytoplasmic antibody (ANCA), 361, 593
Antinuclear antibody (ANA) testing, 356-359
Antiphospholipid antibodies (APA), 281, 359
Antiscorbutic factor, vitamin C deficiency, 1019-1020
Anti-smooth muscle antibody (ASMA), 358-359, 361
Antistreptolysin O (ASO) test, 709*t*, 710
Antithrombin III, 261, 319, 483*t*
Antithrombin III deficiency, 276-278
Antithrombins, natural, 260, 260*t*, 261

Apatite arthropathy, 1011
APC ratio, 278
Aplastic anemia, 117, 119-120, 302, 303
Aplastic crisis, 121, 128, 137
Apolipoprotein AI (apoAI), 472
Apolipoprotein B (apoB), 469, 470, 472
Apolipoprotein B100, 469, 470
Apolipoprotein E (ApoE), 469, 470
Apolipoproteins, 468
APT test, 1048
Arcanobacterium haemolyticum, 674
Arterial blood gas measurement, 509
Arthritis, synovial fluid analysis, 1011-1012
Arthrocentesis, 1008-1009
Arthropod vectors, 605
Artifactual hyperalbuminemia, 388
Artifactual thrombocytopenia, 302
Ascites, 485, 1006
Ascorbate-cyanide test, 75, 76
Ascorbic acid, vitamin C deficiency, 1019-1020
Aseptic technique, blood cultures, 609
Aspartate aminotransferase (AST), 550, 559t
  in liver disorders, 576-578, 576t, 577t
  reference values, 1056t, 1062t
Aspergillosis, 678, 719-720, 720t
Aspirin
  and platelet aggregation, 248, 250
  platelet disorders from, 313, 314
  toxicity and monitoring, 903, 903, 904-905
Ataxia telangiectasia, 338t
Atypical creatine kinase isoenzymes, 538
Atypical lymphocyte, 89
Autoantibodies, 592-593
  association with rheumatic diseases, 355t
  and hemolytic anemia, 155
  liver, 592-593
  measurement of, 355-362
  organ-specific, 359-362, 360t
  thrombocytopenia from, 305
  thyroid, 791-792, 793t
Autohemolysis, 72-73, 130
Autoimmune chronic active hepatitis
  (AICAH), 592
Autoimmune diseases, 439, 592, 797
Autoimmune hemolytic anemia (AIHA),
  155-156, 157, 158-160
  classification of causes of, 156t
  DAT in, 381-382
  and thrombocytopenia, 309
Autoimmune neutropenia, 178
Autoimmune thrombocytopenia, 302, 307-309,
  308t
Autoimmunity, 339, 360
Autologous transfusion, 404-405
Autosomal aneuploidy, 858
Avidin-enzyme conjugate, 624
Azo dye reaction, bilirubin, 939t
Azotemia, 454, 456t, 530
Azurophilic granules, leukocytes, 86

Bacterial catalase and oxidase reactions, 631,
  632-636t
Bacterial contamination of transfused blood,
  409, 410

Bacterial cultures, 630-641, 632-636t
Bacterial diarrhea, mechanisms of, 687t
Bacterial gram stain morphology, 631, 632-636t
Bacterial infections
  respiratory specimens for optimal diagnosis,
    994t
  serology, 709-716, 709t, 714t, 715
  susceptibility testing, 650
Bacteriocins, 604
Band cells, 39, 43t, 83
B antigen, 367, 368, 373
Barbiturates, 892, 892, 894-895
Base, defined, 501
Basophil cells, 744
Basophilia, conditions causing, 93t
Basophilic erythroblast, 44
Basophilic stippling, 45, 67
Basophils, 38, 43t, 85
B-cell ALL, 208
B-cell growth factors, liver disease and, 583
Bence-Jones protein test, 227, 349
Benign chronic neutropenia, 178
Benign monoclonal gammopathy, 233
Bentiromide urinary excretion tests, 990-991
Bentonite flocculation test, 723t, 725
Benzidine, 937t, 982, 984
Benzodiazepines, 894, 907
Bernard-Soulier syndrome, 243, 249
Beta-adrenergic agents, theophylline with, 883
Beta globulins, 481-482, 481, 482t
Beta-hydroxybutyric acid, 521
Beta-lactamase test, 653
Beta lipoprotein, 492
  abetalipoproteinemia, hemolysis with, 154
  liver disease and, 583
  serum analysis, 493
Beta-lipotropin, 745
Beta-thalassemia, 108t, 141-148
Beta-thromboglobulin, 242, 249
Bicarbonate
  acid-base disturbances, compensations for,
    526t
  anion gap, 514-515, 515t
  critical value of, 24t
  laboratory measurement, 505-512, 508, 508t
  metabolic acidosis, hyperchloremic, 520,
    521t
  metabolic alkalosis, 523
  nutritional status assessment, 1025
  reference values, 508t, 1062t
  respiratory acidosis, 523-524
  secretin and, 1001-1002
Bicarbonate/carbonic acid buffering system,
  503, 523-524
Bicarbonate ion concentration, 505-506
Bile acids, liver function tests, 567t
Bile salts, 571-573, 572
Bile staining, ascites, 1006, 1008
Biliary obstruction, serum protein changes, 584
Biliary secretions, duodenal fluid, 1002
Biliary system, 566, 568-569
  bile salts, 571-573
  bilirubin, 568-569
  obstructive disease enzymes, 573-575, 575t

pathophysiologic changes, 569-571, *570, 572*
physiology, 566, 568, *568*
Bilirubin, 459-462, 461*t*, 1062*t*
  and albumin, 489
  biliary physiology, 566, 567*t*, 568-569
  critical value of, 24*t*
  CSF, 967
  direct (conjugated), 81, 460, 461, 461*t*, 566, 567*t*, 568-569
  fetal, 855, 866-867
  hepatocyte dysfunction and, 575
  indirect (unconjugated), 81, 460, 461, 461*t*, 568-569
  intravascular hemolysis and, 81
  liver function tests, 567*t*
  liver transplant monitoring, 598, 598, 599
  measurement of, 460-461
  neonate, hemolytic disease of newborn, 427
  nutritional status assessment, 1027
  urinalysis, 931t, 939t, 954, 954t
Bilirubinuria, tests for, 939t
Binet staging system, for chronic lymphocytic leukemia, 211t
Bioassays, antimicrobial agent levels, 658-659
Biochemical testing, fungi, 642-643
Biopsy, 41-42, 586-587, 611
Biotinylated antibody, 624
Biphasic agar/broth culture, 665-666
Bisalbuminemia, 488
Bladder tumor antigen, 1040-1041
Blastomycosis, serology, 720, 720t
Bleeding
  chronic, and iron deficiency, 106
  platelet function and, 245-246
  traumatic, CSF, 971
Bleeding disorders, 314-315, 316t, 317-320
Bleeding time test, 249-257, 272t
Blister cell, in G-6-PD deficiency, 133
Blood
  composition of, 31
  in CSF, 969-970, 971, 972t
  microbiology specimen collection and transport, 609-610
  in serous fluid, 1003, 1005
  in stool, 982, 984, 985-986t, 987
  in urine, 669-670, 930, 933t, 934, 965
Blood-brain barrier, 967
Blood coagulation, 446, 494
Blood component therapy, 389, 394-406
  cellular components in, 389, 394-400, 395t
  indications and complications of, 391-393t, 396t
  irradiated blood products in, 405-406
  plasma components in, 400-404, 402t, 403t
Blood gases
  acid-base disturbances, compensations for, 526t
  laboratory measurement, 505-510, 508, 508t
  reference values for, 508t, 1062t
Blood groups, 367-387, 366t
  ABO, 367-371, 370t, 373
  antibody formation without known stimulation and, 378-379
  antibody screening test and, 383-384, 383t, 384t, 386-387
  Coombs' test and, 379-380, 380
  direct antiglobulin test and, 381-383, 381t
  red cell alloimmunization and, 378
  Rh, 373-374, 376-377
Blood loss, and anemia, 124-125
Blood order schedule, 385t
Blood products, selection of, 388-389
Blood samples
  anticoagulant, and fibrinogen, 494
  plasma and serum, 446
  pre- and posttransfusion, 413
Bloodstream infections
  specimen collection and transport, 609-610
  microbiology, 609-610, 661-667
Blood urea nitrogen (BUN), 454-454, 454t, 1062t
  in liver disease, 567t, 581-582
  normal values, neonates, 1055t
  nutritional status assessment, 1025
  prerenal causes of uremia, 946-947
Blood urea nitrogen (BUN):creatinine ratio, 947-948
B lymphocytes, 39, 88, 205, 606
  disorders of, 204
  HLA antigens and, 431
  humoral immunity, 87, 88, 328-330
BMC chemstrip test for bilirubinuria, 939t
Body cavity (parietal) membrane, 1002
Body fluids, 924-1013. See also specific body fluids
  bactericidal activity determination, 655-658
  microbiology specimen collection and transport, 610
  serous fluids, 1002-1013
  specimens, 662t, 667-669, 668t
Body water regulation, 751-753, *752*
BOHB (beta-hydroxybutyric acid), 521, 522
Bombay phenotype, 369
Bone
  alkaline phosphatase, 548-549, 548t
  hormonal regulation of mineral turnover in, 799, *799*
  vitamin D deficiency and, 1020-1021
Bone disorders, 464-465, 465t, *559t, 805*, 806
Bone marrow
  aspiration and biopsy, 41-42
  cell-to-fat ratio of, 42
  cytologic evaluation of, 43-44
  differential cell counts of, 43t
  direct sampling of, 40-43
  response to acute blood loss, 124
Bone marrow examination
  ALL, 206
  anemia classification, 103
  hairy cell leukemia, 212
  neutropenia evaluation, 177-178
  thrombocytopenia, 302
Bone marrow failure syndromes, 117, 118t, 119-121, 302
Bone marrow iron, in iron deficiency, 107
Bone marrow replacement, and pancytopenia, 120

Bone marrow transplantation, cyclosporine for, 437, 900-901
Bone mineral density (BMD), 810, 811
Bordetella pertussis culture, 674-675
Borrelia burgdorferi, 709t, 714t, 715-716
Bradykinin, in coagulation cascade, 253
Brain, marker enzymes, 536, 538, 559t
Bromosulphophthalein (BSP) test, 567t
Bronchoalveolar lavage (BAL), 611, 993
Bronze skin, in hemochromatosis, 164
Broth culture, blood, 663-666
Broth-disk elution procedure, 654
Brown recluse spider bite, hemolysis in, 153
BSP excretion test, 567t
Buffering acid solution, 502-504
Buffering system, respiratory acidosis, 523-524
Buffer pair, defined, 501
BUN:creatinine ratio, 456, 456t, 947-948
Burkitt's lymphoma, 206, 220, 222
Burns, hemolytic anemia with, 152-153
Burst-forming unit-erythroid (BFU-E), 35
Burst-promoting activity (BPA), 35
B variant, in G-6-PD deficiency, 131

Cachectin (tumor necrosis factor), 608-609, 1029, 1032
Cachexia, albumin in, 485, 487
Calcitonin, 464, 800, 803-804, 1033
Calcium, 462-467, *463*, 465t, 1062t
  albumin binding, 489
  anion gap, 514-515, 515t
  clinical consideration, 464-466, 465t
  conditions affecting, 465t
  critical value of, 24t
  CSF, 976
  disorders causing decreased, 806-808, 808t, 809t
  disorders causing increased, 804-806, *805*, 808t, 809t
  ionized, 256, 801
  measurement, 466-467
  metabolism, 464, 798, 803t, 809t
  neonate reference values, 1055t
  nutritional status assessment, 1025-1026
  vitamin D deficiency and, 1020-1021
Calcium infusion, calcitonin secretion, 1033
Calcium oxalate stones, 963, 964t, 965t, 966
Calcium phosphate stones, 963, 964t, 965t, 966
Calcium pyrophosphate crystals, synovial fluid, *1013*
Calcofluor white stain, 617-618
Calorie deficiency, 1015
cAMP, 802-803, 883
cAMP-dependent protein kinases, 739, *740*
Campylobacter jejuni culture, 691-692
Cancer, 550, 806
Cancer antigens, 1039-1040
Candida albicans, 678, 681, *682*, 686
Candida serology, 720t, 721
Cannabinoids, 916-917
Carbamazepine, 1066t
  and agranulocytosis, 179
  monitoring and toxicology, 892, 896

Carbohydrate antigens, tumor markers, 1039-1040
Carbohydrate challenge, 451-452
Carbohydrate malabsorption, screening test for, 989
Carbohydrate metabolism, 447-452, 584, 851
Carbon dioxide partial pressure, 506.
  acid-base disturbances, 526t
  reference values, 508t, 1062t
  respiratory control of, 503-504
Carbon monoxide, 917-918
Carcinoembryonic antigen (CEA), 588, 1035-1037
Carcinoid syndrome, 962
Cardiac glycosides, 884-887, *885*
Cardiac injury indicators, 535-545
Cardiac troponin, 543-544
Cardiolipin antigen, in syphilis, 712-713
Carotene, 988-989, *989*, 990, 1017
Carrier proteins, serum analysis, 497
Cary-Blair transport medium, 611
Castenada bottle, 665-666
Casts, urinalysis, 934, 939, 940, 941t, 942
Catecholamine metabolism, 778-779, *778*, 779t
Catecholamines, 777-781
Catheterized specimens, urine, 610
Cations, 500, 504-505.
CD antigens, acute leukemias, 185t, 191t
Celiac disease, 116, 361, 989
Celite, 263
Cell culture passage, viruses, 644-646
Cell-mediated immunity, 88, 604
  and autoantibodies, 360
  deficiencies of, 337, 338t
  measurement of, 352
  principles of, 334-336
Cellular adhesion molecules, and neutrophils, 38
Cellular assays for HLAs, 434
Central nervous system, 525, 757t
Cephalosporins, 890
Cerebrospinal fluid (CSF), 966-978, 1064t
  anatomy and physiology, 966-967
  antigen detection tests, 667-668
  bloody tap, 971-972
  cell count, 971, 972t
  chemistry, 973-976, 974t
  clotting, 970
  cryptococcus, 972-973
  electrophoresis, 484
  general appearance, 969
  indications for lumbar puncture, 967-978
  leukocyte differential, 972, 972t
  microorganisms, 976-977
  normal, 969t
  oligoclonal banding in, 495-496
  patient-care considerations, 977
  pressure, 967, 968, 969t, 970-971
  specimen collection, 977-978
  transferrin, 494
Ceruloplasmin, 497, 589-590
  diagnostic significance of, 483t
  liver function tests, 567t
  in pregnancy, 849

Chain of custody, drug screening, 911
Checkerboard titration method, 655, *656*
Chediak-Higashi syndrome, 87, 172, 173-174
Chemiluminescence, in phagocytosis assessment, 172
Chemistry
    bilirubin, 459-462, 461*t*
    calcium, magnesium, and phosphorus, 462-467, *463*, 465*t*
    carbohydrate metabolism, 447-452
    critical values, 24*t*
    CSF, 973-976
    lipids, 472-480
    nonprotein nitrogenous compounds, 452-459, 454*t*, *455*, 456*t*, 459*t*
    nutritional status assessment, 1024-1027
    panel testing, 19-21, 20*t*, 21*t*
    proteins, 480-498
    reference ranges, 1062-1064*t*
    serous fluids, 1005
    serum analysis, 445-447
Chemokines, and granulopoiesis, 37
Chemotactic factors, and neutrophils, 38
Chemotaxis, neutrophil, 84
    defective, 169-172
    stages of adherence to vascular endothelial cells, *171*
Chemotherapeutic and immunosuppressive agents
    cyclosporine, 900-903, *901*
    methotrexate, 116, 339, 898-900, *899*, 1066*t*
Chemotherapy
    for ALL, 209
    for ANLL, 190, 192
    for CLL, 212
    and immunosuppression, 339
CH50 hemolytic assay, 350
Chlamydia, 612, 646-647
    cultures, 643-647, *645*, *646*, 676, 683-685
    respiratory specimens for optimal diagnosis, 994*t*
Chlordiazepoxide, 907
Chloride
    anion gap, 514-515, 515*t*
    CSF, 976
    hyperchloremic acidosis, 520
    measurement of, 510-512
    metabolic alkalosis, 523
    reference values, 508*t*, 1062*t*
Chloroacetate esterase, 97
Chlorpromazine, 907
Cholecystokinin, 1002
Cholesterol, 467
    diet and, 478
    exogenous pathway, 469
    lipoprotein phenotypes, 476*t*
    measurement of, 472
    reference values, 1057*t*, 1062-1063*t*
    thyroid hormones and, 785, 786
Cholesterol fractionation, 472-478, *473*, *475*, 476*t*, 477*t*
Cholesterol gallstones, 571, 1002
Cholinesterase, 555-557
Chorionic gonadotropin, 794, 831

Chorionic villus sampling (CVS), 855-856
Christmas disease, 253, 257, 287, 289*t*, 293*t*
Chromatography, 703, 879
Chromium labeling, red cell survival measurement, 78-79
Chromogenic cephalosporin test, 653
Chromophobe cells, 744
Chromosomal abnormalities/studies
    fetal karyotyping, 857-858, 857*t*
    in leukemias, 98-100, *99*, 192*t*
    in myelodysplastic syndromes, 204
Chronic granulocytic leukemia (CGL), 193
Chronic granulomatous disease (CGD), 172-173
Chronic hemolytic anemia, in favism, 133
Chronic lymphocytic leukemia (CLL), 210-212, 223
Chronic myelogenous leukemia (CML), 184*t*, 193-196, 205
Chronic myelomonocytic leukemia, 184*t*, 203-204
Chronic respiratory disease, respiratory acidosis, 524
Chylomicrons, 468, 469, *469*, 472, 493
    composition of, 473*t*, 474
    diet and, 478
    lipoprotein phenotypes, 476*t*
Ciliated epithelial cells, 604
Cinchonism, 889
Circulating immune complexes (CICs), measurement of, 351
Circulating pool, in granulopoiesis, 38
Circulatory system
    adrenal hormones, measurement of, 760-761
    hepatic lactate dehydrogenase release, 580
    liver disorders, 565-566
    overload, as transfusion complication, 409
Cirrhosis
    alkaline phosphatase, 575*t*
    aminotransferases in, 578*t*
    defined, 586
    serum protein changes, 584
Citrate, and hypocalcemia, 806
Class I HLA antigens, 430, *432*
Class II HLA antigens, 430-431, *432*, 433
Clear agar-based media, mycobacteria, 641
Clearance tests, urinalysis, 942, 943-947, 945*t*, 946*t*, 947*t*
Clonal line of plasma cells, 328
Clonidine suppression test, 780-781
Clostridial infections, hemolysis in, 153
Clostridium difficile, 629, 690, 692, 891
Clotting, 446, 494, 970
Coagulase test, 635*t*, 637
Coagulation factor disorders, 284-301, 401-404, 1051*t*
Coagulation factors, 256-258
    contact (factor XI, factor XII), 252
    detection by PCR, *280*
    factor I (fibrinogen), 256, 288*t*
    factor II (prothrombin), 238-239*t*, 254, 288*t*, 317*t*, 584, 585
    factor III (tissue factor/tissue thromboplastin), 238-239*t*, 253, 255, *255*, 256
    factor IV (ionized calcium), 256

Coagulation factors (*Continued*)
  factor V, 256-257, 288*t*
  factor V Leiden, 257, 262, *280*
  factor VII (proconvertin), 253, *255*, 267, 288*t*, 317*t*, 584, 585
  factor VIII, 253, 298, 299*t*, 301*t*, 320
  factor VIII concentrates, 292*t*, 293*t*, 294, 295*t*, 401, 402-403
  factor VIII deficiency (hemophilia A), 287, 289*t*, 292*t*
  factor IXa, 253
  factor IX (Christmas factor), 238-239*t*, 253, 255, 257, 287, 289*t*, 293*t*, 584, 585
  factor IX products, 293*t*, 294, 295*t*, 404
  factor X (Stuart factor/Stuart-Prower factor), 238-239*t*, 253-258, 289*t*, 317*t*, 584, 585
  factor XI, 252, 253, 258, 289*t*, 297
  factor XII (Hageman factor), 238-239*t*, 252, 253, 290*t*, 297, 317*t*
  factor XIII (fibrin stabilizing factor), 238-239*t*, 258, 268, 290*t*
  inhibitory antibodies to, 320
  nomenclature and characteristics of, 238-239*t*
Coagulation studies, 262-268, 286-287, 1028, 1061*t*
Coagulation system
  calcium and, 463
  coagulation cascade, *251*, 252-259
  fibrinogen, 494-495
  Lp(a) and, 472
  vitamin K, 1021-1022
Coagulopathies, 272*t*
Coccidioidomycosis, serology, 720*t*, 721-722
Colchicine, in gout, 458
Cold agglutinins (CA) test, mycoplasmal infections, 709*t*, 717
Cold antibodies, 158, 159
Cold autoantibody hemolytic syndromes, 159-160
Cold reactive autoimmune hemolytic anemia, DAT test in, 381, 382
Collagen-vascular disorders, thrombocytopenia in, 309
Colony-count streaking method, 638
Colony-forming units (CFUs), 33, 35, 37
Colony-stimulating factors (CSFs), 35, 37
Color, urine, 927, 928*t*, 929, 930
Colorimetric filtration, urine, 670
Comatose patient, 820*t*, 909-911
Complement, 84, 333-334, 350-351, 494, 605, 606
Complement fixation (CF) tests, 704-705, *705*, 709*t*, 717, 720*t*, 722
Complete blood count (CBC), 62*t*, 1060*t*, 1027
Congenital adrenal hyperplasia, 774-775
Congenital infection, 701, 729
Conjugated (direct) bilirubin, 81, 460, 461, 461*t*, 566, 567*t*, 568-569
Conn's syndrome, 759, 764-765, 770
Consumption coagulopathy, 314, 316*t*
Continuously monitored broth culture, blood, 665
Control suspension, PA antigen detection assay, 622

Cooley's anemia, 146-147
Coombs-negative immune-mediated hemolytic anemia, 158
Coombs' test, 379-380, *380*
  for hemolytic anemia, 158, 159-160
  indirect, 383-384, 383*t*, 384*t*, 386-387
Copper, ceruloplasmin, 589-590
Coproporphyrin, 160
Coproporphyrinogen, 49
Coronary artery disease (CAD), lipids and, 478-479
Corpuscular indices, 64-65
Cortex, renal, 925-926
Cortisol, 758, *758*
  adrenal virilism, 774-775
  binding proteins, 758, 850
  Cushing's syndrome, 765, 766*t*, 767
  metabolic effect of, 448*t*
  pregnancy and, 850
Corynebacterium diphtheriae culture, 674
Counterimmunoelectrophoresis (CIE), 343, 703-704
C-reactive protein (CRP), 359, 497*t*, *608*
Creatine kinase (CK), 534, 535-539, 536*t*, *537*, 559*t*, 1063*t*
  cardiac injury markers, 544, 545
  creatinine clearance, 944
  neonate and pediatric patient normal values, 1056*t*
  during pregnancy, 852, 853
  tumor markers, 1033-1034
Creatine phosphate (CP), 455, *455*, 535
Creatine phosphokinase (CPK), 535, 944. *See also* Creatine kinase
Creatinine, 455-456, *455*, 456*t*, 956, 1063*t*
  amniotic fluid, 869
  BUN/creatinine ratio, 947-948
  nutritional status assessment, 1025
  urinalysis, 958
Creatinine clearance, 456, 946*t*
Cretinism, 785, 792
Crigler-Najjar syndrome, 460, 461*t*
Crossmatching, transfusion medicine, 384, 384*t*, 386-387
Cryoglobulins, in multiple myeloma, 231, *231*
Cryoprecipitate, 294, 402*t*
Cryoprecipitated antihemophilic factor (AHF), 401-402
Cryptococcus, CSF, 972-973
Cryptococcus neoformans, 618, 678
Cryptosporidium parvum, 688
Crystal-induced arthritis, 1011
Crystals, 927, 930, 934, 1012*t*
Cultures, 630-647
  bloodstream pathogens, 663-667
  body fluids, 668-669
  cutaneous specimen, 694-695
  for cytomegalovirus, 729
  eye/ear infections, 697-698
  genital tract specimens, 684-685
  respiratory tract specimen, 673-679
  specimen collection and transport, 609-613
  sputum, 995*t*

urine, 670
wound, tissue/biopsy specimens, 695-696
Cushing's syndrome, 763, 764, 765-767, 766*t*
Cutaneous specimens, 662, 693-695
Cyanide nitroprusside test, 961
Cyanocobalamin, 51. *See also* Vitamin B$_{12}$
Cyclic adenosine monophosphate, 802-803, 883
Cyclic neutropenia, 178
Cycloheximide, 642
Cyclospora cayetanensis, microscopy, 688
Cyclosporine, 900-903, *901*, 1066*t*
Cystathionine beta-synthase, 961
Cysticercosis, serology, 723*t*, 724
Cystic fibrosis, 675, 863-864, 1012-1013
Cystine stones, 964, 964*t*, 965*t*, 966
Cystinosis, 962
Cystinuria, 959-960, 961, 966
Cytapheresis, 406-408*t*
Cytochrome oxidase, 631
Cytokines, 608-609
  and granulopoiesis, *37*
  in hematopoiesis, 34, 34*t*
  in transfusion reactions, 413, 414
Cytomegalovirus
  serology, 727*t*, 729
  transfusion-transmitted, 420, 421*t*
Cytopathic effect (CPE), 645-646, *645*
Cytotoxicity testing, for HLAs, 433
Cytotoxicity toxin assay, 629, 629*t*
Cytotoxic killer lymphocytes, 88, 334

Delayed transfusion reactions, 382-383, 408, 409*t*, 415-416
Delta OD 450*t* test, 425-426, *426*
Demyelinating disorders, oligoclonal banding in, 495-496
Deoxyadenosylcobalamin, 51, *52*
Dermatophytes, 641, 693-694
Desipramine, 908
Desmopressin, hemophilia, 293*t*
Dexamethasone suppression test, 761, 762*t*, 763-764, 767
Diabetes insipidus, 753-754, 755*t*, 756
Diabetes mellitus, 812-823
  abnormalities of diabetic control, 521, 818-823
  classification, 813-814, 814*t*
  diagnosis, 814-817
  glycosylated albumin, 490
  in hemochromatosis, 164
  HLA antigens in, 439
  infection, fungal, 678-679
  monitoring control, 817-818
  pregnancy, estriol fluctuations, 845-846
Diabetic ketoacidosis, 521, 819, 820*t*
Diagnostic peritoneal lavage (DPL), 1008
Diarrhea, 687*t*, 980, 982, 983*t*
Diastase (amylase), 552-555, 554*t*, 1007*t*, 1062*t*
Diazepam, 892, 894, *895*, 907
Diazo reaction, for bilirubinuria, 939*t*
Diet, 469, 480, 558, 988-991
Dietary lipid pathway, 469
Differential media, 630
Diffuse basophilia (polychromasia), 67

Diffuse histiocytic lymphoma, 218, 220
Diffuse large-cell lymphoma, 218, 220
Digoxin, 306, 884-887, *885*, 1066*t*
2,3-Diphosphoglycerate (2,3-DPG), *74*, 77, 507-508, *507*
Direct antiglobulin test (DAT), 380-383
Direct (conjugated) bilirubin, 460, 461, 461*t*, 569
Direct fluorescent antibody (DFA) assays, 706-707
Direct immunofluorescence assays (DFA), 347, 621
Disease association with HLA antigens, 438-439
Disopyramide, 887, 888
Disseminated intravascular coagulation (DIC), 151, 314-315, 317-318, 495
  as acute transfusion reaction, 412
  clinical findings in, 315
  inciting events of, 315, 317, 317*t*
  lab diagnosis of, 317-318
  management of, 318
  pathophysiology of, 315
  profile of, 316*t*
Dissociation, 500-502
Distal convoluted tubule, 925
Distribution space, 874
Diuretics, and urate excretion, 458, 459*t*
Diurnal variation, 17
Diversity (D) encoding regions, immuno-globulin, 326
DNA-based methods
  fetal cells, 1049, 1049*t*
  for HLAs, 434
  in oncology, 1043-1046, *1044*, *1045*, 1046*t*
  prenatal diagnosis, 862
  RFLP, paternity testing, *440*
DNA probe, mycobacteria, 677
Döhle bodies, 86
Donath-Landsteiner test, 160
Dopamine, 779, 779*t*
Double diffusion, 341
Double-stranded nucleic acids, viral, 643
Downey cells, 89, 181
Down syndrome (trisomy 21), 857*t*, 858, 866
Drug monitoring and toxicology, 873-921
  analgesics, 903-907
  antiasthmatic drugs, 881-884, *882*
  antibiotics, 890-892
  antiepileptic drugs, 892-898
  cardiac drugs, 884-890
  chemotherapeutic and immunosuppressive agents, 898-903
  drugs of abuse, 909-917
  methods of drug analysis, 878-881
  patient evaluation and specimen collection, 909-911
  poisoning, 917-921
  principles of drug kinetics, 873-876, *874*, *875*
  psychiatric drugs, 907-909, *910*
  reasons for monitoring, 876-878, *877*
  reference ranges, 1066*t*
Drugs
  and adrenal function tests, 763, 764, 775, 776, 781-782
  albumin binding, 489

Drugs *(Continued)*
  antibodies, and DAT result, 382
  drug-induced hemolysis, 155-159
  and ferric chloride test, 960*t*
  hematologic complications
    and agranulocytosis, 179
    aplastic anemia from, 117, 118*t*, 119
    causing hemolytic anemia, 153, 156*t*
    causing neutropenia and agranulocytosis,
      180*t*
    platelet disorders from, 285, 312-313,
      313*t*, 314
    and thrombocytopenia from, 306-307,
      303-304
  and hypocalcemia, 807
  lipid control, 480
  metabolites, urinalysis, 963
  and neutrophil chemotaxis, 172
  for osteoporosis, 811
  and prolactin levels, 749
  serum chemistry, 445-446
  and sexual function, 840*t*
  and SIADH, 757*t*
  and thyroid hormones, 785, 796*t*
  and urate excretion, 458, 459*t*
Drug screening, 914-917, 914*t*
Dubin-Johnson syndrome, 460, 461*t*
Duffy antigen, malaria, 153
Duodenal fluid, 1001-1002
Dysfibrinogenemias, 288*t*, 296-297, 495
Dysmorphic red cells, in urine, 934
Dysproteinemias, platelet disorders
  from, 314

Ear infections, 696-698
Eating disorders, 1016
Ecchymoses, 237, 286
Echinococcosis serology, 724-725
Ectopic hormone secretion, 1032
Effusion, fluid accumulation, 1003, *1004*
Ehrlichia spp. serology, 718
Ehrlich's aldehyde reaction test, 939*t*
Ehrlich's reagent, 163, 954
Electrolytes
  antidiuretic hormone and, 505
  digoxin and, 886
  excretion of, 949*t*
  ions and dissociation, 500
  laboratory measurement, 510-515, 515*t*
  measurement of, 510-512
  normal reference values for, 508*t*
  nutritional status assessment, 1025
  panel composition, 22*t*
  sweat, 1013
  transfusions and, 411
Electrophoresis
  hemoglobin, 149-150
  lipoprotein, *475*
  lysozyme, 560
  serum proteins, 481-482, *481, 482*, 482*t*, 484*t*
Elementary body, chlamydiae, 646
Elliptical cells, 68*t*, 130
Embden-Meyerhof glycolytic pathway,
  73, 74, 75

Emphysema, alpha-1-antitrypsin and, 490,
  491, 589
Endocrine markers of malignancy, 1032-1033
Endocrine tests, 739-823
  adrenal, 757-783
  adrenal cortical malfunction, 764-777
  adrenal medulla, 777-783, 777*t*, *778, 779t*
  anterior pituitary hormones, 744-749
  general principles, 739-742
  hypothalamic hormones, 743-744, 744*t*
  neonates, 1057
  pancreas, 811-823
  panhypopituitarism, 749-751
  parathyroid gland, 798-811
  pituitary-hypothalamic axis, 742-743, *743*
  posterior pituitary hormones, 751-757*t*
  reproductive system, 849-851, 850*t*, 854*t*
  thyroid gland, 783-798
Endogenous flora, 606
  GI tract, 460, 604, 1022
  vaginal, 605, 685
Endogenous infectious agents, 604
Endogenous lipid pathway, 469-470, *470*
Endoscopic retrograde cholangiopancreatography (ERCP), 1002
Endotracheal aspirate collection and transport, 611
Energy metabolism, 464, 746
Enterococcus, antimicrobial susceptibility tests,
  649, 651, 652
Entry routes of infection, 603-605
Enzymatic assays, 450, 913-914
Enzyme immunoassays (EIAs), 346, 707-708
  blastomycosis, 720, 720*t*
  GI specimens, 688-690
  microbial antigens, 623-625, 624*t*
  microbial toxins, 629
  mycoplasmal infections, 709*t*, 717
  parasite infections, 723-725
  varicella virus infections, 728
  virus infections, 727*t*, 729, 731, 734
Enzyme-linked immunosorbent assay (ELISA),
  60, 345-346, 417-418
Enzymes
  CSF, 974*t*, 976
  fructose deficiency, 452
  neonate and pediatric normal values,
    1056*t*
  nutritional status assessment, 1026
Enzymes, diagnostic markers, 445, 533-560
  cardiac injury indicators, 535-545
  general principles, 533-534
  liver disease, 547-551*t*, 559*t*, 575-580
  malignancy/tumor markers, 545-546, 1032
  miscellaneous, 545-560
Enzymopathies, 130-134. *See also specific entities*
Eosinophils, 38, 43*t*, 84-85, 93*t*, 1050*t*, 1060*t*
Epinephrine
  functions, 777, 777*t*
  metabolic effect of, 448*t*
  normal lab values for, 779*t*
  theophylline with, 883
Epithelial cells, 869, 930, 988
Epitope, 330, 331

Epstein-Barr virus (EBV)
  antigens, 727*t*, 730, *730*
  and infectious mononucleosis, 181
  serology, 727*t*, 729-730, *730*
  transfusion-transmitted, 420
Equivalence, antigen-antibody, 332, 341, *342*
Error, sources of, 17-19
Erythroblastosis fetalis, 421, 422
Erythrocytapheresis, defined, 406
Erythrocyte sedimentation rate (ESR), 93-95,
  94*t*, 608, 1060*t*
Erythrocytosis, 160, 161*t*, 196, 197
Erythroleukemia, 188
Erythromycin, 890
Erythron, 36, 47
Erythropoiesis, 35-36
  ineffective, 36, 46, 121-123
  laboratory evaluation of, 44-47
  stem cells in, 35
Erythropoietic porphyrias, 161, 162*t*, 163, 955,
  956*t*, 957*t*
Erythropoietin, 35, 37, 46-47
Escherichia coli, 690, 692-693
Essential thrombocythemia (ET), 184*t*, 193*t*,
  200-202
Esterase, leukocyte, 97
Esterase stains, 89
Estradiol, 828, 829*t*, 833-835*t*
Estriol, 828, 829*t*, 845
Estrogen, 826, 828, 830
Estrogen receptors (ER) as tumor markers,
  1041-1042
Estrone, 828, 829*t*
Ethanol toxicity and monitoring, 911-914, *913*,
  1066*t*
Ethosuximide, *892*, 894-895, 1066*t*
Euglobulin lysis time, 270-271
Euthyroid sick syndrome, 795-796
Exchange transfusion, neonatal, 427-428, 428*t*
Exercise, and creatine kinase, 536
Exposure routes, 603-605
Extractable nuclear antigen (ENA) testing,
  356, 357
Extramedullary hematopoiesis, 70
Extrinsic coagulation, 251, 253-254
Exudates, 1003, *1004*, 1004*t*, 1007*t*, 1008, 1009*t*

FAB classification of lymphoblastic leuke-
  mias, 206, 207*t*
Facultative anaerobes, 631, 633-635*t*
Fanconi's syndrome, 948, 959-960, 962
Fasting hypoglycemia, 822-823
Fatty acids, 447, 467, 468, 489
Febrile nonhemolytic transfusion reaction
  (FNHTR), 395-396, 413-414
Fecal analysis, 978-991
Feedback control of hormone secretion, 742
Female gonadal function, 826-835*t*
Ferric chloride test, 939*t*, 960, 960*t*
Ferritin, 57, 59, 493
  in differential diagnosis of hypochromic mi-
    crocytic anemia, 108*t*
  hemochromatosis, 165*t*
  in iron deficiency, *106*, 107

liver function tests, 567*t*
  normal values of, 58*t*, 1063*t*
Fetal blood, percutaneous umbilical cord sampling, 855, 1048-1051, 1049*t*, 1050*t*, 1053*t*
Fetal hemoglobin (hemoglobin F), 50, 508
  developmental changes in, *144*
  elevated, conditions associated with, 140*t*
  hereditary persistence of, 139-140
Fetal lung maturity, 426, 867-868, 869
Fetomaternal hemorrhage (FMH), 425
Fetus, prenatal assessment of, 854-869
Fever, and theophylline metabolism, 884
Fibrin
  coagulation cascade and, 252
  degradation products, 269, 314, 318
  in hemostasis, 237
Fibrin-fibrinogen split products, 314, 495
Fibrin monomer, 252, 266-267
Fibrinogen (factor I), 256, 266, 288*t*
  degradation products (FDPs), 269-270,
    314, 318
  disorders of, 296-297
  in hemostasis, 237
  nomenclature and characteristics of, 238-239*t*
  serum analysis, 494-495
Fibrinolysis, 259-260
  in DIC, 318
  in hemostasis, 237
  tests of, 269-271, 269*t*, 273
Fibrinopeptides, 252, 266-267, 318
Fibrin split products (FSP), 314, 495
Fibrin stabilizing factor (FSF), 238-239*t*, 258,
  268, 290*t*
Fibronectin, 605, 606
Fitzgerald factor, 238-239*t*, 253, 290*t*, 297
FK506 binding protein, 901, *901*
Flavin adenine dinucleotide (FAD), 1018
Fletcher factor, 238-239*t*, 290*t*, 297
Flow cytometry, 188, *189*, 353, *354*
Fluorescence polarization assay, 868, 880-881
Fluorescent in situ hybridization (FISH),
  857, 1045-1046
Fluorescent treponemal antibody-absorbed
  double stain (FTA-ABS DS) test, 709*t*,
  713, 714, *715*
Fluorochrome stain, 616-617
Fluoxetine, 909, *910*
Foam stability index (FSI), fetal lung matu-
  rity, 868
Folic acid, 51-56, 1019
Folic acid antagonists, 116
Folic acid deficiency, 54-55, 111-117,
  899-890, *899*
Folinic acid (leucovorin), 116, 899-900, *899*
Follicle-stimulating hormone (FSH), 742, *743*,
  825, 1063*t*
  in females, 826-827, 833-835*t*
  in males, 826, 836-837*t*
  normal serum levels, 829*t*
  pubertal and senescent changes, 828, 829*t*
Follicular lymphomas, 217-218, 220
Formed elements, urinalysis, 930, 934, 939-942*t*
Formiminoglutamic acid (FIGLU), 55, 55*t*
Fouchet's test for bilirubinuria, 939*t*

Four-quadrant streaking method, 638
Free erythrocyte protoporphyrin (FEP), 60, 107, 108*t*
Free thyroxine index (FTI), 788, *789*, 794, 795
Fresh frozen plasma (FFP), indications for, 401, 402*t*
Fungal infections, 641-643, *643*, *644*, 694
   microscopic examination of specimens, 617, 618
   respiratory, 677-679, 994*t*
   serology, 718-722, 720*t*
   skin, 693
   susceptibility testing, 654-655

Galactosemia, 452
Gallbladder, 564
Gallstones, 571, 1002
Gamma globulins, 481-482, *481*, *482*, 482*t*
Gamma-glutamyl transferase/transpeptidase (GGT), 557, 574
   in cadmium toxicity, 921
   in liver disorders, 578*t*, 579
   reference values, 1056*t*, 1063*t*
Gardnerella vaginalis cultures, 685-686
Gas chromatography (GC), drug analysis, 879
Gases, poisoning, 917-918
Gas liquid chromatography (GLC), alcohol assay, 913
Gastrectomy, and B$_{12}$ deficiency, 116
Gastrin, 997, 999, 1000, 1000*t*
Gastrointestinal tract
   bleeding, conditions associated with, 985-986*t*
   disease, 116, 520, 521*t*, 361, 549, 553, 554*t*, 688
   infection via, 603, 604-605
   protein loss via, 487-488
Gastrointestinal tract specimens, 662*t*, 686-693, 687*t*
   antigen detection, 688-690
   cultures, 691-693
   duodenal fluid, 1001-1002
   gastric contents analysis, 611, 996-1002, 999*t*, 1000*t*
   microscopy, 687-688, *689*
   serology, *Helicobacter pylori*, 716
   toxin detection, 690-691
Gaucher's disease, 176
Genetic code, progression to peptide, *142*
Genetic disorders, 857-858, 857*t*, 859-861*t*, 1049*t*, 1051, 1051*t*
Genital tract specimens, 662*t*, 679-686
   antigen detection, 682-683
   collection of, 612
   culture, 684-686
   microscopy, 680-681, *681*, *682*
   nucleic acid probes, 683-684
Genitourinary tract, infection via, 603, 605
Gentamicin, 890, 891, 1066*t*
Gestational diabetes mellitus (GDM), 814, 815-816
Giardia lamblia antigen detection, 689-690
Gibson and Cook method, 1013
Giemsa (G-banding), 857

Giemsa stain, 615, 619-620, 620*t*
Gilbert's syndrome, 460, 461*t*, 462, 571
Glanzmann's thrombasthenia, 248
Globin, 47, 50
Globulin, 404, 567*t*, 583
Globulin fraction, 480
Glomerular filtrate, substances in, 945*t*
Glomerular filtration rate (GFR), 943
Glomerular pores, 925
Glomerulonephritis, autoantibodies and, 361
Glomerulus, 925
Glucagon, 448*t*, 812
Glucocorticoids, 758-759, *758*
Gluconeogenesis, 468
Glucose
   abnormal levels, causes of, 451, 451*t*
   critical value of, 24*t*
   CSF, 974-975, 974*t*, 975*t*
   diabetic control, 817
   factors affecting control, 813*t*
   growth hormone studies, 748
   liver function tests, 567*t*
   measurement of, 447, 449
   monitoring during pregnancy, 851
   normal values, 1063*t*
   nutritional status assessment, 1024-1025
   pleural fluid, 1007*t*
   urinalysis, 851, 931*t*, 935*t*, 948
Glucose metabolism, 447
Glucose oxidase, 450, 935*t*
Glucose-6-phosphate dehydrogenase (G-6-PD), 73, 75
Glucose-6-phosphate dehydrogenase (G-6-PD) deficiency, 72-76, 131-133
Glucose tolerance tests (GTTs), 452, 815, 816-817, 1063*t*
Glucosteroids, 758, *758*
Glutamine, CSF, 975-976
Glutethimide, 907
Glycogen storage, 584, 823
Glycogen storage diseases, 452
Glycophorin, 71
Glycoproteins, 745
Glycosphingolipids, red cell antigens as, 367
Glycosuria, 931*t*, 935*t*, 851, 948
Glycosylated hemoglobin, 450-451, 817, 851
Glycosylation, tissue, 818
Goiter, toxic nodular, 794
Gonadal function, 831-841
Gonadotropin-releasing hormone (GnRH), 825
Goodpasture's syndrome, 361
Gout, 457-458, 1011
G protein, 739, *740*
Graft vs. host disease (GVHD), 405-406, 415, 437
Grain alcohol, 911-914, *913*
Gram stain, 614-615, 614*t*
   body fluids, 667
   chancroid, 681
   morphology, 631
   respiratory tract specimen, 672
   sputum, 993
   vaginal discharge, 680-681
Granular casts, 940, 941*t*

Granulation, in neutrophils, 86
Granulocyte colony-stimulating factor, 37
Granulocytes, 43t, 83-87, 178, 400
Granulocyte transfusions, 400
Granulocytopenia, 178, 400
Granulomatous inflammation, monocytes in, 89
Granulopoiesis, 36-39
  growth factors in, 37
  myeloid growth and distribution in, 38-39
Graves' disease, 791, 794
Growth factors, 32-35, 34t, 37
Growth hormone, 448t, 742, 743, 745-748
Guaiac testing, 984, 987

Haemophilus ducreyi, 681, 686
Haemophilus influenzae, 649, 651, 652
Hairy cell leukemia, 212, 213
Haplotype, 374, 430, 431, 436-437
Haptoglobin, 1063t
  diagnostic significance of, 483t
  and hemoglobin catabolism, 79, 80
  serum analysis, 492-493
hCG. See Human chorionic gonadotropin
HCV. See Hepatitis C virus
HDL. See High-density lipoprotein
HDN. See Hemolytic disease of the newborn
Heart disease, 559t, 577, 884-890
Heat fractionation, alkaline phosphatases, 547
Heat precipitation tests, 227, 266
Heavy chain diseases, 224, 234
Heavy metal poisoning/toxicity, 919-921
Heinz bodies, 69-70, 75, 133, 141, 146
Helicobacter pylori serology, 709t, 716
Hemagglutination inhibition (HI), rubella virus, 731
Hemagglutination treponemal test for syphilis (HATTS), 713, 714
Hemapheresis, therapeutic, 406, 407-408t
Hemarthroses, 291, 286, 1011
Hematocrit, 62
  and anemia classification, 103
  in corpuscular indices, 64
  critical value of, 24t
  fetal, normal values, 1050t
  and glucose measurement, 450
  measurement of, 63
  normal values for, 62t
Hematologic diseases, and thrombocytopenia, 303, 309
Hematology, 847-848, 853t, 1027-1028, 1049, 1050t, 1060t
Hematomas, 286, 291
Hematopoiesis, 32-44, 302
Hematuria, 286, 669-670, 930, 932t, 933t, 934, 965
Heme, 47-50, 160-161, 162t, 163, 459
Hemochromatosis, 163-165t, 590-592
Hemoglobin, 31
  in acute transfusion reaction, 412
  and anemia classification, 103
  bilirubin, 459
  binding with haptoglobin, 492
  buffering effect, 503

catabolism of, 77, 79-81, 81
developmental changes in, 144
electrophoresis, 135, 148, 149-150, 149
glycosylated, 450-451, 817-818
increased turnover, 569
normal values for, 62t, 1050t, 1060t
production and control of, 47-50
in RBC evaluation, 61-62
in RBC staining, 65, 67
references ranges of, 14, 15, 1060t
reticulocyte count and, 45, 46
sickle, 134-135
synthesis of, 134
unstable, 141, 150
urinalysis, 937-938t
Hemoglobin A (HbA), 50, 77, 108t, 134, 135, 144
Hemoglobin C disease, 139, 149
Hemoglobinemia, 79, 80-81, 81
Hemoglobin F, 50, 508
  acid-resistant assay for, 150
  and beta-thalassemia, 145-146
  in differential diagnosis of hypochromic microcytic anemia, 108t
  2,3-DPG and, 77
  in globin chain production, 143
  normal values, 1050t
  and sickle cell disease, 136, 137
  testing, 1048
Hemoglobin H, 143, 144
Hemoglobin H bodies/crystals, 145
Hemoglobin M, 141
Hemoglobinopathies, 134-150
Hemoglobin precursors, urinalysis, 955-956, 956t, 957t
Hemoglobin S, 134-137, 138t, 863
Hemoglobin SC disease, 139
Hemoglobin synthesis, 51-61, 141-143, 142, 144
Hemoglobinuria
  causes of, 937-938t
  haptoglobin and, 80
  march, 152
  paroxysmal nocturnal, 151
Hemolysis
  blood sample, 446, 511
  chromium labeling and, 79
  extravascular, and haptoglobin levels, 79
  intravascular, 79, 80-81, 81
  lactate dehydrogenase isoenzymes, 580
  in PNH, 122-123
Hemolytic anemia(s), 125-160, 152t
Hemolytic crises, 128, 137
Hemolytic disease, 569, 866-867
Hemolytic disease of the newborn (HDN), 421-429
  and DAT result, 382
  definition and pathophysiology of, 421-422
  lab management of, 427-428
  other maternal antibodies and, 428-429
  Rh disease, 422-428
  routine antenatal testing for, 429
Hemolytic transfusion reactions, 378
  antibody-mediated, 411-413
  delayed, 415

Hemolytic transfusion reactions *(Continued)*
  nonimmune, 410
Hemolytic-uremic syndrome, 152, 309, 310, 690
Hemopexin, 79, 497
Hemophagocytosis, 222-223
Hemophilia(s), 287, 289*t*, 291-293*t*, 294, 295*t*
Hemophilia A, 253, 257, 287, 289*t*, 292*t*
Hemophilia B, 253, 257, 287, 289*t*, 293*t*
Hemophilia C, 289*t*
Hemorrhage, 236, 291, 421-422, 423-425
Hemosiderin, 59, 61, 80, 416
Hemosiderosis, 164, 416
Hemostasis, 236-282
  antithrombins/anticoagulants in, 260-262,
    260*t*
  coagulation cascade in, *251*, 252-259, 262-268
  definition of, 236
  disorders of, 272*t*, 314-320, 316*t*
  fibrinolysis in, 259-260, 269-271, 269*t*, 273
  hypercoagulable states and, 273-282
  mechanisms of, 236-237
  platelets in, 240-251
  vascular system in, 240
Heparin, 258-259, 306, 558-559
Heparin-induced thrombocytopenia (HIT)
    syndrome, 306-307, 307*t*
Hepatic porphyrias, 955, 956*t*, 957*t*
Hepatitis, 575*t*, 578, 578*t*
Hepatitis A virus (HAV), 421, 593-594, 596*t*,
    727*t*, 731-732
Hepatitis B virus (HBV), 420, 594-595, 596*t*,
    727*t*, 732-733, *732*
Hepatitis C virus (HCV), 419-420, 595, 596*t*,
    727*t*, 733
Hepatitis D virus, 596*t*, 597, 727*t*, 733
Hepatitis E virus, 596*t*, 597
Hepatitis G virus, 597
Hepatitis viruses, 593-597, 596*t*
  serology, 727*t*, 731-733, *732*
  tests in, 567*t*
  transfusion, transmission via, 419-421
Hepatocellular function, 566, 575-580
Hepatolenticular degeneration, 589
Hereditary acanthocytosis, hemolysis
    with, 154
Hereditary angioedema, 333
Hereditary coproporphyria, 161, 162*t*, 163
Hereditary disorders, 857-861*t*
Hereditary spherocytosis (HS), 72, 127-128,
    129*t*, *129*, 130
Hereditary stomatocytosis, 130
Hereditary xerocytosis, 130
Herpes simplex virus
  cutaneous samples, 694-695
  genital tract specimens, 680, 683, 685
  serology, 726, 727*t*
Heterophile antibodies, EBV, 727*t*, 729-730
High-density lipoprotein (HDL), 468, *471*
  composition of, 473*t*, 474
  lipoprotein phenotypes, 476*t*
  nascent particles, 470, *471*
High-dose dexamethasone testing, 767
High-molecular weight (HMW) kininogen,
    238-239*t*, 253, 290*t*, 297

High-performance liquid chromatography
    (HPLC)
  antimicrobial agent levels, 658, 659
  catecholamines, 780-781
  drug analysis, 879
Histidine catabolism, folic acid and, 55
Histiocytes, 174, 176
Histiocytosis, malignant, 222-223
Histocompatibility antigens, 336
  in hemochromatosis, 164
  measurement of, 353-354
  and rheumatologic disorders, 439
Histoplasmosis, serology, 720*t*, 722
Hodgkin's disease, 213-214, *214*, 216-217*t*
Homocysteine, *53*, *281*, 1019
Homocystinuria, 961
Homogeneous assays, 880
Hormones. *See also* Endocrine tests
  albumin binding, 489
  carbohydrate metabolism, 447, 448*t*
  and glucose levels, 448*t*
  mechanisms of action, 739-740
  as tumor markers, 1032-1035, 1041-1042
Howell-Jolly bodies, 67, 69
HTLV type I serology, 727*t*, 735, *735*
Human chorionic gonadotropin (hCG), 794,
    831, 1062*t*
  in pregnancy, 841-844, *843*
  as tumor marker, 1034-1035
Human herpesvirus types 6, 7, and 8, serology,
    727*t*, 728
Human immunodeficiency virus (HIV-1;
    HIV-2), 174, 337
  and albumin, 400
  evaluation of, 363
  seroconversion window, *418*, 419
  serology, 727*t*, 733-735, *734*
  transmission by transfusion, 417-418, *418*
Human leukocyte antigens (HLAs), 336,
    429-431, 433-439
  classes of, 430-431, 433
  linkage disequilibrium and distribution
    of, 435
  and platelets, 398-399
  structure of, *432*
  testing/typing, 336, 353-354, 433-438, *440*
Human papilloma virus (HPV), 683-684, 1042
Human placental lactogen, 844, 845, 846
Human T-lymphotrophic virus type I, serology,
    727*t*, 735, *735*
Humoral immunity, 87, 88, 328-330, 605, 606
Hybridization assays, microbial antigens,
    627-628, *627*
Hydrops fetalis, 143, 422
Hydroxyl ion, defined, 501
Hydroxyproline, bone metabolism, 802
Hyperaldosteronism, 523, 764-765, 770-774,
    771*t*, *772*, 773*t*
Hyperbilirubinemia, 461*t*, 489
Hypercalcemia, 804-806, *805*, 808*t*
Hypercellularity of bone marrow, 42
Hyperchloremic acidosis, 520, 521*t*
Hyperglycemia, 451*t*, 530, 748
Hyperhomocysteinemia, 279

Hypersegmentation, in leukocytes, 86
Hypersensitivity, 339-340, 340t
Hypersplenism, 153-154
Hypertension, 772, 774, 780, 781
Hyperthyroidism, 786t, 791, 794, 798, 806
Hyperuricemia, 457
Hyperventilation, and respiratory alkalosis, 525
Hyperviscosity syndrome, 230, 406
Hypoalbuminemia, 485, 486t, 495, 496
Hypocalcemia, 256, 465, 800, 806-807, 808t
Hypochromia, 59, 65, 67, 68t
Hypochromic microcytic anemias, 103-111, 108t, 109t
Hypoglycemia, 821-823, 821t
  causes of, 451t, 821t
  in differential diagnosis of diabetic coma, 820t
  growth hormone studies, 748
Hypothalamic-pituitary axis, 742-743, 743, 784-785
Hypothalamic-pituitary-gonadal axis, 825, 830-831, 839
Hypothalamic stimulation, 790
Hypothyroidism, 785, 786t, 792

Ibuprofen toxicity, 903, 903, 904, 906
Idiopathic thrombocytopenic purpura (ITP), 307-309
Imipramine, 908
Immune complexes, 306-307, 331-332, 351
Immune-mediated hemolytic anemia, 154-156, 156t, 158-160, 157
Immune thrombocytopenia, 305-309, 307t, 308t
Immune thrombocytopenic purpura (ITP), 250, 307-309, 308t
Immunity
  diagnostic test procedures for, 340-363
  disorders of, 337, 338t, 339-340
  host defense, 604-609
  principles of, 325-336
Immunoassays, 620-626, 622t, 623, 623t, 624t, 625, 626
  antimicrobial agent levels, 658-659
  drug analysis, 880-881
  fibrinogen measurement, 266
  hCG, 841-843
  microbial antigen, 621-626, 623, 623t, 624t, 625
  pituitary hormones, 745
  synovial fluid, 1011
  for TSH, 789-790
Immunochromatography, 625-626, 625
Immunodeficiency disorders/states, 174, 175t, 337, 338t
  bloodstream infections in, 662
  candidiasis, 721
  fungal infections, 718-719
Immunodiffusion assays, 341-343, 722
  candidiasis, 720t, 721
  coccidioidomycosis, 720t, 721, 722
  histoplasmosis, 722
  precipitin bands, 703, 704
Immunoelectrophoresis (IEP), 343, 703-704
  candidiasis, 720t, 721

  in monoclonal gammopathies, 227, 228
  in multiple myeloma, 232
  types of, 343-345, 344
Immunofluorescence assays, 347, 706-707
  coccidioidomycosis, 720t, 721, 722
  FTA-ABS DS test, 709t, 713, 714, 715
  histoplasmosis, 720t, 722
  microbial antigens, 621, 622t
  rickettsial infections, 718
Immunoglobulins
  characteristics of, 326, 327, 328-330
  classes of, 701-702
  deficiencies of, 337, 338t
  heavy chain gene map, 328
  IgA, 329-330, 338t, 348, 414, 604, 701, 702
  IgD, 701
  IgE, 339-340, 362-363, 414, 707
  IgG, 159, 160, 223-225, 225t, 226, 228, 229, 330, 338t, 412, 606, 701, 701, 702-703, 726
  IgM, 159, 230, 329, 330, 379, 606, 701-702, 701
  IgM-IgG separation, 702-703, 724, 726
  liver disease and, 583, 584t
  measurements of, 347-350
  serum analysis, 495-497, 496
  thyroid-stimulating (TSIg), 792, 793t, 794
Immunophenotyping, 188-189, 190t
Immunoproliferative disorders, 223-234, 231
Immunosuppressive agents, 116, 339, 898-903, 899, 901, 1066t
Indirect antiglobulin test, 380
Indirect (unconjugated) bilirubin, 460, 461, 461t, 569
Indirect fluorescent antibody (IFA), 347, 355, 706-707
  GI specimen, 689-690
  legionellosis, 709t, 711-712
  microbial antigens, 621
  rickettsial infections, 718
Indirect hemagglutination (IHA) assays, parasites, 723, 724, 725
Indirect immunofluorescence (IIF), 723, 724, 729
Infections/infectious diseases
  adrenal dysfunction and, 776-777
  hemolysis associated with, 153
  causing hemolytic anemia, 156t
  perinatal, 1049, 1049t, 1051
  transfusion transmission, 416-421, 417t
Infectious mononucleosis (IM), 89, 159, 181
Infrared spectroscopic broth culture, blood, 664-665
Insulin, 448t, 746, 812, 821, 821t, 851
Integrins, neutrophil adherence to vascular endothelial cells, 171, 171, 172
Interferons, 608
Interleukins, 37, 85, 89, 608-609, 900
Intermediate density lipoprotein (IDL), 468, 469, 470
International Normalized Ratio (INR), 264-265, 265t
Intestinal flora, 460, 640, 1022
Intracellular parasites, viral and chlamydial culture, 643-647, 645, 646t

Intramuscular (IM) administration, 873, 874-875
Intrauterine transfusions, 426-427
Intrinsic coagulation, 251, 252-253
Intrinsic factor (IF-B$_{12}$), 51, *54*, 114, 115
Intrinsic factor deficiency, 56, 116
Ion exchange chromatography, IgM-IgG separation, 703
Ionized calcium measurements, 466-467
Ionizing radiation, and amylase, 553, 554*t*
Ions, serum chemistry, 500-502
Iron
  bone marrow, 60-61
  daily requirements of, 57
  evaluation of, 59
  metabolism of, 57, *58*, 58*t*, 59-61
  normal values for, 58*t*, 1063*t*
  requirements of, 105-106
  transferrin, 493-494, 590-592, 1028
Iron chelation therapy, for severe thalassemia syndrome, 147
Iron deficiency, 46, *106*, 107, 1022
Iron deficiency anemia, 72, 103-108, 148
Iron overload syndromes of, 163-165, 165*t*, 416
Irradiated blood products, 405-406, 405*t*
Isoenzymes, 132, 534
IVY technique, bleeding time, 250-251

Jaundice, 420, 461, 569, 570, *570*
Joint disorders, synovial fluid, 1008-1012, 1010*t*, 1012*t*, *1013*

Kanamycin, 890, 891
Karyotyping, 856-862, 857*t*, 859-860*t*, 861*t*
Kernicterus, 427, 489
Ketoacidosis, 521, 818-819, *819*, 820*t*
17-Ketogenic steroids (17-KGS), 760
Ketones, urine dipstick interpretation, 931*t*
17-Ketosteroids (17-KS), 760, 828, 833-837*t*
Kidney disease
  autoantibodies in, 361
  BUN/creatinine ratio, 456, 456*t*
  and calcium levels, 465
  hemolysis with, 154
  nephrotic syndrome, 232, 234, 487, 492
  protein loss, 486*t*, 487, 492, 936*t*
  uremia, causes of, 453-454, 454*t*
Kidney failure, 412, 804, 805
Kidney function
  ADH and, 751-752, 754
  and alkaline phosphatase, 549
  amylase clearance, 554
  electrolyte regulation, 504, 505
  nephrogenic diabetes insipidus, 756
  panel composition, 22*t*
  pregnancy, 851-852, 854*t*
  renal blood flow, 851, 949, 949*t*
  urinalysis, 942-953*t*
  urine formation, 924-926
Kidney stones, 1020
  analysis of, 963-966, 964*t*, 965*t*
  calcium excretion in, 958-959, 959*t*
Kidney toxicity, 891, 901-902, 903
Kirby-Bauer method, 652-653

Kleihauer-Betke test, 150, 423, 424-425, 1048
Kwashiorkor, 1015

Labile factor proaccelerin, 238-239*t*
Lactate dehydrogenase (LDH), 539-542, 539*t*, *540*, 541*t*, 559*t*, 1063*t*
  biochemistry and tissue sources, 539-540, 539*t*, *540*
  cardiac injury markers, 544, 545
  diagnostic applications, 541-542, 541*t*
  intravascular hemolysis and, 81
  liver disorders, 580
  neonates and pediatric patients, normal values, 1056*t*
  pleural fluid, 1007*t*
  serous fluids, 1005
Lactic acid, 521-522, 974*t*, 975, 1063*t*
Lamotrigine, 898
Latex particle agglutination (LPA), 345, 618, 622, *623*, 720*t*, 721, 722
Lead poisoning, 110-111, 919-920
  compounds present in, 162*t*
  lab findings in, 111*t*
  and porphyrin metabolism, 163, 955-956, 957*t*
Lecithin cholesterol acyl transferase (LCAT), 470
Lecithin/sphingomyelin ratio, 867-868
Left shift, differential white count, 92-93, 608
Legionella sp., 675, 709*t*, 711-712, 994*t*
Leucine aminopeptidase (LAP), 574
Leucovorin, 116, 899-900, *899*
Leukemias
  acute, 186-190, 187*t*
  categorization of, 204
  chromosome studies in, 98-100
  cytochemistry in, 96-98
  cytogenetic abnormalities in, 192*t*
  immunophenotypic and cytogenetic characterization of, 188-189, *189*, 190*t*
  lysozyme in, 559
  Philadelphia chromosome and, 1043-1046, *1044*
  and thrombocytopenia, 302
  undifferentiated, 205
Leukemic reticuloendotheliosis, 212
Leukemoid reactions, 169, 180-181, 181*t*
Leukocyte depletion filters, 413-414
Leukocyte differentiation antigens, nomenclature for, 335*t*
Leukocyte esterase (LE), 97, 669-670
Leukocyte reduced platelets, 400
Leukoerythroblastic (myelophthistic) reaction, 200*t*, 303
Lidocaine, 887, 888, 1066*t*
Lipases, 469, 553, 558-559, 559*t*, 1032, 1063*t*
Lipids, 492, 583-584
  bile salts, 571
  carbohydrate metabolism, 447
  and fatty stools, 987-988
  malabsorption, 988-989, *989*, 990
  and hemolysis, 154
  nutritional status assessment, 1027

serum analysis, 467-480
thyroid hormones and, 785-786
Lipoprotein lipase (LPL), 469, 558-559, 1032
Lipoproteins, 468, 470, *471*, 473*t*, 474, 476*t*, 477*t*
Listeria, antimicrobial susceptibility tests, 649
Liver
 bilirubin formation, 459-460
 carbohydrate metabolism, 447, 583-584
 cyclosporine excretion, 903
 drug metabolism, 876
 glucocorticoid metabolism, 759
 lipid metabolism, 470-471, *471*, 583-584
 lipid synthesis, 469-470, *470*
 metastasis, markers of, 1032
 porphyrias, 955, 956*t*, 957*t*
 during pregnancy, 852
 protein metabolism, 580-583, 584*t*
 protein synthesis, 484-485
 theophylline metabolism, 884
Liver disease
 alkaline phosphatase in, 547-548, 548*t*
 alpha-1-antitrypsin deficiency and, 491
 BUN/creatinine ratio, 456*t*
 jaundice/hyperbilirubinemia, causes of,
  461-462, 461*t*
 marker enzymes, 547-548, 551, 551*t*, 548*t*,
  559*t*, 575-580
Liver function tests, 562-599
 bilirubin and biliary system, 566,
  568-575*t*
 composition of, 22*t*
 hepatocellular function, 551, 575-580
 special tests, 586-599
 structure and function of liver, 563-567*t*
 synthetic function, 580-586
Lung biopsy, specimen collection and transport, 611
Lupus anticoagulant (LAC), 279-282
Luteinizing hormone (LH), 742, *743*, 825-829*t*,
  836-837*t*, 1063*t*
Lymphocyte counts, 91-92, 92*t*
Lymphocytes, 39, 87-89
 CSF, 971, 972*t*
 normal values, 43*t*, 1050*t*, 1060*t*
 plasmacytoid, in Waldenström's macroglobulinemia, 230
 surface markers, measurement of,
  352-353, *354*
Lymphocytic thyroiditis, 794-795
Lymphokines, 87, 606, 608
Lymphomas, *189*, 213-223, *214*, 215*t*-221*t*
Lymphoproliferative disorders, 204-223
 acute, 205-206, 207*t*, 208-209
 chronic, 209-212, 211*t*, *213*
 lymphomas, 213-223
Lysis centrifugation/direct plating, blood,
  666-667
Lysozyme, 84, 559-560

Macroangiopathic hemolytic anemia, 151
Macrocytic red cells, 65
Macrocytosis, 65, 67, 68*t*, 111-112
Macrophages, 89, 174-176, 604, 606, 607
Macropolycytes, 86

Magnesium, 1064*t*
 albumin binding, 489
 anion gap, 514-515, 515*t*
 homeostasis disorders, 466
 measurement of, 467
 nutritional status assessment, 1025-1026
 and PTH, 807
Malabsorption, 487, 988-991, *989*
Malignancy, hypercalcemia of, *805*, 806
Malignant histiocytosis, 222-223
Marginating pool, in granulopoiesis, 38
Mass spectrometer (MS), drug analysis, 879
Maternal antibodies, 154-155, 376-377,
  428-429
Maximal acid output (MAO), 998, 999, 999*t*
May-Hegglin anomaly, WBCs in, 87
Mean corpusclar volume (MCV), 62*t*, 64, 65,
  1050*t*, 1060*t*
Mediterranean anemia, 141, 146-147
Mediterranean enzyme variant of G-6-PD,
  132-133
Mediterranean lymphoma, 234
Megakaryocytes, 39, 40, 240, 304
Megakaryopoiesis, 39-40
Megaloblastic anemia
 laboratory findings in, 113*t*
 during pregnancy, 848
 and Schilling test, 56
 and thrombocytopenia, 302, 303
 from vitamin B$_{12}$ and folic acid deficiency,
  53, 111, 112, 114-115
Melanocyte-stimulating hormone (MSH), 745
Melena, 982, 984
Meningitis, 973, 974*t*
Meningococcemia, 304
Meningomyelocele, 863
Menstrual cycle
 hormone levels, 826-827, *827*
 iron deficiency from blood loss, 106
M:E ratio (myeloid:erythroid ratio),
  42-43, 43*t*
Metabolic abnormalities, 517, 765, 964, 965*t*,
  1051*t*
Metabolic acidosis, 518*t*, 520-522, 521*t*, 526*t*
Metabolic alkalosis, 518*t*, 522-523, 526*t*
Metabolic bone disease, calcium abnormalities,
  464-465, 465*t*
Metabolic panel, composition of, 22*t*
Metabolism, thyroid hormone and, 785
Metabolites, 445, 960*t*
Methemalbumin, intravascular hemolysis and,
  80-81
Methemoglobin reductase pathway, *74*, 76
Methionine, 53, *53*, *281*
Methotrexate, 116, 339, 898-900, *899*, 1066*t*
Methylated xanthine drugs, 881-884, *882*
Methylene blue-methemoglobin test, 76
Metyrapone test, 761, *762*, 764, 770
Microaerophilic aerobes, 631, 633*t*
Microanalysis, in neonatology centers, 1053,
  1054*t*
Microangiopathic hemolytic anemia (MAHA),
  151, 152, 302, 412
Microbial antigen detection, 700

Microbiology, principles of, 603
   antimicrobial susceptibility testing, 647-659, 656, 657
   host interaction with agent, 603-607
   laboratory cultures, 630-647, 636t, 643, 644, 646
   laboratory detection, 607-647
Microbiology, systematic, 661-698
   bloodstream specimens, 661-667
   body fluids, 662t, 667-669, 668t
   cutaneous specimens, 662t, 693-695
   eye/ear specimens, 662t, 696-698
   gastrointestinal tract specimens, 662t, 686-693, 687t
   genital tract specimens, 662t, 679-686
   respiratory specimens, 662t, 671-679
   urine, 662t, 669-671
   wound, tissue/biopsy specimens, 662t, 695-696
Microcytosis, 59, 68t
Microhemagglutination-T. pallidum test (MHA-TP), 713, 714, 715
Microhematocrit method, 63
Microorganisms, 460, 604-606, 976-977, 1022
Microscopy
   bloodstream infections, 662-663
   body fluids, 667
   cutaneous specimens, 693-694
   eye/ear infections, 697
   genital tract specimens, 680
   microbiology specimen preparation and staining, 614-620, 620t
   respiratory tract specimens, 672
   sputum, 992-996, 994-995t, 996t
   stool, 987-988
   urine, 669, 930
   wound, tissue/biopsy specimens, 695
Microtubules, in platelets, 242
Minimum bactericidal concentration (MBC) determination, 650
Minimum inhibitory concentration (MIC) determination, 648-650
Mixed casts, 940, 941t
Mixed lymphocyte culture (MLC), 352, 434
Mobiluncus cultures, 685
Modified acid-fast stain, 617
Modified trichrome stain, 619
Molecular probe analysis, 99-100
Monoblasts, 39, 89
Monoclonal antibodies, 328, 329, 330
Monoclonal gammopathies, 224-233t
Monoclonal immunoglobulin, 495, 496
Monoclonal protein (M protein), 225, 226, 232, 233
Monocytes, 39, 89-90, 607
   conditions causing monocytosis, 93t
   disorders of, 174-176
   normal range of, 43t, 1050t, 1060t
Mononucleosis, infectious (IM), 89, 159, 181
Mucin clot test, 1009, 1011
Multiple endocrine neoplasia (MEN)
   type 2, 804

Multiple myeloma, 223, 224-228, 230-232, 465, 495
   clinical features of, 231, 231
   complications of, 231
   immunoelectrophoretic serum patterns of, 228
   lab features of, 232
   platelet disorders from, 314
   serum protein electrophoresis, 226
Mycobacteria, 639-641, 649, 654, 677, 693, 694, 696, 994t
Mycobacterium chelonei, 649
Mycobacterium fortuitum, 649
Mycoplasma, 717, 994t
Mycoplasma hominis culture, 685
Mycoplasma pneumoniae, 159, 675-676, 709t, 717
Myelocytes, 39, 43t
Myelodysplasias/myelodysplastic syndromes, 121, 122, 148, 182, 184t, 202-204, 303
Myeloid:erythroid ratio (M:E), 42-43, 43t
Myelomonocytic leukemia, 186
Myeloperoxidase, neutrophil, 84
Myeloperoxidase deficiency, 172, 174
Myelophthistic (leukoerythroblastic) reaction, 200t, 303
Myeloproliferative disorders, 182-204
   ANLL, 183t, 184-190, 187t, 189, 190t, 192
   chronic, 192-202, 193t, 197t
   histiocytes in, 176
   myelodysplastic syndromes, 184t, 202-204
Myoglobin, 542-543, 545, 559t
Myxedema, 792

NADPH fluorescent test, 75-76
Naloxone, 910
Naproxen, 904, 906-907
Narcolepsy, and HLA antigens, 439
Neisseria gonorrhoeae
   antimicrobial susceptibility tests, 651, 652, 652
   genital tract specimens, 600, 680, 684, 693
   respiratory tract specimen culture, 674
   specimen collection, 612
Neisseria meningitidis, antimicrobial susceptibility tests, 649, 651
Neonatal alloimmune thrombocytopenia, 306
Neonates
   Chlamydia trachomatis, 676
   congenital hypothyroidism in, 792
   congenital infections in, 701-702, 715, 726
   laboratory tests, 1053-1057, 1055t, 1056t, 1057t
   respiratory infections, yeast, 678
   toxoplasmosis tests, 724
Nephrotic syndrome, 232, 234, 487, 492
Nephrotoxicity, aminoglycoside, 891
Neuropathies, autoimmune, 362
Neutropenia, 176-178, 177t
Neutrophils, 38, 83-84, 604, 607
   disorders of, 169-174, 170t
   neutropenia classification, 176, 177t
   normal range of, 43t, 1050t, 1060t
Nitroblue tetrazolium (NBT) test, 172, 363
Nitrogenous compounds, urinalysis, 956, 958

Nitroprusside tests, 521, 961
Nitrosoureas, and thrombocytopenia, 303
Nocardia sp. respiratory infections, 994*t*
Nonchromogens, 640
Non-Hodgkin's lymphomas, 217-223, 218*t*, 219-220*t*, 221*t*
  angio-immunoblastic lymphadenopathy, 222
  Burkitt's, 220, 222
  classifications of, 218*t*, 219-220*t*
  clinical lab findings in, 223
  flow cytometric immunophenotyping of, *189*
  high-grade, 220
  intermediate-grade, 218, 220
  low-grade malignant, 217-218
  malignant histiocytosis/hemophagocytic syndromes, 222-223
  morphologic features in differential diagnosis of, 221*t*
  mycosis fungoides, 222
  Sezary syndrome, 222
Nonimmune hemolytic anemias, 151-154, 152*t*
Nonimmune thrombocytopenia, 308*t*, 309-310
Non-insulin-dependent diabetes mellitus (NIDDM), 813, 814*t*
Nonketotic hyperosmolar syndrome, 819, 820*t*, 821
Nonprotein nitrogenous compounds, 452-459, 454*t*, *455*, 456*t*, 459*t*
Nordiazepam, 894, 907
Norepinephrine, 777, 777*t*, 779*t*
Normochromic RBCs, 65
Normocytic RBCs, 65
Nucleic acids, 464, 627-628, *627*, 673, 995*t*
Nutrition
  assessment formulas, 1029-1030, 1030*t*
  disorders of, 1015-1030
  laboratory assessment, 1024-1029
  serum proteins as indicator, 485

Obstructive jaundice, 570, *570*
Occult blood tests, 982, 1041
Oncotic pressure, 485, 1003, *1004*
Opsonization, 172, 337, 605, 606
Orthochromatic erythroblast, 44
Orthostatic proteinuria, 487
Osmolality
  antidiuretic hormone and, 753-754, 755*t*
  defined, 501
  laboratory measurement, 515-517
  nonketotic hyperosmolar syndrome, 819, 820*t*
  pregnancy and, 850
  reference values, 508*t*, 1064*t*
  serum, 516, 517
  SIADH, 754, 755*t*
  urinalysis, 948, 950-952, 951*t*
  water and electrolyte metabolism, 527-531, 528*t*, 529*t*, 530*t*
Osmolarity, 1064*t*
  antidiuretic hormone and, 505
  sweat, 1013
  urinalysis, 948, 950-952, 951*t*
Osmotic fragility test, 128, 129*t*
Osmotic pressure, defined, 501-502

Ototoxicity, aminoglycoside, 891
Ouchterlony assays, 341, 703, *704*
Ova and parasite examination, 611
Oxazepam, 907
Oxygen, 521-522, 613, 638-639, 654
Oxytocin, 742, 743, *743*, 751

Pancreas, 811-823
  diabetes mellitus, 812-823, 813*t*, 814*t*, 820*t*, 821*t*
  hormones, 811-812
  enzymes, 469, 553, 558-559*t*, 1001, 1032, 1063*t*
Pancreatitis, 465, 465*t*, 553, 554*t*, 1002
Pancytopenia, 117
  bone marrow replacement and, 120
  causes of, 118*t*
  in hairy cell leukemia, 212
  in hypoproliferative anemia, 117, 119, 121
Panel reactive antibodies (PRA), 434
Panel testing, 19-21, 20*t*, 21*t*, 22*t*
Panhypopituitarism, 749-751
Panic values, 23, 24*t*
Para-aminohippuric acid test (PAHA), 948, 949*t*
Paraneoplastic syndromes, autoantibodies and, 362
Paraphenomenon, in drug-induced hemolysis, 155
Parasites
  serology, 722-725, 723*t*
  stool examination, 611, 687-688, 987
  and vitamin B_{12}, 116, 1019
Parathyroid gland, 798-811
  calcitonin, 800
  calcium and phosphorus metabolism, 798
  disorders causing decreased calcium, 806-808, 808*t*, 809*t*
  disorders causing increased calcium, 804-806, *805*, 808*t*, 809*t*
  osteoporosis, evaluation of, 810-811
  parathyroid hormone, 464-465, 465*t*, 798-799, *799*, 800*t*, 804, 806-807
  phosphate metabolism, disorders of, 808, 809*t*, 810
Paroxysmal cold hemoglobuinuria, 159-160
Paroxysmal nocturnal hemoglobinuria (PNH), 122-123, 151, 303
Partial thromboplastin time (PTT), 264, 585-586
  in hemostatic disorders lab evaluation, 272*t*
  in liver disease, 319
  prolongation of, 267, 268
Particle agglutination/agglutination inhibition (PA/PAI) assays, 706
Particle agglutination assays (PAA), 622-623, 623*t*, *623*, 688-689
Parvovirus, 421, 727*t*, 731
Passive hemagglutination (PHA), rubella virus, 731
Peak acid output (PAO), 998, 999, 999*t*
Peak level, drug, 874-876, *874*, *875*
Pelger-Huet phenomenon, 87
Penicillins, 155, 156*t*, 489, 890
Percutaneous needle aspiration, microbiology specimen collection and transport, 611

Percutaneous umbilical cord blood sampling (PUBS), 855, 1048-1051, 1049*t*, 1050*t*, 1053*t*
Perinatal laboratory testing, 1048-1051, 1049, 1050*t*, 1053*t*
Periodic acid-Schiff (PAS) stain, 97-98
Peripheral blood smear
  critical value of, 24*t*
  Giemsa stain, 619-620, 620*t*
  red blood cell morphology, 65, 67, 68*t*, 69-70, *69*
Peritoneal fluid, 1006, 1008, 1009*t*
Pernicious anemia, 56, 115-116, 997
Petechiae, 237, 245, 286
pH
  blood, 526*t*
  CSF, 969, 969*t*
  defined, 501
  pleural fluid, 1007*t*
  reference values, 508*t*, 1062*t*
Phagocytosis, 38, 84, 170*t*, 172-174, *173*, 605, 606, 607
Phenolphthalein test, 1016
Phenylketonuria (PKU), 959, 960-961
Phenytoin, 116, 892-894, *892*, 1066*t*
Pheochromocytoma, 780
  clonidine suppression test and, 780
  patient-care considerations, 781-783, 781*t*
  symptoms, 781, 781*t*
Philadelphia chromosome, *99*, 195, 196, 206, 209
Phlebotomy, for hemochromatosis, 164-165, 591
Phosphates
  critical value of, 24*t*
  homeostasis disorders, 466
  laboratory testing, 801
  measurement, 466
  metabolic disorders, 808, 809*t*, 810
  nutritional status assessment, 1026
Phosphatidylglycerol (PG), 867, 868-869
Phosphatidylinositol (PI), 868-869
Phosphodiesterase, 739, *740*
6-Phosphogluconate, 73, *74*
Phospholipase, platelet aggregation, 244
Physical trauma, and hemolytic anemia, 151-152, 152*t*
Pituitary, 741-742, 825
Pituitary-adrenal axis, 767
  Addison's disease, 768-769, 770
  pituitary tumors and Cushing's syndrome, 765
  tests of, 761-764, 761*t*, *762*, 762*t*
Pituitary-hypothalamic axis, 742-743, *743*, 784-785
pK, defined, 502
Placental hormones, 844-846
Plasma, 31, 258-259, 446
Plasma cell dyscrasias, 223, 229-234
Plasma cell leukemia, 232
Plasma cells, 39, 43*t*, 223-224, 328, 606
Plasma components, 400-404, 401*t*
Plasmacytoid lymphocytes, 230, 223
Plasma exchange, guidelines for, 407*t*, 408*t*
Plasmapheresis, defined, 406

Plasma protease inhibitors, in transfusion medicine, 404
Plasma thromboplastin antecedent (PTA), 238-239*t*
Plasmin, 237, 259-260, 318
Plasminogen, 259, 260, 271, 273
Platelet adhesion, 240, 242-243, *243*
Platelet aggregation, 240, *243*, 244, *245*, 247-249
Platelet concentrates, 389, 397-400
Platelet count, 246-247
  counting methods, 247
  fetal, 1049
  interpretation of, 247
Platelet counters, 302
Platelet disorders, 301-314
  lab evaluation of, 272*t*
  qualitative, 312-313, 313*t*
  quantitative, 302-312
  secondary to other diseases, 314
Platelet function, thrombopathy, 245, 246
Platelet retention, testing of, 249
Platelets, 31, 39-40, 240-251
  critical value of, 24*t*
  functions of, 240
  in hemostasis, 236-237
  laboratory studies, 245-251, 272*t*
  leukocyte reduced, 400
  normal values for, 62*t*, 1050*t*, 1060*t*
  production and structure of, 240-242, *241*
Platelet studies, normal values for, 237*t*
Platelet therapy, 399*t*, 437-438
Pleural fluid, 542, 1004*t*, 1005-1006, 1007*t*
Pneumocystis carinii, 993, 996, 996*t*
Polychromasia, 45, 67
Polychromatophilia, 68*t*, 128
Polyclonal hypergammaglobulinemia, *226*, 495, *496*
Polycythemia vera, 160, 184*t*, 196-198
Polymerase chain reaction (PCR) sequencing, HLAs, 434
Polymerization, in coagulation cascade, 252, 254
Polypeptides, 744-745
Polyuria, 755*t*, 950*t*
Poorly differentiated lymphocytic lymphoma, 220
Porphobilinogen (PBG), 49, 160, 163
Porphyria cutanea tarda (PCT), 161, 162*t*, 163, 956*t*, 957*t*
Porphyrias, 49, 160-163, 162*t*, 955-956, 956*t*, 957*t*
Porphyria variegata (PV), 161, 163, 162*t*
Porphyrin ring, 47-48, *48*
Porphyromonas spp. culture, 639
Porter-Silber reaction, 759, 775
Posterior pituitary hormones, 751-756, 755*t*, 757*t*
Postheparin lipolytic activity (PHLA), 558
Postpartum hemolytic-uremic syndrome, 310
Postpartum pituitary necrosis, 749-750
Posttransfusion purpura, 306, 416
Potassium, 513
  anion gap, 514-515, 515*t*
  critical value of, 24*t*

deficiency of, 513-514
diabetic ketoacidosis, 819
measurement of, 510-512
reference values, 508*t*, 1062*t*
thrombocytosis and, 312
water and electrolyte metabolism, 527, 529*t*
Prealbumin, 481-485, *481*, 482*t*, 484, 582, 1028, 1064*t*
Precipitates, urine, 930, 934
Pregnancy, 841-869
  alpha-fetoprotein during, 587
  antibody screening tests in, 383, 429
  anti-factor VIII in, 320
  diagnosis of, 841-844, *843*, 854-869
  gestational diabetes in, 814, 815-816
  normal physiologic changes in, 847-854
  physiology, 841
  placental ALP in, 549
  placental hormones, 844-846
  prolactin, 846-847
  toxoplasma screening in, 723
  vitamin A teratogenicity, 1017
Preleukemic syndromes, 121, 148, 202-204
Prenatal laboratory testing, 723, 855, 1048-1051, 1049*t*, 1050*t*, 1053*t*
Pretransfusion testing, *386*, 387-389
Procainamide, 887, 889, 1066*t*
Proconvertin (factor VII), 584. *See also* Coagulation factors, factor VII
Profile testing, 19-21, 20*t*, 21*t*, 22*t*
Progesterone, 826, 827-828, 846
  in female gonadal function disorders, 833-835*t*
  hypothalamic-pituitary-gonadal axis stimulation tests, 830
  normal serum levels, 829*t*
  receptors, as tumor markers, 1041-1042
Prolactin, 742, *743*, 749, 829*t*, 1064*t*
Pronormoblast, 43*t*
Propoxyphene, 904, 915
Prostaglandin pathway, 244, *246*
Prostate-specific antigen (PSA), 559*t*, 1033, 1037-1038, 1064*t*
Protease inhibitors, 490-491
Protein(s)
  acute phase reactants, 497-498, 498*t*
  albumin, 485-490, 486*t*
  alpha-1-antitrypsin, 490-491
  alpha-2-macroglobulin, 491-492
  analysis methods, 480-484, *481*, *482*, 482*t*, 483*t*, 484*t*
  betalipoprotein, 493
  buffering effect, 503
  carrier proteins, 497
  complement C3, 494
  CSF, 971, 973-974, 974*t*, 1064*t*
  fibrinogen, 494-495
  haptoglobin, 492-493
  immunoglobulins, 495-497, *496*
  liver metabolism, 580-583, 584*t*
  loss via digestive tract, 990
  pleural fluid, 1007*t*
  prealbumin, 484-485
  RBC membrane, 127

serum, *226*, 232, 314, 567*t*, 1027
transferrin, 493-494
Protein-bound iodine (PBI), 795
Protein C, 261, 262, 319
Protein C1 esterase inhibitor deficiency, 333
Protein kinases, 739, *740*
Protein-losing enteropathy, 990
Protein matrix, urine casts, 934, 939
Protein S, 261, 278, 319
Proteus strains, 718, 719*t*
Prothrombin (factor II), 238-239*t*, 288*t*, 317*t*, 584, 585
  in coagulation cascade, 254
  nomenclature and characteristics of, 256
Prothrombin time (PT), 264-265, 585-586
  critical value of, 24*t*
  liver function tests, 567*t*
  prolongation of, 267, 268
Protoporphyrin, 48, *48*, 60, 111, 160
Protozoan parasites, 688, 980
Psychiatric drugs, 907-909, *910*
Psychologic factors, endocrine and sexual function evaluation, 839
Psychophysiologic problems, pheochromocytoma, 782-783
Pteroylglutamic acid. *See* Folic acid
Pulmonary/respiratory disease, 361, 517, 756, 1007*t*
Pulmonary infections, specimens for diagnosis of, 994*t*
Pulmonary surfactant, lecithin/sphingomyelin ratio, 867-868
Purpura, 237, 286, 306, 416
Pyrogens, and transfusion reactions, 409
Pyruvate kinase (PK) deficiency, 73, 133-134

Queckenstedt procedure, 970-971
Quinidine, 888-889
  and hemolysis, 155, 156*t*
  and thrombocytopenia, 306
Quinine, and thrombocytopenia, 306
Quinine derivatives, and hemolysis, 155, 156*t*

Radial immunodiffusion (RID), 341-343
Radioactive iodine uptake (RAIU), 796
Radioallergosorbent tests (RAST), 363
Radioimmunoassays (RIAs), 346, 708, 745, 880
Radioiodine uptake testing, thyroid, 790-791
Radiometry, mycobacterial susceptibility testing, 654
Rapid dexamethasone test, 763-764
Rapid plasma reagin (RPR) test, 709*t*, 712, *715*
Receiver operating characteristic (ROC) curve, 10, *11*, *12*
Receptors, hormone, 739, *740*
Recombinant immunoblot assay (RIBA), 733
Red blood cell diseases, 102-165, 161*t*, 162*t*, 165*t*
Red blood cell membrane, hereditary defects of, 125, 127-128, 129*t*, 130
Red blood cells, 31
  acetylcholinesterase, 556
  alloimmunization, 378
  anemia classification, 103

Red blood cells *(Continued)*
  antigens of, 365, 366t, 367
  components and structure of, 125, 127
  CSF, 971, 972t
  enumeration/cell count, 63-64, 1060t
  enzyme deficiencies, 130-134
  erythrocytapheresis, 406
  erythrocytosis, 160, 161t, 196, 197
  frozen deglycerolized, 396
  genetic disorders, PUBS and, 1051t
  metabolism, 70-81, 71, 74
  morphology in peripheral smear, 65, 67, 68t,
    69-70, 128
  normal values for, 62t, 1050t, 1060t
  pleural fluid, 1007t
  pregnancy and, 847-848
  protoporphyrin, 106, 111
  staining of, 65, 67
  in stool, 988
  transfusion products, 394-396, 395t
  in urine, 934, 940, 941t, 942t
Red cell distribution width (RDW), 65, 66, 108t
Reference ranges, 10, 13-14, 15, 16, 17,
    1059-1066
Reference research method, 944
Refractory anemia (RA), 121-122, 184t, 202-203
Renal calculi. *See* Kidney stones
Renal tubular acidosis (RTA), 520, 521t
Renal tubular function, 520, 521t, 948, 950t
Renin-angiotensin system, 759, 771-774, 772
Reproductive endocrinology, 825-869
  amenorrhea, 828, 830-831, 833t
  general physiology, 825-827, 825
  gonadal hormones and their metabolism,
    827-828, 829t
  laboratory tests of, 831-841
  pregnancy and lactation, 841-849
Respiratory acidosis, 518t, 523-525, 526t
Respiratory alkalosis, 518t, 525, 526t
Respiratory specimens, 662t, 671-679
  aerobic cultures, 673-676
  anaerobic cultures, 676-677
  collection and transport, 611
  fungi, 677-679
  microscopy, 672-673
  mycobacteria, 677
  nucleic acid probes, 673
  sputum analysis, 991-995, 993t, 994-995t, 996t
  viruses, 679
Restriction endonucleases, 1043
Reticulocyte count, 36, 45-46, 67
  and anemia classification, 103
  critical value of, 24t
  normal values for, 62t
  pregnancy and, 847-848
Reticulocyte production index, 46
Reticulocytes, 36, 45, 67
Reticulocytosis, 46
Retinol-binding protein (RBP), 484, 497
Retinyl ester, 1017
Revised European American Lymphoma
    (REAL) Classification, 217, 219-220t
Rh antibodies, 154-155, 376-377
Rheumatic disorders, 355t, 357-359, 439

Rheumatoid factor (RF), 359, 702, 1064t
Rh hemolytic disease of the newborn
    (Rh-HDN), 421, 422-428
  diagnosing transplacental hemorrhage and,
    423-425
  lab management of, 425-427
  prevention of, 423, 424t
Rh immunoprophylaxis, 377, 423, 424t, 425
Rh system, 373-374, 376-377
Rickettsial infections, serology, 717-718, 719t
Ring sideroblasts, 61, 109, 110, 203
Ristocetin cofactor (vWF activity), 248, 249,
    257, 298
Rocky Mountain Spotted Fever (RMSF),
    304, 718
Rubella virus serology, 727t, 730-731
Russells viper venom (RVV), 282

Salicylates, 820t, 1066t
Salmonella, 691, 709t, 711
Sarcoidosis, 465, 465t
Schilling test, 55t, 55-56
Schistocytes, 68t, 151, 302
Scleroderma, autoantibodies in, 358
Secretin, 1001
Secretin test, 1001-1002
Secretor (Se) gene, 371, 373
Secretory IgA, 330, 604, 702
Sedimentation rate, erythrocyte, 93-95, 94t, 608,
    1060t
Selectins, 171, 171
Selective media, 630
Semen analysis, 832, 838, 838t
Senescence, erythrocyte, 72-79
Senescent changes, gonadal function, 828, 829t
Sensitivity, 4, 6-7
Serology, 700-735
  antibody detection, 700-708, 704, 705
  bacterial infections, 709-718, 709t, 714t,
    715, 715
  CSF, 977
  fungal infections, 718-722, 720t
  hepatitis viruses, 596t
  HLA tests, 433-434, 700
  parasite infections, 772-725, 723t
  viral infections, 726-735
Serotonin uptake inhibitors, 909, 910
Serous fluids, 1002-1013, 1004t
Sertraline, 909, 910
Serum, 446
  coagulation factors in, 259
  critical values, 24t
  normal values of, 58t
Serum inhibitory titer, 656-657
Serum osmolality, 516, 517
Sex chromosome abnormalities, 857, 857t, 858
Sex-linked diseases, 858, 859t, 860
Sex-related reference range, 14, 15, 16
Shell vial technique, 646
Shift to the left, differential white count,
    92-93, 608
Sickle cell disease, 72, 136-137, 138t, 863
Sickle cell syndromes, 135-139, 138t
Sideroblastic anemias, 108t, 109-110

Sideroblasts, 61, 109, 110, 203
Signal amplification techniques, 628
Simplate II method, bleeding time, 250-251
Single-stranded nucleic acids, viral, 643
Skeletal muscle enzymes, 536, 559t, 578, 580
Skin, 603-605, 695-696
Skin reaction testing, for Hodgkin's lymphoma, 216
Skin tests, 352, 362-363
Small-cell lymphocytic lymphoma, 217, 218
Smoking, and theophylline metabolism, 884
Snake venom test for dysfibrinogenemia, 297
Sodium, 513
    critical value, 24t
    diabetic ketoacidosis, 819
    excretion of, 953, 953t
    measurement of, 510-512
    reference values, 508t, 1064t
Solute loads, 505
Southern blot analysis, 329, 1043, 1044, 1045, 1046t
Spectrin, RBC membrane, 71, 71-72, 127
Spherocytes, 72, 127, 128
Spherocytosis, 68t
Sphingomyelin, 468, 867
Spironolactone, hyperaldosteronism and, 770-771, 771t
Splenomegaly, diseases producing, 194t
Spur cell anemia, 154
Spurious hyperkalemia, 312
Spurious macrocytosis, 112
Sputum
    blood, 992, 993t
    gross appearance, 992
    laboratory assessment, 991-996, 993t, 994t, 995t, 996t
    microscopic examination, 992-996, 994-995t, 996t
    normal physiology, 991-992
Standard deviation (SD), 13-14
Staphylococcal coagulase reaction, 635t, 637
Staphylococcus sp., antimicrobial susceptibility tests, 649, 651, 652
Steroid hormones, 757-759, 758. See also Reproductive endocrinology
Stimulation tests, gonadal steroids, 830
Stomatocytosis, 68t
Stool/fecal analysis, 611. See also Gastrointestinal specimens
    general considerations, 978-979
    laboratory examination, 980-991
    microbial toxin assay, 629t
    microscopy, 687-688
    normal specimen, 979
    specimen collection, 980
Storage lesion, 389, 411
Streaking methods, 638
Streptococcal infections, 649, 651, 652, 709t, 710-711
Streptococcus pneumoniae, 649, 651, 652, 675
Streptokinase, in fibrinolysis, 259-260
Stress, 447, 448t, 768, 776
Strong acid, defined, 501

Succinylcholine, 556
Sudan Black B stains, 96-97
Sugars, 447, 935t. See also Glucose
Sulfosalicylic acid test, for immunoglobulin light chains, 227
Surface glycoproteins, intravascular cell adhesion, 171, 171, 172
Swab specimens, collection and transport, 612-613
Sweat, laboratory assessment, 1012-1013
Syndrome of inappropriate antidiuretic hormone secretion (SIADH), 531, 754, 756, 757t
Synergistic effect, 655, 656, 657
Synovial fluid, laboratory assessment, 1008-1012, 1010t, 1012t, 1013
Syphilis
    CSF tests, 977
    microscopy, 680, 681
    serology, 709t, 712-715, 714t, 715
Systemic lupus erythematosus (SLE), 339, 356, 357, 358

Taenia solium, 724
Tapeworms, and B_{12}, 116, 1019
Target amplification techniques, 628
Target cells, in hemoglobinopathies, 149
Tease preparations, 643, 644
Template method, of bleeding time, 250-251
Test suspension, PA antigen detection assay, 622
Tetany, 525, 807
Tetrahydrofolate, 53, 53, 54
Thalassemia intermedia, 144, 147
Thalassemia syndromes, 108t, 141-148, 146t, 863
Theophylline, 881-884, 882, 1066t
Therapeutic hemapheresis, 406, 407-408t
Therapeutic index, 877, 877
Therapeutic range, 877, 877
Thermal damage, causing hemolytic anemia, 152-153
Thiazides, and thrombocytopenia, 306
Thin-layer chromatography (TLC), 868, 879
Thioridazine, 907
Thrombin clotting time (TCT), 265-266
Thrombin time (TT), 269, 272t
Thrombocytapheresis, defined, 406
Thrombocytes, 31. See also Platelets
Thrombocythemia, essential, 200-202
Thrombocytopenia, 245, 302-310, 303t, 308t, 309-310, 398, 401
Thrombocytosis, 201-202, 311-312, 311t, 312
Thrombophilia
    acquired, 282
    activated protein C resistance, 278-279
    antithrombin III deficiency, 276-278
    classification of, 273-274, 275t
    factors favoring, 274t
    hyperhomocysteinemia, 279
    inherited, 276t
    lab tests for, 274-276, 277t
    lupus anticoagulant, 279-282
Thrombosthenin, in platelets, 241-242

Thrombotic thrombocytopenic purpura (TTP),
151-152, 309-310, 401
Thrombus, 273
Thyroid function tests, 786-792, 793*t*
Thyroid gland, 783-798
    disorders of, 775, 792, 794-798, 1033
    effects of hormones, 785
    factors decreasing activity of, 785-786
    laboratory findings affected by, 78*t*
    measurement of hormone activity, 786-792,
        793*t*
    mechanism of hormone action, 740
    metabolism of thyroid hormones, 783, *784*
    pituitary-hypothalamic relationship, 784-785
    pregnancy and, 849-850, 850*t*
    T_3 and T_4, 783-784
Thyroid-pituitary-hypothalamus feedback loop,
    TRH administration, 790
Thyroid-stimulating hormone (TSH), 742, *743*,
    1064*t*
    euthyroid sick syndrome, 795-796
    in hyperthyroidism, 794
    hypothyroidism and, 792
    stimulation of, 788-790, *789*
    T_3/T_4 and, 784-785
Thyrotropin releasing hormone (TRH), 784-785
Thyroxine (T_4), 783-784, 1064*t*
    assays, 786
    euthyroid sick syndrome, 795
    factors affecting, 796-797, 796*t*
    free thyroxine index, 788, *789*, 794, 795
    in hyperthyroidism, 794
    hypothyroidism and, 792
    metabolic effect of, 448*t*
    prealbumin assays, 1028
    thyroxine-binding globulin, 497
Thyroxine-binding globulin (TBG), 497,
    787-788, *789*
Thyroxine-binding prealbumin (TBPA), 484
Tissue/biopsy material, microbiology specimen
    collection and transport, 612
Tissue factor pathway inhibitor (TFPI), 255, 262
Tissue factor (TF), 238-239*t*, 253, 255, *255*, 256
Tissue glycosylation, 818
Tissue thromboplastin, 238-239*t*, 253, 255,
    255, 256
Tissue typing, 353-354
Tobramycin, 890
alpha-Tocopherol, 1021
Toluidine blue O stain, 618-619
Total iron-binding capacity (TIBC), 59, *106*, 107
Toxins
    detection of, 628-630, 629*t*
    microbial, 604, 607, 687*t*, 690-692
    neutralization assays, 705-706, *705*
    serum measurement, 445-446
Toxocariasis, serology, 723*t*, 725
Toxoplasmosis, serology, 723-724, 723*t*
Transferrin, 57, 497, 590-592, 1028
    binding sites, 59
    diagnostic significance of, 483*t*
    hemochromatosis, 165*t*
    nutritional status assessment, 1028
    saturation, 59-60 *106*, 107, 493-494

Transfusion-related acute lung injury (TRALI),
    414-415
Transfusion-related infections, 397*t*,
    419-421, 729
Transfusion-related noncardiogenic pulmonary
    edema, 414-415
Transient erythroblastopenia of childhood
    (TEC), 121
Transplacental hemorrhage (TPH), 421-422,
    423-425
Transplantation
    bone marrow, 900-901
    cytomegalovirus infections, 729
    HLA typing in, 436-437
    immunosuppressive drugs, 900-903, *901*
    kidney, 437
    liver, 597-599, *598*
    pancreas, 554-555
Transudates, 1003, *1004*, 1004*t*, 1007*t*, 1008,
    1009*t*
Trauma, and hemolytic anemia, 151-152, 152*t*
TRH. *See* Thyrotropin releasing hormone
Trichinellosis serology, 723*t*, 725
Trichomoniasis, 680, 683, 686
Trichrome stain, 619
Triglycerides (TG), 467
    cholesterol fractionation, 474
    exogenous pathway, 469
    lipoprotein phenotypes, 476*t*
    measurement of, 472
Tri-iodothyronine (T_3), 783-784, 1064*t*
    assays, 786-787
    euthyroid sick syndrome, 795, 796
    thyroxine-binding globulin, 497
Trypan blue dye exclusion technique, 433
Tube coagulase test, 637
Tumor(s)
    adrenal, 759, 769, 775
    alpha-fetoprotein production, 588
    and lactate dehydrogenase, 542
    pituitary, 747-748, 763, 765
    causing SIADH, 757*t*
    thyroid, 794, 1033
Tumor markers, 1031-1046
    alpha fetoprotein, 1037
    bladder tumor antigen, 1040-1041
    cancer antigen, 1039-1040
    carcinoembryonic antigen, 1035-1037
    endocrine, 1032-1033
    enzymes, 1033-1034
    estrogen and progesterone receptors,
        1041-1042
    fecal occult blood, 1041
    gene rearrangements, 1043-1046, *1044*, *1045*,
        1046*t*
    human chorionic gonadotropin, 1034-1035
    human papilloma virus, 1042
    metabolic, 1031-1032
    prostate-specific antigen, 1037-1038
Tumor necrosis factor (TNF), 608-609, 1029,
    1032
Turner's syndrome, 857*t*, 858
Two-hour postload glucose (2hPG), 814
Tzanck prep, 680

Ultrafiltration, 925
Umbilical cord blood sampling, 855, 1048-1051, 1049*t*, 1050*t*, 1053*t*
Unconjugated (indirect) bilirubin, 427, 566, 567*t*, 568-569
Urea, 453, 581, 956, 975, 1055*t*, 1064*t*
Ureaplasma urealyticum culture, 685
Uremia, 314, 454, 454*t*, 456*t*, 946-947
Uric acid, 457-458, 459*t*
  malignancy and, 1031
  normal values, neonates and pediatric patients, 1057*t*
  nutritional status assessment, 1025
Urinalysis
  appearance, 927-929, 928*t*
  artifacts, 927
  dipsticks, 929-936, 929*t*, 931-933*t*, 934*t*, 935*t*, 936*t*, 940*t*
  formed elements, 930, 934, 939-940, 941*t*, 942*t*
  kidney stones, analysis of, 963-966, 964*t*, 965*t*
  laboratory assessment, 924-966
  physiology of urine formation, 924-925
  reference ranges, 1065*t*
  renal function assessment, 942-953
  special measurements, 953-963
  specimen collection, 927
Urine
  adrenal hormones, 760-761
  calcium and phosphorus levels, 801
  diabetes, monitoring in, 817
  drug screening, 911
  glucocorticoid excretion, 759
  gram-stained smears, 615
  immunoelectrophoresis, for immunoglobulin light chains, 227
  microbiology, specimen collection and transport, 610-611
  nitrite, 670
  osmolality, 516-517, 755*t*
  polyuria, differential diagnosis of, 755*t*
  porphyrias, ALA in, 163
  proteinuria, 936*t*
  sex steroid metabolites, 828, 829*t*
  specimens, 662*t*, 669-671
  volume, conditions affecting, 950*t*
Urobilinogen, 460, 568, *568*, 571
  in hemoglobin catabolism, 77, *78*
  liver function tests, 567*t*
  urinalysis, 932*t*, 954, 954*t*
Urobilistix test for bilirubinuria, 939*t*
Urokinase, fibrinolysis, 259-260
Uroporphyrinogen, in heme synthesis, 49

Vacuolization, neutrophil, 86
Vaginosis, 681, 685
Valproic acid, 892, 897, 1066*t*
Vancomycin monitoring, 891-892, 1066*t*
Vanillylmandelic acid (VMA), 779, 781, 782
Varicella zoster virus serology, 727*t*, 728
Vascular system, 236, 240, 304, 577
Venereal Disease Research Laboratory (VDRL) test, 709*t*, 712-713
Very low-density lipoprotein (VLDL), 468

Viral inactivation methods, for plasma components, 401*t*
Viral infections
  blood transfusion, transmission via, 397*t*, 416-421, 417*t*
  cultures, 643-647, *645*, *646*
  enteric, 688
  eye, 698
  hemolytic anemia from, 159
  immune globulins, 404
  respiratory tract, 679, 994*t*
  serology, 726-735
Virilism, adrenal, 774-775
Virulence factors, 606-607
Vitamin(s), 584, 1017-1019, 1029
Vitamin B_{12}, deficiency of, 53, 111-116
  dietary requirements of, 51
  replacement therapy, 46, 115-116
Vitamin B complex deficiency, 1018-1019
Vitamin C, 965-966, 1019-1020
Vitamin D, 799-800
  calcium metabolism, 464-465, 806, 807
  deficiency, 806, 807, 1020-1021
  metabolites, 803
Vitamin D-resistant rickets, 807
Vitamin E deficiency, 1021
Vitamin K
  deficiency of, 585, 1021-1022
  and liver disease, 319
  and prothrombin time abnormalities, 585-586
Volume changes, and metabolic alkalosis, 522-523
von Willebrand factor (vWF), 238-239*t*, 242-243, 257, 299*t*, 301*t*
von Willebrand's disease (vWD), 243, 297-298, 301, 751
  features of, 289*t*
  lab findings in, 298, 301
  multimers in, *300*
  as platelet disorder, 312, 313
  platelet function tests of, 248, 249

Warm-reactive autoimmune hemolytic anemia, 158-159, 381, 382
Warthin-Starry stains of lymph node biopsies, 718
Water and electrolyte metabolism, 526-531, 528*t*, 529*t*, 530*t*
  nonketotic hyperosmolar syndrome, 819, 820*t*, 821
  physiology, 500-505
  water deficit, causes of, 530-531, 530*t*
  water excess, clinical manifestations of, 530*t*, 531
  water loading, SIADH diagnosis, 756
Watson-Schwartz test, 955
Weil-Felix (WF) test, 718, 719*t*
Wet mount preparations, 614, 680-681
Wheatley trichrome stain, 619
White blood cell casts, 940, 941*t*, 942*t*
White blood cell concentrates, 400
White blood cell counts, 82-83, 608, 1060*t*
  CSF, 972
  differential, 82, 91-93, 608, 972, 972*t*

White blood cell counts *(Continued)*
  abnormal, 91-93
  bone marrow, 43*t*
  in neutropenia evaluation, 177
  reference ranges, 1060*t*
  serous fluids, 1005
  shift to left in, 92-93, 608
White blood cell diseases, 167-234
  classification of, 167-169, 168*t*
  immunoproliferative and plasma call dyscra-
    sias, 223-234, 225*t*, 229-234
  lymphoproliferative, 204-223
  myeloproliferative disorders, 183*t*, 184-190,
    185*t*, 187*t*, 190*t*, 192-204
  nonclonal, 169-181
White blood cells, 31, 82-93
  and alkaline phosphatase, 549
  blood components, 395*t*
  conditions affecting, 93*t*
  fetal, normal values, 1050*t*
  granulocytes, 83-85
  lymphocytes, 87-89
  monocytes, 89-90

normal values for, 62*t*, 1050*t*, 1060*t*
  pools of, 36, 37, 38
  production of, 36-39
  removal from red cell concentrates, 395, 396*t*
  sputum, 993
  uric acid crystals, 457
  in urine, 930, 933*t*
White clot syndrome, 307
Whole blood, 394
Widal test, 709*t*, 711
Wintrobe method for ESR, 94-95
Wound, tissue/biopsy specimens, 662*t*, 695-696

Xanthochromia, 967
D-Xylose test, 989

Yeast infections, 641, 678
Yersinia enterocolitica culture, 691

Ziehl-Neelsen stain, 616
Zinc protoporphyrin (ZPP), 60
Zona glomerulosa, 759
Zygomycetes, respiratory tract, 678-679